Apert Syndrome

John G. Meara • Mark R. Proctor
Nivaldo Alonso
Editors

Jay G. Berry • Eric Arnaud
Fernando Molina • Katelynn Porto
Section Editors

Apert Syndrome

Comprehensive Care of the Patient and Family

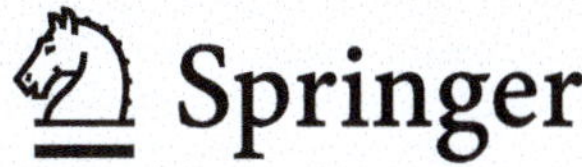

Editors
John G. Meara
Department of Plastic and Oral Surgery
Boston Children's Hospital
Boston, MA, USA

Mark R. Proctor
Department of Neurosurgery
Boston Children's Hospital
Boston, MA, USA

Nivaldo Alonso
Department of Plastic Surgery
Faculdade de Medicina da Universidade
de São Paulo
São Paulo, São Paulo, Brazil

Section Editors
Jay G. Berry
Department of Pediatrics
Department of Plastic and Oral Surgery
Boston Children's Hospital
Boston, MA, USA

Fernando Molina
Plastic Surgery and Craniofacial Surgery
Universidad Nacional Autònoma
de Mexico
Mexico City, Mexico

Eric Arnaud
Craniofacial Unit
Hôpital Necker–Enfants malades
Paris, France

Katelynn Porto
Department of Psychiatry and
Behavioral Sciences
Department of Plastic and Oral Surgery
Boston Children's Hospital
Boston, MA, USA

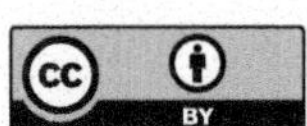

ISBN 978-3-032-12550-7 ISBN 978-3-032-12551-4 (eBook)
https://doi.org/10.1007/978-3-032-12551-4

This work was supported by the Department of Plastic and Oral Surgery, Boston Children's Hospital

This Springer imprint is published by the registered company Springer Nature Switzerland AG
The registered company address is: Gewerbestrasse 11, 6330 Cham, Switzerland

Preface

Caring for individuals with Apert syndrome is as intricate and multifaceted as the condition itself. It presents a unique set of challenges that span the medical, surgical, psychological, and social domains. As healthcare professionals, we often find ourselves navigating a labyrinth of information across various specialties. Indeed, our patients and families must also navigate this maze, often without readily available information or professional expertise. This book, *Apert Syndrome: Comprehensive Care of the Patient and Family*, was conceived in response to a pressing need to consolidate vast knowledge, experiences, and best practices into an accessible resource for doctors and patients alike.

The volume brings together over 100 contributors: surgeons, pediatricians, geneticists, therapists, psychologists, parents, patients, and advocates. Each offers distinct regional insights, clinical experiences, and cultural perspectives in the care of patients with Apert syndrome. Over the years, advancements in medical science have significantly improved the prognosis and quality of life for those affected. However, the complexity of the syndrome necessitates a comprehensive, multidisciplinary approach to care—one that addresses not only the physical manifestations but also the emotional and developmental needs of the patient.

We aim to bridge knowledge gaps, encourage integrated care models, and ultimately improve patient outcomes. Our goal is not simply to present surgical techniques or genetic pathways but to provide a holistic, practical, and compassionate guide to caring for children and adults with Apert syndrome. The book addresses a wide range of topics, including early diagnosis and surgical sequencing, psychosocial development, advocacy, and global health policy. By integrating both high-resource and limited-resource perspectives, it serves as a reference for professionals, patients, and families worldwide.

This work is also a tribute to the patients and families who have shared their lives with us. They have influenced our research, informed our practices, and always reminded us that Apert syndrome is not just a medical diagnosis but a lived experience.

We hope this volume will become a cornerstone for clinicians, trainees, health system leaders, policymakers, and advocates committed to excellence in Apert care. May it inspire future collaboration, spark innovation, and reinforce the idea that shared knowledge—across disciplines and borders—is our most powerful tool. The complexity and diversity of treatment represent a grand challenge for all involved; this textbook demonstrates that surgical intervention is a small component of the overall management of patients with Apert syndrome.

Furthermore, we hope that governments and policymakers will prioritize rare diseases, such as Apert syndrome, in their national health planning and care delivery processes. This approach is the only way to achieve strong, resilient health systems and true global health equity.

We invite readers to engage critically with this work and to center compassion in the ongoing effort to improve the lives of those affected by Apert syndrome.

John G. Meara Boston, MA, USA
Mark R. Proctor Boston, MA, USA
Nivaldo Alonso São Paulo, Brazil

Acknowledgments

This volume reflects a global effort. We are grateful to our editorial and production teams at Springer, particularly Kristopher Spring and Nishanthini Vetrivel, as well as to our co-authors from around the world. In addition, we thank the following individuals for their thoughtful and thorough assistance in managing the project's many details:

Copyeditors
Joseph M. Firriolo, MD
Tamara Haag, MSW
Madelyn Mulreaney
Anna W. Nicholson, PhD, MPhil, MA
Alicia Potter
Dionna Santucci
David C. Thean, MD, BDS

Administrative and Research Support
Marshalee Bowens
Catherine T. McNamara, MPH
Ava G. White

Contents

Contributors

Khalid Al-Dasuqi Department of Radiology, Sidra Medicine, Doha, Qatar

Department of Radiology, Boston Children's Hospital, Boston, MA, USA

Nivaldo Alonso Department of Plastic Surgery, Faculdade de Medicina da Universidade de São Paulo, São Paulo, São Paulo, Brazil

Craniofacial Division, Hospital for Rehabilitation of Craniofacial Anomalies and University of São Paulo, São Paulo, Brazil

Michael Alperovich Division of Plastic and Reconstructive Surgery, Department of Surgery, Yale University School of Medicine, New Haven, CT, USA

Melissa Zattoni Antonelli Speech and Hearing Department, Hospital for Rehabilitation of Craniofacial Anomalies and University of São Paulo, São Paulo, Brazil

Eric Arnaud Craniofacial Unit, Hôpital Necker–Enfants malades, Paris, France

Craniofacial Rare Diseases Competence Center, Clinique Marcel Sembat, Ramsay, Boulogne Billancourt, France

French National Reference Center for Rare Disease (CRANIOST) and European Rare Disease Network member (ERN CRANIO), Paris, France

Jay G. Berry Department of Pediatrics, Department of Plastic and Oral Surgery, Boston Children's Hospital Boston, Boston, MA, USA

Edgard Novaes França Bisneto Department of Orthopedics and Traumatology, Universidade de São Paulo, São Paulo, Brazil

Thomas Bondi Department of Maxillofacial Surgery and Plastic Surgery, and Craniofacial Unit, Hôpital Necker–Enfants malades, Assistance publique–Hôpitaux de Paris, Paris, France

Alice Briozzo Pediatric Otorhinolaryngology and Head and Neck Department, AP-HP, Hôpital Necker–Enfants malades, Paris, France

Letícia Nunes Campos Faculdade de Ciências Médicas, Universidade de Pernambuco, Recife, Pernambuco, Brazil

Department of Clinical Research, Fundación SPINE, Buenos Aires, Argentina

Martin Catala Laboratoire de Biologie du Développement, Institut de Biologie Paris Seine (IBPS), Sorbonne Université, CNRS, INSERM, Paris, France

Charlotte Celerier Pediatric Otorhinolaryngology and Head and Neck Department, AP-HP, Hôpital Necker–Enfants malades, Paris, France

Yoon-Hee Chang Department of Ophthalmology, Boston Children's Hospital, Boston, MA, USA

William Cobb Department of General Surgery, AdventHealth Orlando, Orlando, FL, USA

Vincent Couloigner Pediatric Otorhinolaryngology and Head and Neck Department, AP-HP, Hôpital Necker–Enfants malades, Paris, France

Michael L. Cunningham Division of Craniofacial Medicine, Department of Pediatrics, University of Washington School of Medicine, Craniofacial Center, Seattle Children's Hospital, Seattle, WA, USA

Annette C. Da Costa The Royal Children's Hospital, Melbourne, VIC, Australia

Murdoch Children's Research Institute, Melbourne, VIC, Australia

Linda R. Dagi Department of Ophthalmology, Boston Children's Hospital, Boston, MA, USA

Harvard Medical School, Boston, MA, USA

Isabela Toledo Teixeira da Silveira Department of Oral Surgery, Faculdade de Odontologia Universidade de São Paulo, São Paulo, Brazil

Greta Davis Division of Plastic and Reconstructive Surgery, Center for Health Equity in Surgery and Anesthesia, UC San Francisco Medical Center, San Francisco, CA, USA

Caroline de Paula Oliveira Gringo Department of Oral Surgery, Hospital de Reabilitação de Anomalias Craniofaciais HRAC, Universidade de São Paulo (HRAC-USP), São Paulo, Brazil

Raul Gonçalves de Paula Department of Craniofacial Surgery Hospital de Reabilitação de Anomalias Craniofaciais HRAC, Universidade de São Paulo, São Paulo, Brazil

Luiza do Amaral Virmond Department of Clinical Genetics, Hospital for Rehabilitation of Craniofacial Anomalies, University of São Paulo, Bauru, São Paulo, Brazil

Brigitte Fauroux Pediatric Noninvasive Ventilation and Sleep Unit, AP-HP, Hôpital Necker–Enfants malades, Paris, France

EA 7330 VIFASOM (Vigilance Fatigue Sommeil et Santé Publique), Paris University, Paris, France

Roberto L. Flores Hansjorg Wyss Department of Plastic Surgery, NYU Langone Health, New York, NY, USA

Ingrid M. Ganske Department of Plastic and Oral Surgery, Boston Children's Hospital, Boston, MA, USA

Harvard Medical School, Boston, MA, USA

Ayla Gerk Harvey E. Beardmore Division of Pediatric Surgery, The Montreal Children's Hospital, McGill University Health Centre, Montreal, QC, Canada

Faculty of Medicine and Health Sciences, McGill University, Montreal, QC, Canada

Enrico Ghizoni Institute of Plastic and Craniofacial Surgery, SOBRAPAR Hospital, Campinas, São Paulo, Brazil

Department of Neurology, University of Campinas (UNICAMP), Campinas, São Paulo, Brazil

Marisol Zuluaga Giraldo Consultant Pediatric Anesthesia, King Abdullah Children's Hospital, Riyadh, Saudi Arabia

Susan M. Goobie Department of Anesthesiology, Critical Care and Pain Medicine, Boston Children's Hospital, Boston, MA, USA

Harvard Medical School, Boston, MA, USA

Jeremy A. Goss Division of Plastic and Reconstructive Surgery, Department of Surgery, Yale University School of Medicine, New Haven, CT, USA

Stéphane Guero Institut de la Main, Paris, France

Hôpital Necker–Enfants malades, Université Paris Centre, Paris, France

Samer E. Haber Craniofacial Surgery Unit, CRMR CRANIOST, Hôpital Necker–Enfants malades, Assistance publique–Hôpitaux de Paris, Paris, France

Nicholas A. Han Division of Plastic, Reconstructive, and Oral Surgery, Children's Hospital of Philadelphia, Philadelphia, PA, USA

Emma K. Hartman Department of Neurosurgery, Boston Children's Hospital, Boston, MA, USA

Quentin Hennocq Hôpital Necker–Enfants malades, Assistance publique–Hôpitaux de Paris, Paris, France

Laboratoire Forme et Croissance du Crâne, Institut Imagine, Paris, France

Richard A. Hopper Department of Surgery, Baylor College of Medicine, Houston, TX, USA

Texas Children's Hospital, Austin, TX, USA

Allison C. Hu Division of Plastic, Reconstructive, and Oral Surgery, Children's Hospital of Philadelphia, Philadelphia, PA, USA

Syril James Clinique Marcel Sembat, Centre de Competence Maladies Rares CRANIOST, Ramsay-Generale de Santé, Boulogne Billancourt, France

Hôpital Universitaire Necker–Enfants malades, Paris, France

Kathleen A. Kapp-Simon Shriner's Children's Hospital Chicago, Chicago, IL, USA

University of Illinois at Chicago, Chicago, IL, USA

Sonia Khirani Pediatric Noninvasive Ventilation and Sleep Unit, AP-HP, Hôpital Necker–Enfants malades, Paris, France

ASV Santé, Gennevilliers, France

Roman H. Khonsari Department of Maxillofacial Surgery and Plastic Surgery, and Craniofacial Unit, Hôpital Necker–Enfants malades, Assistance publique–Hôpitaux de Paris, Paris, France

Nancy Mizue Kokitsu-Nakata Department of Clinical Genetics, Hospital for Rehabilitation of Craniofacial Anomalies, University of São Paulo, Bauru, São Paulo, Brazil

Shreenik Kundu Harvey E. Beardmore Division of Pediatric Surgery, The Montreal Children's Hospital, McGill University Health Centre, Montreal, QC, Canada

Faculty of Medicine and Health Sciences, McGill University, Montreal, QC, Canada

Brian I. Labow Department of Plastic and Oral Surgery, Boston Children's Hospital, Boston, MA, USA

Harvard Medical School, Boston, MA, USA

Solomon Lee Division of Plastic and Reconstructive Surgery, UC San Francisco Medical Center, San Francisco, CA, USA

Katelyn Lewis Division of Plastic and Reconstructive Surgery, Department of Surgery, Yale University School of Medicine, New Haven, CT, USA

Beatriz Laus Pereira Lima Universidade São Francisco, Campus Bragança Paulista, São Paulo, São Paulo, Brazil

Romain Luscan Pediatric Otorhinolaryngology and Head and Neck Department, AP-HP, Hôpital Necker–Enfants malades, Paris, France

Ting-Chen Lu Department of Plastic and Reconstructive Surgery and Craniofacial Research Center, Chang Gung Memorial Hospital, Linkou, Taiwan

Luciano Brandao Machado Division of Anesthesia, Hospital for Rehabilitation of Craniofacial, Anomalies Vila Nova Cidade Universitária, Bauru, São Paulo, Brazil

Ben B. Massenburg Division of Plastic, Reconstructive, and Oral Surgery, Children's Hospital of Philadelphia, Philadelphia, PA, USA

Irene M. J. Mathijssen Department of Plastic and Reconstructive Surgery and Hand Surgery, Erasmus Medical Center, Rotterdam, The Netherlands

Hamilton Matushita Department of Neurosurgery, Division of Pediatric Neurosurgery, University of São Paulo, São Paulo, Brazil

John G. Meara Department of Plastic and Oral Surgery, Boston Children's Hospital, Boston, MA, USA

Harvard Medical School, Boston, MA, USA

Rose Meltzer University of Central Florida School of Medicine, Orlando, FL, USA

Fernando Molina Plastic Surgery and Craniofacial Surgery, Universidad Nacional Autònoma de Mexico, Mexico City, Mexico

Medicine Faculty, Postgraduate Division, Fundaciòn Fernando Ortiz Monasterio for Craniofacial Anomalies at Hospital Angeles del Pedregal, CDMX, Mexico City, Mexico

Madelyn Mulreaney Department of Plastic and Oral Surgery, Boston Children's Hospital, Boston, MA, USA

Hugo Nakamoto Department of Orthopedics, Hand and Microsurgery Group, Hospital das Clinicas, University of São Paulo, São Paulo, Brazil

Marine Parodi Pediatric Otorhinolaryngology and Head and Neck Department, AP-HP, Hôpital Necker–Enfants malades, Paris, France

Giovanna Paternoster Pediatric Neurosurgical Department, Craniofacial Unit of Necker Hospital, Paris, France

French National Reference Center for Rare Disease (CRANIOST) and European Rare Disease Network member (ERN CRANIO), Paris, France

Isabella de Oliveira Lima Parizotto Paula Department of Craniofacial Surgery, Hospital for Rehabilitation of Craniofacial Anomalies, University of São Paulo, Bauru, São Paulo, Brazil

Bauru Eye Hospital, Bauru, São Paulo, Brazil

Mariela Peralta-Mamani Department of Oral Surgery, Hospital de Reabilitação de Anomalias Craniofaciais HRAC, São Paulo, Brazil

Marielle Pillon Department of Maxillofacial Surgery and Plastic Surgery, and Craniofacial Unit, Hôpital Necker–Enfants malades, Assistance publique–Hôpitaux de Paris, Paris, France

Natalie M. Plana Hansjorg Wyss Department of Plastic Surgery, NYU Langone Health, New York, NY, USA

Hanna Face and Jaw, New York, NY, USA

Katelynn Porto Department of Psychiatry and Behavioral Sciences, Department of Plastic and Oral Surgery, Boston Children's Hospital, Boston, MA, USA

Harvard Medical School, Boston, MA, USA

Alicia Potter Department of Plastic and Oral Surgery, Boston Children's Hospital, Boston, MA, USA

Mark R. Proctor Department of Neurosurgery, Boston Children's Hospital, Boston, MA, USA

Harvard Medical School, Boston, MA, USA

Tatiana Protzenko National Institute of Health for Women, Children and Adolescents Fernandes Figueira/Osvaldo Cruz Foundation, Rio de Janeiro, Brazil

Cassio Eduardo Raposo-Amaral Institute of Plastic and Craniofacial Surgery, SOBRAPAR Hospital, Campinas, São Paulo, Brazil

Department of Neurology, University of Campinas (UNICAMP), Campinas, São Paulo, Brazil

Cesar Augusto Raposo-Amaral Institute of Plastic and Craniofacial Surgery, SOBRAPAR Hospital, Campinas, São Paulo, Brazil

Marcelo Rosa Rezende Department of Orthopedics, Hand and Microsurgery Group, Hospital das Clinicas, Universidade de São Paulo, São Paulo, Brazil

Joanne M. Rispoli Department of Radiology, Boston Children's Hospital, Boston, MA, USA

Harvard Medical School, Boston, MA, USA

Matthieu Robert Department of Pediatric Ophthalmology, Hôpital Necker–Enfants malades, Paris, France

Caroline D. Robson Department of Radiology, Boston Children's Hospital, Boston, MA, USA

Harvard Medical School, Boston, MA, USA

John Rose Division of Plastic and Reconstructive Surgery, Center for Health Equity in Surgery and Anesthesia, Philip R. Lee Institute for Health Policy Studies, UC San Francisco Medical Center, San Francisco, CA, USA

Isabel A. Ryan Division of Plastic, Reconstructive, and Oral Surgery, Children's Hospital of Philadelphia, Philadelphia, PA, USA

Dionna Santucci Department of Plastic and Oral Surgery, Boston Children's Hospital, Boston, MA, USA

Rajendra Sawh-Martinez Department of General Surgery, AdventHealth, Orlando, FL, USA

University of Central Florida School of Medicine, Orlando, FL, USA

Plastic and Reconstructive Surgery, AdventHealth for Children, Orlando, FL, USA

Henrique Regonaschi Serigatto Department of Clinical Genetics, Hospital for Rehabilitation of Craniofacial Anomalies, University of São Paulo, Bauru, São Paulo, Brazil

Pradip R. Shetye Hansjorg Wyss Department of Plastic Surgery, NYU Langone Health, New York, NY, USA

Matthew L. Speltz Department of Psychiatry and Behavioral Sciences, University of Washington, Seattle, WA, USA

Nicola M. Stock Centre for Appearance Research, University of the West of England, Bristol, UK

Jordan W. Swanson Division of Plastic, Reconstructive, and Oral Surgery, Children's Hospital of Philadelphia, Philadelphia, PA, USA

Amir Taghinia Department of Plastic and Oral Surgery, Boston Children's Hospital, Boston, MA, USA

Harvard Medical School, Boston, MA, USA

Jesse A. Taylor Division of Plastic, Reconstructive, and Oral Surgery, Children's Hospital of Philadelphia, Philadelphia, PA, USA

Luiza Telles Instituto de Educação Médica (IDOMED/Estácio), Vista Carioca Campus, Rio de Janeiro, RJ, Brazil

Briac Thierry Pediatric Otorhinolaryngology and Head and Neck Department, AP-HP, Hôpital Necker–Enfants malades, Paris, France

Catherine Tomat Department of Maxillofacial Surgery and Plastic Surgery, and Craniofacial Unit, Hôpital Necker–Enfants malades, Assistance publique–Hôpitaux de Paris, Paris, France

Cristiano Tonello Department of Surgery, Faculdade de Medicina Universidade de São Paulo, São Paulo, Brazil

Division Craniofacial Hospital de Reabilitação de Anomalias Craniofaciais HRAC, São Paulo, Brazil

Romain Touzé Department of Pediatric Ophthalmology, Hôpital Necker–Enfants malades, Paris, France

Mark Urata Children's Hospital of Los Angeles, University of Southern California, Los Angeles, CA, USA

Elle Vandervord Children's Hospital Westmead, Sydney, NSW, Australia

Marie-Lise C. van Veelen Department of Neurosurgery, Erasmus Medical Center, Rotterdam, The Netherlands

Brigitte Vi-Fane Department of Maxillofacial Surgery and Plastic Surgery, and Craniofacial Unit, Hôpital Necker–Enfants malades, Assistance publique–Hôpitaux de Paris, Paris, France

Andrew O. M. Wilkie MRC Weatherall Institute of Molecular Medicine, University of Oxford, John Radcliffe Hospital, Headington, Oxford, UK

Oxford Craniofacial Unit, Oxford University Hospitals NHS Foundation Trust, John Radcliffe Hospital, Headington, Oxford, UK

Oxford Centre for Genomic Medicine, Oxford University Hospitals NHS Foundation Trust, Nuffield Orthopaedic Centre, Headington, Oxford, UK

Andrew Willmer University of Central Florida School of Medicine, Orlando, FL, USA

Renato Yassutaka Faria Yaedú Department of Oral Surgery Faculdade de Odontologia and Hospital de Reabilitação de Anomalias Craniofaciais HRAC, University of São Paulo, São Paulo, Brazil

Part I

General Principles

Introduction

1

Jay G. Berry and Michael L. Cunningham

Definition and Core Clinical Characteristics of Apert Syndrome

Apert syndrome—also known as type 1 acrocephalosyndactyly—is a rare genetic disorder characterized primarily by synostosis (i.e., bony fusion) of multiple bones, including those in the axial and appendicular skeleton [1, 2]. Gain-of-function mutations in fibroblast growth factor receptor 2 (FGFR-2) cause the majority of cases of Apert syndrome [3–5]. Although the cellular impact of these mutations is not completely understood, enhanced activation of FGFR-2 affects the osteoprogenitor cells of the intra-sutural mesenchyme, resulting in both premature fusion of the sutures of the calvaria and premature ossification of the skull base synchondroses (see Chap. 4 on Molecular Genetics and Chap. 5 on Clinical Genetics for comprehensive accounts of the genetics of Apert syndrome).

J. G. Berry (✉)
Department of Pediatrics, Department of Plastic and Oral Surgery, Boston Children's Hospital, Boston, MA, USA
e-mail: Jay.Berry@childrens.harvard.edu

M. L. Cunningham
Division of Craniofacial Medicine, Department of Pediatrics, University of Washington School of Medicine, Craniofacial Center, Seattle Children's Hospital, Seattle, WA, USA

Craniosynostosis in Apert Syndrome Bilateral fusion of coronal sutures occurs in nearly 100% of infants with Apert syndrome. Bilateral coronal craniosynostosis leads to a high, steep forehead, a tall cranium (i.e., turricephaly), and a shortened anteroposterior skull length (i.e., brachycephaly). Collectively, these findings result in a vertically prominent and short (i.e., turribrachycephalic) skull. The skull deformities associated with Apert syndrome are difficult to diagnose with prenatal ultrasound, especially for de novo cases [6]. Therefore, Apert syndrome is typically diagnosed after birth (see Chap. 3 on Head, Neck, and Extremity Anatomy as well as Chap. 6 on Diagnosis and Imaging for extensive coverage of Apert syndrome findings).

Midfacial Hypoplasia in Apert Syndrome Infants with Apert syndrome exhibit maxillary hypoplasia, a short nose with a depressed nasal bridge, deviated nasal septum, and anterior bulbous tip as well as cathedral-ceiling and/or cleft palate, prominent mandible, and inferior displacement of the oral commissures [7]. Aside from cleft palate, these features relate in part to premature ossification of the sphenooccipital, sphenoethmoid, frontoethmoidal synchondroses and facial sutures, which result in a shortened skull base and midfacial sutures [8]. The constellation of midface abnormalities in Apert syndrome contributes to the high prevalence of chronic rhinosinusitis and obstructive sleep apnea (OSA). Hypertelorism

J. G. Meara et al. (eds.), *Apert Syndrome*, https://doi.org/10.1007/978-3-032-12551-4_1

and proptosis are present in all patients with Apert syndrome and are due to a shallow bony orbit and exotropia.

Syndactyly in Apert Syndrome Syndactyly in Apert syndrome commonly affects both the hands and feet, and can present with a variety of findings, including—but not limited to—bony fusion (involving the second, third, and fourth digits), brachydactyly (short fingers), clinodactyly (curved fingers), symphalangism (fusion of the phalanges), and cutaneous syndactyly of the web spaces [9–11]. Syndactyly is a complex phenomenon affecting the bones, tendons, muscular, and neurovascular bundles. It sometimes involves the first and fifth fingers, can be complete or partial, and varies in severity. Upton's classification of syndactyly in Apert syndrome includes three types [9]. The Type I "spade hand" is the most common and least severe, Type II "mitten hand" is less common and more severe, and Type III "rosebud hand" is the least common and most severe, with osseous/cartilaginous union of the thumb and fingers with fused nail plates (see Surgical Treatment of the Apert Hand, Chap. 31).

Individuals with Apert Syndrome—People First Although healthcare professionals typically diagnose Apert syndrome by craniosynostosis, midfacial hypoplasia, and syndactyly, it is imperative to recognize that these physical manifestations do not define a person. Individuals with Apert syndrome are people, first and foremost. They deserve dignity, respect, and equal opportunity to define and dictate their own interests, abilities, aspirations, contributions, and well-being. Healthcare professionals, teachers, family members, friends, and all of society should embrace the richness of the lives of individuals with Apert syndrome without invalid judgments about cognition and functioning. Seeing the person before the syndrome fosters inclusivity and compassion as well as patient- and-family-centered care (Fig. 1.1).

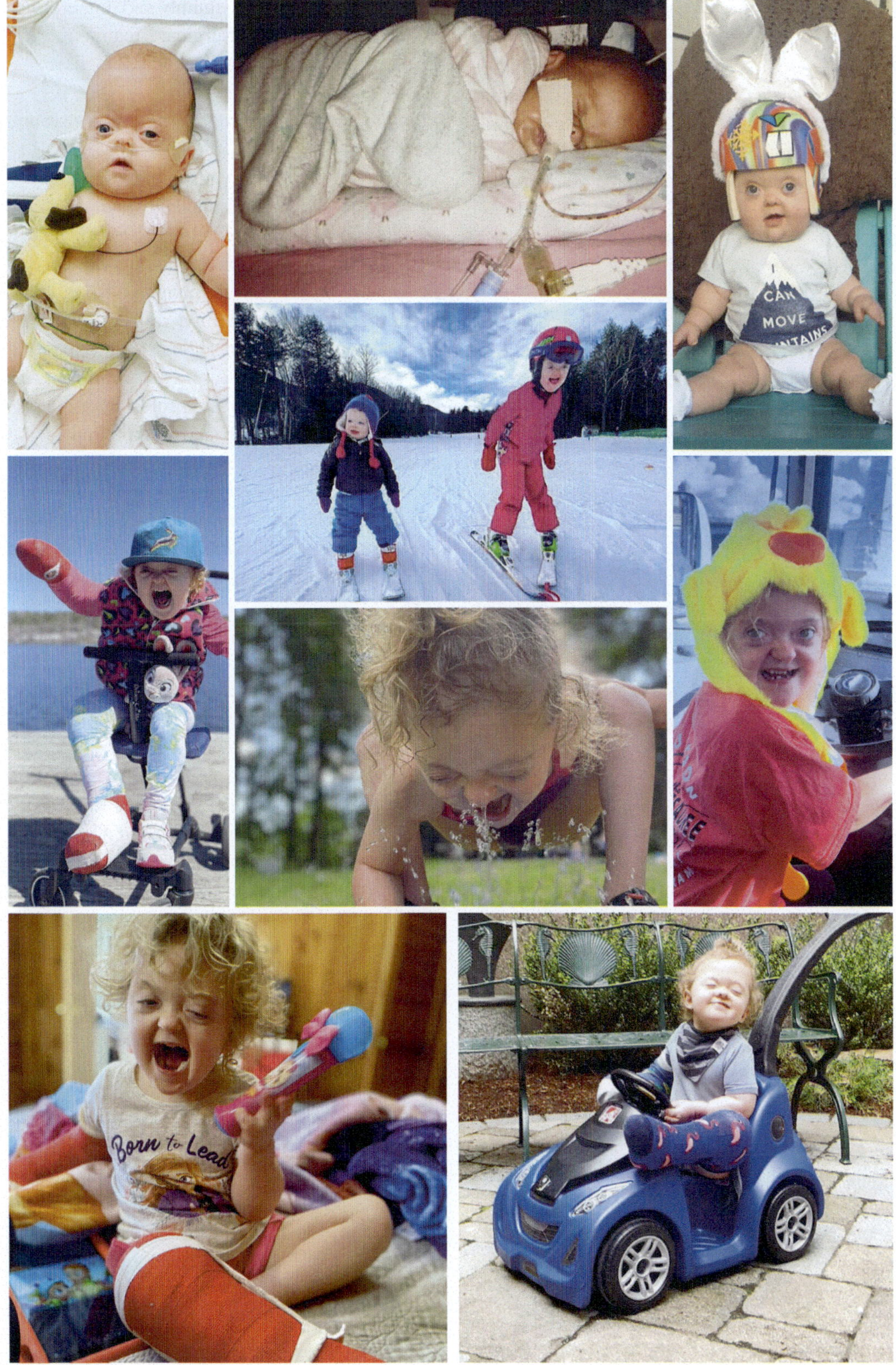

Fig. 1.1 Shown are pictures of a child with Apert syndrome participating in fulfilling, life activities

Epidemiology of Apert Syndrome

Although findings vary across epidemiologic studies, the prevalence of Apert syndrome is estimated as 1 in 65,000 births, with no predilection for females over males [12–14]. Research shows that the prevalence of Apert syndrome increases with paternal age [15]. Although inherited as autosomal dominant, a de novo pathogenic variant of FGFR-2 is responsible for most cases [4, 16].

Systemic Manifestations

In addition to its core clinical features, Apert syndrome is a multisystem condition, with a high prevalence of musculoskeletal, respiratory, neurologic, ophthalmic, dermatologic, and other end-organ health problems. As a result, individuals with Apert syndrome need interdisciplinary care from several medical and surgical specialists to optimize their health and well-being.

Musculoskeletal As many as two-thirds of individuals with Apert syndrome exhibit single- or multilevel fusion of the cervical vertebrae, with variable points of fusion (e.g., articular facets, transverse processes, or block fusion of the vertebral bodies) [17, 18]. C5–C6 fusion is the most common [18]. C1 spina bifida occulta and C1–C2 atlanto-axial subluxation are reported [17]. Upper limb abnormalities can occur [19]. Glenoid dysplasia and progressive loss of range of motion of the glenohumeral joint (particularly abduction) can emerge with age [20]. Additional upper limb abnormalities include epiphyseal dysplasia of the humeral head, greater tuberosity, capitulum, radial head, and radioulnar synostosis [19, 21].

Respiratory Apert syndrome can significantly compromise the airway [22]. Obstructive sleep apnea (OSA) is a significant, prevalent respiratory comorbidity with Apert syndrome [23, 24]. We suspect that most individuals experience OSA to some degree, manifested by loud snoring, recurrent episodes of apnea, frequent wakening, and/or excessive daytime somnolence. Among individuals with Apert syndrome exhibiting these symptoms, 80% are diagnosed with OSA by polysomnogram. Studies suggest that OSA in individuals with Apert syndrome is typically moderate but can range from mild to severe.

The etiology of OSA with Apert syndrome is multilevel, including midfacial hypoplasia, acute angulation of nasal and frontal bones, choanal stenosis, and tongue-based airway obstruction [23]. OSA in Apert syndrome is suspected to occur mainly during rapid eye movement (REM) sleep when the pharyngeal musculature is the most relaxed. In many cases, cleft palate in Apert syndrome mitigates OSA, and closure of the palate significantly exacerbates obstruction at the level of the pharynx. Beyond the midface, anomalies of the trachea are also associated with Apert syndrome. These anomalies include fused tracheal tings, tracheal cartilaginous sleeves, and tracheobronchomalacia and can contribute to OSA [25].

Untreated OSA in Apert syndrome is physiologically detrimental to multiple organ systems. Sequelae include hypercapnia, cor pulmonale, and vasodilation of the cerebral vasculature. Options for OSA treatment include dilatation of the nasal airways and choanal stenosis repair, adenoidectomy, tonsillectomy, midface advancement, noninvasive ventilation, and tracheostomy. Central apnea can occur in Apert syndrome, arising from raised intracranial pressure. Cerebrospinal fluid diversion surgery (e.g., ventriculoperitoneal shunt placement), fronto-orbital advancement, and Chiari decompression aid in managing increased intracranial pressure.

Neurologic and Neurodevelopment Neurologic comorbidities are reported in over 50% of individuals with Apert syndrome, and can be classified as primary malformations and secondary to cranial deformity [26, 27]. Primary ventriculomegaly is common but is typically stable, nonprogressive, and not related to increased intracranial pressure [28, 29]. Progressive and/or pathologic hydrocephalus is rare in individuals with Apert syndrome [30]. Other primary neurologic malformations reported with Apert syndrome include defects of the corpus callosum (e.g., thinning or absence), septum pellucidum, limbic system, and hypoplastic pyramidal tract structures, as well as encephalocele, heterotopic gray matter, hypoplasia of white matter, and gyral anomalies [30–32]. Chiari malformation is cerebellar tonsil extension below the foramen magnum and into the spinal canal, which can be associated with central apnea and bradypnea. Chiari malformation is a secondary neurologic comorbidity that can occur with Apert syndrome, with mixed etiology, including jugular foramen stenosis, small volume of the posterior fossa, and increased intracranial pressure from craniosynostosis [33].

Neurodevelopmental capabilities and outcomes are diverse in Apert syndrome, ranging from normal to significantly impaired [34]. Most of the patients with Apert syndrome in our clinical practice have mild to moderate intellectual deficits. Risk factors for deficits have been inconsistent across studies but include neurologic malformation (especially septum pellucidum), older age at surgery for craniosynostosis, lower education level of family/caregiver, and lower quality of home environment [27]. A detailed neuropsychological evaluation of patients with Apert syndrome is recommended to manage and optimize neurodevelopment [26, 34].

Ophthalmic Nearly all patients with Apert syndrome encounter ocular problems [35, 36]. Examples include amblyopia (lazy eye), anisometropia (asymmetric refraction between the two eyes), and strabismus (deviation of one eye inward or outward). Proptosis (bulging eyes with protrusion from the orbit) can also occur and may lead to exposure keratopathy and/or corneal scarring. Strabismus may worsen after craniofacial surgery [37]. Increased intracranial pressure from craniosynostosis can cause papilledema and vision loss [37].

Dermatologic Apert syndrome is associated with a variety of cutaneous manifestations, including hyperhidrosis and severe acne [38–40]. Acne can occur in atypical locations such as the forearm and upper arm [41]. Skin hypopigmentation, hyperkeratosis, wrinkling (forehead), and dimpling (knuckles, shoulders, and elbows) have also been reported. Nail abnormalities, including brittleness, synonychia, and paronychia, are common. We recommend adding a dermatologist to the care team to manage these conditions.

Cardiac Congenital heart malformations occur in ~10% of individuals with Apert syndrome [42]. These malformations range from mild to severe. Examples of cardiac abnormalities observed in Apert syndrome include atrial septal defect, ventricular septal defect, patent ductus arteriosus, conotruncal defects (e.g., tetralogy of Fallot), and aortic arch anomalies (e.g., aortic coarctation, overriding aorta, and right aortic arch). The clinical presentation of congenital heart malformations in Apert syndrome varies depending on the type, location, and severity of the anomaly. A thorough cardiac physical examination during infancy is paramount for screening and diagnosis. It should cover auscultation for heart murmur, palpation of pulses, and measurement of oxygen saturation and blood pressure.

When congenital cardiac malformations are clinically significant in Apert syndrome, signs and symptoms such as poor feeding, fatigue, failure to thrive, tachypnea, respiratory distress, and cyanosis may arise. Echocardiogram, electrocardiogram, and evaluation by a pediatric cardiologist should be considered for any child with Apert syndrome with an abnormal cardiac examination or systemic signs suggesting cardiac dysfunction. Surgical intervention and/or medical management may be necessary. Careful perioperative planning for these infants should involve collaboration with cardiothoracic surgeons, cardiologists, craniofacial surgeons, and anesthesiologists. Infants with Apert syndrome who need cardiac operations should receive special attention for the timing and order of all surgeries.

Gastrointestinal Problems throughout the gastrointestinal system can occur in infants and children with Apert syndrome. The prevalence of gastrointestinal problems with Apert syndrome is unknown but is likely nontrivial. Craniofacial abnormalities associated with Apert syndrome can affect the functioning of the upper gastrointestinal system. Midface hypoplasia, cleft palate, and/or dental malocclusion can impair feeding and swallowing. These structural anomalies can lead to poor sucking ability, difficulty breathing while eating and drinking, and increased effort and time for nutritional intake. The anomalies, in conjunction with possible neuromuscular impairment, can also contribute to additional oromotor dysfunction and dysphagia, increasing the risk of aspiration.

Although less common, malformations of the mid and lower gastrointestinal system have been reported with Apert syndrome [42]. Examples include esophageal stenosis and atresia, pyloric stenosis, intestinal malrotation with volvulus, and ectopic anus [43, 44]. As with any infant or child, gastroesophageal reflux disease (GERD) and constipation can occur with Apert syndrome.

Other Conditions and Considerations Nearly one in ten children with Apert syndrome is reported to have a genitourinary malformation [45]. The most common are cryptorchidism and obstruction of the urinary collecting system resulting in hydronephrosis [42]. In addition, personal hygiene can be problematic in children with Apert syndrome. Insufficient dental and oral hygiene is common. Inadequate toothbrushing can result in significant plaque accumulation [46]. In addition, elbow fusion can limit effective toileting.

Patient- and Family-Centered, Comprehensive Care

Apert syndrome is thus a complex-form synostosis that can affect several organ systems. Interdisciplinary management by clinical teams with experience diagnosing and treating the various manifestations of Apert syndrome is critical, as highlighted by the European Reference Network of Craniofacial Anomalies and Ear-Nose-Throat Disorders (ERN CRANIO) [47]. Coordinated care can be effective to screen and manage the craniofacial, extremity, pulmonary, cognitive, and other coexisting conditions. Although treatment options and trajectories of medical and surgical management vary across institutions and countries, the need for patient- and family-centered, organized, and proactive care-planning is universal (see Table 1.1 for considerations of care management activities with Apert syndrome). As the subsequent sections and chapters of this book will convey, there are anticipated exposures to medical and surgical interventions that will evolve over time for individuals with Apert syndrome. For example, infancy can be associated with craniosynostosis intervention, early toddler years with syndactyly release, and adolescence with midface optimization. Apnea screening and management (as well as screening for other comorbidities) may occur throughout childhood.

It is beneficial to designate at least one clinician to take a comprehensive view of each patient with Apert syndrome and to help integrate and oversee the various pediatric specialists on the care team. When ideally positioned, this clinician can help (1) educate and navigate children and their families through anticipated and upcoming medical events; (2) orchestrate the order and timing of proposed interventions; and (3) optimize health and safety, especially before major surgical interventions and anesthetic exposures. Regardless of team structure, clinicians caring for individuals with Apert syndrome should strive to include the children and families as full partners in medical decision-making and proactive care-planning. This will ensure that the children, families, and providers agree on the goals of care and the expectations and benefits of treatments.

Table 1.1 Considerations for care management with apert syndrome

Clinical topic	Care management activities
Ophthalmologic	Recurrent, comprehensive examinations by an ophthalmologist, including but not limited to assessments of visual acuity, pupil alignment, proptosis, lid closure, and optic nerves (e.g., with fundoscopy or optical coherence tomography [OCT])
Increased intracranial pressure	Symptom screening for headache, irritability, and vision changes Head circumference measurement and trend Ophthalmology evaluation including fundoscopy/OCT Extra-axial space and ventricle assessment on brain/cranial imaging Consideration of neurosurgeon assessment for placement of an intracranial pressure monitor *Recurrently assess for increased intracranial pressure at least through age six years*
Hydrocephalus	Evaluation with magnetic resonance imaging (MRI) of the brain, and assessment by a neurosurgeon to distinguish hydrocephalus from benign ventriculomegaly
Chiari malformation and spine	Symptom assessment for Chiari, including headaches (posterior, with coughing, sneezing, etc.), impairment with balance, and difficulty swallowing Assessment of severity of Chiari (and possible syrinx) with MRI brain and spine imaging and assessment by a neurosurgeon Plain radiograph and/or MRI spine to assess cervical vertebrae fusion and subluxation
Sleep apnea and airway obstruction	Symptom assessment for sleep apnea, including snoring, pauses in breathing, gasping, excessive daytime somnolence, etc. Upper airway assessment by an otolaryngologist, including upper airway endoscopy to visualize nasal septum and turbinates, adenoids, tonsils, trachea, etc. Sleep medicine assessment, including polysomnogram
Hearing and speech/language	Neonatal hearing screen Recurrent audiology and otolaryngology assessments for external auditory canals and tympanic membranes as well as conductive and sensorineural hearing loss Parent/caregiver and school assessments of hearing and speech/language Neuropsychology assessment for delays or problems in speech/language
Orthodontic	Assessment of dental hygiene, development, enamel, malocclusion, growth of the mandible, etc.
Cognition and behavioral development	Early intervention Screening for cognitive and/or behavioral deficits Neuropsychology assessment for any delays or problems MRI brain to assess for primary brain parenchymal malformations
Psychosocial	Screen for psychosocial adaptation, self-image, and social skills Refer to psychologist or psychiatrist if indicated
Syndactyly	Assessment and categorization of syndactyly type Surgical planning for correction by a hand surgery specialist
Midface and mandible	Assessment by oral and maxillofacial surgeon for utility, timing, and approach to midface advancement
Bony dysplasia of shoulder and elbow	Range of motion assessment of upper extremity and shoulder Consideration for referral to orthopedic surgeon, including radiographic imaging of the arm and shoulder
Skin	Assessment by a dermatologist for hyperhidrosis and severe acne

References

1. Alam MK, Alfawzan AA, Srivastava KC, Shrivastava D, Ganji KK, Manay SM. Craniofacial morphology in Apert syndrome: a systematic review and meta-analysis. Sci Rep. 2022;12(1):5708. https://doi.org/10.1038/s41598-022-09764-y.
2. Conrady CD, Patel BC, Sharma S. Apert syndrome. StatPearls. 2024.
3. Wilkie AO, Morriss-Kay GM. Genetics of craniofacial development and malformation. Nat Rev Genet. 2001;2(6):458–68. https://doi.org/10.1038/35076601.
4. Wilkie AO, Slaney SF, Oldridge M, et al. Apert syndrome results from localized mutations of FGFR2 and is allelic with Crouzon syndrome. Nat Genet. 1995;9(2):165–72. https://doi.org/10.1038/ng0295-165.
5. Slaney SF, Oldridge M, Hurst JA, et al. Differential effects of FGFR2 mutations on syndactyly and cleft palate in Apert syndrome. Am J Hum Genet. 1996;58(5):923–32.
6. Hill LM, Thomas ML, Peterson CS. The ultrasonic detection of Apert syndrome. J Ultrasound Med. 1987;6(10):601–4. https://doi.org/10.7863/jum.1987.6.10.601.
7. Turgut NF, Hogg ES, De S, Sharma SD, Avula S. Variations in paranasal sinus anatomy in children with Apert syndrome: a radiological analysis. J Craniofac Surg. 2022;33(2):707–9. https://doi.org/10.1097/SCS.0000000000008248.
8. Wang MM, Haveles CS, Zukotynski BK, Reid RR, Lee JC. Facial suture pathology in syndromic craniosynostosis: human and animal studies. Ann Plast Surg. 2021;87(5):589–99. https://doi.org/10.1097/SAP.0000000000002822.
9. Upton J. Apert syndrome. Classification and pathologic anatomy of limb anomalies. Clin Plast Surg. 1991;18(2):321–55.
10. Fereshetian S, Upton J. The anatomy and management of the thumb in Apert syndrome. Clin Plast Surg. 1991;18(2):365–80.
11. Mah J, Kasser J, Upton J. The foot in Apert syndrome. Clin Plast Surg. 1991;18(2):391–7.
12. Cohen MM Jr, Kreiborg S, Lammer EJ, et al. Birth prevalence study of the Apert syndrome. Am J Med Genet. 1992;42(5):655–9. https://doi.org/10.1002/ajmg.1320420505.
13. Tolarova MM, Harris JA, Ordway DE, Vargervik K. Birth prevalence, mutation rate, sex ratio, parents' age, and ethnicity in Apert syndrome. Am J Med Genet. 1997;72(4):394–8. https://doi.org/10.1002/(sici)1096-8628(19971112)72:4<394::aid-ajmg4>3.0.co;2-r
14. Czeizel AE, Elek C, Susanszky E. Birth prevalence study of the Apert syndrome. Am J Med Genet. 1993;45(3):392–3. https://doi.org/10.1002/ajmg.1320450322.
15. Glaser RL, Broman KW, Schulman RL, Eskenazi B, Wyrobek AJ, Jabs EW. The paternal-age effect in Apert syndrome is due, in part, to the increased frequency of mutations in sperm. Am J Hum Genet. 2003;73(4):939–47. https://doi.org/10.1086/378419.
16. Mantilla-Capacho JM, Arnaud L, Diaz-Rodriguez M, Barros-Nunez P. Apert syndrome with preaxial polydactyly showing the typical mutation Ser252Trp in the FGFR2 gene. Genet Couns. 2005;16(4):403–6.
17. Breik O, Mahindu A, Moore MH, Molloy CJ, Santoreneos S, David DJ. Central nervous system and cervical spine abnormalities in Apert syndrome. Childs Nerv Syst. 2016;32(5):833–8. https://doi.org/10.1007/s00381-016-3036-z.
18. Kreiborg S, Barr M Jr, Cohen MM Jr. Cervical spine in the Apert syndrome. Am J Med Genet. 1992;43(4):704–8. https://doi.org/10.1002/ajmg.1320430411.
19. Khabyeh-Hasbani N, Lu YH, Baumgartner W, Mendenhall SD, Koehler SM. Contemporary management of the upper limb in Apert syndrome: a review. Plast Reconstr Surg Glob Open. 2024;12(8):e6067. https://doi.org/10.1097/GOX.0000000000006067.
20. Kasser J, Upton J. The shoulder, elbow, and forearm in Apert syndrome. Clin Plast Surg. 1991;18(2):381–9.
21. Cohen MM Jr, Kreiborg S. Skeletal abnormalities in the Apert syndrome. Am J Med Genet. 1993;47(5):624–32. https://doi.org/10.1002/ajmg.1320470509.
22. Xie C, De S, Selby A. Management of the airway in Apert syndrome. J Craniofac Surg. 2016;27(1):137–41. https://doi.org/10.1097/SCS.0000000000002333.
23. Doerga PN, Spruijt B, Mathijssen IM, Wolvius EB, Joosten KF, van der Schroeff MP. Upper airway endoscopy to optimize obstructive sleep apnea treatment in Apert and Crouzon syndromes. J Craniomaxillofac Surg. 2016;44(2):191–6. https://doi.org/10.1016/j.jcms.2015.11.004.
24. Inverso G, Brustowicz KA, Katz E, Padwa BL. The prevalence of obstructive sleep apnea in symptomatic patients with syndromic craniosynostosis. Int J Oral Maxillofac Surg. 2016;45(2):167–9. https://doi.org/10.1016/j.ijom.2015.10.003.
25. Wenger TL, Dahl J, Bhoj EJ, et al. Tracheal cartilaginous sleeves in children with syndromic craniosynostosis. Genet Med. 2017;19(1):62–8. https://doi.org/10.1038/gim.2016.60.
26. Tan AP, Mankad K. Apert syndrome: magnetic resonance imaging (MRI) of associated intracranial anomalies. Childs Nerv Syst. 2018;34(2):205–16. https://doi.org/10.1007/s00381-017-3670-0.
27. Yacubian-Fernandes A, Palhares A, Giglio A, et al. Apert syndrome: factors involved in the cognitive development. Arq Neuropsiquiatr. 2005;63(4):963–8. https://doi.org/10.1590/s0004-282x2005000600011.
28. Hanieh A, David DJ. Apert's syndrome. Childs Nerv Syst. 1993;9(5):289–91. https://doi.org/10.1007/BF00306277.
29. Collmann H, Sorensen N, Krauss J. Hydrocephalus in craniosynostosis: a review. Childs Nerv Syst. 2005;21(10):902–12. https://doi.org/10.1007/s00381-004-1116-y.

30. Cohen MM Jr, Kreiborg S. The central nervous system in the Apert syndrome. Am J Med Genet. 1990;35(1):36–45. https://doi.org/10.1002/ajmg.1320350108.
31. Cohen MM Jr, Kreiborg S. Agenesis of the corpus callosum. Its associated anomalies and syndromes with special reference to the Apert syndrome. Neurosurg Clin N Am. 1991;2(3):565–8.
32. Raybaud C, Di Rocco C. Brain malformation in syndromic craniosynostoses, a primary disorder of white matter: a review. Childs Nerv Syst. 2007;23(12):1379–88. https://doi.org/10.1007/s00381-007-0474-7.
33. Coll G, El Ouadih Y, Abed Rabbo F, Jecko V, Sakka L, Di Rocco F. Hydrocephalus and Chiari malformation pathophysiology in FGFR2-related faciocraniosynostosis: a review. Neurochirurgie. 2019;65(5):264–8. https://doi.org/10.1016/j.neuchi.2019.09.001.
34. Da Costa AC, Savarirayan R, Wrennall JA, et al. Neuropsychological diversity in Apert syndrome: a comparison of cognitive profiles. Ann Plast Surg. 2005;54(4):450–5. https://doi.org/10.1097/01.sap.0000149387.95212.df.
35. Buncic JR. Ocular aspects of Apert syndrome. Clin Plast Surg. 1991;18(2):315–9.
36. Khong JJ, Anderson P, Gray TL, Hammerton M, Selva D, David D. Ophthalmic findings in apert syndrome prior to craniofacial surgery. Am J Ophthalmol. 2006;142(2):328–30. https://doi.org/10.1016/j.ajo.2006.02.046.
37. Khong JJ, Anderson P, Gray TL, Hammerton M, Selva D, David D. Ophthalmic findings in Apert's syndrome after craniofacial surgery: twenty-nine years' experience. Ophthalmology. 2006;113(2):347–52. https://doi.org/10.1016/j.ophtha.2005.10.011.
38. Verma S, Draznin M. Apert syndrome. Dermatol Online J. 2005;11(1):15.
39. Cohen MM Jr, Kreiborg S. Cutaneous manifestations of Apert syndrome. Am J Med Genet. 1995;58(1):94–6. https://doi.org/10.1002/ajmg.1320580119.
40. Cohn MS, Mahon MJ. Apert's syndrome (acrocephalosyndactyly) in a patient with hyperhidrosis. Cutis. 1993;52(4):205–8.
41. Solomon LM, Cohen MM Jr, Pruzansky S. Pilosebaceous abnormalities in Apert type acrocephalosyndactyly. Birth Defects Orig Artic Ser. 1971;7(8):193–5.
42. Cohen MM Jr, Kreiborg S. Visceral anomalies in the Apert syndrome. Am J Med Genet. 1993;45(6):758–60. https://doi.org/10.1002/ajmg.1320450618.
43. Pelz L, Unger K, Radke M. Esophageal stenosis in acrocephalosyndactyly type I. Am J Med Genet. 1994;53(1):91. https://doi.org/10.1002/ajmg.1320530123.
44. Hibberd CE, Bowdin S, Arudchelvan Y, et al. FGFR-associated craniosynostosis syndromes and gastrointestinal defects. Am J Med Genet A. 2016;170(12):3215–21. https://doi.org/10.1002/ajmg.a.37862.
45. Wenger TL, Hing AV, Evans KN. Apert syndrome. In: Adam MP, Feldman J, Mirzaa GM, et al., editors. GeneReviews((R)); 1993.
46. Dalben Gda S, Costa B, Gomide MR. Oral health status of children with syndromic craniosynostosis. Oral Health Prev Dent. 2006;4(3):173–9.
47. Faasse M, Mathijssen IMJ, Craniosynostosis ECWGo. Guideline on treatment and management of craniosynostosis: patient and family version. J Craniofac Surg. 2023;34(1):418–33. https://doi.org/10.1097/SCS.0000000000009143.

2 Eugène Apert: More than a Simple Syndrome

Martin Catala

For most doctors involved in treating congenital malformations, Apert is the name of a syndrome associated with craniofacial and extremity anomalies. They know little of the man who first described this syndrome, so it is important to present his biography in this book dealing with Apert syndrome. Eugène Apert (1868–1940) (Fig. 2.1) was born during the French Second Empire (1852–1870), but lived most of his lifetime during the Third French Republic (1870–1940). Traumatized by defeat in the Franco-Prussian war (1870–1871), France was consumed with desire for revenge against the Germans. Furthermore, the rise of the concept of Western European superiority marked this period and led to the legitimization of colonization. Apert experienced the trauma of the First World War and the Spanish influenza epidemic, both of which caused massive death tolls in France. After the destruction of the war, it was necessary to rebuild the country by appealing to a foreign workforce to replace the personnel shortages due to the dead. The final years of Apert's life were marked by the rise of extremism in Europe that culminated with World War II. Apert died in February 1940, before the French defeat by the Nazis.

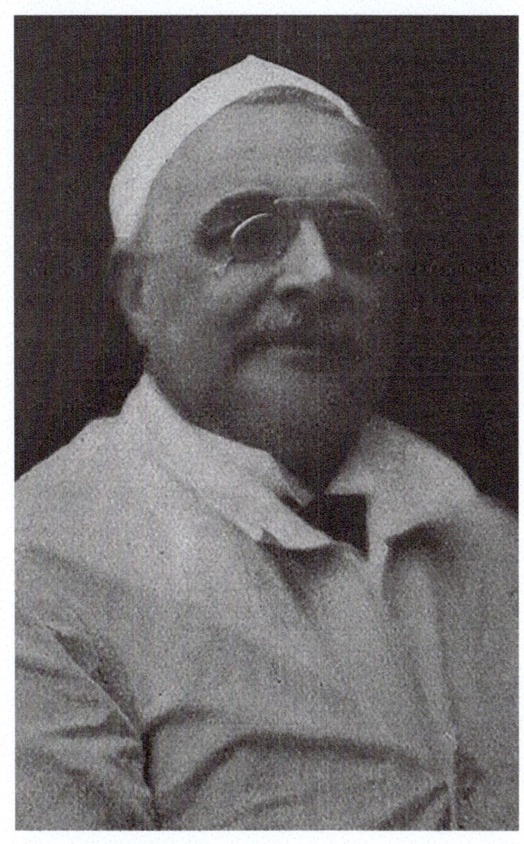

Fig. 2.1 Eugène Apert physician of the hospital. Date unknown. (From: Marfan [80])

M. Catala (✉)
Laboratoire de Biologie du Développement,
Institut de Biologie Paris Seine (IBPS),
Sorbonne Université, CNRS, INSERM, Paris, France
e-mail: martin.catala@sorbonne-universite.fr

J. G. Meara et al. (eds.), *Apert Syndrome*, https://doi.org/10.1007/978-3-032-12551-4_2

The Apert Family and Eugène's Early Years

As is customary in France, surnames do not have fixed spellings. Thus, the Apert family is found under the names Appert and Hapert. The Apert family tree was reconstructed by Mrs. Brigitte Poujade, whom I had the chance to contact. Additional information was provided to me by Mrs. Anne-Marie Driancourt, granddaughter of Eugène Apert's sister, Marie-Laurence Apert (1869–1935). The simplified family tree is presented in Fig. 2.2. Eugène's oldest identified ancestor is a man called Denis, who was born in Saint-Cyr-sur-Morin (Seine-et-Marne) and who died in Nanteuil-sur-Marne (Seine-et-Marne) on March 21, 1694. The Apert family left Seine-et-Marne and settled in the Val d'Oise (first in Survilliers, then in Mareil-en-France) around 1708, when Denis's son, François, was born. Etienne Dominique, who was the first in the family to learn to write, was a schoolmaster in the Val d'Oise (Luzarches).

Although I have not found the exact date of the Apert family's arrival in Paris, the study of directories and/or almanacs associated with the data of the Civil Registry allows us to establish the following facts. Dominique Laurent Apert, grandfather of Eugène, was born in Mariel-en-France in 1814 and married Victoire Caroline Heuzé (1817–1861) in Vaugirard on June 1, 1836. He worked in a grocery store and lived at the time at 47 rue de Sèvres in the village of Vaugirard. This village located in the Southwest of Paris was later integrated into the French capital in 1860 to become Paris's current 15th arrondissement. Gustave Émile, Eugène's father, was born in Paris the following year on November 18, 1837, at his parents' home, 39 rue du Faubourg du Temple (now in the tenth arrondissement). The couple had four more children, but I will only mention Albert Victor (1839–1863). The latter was born in Coulommiers (Seine-et-Marne) at his maternal grandparents' home.

The two brothers, Dominique Laurent and Albert Victor, both became grocers. Albert Victor

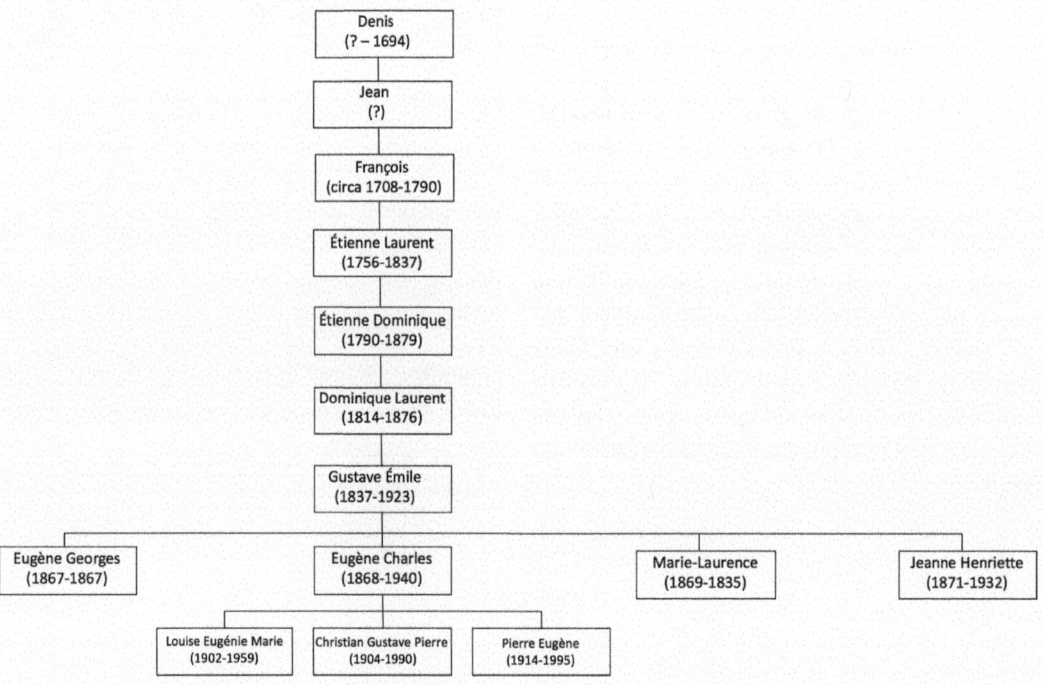

Fig. 2.2 Simplified genealogical tree of Apert's family

set up as a grocer at 23 rue du Chantre (near Notre-Dame Cathedral) from 1842 until his death in 1863. On the other hand, Dominique Laurent's establishment had a longer lifespan. From 1837 to 1840, he was established as a grocer at 39 rue du Faubourg du Temple before moving to Vaugirard (65 rue de Sèvres) in 1841. From 1842 to 1862, the grocery store took the name Apert-Heuzé and was shortened to Apert after the death of Dominique Laurent's wife; only the name Apert persisted until 1865. In 1863, the business diversified by developing a jam factory. Eugène's father, Gustave Émile (see Fig. 2.3a), took over the business in 1866, at the time of his marriage to Eugénie Joséphine Antoinette Hortense Huré (1846–1893) (see Fig. 2.3b). The company moved to 73 rue Lecourbe (15th arrondissement) where the Apert–Huré couple lived.

The Apert–Huré couple's first child, Georges Eugène, was born on January 30, 1867, and died the following February 18. Such early deaths were not unusual at the time, and it is not certain that the memory of this child remained in the family. Subsequently, the couple had three children: Eugène Charles (born July 27, 1868), Marie Laurence (born August 12, 1869), and Jeanne Henriette (born July 8, 1871). The family business must have flourished, because in 1874, it expanded and occupied 71, 73, and 75 rue Lecourbe. In 1875, a tragedy disrupted the lives of Eugène's parents, according to a *Le National* newspaper report dated Saturday, June 26, 1875. Miss Rey, a servant at the Aperts, concealed her pregnancy and gave birth to a live child on the night of March 5–6, 1875. The next day, Gustave Émile visited the room where Miss Rey was staying and found this child who had been suffocated by his mother. The court sentenced Miss Rey to seven years of forced labor on June 25, 1875. We do not know whether Eugène was aware of this. Dominique Laurent remarried in 1868 and died in Paris on July 4, 1876. The company was sold in 1880 to Mr. Brivain and the couple, who were sufficiently wealthy, lived off their income.

We have no information on Eugène's early schooling. However, we know that he attended

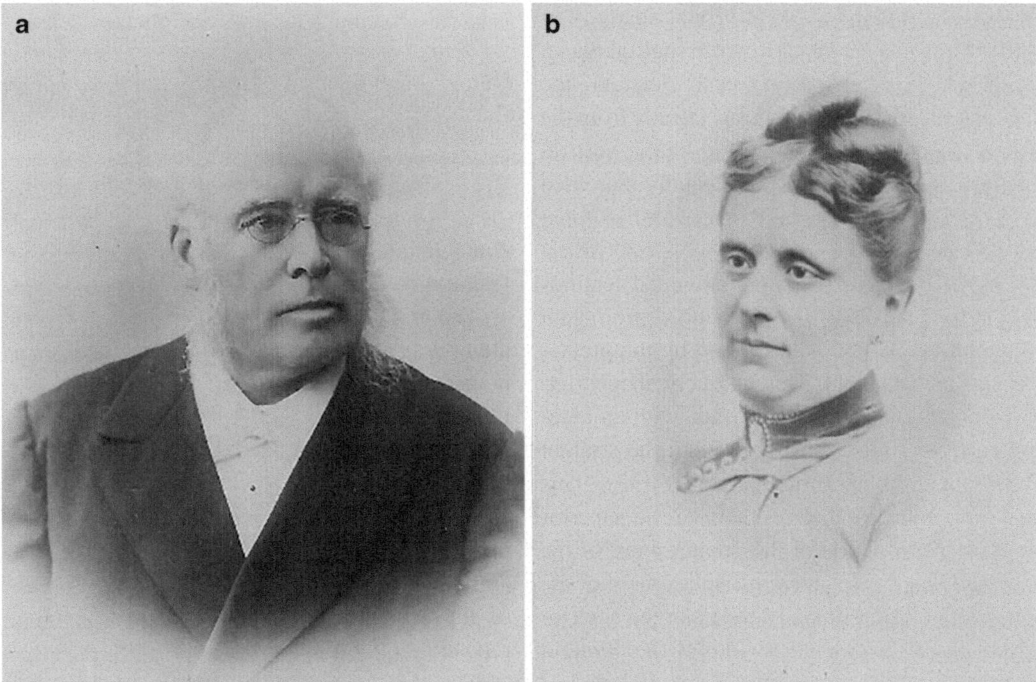

Fig. 2.3 The parents of Eugène Apert. (**a**) Gustave Émile [2] Eugénie Hortense Antoinette Huré. (Photographs courtesy of Mrs. Brigitte Poujade; *fond familial Bertin-Driancourt*)

the *Lycée de Vanves* high school (now *Lycée Michelet* in the southern suburbs of Paris) [80]. He was a brilliant student there, obtaining several high school prizes in 1884, 1885, and 1886. In addition, Eugène was awarded two prizes by *accessit* (distinction) at the *Concours Général des lycées de Paris et Versailles,* a competition between all students attending the high schools of Paris and Versailles. He received the sixth accessit in Algebra and Geometry in 1884 and the fifth *accessit* in Mathematics in 1886.

Medical Education

After studying at the *Lycée de Vanves*, Eugène Apert began his studies at the Faculty of Medicine in Paris. From November 15, 1887, to November 14, 1888, Apert performed his military duties in the 82nd Infantry Regiment. His file gives us some physical information including his height (1.76 m or 5′9″) and the color of his eyes (gray). Subsequently, he did several military stints and was removed from the force on October 28, 1912. We have very little information about Apert's education at the Faculty of Medicine, but the dedications of Apert's thesis (1897) tell us more about his academic career. His first masters in hospitals were Augustin Gilbert (1858–1927) and Albert Brault (1852–1939). At that time, French medical studies were punctuated by competitive examinations that allowed access to hospital positions. The first competition was that of the *externat* (i.e., clinical internship), and then the externs or former externs could take the second competition corresponding to the *internat* (i.e., residency), which lasted four years. The residency ended automatically once the student defended his thesis as a Doctor of Medicine. Young doctors could then continue at both the Faculty of Medicine and the hospital by competing to become *chef de clinique* and *chef de clinique adjoint* (assistant of the former), positions in hospital departments directed by faculty professors.

The first competitive examination was that of the *externat des hôpitaux de Paris*, which Apert passed in January 1890; Apert was ranked 140th out of 307 candidates in the competition. From February 1, 1890, to January 31, 1891, Apert was an *externe* in the department of Ange Ferrand (1835–1899) at Laënnec hospital (rue de Sèvres in the 15th arrondissement of Paris). Ferrand was a former student of Claude Bernard (1813–1878) and an anti-Darwinian [65]. From February 1, 1891, to January 31, 1892, Apert served as *externe* in the department of Joseph Grancher (1843–1907) at the Hospital for Sick Children (*Hôpital des Enfants-Malades,* rue de Sèvres in the 15th arrondissement of Paris). Apert was highly regarded by these two supervisors (he was very good according to Ferrand and excellent according to Grancher). It should be noted that Joseph Grancher was a personal friend of Louis Pasteur (1822–1895) and was involved with Alfred Vulpian (1826–1887) in the first anti-rabies vaccination, which was administered to Joseph Meister (1876–1940). In Grancher's department, Apert received instruction from Jules Louis Alexandre Martin de Gimard (1858–1894), *chef de clinique*, and his *chef de clinique adjoint,* Louis Guinon (1860–1929). Martin de Gimard was considered to have a very bright future due to his work on *Purpura fulminans*. Unfortunately, he was struck down and died during a mountain vacation at only 34 years old.

Eugène Apert applied for the Paris *internat des hôpitaux de Paris* hospital internship competition in 1891 but failed in this attempt. Nevertheless, his ranking of 24th out of 66 in the complementary list allowed him to obtain a temporary intern position. Apert was assigned to the retirement home of *Les Ménages* in the department of André Chantemesse (1851–1919), who studied infectious diseases. The director of this establishment mentioned that Apert was very popular with the patients. At the Aurillac high school, Chantemesse met Émile Roux (1853–1933), the future director of Pasteur Institute, who became his friend. Chantemesse studied bacteriology with both Robert Koch (1843–1910) and Louis Pasteur (1822–1895); he also developed the anti-typhoid serum with Fernand Widal (1862–1929). In his thesis, Apert paid tribute to Chantemesse and Roux for his training in bacteriology. In addition, he thanked Mr. Chautard for teaching him the first lessons in bacteriology. This may have been Paul Chautard, who at the time served as assistant in chemistry and bacteriology at the laboratory of the clinic of the Hospital for Sick Children.

Apert was finally accepted as an intern in the 1892 competition, the results of which were announced on January 24, 1893; he ranked 28th out of 66 accepted. Unfortunately, Eugène Apert's mother died in Paris on January 30, 1893, only six days after this success. From February 1, 1893, to March 10, 1894, Apert chose to work in the surgical department of Dr. Louis-Pierre Prengrueber (1845–1896) at *the Maison Municipale de Santé* (Fernand Widal hospital, *rue du Faubourg Saint-Denis*, Paris tenth arrondissement). It was at this time that Apert published his first work in the *Bulletin Médical*, a journal whose chief editor was Prengrueber. This first paper [1] was a review of the nutrition of young children and therefore foreshadowed his future career as a pediatrician in Paris hospitals. His second paper, published in the *Bulletin Médical* the same year, described four case studies of anal fistulas [2]. Apert wrote that three of these patients were operated on by the head of the department, and the fourth was operated on by Apert himself under the supervision of his chief. Thus, Apert began his internship by practicing surgery. It should also be noted that Apert published a lesson by Professor Stéphane Tarnier (1828–1897) in the same journal [86].

On February 17, 1894, Apert joined forces with three other interns—Maurice Savariaud (1870–1961), Henri Claude (1869–1945), and Raoul-Pierre Baudet (1864–1941)—to give internship lectures. This unofficial teaching was very important for young externs to prepare for the internship competition. From March 1 to November 1, 1894, Apert chose to work in the service of Ange Ferrand, who was now at the *Hôtel-Dieu*. From November 1, 1894, to April 30, 1895, he chose to work at the Maternity (Boulevard de Port-Royal) in the service of Alexandre Guéniot (1832–1935), who was later replaced by Pierre Constant Budin (1846–1907). The assessments of Apert by the heads of department were very good. Guéniot specified that Apert was "…of a kind and circumspect character, he is educated, attentive and seems to me to be a doctor of the future" (774/FOSS/5/36, Assistance Publique-Hôpitaux de Paris APHP archives). With Budin, Apert took charge of the *service des débiles* (which corresponds to premature neonates).

Apert returned as an intern in Joseph Grancher's department at the Hospital for Sick Children from May 1, 1895, to January 31, 1896. Grancher served during the summer semester and was replaced by Antoine Marfan (1858–1942) during the winter semester. Marfan is generally considered to be a principal founder of French pediatrics. Apert was influenced by Marfan, whom he considered one of his masters; they were also close friends [80]. From February 1, 1896, to January 31, 1897, Apert served as an intern under Georges Dieulafoy (1839–1911). He was first at the Necker Hospital until the beginning of November 1896, when he followed his master to the *Hôtel-Dieu*. During his final year of residency, Apert was an instructor for tubing and tracheotomy for Louis Arthur Sevestre (1843–1907) at the Hospital for Sick Children. This extension of activity at the pediatric hospital shows Apert's interest in this specialty of medicine.

Apert prepared his thesis at Dieulafoy's department, directed by Paul Charrier (1862–1903), *chef de clinique*, entitled "Pathogenesis of Purpura and Its Various Clinical Varieties." He defended his thesis [10] on February 18, 1897, before a jury composed of Dieulafoy (president), Mathias Duval (1844–1907), Chantemesse, and Pierre Ménétrier (1859–1935). In the acknowledgments of his thesis, we note that Apert referred not only to his heads of department but also to people who had provided interim services: Fernand Widal (1862–1929) in 1892, Georges Gilles de la Tourette (1857–1904) in 1894, Antoine Marfan in 1895, and Paul de Gennes (1853–1901) in

1896. The latter is the grandfather of Pierre-Gilles de Gennes (1932–2007), winner of the 1991 Nobel Prize in physics. Apert also thanked Charles Walther (1855–1935) for teaching dissections and Albert Gombault (1844–1904) for his training in histology and pathology.

Eugène Apert: Paris Hospital Physician

Beginning March 1, 1898, Apert served as *chef de clinique adjoint* (a contractual position under the supervision of a professor of the faculty and reserved for a Doctor of Medicine) under Dieulafoy at *Hôtel-Dieu*. He then served as *chef de clinique* from March 1, 1900, to February 27, 1902. Apert met Octave Crouzon (1874–1938) in Dieulafoy's department (see Fig. 2.4) and a friendship was established and maintained until the latter's death.

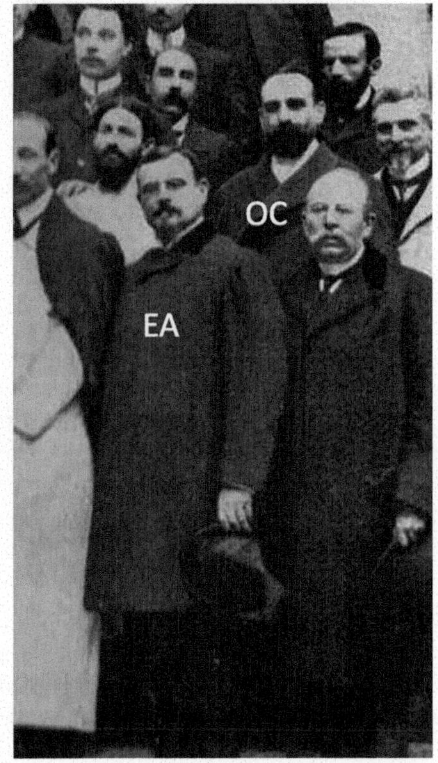

Fig. 2.4 Eugène Apert (EA) and Octave Crouzon (OC) in Dieulafoy's department (*Hôtel-Dieu*) in 1905. (Detail from figure 59 [37]

At the time, acquiring a permanent position at the hospital required passing the competitive examination for *Médecin des Hôpitaux* (i.e., physician of the hospitals). Apert unsuccessfully participated in this competition twice in 1898 and once in 1899. On February 26, 1902, Apert competed to obtain one of six available *Médecin des Hôpitaux* positions. That day, 60 competitors addressed the examination topic of "peritonitis in typhoid fever." To ensure anonymity, the responses were read before the jury gathered at the Charité hospital (6th arrondissement). The results were announced on June 15, 1902, in the following order: René Charles Marie (1868–1952), Jules Auclair (1865–1930), Ernest Marcel Labbé (1870–1939), Louis Joseph Fournier (1867–1930), Eugène Apert, and Alfred André Marie Bergé (1863–1924). Only Labbé was accepted as professor of the faculty of medicine (in 1929); all the others remained hospital doctors.

From 1902 to 1910, Apert replaced several of his colleagues in different hospitals—Tenon, Hérold, Trousseau, and Bretonneau—before assuming the role of head of the department of convalescent children at Saint-Louis hospital (1908–1909). On January 1, 1910, Apert was appointed head of department at Andral Hospital. This hospital opened on January 1, 1903, in place of the former toll barracks of Bastion 27 at 2 Bd MacDonald (19th arrondissement). In 1906, it became a general hospital and took the name of Gabriel Andral (1797–1876), professor of the Faculty of Medicine of Paris; the facility closed definitively in 1933.

In 1915, the army requisitioned Andral hospital to care for contagious soldiers. Although Apert was released from his military obligations due to his age, he placed himself at the disposal of the army health service and was attached to the temporary hospital of the *Grand Palais*. The chief physician, René-Charles Coppin (1861–1926), commanded the temporary hospital and requested that Apert be made a knight of the Legion of Honor in a letter dated January 17, 1919. This request was not granted until May 7, 1921, and the decoration was presented to the recipient on July 2, 1921, by the senator and physician Henri Pottevin (1865–1928).

Apert was appointed head of department at the Hospital for Sick Children (*Hôpital des Enfants Malades*) on February 1, 1919, a position he held until his retirement on January 1, 1935. His student and former intern, Cambessédès [52], specified that Apert refused any gift upon his departure. After his retirement, Apert continued to assiduously attend the sessions of the Paris Pediatric Society and the Hospital Medical Society. He also published several reference books.

Apert remained a hospital doctor throughout his career. Although he took three competitive examinations for the *agrégation* to become a professor at the Faculty of Medicine and failed each time (1901, 1904, and 1907), these failures did not prevent him from teaching brilliantly. Comby [54] wrote, "His bedside teaching, the best of all and which no other could surpass, attracted many students to him." He always preferred teaching directly at the patient's bedside to teaching in lecture halls [52].

It was difficult for us to find the list of young students who passed through Apert's service. However, we know that Gaston Joseph Froget (1879–?), Maurice Dubosc (1881–1944), Georges Marie Joseph Brac (1879–1936), and Marie Jacques Odinet (1903–1998) were *internes provisoires*. His *internes* included Jean Lhermitte (1877–1959), Jules Milhit (1880–1943), Arthur Désiré Delille (1876–1950), Henri Stévenin (1880–1968), Jacques-Marie Rouillard (1887–1937), René Le Maux (1887–?), Robert-Charles Michel (1888–1933), Henri Cambessédès (1885–1945), Pierre Vallery-Radot (1889–1975), Francis Bordet (1890–1981), Charles Bigot (1890–1957), Robert Broca (1888–1964), Henry Chabanier (1891–1966), Raymond Garcin (1897–1971), Yves Gaston Kermorgant (1892–1966), Elie Azerad (1898–1989), Jean Eugène Théodore Lerond (1897–?), Fernand Misaël Benoist (1900–1958), Marie Suzanne Tisserand (1897–?), Madeleine Mornet née Cros (1900–1976), Lucie Madeleine Abricossoff (1894–1944), Elisabeth Anchel née Bach (1899–1989), Fanny Rappoport (1901–?), Charles Peytavin (1899–1969), Roger Louis Goldberg (1903–?), Pierre Charles Alfred Baillet (1904–?), Pierre Robert Edouard Garnier (1903–?), Dolphi Lichtenberg (1904–?), and Jean Eugène Ferroir (1908–1978). Some of these individuals succeeded in competitive examination and went on to become *médecin des hôpitaux* (Benoist, Leblanc, Milhit, Rouillard, Stévenin), professors in Paris (Garcin, Lhermitte), and a professor in Angers (Bigot). Pierre Vallery-Radot was the first cousin of Louis Pasteur-Vallery-Radot (1886–1970), grandson of Louis Pasteur. Robert Broca was related to Paul Broca (1824–1880), who was the first cousin of Robert's grandfather, Nicolas-Élie Broca (1814–?). Louise Madeleine Abricossoff was a natural daughter of Charles Richet (1850–1935), who was a proponent of eugenics.

Family Life

Eugène Apert remained close to his family throughout his life. His sister, Marie-Laurence (1869–1935), married Victor Jules Driancourt (1861–1947) on May 16, 1891 (see Fig. 2.5). The couple had four children: Raymond (1892–1968), Pierre (1893–1914), Jeanne (1894–1978), and Jacques (1895–1965). Eugène's mother died in Paris on January 30, 1893. She was only 47 years old. Apert loved his mother very much, as reflected in his thesis dedication: "…in memory of my holy mother." Given that his mother's death occurred six days after Apert received the results of the internship competition, the joy of the medical graduate was undoubtedly eclipsed by mourning. Apert's thesis dedications also include his externship supervisor: "Mr. Ferrand also knows how grateful I am to him for his valuable assistance in sad circumstances." Although it is not clear that this dedication concerns his mourning of his mother, Apert had known Ferrand since his externship and joined his service on March 1, 1894, in a hospital located on *rue de Sèvres* very close to the family home. Apert's younger sister, Jeanne Henriette, married Léon Auguste Jeulin (1864–1934) on November

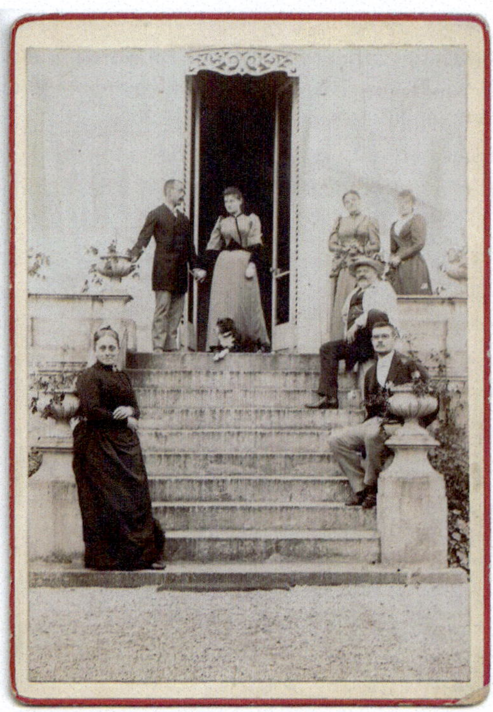

Fig. 2.5 August 6, 1891, in Saint-Brice-sous-Forêt (Val d'Oise): Eugène is seated in the first row on the right. (Photograph courtesy of Mrs. Brigitte Poujade; © *fond familial Bertin-Driancourt*)

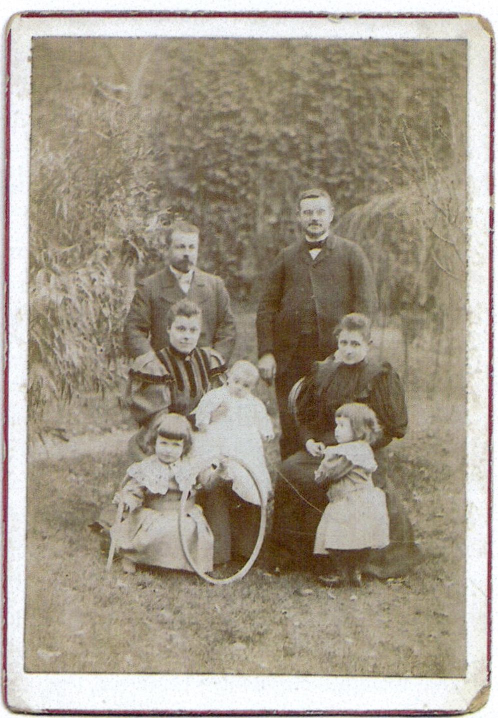

Fig. 2.6 With family in 1894: in the last row, Eugène Apert is standing on the right, Léon Jeulin on the left; the two sisters of Eugène are seated (Jeanne on the left holding her son, André Jeulin, on her knees, Marie-Laurence on the right); in the first row, two children of Marie-Laurence (Raymond with the hoop and Pierre on the right). (Photograph courtesy of Mrs. Brigitte Poujade; © *fond familial Bertin-Driancourt*)

4, 1893. The couple had three children: André Auguste (1894–1915), Henri Gustave Edmond (1898–1987), and Jean Edmond (1907–?).

Apert always remained very close to his sisters, nephews, and nieces (see Fig. 2.6). World War I dramatically affected his family, as was the case for many European families. The lives of Apert's nephews were profoundly disrupted by the war. Pierre Driancourt disappeared on September 29, 1914, while Raymond Driancourt was wounded in October 1914 and remained a German prisoner until the end of the war. Jacques Driancourt was wounded in the right arm in 1915 and remained disabled. Jeanne Driancourt served as a nurse. Apert's nephew, André Jeulin, died in March 1915. Apert was very affected by these familial misfortunes (Anne-Marie Driancourt, personal communication).

On October 28, 1900, Apert married Claire Caroline Estelle Noël (1875–1959) at the castle of Terrides near Labourgade (Tarn-et-Garonne). The bride was the daughter of Louis Hugues Noël, a lawyer, and Jeanne Marie Louise Théodora Magre (?–1922). Claire's aunt, Jane (1851–1916), was the wife of Marcel Dieulafoy (1844–1920), whose brother, Georges Dieulafoy, mentored Apert. Jane and Marcel were both very famous archaeologists; they carried out excavations in Susa (Iran) and brought the Frieze of the Archers and other wonders to the Louvre. It is very likely that the Apert–Noël couple met at Georges Dieulafoy's house. Thus, Apert was linked to Georges Dieulafoy not only by his medical training, but also by family ties. Apert wrote biographies of Dieulafoy [37] and of Pierre Bretonneau (1778–1862) [38], Dieulafoy's master. The castle of Terrides where Apert was married belonged to the Magre family. The Apert couple had the privilege of spending many holidays at the castle, which has since become a luxury hotel. The couple had three children: Louise Eugénie Marie (1902–1959), Christian Gustave Pierre (1904–1990), and Pierre Eugène (1914–1995). None of Apert's children had any descendants.

Eugène Apert as a Pediatrician

Apert became oriented to pediatrics during his internships with Grancher [47, 80] and his time spent in the maternity ward [80]. In the maternity ward, he saw and reported his first case of malformative pathology in a fetus [5] (see Fig. 2.7). Furthermore, his master, Budin, was the first to develop infant consultations. Apert perfectly integrated Budin's teaching and continued providing care for very young children throughout his life. Apert was a member of the Paris Pediatric Society from 1901 until his death. He presented many communications, the first in 1900 and the last in December 1934. He was very assiduous at the sessions and frequently participated until 1939, when the meetings were interrupted during World War II (Martin Catala, unpublished data). Apert's discussions demonstrated his great erudition and immense clinical experience.

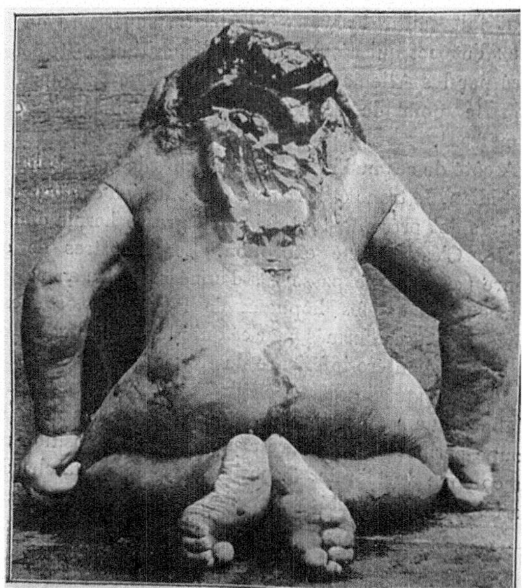

Fig. 2.7 Photograph of the first case of fetal malformation, a craniorachischisis, reported by Apert [5]. The article was not illustrated but the fetus was represented later. (From: Apert [19])

Apert participated in the dissemination of pediatric knowledge among his colleagues. For instance, he translated the *Atlas-Manual of Children's Diseases* (*Atlas-manuel des maladies de enfants*) from German [73]. He wrote the *Compendium of Children's Diseases* (*Précis des maladies des enfants*) [20], which had three subsequent editions in 1914, 1920, and 1926. In addition, Apert wrote a reference treatise on child hygiene [24, 25]. This treatise disseminated the knowledge necessary for the proper care of children to the general public, and was very successful among mothers. The author insisted on the need to respect the quality of sleep (pp. 128–131), described in detail the intellectual development of the child (pp. 203–207), and emphasized the importance of education. Apert also recognized the importance of vacations (p. 217). The second part of the work described behavior to adopt when faced with a sick child. The book was such a success that a second edition was published in 1924. Mrs. Anne-Marie Driancourt told me that when her older sister was born, Eugène Apert gave a copy of this book to her mother (who was married to one of his nephews). Mrs. Driancourt told me that, like her mother, she took great pleasure in reading it herself.

Eugène Apert and Genetics

For a long time, diseases transmitted from one generation to the next were called hereditary diseases. The term "heredity" was conceived according to its legal meaning: inheritance from one of the parents. The word "genetics," which is infinitely more familiar to us, was proposed by William Bateson (1861–1926) in a private letter dated April 18, 1905. Then, this term was used at the third international conference organized by the Royal Horticultural Society in London. The word "gene" was first defined by Wilhelm Ludwig Johanssen (1857–1927) in 1909.

The science of genetics presupposes knowledge of the laws governing the transmission of characteristics during reproduction. These laws, discovered in 1866 by Gregor Mendel (1822–1884), were largely ignored at the time. In 1900, three botanists—Hugo De Vries (1848–1935), Carl Correns (1864–1933), and Erich Tschermak (1871–1962)—rediscovered these laws and disseminated them throughout the scientific world. It is interesting to note that the laws of genetics were first established in plants. Very quickly after their rediscovery, these laws were applied to animals.

In France, these notions of transmission obeying defined laws were well accepted by botanists and some scientists, but adoption within the medical world was slow [23]. In 1907, Apert published *The Treatise on Familial Diseases and Congenital Diseases* (*Traité des maladies familiales et des maladies congénitales*), which can be considered to be the first book on medical genetics published in French. His definition of familial disease was very strict (p. 1): (1) several subjects are affected in the same family, (2) the disease presents the same form and the same evolution in all affected subjects, and (3) the condition occurs in the absence of external causes. Apert's sentence (p. 1) is unambiguous: "These are therefore diseases of the germ itself; the ovum or spermatozoon from which the subject is derived already has, from its origin, a latent defect; the external evolution of the subject only allows the original defect to manifest itself." In our eyes, this definition corresponds to our current genetic diseases. It is important to note that Apert excluded diseases caused by external events, including those occurring during the intrauterine period. Thus, he separated prenatal infections from familial diseases. He admitted that these infections could generate congenital diseases, hence the terms widely used in the nineteenth century and at the beginning of the twentieth century such as "heredo-syphilis" or "heredo-tuberculosis." In this same book (pp. 327–338), Apert explained the laws of heredity as discovered by Mendel and then rediscovered by De Vries. He supplemented this data with the experiments of Lucien Cuénot (1866–1951) on mice. Apert's chapter constitutes the first didactic presentation of the laws of heredity for a medical environment.

Apert's book includes a description of different modes of genetic transmission (pp. 320–327). In direct inheritance, the disease is transmitted from the patient to his descendants. Apert defined "continuous direct inheritance" as transmission in which all generations are affected (now referred to as "autosomal dominant inheritance") and "discontinuous direct inheritance" as transmission in which some generations are unaffected (corresponding to the notion of incomplete penetrance). Apert discussed another mode of transmission that he called "collateral inheritance," which involves a sudden appearance of a disease in a subject who then transmits it via a continuous, direct mode (now referred to as "neomutation"). Apert also described a mode of transmission in which only men are affected, and in which unaffected women transmit the disease. He noted that this mode of transmission is associated with conditions such as hemophilia, Duchenne's myopathy, and Daltonism, among others. Drawing an analogy with the transmission of inheritance in some societies, Apert called this mode "matriarchal transmission" (now referred to as "X-linked transmission"). In the final mode of transmission, Apert described: "Transmission can also occur exclusively through women for diseases that affect not only men, but also men and women. In affected families, there are about as many men as women affected; but the former do not transmit their affliction to their descendants, and it is only in the descendants of the latter that the disease is found" (p. 324). This mode of transmission is now well known as "mitochondrial transmission," but Apert could not have had the slightest intuition of this at his time.

Apert used the term "dominant trait," but it is curious to note that he did not use the word "recessive" (first used by Gregor Mendel). Instead, he wrote of a "dominated trait," and he did not use the term "recessive" until years later in his work on morbid heredity [26]. This can be explained by Apert's acknowledgment that he was not initially well trained in genetics. As he later explained [23], his interest in genetics was ignited by his work on achondroplasia [11]. At that time, he associated this disease with the concept of mutation developed by Hugo De Vries [62] to account for the evolution of species. According to De Vries, a mutation suddenly causes a new characteristic to appear and is thus opposed to the concept of progressive variability proposed by Charles Darwin (1809–1882). Later, and with humor, Apert wrote that he was doing genetics without knowing it [23]; he drew an analogy with Molière's Monsieur Jourdain who wrote prose without knowing it in *Le Bourgeois Gentilhomme*.

Apert [25] recognized the heredity of not only physical characteristics such as height and facial features, but also intellectual abilities. However, he held a nuanced view of the role of heredity in intelligence: "Such observations prove the enormous importance of the hereditary fund, but do not invalidate the no less enormous importance of education, provided that it is rational and does not fail to take into account the primordial innate differences between the various temperaments" ([30], p. 247). He concluded that education should not be homogeneous for all children, but instead adapted according to their innate abilities. This concept is currently the subject of discussion on establishing differentiated classes according to the academic levels of the pupils. Apert also believed in the heredity of moral qualities [25]. In particular, he affirmed the heredity of bad instincts by referring to the "born-criminal," a subject studied and disseminated by Cesare Lumbroso (1835–1909). Of course, he did not exclude the importance of the environment to a person's morality. These notions naturally led him to evoke the problem of free will, specifying that he could not resolve such a subject. The problem of genetic transmission of intellectual traits is still present in our society. In the early 1980s, when I was a student in a pediatric department at Montpellier Hospital, the head of the department advised students not to marry someone whose parents they did not know because heredity was fundamental in avoiding surprises that could affect offspring.

It is impossible to present all of Apert's work on genetics here. Nevertheless, I would like to discuss his hypotheses regarding the toxic action of exogenous substances [26]. Thus, Apert distinguished direct actions on spermatozoa or oocytes and, later, actions on cells of the fertilized egg. This is, therefore, the beginning of fetal medicine as we know it today. Finally, Apert was interested in twin pregnancies [28, 30]. He distinguished between monozygotic and dizygotic pregnancies, and he specified that study of the former could provide information on genetic factors and study of the latter could further understanding of environmental factors. Unfortunately, during his time it was not always possible to affirm the genetic status of twinning.

Eugène Apert and Infectious Diseases

With masters such as Joseph Grancher, André Chantemesse, and Émile Roux, Apert could not help but be interested in infectious pathology. His first works dealing with this subject were communications to the Anatomical Society of Paris in 1894 [3, 4]. These detailed cases of infective endocarditis were seen during his internship with Ange Ferrand. It is, of course, impossible for us to cite all of Apert's publications concerning infectious diseases. Nevertheless, we note his descriptions of certain epidemics of scarlet fever [9], rubella [48], and measles [31, 45], as well as his description of infantile forms of lethargic encephalitis [41].

During his studies, Apert witnessed the therapeutic revolution of vaccines and serums. In an article entitled "Death Is Retreating" [30, 31], Apert reported on these advances by observing that he had not seen a case of smallpox for 20 years. Diphtheria—so fearsome when he was an intern—was defeated by Roux's antitoxin serum, and the anti-typhoid vaccine was a great success in the fight against that disease. With Jean Lhermitte, then an intern, Apert treated tetanus by injecting serum into the epidural space to concentrate the serum at the level of the nerve roots [43]. Finally, faithful to his educational mission, Apert wrote a book on vaccines and serums [27], presenting the different types of therapeutic agents and acknowledging their potential side effects.

Eugène Apert and Acrocephalosyndactyly

Apert presented a case associating skull anomalies and syndactyly at the *Société Médicale des Hôpitaux de Paris* (Medical Society of Paris Hospitals) on December 21, 1906 [18]. This patient was a 15-month-old girl Apert received at the *Hôpital des Enfants-Malades* in 1896. Why did he take so long to publish this observation? We have no definite explanation. Maurice Camus (1877–1960), an intern at Paris hospitals, presented a similar case to the Biological Society on December 5, 1903 [53]. Apert had presented a botanical observation to the same society in November 1903. Was he present in December? Did this presentation force him to publish his case with a literature review? In the absence of primary documents, this is not clear. In the 1906 presentation, Apert referred to eight similar cases in the literature:

- Robert Troquart (1852–?) presented a case on February 12, 1886, at the Medico-Surgical Society of Bordeaux in a one-day-old newborn [87]. This case was not illustrated.
- Joseph Beno (1862–1894) reported a case of an 18-month-old girl (born in August 1884) (observation 29) in his medical thesis [50]. This case had been communicated to him by Professor Joseph Rohmer (1856–1921) of Nancy. Only the appearance of the hands was illustrated (see Fig. 2.8). This case is also the first for which the hands were operated on with reconstruction of a thumb (see Fig. 2.8b, c).
- Valentin Magnan (1835–1916) and Victor Galippe (1848–1922) presented the case of a 35-year-old man living at Sainte-Anne Hospital (Paris) with both typical dysmorphia and hand and foot syndactyly [79]. This was the first reported case in an adult and for which the dysmorphia was illustrated (see Fig. 2.9).
- Samuel Walton Wheaton (1861–1948) of the Royal Hospital for Children and Women in London reported two pathological cases in children who died at two and three months of age [91]. These two cases are the first for which a complete study could be carried out and for which anomalies of the base of the skull were described. Unfortunately, the article is not illustrated.
- Eugène Charles Maygrier (1849–1926) presented another case in a newborn girl (Maygier 1898). The observation was accompanied by the first photograph of a case of Apert syndrome and the first hand X-ray (see Fig. 2.10). This case was taken up by Edmond Fournier (1864–1938) in his medical thesis (observation 328). It is interesting to note that Apert gave two observations of congenital syphilis

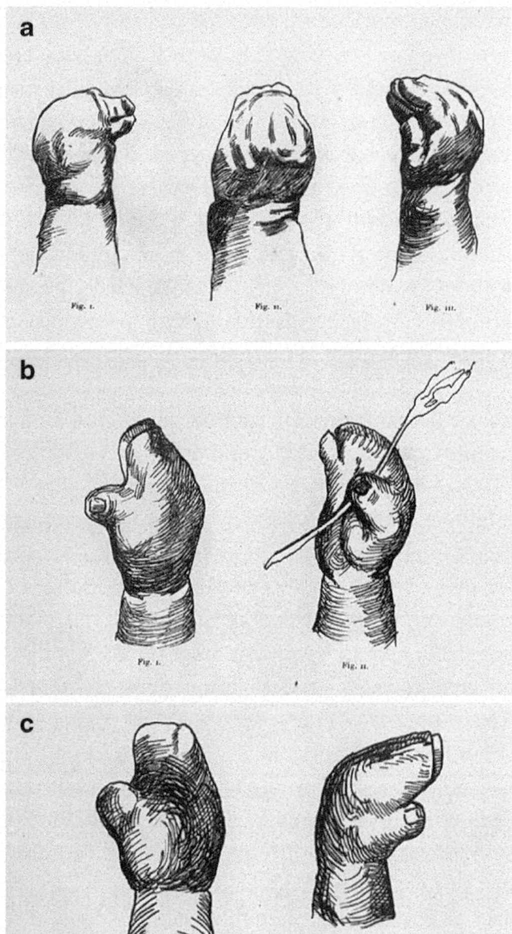

Fig. 2.8 (**a**) The left hand before surgery based on a hand cast of the patient at 18 months old. (**b**) The right hand after thumb release surgery (8 months later). (**c**) The left hand after surgery. (Reproduced from: Beno [50])

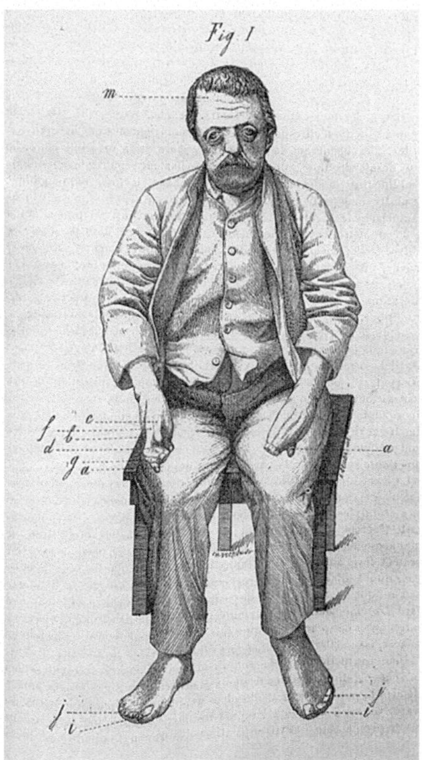

Fig. 2.9 The patient seen by Magnan and Galippe [79] at the age of 35. Note the craniofacial dysmorphia as well as the syndactyly of the hands and feet

(numbers 274 and 319) to Fournier in this thesis. Thus, we can be certain that Apert was familiar with Fournier's work.

- The same year, Louis Dubrisay (1863–1929) published another case in a newborn girl [64] (see Fig. 2.11).
- Maurice Camus presented a case in a boy aged 10.5 years [53]. This last observation was not illustrated.

Apert referred to another case that he considered to be different from the others, in that the craniofacial dysmorphia was associated with limb anomaly characterized by polysyndactyly. Today, this case seems more compatible with Greig syndrome than Apert syndrome. Apert did not illustrate his case in the article published in 1906, but he illustrated the limb anomalies the following year in his book on familial diseases [19] (see Fig. 2.12).

Using the eight published observations and his personal case, Apert defined the common features of a syndrome that he called "acrocephalosyndactyly." These features include a skull deformed with flattening of the occipital bone, domed forehead, brachycephaly, and elongated skull resembling a helmet. Newborns present a widening of the sagittal sutures and fontanelles. The skull and face are usually symmetrical, but this is not constant. The face is affected with depressed nasal bones and exorbitism of the eyes. The palate is abnormal, with a cleft and a bifid uvula. Sometimes, the upper jaws are fused at their anterior portion (see Fig. 2.13). In some cases, the number of fingers and toes is reduced. Syndactyly affects all or only some of the fingers and toes. The mechanism of craniofacial deformity is the premature fusion of the coronal suture and fusion of some synchondroses of the base of the skull. According to Apert, the origin of this malformation was unknown, and he invited his readers to be very cautious before concluding that syphilis was responsible, an etiology suggested by several authors before him. Thus, even if Apert was not the first to describe such patients, Apert was certainly the author who defined the syndrome and thus it is fair to give his name to this nosological entity. Initially, Apert considered this syndrome a nongenetic one, but later descriptions of familial recurrence led to his reconsidering this assertion [32, 35].

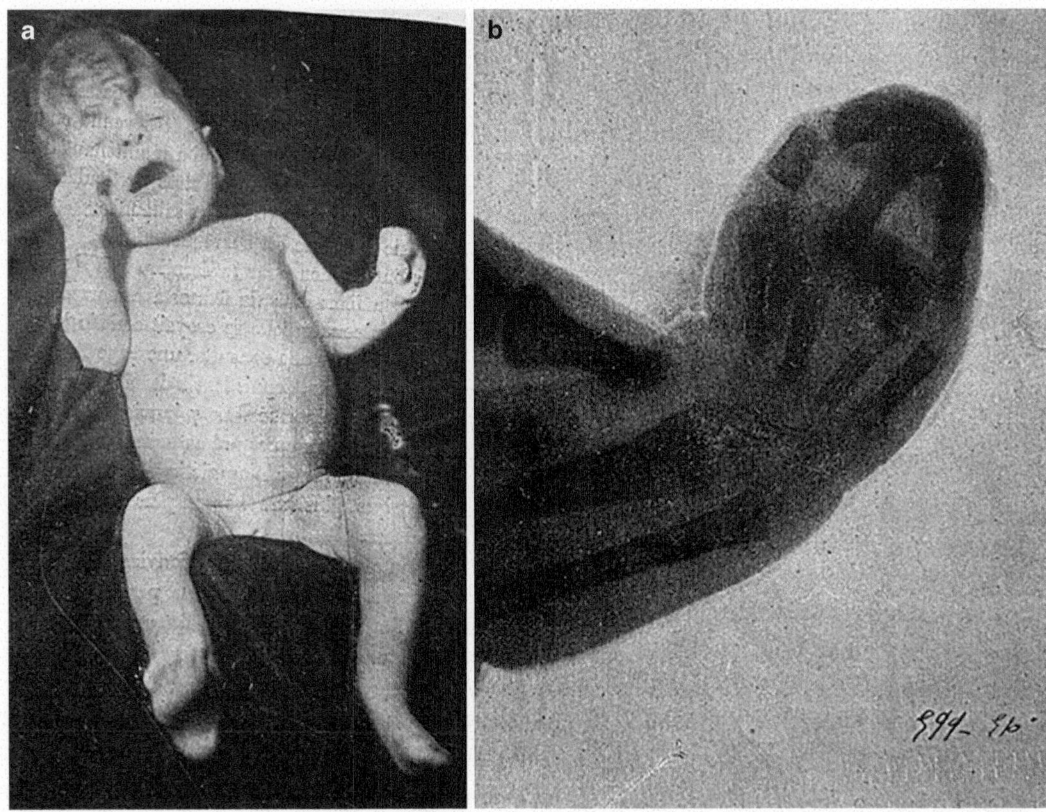

Fig. 2.10 (**a**) Photograph showing a newborn girl affected with Apert's syndrome. (**b**) Hand radiography performed in such a syndrome. (Reproduced from: Maygrier [81])

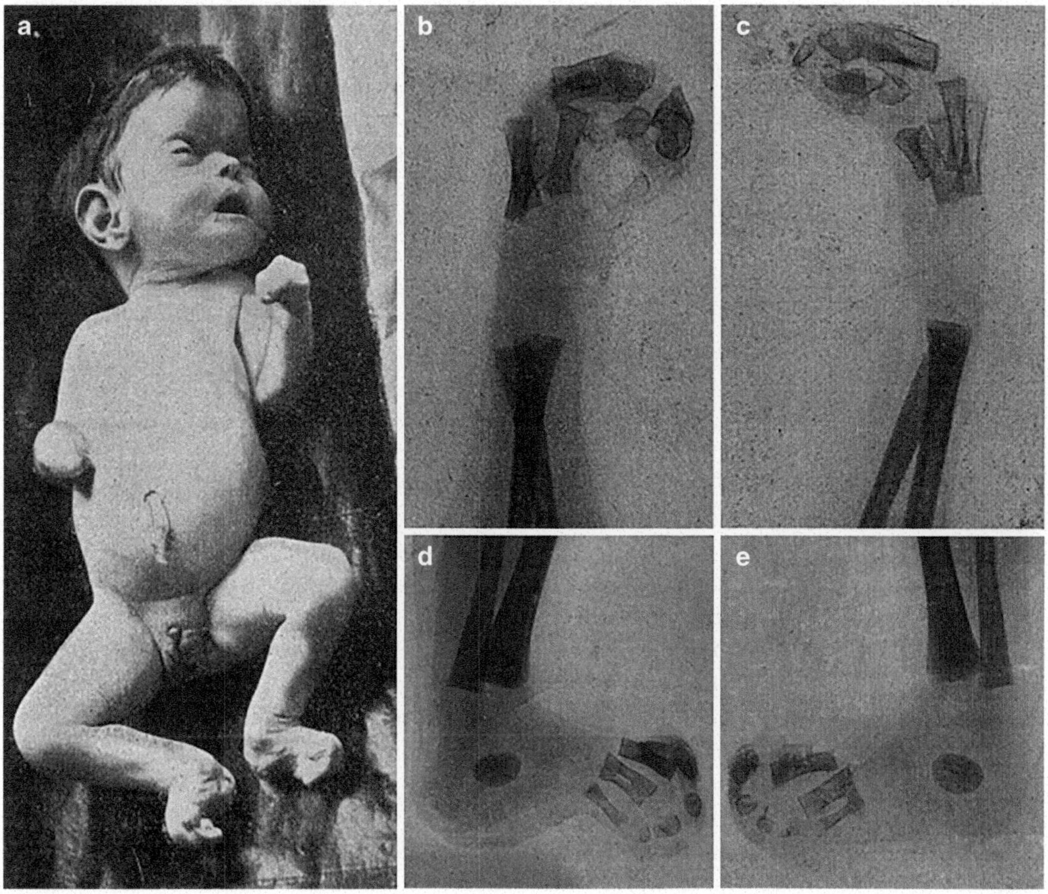

Fig. 2.11 (**a**) Photograph of the neonate. Radiographies of the right hand (**b**), left hand (**c**), right foot (**d**), and left foot (**e**). (Reproduced from: Dubrisay [64])

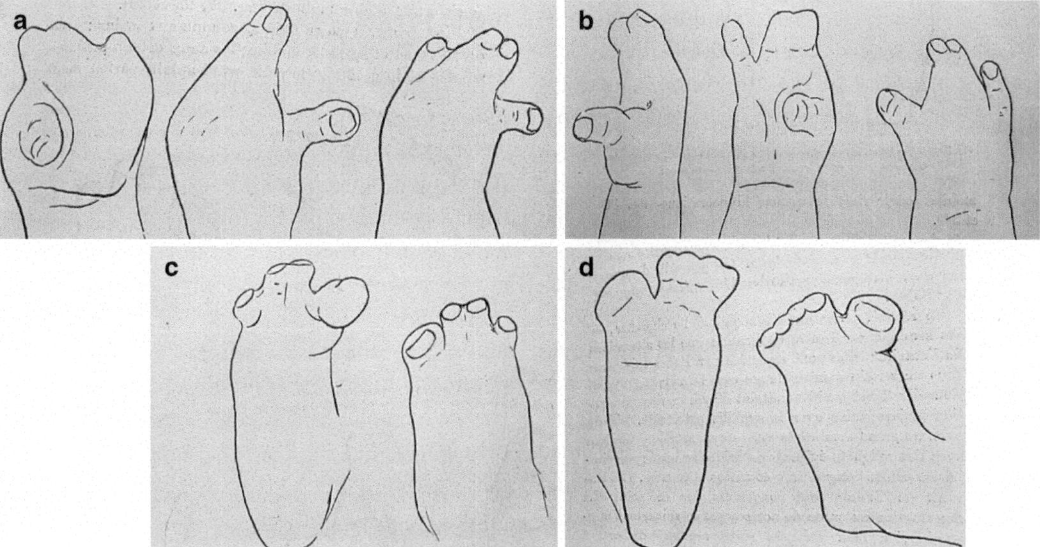

Fig. 2.12 Illustration of limb anomalies. (**a**) Left hand. (**b**) Right hand. (**c**) Right foot. (**d**) Left foot. (Reproduced from: Apert [19])

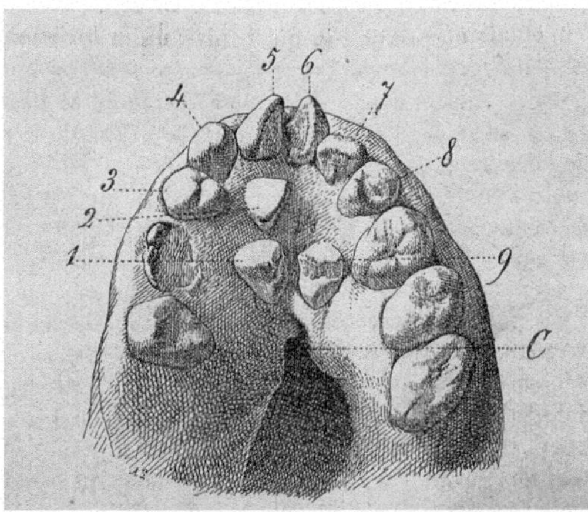

Fig. 2.13 Abnormal palate with fusion of the anterior region of the maxillary bones. (Reproduced from: Magnan and Galippe [79])

Eugène Apert: Achondroplasia and Other Dwarfisms

The representation of people with dwarfism has long existed in art. For example, Seneb of the ancient Egyptian Empire probably suffered from achondroplasia, and the painter Velásquez (1599–1660), at the Court of the King of Spain, depicted figures with dwarfism. However, the medical diagnosis was not specified in these old illustrations. At the Academy of Medicine in 1851, the obstetrician Jean Depaul (1811–1883) reported the case of a fetus suffering from dwarfism [63]. Until then, such cases had been described as fetal rickets. Depaul described the bones of this fetus and showed that the anomalies were not those of rickets. He thereby identified a new condition. The pediatrician Joseph Parrot (1829–1883) gave it the name "achondroplasia" because of the cartilage lesions found in this type of dwarfism [82].

The first observation of achondroplasia reported by Apert was a neonatal case observed on December 8, 1894, at the Maternity where he was then an intern of Guéniot [6]. The child was born and died after a few respiratory movements. The four limbs were abnormally small (see Fig. 2.14), contrasting with a normal head and trunk. The bones of the limbs were very abnormal (see Fig. 2.8) but did not resemble the deformations of rickets. In 1902 at the Biological Society, Apert responded to the veterinarian Louis Camille Leblanc (1827–1903) who considered bulldog calves (bovine achondroplasia) as suffering from myxedema. Apert [16] refuted Leblanc's conclusion by developing robust evidence obtained by studying these human conditions.

Apert reported two new cases of achondroplasia observed in adult males [11]. He noted that the external genitalia were well developed and sexual functions were normal. He recalled cases of transmission of the pathology by the mother, and his conclusion was unambiguous: "Achondroplasia, therefore, has an undeniable tendency to be transmitted by heredity" ([11], p. 296). Launois and Apert described another family affected by achondroplasia [75, 76]. They combined all the familial cases of this condition, reinforcing their conclusion of a genetic origin of this disease. Furthermore, they referred to the daughter of one of the patients presented by Apert previously [11], whose existence had been hidden by the father in 1901. The pediatrician Louis Arthur Sevestre (1843–1907) followed this child and informed Apert of her existence. This demonstrates that parents sometimes hide familial details from their doctors, posing challenges to genetic disease interviews. Later, other affected children were born from this man [21]. Another new case, observed in 1911 and reported in March 1914, was a woman who died at the age of 78 [42]. The authors described some particularities suggesting the coexistence of Paget's disease with achondroplasia.

Interestingly, Apert referred to animal pathologies resembling achondroplasia [11, 75, 76]. He even urged veterinarians to study the cartilage of these animals [76]. Thus, from the beginning of the twentieth century, Apert recognized the importance of what we now call "animal models." Apert referred to Hugo De Vries' theory of mutations [62], which proposed that speciation was due to genetic mutation. This led Apert to an original hypothesis. Drawing an analogy to animal pathologies resembling achondroplasia, Apert proposed that this condition could be the beginning of the emergence of a new variety of

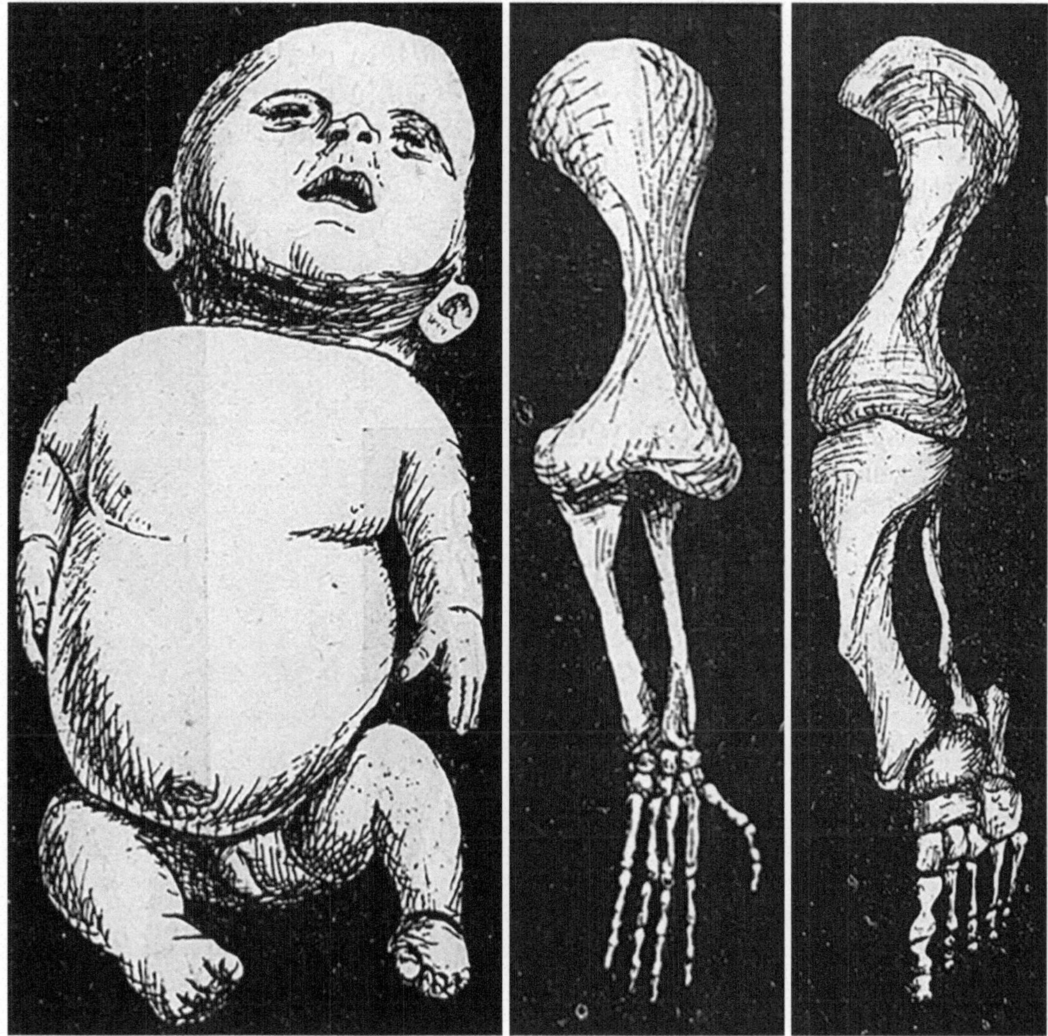

Fig. 2.14 A case of achondroplasia observed by Apert in 1894 [6]. General aspect of the fetus and of the limb bones

human beings. However, he noted that this new trait led to difficulty in childbirth, which entailed a selective disadvantage harmful to evolution. Apert deserves credit for his early imagining of the phenomena of island dwarfism long before the discovery of the famous Flores Man (*Homo floresiensis*). Apert described renal dwarfism as a growth arrest secondary to chronic renal failure in children [33, 44]. Additionally, he mentioned a growth retardation related to endocrine disorders—particularly thyroid disorders—that is reversible by hormonal treatment, differentiating it from true dwarfism [17].

Apert and Malformative Syndromes

Apert oriented early toward the study of malformations, as indicated by one of his first publications about a case of craniorachischisis [5] (see

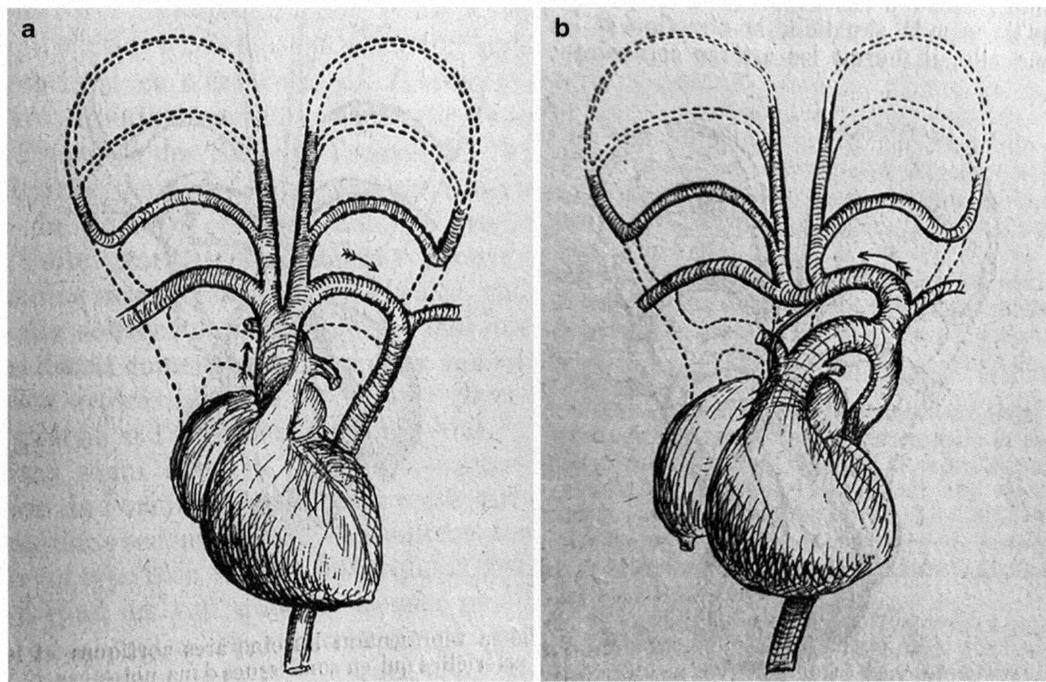

Fig. 2.15 A case of hypoplastic left heart syndrome. (**a**) Normal vessels derived from aortic arches. (**b**) Abnormal features of the vessels due to hypoplasia of the left heart. (Reproduced from: Apert [7])

Fig. 2.7). Apert described one case of what is now called hypoplastic left heart syndrome [7]. He attributed this lesion to a primary absence of the orifice of the aorta, and he analyzed the consequences in vessel morphogenesis (see Fig. 2.15). This case and the literature review demonstrate Apert's mode of analysis based upon physiology. Although it is impossible to reference all the observations of malformative syndromes published by Apert, it is interesting to note that he distinguished these processes according to their possible causes. For example, he reported limb deformations (arthrogryposis) linked to oligoamnios [8] (see Fig. 2.16).

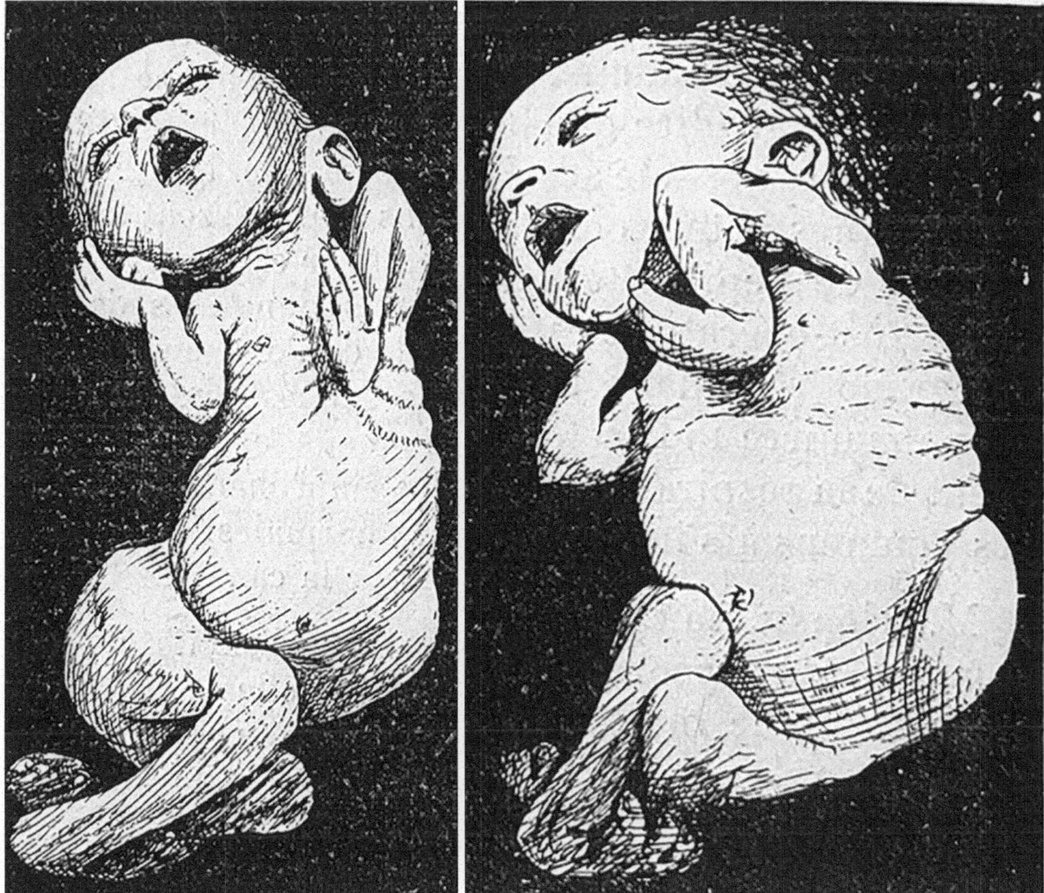

Fig. 2.16 Fetus affected by arthrogryposis secondary to oligoamnios. (Reproduced from: Apert [8])

Apert and Endocrinology

Apert's first patients with endocrine disorders were received at the Hôtel-Dieu in 1899 and 1900 [12–14]. They were adolescents or young adults aged 15.5–21 years with delayed puberty, delayed psychological development, and delayed growth. Their appearance was that of adults or young adults who had remained childlike (*infantilisme*). The obesity in the first case [12] led him to suggest myxedema, and Apert consulted Édouard Brissaud (1852–1909), a specialist in these problems, for his opinion. Brissaud confirmed Apert's clinical diagnosis and encouraged him to implement the substitution treatment that Apert wanted to try. In addition, Brissaud advised Apert to take photographs of the patient before and during the treatment to judge its effectiveness. Apert reported the positive results of the opotherapy treatment, effects that were confirmed in a second case [13]. The third case reported by Apert died, thus allowing a histological analysis of the principal glands. The thyroid was analyzed with the help of Brissaud, Marcel Garnier (1870–1940) [14], and Victor Cornil (1827–1908) [15]. Cornil confirmed the definitive diagnosis of thyroid adenomas [15]. The testes were prepubertal and the pituitary gland was normal. Later, Apert made a synthesis of the "retarded child" (*enfants retardaires*) [17] or the *infantilisme* [34]. He insisted that the condition was a treatable global developmental delay, unlike fixed mental retardation.

At the meeting of the Paris Pediatric Society held on June 20, 1939, Apert demanded that

Cushing's syndrome of adrenal origin be named Apert–Gallais syndrome [39]. Apert referred to a literature review that he presented to the Paris Pediatric Society during the December 20, 1910, session in which he grouped and analyzed 31 autopsy cases of adrenal tumor or hyperplastic anomalies [22]. This allowed him to isolate a clinical syndrome in certain patients, now known as Cushing's syndrome. On this occasion, Apert proposed the term *hirustisme* to define the hypertrichosis associated with the syndrome. This work led Pierre-Émile Launois (1856–1914), Marcel Pinard (1881–1939), and Alfred Gallais (1881–?) to describe a patient presenting this symptomatology due to adrenal tumors [77]. Meanwhile, Harvey Cushing (1869–1939) delivered a lecture on dyspituitarism to the Harvey Society on December 10, 1910 [56]. He described a polyglandular syndrome explained by an impairment of several endocrine glands. Unfortunately, this lecture has not reached us in its entirety. Two years later, Cushing published a monograph on the pituitary gland and its disorders [57]. This work constituted an expanded edition of his Harvey lecture. Cushing reported the case of 23-year-old Miss M. G., seen by him on December 29, 1910 [57]. This patient presented clinical features of hypercortisolism. Cushing suspected a pituitary disorder that he was unable to identify at that time. Of note, Cushing saw this patient after giving his Harvey lecture on December 10, and therefore the case was not included in his talk. Cushing wrote that this case could be secondary to an adrenal anomaly, and he reported on the publication of Launois et al. [77]. Finally, he described pituitary Cushing's disease in 1932 [58]. Although Apert played a role in the individualization of this syndrome, Cushing's nomenclature became established, as it would not be desirable to us today to have two different names for the same clinical syndrome. The distinction between Cushing's disease (of pituitary origin) and Cushing's syndrome (in other cases) seems much more educational. Sic transit gloria mundi.

Apert was the first to study the blood cholesterol level in people with diabetes [46]. In 1910, Adrien Grigaut (1884–1960), chemist and chief of the chemistry laboratory of medical doctor Anatole Chauffard (1855–1932), developed a technique for measuring cholesterol levels in 1910 [71]. Apert's study was preliminary and imperfect in only including nine patients with diabetes, two subjects with xanthomas, and two "controls" without glycosuria (one with advanced heart failure and the other with senility). The authors concluded that the blood level was not significantly higher in people with diabetes than in healthy subjects. Even if the methodology is far from perfect, it is noteworthy that Apert was the first to study cholesterol in diabetic patients. World War I disrupted these studies, and Apert abandoned this clinical field to focus on pediatrics with his appointment to the Hospital for Sick Children.

Apert and Eugenics

Francis Galton (1822–1911), a cousin of Charles Darwin (1809–1882), wanted to study heredity in "illustrious" men using statistical methods [68]. To do this, he analyzed data from over 1000 individuals in 300 families, 415 of whom were categorized as illustrious (p. 316). His study included subjects from diverse professions, such as judges, statesmen, high-ranking military men, literary figures, scientists, poets, artists, and religious men. Obviously, the results differed according to the groups (p. 317). Nevertheless, Galton found eminent men among the ancestors and the descendants of illustrious subjects, and he concluded that genius was hereditary. This work presents many biases and could no longer be considered valid. For instance, there is no control group. Moreover, a detailed analysis of Galton's data shows that he found illustrious ancestors among great-grandfathers in all categories except literary, scientific, and artistic ones. To our current eyes, the advantages of class appear more relevant than hereditary acquisition. Finally, let us not forget that Galton was only interested in male subjects in these studies.

In 1874, Galton published a book about prominent British scientists [69]. In this work, he proposed the expression "nature versus nurture" to discriminate between what is intrinsic to the subject (nature) and what is acquired after birth in response to external influences (nurture) (pp. 12–16). Galton expressed no doubt that what he called nature played a role in relation to nurture. However, he acknowledged that it was difficult for him to study hereditary characteristics (pp. 39–40) and that interest in science was not highly heritable (pp. 196–197). Galton lamented that branches of science led to less financially lucrative professions (p. 259). Finally, he attempted to establish the best educational system (p. 256) that would emphasize teachings in (1) mathematics, (2) logic, (3) observation, theory, and experimentation, (4) accurate drawing, and (5) mechanical manipulation. Galton's studies were very well received at the end of the nineteenth century, especially in conservative circles. Galton then proposed:

> We greatly want a brief word to express the science of improving stock, which is by no means confined to questions of judicious mating, but which, especially in the case of man, takes cognisance of all influences that tend in however remote degree to give to more suitable races or strains of blood a better chance of prevailing speedily over the less suitable than they otherwise would have had. The word eugenics would sufficiently express the idea (p. 25) …. [70]

Several eugenics societies were created throughout the world, and the first International Eugenics Congress was held in London in July 1912. Among the vice-presidents of this congress were Jules Dejerine (1849–1917) and Valentin Magnan. The French delegation included five pediatricians (including Apert), three alienists, one dermatologist, one demographer, and one biologist. A few months later, the French Eugenics Society was created in January 1913. However, World War I interrupted the work of this society and after the war, the main concern in France was promoting birth rate, not optimizing eugenics. The French Eugenics Society was in fact very ideologically heterogeneous [78]. Some members were extremists, such as Charles Richet (1850–1935), who advocated the infanticide of abnormal newborns on the pretext that they did not yet have a psyche [85]. In contrast, Apert was more moderate [78]. He was against sterilization [90], abortion, and, of course, infanticide. He only advocated the education of families in cases of recessive diseases [89]. Apert specified, "We do not claim to be directors of people or legislators" ([36], p. 8). Furthermore, he stated, "It remains that with regard to harmful, pathological genetic characteristics, we know which unions should be discouraged or even forbidden. This is negative eugenics. Positive eugenics would aim at the conservation of qualities" ([36], p. 9). However, let us note that Apert did not espouse an absolute ideal of the human species [89]. Apert was always cautious, asking that scientific studies reinforce knowledge of hereditary transmission before applying it in legislation [89]. Apert was only in favor of prohibiting consanguineous marriage in the case of a recessive disease or marriage between descendants of subjects suffering from the same recessive disease [89]. Thus, Apert was a moderate eugenicist who wanted to develop research and education before proposing more drastic legislative measures. Let us remember that such measures—including compulsory sterilization—were in force at this time in many countries.

The Eugenics Society in France proposed measures to encourage births, but few were the subject of laws [40]. These included family allowances to help families with more than three children (a measure that was the subject of various laws between 1923 and 1938) and the establishment of a family quotient allowing income tax to be reduced according to the number of children (not implemented until the *Libération* in 1945). Additionally, we should note that the French Eugenics Society suggested the introduction of the prenuptial certificate [40]. This certificate, still in use in France, was introduced by the collaborationist regime of Philippe Pétain (1856–1951) in 1942.

Eugène Apert and Immigration

Apert developed racist theses in several of his publications. In my opinion, his theses are to be condemned. Nevertheless, the work of a biographer requires an attempt to place the concepts in the currents of thought at the time they were written, not to excuse the ideas, but rather trying to analyze the historical context. At the beginning of the twentieth century, France was experiencing a low birth rate, in contrast to its neighbors. Such a low birth rate had been noted in France since at least the beginning of the nineteenth century [83]. After disastrous defeat in the Franco-Prussian War of 1870–1871, France developed a spirit of revenge against its natural enemy, Germany. After World War I, the French population declined, with 1.4 million deaths caused directly by the war and another 240,000 deaths related to Spanish influenza. This demographic loss led to using foreign labor to rebuild the country. In addition, soldiers from the various colonies were stationed in France. These factors led to a national shift in perspective on immigration.

The heterogeneity of human populations has long been noted in religious books, with the Bible describing the three sons of Noah whose descendants share the Earth. However, the concept of human races was not developed until the seventeenth century. This concept was described by Englishman William Petty (1623–1687) in an unpublished manuscript and by the Frenchman François Bernier (1620–1688) in an article published on April 24, 1684, in the *Journal des Sçavans*. Bernier recognized at least four different races, but he admitted having difficulty classifying certain populations. It is interesting to note that Bernier did not in any way hierarchize the members of these classes. Subsequent discussion focused on the number of races, each being subdivided into varieties. Georges Cuvier (1769–1832) recognized three races based on skin color (1817): "white," "yellow," and "black." I will use this nineteenth-century terminology in this chapter because it underlies the conceptions of the various authors I quote. From that time onward, Cuvier associated each race with a hierarchy, ranking the white race superior to the yellow, and ranking both as superior to the black race. But the foundation of biological racism came from the writings of Robert Knox (1791–1862) in his book on the races of men [74] and of Count Arthur de Gobineau (1816–1882) in his writing on the inequalities of human races [60]. In 1859, Paul Broca (1824–1880) created the Anthropological Society with 18 colleagues. He published his work on the volume and shape of the brain in 1861, in which he stated that the brain was larger in white subjects than in yellow subjects and smallest in black subjects. The birth of a science or pseudoscience justifying racial inequality led to the biological racism of the nineteenth and mid-twentieth centuries. However, it is necessary to note the work of the Haitian anthropologist Joseph Anténor Firmin (1850–1911), who published a book criticizing the concept of racial inequality [66]. Nevertheless, inegalitarian currents were preponderant in Europe and in the United States. Apert was a supporter of this inequality of the human population. In this sense, immigration and miscegenation (i.e., marriage, cohabitation, or sexual intercourse between a white person and a member of another race) posed a problem to his ideology.

Apert reported the increasing number of children of foreign origin treated in his department at the Children's Hospital [29]. For him, one of the causes of this increase was that health care was free of charge for this foreign-born population, while the French population had to pay for consultation. For Apert, a second cause of immigration was the deficit of the native French population, which had been exacerbated by the war, and he recognized that using foreign labor was essential [29]. Apert noted that a third source of immigration was the presence of colonial soldiers who had come to metropolitan France. This influx of foreigners led Apert to consider the problem of miscegenation [29], and he differentiated several cases. Aligned with the racist ideas of Charles Richet [85], Apert considered the miscegenation between white individuals with black or yellow people to be harmful. He recalled with satisfaction the American laws at the time that prohibited mixed marriages and encouraged segregation. The second case concerned marriages between white populations. Apert recognized the absence of pure races in Europe due to its history marked by multiple migrations [29, 36]. According to him, populations close to France—Belgians, Italians, Spanish, and Portuguese—integrated easily [29, 40]. Apert considered the influx of people from the East—Armenians, Syrians, Greeks, and Anatolians—to be a radically different problem [29]. Indeed, for him these populations were not inclined to agricultural work. While Apert believed Russians had a tendency toward alcoholism, he considered the Czechs and Poles to be better suited to hard labor. Nevertheless, he was concerned that their mixing with the French population could yield potentially unfortunate consequences. Finally, Apert [29] considered the issue of Jewish immigration from Central Europe. Although he acknowledged the possible success of Jewish people in France, he lamented their endogamy and the maintenance of their traditions. Thus, Apert, who feared miscegenation in some cases, regretted its absence in others. It is interesting to note that Apert did not refer to Jewish populations in his 1940 article. Was this a reaction against Nazi discriminatory policy? We have found no reference to this. Apert recommended a limitation on immigration and again referred to American legislation that had led to a restriction of the influx of populations from southern and central Europe.

Conclusion

Eugène Apert was one of the precursors of modern pediatrics in France. He introduced the laws of Mendelian genetics into the French medical field. Apert developed the analysis of fetal malformations and described several syndromes, including the one that bears his name. Like other prominent doctors at the time, he was a fervent follower of moderate eugenics, and he supported xenophobic views. His clinical activity and dissemination of knowledge were very important, as reflected in his considerable number of publications.

Acknowledgments I dedicate this chapter to my friend Dominique Renier who introduced me to craniofacial malformations in 1985. I acknowledge the valuable information on Apert's family obtained by Anne-Marie Driancourt and Brigitte Poujade. This chapter was suggested to me by Eric Arnaud, who is more than a colleague.

References

1. Apert E. De l'alimentation des enfants du premier âge. Bull Med. 1893a;7:843–4.
2. Apert E. Traitement des fistules à l'anus par la Réunion primitive. Bull Med. 1893b;7:1124–6.
3. Apert E. Deux cas d'endocardite végétante. Bulletins de la Société Anatomique de Paris. 1894a;69:305–8.
4. Apert E. 1° Endocardite végétante mitrale d'origine puerpérale. 2° Endocardite végétante tricuspidienne d'origine biliaire. Bull Soc Anat Paris. 1894b;69:427–30.
5. Apert E. Monstre pseudencéphale avec hernie ombilicale et malformations génitales. Naissance au terme de 7 mois.—Mort peu après la naissance. Bulletins et Mémoires de la Société Obstétricale et Gynécologique de Paris. 1894c;10:285–9.
6. Apert E. Achondroplasie. Bull Soc Anat Paris. 1895a;70:772–5.
7. Apert E. Absence congénitale d'orifice aortique. Atrophie du cœur gauche et de l'aorte ; système artériel entièrement fourni par l'artère pulmonaire. Bull Soc Anat Paris. 1895b;70:683–91.
8. Apert E. Malformations congénitales multiples par oligoamnios. Bulletins de la Société Anatomique de Paris. 1895c;70:762–72.
9. Apert E. La scarlatine à l'hôpital des Enfants-Malades en 1895. Bull Mem Soc Med Hop Paris. 1896;13(3e série):424–41.
10. Apert E. Le purpura, sa pathogénie et celle de ses diverses variétés cliniques. G Steinheil, Paris: Thèse de médecine de Paris; 1897.
11. Apert E. Quelques remarques sur l'achondroplasie (deux observations nouvelles d'achondroplases adultes). Nouvelle Iconographie de la Salpêtrière. 1901a;14:290–8.
12. Apert E. Obésité, état énuchoïde, cryptorchidie, traitement thyroïdien, guérison. Bulletins de la Société de Pédiatrie de Paris. 1901b;3:108–14.
13. Apert E. Infantilisme dysthyroïdien ; traitement par le corps thyroïde ; guérison. Bulletins de la Société de Pédiatrie de Paris. 1901c;3:114–7.
14. Apert E. Infantilisme très accentué ; autopsie ; examen histologique du corps thyroïde, du corps pituitaire, des capsules surrénales et des testicules. Bulletins de la Société de Pédiatrie de Paris. 1901d;3:118–26.
15. Apert E. Examen histologique du corps thyroïde et d'autres organes d'un sujet atteint d'infantilisme. Bulletins de la Société de Pédiatrie de Paris. 1901e;3:200–2.
16. Apert E. Le myxœdème et l'achondroplasie sont deux affections totalement différentes. Comptes Rendus des Séances de la Société de Biologie. 1902a;54:127–9.
17. Apert E. Les enfants retardataires. J-B Baillière & Fils, Paris. 1902b. 95 pages.
18. Apert E. De l'acrocéphalosyndactylie. Bull Mem Soc Med Hop Paris. 1906;23(3e série):1310–30.

19. Apert E. Traité des maladies familiales et des maladies congénitales. Paris: J-B Baillière et Fils; 1907. 364 pages.
20. Apert E. Précis des maladies des enfants. Paris: J-B Baillière et Fils; 1909a. 524 pages.
21. Apert E. Une famille d'achondroplases (présentation de malades). Bulletins de la Société de Pédiatrie de Paris. 1909b;11:35–7.
22. Apert E. Dystrophies en relation avec des lésions des capsules surrénales. Hirsutisme et progeria. Bulletins de la Société de Pédiatrie de Paris. 1910;12:501–18.
23. Apert E. La génétique. Lois de Mendel et descendances morbides. Paris Med. 1912;5:81–6.
24. Apert E. Hygiène de l'enfance. L'enfant bien portant—L'enfant malade. J-B Baillière, Paris. 1913a. 416 pages.
25. Apert E. Les problèmes de l'hérédité. Rev Sci. 1913b;51:39–48.
26. Apert E. L'hérédité morbide. Paris: Ernest Flammarion; 1919. p. 306.
27. Apert E. Vaccins et sérums. Paris: Ernest Flammarion; 1922. 282 pages.
28. Apert E. Les jumeaux, étude biologique, physiologique et médicale. Paris: Ernest Flammarion; 1923a. 264 pages.
29. Apert E. Immigration et métissage. Leur influence sur la santé de la Nation. Presse Med. 1923b;36:1565–9.
30. Apert E. Maladies gémellaires. Revue Anthropologique. 1925a;35:252–7.
31. Apert E. L'épidémie de rougeole actuelle ; sa prédominance chez les tout-petits. Bulletins Société de Pédiatrie de Paris. 1925b;23:138–40.
32. Apert E. Discussion. Bulletin de la Société de Pédiatrie de Paris. 1928a;26:494–5.
33. Apert E. Les altérations osseuses sans les néphrites atrophiques infantiles. Nanisme rénal Pseudo-rachitisme rénal. Presse Med. 1928b;36:577–9.
34. Apert E. L'infantilisme. Doin, Paris. 1931. 69 pages.
35. Apert E. Discussion. Bulletins de la Société de Pédiatrie de Paris. 1937a;35:145–6.
36. Apert E. L'importance sociale des études eugéniques. In: Premier Congrès Latin d'Eugénique (Paris). Paris: Masson et Cie; 1937b. p. 7–12.
37. Apert E. Georges Dieulafoy (1839–1911). In: Les Biographies Médicales. Paris: J-B Baillière; 1938a.
38. Apert E. Pierre Bretonneau (1778–1862). In: Les Biographies Médicales. Paris: J-B Baillière; 1938b.
39. Apert E. Discussion. Bulletins de la Société de Pédiatrie de Paris. 1939;37:331–3.
40. Apert E. L'Eugénique en France. Le Nourrisson. 1940;28–29:89–102.
41. Apert E, Broca R, Chabanier. L'encéphalite léthargique chez les enfants des premières années. Bulletins de la Société de Pédiatrie de Paris. 1923;21:74–80.
42. Apert E, Le Maux R. Étude du squelette d'une achondroplase morte à 78 ans avec un état de certains os rappelant la maladie de Paget. Bulletins et Mémoires de la Société Anatomique de Paris. 1914–1919;89:127–36.
43. Apert E, Lhermitte J. Tétanos par infection d'un ulcère de jambe. Injection épidurales (para-radiculaires) de sérum antitétanique. Guérison. Bull Mem Soc Med Hop Paris. 1904;21:482–6.
44. Apert E, Peytavin C. Arrêt de croissance et déformations osseuses par néphrite interstitielle. Bulletins de la Société de Pédiatrie. 1929;27:307–14.
45. Apert E, Vallery-Radot P. La rougeole à l'Hôpital des Enfants-Malades en 1920. Bulletins de la Société de Pédiatrie de Paris. 1921;19:24–9.
46. Apert E, Péchery R, Rouillard J-M. Mesure de la cholestérinémie chez les diabétiques. Comptes Rendus Hebdomadaires des Séances et Mémoires de la Société de Biologie. 1912;72:822–4.
47. Armand-Delille P. Nécrologie. M E Apert et M Ed Pichon. Bulletins de la Société de Pédiatrie de Paris. 1940;37:505–7.
48. Aviragnet EC, Apert E. Relation de deux épidémies de rubéole avec remarques sur la symptomatologie et le diagnostic de cette maladie. Bulletins de la Société de Pédiatrie de Paris. 1906;8:33–49.
49. Babonneix L. Eugène Apert. Gazette des Hôpitaux Civils et Militaires. 1940;113:169.
50. Beno J. Essai sur la syndactylie congénitale. Observation 29. Thèse de Médecine (Nancy) n°238. 1886. pp. 43–9.
51. Broca P. Sur le volume et la forme du cerveau suivant les individus et suivant les races. Paris: Hennuyer; 1861. 75 pages.
52. Cambessédès H. Nécrologie : Eugène Apert. Paris Médical (partie paramédicale). 1940;116–117:235–6.
53. Camus M. Accumulation de stigmates physiques chez un dégénéré. Compte Rendus Hebdomadaires des Séances et Mémoires de la Société de Biologie. 1903;55:1555–7.
54. Comby J. Nécrologie (E. Apert). Archives de Médecine des Enfants. 1940;43:191–2.
55. Correns C. G Mendels Regel über das Verhalten der Nachkommenschaft der Rassenbastarde. Berichte der deutschen botanischen Gesellschaft. 1900;18:158–68.
56. Cushing H. Dyspituitarism. The Harvey lectures 1910–1911. Philadelphia and London: JB Lippincott Company; 1911. p. 31–45.
57. Cushing H. The pituitary body and its disorders. Clinical states produced by disorders oft he hypophysis cerebri. Philadelphia & London: JB Lippincott Company; 1912. 341 pages.
58. Cushing H. The basophil adenomas of the pituitary body and their clinical manifestations (pituitary basophilism). Bull Johns Hopkins Hosp. 1932;50:137–95.
59. Cuvier G. Le règne animal distribué d'après son organisation pour servir de base à l'histoire naturelle des animaux et d'introduction à l'anatomie comparée, vol. 1. Paris: Deterville; 1817. p. 94–5.
60. de Gobineau A. Essai sur l'inégalité des races humaines. Vol 1. Paris: Firmin Didot frères; 1853. 492 pages.

61. De Vries H. Das Spaltungsgesetz der Bastarde. Berichte der deutschen botanischen Gesellschaft. 1900;18:83–90.
62. De Vries H. Die Mutationstheorie. Versuche und Beobachtungen über die Entstehung von Arten im Pflanzenreich, vol. 1. Leipzig: Veit & Comp; 1901. 648 pages.
63. Depaul J. Sur une maladie spéciale du système osseux, développée pendant la vie intra-utérine, et qui est généralement décrite sous le nom de rachitisme. Bulletins de l'Académie Nationale de Médecine. 1851;16:378–9.
64. Dubrisay L. Enfant atteint de proencéphalie et de syndactylie, issu d'une mère syphilitique—Présentation de pièces et photographies radiographiques. Bulletin de la Société d'Obstétrique de Paris. 1898;1:81–7.
65. Ferrand A. L'homme et la thèse de l'évolutionnisme. Union Médicale. 1879;27:41–144.
66. Firmin JA. De l'égalité des races humaines. Cotillon, F Pichon, Paris. 1885. 665 pages.
67. Fournier E. Stigmates dystrophiques de l'hérédo-syphilis. Paris: Thèse de Médecine; 1898. p. 244–6.
68. Galton F. Hereditary genius: an inquiry into its laws and consequences. London: Macmillan and CO.; 1869. 390 pages.
69. Galton F. English men of science. Their nature and nurture. London: Macmillan & Co.; 1874. 270 pages.
70. Galton F. Inquiries into human faculty and its development. London: Macmillan and Co.; 1883. 387 pages 25.
71. Grigaut A. Procédé colorimétrique de dosage de la cholestérolémie dans l'organisme note préliminaire. Comptes Rendus Hebdomadaires des Séances et Mémoires de la Société de Biologie. 1910;68:791–3.
72. H. Eugène Apert (1868-1940). Presse Med. 1940;48:566–7.
73. Hecker R, Trumpp J. Atlas-Manuel des maladies de enfants. Traduction d'E. Apert J-B Baillière et Fils Paris; 1906. 423 pages.
74. Knox R. The races of men: a fragment. London: Henry Renshaw; 1850. 479 pages.
75. Launois PE, Apert E. Achondroplasie héréditaire. Bull Mem Soc Med Hop Paris. 1905a;22(3e série):606–13.
76. Launois EP, Apert E. L'hérédité de l'achondroplasie chez l'homme et les animaux. Bulletin de la Société de Pathologie Comparée. 1905b;4:18–21.
77. Launois PE, Pinard M, Gallais A. Syndrome adiposo-génital, avec hypertrichose, troubles nerveux et mentaux d'origine surrénale. Gazette Hôpitaux Civils et Militaires. 1911;84:649–54.
78. Léonard J. Les origines et les conséquences de l'eugénique en France. Annales de Démographie Historique. 1986;1:203–14.
79. Magnan V, Galippe V. Accumulation de stigmates physiques chez un débile. Brachycéphalie, plagiocéphalie, acrocéphalie, asymétrie faciale, atrésie buccale, syndactylie des quatre extrémités. Comptes Rendus Hebdomadaires des Séances et Mémoires de la Société de Biologie. 1892;44:277–87.
80. Marfan A-M. Nécrologie. Eugène Apert (1868-1940). Le Nourrisson. 1940;28–29:134–6.
81. Maygrier EC. Présentation d'un enfant atteint de malformations du crâne (proencéphalie) et des extrémités (syndactylie) par hérédo-syphilis. Bulletin de la Société d'Obstétrique de Paris. 1898;1:28–33.
82. Parrot J. Sur la malformation achondroplasique et le Dieu Phtah. Bulletins de la Société Anthropologique de Paris. 1878;17:296–308.
83. Pison G. France-Allemagne: histoire d'un chassé-croisé démographique. Population & Sociétés; 2012. https://www.ined.fr/fichier/s_rubrique/19155/487.fr.pdf
84. Punnett RC. Mendelism. London: Macmillan and Bowes. 1905. 63 pages.
85. Richet C. La sélection humaine. Paris: Félix Alcan; 1919. 262 pages.
86. Tarnier S. De l'inertie utérine primitive. Leçon prise par E. Apert Bulletin Médical. Bull Méd. 1893;7:1155–6.
87. Troquart R. Syndactylie et malformations diverses. Mémoires et Bulletins de la Société de Médecine et de Chirurgie de Bordeaux. 1886;15:69–71.
88. Tschermak E. Ueber künstliche Kreuzung bei *Pisum staivum*. Berichte der deutschen botanischen Gesellschaft. 1900;18:232–9.
89. Vignes H. Certificat de mariage et vulgarisation des notions d'eugénique. In: IIe Session de l'Institut International d'Anthropologie (Prague). Paris: E Nourry; 1924. p. 455–9.
90. Vignes H. Stérilisation des inadaptés sociaux. Revue Anthropologique. 1932;42:228–43.
91. Wheaton SW. Two specimens of congenital cranial deformity in infants associated with fusion of the fingers and toes. Trans Pathol Soc London. 1894;45:238–41.

3 Head and Neck and Extremity Anatomy

Katelyn Lewis, Jeremy A. Goss, and Michael Alperovich

Introduction

Apert syndrome is a form of acrocephalosyndactyly resulting from an autosomal dominant mutation in the FGFR2 gene (fibroblast growth factor receptor 2), a gene essential for embryonic development, particularly in the formation of bones, connective tissue, and skin. In 1906, French physician Eugene Apert published a paper titled *De l'acrocephalosyndactylie*, initially describing nine patients with a distinctive combination of craniofacial, hand, and foot deformities [4]. Figure 3.1 includes a representative patient with Apert syndrome.

Apert's detailed descriptions laid the groundwork for modern diagnostic criteria. In 1920, Park and Powers published the first comprehensive evaluation of Apert's condition, arguing that rather than being a single clinical entity, there was significant variability in the syndrome's clinical presentations [43]. It was not until 1960 that C.E. Blank confirmed Apert's original hypothesis and identified the heterozygous gene mutation, leading to the ubiquitous use of "Apert's syndrome" rather than "acrocephalosyndactyly" in the medical literature [5]. Over the past century, numerous studies have examined the unique anatomical features associated with Apert syndrome.

K. Lewis · J. A. Goss · M. Alperovich (✉)
Division of Plastic and Reconstructive Surgery, Department of Surgery, Yale University School of Medicine, New Haven, CT, USA
e-mail: Michael.Alperovich@yale.edu

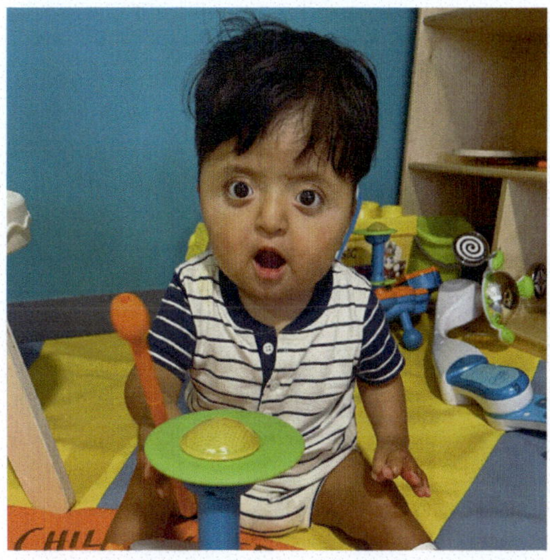

Fig. 3.1 Apert syndrome patient treated at Yale University

This chapter will provide a comprehensive overview of the anatomical differences observed in individuals with this condition.

Skull (Apert Skull Figs. 3.1, 3.2, 3.3, 3.4, 3.5, and 3.6)

As nearly all Apert syndrome patients have craniosynostosis, patients with Apert syndrome account for roughly 5% of all craniosynostosis cases. The congenital, progressive fusion of the cranial sutures contributes to the characteristic brachycephalic skull deformity, intracranial hypertension, restricted brain

J. G. Meara et al. (eds.), *Apert Syndrome*, https://doi.org/10.1007/978-3-032-12551-4_3

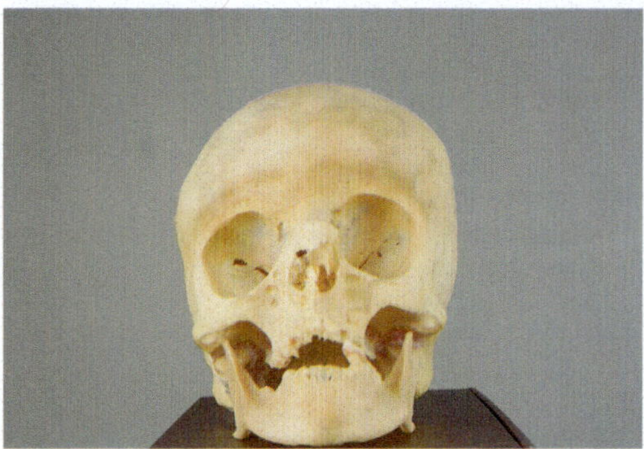

Apert Skull Fig. 3.1 Front view of the skull. Observe the ascension of the left orbit and the width of the forehead

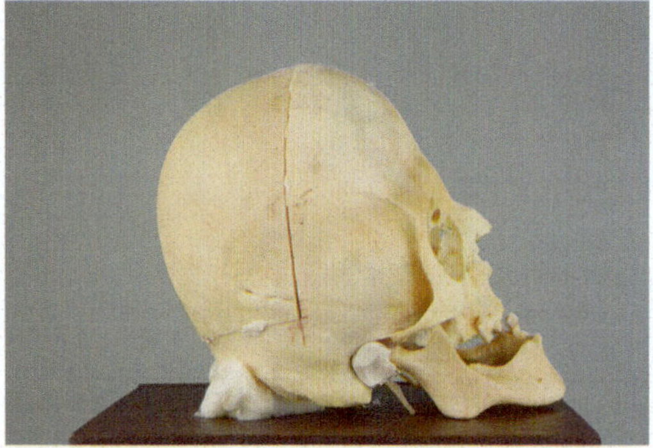

Apert Skull Fig. 3.2 Right lateral view. Note brachycephaly and maxillary retrusion

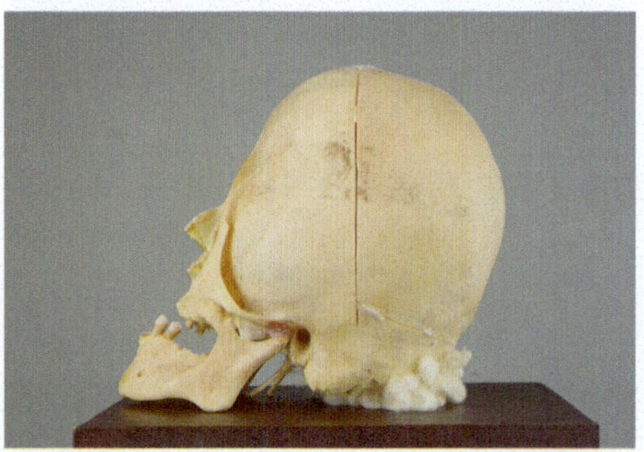

Apert Skull Fig. 3.3 Left lateral view. Note brachycephaly and maxillary retrusion

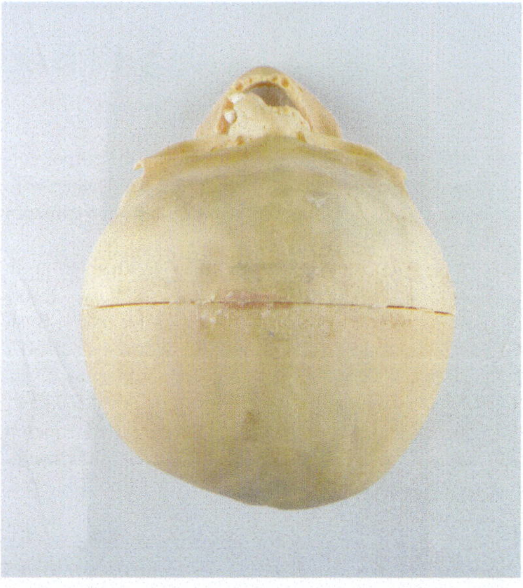

Apert Skull Fig. 3.4 Vertex view. Note relatively symmetric frontal bones. This most likely represents early left coronal synostosis with subsequent bilateral coronal fusion. Note left occipital flattening

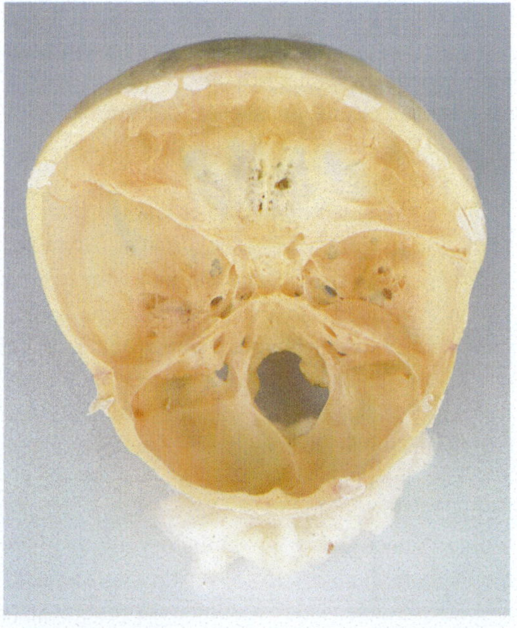

Apert Skull Fig. 3.5 Internal view of skull base. Ascension of the left greater sphenoid wing correlated to early left coronal suture fusion. The temporal lobes were highly asymmetric. There are no signs of fingerprinting, and the bone is thick, indicating the absence of raised intracranial pressure

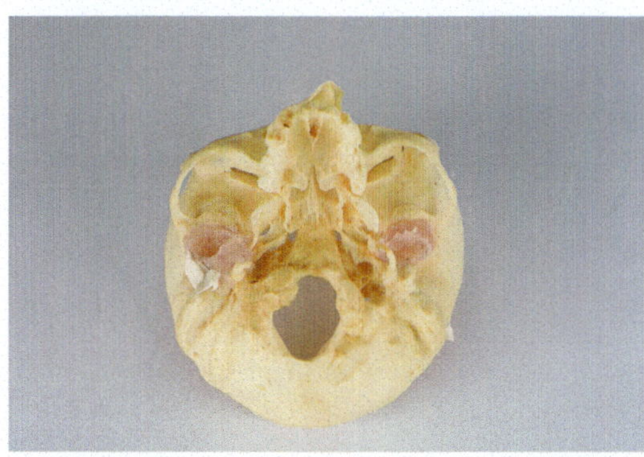

Apert Skull Fig. 3.6 External view of skull base (Wax was added to replace condyles)

growth, and impaired cognitive and behavioral development. On rare occasions, patients with Apert syndrome may develop midface retrusion and syndactyly without major suture craniosynostosis.

The Apert skull (Fig. 3.1 to 3.6) of an adult female patient 40 to 50 years of age, with no history of craniofacial surgical correction, is from the private collection of Dr. Eric Arnaud from the donation of Dr. Françoise Firman. No clinical pictures are available.

The most common skull pathology in Apert syndrome is bicoronal craniosynostosis resulting in a short, wide skull with pronounced vertical growth (turribrachycephaly). Whereas the coronal sutures are invariably involved, the sagittal and lambdoid sutures may also be implicated (85 and 81%, respectively) in multi-suture craniosynostosis or pansynostosis leading to a cloverleaf skull shape. As demonstrated in Fig. 3.2, variations in affected cranial sutures, cranial base, and facial morphology help stratify Apert skulls into one of three subtypes: Class I—bilateral coronal synostosis; Class II—pansynostosis; and Class III—perpendicular combination synostosis (including IIIA, unilateral coronal and metopic synostosis; IIIB, sagittal with bilateral/unilateral lambdoid synostosis; and IIIC, other synostosis) [36]. Depending on cranial suture involvement, children with Apert syndrome can also present with oversized anterior fontanelles that are displaced onto the forehead [13].

The cranial base angle in patients with Apert syndrome was initially reported to be more obtuse than normative controls [18, 29]. However, more recent studies suggest that cranial base angles in these patients may be nearly normal [18, 34]. The cranial base length is shortened due to the fusion of the cranial base synchondroses. Bicoronal synostosis restricts the anterior–posterior length of the cranial vault, which in turn affects the length of the anterior cranial fossa [8, 45]. Additionally, the posterior fossa is shortened due to early fusion of the spheno-occipital synchondrosis, typically occurring around four years of age [23]. In contrast, there is compensatory height increases in all cranial fossae leading to the characteristic head shape seen in Apert syndrome, turricephaly, and brachycephaly [34].

Apert syndrome differs from many other syndromic and nonsyndromic craniosynostoses by typically preserving or increasing intracranial volume [6]. Research has shown that their intracranial volume often exceeds normal ranges as these patients age, particularly between six and eight [6, 21]. Recent studies suggest that this increased volume is primarily due to distortions in the middle cranial fossa, affecting both the anterior and posterior cranial fossae [37]. These volumetric changes, reaching up to 77%, are primarily linked to known sphenoidal malformations in Apert syndrome [37]. This indicates that malformations in the middle cranial fossa may be a key initiating factor in the series of cranial morphological abnormalities seen in the syndrome, highlighting the value of procedures that expand the posterior vault.

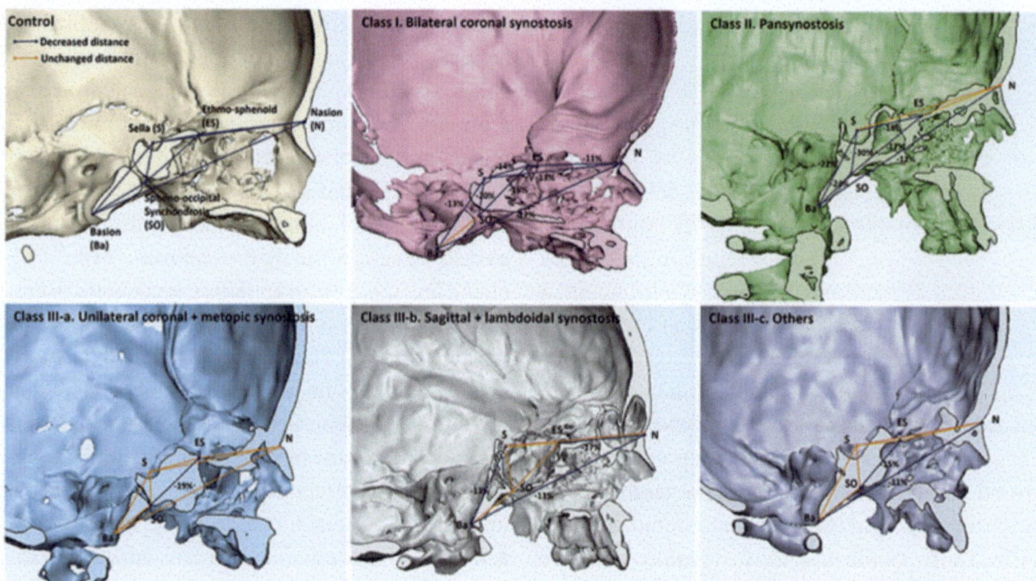

Fig. 3.2 Cranial base inner distances represented on sagittal view show the different changes in each subtype of Apert syndrome. Class I has a more evident shortened anteroposterior length of middle cranial base. Class II has a significantly shortened posterior cranial base. Three subtypes of class III have an inconsistently decreased cranial base length. (Source: Lu et al. [36])

Midface

The Apert midface is distinctly different from other syndromic midface deficiencies. There is severe growth restriction in both the sagittal and vertical dimensions, leading to a central concavity. It has been said that it is an abnormal face in an abnormal position. A retruded maxilla and bilateral posteriorly oriented zygomas are typical facial features in Apert syndrome. Restricted maxillary growth may manifest as malocclusion and/or mandibular prognathism and retrusion of the zygomas in an anteroposterior position at birth, which will persist into adulthood if left uncorrected [13]. The zygoma is perhaps the most affected facial structure in infancy in Apert syndrome and may contribute malforming stresses to other facial structures influencing the maxilla's development [35].

In Apert syndrome, the sphenoid bone is often underdeveloped, with the greater wing displaying a narrowed, rotated alignment. This deformity likely contributes to the restricted growth of the midface, along with the narrowed relationship between the sphenoid's greater wing and the pterygoid process. As the sphenoid forms the lateral wall of the nasal cavity and the pterygoid process connects to the palatine bone, this narrowing can severely limit midfacial development and lead to significant respiratory issues [39].

Half of all patients with Apert syndrome have high-arched palates, some have clefts of the palate, and one-third have bifid uvulas [50]. While cleft lip is rare in Apert syndrome, the lips of these patients may be trapezoidal shaped with a protuberant lower lip. Dentofacial anomalies abound in Apert syndrome, with patients experiencing delayed and/or ectopic tooth eruption (most often maxillary first molars), dental agenesis (typically maxillary canines), anterior open bites, and dental overcrowding [42]. The mandible of patients with Apert syndrome is thought to be relatively unaffected [51].

Airway

Patients with Apert syndrome may experience respiratory insufficiency and obstructive sleep apnea resulting from multilevel structural abnormalities, including choanal atresia, midface retrusion, mandibular hypoplasia, abnormalities in the hypopharynx and larynx, and palatal anomalies [10, 20, 32, 38, 44]. To comprehend the airway challenges in these patients, it is essential to examine both the bony and soft tissue abnormalities associated with Apert syndrome.

In anatomical studies, Apert syndrome children have normal nasal length, width, and projection and similar airway volume compared with normal controls [20]. However, as air progresses, the respiratory impingement seen in Apert syndrome becomes more apparent due to the degree of respiratory compromise and obstructive sleep apnea being directly correlated to the severity of midface hypoplasia and retrusion [20, 38].

The choanae are a pair of posterior apertures in the nasal cavity that open into the nasopharynx. Functionally, they serve as an internal nostril connecting the nasal airway to the pharyngeal space [32]. Complete obstruction of the choanae, defined as choanal atresia, leads to a blockage in the nasopharyngeal airway, thereby preventing inhalation and exhalation.

In the oropharyngeal area, patients with Apert syndrome can have reduced bony diameter in the mediolateral dimension, which extends to the entire length of the laryngopharyngeal airway (Fig. 3.3). In the anterior–posterior dimension, there is a progressive decrease in the diameter of the airway extending from the pharynx to the larynx, further exacerbating the airway stenosis [20, 38]. Consequently, the pharyngeal airway capacity significantly decreases by as much as 40%, as seen in Fig. 3.3 [20].

Poiseuille's law states that resistance to flow is inversely proportional to the fourth power of the radius and directly proportional to the length of the tube. Consequently, increased airway length, decreased mediolateral diameter, and decreased posterior airway space potentiate the severity of obstructive airway disease [20, 38].

Tracheal cartilaginous sleeves affect up to 22% of patients with syndromic craniosynostosis [49]. A tracheal cartilaginous sleeve (TCS) is associated with absence of the C-shaped tracheal rings. The trachea consists of a long tube of rigid cartilage anterolaterally with a normal membranous wall posteriorly [24]. Without tracheal rings, the mechanism for airway clearance and distension fails resulting in a stenotic airway that places patients at risk for sudden tracheal occlusion. Without a tracheostomy, the risk for sudden death can be as high as 90% in infancy [31].

A recent study has suggested that patients with the Ser252Trp mutation in FGFR2 display a

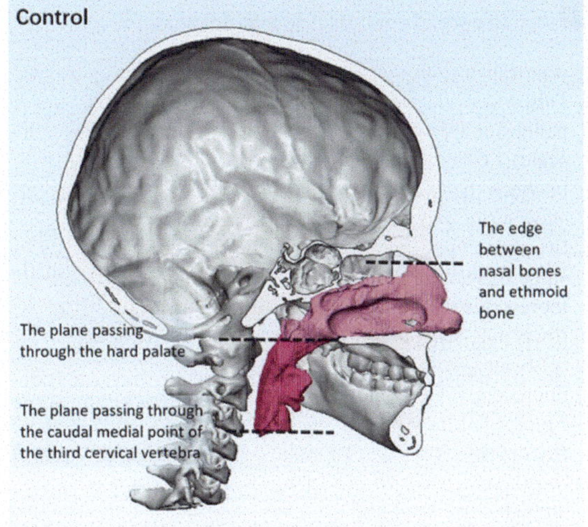

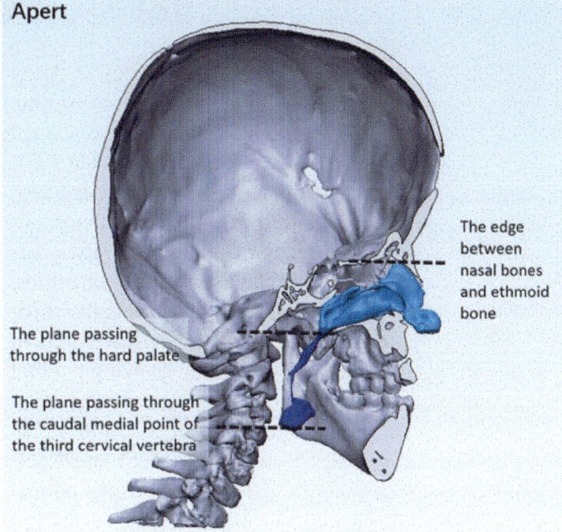

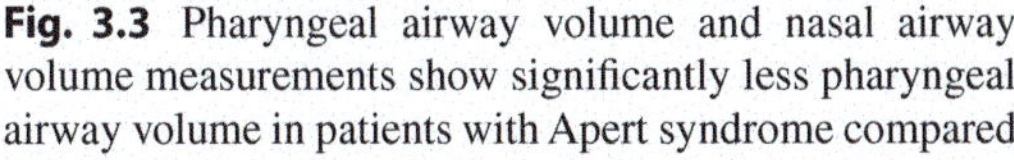

Fig. 3.3 Pharyngeal airway volume and nasal airway volume measurements show significantly less pharyngeal airway volume in patients with Apert syndrome compared to those with normal anatomy. Computed tomographic scans of a six-year-old male control (left) and a patient with Apert syndrome (right). (Source: Forte et al. [20])

higher incidence of obstructive airway physiology due to reduced nasopharyngeal airway volumes and higher incidence of nasopharyngeal airway stenosis [48].

Eyes

Patients with Apert syndrome exhibit a range of ocular abnormalities. These issues stem from a mismatch in the growth rates of the eyes and brain compared to the slower expansion of the cranial base and orbital areas [7]. Due to the early fusion of cranial sutures, the orbits become relatively small in relation to the skull, resulting in the typical conditions of proptosis, hypertelorism, and strabismus observed in these patients. In addition to these primary features, numerous anatomical variations require ophthalmologic interventions to prevent vision loss.

Orbits

Extensive cephalometric analysis has been conducted to define the aberrant orbital anatomy of Apert syndrome [7, 19, 28]. In the sagittal plane, the orbital roof and floor are shorter, and the superior and inferior orbital rims retrude from the cranial base [28, 40] (Fig. 3.4). In the vertical plane, the orbital height is significantly increased along with the interorbital distance in the transverse plane [12, 40].

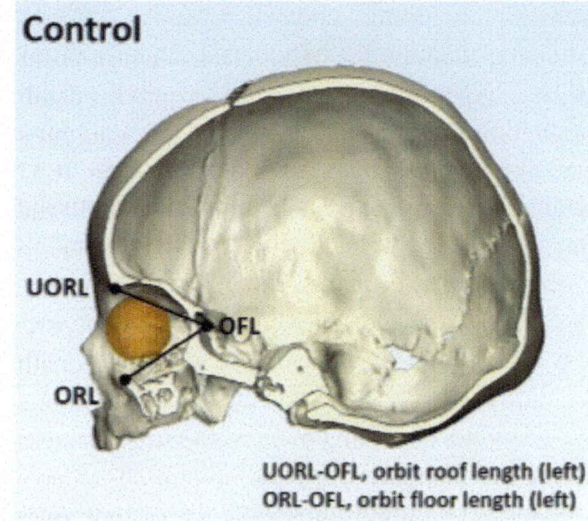

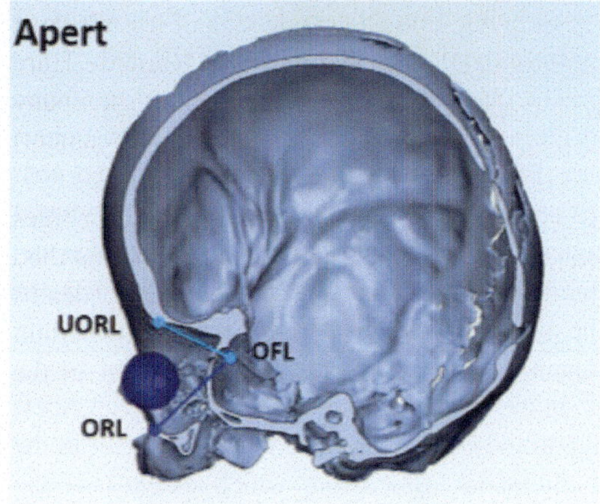

Fig. 3.4 Illustrations of the orbital length changes in Apert syndrome. Patients with Apert syndrome experience a shortened orbital floor and orbital roof length compared to normal controls. (Source: Lu et al. [40])

One of the most striking anatomical features in Apert syndrome is the pronounced protrusion of the lateral orbital wall, formed by the greater wing of the sphenoid. This uniquely shaped lateral wall exhibits a curved surface with an anterior convex profile, contrasting with the straight plane observed in normal controls [33]. This alteration is believed to result from the superior and posterior rotation of the greater wing of the sphenoid, leading to anterior displacement of the sphenoid [33]. Additionally, the enlarged anterior cranial fossa increases the width of the ethmoid sinus, which further broadens the medial wall of the orbit. As a result, there is an increased horizontal diameter between the orbits in the mediolateral direction.

The pronounced protrusion of the lateral wall, along with the shortened orbit and other abnormal anatomical features, restricts the orbit's ability to house the full orbital volume, leading to both exorbitism and enophthalmos. As a result of the exorbitism, patients with Apert characteristically exhibit an "antimongoloid" or downslanting palpebral fissure (Fig. 3.5). This antimongoloid slant often leads to lateral ptosis of the eye, which may require lateral canthal repositioning through a canthoplasty procedure.

The physical manifestations of the underlying bony dysmorphology can lead to detrimental

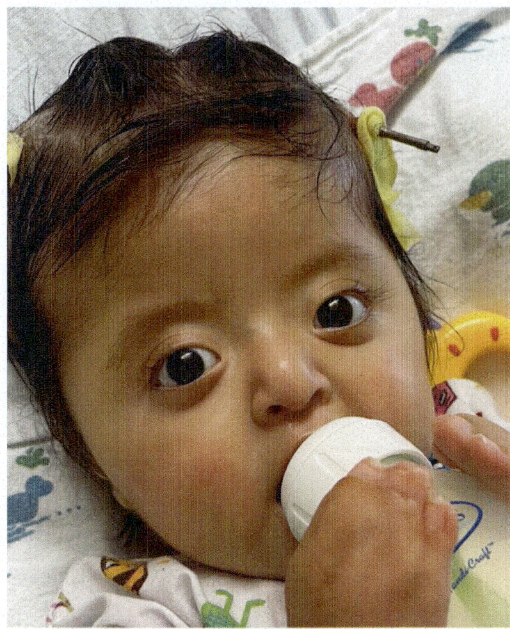

Fig. 3.5 Clinical features of a child with Apert syndrome. Note the proptosis, hypertelorism, downward slanting palpebral fissures, and strabismus in the orbital region. Also of note is the Apert type II hand anomaly in this patient

visual issues. Children with Apert syndrome are often unable to completely close their eyelids and sleep with their eyes open when lying flat. Significant exposure to keratitis can result in corneal scars and opacifications [26]. An extreme complication of exorbitism is the actual subluxation of the globe beyond the orbit and eyelid, which can occlude venous outflow and produce acute blindness.

One of the most prevalent orbital findings in patients with Apert syndrome is strabismus, with approximately two-thirds of patients eventually developing this condition [7, 9, 13, 26, 27]. Exotropia in a V-pattern is common with divergent upgaze and estrotropic downgaze [9, 14]. The exact etiology of strabismus and its increased prevalence in Apert syndrome and in patients with craniosynostosis remain unclear. It has been suggested that a shallow orbit may contribute to excyclotorsion of the eye and its muscles, while posterior rotation of the trochlea due to a dysmorphic bony orbit has been proposed as a mechanism for the characteristic V-pattern strabismus [9]. Recently, it has been observed that bowing of the medial wall into the orbit is associated with strabismus in this patient group [30]. This phenomenon can lead to anomalous anchoring of the extraocular muscle pulleys, altering their paths and contractile forces [30].

Other, less common ocular pathologies in Apert syndrome include lacrimal apparatus dysfunction, absence of extraocular muscles, coloboma, albinism, keratoconus, congenital glaucoma, and cataracts [27].

Ears

External Ear

Numerous otologic manifestations in Apert syndrome primarily arise from broader skeletal abnormalities. The ears are consistently low-set and generally larger [16].

Asymmetric temporal bulging, commonly present in Apert syndrome, produces ear protrusion, giving the appearance of low-set ears [16]. Additionally, the external ear is often rotated posteriorly and may display pinna anomalies, such as lop or constricted ear.

Internal Ear

Internal ear anomalies are less frequently discussed in Apert syndrome but are still significant, as the most prevalent otologic issue is bilateral conductive hearing loss [1]. Frequent middle ear effusions, likely due to eustachian tube dysfunction and cleft palate, often result in recurrent otitis media and subsequent conductive hearing loss. Additional factors contributing to hearing loss in these individuals include tympanic membrane sclerosis and ossicular fixation [1].

Foot

The Apert foot deformity has been well characterized in the literature. At birth and during infancy, there is a simple syndactyly with segmented nails [41] (Fig. 3.6). In comparison to the hands, acro-

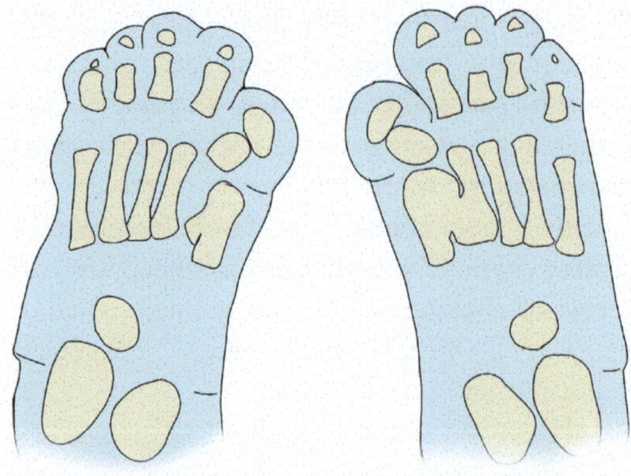

Fig. 3.6 Upton's Apert foot classification. Common foot deformities can be classified into two types determined by the degree of complexity of the fusion between the first two rays. (Source: Upton [47])

syndactyly does not appear to occur in the feet. Radiographic imaging at this stage of life tends to show normal skeletal structures with clear segmentation of ossification centers that begin to coalesce in children by the age of 4 years [41].

The proximal phalanx of the great toe assumes a delta-shaped appearance with a longitudinally bracketed diaphysis medially, leading to progressive medial deviation of the great toe (hallux varus) [41]. As the foot grows, brachymetatarsia is classically seen in the first ray. This leads to a shift of the weight-bearing function from the first metatarsal to the second metatarsal bone with progressive foot supination. This ultimately leads to callus formation and difficulty with shoe fitting as a major complaint. Additional common findings of the first metatarsal include proximal duplication or a bifid metatarsal [3, 41].

Progressive fusions occur in the foot in both a longitudinal and transverse direction [3] with age. The fusion of tarsal bones is characteristically seen, in particular, the calcaneus with the cuboid, along with fusions of the third metatarsal with the lateral cuneiform or medial cuneiform with the navicular bone [46]. All patients experience interphalangeal fusion (synostosis).

Using clinical and radiographic imaging, Upton et al. classified Apert feet into two distinct groups depending on the extent of fusion between the first two rays [47]. In type I feet, the separation between the cuneiform bones and first metatarsal are present at birth. In type II feet, there are more severe skeletal deformities [47]. There is fusion between the cuneiform and navicular bones of which arises a bifid metatarsal. Additionally, there is synostosis of the first and second rays. Growth of the first ray is more restricted, and a greater medial deviation of the toe is appreciated [15, 41, 47].

Hand and Upper Extremity

Introduction

A key clinical characteristic of Apert syndrome is the abnormal structure of the upper limbs. In the 1990s, Dr. Upton conducted the most thorough study of the pathological upper extremity anatomy, examining the hands and upper limbs of 68 individuals with Apert syndrome [47]. Proper identification of the abnormal upper extremity anatomy in this patient group is essential for directing treatment and enhancing functionality.

Shoulder

In individuals with Apert syndrome, motion of the glenohumeral joint is restricted, and this restriction worsens with age. Glenoid dysplasia, a common feature in this population, results in a small glenoid fossa with a central depression or transverse cleft [11, 47]. As the child grows, the humeral head tends to become oblong due to overgrowth of the greater tuberosity and tends to medialize because of hypoplasia [25]. While becoming more prominent due to the medialization of the humeral head, the acromion does not show signs of overgrowth [25]. The combination of these anatomical abnormalities leads to a clinical presentation resembling an inferiorly subluxed glenohumeral joint [47, 52]. Shoulder range of motion with abduction, forward flexion, and external rotation is thereby compromised and becomes more limited with growth [25, 52].

Elbow

The anatomical abnormalities at the elbow in Apert syndrome are less consistent than those seen at the shoulder. Elbow range of motion varies widely, with some individuals maintaining normal motion, while others experience complete loss of movement due to significant ankylosis [2, 25, 52].

Upton identified two recurring patterns in his cohort of patients. The first pattern involved a flat radial head and hypoplasia of the capitellum, predisposing patients to subluxation or even dislocation of the radial head. The second pattern involved a posterior angulation of the radial neck before it articulated with a flat capitellum [25].

Hand

The hands in Apert syndrome display several characteristic features, including (1) a shortened thumb with radial clinodactyly of both the proximal and distal phalanges, (2) complex osseous syndactyly involving the index, middle (long), and ring fingers, (3) symphalangism, and (4) simple syndactyly of the fourth webspace (between the ring and little fingers) (Fig. 3.7) [22, 47]. Upton's classification system for the Apert hand is based on the configuration of the first webspace, providing valuable insight into the severity and specific nature of the hand deformities in this syndrome [47].

Type I Hand The Type I hand is the most common and least severe configuration, often called the "obstetrician hand" or "spade hand." The thumb is separated from the index finger by a shallow webspace, while the index, middle, and ring fingers are fused side-to-side at the level of the distal interphalangeal (DIP) joint. There is no bony connection between the ring and small fingers in the webspace, but they are united by a simple syndactyly, which may be complete or incomplete [47].

Type II Hand The Type II hand is the "mitten" or "spoon hand." In this configuration, the thumb is not fully free as in Type I, but joins the index finger by either complete or incomplete syndactyly. Despite the connection, the thumb has a separate nail matrix, with no bony union. The complex syndactyly at the DIP joint results in a concave palm with splaying of the metacarpals and proximal phalanges. Unlike Type I, the syndactyly between the fourth and fifth fingers is nearly always complete [47].

Type III Hand The Type III hand, often called the "rosebud" hand, represents the rarest and most severe hand configuration due to tight bony fusion of the thumb, index, middle, and ring fin-

Common Features in the Apert Hand
1. Short Deviated Thumb
2. Complex Syndactyly: index/long/ring
3. Symbrachyphalangism
4. Simple Syndactyly: 4th web

Fig. 3.7 Four common features of the hand in Apert syndrome regardless of severity

gers. These digits are joined with a single conjoined nail, which may or may not show longitudinal ridging, indicating partial separation of the distal phalanges. The small finger is not involved in the bony fusion but is attached to the other digits by a complete, simple syndactyly [47].

Metacarpals

The most common abnormality of the metacarpals is synostosis between the index and small finger, which ranges from a small bridge to complete fusion (Fig. 3.8). Synostosis here creates a flattened, rigid metacarpal arch, which greatly reduces carpometacarpal motion and function. At the level of the metacarpophalangeal joint, Upton found that functional motion decreased from the thumb, fifth, ring, long, and index digits, respectively, with growth [47].

Proximal Phalanx/Middle Phalanx/Distal Phalanx

Brachysymphalangism is characteristic of Apert syndrome and is caused by the abnormal anatomy of the phalanges [22, 47]. In Apert syndrome, the proximal phalanx of the thumb is

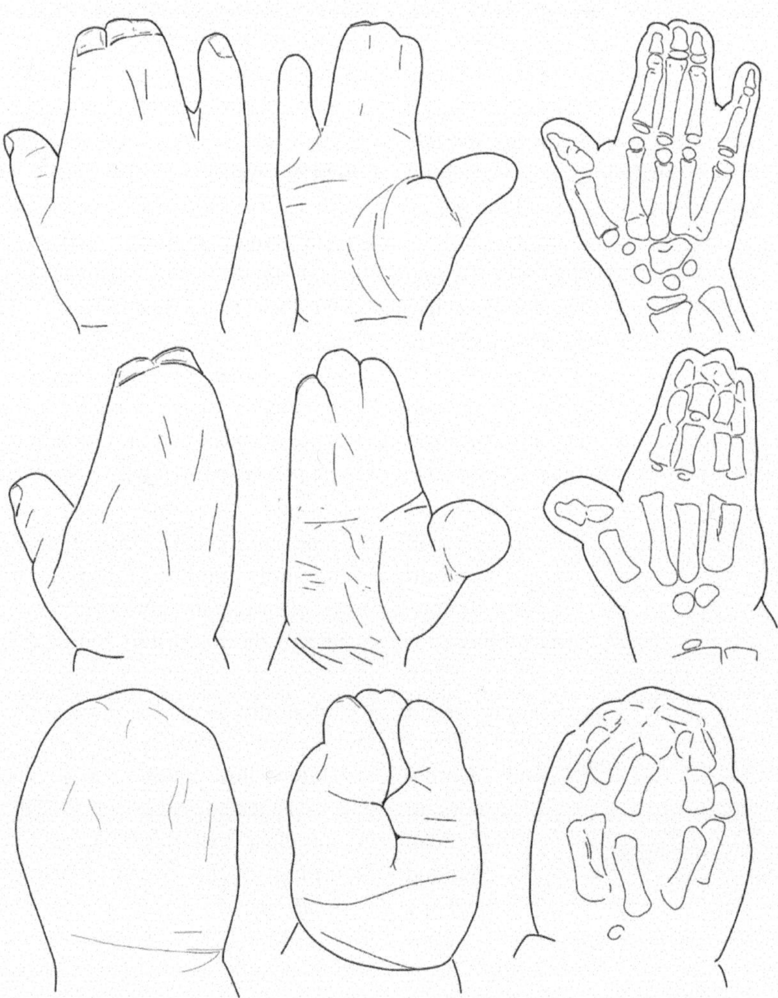

Fig. 3.8 Apert hand classification

always abnormal. This abnormality, often referred to as the "hitchhiker" thumb or radial clinodactyly, results from a C-shaped epiphysis that extends along one side of the phalanx, causing the distal portion of the thumb to deviate toward that side [17]. The thumb also experiences deficient longitudinal growth, leading to its characteristic broad and wide appearance. As the child grows, the proximal phalanx of the thumb continues to deviate, with early closure of the growth plate exacerbating this issue [17]. This abnormal anatomy at the proximal phalanx can result in the loss of motion at the interphalangeal joint, creating significant functional challenges for these patients [17].

In Apert syndrome, the proximal phalanx of the index finger is commonly malformed. Upton described two distinct configurations of this deformity. In the first, the index finger appears straight due to fusion with the long finger [47]. However, after surgical release, the bone develops a delta shape and gradually deviates radially. In the second configuration, the index finger has a bipartite epiphysis, showing progressive radial deviation over time [47].

The middle phalanges are often hypoplastic, or, in extreme cases, congenitally absent. This results in a lack of functional movement at the proximal interphalangeal joint (PIPJ), with some variable motion at the distal interphalangeal joint (DIPJ). As patients approach skeletal maturity, significant phalangeal osseous fusion occurs with complete lack of clinical range of motion at the PIPJ and DIPJ [47].

As noted in Upton's classification, synostosis (fusion) between the distal phalanges is always present in Apert syndrome, with occasional fusion involving other phalanges [47]. The ring and long fingers are most commonly conjoined and are often synostosed with the index finger. A clue to the underlying osseous fusion of digits is the appearance of the nails. In cases of complete synostosis, such as in Type III hands, a single nail plate is typically observed. In contrast, clear demarcation between nail plates is visible when the digits are completely separated, as seen in some Type I hands [47].

Other Hand Findings

Aside from significant osseous anomalies, the soft tissue of the distal upper extremity may be affected. The intrinsic musculature, extrinsic tendons, and neurovascular bundles can be deficient or have anomalous anatomy. For example, the flexor digitorum has been found to insert on the entire length of the unified proximal–middle phalanx [22]. The flexor digitorum profundus normally inserts on the distal phalanx; however, with Apert syndrome, it does so in a fan-like appearance [22]. The intrinsic musculature is often absent in the central rays, but present or even hypertrophied in the radial/ulnar rays [22].

Conclusion

Apert syndrome is an inherently complex craniofacial syndrome characterized by multiple congenital anomalies from the head to the toe. The characteristic malformations, such as craniosynostosis, midface hypoplasia, and syndactyly, are direct results of mutations in the FGFR2 gene. These anatomical variations significantly impact the physical appearance and function of affected individuals, and early intervention is key to improving quality of life. Understanding these anatomical differences is crucial for families and health care providers in effectively managing the condition and improving patient outcomes.

Acknowledgments Dr. Peyton Hull for creating Fig. 3.7 and illustrating Fig. 3.8.

Disclosures Dr. Alperovich consults for Johnson & Johnson.

References

1. Agochukwu NB, Solomon BD, Muenke M. Hearing loss in syndromic craniosynostoses: otologic manifestations and clinical findings. Int J Pediatr Otorhinolaryngol. 2014;78(12):2037–47. https://doi.org/10.1016/j.ijporl.2014.09.019.
2. Anderson PJ, Hall CM, Evans RD, Hayward RD, Jones BM. The elbow in syndromic craniosynosto-

sis. J Craniofac Surg. 1998;9(3):201–6. https://doi.org/10.1097/00001665-199805000-00002.
3. Anderson PJ, Hall CM, Evans RD, Hayward RD, Jones BM. The feet in Apert's syndrome. J Pediatr Orthop. 1999;19(4):504–7. https://doi.org/10.1097/00004694-199907000-00015.
4. Apert E. De l'acrocephalosyndactylie. Bull Soc Med Hop Paris. 1906;23:1310–3.
5. Blank CE. Apert's syndrome (a type of acrocephalosyndactyly)-observations on a British series of thirty-nine cases. Ann Hum Genet. 1960;24:151–64. https://doi.org/10.1111/j.1469-1809.1959.tb01728.x.
6. Breakey RWF, Knoops PGM, Borghi A, Rodriguez-Florez N, O'Hara J, James G, Dunaway DJ, Schievano S, Jeelani NUO. Intracranial volume and head circumference in children with unoperated syndromic craniosynostosis. Plast Reconstr Surg. 2018;142(5):708e–17e. https://doi.org/10.1097/PRS.0000000000004843.
7. Buncic JR. Ocular aspects of Apert syndrome. Clin Plast Surg. 1991;18(2):315–9. https://www.ncbi.nlm.nih.gov/pubmed/2065492.
8. Carinci P, Becchetti E, Bodo M. Role of the extracellular matrix and growth factors in skull morphogenesis and in the pathogenesis of craniosynostosis. Int J Dev Biol. 2000;44(6):715–23.
9. Coats DK, Paysse EA, Stager DR. Surgical management of V-pattern strabismus and oblique dysfunction in craniofacial dysostosis. J AAPOS. 2000;4(6):338–42. https://doi.org/10.1067/mpa.2000.110337.
10. Cohen MM Jr, Kreiborg S. Upper and lower airway compromise in the Apert syndrome. Am J Med Genet. 1992;44(1):90–3. https://doi.org/10.1002/ajmg.1320440121.
11. Cohen MM Jr, Kreiborg S. Skeletal abnormalities in the Apert syndrome. Am J Med Genet. 1993;47(5):624–32. https://doi.org/10.1002/ajmg.1320470509.
12. Cohen MM Jr, Kreiborg S. Cutaneous manifestations of Apert syndrome. Am J Med Genet. 1995;58(1):94–6. https://doi.org/10.1002/ajmg.1320580119.
13. Cohen MM Jr, Kreiborg S. A clinical study of the craniofacial features in Apert syndrome. Int J Oral Maxillofac Surg. 1996;25(1):45–53. https://doi.org/10.1016/s0901-5027(96)80011-7.
14. Dagi LR, MacKinnon S, Zurakowski D, Prabhu SP. Rectus muscle excyclorotation and V-pattern strabismus: a quantitative appraisal of clinical relevance in syndromic craniosynostosis. Br J Ophthalmol. 2017;101(11):1560–5. https://doi.org/10.1136/bjophthalmol-2016-309996.
15. Dell PC, Sheppard JE. Deformities of the great toe in Apert's syndrome. Clin Orthop Relat Res. 1981;157:113–8.
16. Farkas LG. Ear morphology in treacher Collins', apert's, and crouzon's syndromes. Arch Otorhinolaryngol. 1978;220(1):153–7. https://doi.org/10.1007/BF00456310.
17. Fereshetian S, Upton J. The anatomy and management of the thumb in Apert syndrome. Clin Plast Surg. 1991;18(2):365–80.
18. Forte AJ, Alonso N, Persing JA, Pfaff MJ, Brooks ED, Steinbacher DM. Analysis of midface retrusion in Crouzon and Apert syndromes. Plast Reconstr Surg. 2014;134(2):285–93. https://doi.org/10.1097/prs.0000000000000360.
19. Forte AJ, Steinbacher DM, Persing JA, Brooks ED, Andrew TW, Alonso N. Orbital dysmorphology in untreated children with Crouzon and Apert syndromes. Plast Reconstr Surg. 2015;136(5):1054–62. https://doi.org/10.1097/prs.0000000000001693.
20. Forte AJ, Lu X, Hashim PW, Steinbacher DM, Alperovich M, Persing JA, Alonso N. Airway analysis in Apert syndrome. Plast Reconstr Surg. 2019;144(3):704–9. https://doi.org/10.1097/prs.0000000000005937.
21. Gosain AK, McCarthy JG, Glatt P, Staffenberg D, Hoffmann RG. A study of intracranial volume in Apert syndrome. Plast Reconstr Surg. 1995;95(2):284–95. https://doi.org/10.1097/00006534-199502000-00008.
22. Holten IW, Smith AW, Bourne AJ, David DJ. The Apert syndrome hand: pathologic anatomy and clinical manifestations. Plast Reconstr Surg. 1997;99(6):1681–7. https://doi.org/10.1097/00006534-199705000-00031.
23. Hughes DC, Kaduthodil M, Connolly D, Griffiths P. Dimensions and ossification of the normal anterior cranial fossa in children. Am J Neuroradiol. 2010;31(7):1268–72.
24. Inglis AF Jr, Kokesh J, Siebert J, Richardson MA. Vertically fused tracheal cartilage. An under-recognized anomaly. Arch Otolaryngol Head Neck Surg. 1992;118(4):436–8. https://doi.org/10.1001/archotol.1992.01880040102017.
25. Kasser J, Upton J. The shoulder, elbow, and forearm in Apert syndrome. Clin Plast Surg. 1991;18(2):381–9.
26. Khong JJ, Anderson P, Gray TL, Hammerton M, Selva D, David D. Ophthalmic findings in apert syndrome prior to craniofacial surgery. Am J Ophthalmol. 2006a;142(2):328–30. https://doi.org/10.1016/j.ajo.2006.02.046.
27. Khong JJ, Anderson P, Gray TL, Hammerton M, Selva D, David D. Ophthalmic findings in Apert's syndrome after craniofacial surgery: twenty-nine years' experience. Ophthalmology. 2006b;113(2):347–52. https://doi.org/10.1016/j.ophtha.2005.10.011.
28. Kreiborg S, Cohen MM Jr. Ocular manifestations of Apert and Crouzon syndromes: qualitative and quantitative findings. J Craniofac Surg. 2010;21(5):1354–7. https://doi.org/10.1097/SCS.0b013e3181ef2b53.
29. Kreiborg S, Marsh JL, Cohen MM Jr, Liversage M, Pedersen H, Skovby F, Børgesen SE, Vannier MW. Comparative three-dimensional analysis of CT-scans of the calvaria and cranial base in Apert and Crouzon syndromes. J Craniofac Surg. 1993;21(5):181–8.
30. Lee TC, Walker E, Ting MA, Bolar DS, Koning J, Korn BS, Kikkawa DO, Granet D, Robbins SL, Alperin M, Engle EC, Liu CY, Rudell JC. The influence of orbital architecture on strabismus in cranio-

synostosis. J AAPOS. 2024;28(1):103812. https://doi.org/10.1016/j.jaapos.2023.10.006.
31. Lertsburapa K, Schroeder JW Jr, Sullivan C. Tracheal cartilaginous sleeve in patients with craniosynostosis syndromes: a meta-analysis. J Pediatr Surg. 2010;45(7):1438–44. https://doi.org/10.1016/j.jpedsurg.2009.09.005.
32. Lesciotto KM, Heuzé Y, Jabs EW, Bernstein JM, Richtsmeier JT. Choanal atresia and craniosynostosis: development and disease. Plast Reconstr Surg. 2018;141(1):156–68. https://doi.org/10.1097/prs.0000000000003928.
33. Lu X, Forte AJ, Sawh-Martinez R, Wu R, Cabrejo R, Steinbacher DM, Alperovich M, Alonso N, Persing JA. Anterior convex lateral orbital wall: distinctive morphology in Apert syndrome. Br J Oral Maxillofac Surg. 2018a;56(9):864–9. https://doi.org/10.1016/j.bjoms.2018.09.011.
34. Lu X, Forte AJ, Sawh-Martinez R, Wu R, Cabrejo R, Steinbacher DM, Alperovich M, Alonso N, Persing JA. Normal angulation of skull base in Apert syndrome. J Craniomaxillofac Surg. 2018b;46(12):2042–51. https://doi.org/10.1016/j.jcms.2018.09.026.
35. Lu X, Forte AJ, Sawh-Martinez R, Wu R, Cabrejo R, Wilson A, Steinbacher DM, Alperovich M, Alonso N, Persing JA. Spatial and temporal changes of midface in Apert's syndrome. J Plast Surg Hand Surg. 2019a;53(3):130–7. https://doi.org/10.1080/2000656x.2018.1541324.
36. Lu X, Sawh-Martinez R, Jorge Forte A, Wu R, Cabrejo R, Wilson A, Steinbacher DM, Alperovich M, Alonso N, Persing JA. Classification of subtypes of Apert syndrome, based on the type of vault suture synostosis. Plast Reconstr Surg Glob Open. 2019b;7(3):e2158. https://doi.org/10.1097/gox.0000000000002158.
37. Lu X, Forte AJ, Wilson A, Steinbacher DM, Alperovich M, Alonso N, Persing JA. Cranial fossa volume and morphology development in Apert syndrome. Plast Reconstr Surg. 2020;145(4):790e–802e. https://doi.org/10.1097/prs.0000000000006679.
38. Lu X, Forte AJ, Park KE, Allam O, Alperovich M, Steinbacher DM, Tonello C, Alonso N, Persing JA. Morphological basis for airway surgical intervention in Apert syndrome. Ann Plast Surg. 2021a;87(1):59–64. https://doi.org/10.1097/sap.0000000000002601.
39. Lu X, Forte AJ, Park KE, Allam O, Mozaffari MA, Alperovich M, Steinbacher DM, Alonso N, Persing JA. Sphenoid bone structure and its influence on the cranium in syndromic versus nonsyndromic craniosynostosis. J Craniofac Surg. 2021b;32(1):67–72. https://doi.org/10.1097/scs.0000000000006914.
40. Lu X, Forte AJ, Dinis J, Junn A, Alperovich M, Alonso N, Persing JA. Influence of nonsyndromic bicoronal synostosis and syndromic influences on orbit and periorbital malformation. Plast Reconstr Surg. 2022;149(5):930e–42e. https://doi.org/10.1097/prs.0000000000009051.
41. Mah J, Kasser J, Upton J. The foot in Apert syndrome. Clin Plast Surg. 1991;18(2):391–7.
42. Nurko C, Quinones R. Dental and orthodontic management of patients with Apert and Crouzon syndromes. Oral Maxillofac Surg Clin North Am. 2004;16(4):541–53. https://doi.org/10.1016/j.coms.2004.08.003.
43. Park EA. Acrocephaly and scaphocephaly with symmetrically distributed malformations of the extremities. A study of the so called'acrocephalosyndactylism. Am J Dis Child. 1920;20:235–315.
44. Pickrell BB, Meaike JD, Cañadas KT, Chandy BM, Buchanan EP. Tracheal cartilaginous sleeve in syndromic craniosynostosis: an underrecognized source of significant morbidity and mortality. J Craniofac Surg. 2017;28(3):696–9. https://doi.org/10.1097/scs.0000000000003489.
45. Rosenberg P, Arlis HR, Haworth RD, Heier L, Hoffman L, LaTrenta G. The role of the cranial base in facial growth: experimental craniofacial synostosis in the rabbit. Plast Reconstr Surg. 1997;99(4):1396–407.
46. Schauerte EW, St-Aubin PM. Progressive synosteosis in Apert's syndrome (acrocephalosyndactyly), with a description of roentgenographic changes in the feet. Am J Roentgenol Radium Therapy, Nucl Med. 1966;97(1):67–73. https://doi.org/10.2214/ajr.97.1.67.
47. Upton J. Apert syndrome. Classification and pathologic anatomy of limb anomalies. Clin Plast Surg. 1991;18(2):321–55.
48. Wagner CS, Wietlisbach LE, Kota A, Villavisanis DF, Pontell ME, Barrero CE, Salinero LK, Swanson JW, Taylor JA, Bartlett SP. Genetic subtypes of Apert syndrome are associated with differences in airway morphology and early upper airway obstruction. J Craniofac Surg. 2023;34(7):1999–2003. https://doi.org/10.1097/scs.0000000000009583.
49. Wenger TL, Dahl J, Bhoj EJ, Rosen A, McDonald-McGinn D, Zackai E, Jacobs I, Heike CL, Hing A, Santani A, Inglis AF, Sie KC, Cunningham M, Perkins J. Tracheal cartilaginous sleeves in children with syndromic craniosynostosis. Genet Med. 2017;19(1):62–8. https://doi.org/10.1038/gim.2016.60.
50. Willie D, Holmes G, Jabs EW, Wu M. Cleft palate in Apert syndrome. J Dev Biol. 2022;10(3) https://doi.org/10.3390/jdb10030033.
51. Wink JD, Bastidas N, Bartlett SP. Analysis of the long-term growth of the mandible in Apert syndrome. J Craniofac Surg. 2013;24(4):1408–10. https://doi.org/10.1097/SCS.0b013e31828dcf09.
52. Wood VE, Sauser DD, O'Hara RC. The shoulder and elbow in Apert's syndrome. J Pediatr Orthop. 1995;15(5):648–51. https://doi.org/10.1097/01241398-199509000-00020.

Molecular Genetics and Pathophysiology

4

Andrew O. M. Wilkie

Introduction

Few pediatric disorders are as readily clinically diagnosed as Apert syndrome. The combination of characteristic dysmorphic appearance accompanied by syndactyly of the hands and feet (usually in the absence of polydactyly) is shared with very few other conditions. There is correspondingly exquisite specificity in the underlying molecular genetic basis of Apert syndrome; all described mutations occur in a single gene, *FGFR2* (encoding fibroblast growth factor [FGF] receptor type 2), and > 98% of these can be attributed to one of two heterozygous amino acid substitutions, p.Ser252Trp or p.Pro253Arg, the "canonical" Apert syndrome missense mutations that map to adjacent positions of the polypeptide chain.

Alongside this apparently simple pattern, two seemingly paradoxical observations must be explained. First, many of the other 1–2% of Apert syndrome mutations are of a completely different nature from the missense variants, being either large deletions or insertions that affect a different region of *FGFR2* from the canonical substitutions. Second, the amino acid substitutions themselves must be exquisitely specific in their pathological mechanism, because other nearby missense variants (including at the Ser252 and Pro253 residues themselves) are not associated with Apert syndrome.

In fact, putting these observations together is central to understanding the pathophysiological processes underlying Apert syndrome. This chapter will describe how human molecular genetics, biochemistry, cell and structural biology, and mouse models have all played a key role in defining the mechanisms.

This work leads to two other topics explored in this chapter. The first is to explain why the apparent germline mutation rate in *FGFR2* causing the two canonical amino acid substitutions is so high (~1000-fold above background). In fact, the study of Apert syndrome *FGFR2* mutations provided key evidence for defining a newly described pathological phenomenon, termed selfish spermatogonial selection (SSS), to explain this. The second topic is to explore how knowledge of the mechanisms of abnormal signaling in Apert syndrome can help to pinpoint ways to counteract the harmful effects of the mutations on development—although achieving this therapeutically will have many challenges.

A. O. M. Wilkie (✉)
MRC Weatherall Institute of Molecular Medicine, University of Oxford, John Radcliffe Hospital, Headington, Oxford, UK

Oxford Craniofacial Unit, Oxford University Hospitals NHS Foundation Trust, John Radcliffe Hospital, Headington, Oxford, UK

Oxford Centre for Genomic Medicine, Oxford University Hospitals NHS Foundation Trust, Nuffield Orthopaedic Centre, Headington, Oxford, UK
e-mail: andrew.wilkie@imm.ox.ac.uk

J. G. Meara et al. (eds.), *Apert Syndrome*, https://doi.org/10.1007/978-3-032-12551-4_4

Discovery of Canonical *FGFR2* Mutations (p.Ser252Trp, p.Pro253Arg) in Apert Syndrome

By the early 1990s, geneticists were making good progress with mapping the human genome. Several important disease genes had already been found—for example those for Duchenne muscular dystrophy [54] and cystic fibrosis [74]. These successes had come either from identifying a chromosomal rearrangement visible down the microscope (such as a large deletion or translocation), which was postulated to directly disrupt the disease gene in question, or by tracking the disease through large families, enabling the position of the disease gene to be localized by linkage to polymorphic genetic markers. Key early highlights when applying these approaches in the craniofacial field came in 1991, when Greig cephalopolysyndactyly was solved (*GLI3* gene) using chromosome translocations [85], and in 1993, when a linkage and candidate gene approach was used to show that a large family segregating a dominantly inherited form of craniosynostosis ("Boston-type") harbored an amino acid substitution encoded by the *MSX2* gene [31].

For Apert syndrome, 1994 proved to be the key year. Late in 1993 the author had moved to Oxford, England, to join Sarah Slaney (now Smithson), a clinical fellow already working there, with the goal of discovering the genetic basis of Apert syndrome. Adopting one of the strategies described above, we checked the karyotypes of many dozens of individuals with Apert syndrome in the hope of identifying a rare patient harboring a visible chromosome abnormality (an entirely fruitless quest, as it turned out). In parallel, we searched for families in which an individual with Apert syndrome had two or more children (irrespective of whether they were affected or unaffected); this involved sending personal letters by airmail (email was only just becoming popular) to dozens of craniofacial surgeons around the world. The outcome was the identification of just three families (comprising four informative meioses), making feasible a screen of a small number of candidate loci to check whether the segregation of genetic markers transmitted from the affected parent to each of their children was concordant with the presence of the condition.

During 1994, scientific advances moved apace. In June, linkage studies in Crouzon syndrome, a dominantly inherited craniosynostosis disorder sharing similar facial features to Apert syndrome, localized the major Crouzon syndrome locus to the long arm of chromosome 10, where the *FGFR2* gene was known to reside (although this detail was not highlighted by the authors of the paper [68]). The following month, the first disorder caused by mutation in a fibroblast growth factor receptor was reported (achondroplasia with mutation in *FGFR3* [78]). By August 1994, the author's communication with the group working at the Institute of Child Health/Great Ormond Street Hospital, London, England (led by Susan Malcolm, William Reardon, and Robin Winter), confirmed that they had succeeded in identifying *FGFR2* mutations in Crouzon syndrome; this was reported in September 1994 [71].

These developments set the scene for the Oxford group to use samples from their four Apert syndrome meioses for candidate gene exclusion. Of the five genes chosen based on the previous discoveries—the two MSX genes *MSX1* and *MSX2*, and three of the four FGFR genes, *FGFR1*, *FGFR2*, *FGFR3*—four could be excluded based on inconsistent segregation patterns; only *FGFR2* showed consistent segregation, albeit there was a 1-in-16 probability this had occurred entirely by chance [91, 92]. This prompted an intensive search for mutations in the entire coding region of *FGFR2* in a panel of 40 samples from unrelated patients with Apert syndrome that had been collected by this stage. Essential to the success of this endeavor was the availability of fibroblast or lymphoblastoid cell lines from affected individuals, so that complementary DNA (cDNA)—as opposed to genomic DNA—could be screened for mutations. (At this point in time, the intronic sequences flanking the exons of *FGFR2* were not fully catalogued, so that other investigators were using genomic primers for polymerase chain reaction [PCR] designed from sequences at the ends of the exons. Because both canonical Apert syndrome mutations turn out to reside within 10 base pairs of the start of an exon, any primer designed from the genomic DNA sequence would sit directly on top of the Apert syndrome mutations, rendering them physically impossible to detect.)

The first cloned cDNA sequence result pinpointing one of the Apert syndrome mutations in *FGFR2* (c.755C>G encoding the p.Ser252Trp amino acid substitution) is shown in Fig. 4.1a; the c.758C>G (p.Pro253Arg) substitution was identified during the following week. Of the first 40 unrelated samples analyzed, 25 were heterozygous for p.Ser252Trp and 15 for p.Pro253Arg [91, 92]. Indeed, subsequent studies from many different countries have confirmed the predominance of these two canonical mutations, which together account for >98% of patients with Apert syndrome (Table 4.1)—the p.Ser252Trp variant being about twice as common as p.Pro253Arg. Figure 4.1b shows the sequence context of the canonical mutations, located within the linker between the extracellular immunoglobulin-like (Ig) domains IgII and IgIII of FGFR2. Note that both mutations involve C>G transversions at the middle nucleotide of adjacent triplet codons; however, the Ser252 codon (T<u>C</u>G) contains a CG dinucleotide, which is potentially hypermutable [70], whereas the Pro253 codon (C<u>C</u>T) does not (substituted bases underlined). Although this could contribute to the greater prevalence of the Ser252Trp mutation, differential selection is likely to be quantitatively more important (see Section "Apert syndrome and selfish spermatogonial selection: experimental evidence and clinical implications").

To understand the mechanisms whereby just two mutations cause the great majority of cases of Apert syndrome, two questions regarding important pieces of contextual information are essential to answer. First, what is the structure of a fibroblast growth factor receptor (FGFR) and how does it function? Second, what differentiates Apert syndrome mutations from closely adjacent *FGFR2* mutations that, as had become apparent within a short space of time, cause two other classical craniosynostosis syndromes, Crouzon and Pfeiffer syndromes [32, 37, 71, 76]?

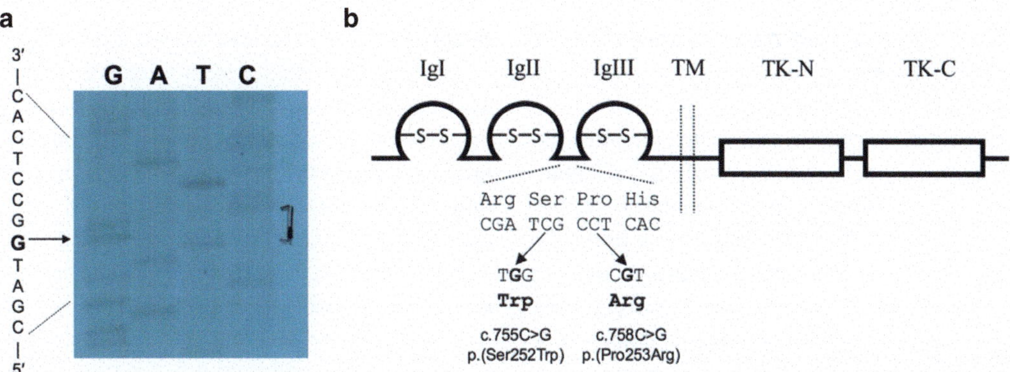

Fig. 4.1 The canonical Apert syndrome mutations in *FGFR2*. (**a**) The first autoradiographic evidence identifying a specific Apert syndrome mutation, which was obtained on September 27, 1994. Dideoxy-DNA sequencing of cloned *FGFR2* cDNA ("clone 73") was undertaken using ^{35}S-labeled dATP (deoxyadenosine triphosphate). The bracket mark is an annotation on the original autoradiograph highlighting the location of the variant nucleotide. Note how G (enlarged and bold in the sequence interpretation) replaces the expected C at this position. This individual has the 755C>G mutation. (**b**) Context of the canonical mutations. The FGFR2 protein comprises extracellular FGF-binding immunoglobulin-like domains (IgI, IgII, IgIII), each including a pair of buried, covalently linked cysteine residues (-S-S-), a single-pass transmembrane region (TM), and a split tyrosine kinase domain (TK-N and TK-C). The canonical Apert syndrome mutations 755C>G and 758C>G encode amino acid substitutions p.(Ser252Trp) and p.(Pro253Arg), respectively, located at adjacent amino acid residues in the linker between the IgII and IgIII domains

Table 4.1 Mutation spectrum in independent studies of Apert syndrome comprising ≥15 unrelated patients

Country of origin	c.755C>G (p.Ser252Trp)	c.758C>G (p.Pro253Arg)	Other mutations (total)	Total	References
UK + international	147	74	6	227	Bochukova et al. [7]
Australia	34	13	2[a]	47	Roscioli et al. [75]
USA	20	18		38	Fearon and Podner [14]
France	23	12	1	36	Lajeunie et al. [38]
USA	26	9	1[a]	35	Park et al. [63]
Brazil	16	10	1	27	Passos-Bueno et al. [65]
Spain	15	8		23	Paumard-Hernandez et al. [66]
Canada	13	3		16	Chun et al. [12]
Taiwan	13	2		15	Tsai et al. [84]
Norway	9	6		15	Tonne et al. [82]
Total	316 (66.0%)	155 (32.4%)	8 (1.7%)	479	

[a]These patients were also reported by Bochukova et al. [7], so are not separately included in the total

Biological and Pathological Context: FGFR2 Structure, Function, and Comparative Mutation Patterns in Apert, Crouzon, and Pfeiffer Syndromes

Some key molecular aspects of FGFR structure and function are illustrated in Fig. 4.2. As the name implies, the classical function of FGFRs (of which there are four major members) is to act as sensors for extracellular fibroblast growth factors (FGFs), which comprise 18 mostly paracrine-acting family members (reviewed by [62]). FGFR molecules traverse the cell membrane, so by detecting the prevailing extracellular FGF milieu they can signal into the cell to modify the cell's activity—for example, instructing it to divide, differentiate, or migrate, according to the particular intracellular pathways activated (reviewed by [16]).

As shown in the upper part of Fig. 4.2, in the presence of an appropriate paracrine FGF and heparan sulfate proteoglycans in the extracellular matrix, a binding complex is formed comprising two FGFs and two FGFRs; binding specificity is achieved through contacts made with the IgII and IgIII domains of the FGFR. This binding event brings the two FGFRs in close apposition, activating the intracellular tyrosine kinase domains through the cumulative phosphorylation of several key tyrosine residues [16]. As illustrated in the lower part of Fig. 4.2, either by phosphorylating other intracellular proteins or through the binding of proteins to the phosphotyrosines (for example Tyr766), several key intracellular signaling pathways (including RAS [rat sarcoma viral oncogene homolog]/MAP [mitogen activated protein] kinase, PI3K [phosphatidylinositol 3 kinase]/AKT [v-AKT murine thymoma viral oncogene homolog], and PKC [protein kinase C]) can be activated (reviewed by [8]). Set in this context, the potential significance of the canonical Apert syndrome substitutions can be appreciated, as they lie at adjacent positions in the linker between the IgII and IgIII domains (Fig. 4.1). This location suggests that they affect the affinity of FGF ligand binding [91, 92].

The second key context is to understand how Apert syndrome mutations differ in type and distribution compared to those causing Crouzon and Pfeiffer syndromes, the majority of which are located in the IgIII domain of FGFR2 just downstream of the canonical Apert syndrome mutations (Fig. 4.3). Like Apert syndrome, Crouzon and Pfeiffer syndromes are also characterized by craniosynostosis (although the pattern of suture fusions is more variable, with the sagittal suture commonly involved whereas there is a predilection for coronal synostosis in Apert syn-

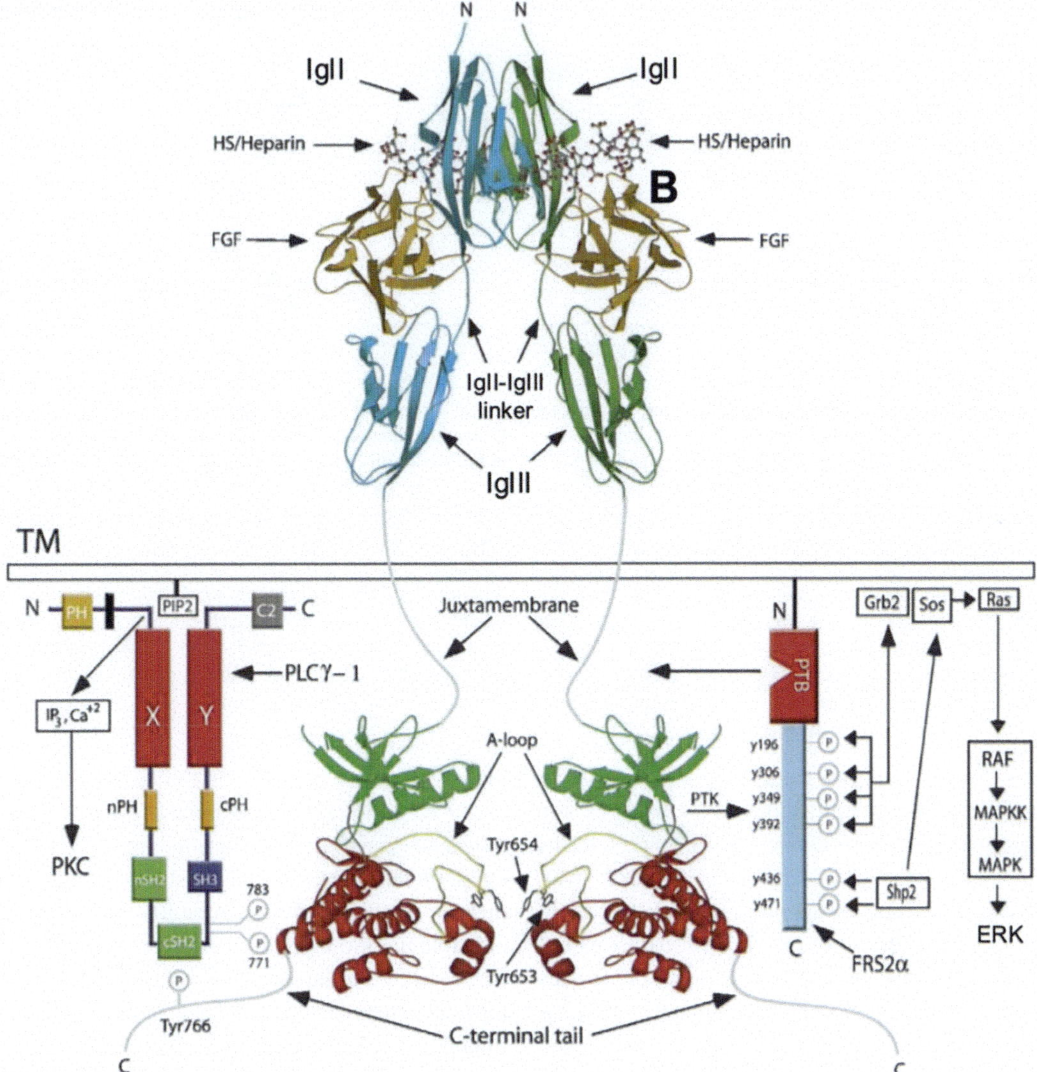

Fig. 4.2 Overview of the structural basis of FGF–FGFR signaling (reproduced in modified form from: [52]). The IgII and IgIII domains of two FGFR monomers (each colored blue or green) are shown in the upper part of the diagram binding to two FGFs (ochre), facilitated by heparan sulfate (HS) or heparin. After crossing the cell membrane (transmembrane, TM), juxtaposition of the two tyrosine kinase domains of the FGFRs promotes phosphorylation at key tyrosine residues (including those labeled Tyr653 and Tyr654), further activating the kinase activity to phosphorylate additional target proteins (denoted by P surrounded by circle). This leads to context-dependent activation of multiple intracellular pathways, including RAS/MAP kinase (MAPK), PKC, and PLCγ (phospholipase C gamma). See main text for further discussion

drome). However, the limb phenotype (by diagnostic definition) is different, varying from extensive cutaneous ± bony syndactyly in Apert syndrome, through broadening and medial deviation of the first digits (sometimes with incomplete cutaneous syndactyly) in Pfeiffer syndrome, to superficially normal limbs in Crouzon syndrome. In all three disorders, mutation hotspots are concentrated around two specific exons of *FGFR2*, exon IIIa and exon IIIc (Fig. 4.3). These exons together encode the IgIII domain; importantly however—and to further complicate mat-

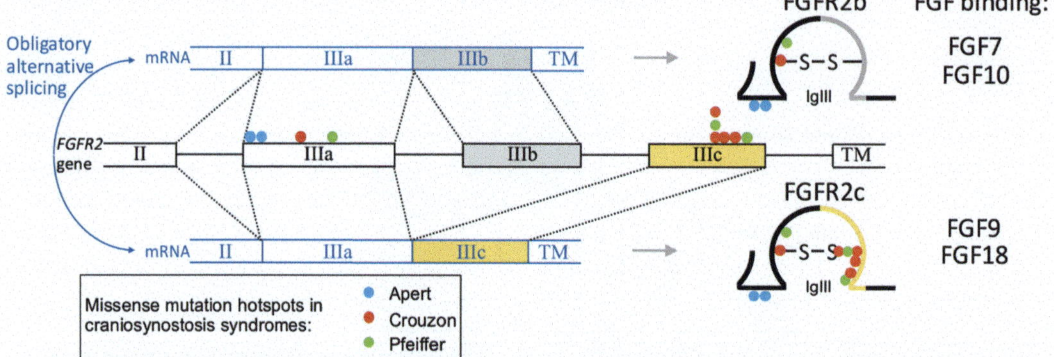

Fig. 4.3 Alternative splicing of *FGFR2* and location of mutation hotspots in craniosynostosis syndromes. A diagrammatic section of the *FGFR2* gene is shown (black type), with exons IgII, IgIIIa, IgIIIb, IgIIIc, and TM labeled and enclosed by boxes. Lines connecting exons are the intervening introns (not drawn to scale). Colored dots (see key) show locations of the ten most frequently occurring missense mutations causing Apert, Crouzon, and Pfeiffer syndromes in the gene and protein models (for clarity, omitted from mRNA models). Following initial transcription of *FGFR2*, developmentally regulated alternative splicing creates two different types of messenger RNA, shown in blue lettering above and below the gene model and depending on tissue-specific inclusion of either exon IIIb (gray) or exon IIIc (ochre). Translation yields two alternative isoforms of the FGFR2 protein termed FGFR2b and FGFR2c (right), which contain IgIII domains that differ in the sequence of the colored region (same coloring scheme as for mRNA) and bind a different repertoire of FGF ligands (only a selection of key ligands is shown). Note that although the canonical Apert syndrome mutations are present in both FGFR2 isoforms, a majority of Crouzon and Pfeiffer mutations are only expressed in the FGFR2c isoform

ters—an unusual obligatory alternative splicing event involving either the IIIc exon or the upstream IIIb exon creates two different forms of the receptor (FGFR2c and FGFR2b, respectively) that have different repertoires of FGF binding (see legend to Fig. 4.3 for further explanation). With some exceptions, the mechanisms by which Crouzon and Pfeiffer syndrome mutations act are qualitatively similar, but more severe quantitatively in Pfeiffer syndrome compared to Crouzon syndrome; hence the distribution and types of mutation overlap substantially between these two disorders. By contrast, Apert syndrome mutations are qualitatively distinct and belong to their own separate category.

A simple experiment, performed not long after the discovery of the molecular basis of Apert and Crouzon syndromes, illustrates the fundamentally contrasting mechanisms underlying the molecular pathology of these two disorders [4]. Isolated extracellular FGFR2 domains (ectodomains) containing wild-type (normal) sequence, the Apert syndrome substitution p. Ser252Trp, and a nearby substitution p.Ser267Pro associated with Crouzon syndrome (Fig. 4.4a) were electrophoresed in a non-denaturing gel in the presence or absence of FGF2, which normally binds to this extracellular region as illustrated in Fig. 4.2. Whereas the result for the Crouzon substitution was grossly abnormal (the mutant protein formed covalently cross-linked ectodomain dimers even in the absence of FGF2, and exhibited no binding to FGF2), the behavior of the Apert syndrome mutant protein was indistinguishable from wild-type (Fig. 4.4b). This shows that the Apert syndrome mutant retains the ability to bind FGF2 and, given the location of the substitutions in the IgII–IgIII linker, is predicted to affect binding affinity for specific FGF ligands. Indeed, this was demonstrated for a limited repertoire of FGFs by Anderson et al. [4]. In summary whereas Crouzon and Pfeiffer syndrome substitutions are mostly *constitutively* acting (meaning they cause FGFR2 activation in the absence of FGF ligand, often through the formation of FGFR2 dimer pairs that are covalently cross-linked by intermolecular cysteine-mediated disulfide bridges and thereby permanently activated; [73]), Apert syndrome mutations are *ligand-dependent*, exerting their pathology through a much more subtle mechanism. Although this answers the question, “why does

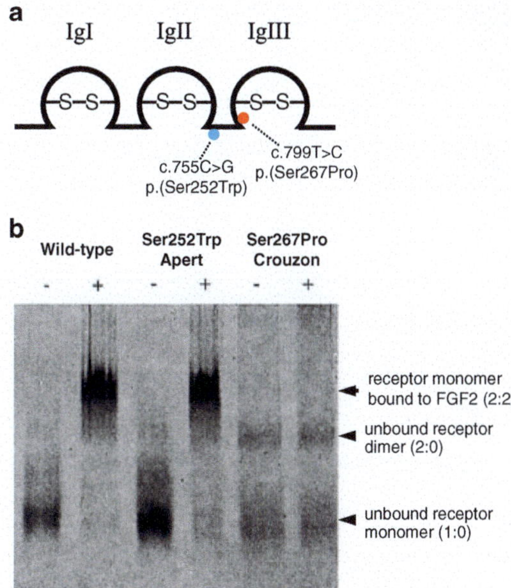

Fig. 4.4 FGF-binding experiment illustrating the fundamentally different nature of FGFR2 mutations causing Apert and Crouzon syndromes. (**a**) Design of the experiment, in which the extracellular part of FGFR2 only ("ectodomain," comprising IgI, IgII, IgIII domains) was synthesized, either in wild-type (normal) form, or containing one or other of the missense substitutions Ser252Trp (causing Apert syndrome) or Ser267Pro (causing Crouzon syndrome). (**b**) Result of non-denaturing polyacrylamide gel electrophoresis of FGFR2 ectodomains in either the absence (−) or presence (+) of a twofold molar excess of FGF2 ligand (reproduced in modified form from: [4]). Coomassie blue staining was used to visualize the protein. The interpretation is shown to the right of the gel, annotated with the ratio of protein species (ectodomain:FGF) present in each band visualized. See text for further commentary

Apert syndrome present differently from Crouzon and Pfeiffer syndromes, when their causative *FGFR2* amino acid substitutions are so close to each other?," it also leads to a new question: "What are the key FGF ligands mediating the Apert syndrome pathology?"

Canonical Substitutions p.Ser252Trp and p.Pro253Arg Result in Increased Binding Affinity and/or Altered Specificity for Specific FGFs

Two publications provided definitive data to explain how the canonical Apert syndrome mutations act in causing abnormal developmental signaling. First, Ibrahimi et al. [29] obtained structures by X-ray crystallography of the two Apert syndrome mutants bound to FGF2 (Fig. 4.5a). This work showed that both bulky amino acid substitutions introduce additional molecular contacts with the FGF, so they bind with higher affinity than normal (essentially, acting as "souped up" versions of the physiological receptor). The legend to Fig. 4.5a provides further details. Ibrahimi et al. [30] then exploited a biophysical method, surface plasmon resonance, to compare the binding affinities of every FGF to wild-type and Apert syndrome mutant receptors. A pathological effect in a given tissue and at a given time in development would be predicted if (i) the FGF ligand shows increased binding affinity to mutant receptor, compared to wild-type and (ii) the FGF ligand is expressed in that tissue. Table 4.2 summarizes the results for some of the ligand/receptor combinations thought to be most pathologically significant.

Perusal of Table 4.2 demonstrates two mechanisms (*increased affinity* and *altered specificity*) by which ligand-dependent Apert syndrome mutations could cause pathology; examples of each mechanism are shown in Fig. 4.5b. In the coronal suture (the most relevant cranial suture to consider in Apert syndrome), a combination of single cell transcriptomic analysis (which demonstrates expression of the relevant gene in the undifferentiated suture during embryogenesis) and mouse genetics (in which mutations of the cognate genes are associated with suture abnormalities) suggests that FGF9 and FGF18 are likely to be key physiological ligands [13, 27, 41, 58]. For both these ligands, the Apert syndrome mutants show enhanced FGF affinity (reflected in lower dissociation constant [K_D]) compared to wild-type FGFR2c, similar to the observation for FGF2 illustrated in the upper panel of Fig. 4.5b.

The effect on enhanced FGF9-mediated signaling is likely to be more important, for two reasons. First, the absolute K_D values are lower and fold-increase values are greater for FGF9 compared with FGF18 (especially for the p.Ser252Trp mutant; Table 4.2); second, for FGF9, the relative fold-increases in affinity, comparing the two mutations, align with the greater severity of the craniofacial phenotype associated with the p. Ser252Trp mutation (see Chap. 5), whereas for

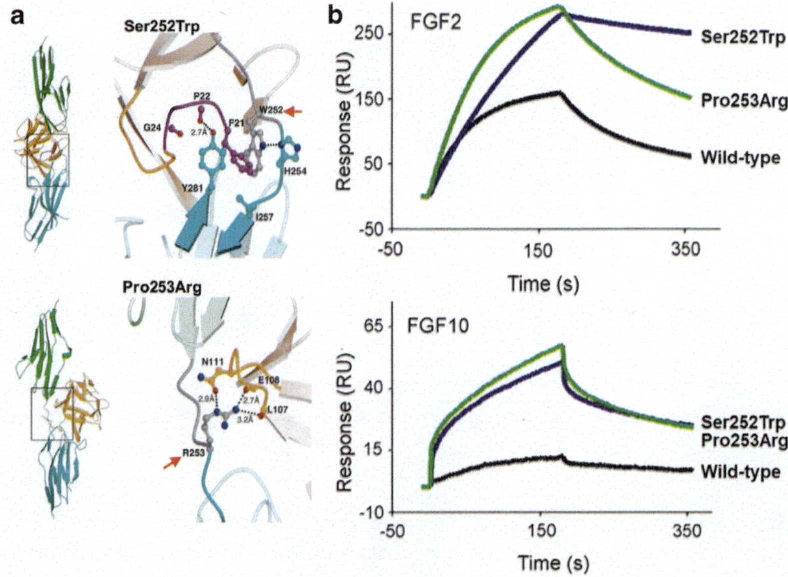

Fig. 4.5 Assessment of canonical Apert syndrome mutations using X-ray crystallography and surface plasmon resonance. (**a**) Structural basis by which canonical Apert syndrome mutations result in increased FGF ligand affinity (upper panel, Ser252Trp; lower panel, Pro253Arg). On the left is an overview of the IgII and IgIII domains (colored green and cyan, respectively) of Apert syndrome-mutant FGFR2c, bound to FGF2 (ochre). Rectangles indicate regions blown up in the images to the right. In the higher-resolution images, mutant residues in FGFR2 are highlighted with red arrows; note use of the single-letter amino acid abbreviation (W252 = Trp252, and R253 = Arg253). Both Apert syndrome mutations introduce additional contacts with FGF2, accounting for the increased binding affinity, but the mechanisms by which they do so are entirely distinct. The large aromatic side chain of Trp252 (gray) engages in a van der Waals (hydrophobic) interaction with the aromatic side chain of Phe21 in FGF2 (labeled F21 and colored purple). By contrast, the Arg253 side chain (gray) forms new hydrogen bonds with three different residues of FGF2, located at Leu107 [L107], Glu108 [E108] (both backbone interactions), and Asn111 [N111] (side chain interaction). Owing to these different mechanisms, the alteration in binding affinity for different FGFs by each Apert syndrome mutant is anticipated to be different (reproduced in modified form from: [29]). (**b**) Representative traces from surface plasmon resonance analysis of binding by FGF2 (above) and FGF10 (below) to wild-type (normal) and Apert syndrome mutants. The time trace shows the progressive binding of FGF to the receptor up to ~170 s, followed by washing off of the ligand. In the upper panel note how the FGFR2c-Ser252Trp mutant shows a very slow rate of FGF2 dissociation, consistent with increased binding affinity compared to wild-type. In the lower panel, the wild-type receptor exhibits almost no binding to FGF10, whereas both Apert syndrome mutants bind this ligand (altered ligand specificity). (Reproduced in modified form from: [52])

Table 4.2 Binding affinities of FGFR2 isoforms to selected FGF ligands[a]

			p.Ser252Trp		p.Pro253Arg		
Ligand	FGFR2 isoform	Wild-type	K_D (M)	Fold increase	K_D (M)	Fold increase	Relevant tissue
FGF2	FGFR2c	1.0×10^{-8}	2.2×10^{-9}	4.7	4.45×10^{-9}	2.3	Spermatogonial stem cell
FGF9	FGFR2c	1.3×10^{-6}	8.0×10^{-8}	15.8	1.0×10^{-7}	12.4	Cranial suture, spermatogonial stem cell
FGF18	FGFR2c	5.0×10^{-7}	1.8×10^{-7}	2.8	1.4×10^{-7}	3.5	Cranial suture
FGF10	FGFR2c	No binding	1.4×10^{-6}	NA[b]	9.4×10^{-7}	NA	Limb bud, cranial suture
FGF10	FGFR2b	6.2×10^{-7}	2.9×10^{-7}	2.1	4.0×10^{-7}	1.6	Limb bud

[a]Data reproduced from Ibrahimi et al. [30]; the lower the K_D (dissociation constant), the higher the binding affinity
[b]*NA* not applicable. Note that binding affinity for FGF10 is 1.5-fold higher for p.Pro253Arg compared to p.Ser252Trp

FGF18, the Pro253Arg substitution exhibits slightly greater fold-increase in affinity. In summary, the mechanism by which craniosynostosis occurs is likely to be through supraphysiological signaling in the cranial sutures, because of enhanced binding affinity of the Apert syndrome mutant receptors for ligands normally present in the suture. The strongest evidence that this effect is mediated through the FGFR2c rather than the FGFR2b isoform, is that many craniosynostosis-associated Crouzon and Pfeiffer syndrome mutations localize to exon IIIc and thereby exclusively affect the FGFR2c isoform (Fig. 4.3).

In the early limb bud, a different FGF signaling system is likely perturbed. Here, a key inductive signaling loop between mesenchymally located FGF10 and ectodermally located FGFR2b is normally essential for limb outgrowth, such that abolition of this signaling causes limblessness. That FGFR2b is clearly the key isoform for this signaling is demonstrated because FGFR2c is unable to bind FGF10 (Table 4.2, see wild-type column). Two publications [29, 30] demonstrated that when the FGFR2c isoform contains a canonical Apert syndrome mutation, it gains the ability to bind FGF10. This sets up a pathological autocrine signaling loop, because both FGFR2c and FGF10 are expressed in the mesenchymal cells of the limb bud (reviewed by [98]). Hence this pathology represents an ectopic or illegitimate signaling process. Although FGF10 binding affinity to Apert syndrome-mutant FGFR2b isoforms was found to be mildly enhanced (Table 4.2), evidence supporting that the syndactyly is FGFR2c-mediated includes: (i) the greater binding affinity of the FGFR2 Pro253Arg mutant, compared with Ser252Trp (Table 4.2), is consistent with the clinical observation that syndactyly tends to be more severe in association with the p.Pro253Arg mutation (see Chap. 5); and (ii) the observation [93] of syndactyly in two generations of a rare family harboring a p.[Ser252Leu;Ala315Ser] double substitution in *cis* on the same *FGFR2* allele (Table 4.3), which could only affect the FGFR2c isoform and was shown, like the canonical Apert syndrome mutations, to lead to illegitimate FGF10 binding. Relevant to understanding the mechanism of the double substitution, structural studies show that swapping Ala to Ser at position 315 switches FGFR2c to having FGFR2b-like binding properties [16, 30].

To end this section on a cautionary note, while the reductionist structural and biophysical methods presented above give satisfying explanations for the molecular pathology of Apert syndrome, by no means does this represent the full story. For example, Schuller et al. [77] and Ahmed et al. [1] used biochemical approaches to uncover several

Table 4.3 Additional molecular causes of Apert syndrome and closely related phenotypes

Category of mutation	DNA change	Amino acid change/Functional effect	References
Amino acid substitution	c.755_756delinsTT	p.Ser252Phe	Oldridge et al. [60]
	c.755_756delinsTT	p.Ser252Phe	Lajeunie et al. [38]
	c.755_756delinsTC	p.Ser252Phe	Goriely et al. [19]
	c.756_758delinsCTT	p.Pro253Phe	Lumaka et al. [42]
	c.[755C>T;943G>T]	p.[Ser252Leu;Ala315Ser][a]	Wilkie et al. [93]
Altered splicing (mostly *Alu* insertions)	c.940-4_940-3insAlu	Disrupted exon IIIc acceptor site	Oldridge et al. [61]
	c.1041_1042insAlu	[Disrupted exon IIIc splicing][b]	Oldridge et al. [61]
	c.1002_1003insAlu	[Disrupted exon IIIc splicing][b]	Bochukova et al. [7]
	c.940-19_940-18insAlu	[Disrupted exon IIIc acceptor site][b]	Topa et al. [83]
	c.940-2A>G[c]	Disrupted exon IIIc acceptor site (mild)	Passos-Bueno et al. [64]
Exon IIIc deletion	c.940-890_1084 + 895del	Complete loss of IgIIIc isoform	Bochukova et al. [7]
	c.940-1290_1021del	Hybrid IgIIIb/c isoform	Fenwick et al. [15]

[a]Syndactyly of hands and feet resembling Apert syndrome; broad forehead; no craniosynostosis
[b]Square brackets indicate predicted functional effect; no experimental data available
[c]Attenuated Apert syndrome phenotype with complete syndactyly of toes and syndactyly of digits 3 and 4 only in hands; patients with this mutation are more commonly diagnosed with Pfeiffer syndrome [61]

additional complexities in the cell biological effects of the canonical Apert syndrome mutations, notably showing that upon FGF9 stimulation, the mutant proteins persisted on the membrane of HEK (human embryonic kidney)-293 T cells in an abnormally glycosylated state, compared with the rapid endocytosis of the wild-type receptor on FGF stimulation. Qualitative differences in behavior between the Ser252Trp and Pro253Arg mutants were also documented [1, 77]. Another paradox—given the virtual ubiquity of FGFR2-mediated signaling for organogenesis in the early human embryo—is that these gain-of-function Apert syndrome mutations are compatible with life. This observation, and the lack of notably progressive natural history disease features in adults with Apert syndrome, both point to poorly understood mechanisms of tight autoregulation of FGF signaling that succeed in keeping in check the harmful effects of these mutations, in most cellular and developmental contexts.

Beyond the Canonical Mutations: Rare Molecular Causes of Apert Syndrome

In every 1–2 of 100 individuals with Apert syndrome, testing for the two common mutations yields negative results (Table 4.1). In all cases reported to date, a different molecular abnormality within the *FGFR2* gene has been identified (Table 4.3). These abnormalities can be divided into three broad groups: (1) amino acid substitutions, (2) variants (mostly insertions of *Alu* repeat sequences) causing altered splicing, and (3) deletions. These different types of molecular lesion are mapped onto the *FGFR2* gene in Fig. 4.6.

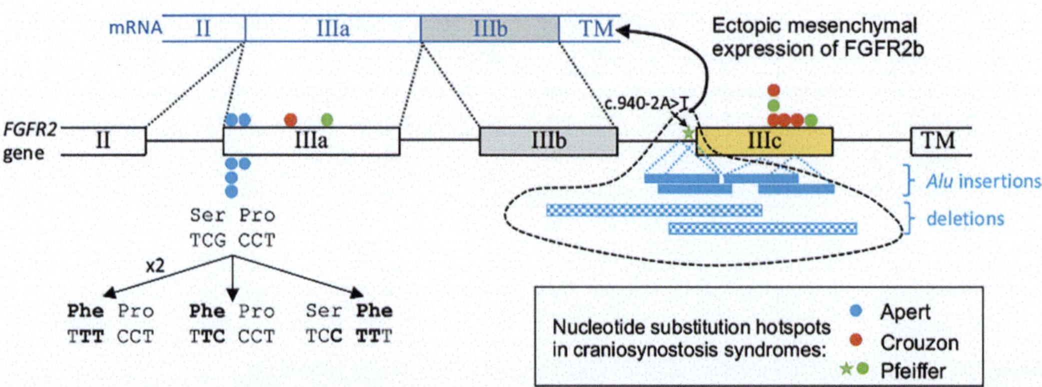

Fig. 4.6 Rare *FGFR2* mutations causing Apert syndrome. The gene model, showing part of *FGFR2* with hotspots of pathogenic missense mutation (filled circles above the gene; see key for color code—the two blue circles represent canonical Apert syndrome mutations), is reproduced from Fig. 4.3. Below the gene model are shown the positions of rare mutations causing Apert syndrome (see Table 4.3 for references). These fall into three classes: (1) (Four blue circles) Rare multinucleotide substitutions (bold type) involving two or three consecutive nucleotides ($n = 4$ cases) that normally encode the Ser252-Pro253 dipeptide; each results in substitution to a bulky phenylalanine (Phe) residue (2). (Four solid blue horizontal bars; dots connect to respective insertion sites) Insertions of mobile *Alu* genetic elements either within ($n = 2$), or immediately upstream of ($n = 2$) exon IIIc. Note that this diagram is not drawn to scale and that the inserted *Alu* elements (size range 214–368 base pairs) are all larger than the IIIc exon itself (145 base pairs) (3). (Two hatched blue bars) Deletions that either create a hybrid IIIb/IIIc exon (upper) or excise the IIIc exon entirely (lower). *Alu* insertions and deletions both functionally eliminate exon IIIc and result in the illegitimate expression of the IIIb exon-containing spliceform in mesenchymal tissues. Also indicated (green star) is the location of the c.940-2A>T mutation usually associated with Pfeiffer syndrome; see text for further details

Non-canonical Amino Acid Substitutions

The explanation for the rarity of the two different non-canonical Apert syndrome-causing amino acid substitutions (p.Ser252Phe and p. Pro253Phe) is straightforward. Each occurs within the same Ser-Pro dipeptide as the canonical substitutions and each encodes a substitution to phenylalanine (Phe), which has a bulky aromatic side chain. It is anticipated (but has not, to the author's knowledge, been experimentally established) that the Phe side chain would make additional contacts with FGF, analogous to those shown in Fig. 4.5a for the two canonical substitutions. The rarity of these events is attributable to the fact that conversion of both the Ser252 and Pro253 codons to Phe requires two bases of the codon to be substituted, an intrinsically rare event. It is important to note that Apert syndrome is not the inevitable consequence of amino acid substitution at this Ser-Pro dipeptide. Notably, p.Ser252Leu (resulting from c.934C > T) occurs at a low frequency in the normal population (1 in every 24,814 alleles in the gnomADv4.1.0 database; [34]) and—although rarely—heterozygous individuals may present with a mild form of Crouzon syndrome [59, 60]. Also, the p. Pro253Leu substitution has been reported in two patients with bicoronal synostosis [75].

Insertions and Deletions

The two other types of mutational event are much more surprising, both because they are completely different in nature (rearrangements involving *Alu* insertions, or deletions, between them varying in size between 214 bp and 1930 bp), and because they involve a different exon, exon IIIc, compared with exon IIIa where all the Apert syndrome-associated missense mutations localize (Table 4.3). As noted previously, exon IIIc contains multiple missense mutation hotspots, but these give rise to Crouzon and Pfeiffer syndrome phenotypes, not to Apert syndrome (see Figs. 4.3 and 4.6).

Although it has only been possible to perform functional analysis on samples from one of the patients harboring an *Alu* insertion, this provides a strong clue to the likely pathogenic mechanism. A skin biopsy from a patient with Apert syndrome heterozygous for a 368 bp *Alu* insertion (located three nucleotides upstream of the exon IIIc splice acceptor site) was cultured to yield keratinocytes (which normally express only the *FGFR2b* spliceform) and fibroblasts (which normally express only the *FGFR2c* spliceform). Whereas the keratinocytes maintained their expected expression pattern, the fibroblasts showed illegitimate expression of *FGFR2b* [61]. This is likely to reflect failure to recognize the exon IIIc splice acceptor, causing breakdown of the normal tissue-specific splice choice between exon IIIb and IIIc and leading to ectopic *FGFR2b* expression in tissues of mesenchymal origin (such as fibroblasts). A similar pathological process has most likely occurred in the other patients with *Alu* insertions. Meanwhile the two deletions, by definition, destroy the normal IIIb/IIIc splice site choice, therefore also driving the illegitimate mesenchymal expression either of the IIIb exon (patient with complete deletion of IIIc exon), or a IIIb/IIIc hybrid (patient with deletion bridging IIIb and IIIc exons). Although no corroborative functional studies were performed in either of the patients with Apert syndrome harboring deletions, cDNA analysis of a mouse model engineered to contain a complete deletion of exon IIIc (*Fgfr2*$^{\Delta IIIc/+}$; further discussed in Section "Mouse models of Apert syndrome") demonstrated that illegitimate expression of the IIIb spliceform indeed occurred in E14.5 whole mouse brains, which normally express the IIIc spliceform [21, 22].

The ectopic mesenchymal expression of the FGFR2b receptor isoform is anticipated to give rise to an autocrine signaling loop driven by FGF10 binding, which is analogous to the autocrine loop generated by FGFR2c isoforms bearing canonical Apert syndrome substitutions that illegitimately bind FGF10 [98]. This provides a neat explanation for how such very different underlying genetic lesions in *FGFR2* each cause the Apert syndrome phenotype. By crossing the exon IIIc-deleted mouse strain, which develops craniosynostosis, with another strain in which the *Fgf10* gene was deleted, Hajihosseini et al. [22] found that in double mutants ($Fgfr2^{\Delta IIIc/+}$; $Fgf10^{-/-}$), normal cranial suture development was restored. In addition, most $Fgfr2^{\Delta IIIc/+}$ and $Fgf10^{+/-}$ mice exhibited amelioration of the abnormal lung lobulation, alveologenesis, and intersternebral cartilage ossification defects usually present in $Fgfr2^{\Delta IIIc/+}$ animals with a normal *Fgf10* genotype. It is therefore likely that in humans, illegitimate FGF10-mediated signal activation underlies craniosynostosis in patients with *Alu* insertions and exon IIIc deletions. By extension of this argument, abnormal FGF10-mediated signaling (as well as FGF9- and FGF18-mediated signaling discussed in Section "Canonical substitutions p.Ser252Trp and p. Pro253Arg result in increased binding affinity and/or altered specificity for specific FGFs") may contribute to craniosynostosis caused by the canonical mutations as well.

A final point to note is that some patients with Pfeiffer syndrome present with cutaneous syndactyly and that this may overlap phenotypically with some individuals with Apert syndrome who have particularly mild syndactyly. For example, Passos-Bueno et al. [64] reported a patient with a diagnostic label of Apert syndrome based on a combination of craniosynostosis, broad thumbs, cutaneous syndactyly of digits 3–4 in the hands, duplication of metatarsal 1 with fusion of the proximal phalanges and absence of the distal phalanges, and complete syndactyly of toes 2–5 in the feet. This individual was heterozygous for the mutation c.940-2A>G, located within the invariant acceptor splice site sequence of exon IIIc and co-located with c.940-2A>T, a mutation hotspot for Pfeiffer syndrome (Fig. 4.6, green starred variant). Indeed, the limb involvement of Pfeiffer syndrome patients with mutations of this splice site tends to be particularly severe and a previous study of two such patients (one each with c.940-2A>G and c.940-2A>T) demonstrated illegitimate expression of the *FGFR2b* spliceform in fibroblasts, that was similar to, but quantitatively less marked than, the patient with Apert syndrome with an *Alu* insertion analyzed in the same publication [61]. Hence the pathogenesis of this particular subtype of Pfeiffer syndrome may be viewed as qualitatively overlapping, but quantitatively less severe, than patients with Apert syndrome caused by *Alu* insertions or deletions involving exon IIIc.

Apert Syndrome and Selfish Spermatogonial Selection: Experimental Evidence and Clinical Implications

The reasons that this entire book is devoted to Apert syndrome are twofold. First, as a multisystem disorder, its clinical management poses many challenges and second, it is one of the most common syndromic causes of craniosynostosis. The multisystem presentation can be attributed to the importance of FGFR2 signaling in many organ systems (developmental pleiotropy). But why is Apert syndrome so common? Birth prevalence studies indicate a frequency of Apert syndrome of ~13.5 per million ([88]; also Chap. 5); nearly all of these cases are the result of new mutation. Given this frequency, what makes Apert syndrome remarkable is the very narrow mutational spectrum, with 98–99% cases accounted for by just two mutations in the human genome, occurring at a ~ 2:1 ratio. This means that the birth prevalence of the c.755C > G mutation is ~1 in 111,000 and the c.758C > G mutation is ~1 in 222,000, per diploid genome. If these figures are contrasted with the background per-allele germline mutation rate of 1.2×10^{-8} (~1 in 83,000,000; [5]), then the rates of the Apert syndrome mutations are elevated several hundred-fold above expectation and occur more frequently than any other de novo mutation in *FGFR2* [17, 33, 46]. The search for the underlying explanation for this remarkable mutation enrichment has led to the identification of a novel genetic phenomenon termed *selfish spermatogonial selection* (SSS; [17]). In fact, this turns out to be another manifestation of the developmental pleiotropy of FGFR2: in the context of a male germ cell, a mutation harmful to the whole organism paradoxically confers a selective advantage to the particular testis cell in which it has randomly arisen.

Experimental Evidence for Selfish Spermatogonial Selection

The elucidation of SSS in Apert syndrome arose from four sequential discoveries that are summarized below and illustrated in Fig. 4.7. First, following the identification of the canonical *FGFR2* mutations causing Apert syndrome, a method was designed to determine, in each affected child/unaffected parent trio, whether the *FGFR2* allele on which the child's Apert syndrome mutation had arisen was the allele transmitted from the mother or the father. This method exploited two common natural variants (single nucleotide polymorphisms or SNPs) in *FGFR2* located within a few hundred base pairs of the Apert syndrome mutations, that could be phased with respect to the mutation and then tracked back to the parents to determine who had transmitted the allele bearing the mutation (see Fig. 4.7a and legend for details). This yielded the striking result that, in all 57 informative families, the mutant allele arose from the healthy father [53]. Relevant to this finding was the previous observation that the parents of children with Apert syndrome tended to be older than average for the population, and this effect appeared stronger for the father's age than the mother's age ([6, 72]; see also Chap. 5). The observation of exclusive paternal origin of Apert syndrome mutations [53], which at the time of writing this chapter remains the largest such study published for any genetic disorder, showed that to investigate the phenomenon of the high apparent mutation rate, it was necessary to develop methods to accurately measure levels of Apert syndrome mutations in men's sperm.

A robust method to measure the level of the more common *FGFR2* 755C > G Apert syndrome mutant molecule down to 1 in one million (based on digesting away the majority of the normal DNA using a restriction enzyme cutting the normal sequence, then quantifying the remaining material using pyrosequencing) was published by Goriely et al. [18]. This work, which studied 99 sperm donors and 6 additional men who had fathered a child with Apert syndrome, reported several key observations (Fig. 4.7b): (1) the 755C>G mutation was detectable in the sperm of a majority (but not all) men, with levels varying considerably from 1 in 6250 to less than 1 in a million; (2) the level in an individual man remained stable over weeks or months, indicating that the mutation source(s) were long-lived cells; (3) levels in sperm of fathers of children with Apert syndrome fell within the envelope of values found in other sperm donors, but tended to cluster in the upper part of the range (>1 in 10^5); and (4) levels of 755G mutant molecules in sperm were strongly positively correlated (r = 0.39) with the age of the donor. An additional unexpected observation, which exploited one of the nearby SNPs mentioned above (rs2071616) to distinguish the two *FGFR2* alleles, was that even in men producing relatively high levels of the Apert syndrome mutation in their sperm, the mutant alleles tended to predominate on just one or other of the two allelic copies, rather than being distributed ~50:50 between them. This key observation suggested that the originating mutations must be rare, but by conferring a selective (growth) advantage to the mutant cell, the cell's progeny become gradually more numerous over the course of time [18].

A prediction of the selective advantage model was that the originating mutations in the testis should be clonal, and hence potentially localized to small regions within a testis. Qin et al. [69] assessed this prediction for the c.755C > G mutation by cutting testis slices from cadaveric donors into ~200 pieces, measuring the level of c.755G in each piece, then constructing a three-dimensional heat map of mutant distribution based on these measurements [69]. This work showed that the Apert syndrome mutations within a given testis indeed tended to be highly localized, with the highest mutant level measured in an individual piece up to 6%, but also with large "deserts" of entirely mutation-negative regions between these hotspots ([69]; Fig. 4.7c). The same group subsequently made similar observations on the distribution of *FGFR2* c.758C>G

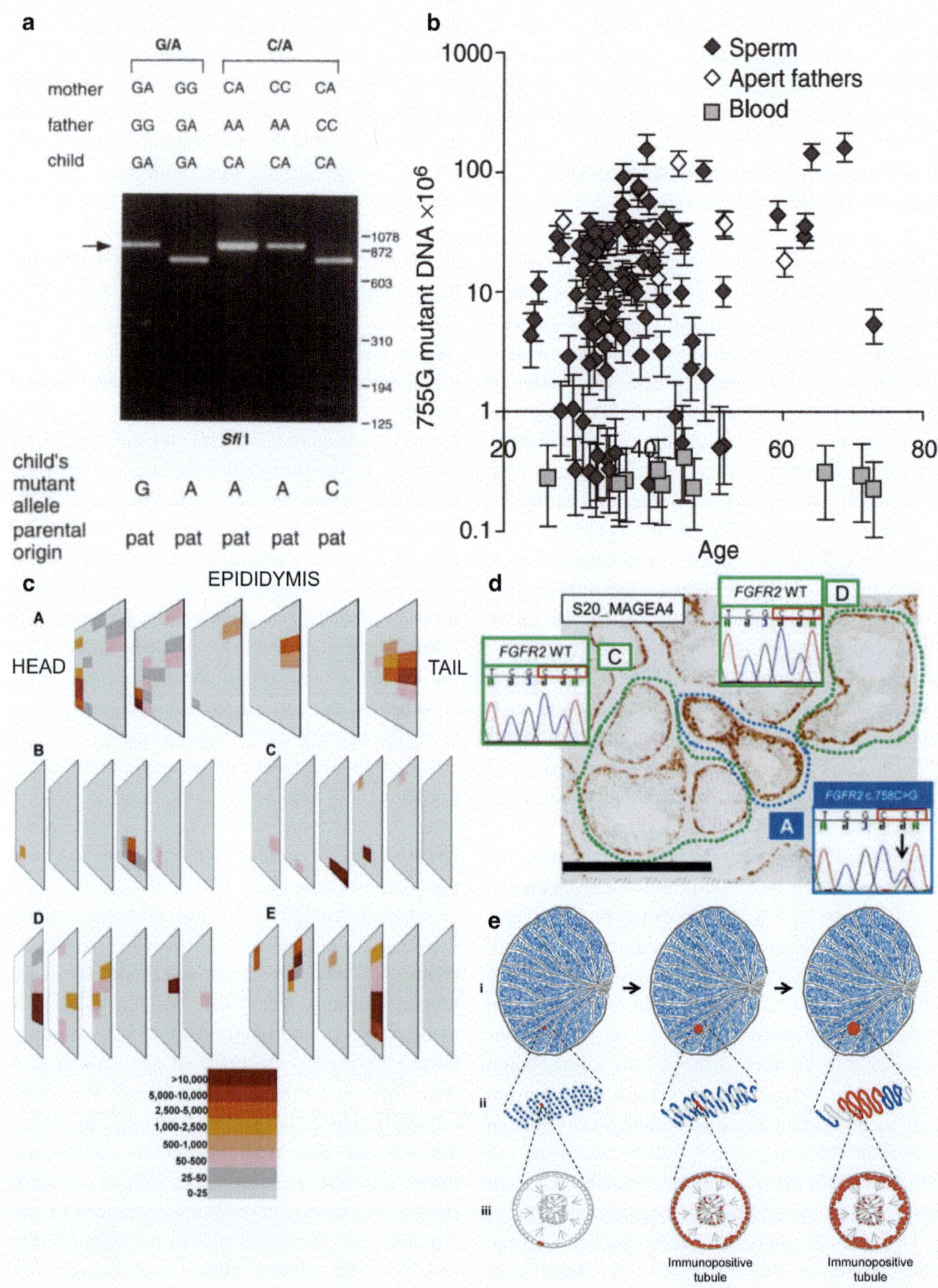

a
G/A
C/A
mother GA GG CA CC CA
father GG GA AA AA CC
child GA GA CA CA CA
-1078
-872
-603
-310
-194
-125
SfiI
child's mutant allele G A A A C
parental origin pat pat pat pat pat
b
Sperm
Apert fathers
Blood
755G mutant DNA ×10^6
Age
c
EPIDIDYMIS
HEAD
TAIL
>10,000
5,000-10,000
2,500-5,000
1,000-2,500
500-1,000
50-500
25-50
0-25
d
S20_MAGEA4
FGFR2 WT
FGFR2 c.758C>G
e
i
ii
iii
Immunopositive tubule
Immunopositive tubule

Fig. 4.7 How the study of Apert syndrome mutations supports the theory of selfish spermatogonial selection. (**a**) Apert syndrome mutations arise exclusively on the *FGFR2* allele transmitted from the father. The top panel shows, for five different Apert syndrome trios (in each of which the child is heterozygous at c.755C>G and the parents are unaffected), the genotypes at one or other of two nearby polymorphic loci—rs2071616 (c.749-112G>A; labelled G/A) or rs2981451 (c.939+579C>A; labelled C/A). In the middle panel, allele-specific PCR was performed on the child's sample using primers designed selectively to amplify the A allele only (G/A variant), or the C allele only (C/A variant). The restriction enzyme *Sfi*I specifically digests the c.755G mutant allele; so if the product digested (yielding a shortened band on electrophoresis), this would indicate that mutant allele had been amplified, and vice-versa. The bottom panel shows the interpretation of the digest result, indicating the allele on which the Apert syndrome mutation must be present. In all cases displayed, the mutation is paternal (pat) in origin; this proved to be the case in all 57 informative families (figure from: [53]). (**b**) Quantitation of the 755C > G Apert syndrome mutation in sperm and blood samples (see key) in relation to age of the donor. Sperm measurements were obtained for 99 men with no family history of Apert syndrome and for 6 men who had fathered a child with Apert syndrome. Note that the mutations are effectively undetectable ($<10^{-6}$) in blood, but are present at measurable levels in sperm of most, but not all men in the population. See text for further discussion (figure from: [18]). (**c**) Spatial analysis of the c.755C > G mutation in four cadaveric testes from two men aged 54 and 62 years, obtained from a tissue bank (C and D are from different parts of the same testis). Each testis was dissected into ≥192 geographically registered pieces, the level of Apert syndrome mutation measured in each piece, and the distribution of mutations reconstructed for each testis according to the position of each piece in the original dissection. The color scale indicates the number of mutant molecules per million genomes (figure from: [69]). (**d**) Direct isolation and identification of an Apert syndrome mutation in a seminiferous tubule. Immunohistochemistry was performed on a testis cross-section with the antibody MAGEA4. Note the stronger peripheral brown staining in the tubule surrounded by blue dotted lines, compared to the tubules surrounded by green dotted lines. Insets show the results of *FGFR2* DNA sequencing of each of the highlighted regions, following microdissection of the corresponding tubule(s) from an adjacent tissue slice. The blue-surrounded tubule labeled A contains the c.758C > G Apert syndrome mutation (indicated by down-pointing arrow), whereas the green-surrounded tubules labeled C and D show only the normal *FGFR2* sequence at this location. Black scale bar indicates 500 μm (figure from: [45]). (**e**) Cartoon illustrating the evolution of a positively selected clone within the testis. Each figure part shows a whole testis at the top, a length of seminiferous tubule in the middle, and a cross-section through an individual seminiferous tubule at the bottom. Mutant cells are colored red. Left: A mutation has randomly arisen in a single spermatogonial stem cell, located adjacent to the basement membrane of the tubule. Middle and right: As a result of preferential proliferation of the cell and its progeny, the mutant cell has first populated the entire circumference of the tubule, then over the course of time the clone has extended along an increasing length of the tubule. Half the sperm produced by the mutant stem cell bear the Apert syndrome mutation, hence the output of mutant sperm increases over the years. Note that the absolute mutation level (hence the recurrence risk for the father) remains very low (<1 in 1000), because mutant cells only constitute a small fraction of the testis as a whole. (Figure from: [44])

mutations within the testis [11], as well as measuring levels of both mutations in sperm samples [96], independently concluding that their data best fitted a selective advantage rather than a mutation hotspot model.

Although these reports supported the occurrence of selective advantage, the underlying evidence for the cellular distribution of mutations was lost because the experimental approach used DNA extracted from testis pieces. Following the discovery [40] that immunohistochemistry on testis sections using an antibody raised to a tumor antigen (MAGEA4 [melanoma antigen gene A4]) highlighted a subset of seminiferous tubules exhibiting an abnormally prominent staining pattern, Maher et al. [45] then used a combination of laser capture microdissection, whole genome amplification of extracted DNA, and next-generation sequencing and targeted dideoxy-sequencing to demonstrate that these unusual-appearing tubules often harbored a specific mutation encoding a gain-of-function protein encoded by one or other of a handful of genes, including *FGFR2* [45]. Indeed, one of the mutations identified [45] was the Apert syndrome *FGFR2* c.758C > G, pinpointed in a seminiferous tubule from a 39-year-old man, whose testis had been removed as part of a hernia operation (Fig. 4.7d). Using cartoon illustrations of a testis, Fig. 4.7e summarizes the conclusions arising from this body of work, showing how, through a process of positive selection, a single cell harboring a rare, randomly occurring mutation forms a slowly expanding clone over the course of time. The process is referred to as "selfish," because although the mutation benefits the spermatogonial stem cell in which it arises (conferring a replicative advantage), it is harmful to any progeny arising from fertilization by progeny mutant sperm (in this case, causing Apert syndrome). Further work has highlighted activation of RAS–MAP kinase, one of the key pathways activated by FGFR2 signaling (Fig. 4.2) as the common thread linking all the major genes for which mutations are enriched by selfish selection [46]. This provides evidence that the RAS–MAP kinase pathway plays a key role in regulating spermatogonial stem cell turnover; we will return to the important role of this pathway in Apert syndrome pathogenesis in Section "Pathways activated in Apert syndrome and approaches to therapeutic inhibition."

The cellular mechanisms of Apert syndrome-mediated selfish spermatogonial selection were investigated by Martin et al. [47] using mouse spermatogonial stem cells transduced with either the Apert syndrome FGFR2-Ser252Trp or wild-type cDNAs using a lentiviral system [47]. Confirming previous work, *FGFR2* was shown to be expressed in putative spermatogonial stem cells adjacent to the basement membrane of the seminiferous tubule. Apert syndrome-mutant cells showed increased proliferation when exposed to low doses of FGF2. Most pertinently, transplantation of labeled mutant or wild-type cells into mouse testes showed preferential population by the mutant cells, consistent with a selective advantage. Several FGFs appear to play physiological roles in the testis including FGF2, FGF5, FGF8, and FGF9, with cells responding to precise doses [36, 94]. Since the Apert syndrome mutations exhibit increased binding to most of these ligands [30], the strong selective advantage might work through a combinatorial effect involving several ligands.

Given the conclusion that, in the appropriate cellular context, an Apert syndrome mutation confers the cell with a proliferative advantage over its wild-type neighbors, it should not come as a surprise that the identical canonical mutations, when arising somatically in specific tissue types, have been identified in several cancers. In fact, the p.Ser252Trp FGFR2 mutation is the single most common somatic mutation occurring in endometrial cancer [67], and the COSMIC database documents the occurrence of the somatic equivalent of Apert syndrome mutations in other cancer types (https://cancer.sanger.ac.uk/cosmic/gene/analysis?ln=FGFR2). While a detailed discussion is outside the scope of this chapter, it is important to note that no strong evidence exists that Apert syndrome itself is associated with a substantially increased cancer risk. This seemingly paradoxical fact may be understood when it is appreciated that the milieu of the Apert syndrome-mutant cell differs according to context. In Apert syndrome itself, all neighboring cells are also mutant, whereas in cancer (as well as in men's testes), the neighboring cells are wild-type, making it more likely in the latter situation that differential selection between cells can occur.

Clinical Implications of Selfish Spermatogonial Selection

An important clinical implication of this body of work is that when a healthy couple has a child affected by Apert syndrome, the recurrence risk for another affected child is likely to be extremely low (< 1 in 1000; [90]). This is because, even though the mutant clone is positively selected (explaining the high mutation rate), it remains diluted out by the large number of non-mutant cells in the entire testis (as illustrated in Fig. 4.7e). This deduction is further supported by quantitation of Apert syndrome mutation levels in individuals who have fathered a child with Apert syndrome (Fig. 4.7b). While high-level germinal mosaicism is theoretically possible, and has been documented in a single instance of a Crouzon *FGFR2* mutation [20], it has not yet been molecularly confirmed in Apert syndrome, although a single sibling recurrence was reported in the historical literature [3]. Owing to this very low recurrence risk it is the author's recommendation, for couples who have had a child affected with Apert syndrome, not to promote use of invasive diagnostic procedures in subsequent pregnancies, as the risk of causing the miscarriage of an unaffected fetus will in nearly all cases exceed the risk of Apert syndrome itself.

An alternative route for the genetic detection of Apert syndrome fetuses during pregnancy is to exploit the fact that small amounts of fetal DNA circulate in the maternal blood. This has led to development of a generalized strategy for noninvasive prenatal screening (NIPS) including multiple genetic disorders, starting with a maternal peripheral blood sample [99]. Among the proof-of-principle cases presented in this series was the confirmation of Apert syndrome in a pregnancy of 20 weeks' gestation, already clinically suspected to be affected based on ultrasound findings. In principle, the approach presented by Zhang et al. [99] would be technically feasible for NIPS of low-risk pregnancies at much earlier (~10 weeks') gestations. However, further technical refinements and demonstration of cost-effectiveness will be required before entering clinical practice.

Mouse Models of Apert Syndrome

Although valuable insights into the pathogenesis of Apert syndrome have been gained from the study of affected fetuses (reviewed by [88]; see also Chap. 5), the use of genetically equivalent mouse models enables substantially more detailed studies of the pathogenesis of malformation. For example, the use of one such model, the *Fgfr2*$^{\Delta IIIc/+}$ mouse, to investigate the pathogenic mechanism of *FGFR2*-exon IIIc deletions was discussed in Section "Beyond the canonical mutations: rare molecular causes of Apert syndrome." Regarding the canonical mutations, an initial barrier to creating mouse models was that heterozygous Apert syndrome mice are more severely affected in their craniofacial development than humans with the equivalent mutations, making it effectively impossible to breed Apert syndrome mouse lines directly. Rather, the mice must be created by first making lines in which the Apert syndrome mutation is present but not expressed at a high level, and then secondarily uncovering the functioning mutation by further genetic manipulation. Using such targeting strategies, the first model of the p.Ser252Trp mutation was made by Chen et al. [9] and the first model of the Pro253Arg was made by Yin et al. [95] (conveniently, the cDNA numbering of human *FGFR2* and orthologous mouse *Fgfr2* genes is identical; with the aim to distinguish more clearly the outcome of work performed on mice and humans, the canonical mutations in mice are denoted S252W and P253R for the remainder of this chapter). Independently generated S252W and P253R models were also subsequently made [86, 87]. These mice have been used to study the developmental origins of the morphological abnormalities that occur in Apert syndrome (summarized in Table 4.4; see [23], for review), and are particularly valuable for studies that address pathways of perturbed FGFR2 signaling in malformation and how these may be therapeutically manipulated (Section "Pathways activated in Apert syndrome and approaches to therapeutic inhibition").

One striking observation from the examination of these Apert syndrome mice is that although they reliably manifest craniosynostosis (Table 4.4), only very rarely do they exhibit digital syndactyly, so that the development of this latter phenotype cannot be fully investigated. More usefully, the coronal sutures are nearly always fused at birth in Apert syndrome model mice, whereas the sagittal suture starts off as patent but with a prominent cartilaginous element. Detailed analysis of the coronal suture [25] found that in E13.5 *Fgfr2*$^{S252W/+}$ mutant mice, the osteogenic fronts of the newly appearing basal coronal sutures are already in a state of incipient fusion. In the mid/upper coronal sutures, the anlage of the frontal and parietal bones is also substantially closer in mutant than wild-type animals, with complete fusion in the mutants by birth (postnatal day [P]0) (Fig. 4.8a). A systematic analysis of markers of proliferation, differentiation, and apoptosis concluded that the primary cause of craniosynostosis in *Fgfr2*$^{S252W/+}$ mice is early (embryonic day [E]12) loss of basal sutural mesenchyme. This represents a differentiation defect involving the osteogenic fronts expressing activated Fgfr2, leading these fronts to unite to form a contiguous skeletogenic membrane. As development proceeds, the superior part of the coronal suture initially forms in mutants, but fuses as a

Table 4.4 Survey of major anatomical features observed in engineered Apert syndrome mouse mutants

	Design	Cranial sutures	Cranial base	Facial	Other organs	Skeleton	Stature	Survival	Fertility	References
S252W	Intronic loxP-*neo* cassette upstream of exon IIIa inhibits expression	Coronal synostosis from E18.5; calvarial bones 25% thinner; primary differentiation defect of sutures; secondary increase in apoptosis; normal proliferation	Normal synchondroses of presphenoid-sphenoidal, basisphenoid-occipital, and basioccipital-exoccipital bones; short presphenoid bone	Midface hypoplasia; malocclusion		Shortened hindlimbs, reduced bone density, sparse trabecular network, and delayed secondary ossification centers in tibial epiphyses; no limb syndactyly	<80% wild-type	Ranging from death at 20 day in severely runted mice to survival to adulthood	Female, infertile; male, much reduced (1 fertile male obtained)	Chen et al. [9, 10], Holmes et al. [25]
S252W	Intronic loxP-*neo* cassette downstream of exon IIIa inhibits expression	Coronal and lambdoid synostosis from E18.5; ectopic cartilage in sagittal suture E16.5–E18.5 and synostosis from P1; widened interfrontal (metopic) suture	Increased cartilage of basicranium	Thickened nasal cartilage	Complete cartilage sleeve of the trachea	No limb syndactyly; fusion of sternal bones; disorganized growth plates of long bones	Birthweight 83% of wild-type	Death at 24–36 h postnatally (respiratory), except with incomplete *neo* excision	Insufficient survival to test	Wang et al. [86]

P253R	Intronic loxP-*neo* cassette upstream of exon IIIa inhibits expression	Coronal synostosis; delayed fusion of posterior frontal suture (cartilage absent compared to controls); ectopic cartilage in sagittal suture	Retardation of cranial base synchondroses	Reduced nasale–nasion distance		Syndactyly present in 3/40 individuals; delayed ossification centers in tibial epiphysis	Birthweight 90% of wild-type; weight 50–60% of controls at 3 weeks	35% death by P20; 45% by 6 months; 20% survived to adulthood	Normal	Yin et al. [95]
P253R	Intronic loxP-*neo* cassette downstream of exon IIIa inhibits expression	Coronal synostosis at P0; increased osteoid in sagittal and lambdoid sutures; ectopic cartilage in sagittal suture	Shortened anterior cranial base	10% reduction of maxilla and nasal region; bilateral incomplete fusion of primary and secondary palatal shelves		Abnormal sternal fusions; no syndactyly	Normal birthweight; 40% reduction in weight by P5	40% death at 24–36 h; 1/20 survived to P14	Insufficient survival to test	Wang et al. [87]
ΔIIIc	Complete deletion of exon IIIc	Coronal synostosis at E18		Truncated maxilla; fused zygomatic arch bones	Abnormal lung lobulation; incomplete alveolarization; small kidneys	Precocious ossification of the intersternebral cartilage; no syndactyly	Mild reduction in birthweight in 90%; severe in 10%	100% death by P9	No survival	Hajihosseini et al. [21]

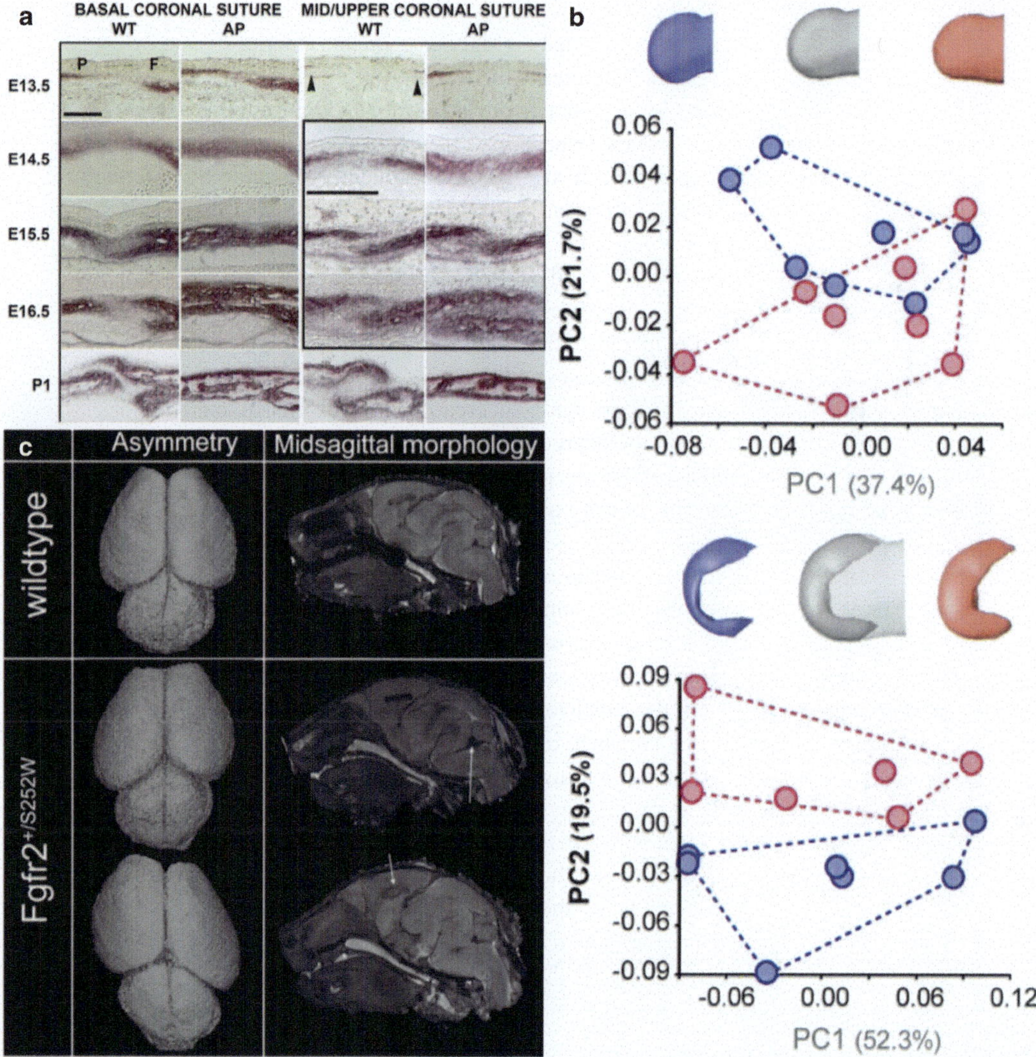

Fig. 4.8 Abnormal developmental phenotypes in Apert syndrome mutant mouse models. (**a**) Coronal suture. Sagittal cross-sections of alkaline phosphatase-stained sutures at two levels (left, basal; right, mid/upper) in wild-type (WT) and *Fgfr2*$^{S252W/+}$ mutant (AP) mice, from E13.5 (top) to postnatal day 1 (P1, bottom). At E13.5, abnormality of the basal suture is already evident, with only a narrow gap in the alkaline phosphatase-stained territories, which have merged 1 day later. At higher levels the coronal suture is initially patent but evidently narrower than in WT, and has closed by P1. Note that the growing parietal bone tip overlaps the frontal bone tip in the normal coronal suture. Scale bars are 100 μm (reproduced from: [25]). (**b**) Limb bud morphology in E11 WT (blue) and Apert syndrome mutant *Fgfr2*$^{P253R/+}$ (red) mice, using optical projection tomography fluorescence scanning to analyze shape (upper panel) and whole-mount in situ hybridization/transmission scanning to analyze expression of *Dusp6*, a direct target of Fgfr2-mediated signaling (lower panel: renditions of limb buds are not shown at the same scale). Gray images represent regions of similarity between the two genotypes. The lower plots in each panel show principal component analyses, indicating that the two genotypes are largely separable at this embryonic stage, particularly based on *Dusp6* expression, which is more extensive in the mutant limb buds that exhibit a narrower but longer shape profile (reproduced from: [50]). (**c**) Brains from P0 mice analyzed by magnetic resonance microscopy. Compared to wild-type, the Apert syndrome *Fgfr2*$^{S252W/+}$ mutant mouse brains more frequently showed asymmetry (two examples at mid/lower left), enlarged fourth ventricle (white arrow in middle right image), and arched corpus callosum (white arrow in bottom right image). (Reproduced from: [2])

result of localized induction of osteogenesis within the narrow margin of mesenchyme separating the adjacent osteogenic fronts [25]. Using a Mesp1-cre driver it was shown that expression of the Apert syndrome mutation in cephalic mesoderm (which includes the mesodermally derived coronal suture) was sufficient to cause coronal suture fusion [24].

Following on from this work, a series of detailed descriptive studies has been published addressing various elements of Apert syndrome mouse morphology, including several aspects of facial and mandibular growth [26, 28, 48, 56] as well as palate development [49]; the interested reader should consult the original articles for further details. Subtle abnormalities of the limbs, including forefoot bones, have been documented using advanced imaging techniques and have been associated with increased expression in *Fgfr2*$^{P253R/+}$ mutants of the target gene *Dusp6*; this first occurred at E10.5, ~12 h before any morphological abnormality (a slightly smaller and dorsoventrally thicker limb paddle in mutant; Fig. 4.7b) became evident [50]. However, as noted above, these early limb bud abnormalities, although consistently present, do not result in syndactyly later in development. Also of particular interest, study of the brain using magnetic resonance microscopy has shown that both Apert syndrome mouse mutants exhibit variable but significant primary abnormalities of brain morphology, for example severe brain asymmetry, arched corpus callosum, and/or fourth ventricle enlargement [2] (Fig. 4.7c). These observations mirror clinical observations of the brain in Apert syndrome and are relevant to the question whether these represent primary neurological abnormalities or are secondary to cranial suture fusion (see Chap. 5).

Pathways Activated in Apert Syndrome and Approaches to Therapeutic Inhibition

As discussed in Section "Biological and pathological context: FGFR2 structure, function, and comparative mutation patterns in Apert, Crouzon and Pfeiffer syndromes" and illustrated in Fig. 4.2, FGFR-mediated signal activation may occur through multiple different pathways according to the cellular and developmental context. This raises the question, "what are the most important signaling pathways perturbed by Apert syndrome mutations?" I will start by presenting a beautiful experiment that helps to address this question.

Analysis of Mouse Models

Using a previously constructed mouse model of the S252W mutation [9] (see previous section), Shukla et al. [81] experimented with two distinct methods to prevent the developmental abnormalities caused by the mutation. One approach used a short hairpin RNA (shRNA) to target the specific Apert syndrome mutant allele. Owing to different codon usage between human and mouse, the substitution required in the mouse to encode S252W is not TCG > T<u>G</u>G (human), but TCA > T<u>GG</u> (substituted bases underlined). This means that there is a dinucleotide difference in the mouse between the normal and Apert syndrome mutant sequence, making direct shRNA-based targeting somewhat more specific. After generating a transgenic mouse containing a specific U6shRNA construct, the authors crossed this to yield mice doubly heterozygous with the Apert syndrome mutation. Remarkably, these mice had normal craniofacial phenotypes [81]. Importantly, comparison of both lung and thymic tissues showed prominently increased phospho-ERK (extracellular signal-related kinase; pERK) in the Apert syndrome mutants, which normalized when the shRNA transgene was additionally present. Phosphorylation of ERK (which is encoded by the genes *MAPK1* and *MAPK3*) is the final step in the activation of the important RAS–MEK–ERK (also referred to as the RAS–MAPK or p42/44) signaling pathway (Fig. 4.9a) [39]. Therefore, this result was consistent with, but did not prove, that craniosynostosis and other malformations resulted from activation of this pathway.

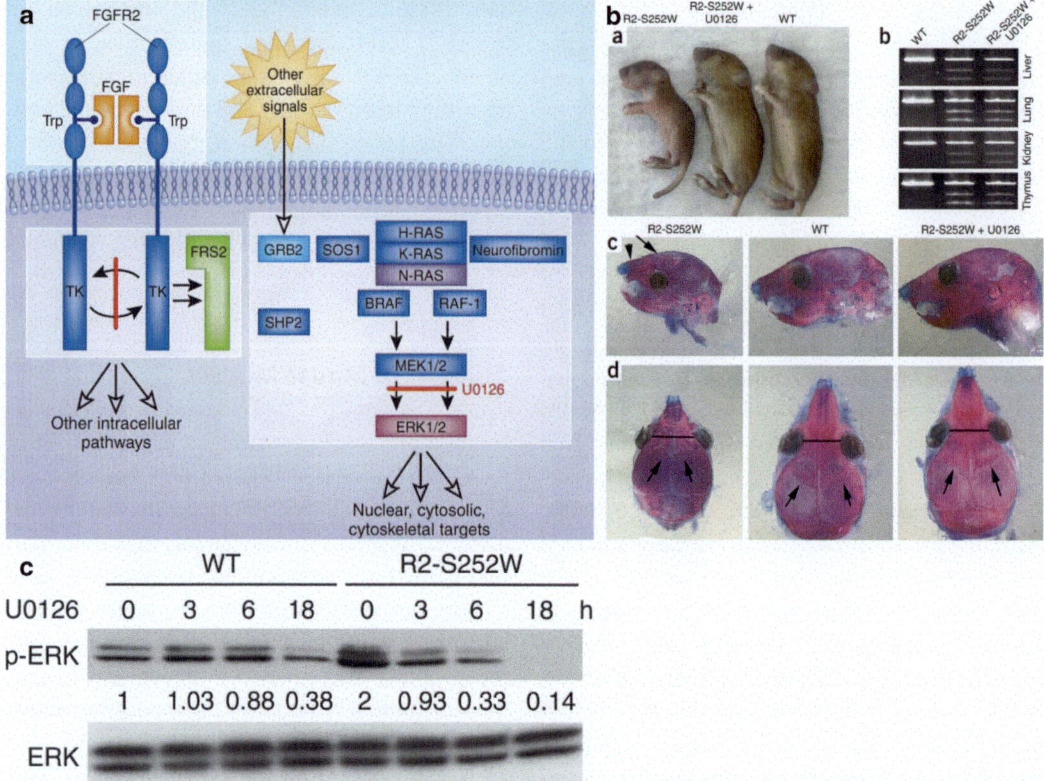

Fig. 4.9 Correction of morphological abnormalities in Apert syndrome mouse using a MEK1/2 inhibitor. (**a**) Schematic of signaling from mutant FGFR2 molecules through the RAS–MAPK pathway. The position of U0126 blockade of MEK1/2 is indicated by the red bar (figure adapted from: [89]). (**b**) Mouse phenotypes and mutation confirmation. Panels a, c, and d show the whole body (a) and cleared Alizarin red/Alcian blue-stained skull (c,d), all at P8, in mice heterozygous for the S252W mutation (R2-S252W) that were either untreated or treated with U0126, and in genotypically normal wild-type controls (WT). Panel b shows a cDNA-based assay for *FGFR2* expression; the pair of lower bands are diagnostic for presence of the engineered mutation. (**c**) Immunoblot measurement of phosphorylation of the downstream effector proteins ERK1/2 in wild-type mice (WT, left) and S252W-mutant mice (right). Note how the total amount of ERK remains unchanged with U0126 treatment (lower panel), but the active phospho-ERK (p-ERK) transitions from a hyperactivated state (time zero) to complete loss (inactivation) by 18 h. (Figure parts b, c from: [81])

To test this possibility directly, Shukla and colleagues [81] injected pregnant female mice bearing embryos heterozygous for the S252W mutation with a chemical, U0126, originally designed as an anti-cancer drug via selective inhibition of MEK1/2, a critical intermediate component of the RAS–MAPK pathway (Fig. 4.9a). The injections started at E13 of gestation, then continued in the postnatal period up to P26. Remarkably, the treated mice were born without craniosynostosis and, unlike genetically identical but untreated pups, several grew up to be fertile (Fig. 4.9b). Tissue analysis confirmed that the U0126 treatment not only corrected the excessive ERK phosphorylation present in mutant mice, but after 18 h it was abolished altogether; in other words, it was overcorrected (Fig. 4.9c). Similar conclusions were obtained for the P253R mouse model, this time using treatments with a different MEK1/2 inhibitor (PD98059), conducted on in vitro cultured calvaria and femur explants [95].

These groundbreaking experiments using pharmacological inhibition convincingly demonstrated that several of the major malformative features of Apert syndrome arise through hyperactivation of the RAS–MAPK signaling pathway, consistent with other genetic data that this pathway is especially important in FGF receptor signal transduction [8]. Moreover, they illustrate a powerful proof-of-principle that Apert syndrome-associated malformations are in theory correctable, if therapy could be introduced early enough during the pregnancy. However, this work also highlights the major challenges of contemplating such an approach. In pregnancy, except in the rare cases at high risk (when one of the parents is affected with the condition), Apert syndrome is only routinely detected (if at all) by the ultrasound-based identification of anatomical abnormality; by definition, this would be too late to start preventative therapy. Another aspect is the potential for intrauterine therapies to cause harm; U0126 was never licensed for clinical use owing to toxicity, and Fig. 4.9c illustrates that overdosing could readily abolish the normal physiological functions of ERK activation. The possibility remains that inhibitory therapies based on the principles illustrated above might be used for secondary prevention of progression following surgery; however, this particular application does not seem to have advanced greatly since the original report by Shukla et al. [81].

Importantly, ERK1/2 activation does not mediate all Apert syndrome-related pathology. Analysis of previously described mouse models (Table 4.4) also demonstrated increased phosphorylation (hence activation) of the p38 serine threonine kinase signaling pathway, mediated by a family of MAPKs (encoded by the genes *MAPK11*, *−12*, *−13* and *−14*) that are activated by cellular stress and/or several growth factors and cytokines [10, 39, 87]. Chen et al. [10] focused on development of the long bones and vertebrae in S252W mice, observing reduced bone density, sparser trabecular network, and delayed secondary ossification centers in the tibial epiphyses of mutants (Table 4.4); this was associated with reduced markers of proliferation and differentiation in mutant tibial growth plates and cells. (These investigators attempted to counter any non-specific effects from malnutrition owing to dental malocclusion in mutants by cutting the overgrown incisor teeth.) In cultured mesenchymal stem cells (MSCs), increased phosphorylation of both pERK1/2 and p38 was observed. Treatment of cultured tibiae with specific inhibitors for the two pathways (PD98059 and SB203580, respectively) showed greater restoration of phenotype using the latter inhibitor, suggesting a greater influence of p38 MAPK function [10]. Excessive osteoclast activation has also been implicated in the abnormal long bone phenotype of Apert syndrome mutants [80].

Downstream from RAS–MAPK signaling, the master osteogenic regulator RUNX2 has been identified as a further potential therapeutic target. Intraperitoneal injection of pregnant female mice with juglone, an inhibitor of PIN1 (peptidyl-prolyl cis–trans isomerase NIMA-interacting 1), prevented the development of craniosynostosis in *Fgfr2*$^{S252W/+}$ mutant offspring. This effect is believed to be mediated through destabilization of RUNX2, antagonizing stabilizing RUNX2 post-translational modifications induced by the activating *Fgfr2*$^{S252W/+}$ mutation [35, 79, 97]. However, given that PIN1 has many other biological targets, use of juglone therapeutically would raise safety concerns analogous to those applying to MEK1 inhibitors. Evidence for activation of the canonical Wnt (wingless-type MMTV integration site family)/β-catenin signaling pathway in the cranial sutures has also been presented [51]. How the FGF and WNT signaling pathways interlink requires further elucidation.

Recent Therapeutic Approaches

In summary, the above studies illustrate the complexity of pharmacological inhibition of signaling downstream of FGFR2 activation, which has led to more targeted approaches. For example, crossing of *Fgfr2*$^{S252W/+}$ mice with a transgenic mouse expressing a soluble (extracellular) portion of the Fgfr2^{S252W} mutant receptor showed modest amelioration of the craniofacial phenotype, attributed to reduction of FGFR2 signaling by acting as a competitive decoy receptor [55]. However, it would be challenging to exploit this approach as a therapeutic owing to likely non-specific effects on other aspects of FGFR-mediated signaling. A more promising strategy, encouraged by the success of the transgenic shRNA experiment described above [81], has been to explore different methods to deliver either an shRNA or short interfering RNA (siRNA) targeting one of the canonical mutations, to achieve specific knockdown of mutant FGFR2. For example, by linking an shRNA construct to AAV9 (adeno-associated virus 9), followed by calvarial injection of virus particles at P0 and P4, reduced expression of the mutant *Fgfr2* mRNA and modest rescue of the suture fusion phenotype of the $Fgfr2^{P253R/+}$ Apert syndrome mouse was achieved [43]. However, systemic delivery would be preferable for wider therapeutic benefit. An exosome-based delivery of siRNA targeting $Fgfr2^{S252W/+}$ tissue has also been explored, but to date only in vitro, by incubation of loaded exosomes with primary calvarial osteoblast-like cells [57].

Concluding Comments

Most of this chapter has been taken up by exploring the pathological consequences of the two canonical Apert syndrome-causing mutations that arise in the *FGFR2* gene. It is hard for the human brain to conceptualize what a tiny proportion of the human genome this represents; a smaller proportion, for example, than the lives elapsed of anyone reading this chapter in relation to the age of the known universe. Although the amount, and detail, that we have learnt about these two canonical mutations over the past three decades is remarkable, this must be tempered with a strong measure of humility, because the information has so far had a rather limited impact on the lives of those affected by Apert syndrome. However, on a positive note, the basic scientific knowledge presented here, combined with ongoing and rapid technological advances, provides optimism that new approaches to both prevention (Section "Clinical Implications of Selfish Spermatogonial Selection") and therapy (Section "Recent Therapeutic Approaches") will emerge before another three decades pass.

Acknowledgments I thank my brilliant colleagues Elena Bochukova, Dominique Davidson, Aimee Fenwick, Anne Goriely, Ruth Hansen, John Heath, Shih-hsin Kan, Jasmine Lim, Geoffrey Maher, Gil McVean, Gillian Morriss-Kay, Michael Oldridge, Susannah Patey, Sarah Smithson and Steve Twigg, who accompanied me during my personal journey of discovery into Apert syndrome and made key contributions to the work presented here. The Wellcome Trust provided the majority of the funding for my laboratory. This chapter is dedicated to the memory of my mentor, Sir David Weatherall FRS, whose steadfast support enabled this research to happen.

References

1. Ahmed Z, Schuller AC, Suhling K, Tregidgo C, Ladbury JE. Extracellular point mutations in FGFR2 elicit unexpected changes in intracellular signalling. Biochem J. 2008;413(1):37–49.
2. Aldridge K, Hill CA, Austin JR, Percival C, Martinez-Abadias N, Neuberger T, Wang Y, Jabs EW, Richtsmeier JT. Brain phenotypes in two FGFR2 mouse models for Apert syndrome. Dev Dyn. 2010;239(3):987–97.
3. Allanson JE. Germinal mosaicism in Apert syndrome. Clin Genet. 1986;29(5):429–33.
4. Anderson J, Burns HD, Enriquez-Harris P, Wilkie AOM, Heath JK. Apert syndrome mutations in fibroblast growth factor receptor 2 exhibit increased affinity for FGF ligand. Hum Mol Genet. 1998;7(9):1475–83.
5. Bergeron LA, Besenbacher S, Turner T, Versoza CJ, Wang RJ, Price AL, Armstrong E, Riera M, Carlson J, Chen HY, Hahn MW, Harris K, Kleppe AS, Lopez-Nandam EH, Moorjani P, Pfeifer SP, Tiley GP, Yoder AD, Zhang G, Schierup MH. The Mutationathon highlights the importance of reaching standardization in estimates of pedigree-based germline mutation rates. eLife. 2022;11:e73577.
6. Blank CE. Apert's syndrome (a type of acrocephalosyndactyly)-observations on a British series of thirty-nine cases. Ann Hum Genet. 1960;24:151–64.
7. Bochukova EG, Roscioli T, Hedges DJ, Taylor IB, Johnson D, David DJ, Deininger PL, Wilkie AOM. Rare mutations of *FGFR2* causing Apert syndrome: identification of the first partial gene deletion, and an *Alu* element insertion from a new subfamily. Hum Mutat. 2009;30(2):204–11.
8. Brewer JR, Mazot P, Soriano P. Genetic insights into the mechanisms of Fgf signaling. Genes Dev. 2016;30(7):751–71.
9. Chen L, Li D, Li C, Engel A, Deng CX. A Ser252Trp [corrected] substitution in mouse fibroblast growth

factor receptor 2 (Fgfr2) results in craniosynostosis. Bone. 2003;33(2):169–78.
10. Chen P, Zhang L, Weng T, Zhang S, Sun S, Chang M, Li Y, Zhang B, Zhang L. A Ser252Trp mutation in fibroblast growth factor receptor 2 (FGFR2) mimicking human Apert syndrome reveals an essential role for FGF signaling in the regulation of endochondral bone formation. PLoS One. 2014;9(1):e87311.
11. Choi SK, Yoon SR, Calabrese P, Arnheim N. A germ-line-selective advantage rather than an increased mutation rate can explain some unexpectedly common human disease mutations. Proc Natl Acad Sci USA. 2008;105(29):10143–8.
12. Chun K, Teebi AS, Azimi C, Steele L, Ray PN. Screening of patients with craniosynostosis: molecular strategy. Am J Med Genet A. 2003;120A(4):470–3.
13. Farmer DT, Mlcochova H, Zhou Y, Koelling N, Wang G, Ashley N, Bugacov H, Chen HJ, Parvez R, Tseng KC, Merrill AE, Maxson RE Jr, Wilkie AOM, Crump JG, Twigg SRF. The developing mouse coronal suture at single-cell resolution. Nat Commun. 2021;12(1):4797.
14. Fearon JA, Podner C. Apert syndrome: evaluation of a treatment algorithm. Plast Reconstr Surg. 2013;131(1):132–42.
15. Fenwick AL, Bowdin SC, Klatt RE, Wilkie AOM. A deletion of *FGFR2* creating a chimeric IIIb/IIIc exon in a child with Apert syndrome. BMC Med Genet. 2011;12:122.
16. Goetz R, Mohammadi M. Exploring mechanisms of FGF signalling through the lens of structural biology. Nat Rev Mol Cell Biol. 2013;14(3):166–80.
17. Goriely A, Wilkie AOM. Paternal age effect mutations and selfish spermatogonial selection: causes and consequences for human disease. Am J Hum Genet. 2012;90(2):175–200.
18. Goriely A, McVean GA, Rojmyr M, Ingemarsson B, Wilkie AOM. Evidence for selective advantage of pathogenic FGFR2 mutations in the male germ line. Science. 2003;301(5633):643–6.
19. Goriely A, McVean GA, van Pelt AM, O'Rourke AW, Wall SA, de Rooij DG, Wilkie AOM. Gain-of-function amino acid substitutions drive positive selection of *FGFR2* mutations in human spermatogonia. Proc Natl Acad Sci USA. 2005;102(17):6051–6.
20. Goriely A, Lord H, Lim J, Johnson D, Lester T, Firth HV, Wilkie AOM. Germline and somatic mosaicism for *FGFR2* mutation in the mother of a child with Crouzon syndrome: Implications for genetic testing in "paternal age-effect" syndromes. Am J Med Genet A. 2010;152A(8):2067–73.
21. Hajihosseini MK, Wilson S, De Moerlooze L, Dickson C. A splicing switch and gain-of-function mutation in *FgfR2-IIIc* hemizygotes causes Apert/Pfeiffer-syndrome-like phenotypes. Proc Natl Acad Sci USA. 2001;98(7):3855–60.
22. Hajihosseini MK, Duarte R, Pegrum J, Donjacour A, Lana-Elola E, Rice DP, Sharpe J, Dickson C. Evidence that Fgf10 contributes to the skeletal and visceral defects of an Apert syndrome mouse model. Dev Dyn. 2009;238(2):376–85.
23. Holmes G. Mouse models of Apert syndrome. Childs Nerv Syst. 2012;28(9):1505–10.
24. Holmes G, Basilico C. Mesodermal expression of *Fgfr2*^{S252W} is necessary and sufficient to induce craniosynostosis in a mouse model of Apert syndrome. Dev Biol. 2012;368(2):283–93.
25. Holmes G, Rothschild G, Roy UB, Deng CX, Mansukhani A, Basilico C. Early onset of craniosynostosis in an Apert mouse model reveals critical features of this pathology. Dev Biol. 2009;328(2):273–84.
26. Holmes G, O'Rourke C, Motch Perrine SM, Lu N, van Bakel H, Richtsmeier JT, Jabs EW. Midface and upper airway dysgenesis in FGFR2-related craniosynostosis involves multiple tissue-specific and cell cycle effects. Development. 2018;145(19):dev166488.
27. Holmes G, Gonzalez-Reiche AS, Saturne M, Motch Perrine SM, Zhou X, Borges AC, Shewale B, Richtsmeier JT, Zhang B, van Bakel H, Jabs EW. Single-cell analysis identifies a key role for *Hhip* in murine coronal suture development. Nat Commun. 2021;12(1):7132.
28. Hoshino Y, Takechi M, Moazen M, Steacy M, Koyabu D, Furutera T, Ninomiya Y, Nuri T, Pauws E, Iseki S. Synchondrosis fusion contributes to the progression of postnatal craniofacial dysmorphology in syndromic craniosynostosis. J Anat. 2023;242(3):387–401.
29. Ibrahimi OA, Eliseenkova AV, Plotnikov AN, Yu K, Ornitz DM, Mohammadi M. Structural basis for fibroblast growth factor receptor 2 activation in Apert syndrome. Proc Natl Acad Sci USA. 2001;98(13):7182–7.
30. Ibrahimi OA, Zhang F, Eliseenkova AV, Itoh N, Linhardt RJ, Mohammadi M. Biochemical analysis of pathogenic ligand-dependent FGFR2 mutations suggests distinct pathophysiological mechanisms for craniofacial and limb abnormalities. Hum Mol Genet. 2004;13(19):2313–24.
31. Jabs EW, Muller U, Li X, Ma L, Luo W, Haworth IS, Klisak I, Sparkes R, Warman ML, Mulliken JB, et al. A mutation in the homeodomain of the human MSX2 gene in a family affected with autosomal dominant craniosynostosis. Cell. 1993;75(3):443–50.
32. Jabs EW, Li X, Scott AF, Meyers G, Chen W, Eccles M, Mao JI, Charnas LR, Jackson CE, Jaye M. Jackson-Weiss and Crouzon syndromes are allelic with mutations in fibroblast growth factor receptor 2. Nat Genet. 1994;8(3):275–9.
33. Kan S-h, Elanko N, Johnson D, Cornejo-Roldan L, Cook J, Reich EW, Tomkins S, Verloes A, Twigg SRF, Rannan-Eliya S, McDonald-McGinn DM, Zackai EH, Wall SA, Muenke M, Wilkie AOM. Genomic screening of fibroblast growth factor receptor 2 reveals a wide spectrum of mutations in patients with syndromic craniosynostosis. Am J Hum Genet. 2002;70(2):472–86.
34. Karczewski KJ, Francioli LC, Tiao G, Cummings BB, Alfoldi J, Wang Q, Collins RL, Laricchia KM, Ganna A, Birnbaum DP, Gauthier LD, Brand H,

Solomonson M, Watts NA, Rhodes D, Singer-Berk M, England EM, Seaby EG, Kosmicki JA, Walters RK, Tashman K, Farjoun Y, Banks E, Poterba T, Wang A, Seed C, Whiffin N, Chong JX, Samocha KE, Pierce-Hoffman E, Zappala Z, O'Donnell-Luria AH, Minikel EV, Weisburd B, Lek M, Ware JS, Vittal C, Armean IM, Bergelson L, Cibulskis K, Connolly KM, Covarrubias M, Donnelly S, Ferriera S, Gabriel S, Gentry J, Gupta N, Jeandet T, Kaplan D, Llanwarne C, Munshi R, Novod S, Petrillo N, Roazen D, Ruano-Rubio V, Saltzman A, Schleicher M, Soto J, Tibbetts K, Tolonen C, Wade G, Talkowski ME, C. Genome Aggregation Database, Neale BM, Daly MJ, MacArthur DG. The mutational constraint spectrum quantified from variation in 141,456 humans. Nature. 2020;581(7809):434–43.

35. Kim B, Shin H, Kim W, Kim H, Cho Y, Yoon H, Baek J, Woo K, Lee Y, Ryoo H. PIN1 attenuation improves midface hypoplasia in a mouse model of Apert syndrome. J Dent Res. 2020;99(2):223–32.
36. Kitadate Y, Jorg DJ, Tokue M, Maruyama A, Ichikawa R, Tsuchiya S, Segi-Nishida E, Nakagawa T, Uchida A, Kimura-Yoshida C, Mizuno S, Sugiyama F, Azami T, Ema M, Noda C, Kobayashi S, Matsuo I, Kanai Y, Nagasawa T, Sugimoto Y, Takahashi S, Simons BD, Yoshida S. Competition for mitogens regulates spermatogenic stem cell homeostasis in an open niche. Cell Stem Cell. 2019;24(1):79–92 e76.
37. Lajeunie E, Ma HW, Bonaventure J, Munnich A, Le Merrer M, Renier D. *FGFR2* mutations in Pfeiffer syndrome. Nat Genet. 1995;9(2):108.
38. Lajeunie E, Cameron R, El Ghouzzi V, de Parseval N, Journeau P, Gonzales M, Delezoide AL, Bonaventure J, Le Merrer M, Renier D. Clinical variability in patients with Apert's syndrome. J Neurosurg. 1999;90(3):443–7.
39. Lavoie H, Gagnon J, Therrien M. ERK signalling: a master regulator of cell behaviour, life and fate. Nat Rev Mol Cell Biol. 2020;21(10):607–32.
40. Lim J, Maher GJ, Turner GD, Dudka-Ruszkowska W, Taylor S, Rajpert-De Meyts E, Goriely A, Wilkie AOM. Selfish spermatogonial selection: evidence from an immunohistochemical screen in testes of elderly men. PLoS One. 2012;7(8):e42382.
41. Liu Z, Xu J, Colvin JS, Ornitz DM. Coordination of chondrogenesis and osteogenesis by fibroblast growth factor 18. Genes Dev. 2002;16(7):859–69.
42. Lumaka A, Mubungu G, Mukaba P, Mutantu P, Luyeye G, Corveleyn A, Tady BP, Lukusa Tshilobo P, Devriendt K. A novel heterozygous mutation of three consecutive nucleotides causing Apert syndrome in a Congolese family. Eur J Med Genet. 2014;57(4):169–73.
43. Luo F, Xie Y, Wang Z, Huang J, Tan Q, Sun X, Li F, Li C, Liu M, Zhang D, Xu M, Su N, Ni Z, Jiang W, Chang J, Chen H, Chen S, Xu X, Deng C, Wang Z, Du X, Chen L. Adeno-associated virus-mediated RNAi against mutant alleles attenuates abnormal calvarial phenotypes in an apert syndrome mouse model. Mol Ther Nucleic Acids. 2018;13:291–302.
44. Maher GJ, Goriely A, Wilkie AOM. Cellular evidence for selfish spermatogonial selection in aged human testes. Andrology. 2014;2(3):304–14.
45. Maher GJ, McGowan SJ, Giannoulatou E, Verrill C, Goriely A, Wilkie AOM. Visualizing the origins of selfish de novo mutations in individual seminiferous tubules of human testes. Proc Natl Acad Sci USA. 2016;113(9):2454–9.
46. Maher GJ, Ralph HK, Ding Z, Koelling N, Mlcochova H, Giannoulatou E, Dhami P, Paul DS, Stricker SH, Beck S, McVean G, Wilkie AOM, Goriely A. Selfish mutations dysregulating RAS-MAPK signaling are pervasive in aged human testes. Genome Res. 2018;28(12):1779–90.
47. Martin LA, Assif N, Gilbert M, Wijewarnasuriya D, Seandel M. Enhanced fitness of adult spermatogonial stem cells bearing a paternal age-associated FGFR2 mutation. Stem Cell Rep. 2014;3(2):219–26.
48. Martinez-Abadias N, Percival C, Aldridge K, Hill CA, Ryan T, Sirivunnabood S, Wang Y, Jabs EW, Richtsmeier JT. Beyond the closed suture in Apert syndrome mouse models: evidence of primary effects of FGFR2 signaling on facial shape at birth. Dev Dyn. 2010;239(11):3058–71.
49. Martinez-Abadias N, Holmes G, Pankratz T, Wang Y, Zhou X, Jabs EW, Richtsmeier JT. From shape to cells: mouse models reveal mechanisms altering palate development in Apert syndrome. Dis Model Mech. 2013;6(3):768–79.
50. Martinez-Abadias N, Mateu Estivill R, Sastre Tomas J, Motch Perrine S, Yoon M, Robert-Moreno A, Swoger J, Russo L, Kawasaki K, Richtsmeier J, Sharpe J. Quantification of gene expression patterns to reveal the origins of abnormal morphogenesis. elife. 2018;7:e36405.
51. Min Swe NM, Kobayashi Y, Kamimoto H, Moriyama K. Aberrantly activated Wnt/beta-catenin pathway co-receptors LRP5 and LRP6 regulate osteoblast differentiation in the developing coronal sutures of an Apert syndrome (*Fgfr2*$^{S252W/+}$) mouse model. Dev Dyn. 2021;250(3):465–76.
52. Mohammadi M, Olsen SK, Ibrahimi OA. Structural basis for fibroblast growth factor receptor activation. Cytokine Growth Factor Rev. 2005;16(2):107–37.
53. Moloney DM, Slaney SF, Oldridge M, Wall SA, Sahlin P, Stenman G, Wilkie AOM. Exclusive paternal origin of new mutations in Apert syndrome. Nat Genet. 1996;13(1):48–53.
54. Monaco AP, Neve RL, Colletti-Feener C, Bertelson CJ, Kurnit DM, Kunkel LM. Isolation of candidate cDNAs for portions of the Duchenne muscular dystrophy gene. Nature. 1986;323(6089):646–50.
55. Morita J, Nakamura M, Kobayashi Y, Deng CX, Funato N, Moriyama K. Soluble form of FGFR2 with S252W partially prevents craniosynostosis of the Apert mouse model. Dev Dyn. 2014;243(4):560–7.
56. Motch Perrine SM, Wu M, Stephens NB, Kriti D, van Bakel H, Jabs EW, Richtsmeier JT. Mandibular dysmorphology due to abnormal embryonic osteogenesis

in FGFR2-related craniosynostosis mice. Dis Model Mech. 2019;12(5)
57. Myo AC, Kobayashi Y, Niki Y, Kamimoto H, Moriyama K. Exosome-mediated small interfering RNA delivery inhibits aberrant osteoblast differentiation in Apert syndrome model mice. Arch Oral Biol. 2023;153:105753.
58. Ohbayashi N, Shibayama M, Kurotaki Y, Imanishi M, Fujimori T, Itoh N, Takada S. FGF18 is required for normal cell proliferation and differentiation during osteogenesis and chondrogenesis. Genes Dev. 2002;16(7):870–9.
59. Ohishi A, Nishimura G, Kato F, Ono H, Maruwaka K, Ago M, Suzumura H, Hirose E, Uchida Y, Fukami M, Ogata T. Mutation analysis of *FGFR1-3* in 11 Japanese patients with syndromic craniosynostoses. Am J Med Genet A. 2017;173(1):157–62.
60. Oldridge M, Lunt PW, Zackai EH, McDonald-McGinn DM, Muenke M, Moloney DM, Twigg SR, Heath JK, Howard TD, Hoganson G, Gagnon DM, Jabs EW, Wilkie AOM. Genotype-phenotype correlation for nucleotide substitutions in the IgII-IgIII linker of *FGFR2*. Hum Mol Genet. 1997;6(1):137–43.
61. Oldridge M, Zackai EH, McDonald-McGinn DM, Iseki S, Morriss-Kay GM, Twigg SR, Johnson D, Wall SA, Jiang W, Theda C, Jabs EW, Wilkie AOM. *De novo Alu*-element insertions in *FGFR2* identify a distinct pathological basis for Apert syndrome. Am J Hum Genet. 1999;64(2):446–61.
62. Ornitz DM, Itoh N. The Fibroblast Growth Factor signaling pathway. Wiley Interdiscip Rev Dev Biol. 2015;4(3):215–66.
63. Park WJ, Theda C, Maestri NE, Meyers GA, Fryburg JS, Dufresne C, Cohen MM Jr, Jabs EW. Analysis of phenotypic features and FGFR2 mutations in Apert syndrome. Am J Hum Genet. 1995;57(2):321–8.
64. Passos-Bueno MR, Sertie AL, Zatz M, Richieri-Costa A. Pfeiffer mutation in an Apert patient: how wide is the spectrum of variability due to mutations in the FGFR2 gene? Am J Med Genet. 1997;71(2):243–5.
65. Passos-Bueno MR, Sertie AL, Richieri-Costa A, Alonso LG, Zatz M, Alonso N, Brunoni D, Ribeiro SFM. Description of a new mutation and characterization of *FGFR1*, *FGFR2*, and *FGFR3* mutations among Brazilian patients with syndromic craniosynostoses. Am J Med Genet. 1998;78(3):237–41.
66. Paumard-Hernandez B, Berges-Soria J, Barroso E, Rivera-Pedroza CI, Perez-Carrizosa V, Benito-Sanz S, Lopez-Messa E, Santos F, Garcia R II, Romance A, Ballesta-Martinez JM, Lopez-Gonzalez V, Campos-Barros A, Cruz J, Guillen-Navarro E, Sanchez Del Pozo J, Lapunzina P, Garcia-Minaur S, Heath KE. Expanding the mutation spectrum in 182 Spanish probands with craniosynostosis: identification and characterization of novel *TCF12* variants. Eur J Hum Genet. 2015;23(7):907–14.
67. Pollock PM, Gartside MG, Dejeza LC, Powell MA, Mallon MA, Cancer Genome Project, Davies H, Mohammadi M, Futreal PA, Stratton MR, Trent JM, Goodfellow PJ. Frequent activating FGFR2 mutations in endometrial carcinomas parallel germline mutations associated with craniosynostosis and skeletal dysplasia syndromes. Oncogene. 2007;26(50):7158–62.
68. Preston RA, Post JC, Keats BJ, Aston CE, Ferrell RE, Priest J, Nouri N, Losken HW, Morris CA, Hurtt MR, et al. A gene for Crouzon craniofacial dysostosis maps to the long arm of chromosome 10. Nat Genet. 1994;7(2):149–53.
69. Qin J, Calabrese P, Tiemann-Boege I, Shinde DN, Yoon SR, Gelfand D, Bauer K, Arnheim N. The molecular anatomy of spontaneous germline mutations in human testes. PLoS Biol. 2007;5(9):e224.
70. Rahbari R, Wuster A, Lindsay SJ, Hardwick RJ, Alexandrov LB, Turki SA, Dominiczak A, Morris A, Porteous D, Smith B, Stratton MR, UK10K Consortium, Hurles ME. Timing, rates and spectra of human germline mutation. Nat Genet. 2016;48(2):126–33.
71. Reardon W, Winter RM, Rutland P, Pulleyn LJ, Jones BM, Malcolm S. Mutations in the fibroblast growth factor receptor 2 gene cause Crouzon syndrome. Nat Genet. 1994;8(1):98–103.
72. Risch N, Reich EW, Wishnick MM, McCarthy JG. Spontaneous mutation and parental age in humans. Am J Hum Genet. 1987;41(2):218–48.
73. Robertson SC, Meyer AN, Hart KC, Galvin BD, Webster MK, Donoghue DJ. Activating mutations in the extracellular domain of the fibroblast growth factor receptor 2 function by disruption of the disulfide bond in the third immunoglobulin-like domain. Proc Natl Acad Sci USA. 1998;95(8):4567–72.
74. Rommens JM, Iannuzzi MC, Kerem B, Drumm ML, Melmer G, Dean M, Rozmahel R, Cole JL, Kennedy D, Hidaka N, et al. Identification of the cystic fibrosis gene: chromosome walking and jumping. Science. 1989;245(4922):1059–65.
75. Roscioli T, Elakis G, Cox TC, Moon DJ, Venselaar H, Turner AM, Le T, Hackett E, Haan E, Colley A, Mowat D, Worgan L, Kirk EP, Sachdev R, Thompson E, Gabbett M, McGaughran J, Gibson K, Gattas M, Freckmann ML, Dixon J, Hoefsloot L, Field M, Hackett A, Kamien B, Edwards M, Ades LC, Collins FA, Wilson MJ, Savarirayan R, Tan TY, Amor DJ, McGillivray G, White SM, Glass IA, David DJ, Anderson PJ, Gianoutsos M, Buckley MF. Genotype and clinical care correlations in craniosynostosis: findings from a cohort of 630 Australian and New Zealand patients. Am J Med Genet C Semin Med Genet. 2013;163C(4):259–70.
76. Rutland P, Pulleyn LJ, Reardon W, Baraitser M, Hayward R, Jones B, Malcolm S, Winter RM, Oldridge M, Slaney SF, Poole MD, Wilkie AOM. Identical mutations in the *FGFR2* gene cause both Pfeiffer and Crouzon syndrome phenotypes. Nat Genet. 1995;9(2):173–6.
77. Schuller AC, Ahmed Z, Ladbury JE. Extracellular point mutations in FGFR2 result in elevated ERK1/2 activation and perturbation of neuronal differentiation. Biochem J. 2008;410(1):205–11.

78. Shiang R, Thompson LM, Zhu YZ, Church DM, Fielder TJ, Bocian M, Winokur ST, Wasmuth JJ. Mutations in the transmembrane domain of FGFR3 cause the most common genetic form of dwarfism, achondroplasia. Cell. 1994;78(2):335–42.
79. Shin HR, Bae HS, Kim BS, Yoon HI, Cho YD, Kim WJ, Choi KY, Lee YS, Woo KM, Baek JH, Ryoo HM. PIN1 is a new therapeutic target of craniosynostosis. Hum Mol Genet. 2018;27(22):3827–39.
80. Shin HR, Kim BS, Kim HJ, Yoon H, Kim WJ, Choi JY, Ryoo HM. Excessive osteoclast activation by osteoblast paracrine factor RANKL is a major cause of the abnormal long bone phenotype in Apert syndrome model mice. J Cell Physiol. 2022;237(4):2155–68.
81. Shukla V, Coumoul X, Wang RH, Kim HS, Deng CX. RNA interference and inhibition of MEK-ERK signaling prevent abnormal skeletal phenotypes in a mouse model of craniosynostosis. Nat Genet. 2007;39(9):1145–50.
82. Tonne E, Due-Tonnessen BJ, Mero IL, Wiig US, Kulseth MA, Vigeland MD, Sheng Y, von der Lippe C, Tveten K, Meling TR, Helseth E, Heimdal KR. Benefits of clinical criteria and high-throughput sequencing for diagnosing children with syndromic craniosynostosis. Eur J Hum Genet. 2021;29(6):920–9.
83. Topa A, Rohlin A, Fehr A, Lovmar L, Stenman G, Tarnow P, Maltese G, Bhatti-Softeland M, Kolby L. The value of genome-wide analysis in craniosynostosis. Front Genet. 2023;14:1322462.
84. Tsai FJ, Tsai CH, Peng CT, Lin SP, Hwu WL, Wang TR, Lee CC, Wu JY. Molecular diagnosis of Apert syndrome in Chinese patients. Acta Paediatr Taiwan. 1999;40(1):31–3.
85. Vortkamp A, Gessler M, Grzeschik KH. GLI3 zinc-finger gene interrupted by translocations in Greig syndrome families. Nature. 1991;352(6335):539–40.
86. Wang Y, Xiao R, Yang F, Karim BO, Iacovelli AJ, Cai J, Lerner CP, Richtsmeier JT, Leszl JM, Hill CA, Yu K, Ornitz DM, Elisseeff J, Huso DL, Jabs EW. Abnormalities in cartilage and bone development in the Apert syndrome FGFR2$^{+/S252W}$ mouse. Development. 2005;132(15):3537–48.
87. Wang Y, Sun M, Uhlhorn VL, Zhou X, Peter I, Martinez-Abadias N, Hill CA, Percival CJ, Richtsmeier JT, Huso DL, Jabs EW. Activation of p38 MAPK pathway in the skull abnormalities of Apert syndrome *Fgfr2*$^{+P253R}$ mice. BMC Dev Biol. 2010;10:22.
88. Wilkie AOM. Bad bones, absent smell, selfish testes: the pleiotropic consequences of human FGF receptor mutations. Cytokine Growth Factor Rev. 2005;16(2):187–203.
89. Wilkie AOM. Cancer drugs to treat birth defects. Nat Genet. 2007;39(9):1057–9.
90. Wilkie AOM, Goriely A. Gonadal mosaicism and non-invasive prenatal diagnosis for 'reassurance' in sporadic paternal age effect (PAE) disorders. Prenat Diagn. 2017;37(9):946–8.
91. Wilkie AOM, Morriss-Kay GM, Jones EY, Heath JK. Functions of fibroblast growth factors and their receptors. Curr Biol. 1995;5(5):500–7.
92. Wilkie AOM, Slaney SF, Oldridge M, Poole MD, Ashworth GJ, Hockley AD, Hayward RD, David DJ, Pulleyn LJ, Rutland P, et al. Apert syndrome results from localized mutations of *FGFR2* and is allelic with Crouzon syndrome. Nat Genet. 1995b;9(2):165–72.
93. Wilkie AOM, Patey SJ, Kan SH, van den Ouweland AMW, Hamel BCJ. FGFs, their receptors, and human limb malformations: clinical and molecular correlations. Am J Med Genet. 2002;112(3):266–78.
94. Yang F, Whelan EC, Guan X, Deng B, Wang S, Sun J, Avarbock MR, Wu X, Brinster RL. FGF9 promotes mouse spermatogonial stem cell proliferation mediated by p38 MAPK signalling. Cell Prolif. 2021;54(1):e12933.
95. Yin L, Du X, Li C, Xu X, Chen Z, Su N, Zhao L, Qi H, Li F, Xue J, Yang J, Jin M, Deng C, Chen L. A Pro253Arg mutation in fibroblast growth factor receptor 2 (Fgfr2) causes skeleton malformation mimicking human Apert syndrome by affecting both chondrogenesis and osteogenesis. Bone. 2008;42(4):631–43.
96. Yoon SR, Qin J, Glaser RL, Jabs EW, Wexler NS, Sokol R, Arnheim N, Calabrese P. The ups and downs of mutation frequencies during aging can account for the Apert syndrome paternal age effect. PLoS Genet. 2009;5(7):e1000558.
97. Yoon WJ, Cho YD, Kim WJ, Bae HS, Islam R, Woo KM, Baek JH, Bae SC, Ryoo HM. Prolyl isomerase Pin1-mediated conformational change and subnuclear focal accumulation of Runx2 are crucial for fibroblast growth factor 2 (FGF2)-induced osteoblast differentiation. J Biol Chem. 2014;289(13):8828–38.
98. Yu K, Ornitz DM. Uncoupling fibroblast growth factor receptor 2 ligand binding specificity leads to Apert syndrome-like phenotypes. Proc Natl Acad Sci USA. 2001;98(7):3641–3.
99. Zhang J, Li J, Saucier JB, Feng Y, Jiang Y, Sinson J, McCombs AK, Schmitt ES, Peacock S, Chen S, Dai H, Ge X, Wang G, Shaw CA, Mei H, Breman A, Xia F, Yang Y, Purgason A, Pourpak A, Chen Z, Wang X, Wang Y, Kulkarni S, Choy KW, Wapner RJ, Van den Veyver IB, Beaudet A, Parmar S, Wong LJ, Eng CM. Non-invasive prenatal sequencing for multiple Mendelian monogenic disorders using circulating cell-free fetal DNA. Nat Med. 2019;25(3):439–47.

Clinical Genetic Aspects

5

Nancy Mizue Kokitsu-Nakata,
Luiza do Amaral Virmond,
and Henrique Regonaschi Serigatto

Introduction

Cranial abnormalities have been known since antiquity, first described by Hippocrates and Galen. In 1851, pathologist Rudolf Virchow was the first to associate the abnormal shape of the skull with premature fusion of the cranial sutures [28]. Posteriorly, in 1906, French physician Eugene Apert identified and documented nine cases with features of acrocephaly and syndactyly in the limbs, naming the condition acrocephalosyndactyly, later recognized as Apert syndrome [3].

There are six genes commonly associated with craniosynostosis: *FGFR2*, *FGFR3*, *TWIST1*, *EFNB1*, *TCF12*, and *ERF*. Variants in *FGFR2*, *FGFR3*, *TWIST1*, and *EFNB1* genes are primarily associated with specific craniofacial syndromes: *FGFR2* correlates with Apert, Crouzon, and Pfeiffer syndromes; *FGFR3* with Muenke syndrome and Crouzon with acanthosis nigricans; *TWIST1* with Saethre-Chotzen syndrome; and *EFNB1* with craniofrontonasal syndrome. The molecular basis of these conditions has allowed extensive documentation of genotype–phenotype correlations [51, 80, 85].

Apert syndrome is a rare genetic condition characterized by craniofacial anomalies (see Fig. 5.1) including craniosynostosis, flat facies, horizontal supraorbital groove, shallow orbits, hypertelorism, strabismus, down-slanting palpebral fissures, maxillary hypoplasia, narrow palate with median groove, cleft palate, and/or bifid uvula [15, 62]. Other organs may be affected, including the brain, heart, trachea, and genitourinary system. Additional skeletal abnormalities are common, and skin involvement may include acneiform lesions [36]. Other features include intellectual disability, obstructive sleep apnea, and recurrent ear infections [12].

Although Apert syndrome is an autosomal dominant condition, most cases occur sporadically and are associated with advanced paternal age, with 98% of cases resulting from de novo mutations [22]. Wilkie et al. [86] identified two recurrent variants (p.Ser252Trp and p.Pro253Arg) in the *FGFR2* (fibroblast growth factor receptor 2) gene, located on chromosome 10q, as causing the syndrome in all patients studied. Subsequent research identified two other de novo insertion variants in the same gene, transmitted by the paternal chromosome, reinforcing the association between advanced paternal age and increased risk for Apert syndrome [34, 61]. The wide phenotypic variability observed among patients suggests the influence of environmental or supplemental genetic factors [9, 10].

This chapter presents a detailed analysis of the craniofacial and extra-craniofacial findings of

N. M. Kokitsu-Nakata (✉) · L. do Amaral Virmond · H. R. Serigatto
Department of Clinical Genetics, Hospital for Rehabilitation of Craniofacial Anomalies, University of São Paulo, Bauru, São Paulo, Brazil
e-mail: nancykn@usp.br

J. G. Meara et al. (eds.), *Apert Syndrome*, https://doi.org/10.1007/978-3-032-12551-4_5

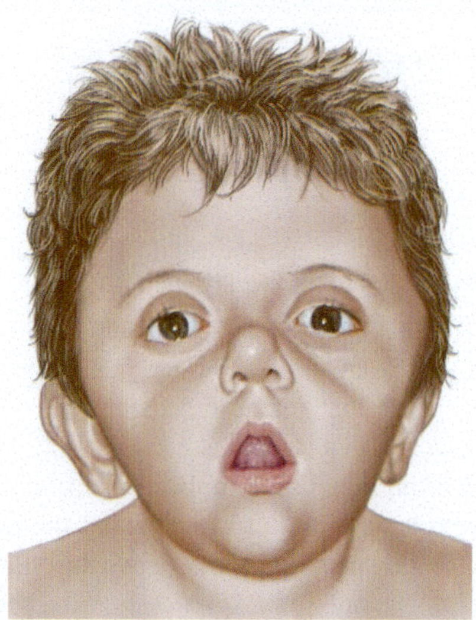
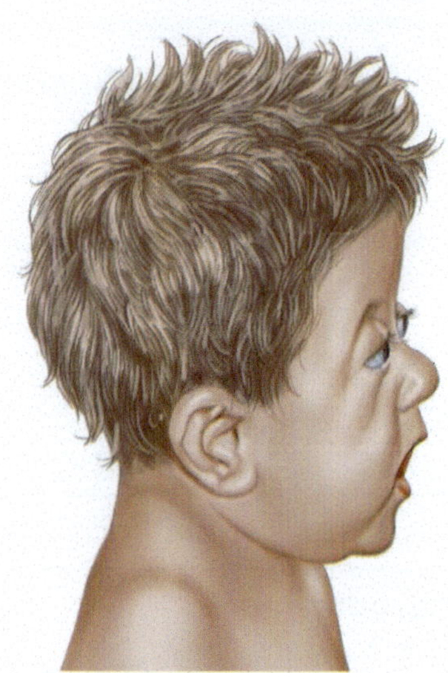

Fig. 5.1 Illustration of a boy with Apert syndrome showing the typical craniofacial appearance. Note brachycephaly, widely spaced eyes, shallow orbits, proptosis, down-slanting palpebral fissures, flat face, and low-set ears

Apert syndrome, highlighting the clinical variability widely documented in the literature and comparing it with observations made at our institution. This approach allows us to assess the spectrum and diversity of the phenotypic manifestations of the syndrome, contributing to a more precise understanding of the clinical and diagnostic aspects of Apert syndrome.

Birth Prevalence of Craniosynostosis and Apert Syndrome

Craniosynostosis is defined as the premature closure of one or more cranial sutures. Its prevalence is variable, depending on the population studied, and ranges from 3 to 8 per 10,000 live births [24, 59, 83, 85], with estimates suggesting that over 80,000 children are born with craniosynostosis globally each year [72]. Clinically, craniosynostosis can be classified as (a) non-syndromic, when it is an isolated defect, or (b) syndromic, when associated with multiple congenital anomalies. Non-syndromic craniosynostosis, usually characterized by the involvement of a single suture, represents 65–90% of cases [24, 29, 85]. Syndromic craniosynostoses are rare, most of them have known genetic causes, and are part of the phenotype of several conditions, including the most common: Apert, Crouzon, Pfeiffer, Muenke, and Saethre-Chotzen syndromes [24, 70, 85]. Apert syndrome is mainly characterized by bicoronal craniosynostosis and syndactyly of the hands and feet. The birth prevalence of Apert syndrome is estimated to be approximately 13–15 per 1,000,000 live births (1 in 65,000), accounting for nearly 4.5% of all craniosynostosis cases [22, 25, 86].

Sex Ratio

The sex ratio of individuals with craniosynostosis depends on the affected suture and, therefore, presents variability. Overall, there is a predilection toward male sex in single suture craniosynostosis, with a ratio of 2.5:1 [24]. For sagittal craniosynostosis, the most common single suture type of craniosynostosis, there is a male predilection with a ratio of 3:1. Additionally, male sex has been considered a risk factor for metopic and lambdoid craniosynostosis. However, when analyzing coronal craniosynostosis, there is a predilection for females. In cases of multiple suture craniosynostosis, sex is not considered a risk factor, although a few studies have shown a male predilection [8, 24, 29, 36, 52, 73].

Regarding Apert syndrome, there is a slight predilection for females, with a ratio of 1:2, which is not surprising considering that coronal craniosynostosis is more common in females [24].

Parental Age Effect in Apert Syndrome

The effects of parental age, mainly paternal age, on Apert syndrome have been suggested and observed over the last few decades [31, 34, 56]. De novo variants associated with Apert syndrome are exclusively of paternal origin [56]. Advanced parental age has been noted in over 20% of cases, with both paternal and maternal ages exceeding 35 years [79]. The same study showed that paternal age was over 35 years in almost half of the cases (46.9%), further corroborating the association of new variants from paternal origin in Apert syndrome rather than maternal [56, 79]. Most, if not all, cases of Apert syndrome arise from paternal variants. Therefore, the effect of parental age is largely attributable to paternal age [56].

Advanced paternal age is associated primarily with an increased frequency of variants in sperm, among other contributing factors [34]. Furthermore, fathers of children with Apert syndrome have been found to present a higher frequency of variants in sperm compared with a control group, even at younger ages [34]. Moreover, the variant frequency and the number of different variants at advanced ages are not observed in white blood cells, suggesting that age effects are cell-type specific. Detailed information about the mechanisms responsible for these observations and paternal-age effects are presented in Chap. 4.

Clinical Diagnosis

Apert syndrome is a well-known condition characterized by a recognizable pattern of anomalies (see Fig. 5.2). The hallmark of this condition is craniosynostosis associated with syndactyly of the hands and feet, an unusual combination of anomalies rarely seen in other syndromes [36, 41]. Therefore, experienced clinicians can promptly diagnose Apert syndrome after a physical examination. The clinical findings described here are based on our experience, supplemented with relevant data from the literature.

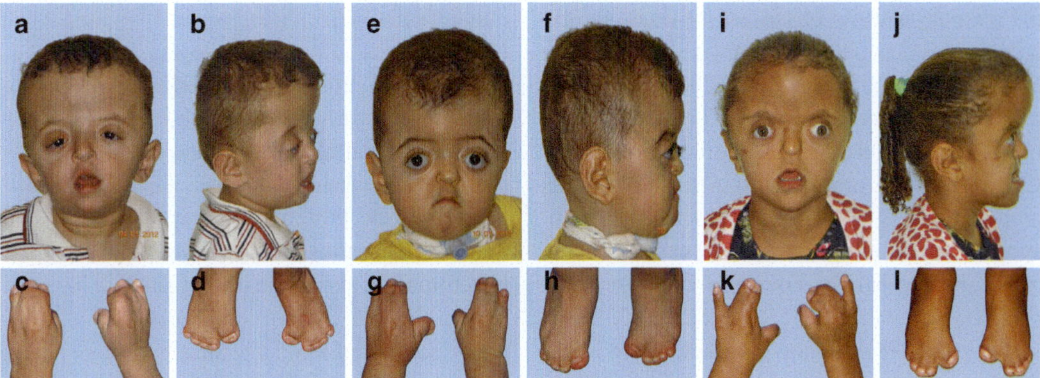

Fig. 5.2 Clinical aspects of patients with typical Apert syndrome phenotype. (**a–d**) Boy with Apert syndrome at age 1 year and 10 months. (**e–h**) Boy with Apert syndrome at age 1 year and 3 months. (**i–l**) Girl with Apert syndrome at age 3 years. Note that all three cases share common craniofacial features (brachycephaly, turricephaly, flat face, midface hypoplasia, proptosis, downslanting palpebral fissures, strabismus, and low-set ears) and discordant hands–feet syndactyly; (**c**) type II hands and (**d**) type I feet; (**g**) type II hands and (**h**) type III feet; (**k**) type I hands and (**l**) type II feet

Craniofacial Features

Skull

One of the main clinical features of Apert syndrome is the premature fusion of the cranial sutures, mainly the coronal. This early fusion prevents proper growth of the skull, resulting in significant craniofacial deformity. The premature closure of the coronal sutures compromises anterior, lateral, and posterior expansion of the skull, resulting in abnormal growth toward other directions. This abnormal development results in a cranial configuration known as brachycephaly, which is typically described by a steep, broad, and flat forehead. The skull base is also affected by growth restriction, leading to alterations in craniofacial proportion and symmetry. Craniosynostosis in Apert syndrome not only affects the aesthetics of the skull, but may also have functional implications, such as increased intracranial pressure, which can compromise neurological development. From a molecular point of view, this condition is associated with variants in the *FGFR2* gene, which affect the regulation of bone development and fusion of the cranial sutures.

The major finding in Apert syndrome is bicoronal craniosynostosis. However, unilateral coronal craniosynostosis or closure of other sutures can also be observed, although it is rare for the coronal sutures to remain unaffected [32, 50, 68].

Although craniosynostosis is a main finding of this condition, de Ângelis Ramos et al. [27] reported a female with Apert syndrome, confirmed by genetic testing, without craniosynostosis. To date, there are few cases without craniosynostosis reported in the literature [23, 50, 68].

Long-term follow-up is essential in these cases, due to the risk of additional bone fusions, which may require surgical intervention. Continuous monitoring allows early detection of new fusions and assessment of the progression of the condition, which is essential for making appropriate therapeutic decisions, thus ensuring effective management and minimizing complications [27].

Ocular

Ocular features are very important in Apert syndrome since most of them are secondary to craniosynostosis. One of the first ocular findings that clinicians should be aware of is proptosis, defined as the protrusion of the eye beyond the plane of the face, resulting in a protuberant ocular globe. Proptosis can range from mild to severe and is usually present in Apert syndrome, observed in 90% of cases [15, 39]. In some cases, proptosis is mild and may be underdiagnosed. The protrusion of the eye globe can lead to another clinical finding known as lagophthalmos, which is the inability to completely close the eyelids while awake or asleep. This often causes corneal and/or conjunctival irritation due to constant eye exposure and dryness. Thus, ophthalmological evaluation is essential for patients with Apert syndrome.

The eyes in Apert syndrome are usually widely spaced, reported in nearly all cases. Measurements of inner and outer canthi, as well as interpupillary distances should be taken to properly assess this feature. The palpebral fissures are down-slanted. Strabismus is present in 50% of cases, which may lead to amblyopia. Shallow orbits with an underdeveloped supraorbital ridge are also frequently observed, in approximately 90% of cases [15, 49, 62].

Nasal

The nose in Apert syndrome is characterized by a short nose with reduced length and a markedly depressed nasal bridge. The nasal tip is usually described as round or bulbous [15]. Anteverted nares may be present in some cases. Choanal atresia or stenosis is a common feature in Apert syndrome and should be investigated.

Oral

The mouth of patients with Apert syndrome is described as having a trapezoidal shape with hypotonic lips. This configuration results from midface hypoplasia, which tends to elevate the hypotonic upper lip [15, 53]. The palate is typically arched and narrow. Cleft palate is common and varies in presentation, ranging from submucous cleft to a complete cleft palate (see Fig. 5.3)

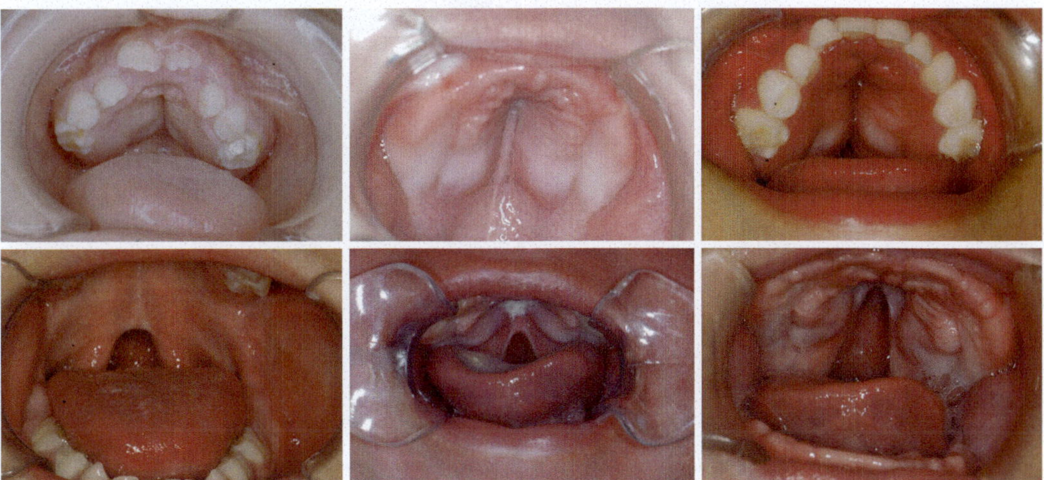

Fig. 5.3 Clinical variability of the palate. Note narrow and highly arched palate, bifid uvula, cleft soft palate, and complete cleft palate

[87]. The uvula can be notched or bifid and may represent an underdiagnosed submucous cleft when associated with other palatal abnormalities. Delayed tooth eruption, crowded teeth, tooth agenesis, anterior open bite, mandibular overjet, and malocclusion are also common in Apert syndrome [2, 15, 53].

Maxillofacial

The face of patients with Apert syndrome is very characteristic and can be recognized during physical examinations. The forehead is broad and prominent, the facial profile is flat, and there is relative mandibular prognathism. Marked midface hypoplasia, resulting from zygomatic and maxillary anomalies, gives the clinical impression that the mandible is projected. This becomes more pronounced over time as the facial bones grow [2, 15].

Auricular

The ears in Apert syndrome generally have no remarkable anomalies. They are typically described as low-set, large, and mildly dysplastic, without major anomalies. The occurrence of low-set and posteriorly rotated ears in Apert syndrome may be related to the degree of skull involvement as secondary defects. Prominent ears are observed in some cases and may also be secondary to skull deformities. Ear tags have been rarely described in Apert syndrome [15]. Middle ear abnormalities are frequently reported, with the most common being chronic middle ear effusion, recurrent otitis media, and fused or malformed ossicles [1]. Inner ear anomalies are also present, including abnormalities of the semicircular canals, cochlear hypoplasia, enlargement of the vestibule, and a high-riding jugular bulb [1, 38, 91]. The protrusion or dehiscence of the jugular in the middle ear (see Fig. 5.4) should be mentioned as an awareness for otological surgeons when performing procedures such as placement of ventilation tubes [4].

Despite the absence of visible anomalies in the external ears, audiological outcomes in Apert syndrome remain a concern and should be further evaluated. Hearing loss is commonly associated with several syndromes involving craniosynostosis. In Apert syndrome, conductive hearing loss is the most frequent type, reported in approximately 80% of cases. Mixed or sensorineural hearing loss can also occur, though it is uncommon [1].

Hands and Feet

Another distinctive feature of the Apert syndrome is the presence of syndactyly, which can manifest in two ways: cutaneous syndactyly, characterized by an anomalous fusion of the skin between the

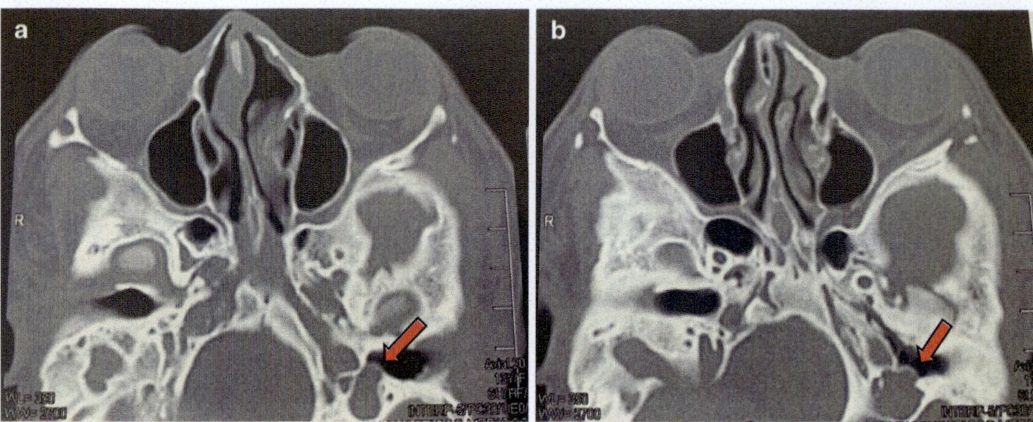

Fig. 5.4 Axial computed tomography (CT) scan (**a**, **b**) showing the jugular vein protruding in the temporal bone (red arrows) in a patient with Apert syndrome

digits/toes, and bony syndactyly, which involves the fusion of adjacent bones of the fingers. These alterations affect both hands and feet, with variations in severity and functional impact, affecting the mobility of the fingers and often requiring surgical intervention to improve both function and aesthetics. In addition to syndactyly, mild postaxial polydactyly was identified in approximately 7% of the cases. Although this pattern is uncommon, it cannot be considered rare [18].

Besides the involvement of the phalanges in syndactyly, progressive fusions of metacarpals/metatarsals, carpal bones, particularly the capitate and hamate, and the tarsal bones have been documented. The latter is associated with functional complications due to decreased mobility of the feet and ankle [18].

Several classification systems have been proposed to categorize the anomalies in the hands and feet of individuals with Apert syndrome, based on radiographic examinations, a combination of clinical and radiographic characteristics, or anatomical criteria [6, 13, 81].

According to Cohen Jr. and Kreiborg [18], complex syndactyly of the hands and feet in Apert syndrome varies considerably and has been classified into three distinct groups (see Figs. 5.5 and 5.6).

This classification system facilitates the identification of the severity and pattern of fusion between the digits and is essential for planning surgical and therapeutic interventions. The variability observed in syndactyly (see Fig. 5.7) reflects the need for individualized therapeutic approaches to optimize hand function and aesthetic results.

Growth

A child's growth is typically evaluated through a series of measurements of weight, length/height, and head size over time. Various factors—physical, social, or emotional—can influence growth [64]. Literature provides limited data on growth in individuals with Apert syndrome. In general, at birth, weight and length are within what is expected for gestational age; however, it has been pointed out by Cohen Jr. and Kreiborg [19] that due to the presence of megalencephaly and turribrachycephaly, they may present with head circumference measurements above the 50th percentile. Regarding nutritional aspects and weight gain, the craniofacial and orofacial anatomy observed in individuals with Apert syndrome (see Chap. 3) may contribute to difficulties in feeding, especially in the first years of life [64]. In addition, cognitive impairment may also be a risk factor for these difficulties [64].

In terms of height, deceleration of linear growth during childhood and adolescence has been observed in some individuals [19, 64]. Additionally, certain skeletal anomalies, such as those affecting the vertebrae and limbs, which

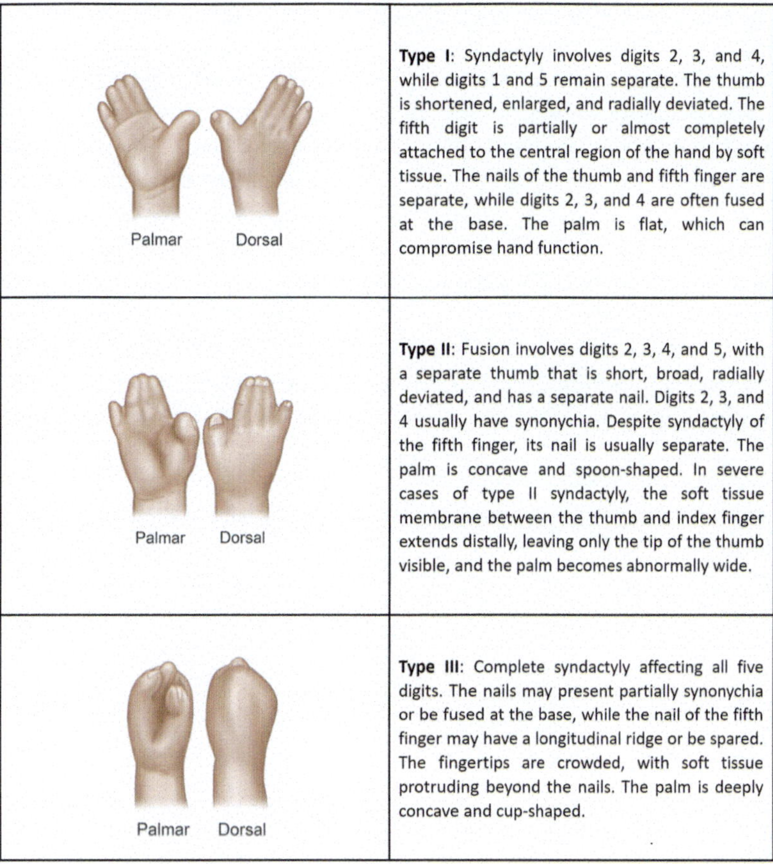

Palmar Dorsal	**Type I**: Syndactyly involves digits 2, 3, and 4, while digits 1 and 5 remain separate. The thumb is shortened, enlarged, and radially deviated. The fifth digit is partially or almost completely attached to the central region of the hand by soft tissue. The nails of the thumb and fifth finger are separate, while digits 2, 3, and 4 are often fused at the base. The palm is flat, which can compromise hand function.
Palmar Dorsal	**Type II**: Fusion involves digits 2, 3, 4, and 5, with a separate thumb that is short, broad, radially deviated, and has a separate nail. Digits 2, 3, and 4 usually have synonychia. Despite syndactyly of the fifth finger, its nail is usually separate. The palm is concave and spoon-shaped. In severe cases of type II syndactyly, the soft tissue membrane between the thumb and index finger extends distally, leaving only the tip of the thumb visible, and the palm becomes abnormally wide.
Palmar Dorsal	**Type III**: Complete syndactyly affecting all five digits. The nails may present partially synonychia or be fused at the base, while the nail of the fifth finger may have a longitudinal ridge or be spared. The fingertips are crowded, with soft tissue protruding beyond the nails. The palm is deeply concave and cup-shaped.

Fig. 5.5 Classification of types of syndactyly in the hands. (Adapted from [18])

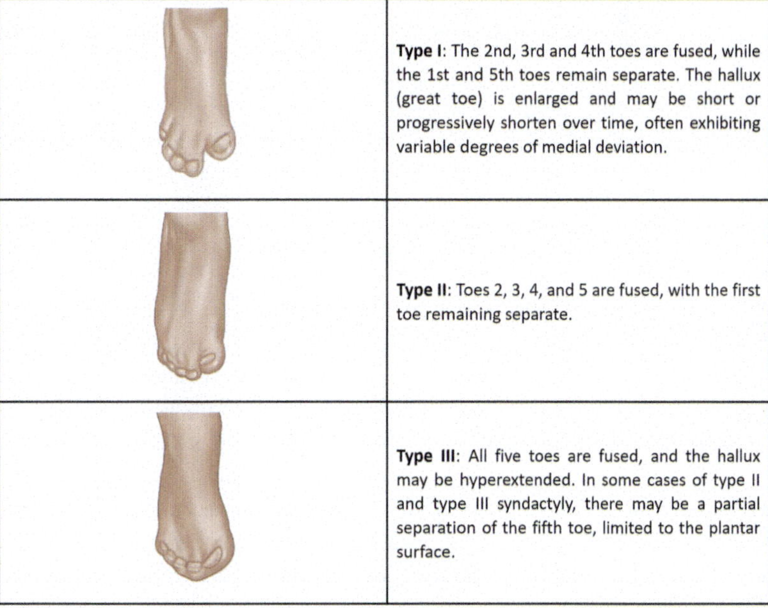

	Type I: The 2nd, 3rd and 4th toes are fused, while the 1st and 5th toes remain separate. The hallux (great toe) is enlarged and may be short or progressively shorten over time, often exhibiting variable degrees of medial deviation.
	Type II: Toes 2, 3, 4, and 5 are fused, with the first toe remaining separate.
	Type III: All five toes are fused, and the hallux may be hyperextended. In some cases of type II and type III syndactyly, there may be a partial separation of the fifth toe, limited to the plantar surface.

Fig. 5.6 Classification of types of syndactyly in the feet. (Adapted from [18])

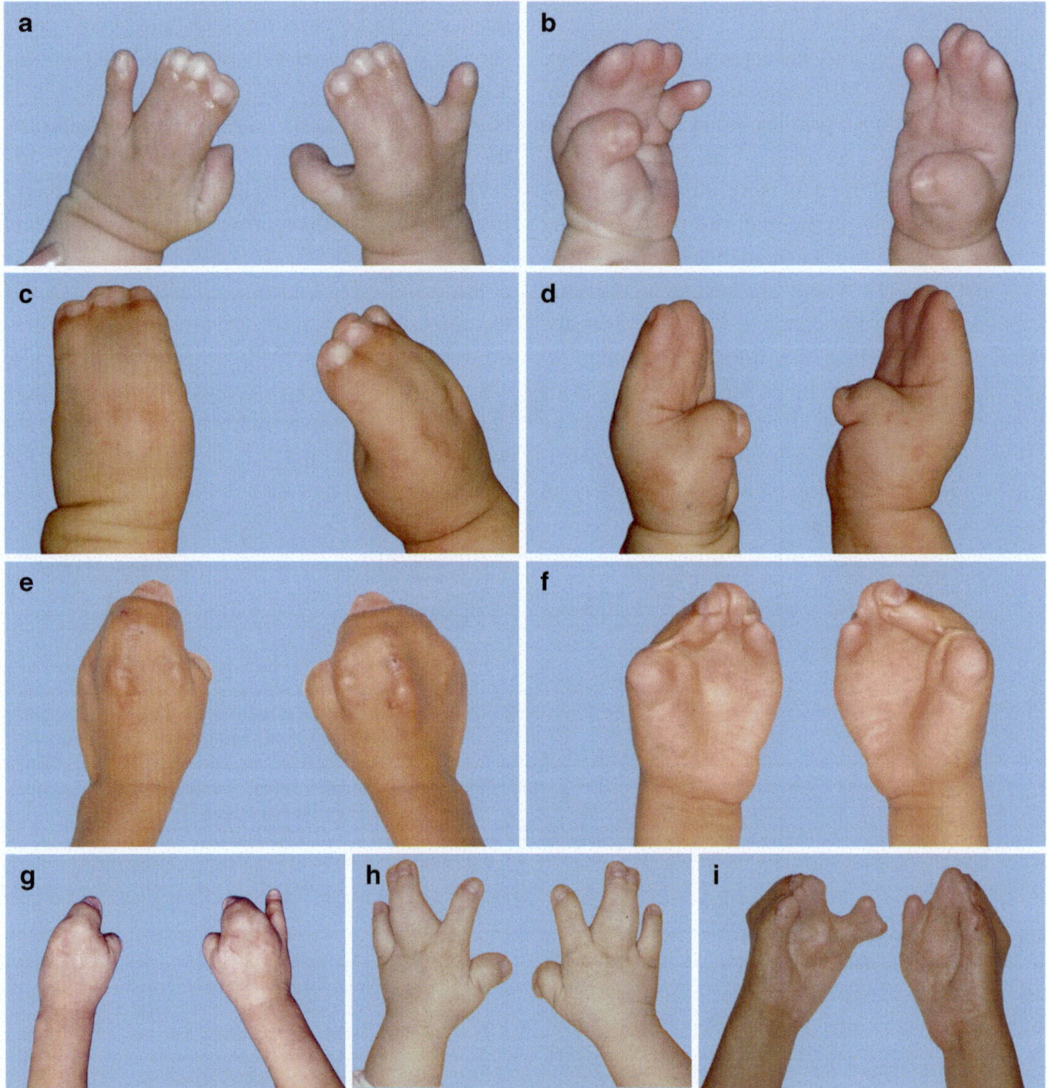

Fig. 5.7 Variability of hand syndactyly. (**a**, **b**) Type I syndactyly. (**c**, **d**) Type II syndactyly. (**e**, **f**) Type III syndactyly. (**g**, **i**) Note atypical hand syndactyly

will be discussed later in this section, may impact final height and posture [21, 48].

Central Nervous System

Several central nervous system (CNS) anomalies have been reported in individuals with Apert syndrome. These anomalies can be classified as either primary or secondary, with the latter being considered a consequence of cranial deformities caused by craniosynostosis [20, 57, 67, 77].

Among the primary CNS anomalies, the most frequently observed is the non-progressive ventriculomegaly, which occurs in 60–76% of cases [66, 67]. Noetzel et al. (1985) suggested that this condition presents a characteristic radiological appearance (see Fig. 5.8), where ventricular enlargement is limited to the lateral ventricles, specifically in the posterior horns. To date, the

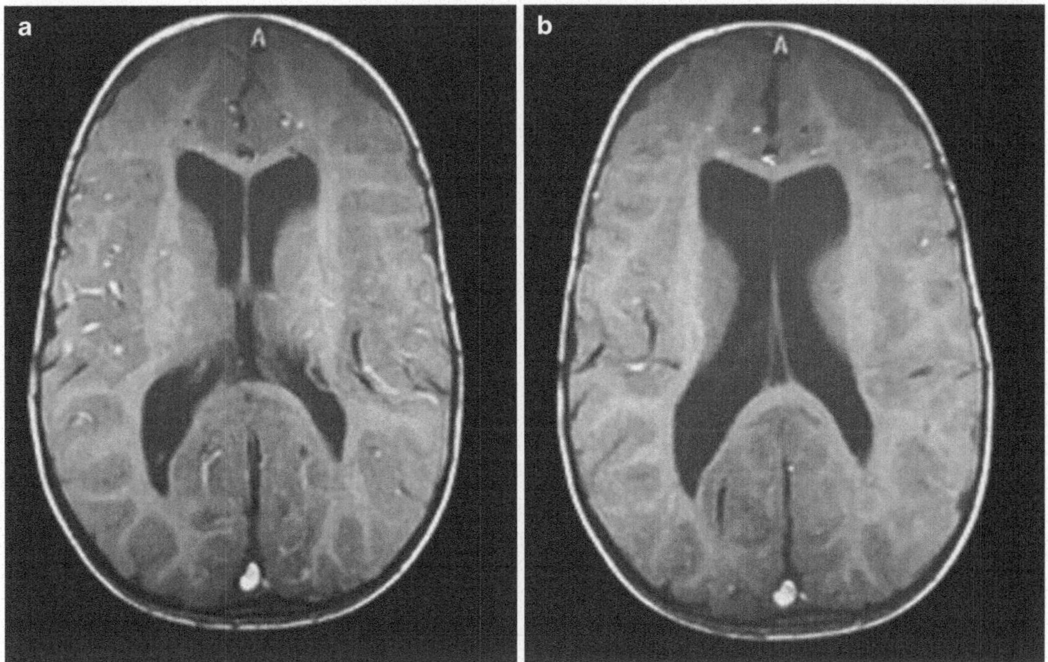

Fig. 5.8 Axial brain magnetic resonance imaging (MRI) (**a**, **b**) showing ventriculomegaly in a patient with Apert syndrome

exact cause of this ventriculomegaly remains debatable. Most believe it to be secondary to a CNS anomaly, although it is also thought to possibly represent a compensated hydrocephalic state [9, 10, 77].

It is critical to distinguish between nonprogressive and progressive ventriculomegaly because the latter may be a sign of hydrocephalus, which requires specific therapeutic interventions. In Apert syndrome, hydrocephalus is less common than in other syndromic craniosynostosis, such as Crouzon and Pfeiffer syndromes [20, 77], but it can still occur in approximately 10% of cases [66]. Munarriz et al. [57] observed in their cohort, where skull magnetic resonance imaging (MRI) scans of individuals with Apert syndrome were evaluated, that most of those who developed hydrocephalus had already undergone cranial vault remodeling surgeries. There are some hypotheses regarding the development of hydrocephalus in these individuals, ranging from anomalies in brain development to venous anomalies or compression [20, 67].

Other CNS anomalies observed include midline development defects [20, 77]. Such anomalies may involve corpus callosum (hypoplasia and agenesis), found in 11% of cases, and septum pellucidum (mainly absence), observed in 13% (see Fig. 5.9). The concurrent involvement of these two structures is frequent, likely due to their common embryonic origin [9, 10, 20, 77]. Limbic system abnormalities, anomalies of the olfactory bulb, and septo-optic dysplasia spectrum have also been described in patients with Apert syndrome. Despite being anomalies found in other clinical conditions [20], they are found with considerable frequency in individuals with Apert syndrome [9, 10, 20, 77]. Other primary anomalies described in individuals with Apert syndrome are related to cortical development, such as polymicrogyria, microgyria, and pachygyria [20].

Yeh et al. [90] conducted a study analyzing the key variant associated with Apert syndrome (p.Ser252Trp), revealing that this variant activates novel signaling pathways that regulate gene

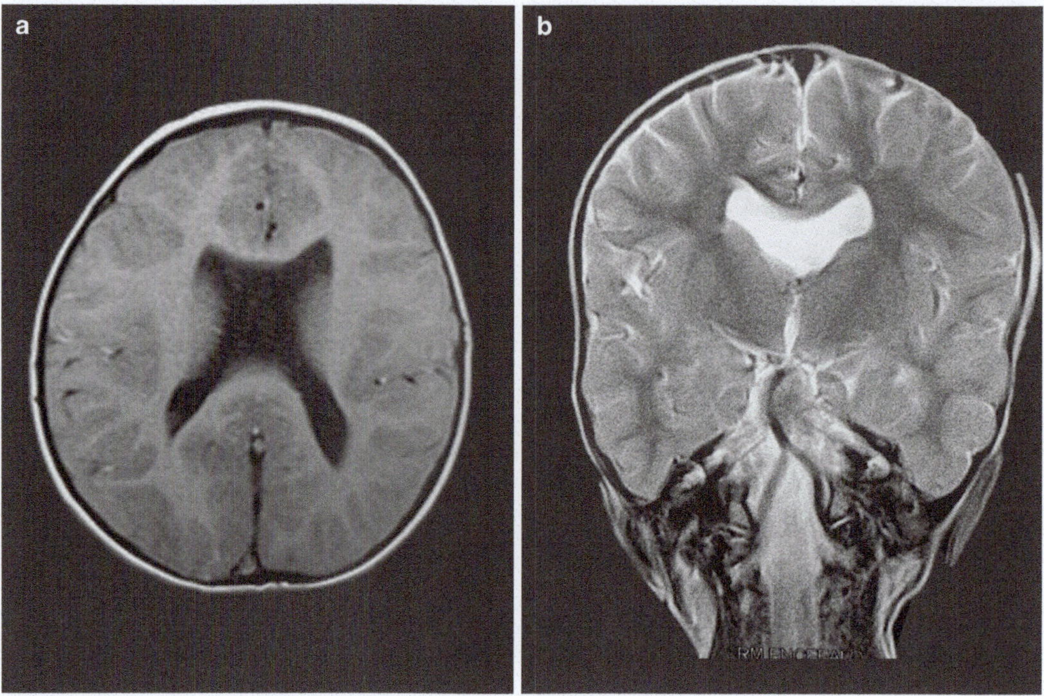

Fig. 5.9 Axial (**a**) and coronal (**b**) brain MRI demonstrating absent septum pellucidum in a patient with Apert syndrome

expression related to CNS development. These results provide evidence for the increased prevalence of CNS anomalies in Apert syndrome compared with other allelic disorders, such as Crouzon syndrome.

Of note, Apert syndrome was previously believed to be closely associated with significant cognitive impairment. However, with advancements in the follow-up and management of these cases, it has been observed that although it is more frequent when compared to other syndromic craniosynostoses, many individuals do not exhibit such impairment [16, 20]. Cognitive deficits in Apert syndrome were once thought to be directly associated with the presence of primary CNS anomalies. However, this correlation is not universal, as the presence of CNS anomalies without corresponding cognitive impairment has been reported [33]. Cognitive development is a multifaceted process influenced by environmental, socioeconomic, and familial factors, as well as genetic and physical aspects, that remains incompletely understood. Further research is necessary to elucidate these correlations.

Among secondary CNS anomalies, Arnold-Chiari malformation type I (characterized by chronic tonsillar herniation) is the most prevalent, observed in 2% of cases. However, its incidence is significantly lower when compared with Crouzon syndrome. This difference can be attributed to the early fusion of the lambdoid sutures, which occurs much earlier in Crouzon syndrome compared with Apert syndrome, resulting in a reduced posterior fossa and consequently limited cerebellar growth [9, 10, 20, 77]. Still, regarding secondary anomalies, encephaloceles are less frequent, although they have been reported in some individuals with Apert syndrome, including cases of frontal, occipital, and temporal encephaloceles. The description of frontal encephalocele is the most frequent in Apert syndrome; however, it has been debated whether it can be considered a “true” encephalocele, as it is secondary to the shortening of the anterior cranial fossa and the presence of a large midline calvarial defect [20].

Skeletal

Skeletal involvement in Apert syndrome can be extensive, ranging from spinal anomalies, mainly cervical, to anomalies of long bones such as the humerus and radius. These findings are underexplored in the literature and may be far more common than reported, as they are frequently not thoroughly investigated [21, 58].

A phenomenon of progressive synostosis (bone fusion) has been reported in Apert syndrome, potentially involving multiple skeletal regions, including progressive craniosynostosis, synchondrosis, and hand, feet, and vertebral fusions [5, 9, 10, 48, 78]. This phenomenon is linked to progressive morphological abnormalities in bone structure, which may lead, with aging, to mobility impairments, contributing to functional decline and a reduction in quality of life [5, 48, 78]. Recognizing this phenomenon is essential for proper periodic evaluation and re-evaluation of these patients to detect potential abnormalities, since these fusions could have significant implications for their health and management.

Cervical anomalies, particularly vertebral fusion, are the most observed, occurring in 50–65% of cases [9, 10, 48, 78]. The extent of vertebral fusion in these individuals can vary by the number of vertebrae involved, the nature of the fusion (whether continuous or segmental), and by location. The fusion of the posterior elements of C5–C6 is the most frequently reported. These anomalies are crucial to assess, as they can complicate intubation procedures due to limited cervical mobility [9, 10, 48]. As previously outlined, the manifestation of bone fusion may be age-related due to ongoing ossification. However, early radiographs can reveal certain characteristics indicative of potential future fusion, as described by Kreiborg et al. [48] and Thompson et al. [78]. These characteristics include irregularities in the vertebral column and narrowing of the affected intervertebral spaces [9, 10, 48, 78].

In addition to cervical fusion, a range of skeletal anomalies have been documented, including thoracic vertebral abnormalities (hemivertebrae and spina bifida) and joint anomalies in the upper limbs, hips, and knees [48]. Upper limb involvement primarily includes abnormalities in the shoulder and elbow joints. These may present as a prominent acromioclavicular joint (see Fig. 5.10), restricted mobility of the glenohumeral joint, and, less commonly, ankylosis of the glenohumeral joint [21, 58, 89]. Over time, this involvement can progress, resulting in limitations in shoulder mobility, particularly affecting abduction, forward flexion, and both internal and external rotation. Other common findings in radiographic studies include hypoplasia/dysplasia of the glenoid cavity and flattening of the humeral head, accompanied by relative overgrowth of the greater tuberosity [21, 58, 89]. Moreover, rhizomelic shortening of the humerus has been observed in some patients (also Fig. 5.10), with severity ranging from mild to severe [21]. Anomalies of the hip and lower limbs, excluding the feet, are seldom documented in the literature [21]. However, cases of hip dysplasia and femorotibial ankylosis have been reported [21, 44].

Other Findings

Clinical findings that are less common in Apert syndrome have been observed in case series or case reports. Congenital heart defects are present in approximately 10% of the cases of Apert syndrome, including ventricular and atrial septal defects, patent ductus arteriosus, patent foramen ovale, coarctation of the aorta, dextrocardia, tetralogy of Fallot, and multiple heart defects [17, 62]. Urogenital anomalies are present in 9%, and the most frequent are cryptorchidism and hydronephrosis [17]. Gastrointestinal anomalies are observed in 1%, including esophageal atresia, pyloric stenosis, and imperforate anus [17]. Anomalies of the respiratory system are present in 1.5%, mainly completely or partially solid cartilaginous trachea [17]. Congenital diaphragmatic hernia is a severe and complex malformation that has been described in five cases [11, 43, 47,

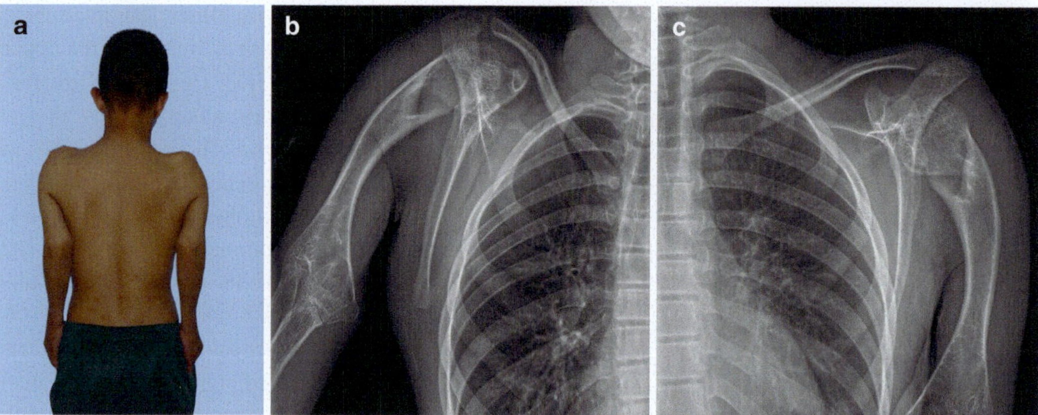

Fig. 5.10 (**a**) Clinical aspects of a patient with Apert syndrome at age 14 years. Note prominent acromioclavicular joint and bilateral rhizomelic shortening. Right (**b**) and left (**c**) radiographs. Note prominent acromion, flattened and irregular humeral head, and short and bowed humeri

75, 88]. Omphalocele has also been reported in two cases of Apert syndrome [30, 37]. Other rare clinical findings include ovarian dysgerminoma, which has been reported in one case with the p.Pro253Arg variant [69].

An intriguing finding that has been associated with Apert syndrome is the presence of moderate to severe acne in the face, chest, and back, but also that unusually extends to the forearms in some cases [18, 76]. Although this feature seems atypical, there is an association between *FGFR2* signaling and the pathogenesis of acne in Apert syndrome [55]. Other cutaneous manifestations in Apert syndrome include hyperhidrosis, oily skin, medially sparse eyebrows, dimples on knuckles, shoulders, and elbows, plantar hyperkeratosis, and forehead with excessive wrinkling [18].

Despite the main clinical features of Apert syndrome being craniofacial and limb anomalies, the complex multisystemic involvement observed in some cases represents a true challenge for patient rehabilitation and clinical management. Therefore, a specialized multidisciplinary team is required to achieve the best results in their treatment.

Differential Diagnosis

Apert syndrome is recognized as one of the most common forms of syndromic craniosynostosis. This group of conditions is highly diverse, encompassing a broad spectrum of disorders. Clinically, many syndromic craniosynostoses exhibit overlapping features; however, certain distinct findings can aid in enhancing differential diagnosis. Additionally, Apert syndrome is associated with allelic clinical conditions—disorders also caused by variants in the *FGFR2* gene—that similarly present craniosynostosis as a key feature. Table 5.1 outlines the primary differential diagnoses of Apert syndrome, including information of associated genes, inheritance patterns, affected sutures, and distinguishing clinical characteristics.

Table 5.1 Overview of craniosynostosis as a differential diagnosis from Apert syndrome

Clinical condition	Gene	Inheritance	Affected sutures	Distinguishing findings	Reference
Crouzon syndrome (OMIM #123500, #612247)	*FGFR2*, *FGFR3*[a]	AD	Coronal (bilateral), multisuture	Extremities *not* involved, acanthosis nigricans[a]	Twigg and Wilkie [80], Katouni et al. [42]
Pfeiffer syndrome (OMIM #101600)	*FGFR2*, *FGFR1*	AD	Coronal (bilateral), multisuture	Broad and deviated thumbs/halluces	Twigg and Wilkie [80], Katouni et al. [42]
Saethre-Chotzen syndrome (OMIM #101400)	*FGFR2*, *TWIST1*	AD	Coronal	Ptosis, small ears with prominent crus	Twigg and Wilkie [80], Katouni et al. [42]
Antley-Bixler syndrome (OMIM #207410[a], #201750)	*FGFR2*[a], *POR*	AD, AR	Coronal, multisuture	Bowed femora, joint contractures, genital abnormalities[a]; abnormal steroidogenesis[a]	Twigg and Wilkie [80]
Beare-Stevenson syndrome (OMIM #123790)	*FGFR2*	AD	Coronal	Cutis gyrata, acanthosis nigricans, skin tags, prominent umbilicus	Twigg and Wilkie [80]
Jackson-Weiss syndrome (OMIM #123150)	*FGFR2*, *FGFR1*	AD	Coronal, multisuture	Broad deviated halluces, normal hands	Cohen Jr. [14]
Muenke syndrome (OMIM #602849)	*FGFR3*	AD	Coronal	Sensorineural hearing loss, mild brachydactyly, cone-shaped epiphyses	Twigg and Wilkie [80], Katouni et al. [42]
Carpenter syndrome (OMIM #201000, #614976)	*RAB23*, *MEGF8*	AR	Coronal, metopic	Brachydactyly	Twigg and Wilkie [80]

AD autosomal dominant, *AR* autosomal recessive
[a]Specific findings related to that gene

Genotype–Phenotype Correlation of the Two Common Variants

Apert syndrome is caused by variants in the fibroblast growth factor receptor 2 (*FGFR2*) gene [86]. Two specific heterozygous missense variants are responsible for more than 98% of cases of Apert syndrome: c.755C>G, p. Ser252Trp (S252W); and c.758C>G, p. Pro253Arg (P253R). The remaining cases result from other rare variants in *FGFR2*, partial gene deletions, and *Alu* element insertions [7, 54, 60, 61, 62, 63, 71, 86].

Since the discovery of the molecular basis, several studies have discussed the genotype–phenotype correlation in Apert syndrome, owing to its clinical variability. One of the first correlations identified was that the p.Pro253Arg variant is associated with greater severity of syndactyly [86], an observation confirmed by other studies [50, 74, 82], although one study did not find this correlation to be statistically significant [62]. Craniofacial variability in Apert syndrome has also been correlated with the frequent occurrence of cleft palate, particularly cleft soft palate, in patients with the p.Ser252Trp variant [46, 50, 62, 74, 82, 87]. Severe midface hypoplasia and dental anomalies have been suggested to be associated with the p.Ser252Trp variant, though no statistical significance has been demonstrated [74, 82]. Additionally, higher severity of obstructive sleep apnea and decreased nasopharyngeal airway volume have been associated with the p.Ser252Trp variant [84]. Differences in the incidence of ocular anomalies between the two common variants have also been reported, with patients carrying the p.Ser252Trp variant presenting more ocular anomalies than those with the p.Pro253Arg variant [39, 45]. Other findings, such as cardiac, urogenital, and central nervous system anomalies, have been studied, but none have been associated with a specific variant [50, 62, 74].

Another study reported that patients with the p.Pro253Arg variant may have had cognitive deficits of higher severity, although other factors may influence the prognosis of these patients [50]. Therefore, further studies are required to confirm this correlation. Difficulties in hearing, speech, language, and communicative participation have been reported in patients with Apert syndrome, and these difficulties tend to be more severe in those with the p. Ser252Trp variant [46]. Autism spectrum disorder has also been reported to be more frequent in patients with the p.Ser252Trp variant [46], but additional studies are needed to clarify this observation.

In addition to research focusing on clinical features, some studies have attempted to establish genotype–phenotype correlations by evaluating surgical outcomes [35, 82]. Prior studies found an association between cleft palate and more severe craniofacial involvement with the p.Ser252Trp variant [50, 62, 74, 82], raising the hypothesis that surgical procedures and outcomes in these patients would be worse than in those with the p.Pro253Arg variant. Craniofacial outcomes following surgery were better in patients with the p.Pro253Arg variant [82]. The outcomes of cranial vault expansion in the two groups were evaluated to determine which group would experience better results, but this hypothesis could not be confirmed due to a small sample size, requiring further studies [35].

All data related to this topic are summarized in Table 5.2.

Table 5.2 Genotype–phenotype correlations in Apert syndrome

Variant	Associated features	References
c.755C>G; p.Ser252Trp (S252W)	Increased incidence of cleft palate (mainly soft palate)	Park et al. [62], Slaney et al. [74], Lajeunie et al. [50], Von Gernet et al. [82], Kilcoyne et al. [46] and Willie et al. [87]
	Possible severe midface hypoplasia and dental anomalies	Slaney et al. [74], Von Gernet et al. [82]
	Higher severity of obstructive sleep apnea and decreased nasopharyngeal airway volume	Wagner et al. [84]
	Higher incidence of ocular anomalies	Jadico et al. [39], Khong et al. [45]
	Hearing, speech, and communication difficulties	Kilcoyne et al. [46]
	Possible higher frequency of autism spectrum disorder	Kilcoyne et al. [46]
c.758C>G; p.Pro253Arg (P253R)	Greater severity of syndactyly	Wilkie et al. [86], Slaney et al. [74], Lajeunie et al. [50] and Von Gernet et al. [82]
	Potentially more severe cognitive outcomes	Lajeunie et al. [50]
	Probably better craniofacial surgical outcomes	Von Gernet et al. [82]
No association	Cardiac, urogenital, or central nervous system anomalies	Park et al. [62], Slaney et al. [74] and Lajeunie et al. [50]
	Cranial vault expansion outcomes	Goodarzi et al. [35]

Genetic Counseling for Unaffected Parents and Affected Individuals

Genetic counseling involves a process of providing comprehensive information to individuals and families regarding genetic disorders and their associated risks. This process empowers them to make informed medical and personal decisions [65].

Apert syndrome is inherited in an autosomal dominant pattern, with most cases being sporadic and considered as likely de novo, meaning that the parents do not carry the variant in their germline. Since Apert syndrome is characterized by complete penetrance, affected parents are expected to exhibit clinical signs of the disorder. Therefore, even in the absence of molecular testing, cases may be considered de novo if the parents are unaffected [40, 56]. Nevertheless, for appropriate genetic counseling, it is important to highlight two findings identified through advances in genetics and genomics: (1) studies have revealed that even sporadic cases may often arise due to increasing paternal age, leading to de novo mutations in the paternal lineage (see Section "Parental age effect in Apert syndrome"); and (2) although rare, gonadal mosaicism has also been reported in Apert syndrome [26, 40, 56].

In summary, unaffected parents of a proband with Apert syndrome have a low probability (<1%) of having another affected child [40]; however, it is important to consider the previously mentioned factors. If a parent of a proband is affected, the risk of having an affected sibling increases to 50%. Furthermore, an affected proband has a 50% risk of having an offspring with Apert syndrome [40].

Our Experience

The clinical findings described here are based on our experience caring for individuals with Apert syndrome in a referral clinical center for treating craniofacial anomalies.

Despite the frequency of distribution between syndromic and non-syndromic craniosynostosis being widely corroborated by many studies, it does not illustrate the picture of our institution. Our service has evaluated more than 500 patients with craniosynostosis over three decades of work in the field of dysmorphology and clinical genetics. Strikingly, data retrieved from the Clinical Genetics and Molecular Biology database show that 90% of our patients with craniosynostosis present with syndromic cases, whereas only 10% are non-syndromic cases, the exact opposite of what is reported in the literature. One hypothesis that could explain this is that our institution is a national referral hospital for the rehabilitation of craniofacial anomalies; hence, many other centers and hospitals refer patients to us, especially those with multiple congenital anomalies characterized by syndromic craniosynostosis. Non-syndromic cases may be underdiagnosed at birth and therefore are not referred to our hospital for treatment and follow-up. Notwithstanding these observations, the most common syndromes with craniosynostosis reported in our records are in accordance with the literature. Thus, Apert syndrome is indeed the most common syndrome among those presenting craniosynostosis as part of the phenotype, followed by Crouzon, Pfeiffer, and Saethre-Chotzen syndrome.

Evaluation of 99 patients with Apert syndrome from our institution showed that 47 are males and 52 females, resulting in no statistically significant difference in the sex ratio.

The parental age at conception is always a key point when evaluating patients with craniosynostosis, either syndromic or non-syndromic. Advanced parental age (i.e., both paternal and maternal age over 35 years) was noted in 12% of our cases with Apert syndrome. Of note, advanced paternal age was noted in 33%, with paternal age ≥ 40 years representing half of these cases.

Radiological analysis performed in a group of 36 patients, out of 99 treated, revealed different frequencies of craniosynostosis when combined with coronal craniosynostosis. Brachycephaly was noted in 90 cases, turricephaly in 61, and turribrachycephaly in 59. Among the exams analyzed, a prevalence of 2.8% for sagittal craniosynostosis, 5.6% for metopic craniosynostosis, and 8.3% for lambdoid craniosynostosis was observed. These data provide valuable insights into the distribution of different forms of craniosynostosis within the Apert syndrome study population, facilitating the identification of specific patterns and the planning of individualized interventions for the effective management of these conditions.

Additionally, of the 99 patients diagnosed with Apert syndrome, our data showed two atypical cases. Both patients presented with type III syndactyly of hands and feet, but there was no clinical or radiological evidence of craniosynostosis (see Fig. 5.11). Unfortunately, both children were evaluated only once and did not return to our institution for follow-up, which made it impossible to perform clinical monitoring and molecular tests.

Regarding craniofacial anomalies, 97% of patients have a broad and high forehead. Flat face and midface hypoplasia were observed in nearly all cases. Some patients evaluated in the perinatal period did not initially present with midface hypoplasia, but reexaminations revealed that this feature became more pronounced as they grew. The same pattern was observed with mandibular prognathism; initial evaluations did not show this

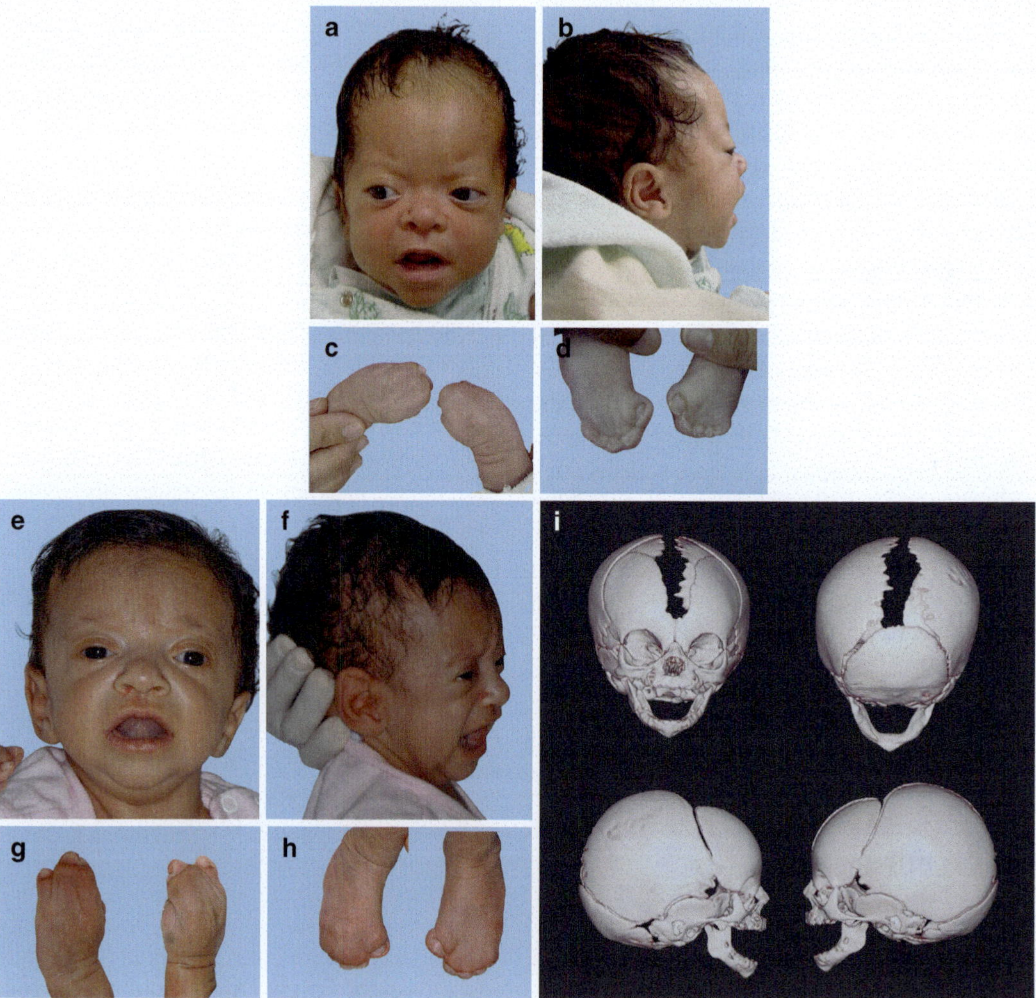

Fig. 5.11 Clinical aspects of two atypical cases of Apert syndrome without craniosynostosis. (**a–d**) Boy at age 2 months. (**e–h**) Girl at age 1 month. (**i**) Three-dimensional reconstruction of CT scan of the girl showing a wide anterior fontanelle without brachycephalic shape of the cranial vault or signs of craniosynostosis

finding, but it later became evident, occurring in 67% of cases. Ocular hypertelorism was observed in 90%. Proptosis was variable in degree but present in nearly all cases. The palpebral fissures were down-slanting in all cases. Strabismus, mainly divergent, was noted in 50%. Atypical ocular findings include unilateral ptosis in one case, pterygium in one, and keratoconus in three. The nose was typical for Apert syndrome, characterized by a short nose with a depressed nasal bridge, although some exceptions were observed. Choanal stenosis or atresia was observed in 50% (16/32) of our cases. The palate was often narrow, and 50% of patients had a cleft palate, mainly involving the soft palate. Submucous cleft was observed in three patients. The uvula was notched or bifid in some cases, leading to further investigation of the presence of a submucous cleft. Major ear anomalies were unremarkable. Low-set, prominent, and large ears were the most common. Additionally, preauricular tag was noted in one case. Chronic otitis media was reported in 55%. Furthermore, 35 out of 46 (76%) patients with Apert syndrome have hearing loss, predominantly conductive. Semicircular canal abnormalities were reported in five of our cases.

Regarding hands and feet, all cases had syndactyly. The type II syndactyly in the hands was the most prevalent among our cases, followed by type I and III with the same frequency. This finding contrasts with the results of the study by Cohen Jr. and Kreiborg [18], who identified type I syndactyly as the most prevalent form in the hands. These differences may reflect population variability, classification methodologies, or distinct genetic factors, contributing to the understanding of the phenotypic presentation of syndactyly in different groups. The predominance of type III syndactyly in the feet was observed in our cohort, as well as in the same study by Cohen Jr. and Kreiborg [18]. Type II syndactyly of the feet was the least prevalent. Of note, the type of syndactyly was asymmetric in a few cases, presenting type I on one hand and type II on the other. The same was observed on the feet.

Concerning growth, most individuals had weight and height measurements appropriate for their age at the time of assessment, reinforcing that, despite limited data, these patients generally do not exhibit growth deficits. Nevertheless, maintaining good physical and nutritional health is essential for proper growth and improving surgical outcomes. Given the complexity of their condition, these patients require monitoring by a multidisciplinary team, including pediatricians and nutritionists.

In our cohort, 36 individuals had available data from central nervous system imaging studies. Ventriculomegaly (see Fig. 5.8) was observed in 50% of cases, hydrocephalus in 19%, corpus callosum anomalies in 30.5%, absence of the septum pellucidum (see Fig. 5.9) in 11%, and porencephaly was present in 2.7%. Additionally, no cases exhibited Arnold-Chiari malformation type 1. Of note, encephalocele was noted in 11%, including two frontal encephaloceles.

Cervical vertebral fusion was present in 17 out of 32 (53%) cases for which cervical radiography images were available. Fusion between C5 and C6 was the most frequently observed, although many cases involved multiple cervical vertebrae segments. Congenital scoliosis was present in three cases. Radiohumeral synostosis was identified in 2 of 14 cases (see Fig. 5.12), and 16 individuals exhibited prominent acromioclavicular joints. Only one individual exhibited rhizomelic shortening of the upper limbs with bending humerus (see Fig. 5.10). These data emphasize the importance of a comprehensive assessment of these individuals, including skeletal radiographic documentation across different ages, to monitor and evaluate congenital or progressive anomalies.

Other findings observed in our cohort include short neck, congenital torticollis, congenital heart defects, umbilical hernia, inguinal hernia, and imperforate anus.

About the genetic investigations of 99 cases from our institution, molecular testing of the *FGFR2* gene was performed in 10 cases (10%). Among these, the classic variants associated with Apert syndrome were observed in 90% of the cases. The p.Ser252Trp variant was found in eight cases (80%), while the p.Pro253Arg was identified in only one. Furthermore, the c.940-

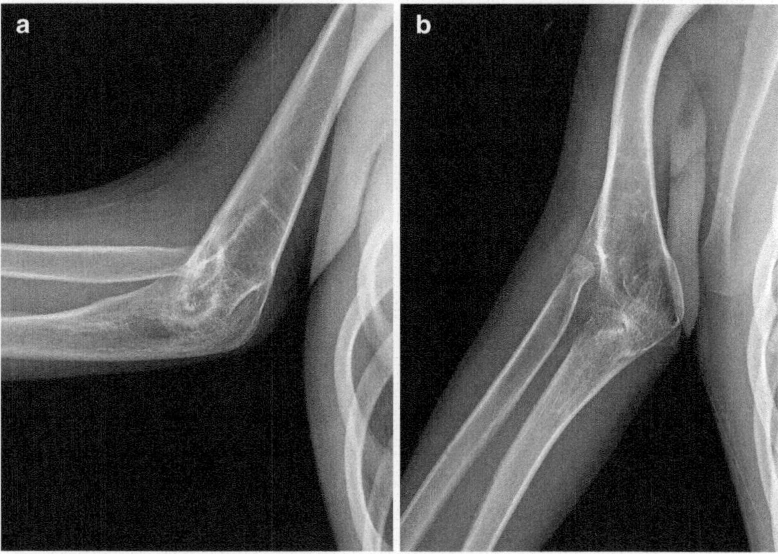

Fig. 5.12 Different incidences of the elbow (**a**, **b**) radiographs of a patient with Apert syndrome presenting radiohumeral synostosis

2A > G variant was detected in one case, which was previously reported by Passos-Bueno et al. [63]. The relatively low number of individuals subjected to molecular testing can be attributed to the limited availability of these tests within Brazil's public health system; molecular investigations are mainly conducted through research initiatives.

Despite the challenges related to complex management in a referral center for treating craniofacial anomalies from the national public health system, significant efforts are made to provide care, treatment, and genetic counseling to individuals with Apert syndrome, along with providing compassionate assistance and advances in clinical and surgical services through a dedicated research program.

Final Considerations

In 1987, the Clinical Genetics Service of the Hospital for Rehabilitation of Craniofacial Anomalies, affectionately called "Centrinho," was established by our dear mentor, neurogeneticist Dr. Antonio Richieri-Costa (in memoriam), who, with his innovative vision, laid the foundations for the development of this field. He was instrumental in advancing diagnostic and research practices, providing a distinctive approach that combined emerging scientific knowledge with a humanized understanding of patients' needs. His pioneering work at our center, recognized to this day for its contributions, helped shape what would become a highly relevant specialty for the treatment of individuals with craniofacial anomalies.

Our experience in a hospital specialized in the rehabilitation of children with craniofacial anomalies has deepened our understanding of the complexity involved in genetic diagnosis, as well as the importance of early diagnosis and rehabilitation for patients with Apert syndrome. In these cases, surgical intervention to correct craniosynostosis is essential at an early age, which aims to minimize complications such as progressive craniofacial deformities, intracranial hypertension, and deficits in neurological development. Additionally, a timely and accurate diagnosis allows for individualized therapeutic planning, adequate genetic counseling, and multidisciplinary rehabilitation to ensure better long-term functional and aesthetic outcomes for our children.

Acknowledgments We would like to express our gratitude to the patients who participated in this chapter and to the team of the Clinical Genetics Service of the Hospital for Rehabilitation of Craniofacial Anomalies of the University of São Paulo: Dr. Antonio Richieri-Costa (in memoriam), Dr. Maria Leine Guion-Almeida, Dr. Roseli

Maria Zechi-Ceide, and Dr. Siulan Vendramini Paulovich Pittoli. We would like to extend our gratitude to the Craniofacial Team, especially to Dr. Nivaldo Alonso for the opportunity to collaborate in this book. We also thank Rosangela Novo dos Santos, who is always available and highly effective in her support. Last but not least, we would like to thank Milton Nakata for the illustrations in this chapter.

Competing Interests The authors have no conflicts of interest to declare that are relevant to the content of this chapter.

Ethical Approval The data presented in this chapter were conducted in accordance with the principles of the Declaration of Helsinki. Written informed consent for the publication of images was obtained from participants or parents/legal guardians in cases involving minors or individuals unable to provide consent independently.

References

1. Agochukwu NB, Solomon BD, Muenke M. Hearing loss in syndromic craniosynostoses: otologic manifestations and clinical findings. Int J Pediatr Otorhinolaryngol. 2014;78:2037–47. https://doi.org/10.1016/j.ijporl.2014.09.019.
2. Alam MK, Alfawzan AA, Srivastava KC, et al. Craniofacial morphology in Apert syndrome: a systematic review and meta-analysis. Sci Rep. 2022;12 https://doi.org/10.1038/s41598-022-09764-y.
3. Apert E. De l'acrocephalosyndactylie. Bull Mem Soc Med Hop Paris. 1906;23:1310–3.
4. Atmaca S, Elmali M, Kucuk H. High and dehiscent jugular bulb: clear and present danger during middle ear surgery. Surg Radiol Anat. 2014;36:369–74. https://doi.org/10.1007/s00276-013-1196-z.
5. Beligere N, Harris V, Pruzansky S. Progressive bony dysplasia in Apert syndrome. Radiology. 1981;139:593–7. https://doi.org/10.1148/radiology.139.3.6785821.
6. Blank CE. Apert's syndrome (a type of acrocephalosyndactyly) – observations on a British series of thirty-nine cases. Ann Hum Genet. 1959;24:151–64. https://doi.org/10.1111/j.1469-1809.1959.tb01728.x.
7. Bochukova EG, Roscioli T, Hedges DJ, et al. Rare mutations of FGFR2 causing Apert syndrome: identification of the first partial gene deletion, and an Alu element insertion from a new subfamily. Hum Mutat. 2009;30:204–11. https://doi.org/10.1002/humu.20825.
8. Boulet SL, Rasmussen SA, Honein MA. A population-based study of craniosynostosis in metropolitan Atlanta, 1989–2003. Am J Med Genet A. 2008;146A:984–91. https://doi.org/10.1002/ajmg.a.32208.
9. Breik O, Mahindu A, Moore MH, et al. Apert syndrome: surgical outcomes and perspectives. J Craniofac Surg. 2016a;44:1238–45. https://doi.org/10.1016/j.jcms.2016.06.001.
10. Breik O, Mahindu A, Moore MH, et al. Central nervous system and cervical spine abnormalities in Apert syndrome. Childs Nerv Syst. 2016b;32:833–8. https://doi.org/10.1007/s00381-016-3036-z.
11. Bulfamante G, Gana S, Avagliano L, et al. Congenital diaphragmatic hernia as prenatal presentation of Apert syndrome. Prenat Diagn. 2011;31:910–1. https://doi.org/10.1002/pd.2788.
12. Carpentier S, Schoenaers J, Carels C, Verdonck A. Cranio-maxillofacial, orthodontic and dental treatment in three patients with Apert syndrome. Eur Arch Paediatr Dent. 2014;15:281–9. https://doi.org/10.1007/s40368-013-0105-9.
13. Cohen MM Jr. An etiologic and nosologic overview of craniosynostosis syndromes. Birth Defects Orig Artic Ser. 1975;11:137–89.
14. Cohen MM Jr. Jackson-Weiss syndrome. Am J Med Genet. 2001;100:325–9. https://doi.org/10.1002/ajmg.1271.
15. Cohen MM Jr, Kreiborg S. A clinical study of the craniofacial features in apert syndrome. Int J Oral Maxillofac Surg. 1996;25:45–53. https://doi.org/10.1016/s0901-5027(96)80011-7.
16. Cohen MM Jr, Kreiborg S. An updated pediatric perspective on the Apert syndrome. Am J Dis Child. 1993a;147:989. https://doi.org/10.1001/archpedi.1993.02160330079025.
17. Cohen MM Jr, Kreiborg S. Visceral anomalies in the Apert syndrome. Am J Med Genet. 1993b;45:758–60. https://doi.org/10.1002/ajmg.1320450618.
18. Cohen MM Jr, Kreiborg S. Cutaneous manifestations of Apert syndrome. Am J Med Genet. 1995;58:94–6. https://doi.org/10.1002/ajmg.1320580119.
19. Cohen MM Jr, Kreiborg S. Growth pattern in the Apert syndrome. Am J Med Genet. 1993c;47:617–23. https://doi.org/10.1002/ajmg.1320470508.
20. Cohen MM Jr, Kreiborg S. The central nervous system in the Apert syndrome. Am J Med Genet. 1990;35:36–45. https://doi.org/10.1002/ajmg.1320350108.
21. Cohen MM Jr, Kreiborg S. Skeletal abnormalities in the Apert syndrome. Am J Med Genet. 1993d;47:624–32. https://doi.org/10.1002/ajmg.1320470509.
22. Cohen JMM, Kreiborg S, Lammer E, et al. Birth prevalence study of the Apert syndrome. Am J Med Genet. 1992;42:655–9.
23. Coomaralingam S, Roth P. Apert syndrome in a newborn infant without Craniosynostosis. J Craniofac Surg. 2012;23:e209–11. https://doi.org/10.1097/scs.0b013e31824de344.
24. Cornelissen M, den Ottelander B, Rizopoulos D, et al. Increase of prevalence of craniosynostosis. J Craniofac Surg. 2016;44:1273–9. https://doi.org/10.1016/j.jcms.2016.07.007.

25. Czeizel AE, Elek C, Susánszky É. Birth prevalence study of the Apert syndrome. Am J Med Genet. 1993;45:392. https://doi.org/10.1002/ajmg.1320450322.
26. Das S, Munshi A. Research advances in Apert syndrome. J Oral Biol Craniofac Res. 2018;8:194–9. https://doi.org/10.1016/j.jobcr.2017.05.006.
27. de Ângelis Ramos D, Matushita H, Cardeal DD, et al. Apert syndrome without craniosynostosis. Childs Nerv Syst. 2019;35:565–7. https://doi.org/10.1007/s00381-019-04050-1.
28. Delashaw JB, Persing JA, Jane JA. Cranial deformation in craniosynostosis. A new explanation. Neurosurg Clin N Am. 1991;2:611–20.
29. Dempsey RF, Monson LA, Maricevich RS, et al. Nonsyndromic Craniosynostosis. Clin Plast Surg. 2019;46:123–39. https://doi.org/10.1016/j.cps.2018.11.001.
30. Ercoli G, Bidondo MP, Senra BC, Groisman B. Apert syndrome with omphalocele: a case report. Birth Defects Res A Clin Mol Teratol. 2014;100:726–9. https://doi.org/10.1002/bdra.23270.
31. Erickson JD, Cohen MM Jr. A study of parental age effects on the occurrence of fresh mutations for the Apert syndrome. Ann Hum Genet. 1974;38:89–96. https://doi.org/10.1111/j.1469-1809.1974.tb01996.x.
32. Fearon JA, Podner C. Apert syndrome: evaluation of a treatment algorithm. Plast Reconstr Surg. 2013;131:132–42. https://doi.org/10.1097/prs.0b013e3182729f42.
33. Fernandes MBL, Maximino LP, Perosa GB, et al. Apert and Crouzon syndromes-cognitive development, brain abnormalities, and molecular aspects. Am J Med Genet A. 2016;170:1532–7. https://doi.org/10.1002/ajmg.a.37640.
34. Glaser RL, Broman KW, Schulman RL, et al. The paternal-age effect in Apert syndrome is due, in part, to the increased frequency of mutations in sperm. Am J Hum Genet. 2003;73:939–47. https://doi.org/10.1086/378419.
35. Goodarzi MR, Breakey WF, van de Lande LS, et al. Does the mutation type affect the response to cranial vault expansion in children with Apert syndrome? J Craniofac Surg. 2023;34:910–5. https://doi.org/10.1097/scs.0000000000009126.
36. Gorlin RJ, Cohen MM Jr, Hennekam RCM. Syndromes with Craniosynostosis: general aspects and well-known syndromes. In: Syndromes of the head and neck. Oxford University Press; 2001. p. 654–70.
37. Herman TE, Siegel MJ. Apert syndrome with omphalocele. J Perinatol. 2010;30:695–7. https://doi.org/10.1038/jp.2010.72.
38. Hogg ES, Turgut NF, McCann E, et al. Inner ear anomalies in children with Apert syndrome: a radiological and Audiological analysis. J Craniofac Surg. 2022;33:1428–30. https://doi.org/10.1097/scs.0000000000008636.
39. Jadico SK, Young DA, Huebner A, et al. Ocular abnormalities in Apert syndrome: genotype/phenotype correlations with fibroblast growth factor receptor type 2 mutations. J Am Assoc Pediatr Ophthalmol Strabismus. 2006;10:521–7. https://doi.org/10.1016/j.jaapos.2006.07.012.
40. Johnson D, Wilkie AOM. Craniosynostosis. Eur J Hum Genet. 2011;19:369–76. https://doi.org/10.1038/ejhg.2010.235.
41. Jones KL, Jones MC, del Campo M. Smith's recognizable patterns of human malformation. 8th ed. Philadelphia: Elsevier; 2022.
42. Katouni K, Nikolaou A, Mariolis T, et al. Syndromic craniosynostosis: a comprehensive review. Cureus. 2023;15:e50448. https://doi.org/10.7759/cureus.50448.
43. Kaur R, Mishra P, Kumar S, et al. Apert syndrome with congenital diaphragmatic hernia: another case report and review of the literature. Clin Dysmorphol. 2019;28:78–80. https://doi.org/10.1097/mcd.0000000000000261.
44. Khan SA, Moores TS, Docker C. Apert syndrome: be aware of the "dodgy" hip! BMJ Case Rep. 2018:bcr-221789. https://doi.org/10.1136/bcr-2017-221789.
45. Khong JJ, Anderson PJ, Hammerton M, et al. Differential effects of FGFR2 mutation in ophthalmic findings in Apert syndrome. J Craniofac Surg. 2007;18:39–42. https://doi.org/10.1097/01.scs.0000249358.74343.70.
46. Kilcoyne S, Luscombe C, Scully P, et al. Hearing, speech, language, and communicative participation in patients with Apert syndrome: analysis of correlation with fibroblast growth factor receptor 2 mutation. J Craniofac Surg. 2021;33:243–50. https://doi.org/10.1097/scs.0000000000008019.
47. Kosiński P, Luterek K, Wielgoś M. Diaphragmatic hernia as an early ultrasound manifestation of Apert syndrome. Ginekol Pol. 2016;87:830. https://doi.org/10.5603/gp.2016.0097.
48. Kreiborg S, Barr M, Cohen MM Jr. Cervical spine in the Apert syndrome. Am J Med Genet. 1992;43:704–8. https://doi.org/10.1002/ajmg.1320430411.
49. Kreiborg S, Cohen MM Jr. Ocular manifestations of Apert and Crouzon syndromes. J Craniofac Surg. 2010;21:1354–7. https://doi.org/10.1097/scs.0b013e3181ef2b53.
50. Lajeunie E, Cameron R, Ghouzzi VE, et al. Clinical variability in patients with Apert's syndrome. J Neurosurg. 1999;90:443–7. https://doi.org/10.3171/jns.1999.90.3.0443.
51. Lattanzi W, Barba M, Di Pietro L, Boyadjiev SA. Genetic advances in craniosynostosis. Am J Med Genet A. 2017;173:1406–29. https://doi.org/10.1002/ajmg.a.38159.
52. Lee HQ, Hutson JM, Wray AC, et al. Changing epidemiology of nonsyndromic Craniosynostosis and revisiting the risk factors. J Craniofac Surg.

2012;23:1245–51. https://doi.org/10.1097/scs.0b013e318252d893.
53. Letra A, de Almeida ALPF, Kaizer R, et al. Intraoral features of Apert's syndrome. Oral Surg Oral Med Oral Pathol Oral Radiol Endod. 2007;103:e38–41. https://doi.org/10.1016/j.tripleo.2006.04.006.
54. Lumaka A, Mubungu G, Mukaba P, et al. Clinical report a novel heterozygous mutation of three consecutive nucleotides causing Apert syndrome in a Congolese family. Eur J Med Genet. 2014;57:169–73. https://doi.org/10.1016/j.ejmg.2014.01.004.
55. Melnik B, Schmitz G. FGFR2 signaling and the pathogenesis of acne. J Dtsch Dermatol Ges. 2008;6:721–8. https://doi.org/10.1111/j.1610-0387.2008.06822.x.
56. Moloney DM, Slaney SF, Oldridge M, et al. Exclusive paternal origin of new mutations in Apert syndrome. Nat Genet. 1996;13:48–53. https://doi.org/10.1038/ng0596-48.
57. Munarriz PM, Pascual B, Castaño-Leon AM, et al. Apert syndrome: cranial procedures and brain malformations in a series of patients. Surg Neurol Int. 2020;11:361. https://doi.org/10.25259/sni_413_2020.
58. Murnaghan LM, Thurgur CH, Forster BB, et al. A Clinicoradiologic study of the shoulder in Apert syndrome. J Pediatr Orthop. 2007;27:838–43. https://doi.org/10.1097/bpo.0b013e3181455886a.
59. Neusel C, Class D, Eckert AW, et al. Multicentre approach to epidemiological aspects of craniosynostosis in Germany. Br J Oral Maxillofac Surg. 2018;56:881–6. https://doi.org/10.1016/j.bjoms.2018.10.003.
60. Oldridge M, Lunt PW, Zackai EH, et al. Genotype-phenotype correlation for nucleotide substitutions in the IgII- IgIII linker of FGFR2. Hum Mol Genet. 1997;6:137–43. https://doi.org/10.1093/hmg/6.1.137.
61. Oldridge M, Zackai EH, McDonald-McGinn DM, et al. De novo Alu-element insertions in FGFR2 identify a distinct pathological basis for Apert syndrome. Am J Hum Genet. 1999;64:446–61. https://doi.org/10.1086/302245.
62. Park W, Theda C, Maestri NE, et al. Analysis of phenotypic features and FGFR2 mutations in Apert syndrome. Am J Hum Genet. 1995;57:321–8.
63. Passos-Bueno MR, Sertié AL, Zatz M, Richieri-Costa A. Pfeiffer mutation in an Apert patient: how wide is the spectrum of variability due to mutations in the FGFR2 gene? Am J Med Genet. 1997;71:243–5.
64. Pereira V, Sacher PM, Ryan M, Hayward RD. Dysphagia and nutrition problems in infants with Apert syndrome. Cleft Palate Craniofac J. 2009;46:285–91. https://doi.org/10.1597/08-010.1.
65. Pina-Neto JM. Genetic counseling. J Pediatr. 2008; https://doi.org/10.2223/jped.1782.
66. Quintero-Rivera F, Robson CD, Reiss R, et al. Intracranial anomalies detected by imaging studies in 30 patients with Apert syndrome. Am J Med Genet. 2006;140A:1337–8. https://doi.org/10.1002/ajmg.a.31277.
67. Raybaud C, Di Rocco C. Brain malformation in syndromic craniosynostoses, a primary disorder of white matter: a review. Childs Nerv Syst. 2007;23:1379–88. https://doi.org/10.1007/s00381-007-0474-7.
68. Renier D, Lajeunie E, Arnaud E, Marchac D. Management of craniosynostoses. Child's Nervous Syst. 2000;16:645–58. https://doi.org/10.1007/s003810000320.
69. Rouzier C, Soler C, Hofman P, et al. Ovarian dysgerminoma and Apert syndrome. Pediatr Blood Cancer. 2007;50:696–8. https://doi.org/10.1002/pbc.21156.
70. Sawh-Martinez R, Steinbacher DM. Syndromic Craniosynostosis. Clin Plast Surg. 2019;46:141–55. https://doi.org/10.1016/j.cps.2018.11.009.
71. Shi Q, Dai R, Wang R, et al. A novel FGFR2 (S137W) mutation resulting in Apert syndrome. Medicine (Baltimore). 2020;99:e22340. https://doi.org/10.1097/md.0000000000022340.
72. Shlobin NA, Baticulon RE, Ortega CA, et al. Global epidemiology of Craniosynostosis: a systematic review and meta-analysis. World Neurosurg. 2022;164:413–423.e3. https://doi.org/10.1016/j.wneu.2022.05.093.
73. Singer S, Bower C, Southall P, Goldblatt J. Craniosynostosis in Western Australia, 1980–1994: a population-based study. Am J Med Genet. 1999;83:382–7.
74. Slaney SF, Oldridge M, Hurst J, et al. Differential effects of FGFR2 mutations on syndactyly and cleft palate in Apert syndrome. Am J Hum Genet. 1996;58:923–32.
75. Sobaih BH, Al Ali AA. A third report of Apert syndrome in association with diaphragmatic hernia. Clin Dysmorphol. 2015;24:106–8. https://doi.org/10.1097/mcd.0000000000000083.
76. Solomon LM, Fretzin D, Pruzansky S. Pilosebaceous abnormalities in Apert's syndrome. Arch Dermatol. 1970;102:381. https://doi.org/10.1001/archderm.1970.04000100029007.
77. Tan AP, Mankad K. Apert syndrome: magnetic resonance imaging (MRI) of associated intracranial anomalies. Childs Nerv Syst. 2017;34:205–16. https://doi.org/10.1007/s00381-017-3670-0.
78. Thompson DN, Slaney SF, Hall CM, et al. Congenital cervical spinal fusion; a study in Apert syndrome. Pediatr Neurosurg. 1996;25:20–7. https://doi.org/10.1159/000121091.
79. Tolarova M, Harris J, Ordway D, Vargervik K. Birth prevalence, mutation rate, sex ratio, parents' age, and ethnicity in Apert syndrome. Am J Med Genet. 1997;72:394–8.
80. Twigg Stephen RF, Wilkie Andrew OM. A genetic-pathophysiological framework for Craniosynostosis. Am J Hum Genet. 2015;97:359–77. https://doi.org/10.1016/j.ajhg.2015.07.006.
81. Upton J. Apert syndrome. Classification and pathologic anatomy of limb anomalies. Clin Plast Surg. 1991;18:321–55.
82. Von Gernet S, Golla A, Ehrenfels Y, et al. Genotype–phenotype analysis in Apert syndrome suggests

opposite effects of the two recurrent mutations on syndactyly and outcome of craniofacial surgery. Clin Genet. 2000;57:137–9. https://doi.org/10.1034/j.1399-0004.2000.570208.x.
83. Vuola P, Pakkasjärvi N, Ritvanen A, et al. Prevalence of craniosynostosis in Finland, 1987–2010: a population-based study. Birth Defects Res. 2024;116 https://doi.org/10.1002/bdr2.2319.
84. Wagner CS, Wietlisbach LE, Kota A, et al. Genetic subtypes of Apert syndrome are associated with differences in airway morphology and early upper airway obstruction. J Craniofac Surg. 2023;34:1999–2003. https://doi.org/10.1097/scs.0000000000009583.
85. Wilkie AOM, Johnson D, Wall SA. Clinical genetics of craniosynostosis. Curr Opin Pediatr. 2017;29:622–8. https://doi.org/10.1097/mop.0000000000000542.
86. Wilkie AOM, Slaney SF, Oldridge M, et al. Apert syndrome results from localized mutations of FGFR2 and is allelic with Crouzon syndrome. Nat Genet. 1995;9:165–72. https://doi.org/10.1038/ng0295-165.
87. Willie D, Holmes G, Jabs EW, Wu M. Cleft palate in Apert syndrome. J Dev Biol. 2022;10:33. https://doi.org/10.3390/jdb10030033.
88. Witters I, Devriendt K, Moerman P, et al. Diaphragmatic hernia as the first echographic sign in Apert syndrome. Prenat Diagn. 2000;20:404–6.
89. Wood VE, Sauser DD, RC OH. The shoulder and elbow in Apert's syndrome. J Pediatr Orthop. 1995;15:648–51. https://doi.org/10.1097/01241398-199509000-00020.
90. Yeh E, Fanganiello RD, Sunaga DY, et al. Novel molecular pathways elicited by mutant FGFR2 may account for brain abnormalities in Apert syndrome. PLoS One. 2013;8:e60439. https://doi.org/10.1371/journal.pone.0060439.
91. Zhou G, Schwartz LT, Gopen Q. Inner ear anomalies and conductive hearing loss in children with Apert syndrome. Otol Neurotol. 2009;30:184–9. https://doi.org/10.1097/mao.ob013e318191a352.

Diagnosis and Imaging

6

Khalid Al-Dasuqi, Quentin Hennocq,
Roman H. Khonsari, Syril James,
Caroline D. Robson, and Joanne M. Rispoli

Introduction

Although clinical evaluation is paramount for diagnosis in Apert syndrome, imaging plays a crucial role in prenatal detection, confirming the diagnosis, managing associated complications, and aiding in surgical planning. The imaging evaluation of Apert syndrome requires a multimodality approach, as each imaging technique provides unique insights. The major imaging modalities used include:

- Plain radiography: Widely used for initial assessments, particularly for identifying skeletal deformities in the hands, feet, cranium, and spine.
- Computed tomography (CT): The gold standard for detailed evaluation of craniosynostosis, midface anomalies, and other osseous abnormalities. CT provides detailed anatomic assessment and enables three-dimensional (3D) reconstructions, critical for surgical planning. When the primary objective is to image craniosynostosis and osseous abnormalities, a low-dose CT technique should be used to reduce radiation dosage [1].
- Magnetic resonance imaging (MRI): Particularly useful for assessing ventriculomegaly, brain malformations, Chiari deformity, and spinal cord abnormalities. While many younger patients may require sedation for a detailed MRI examination, fast imaging with abbreviated protocols can be used to assess ventriculomegaly to avoid sedation. Typically, this protocol includes multiplanar T2-weighted half-Fourier acquisition with single-shot turbo spin-echo (HASTE) images [2].
- Ultrasound (US): Important for prenatal sonographic evaluation of the common structural abnormalities seen in Apert syndrome. Ultrasound is also used in neonates for the sequential assessment of ventricular size and craniosynostosis.

This chapter will review the essential radiologic features of Apert syndrome, focusing on the associated craniofacial, spinal, and limb abnormalities. We begin by discussing the prenatal evaluation of Apert syndrome before moving on to the spinal and musculoskeletal findings, emphasizing the radiographic evaluation. Lastly, we provide an overview of the craniofacial imaging findings using a modality-based approach.

K. Al-Dasuqi · C. D. Robson · J. M. Rispoli (✉)
Boston Children's Hospital, Boston, MA, USA
e-mail: Joanne.Rispoli@childrens.harvard.edu

Q. Hennocq · R. H. Khonsari
Hôpital Necker–Enfants malades, Assistance publique–Hôpitaux de Paris, Paris, France

Laboratoire Forme et Croissance du Crâne, Institut Imagine, Paris, France

S. James
Hôpital Universitaire Necker–Enfants malades, Paris, France

J. G. Meara et al. (eds.), *Apert Syndrome*, https://doi.org/10.1007/978-3-032-12551-4_6

Fetal Assessment

The diagnosis of Apert syndrome can be made prenatally, although the findings may be subtle. Craniosynostosis may not be suspected until late into the second or third trimester with sutures forming around 16 weeks in pregnancy [3]. Furthermore, distinguishing between different syndromic causes of synostosis prenatally may be challenging; however, features such as cranial deformity, midface hypoplasia, hypertelorism, exorbitism, and syndactyly should be recognized and help to suggest the diagnosis. Importantly, abnormal in-utero calvarial morphology does not always signify craniosynostosis and can be associated with positional plagiocephaly or normal postnatal calvarial morphology [4].

Features of Apert syndrome will first be identified on fetal ultrasound, often prompting MRI for confirmation of additional findings. Consensus guidelines from the American College of Radiology and the American College of Obstetricians and Gynecologists state that evaluation of the head, neck, and face are a required part of the fetal anatomic survey to be performed in the second trimester of pregnancy [5]. On conventional two-dimensional (2D) ultrasound, craniosynostosis may be suspected in the setting of abnormal calvarial morphology with bicoronal synostosis resulting in foreshortening of the anterior cranial fossa with brachycephaly or turribrachycephaly with variable severity of involvement of multiple sutures (Fig. 6.1). In the setting of craniosynostosis, sutures may have an indentation along the expected course of the suture [6]. In the presence of these calvarial findings, it is important to assess the fetus for additional craniofacial features as well as the presence of syndactyly (Fig. 6.2), with a combination of findings being suggestive of the diagnosis of Apert syndrome. Hypertelorism can be appreciated on MR or US, with exorbitism best assessed on MR examination (Fig. 6.3). Craniofacial features such as maxillary hypoplasia with a flat midface, low set ears, and cleft lip and palate are also characteristic [7]. Three-dimensional ultrasound can be used in conjunction with 2D ultrasound for improved visualization of craniofacial features and extremities [8] with prior studies reporting that 3D ultrasound can play a key role in parental counseling. On ultrasound, intracranial findings such as ventriculomegaly, deficient septal leaflets, or callosal agenesis should prompt further investigation with MR, which provides more detailed assessment of the brain in fetal life.

Following abnormal US findings, patients are often referred for fetal MR exam to assess for

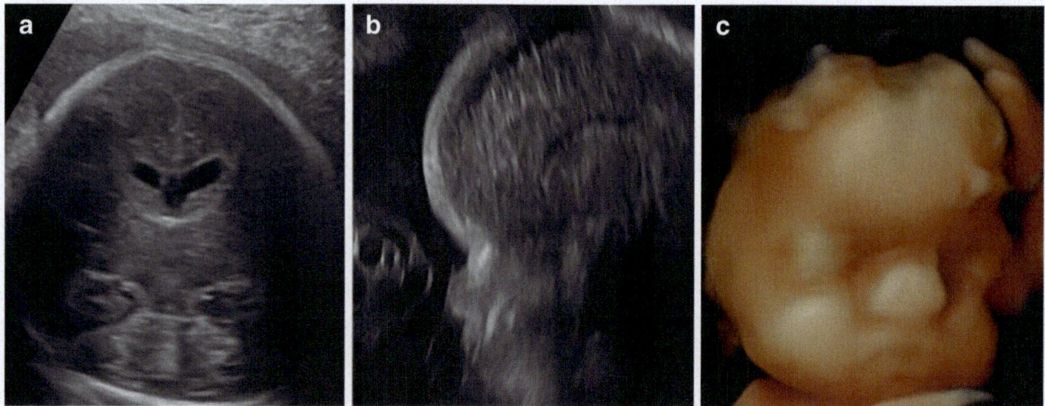

Fig. 6.1 Twenty-seven weeks gestational age fetus with ultrasound images in coronal (**a**) and sagittal (**b**) demonstrating turribrachycephaly, flattened nasal bridge, and midface hypoplasia. 3D Ultrasound images (**c**) allows for improved visualization of facial features

any additional abnormalities. MR examination allows for more optimal assessment of the brain parenchyma, possible temporal lobe anomalies, and craniofacial features. MRI protocols typically include fast T2-weighted imaging including Half Fourier single-shot turbo spin-echo (HASTE) and balanced steady-state free precession (SSFP) in three orthogonal planes for the evaluation of craniofacial features and brain parenchyma [9]. Key features to observe on MR include abnormal calvarial morphology, frontal bossing, shortened anterior cranial fossa, ridging of the sutures, and possible convolutional markings along the inner table of the calvarium (Fig. 6.4a, b) [10]. Although midline brain anomalies can be initially identified on US, MR offers superior evaluation of the brain parenchyma. In addition to callosal and septal anomalies, there are characteristic temporal lobe anomalies that have been described in Apert syndrome and fibroblast growth factor receptor (FGFR) mutations including temporal lobe overexpansion and over convolution with temporal lobe clefts (Fig. 6.4c) [11, 12]. Evaluation of the temporal bones on fetal MR is often challenging due to fetal motion; however, with thin section 3T imaging, temporal bone anomalies may be identified and although non-specific can support a diagnosis of Apert syndrome in association with other typical findings. Temporal bone findings include malformation of the lateral semicircular canal and vestibule with absence of the intervening bony island. As with ultrasound, MR imaging can confirm midface hypoplasia and exorbitism.

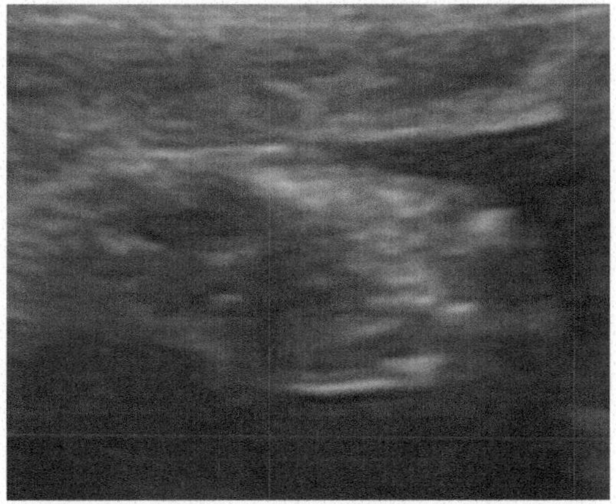

Fig. 6.2 Ultrasound image of the right upper extremity with soft tissue syndactyly of multiple digits

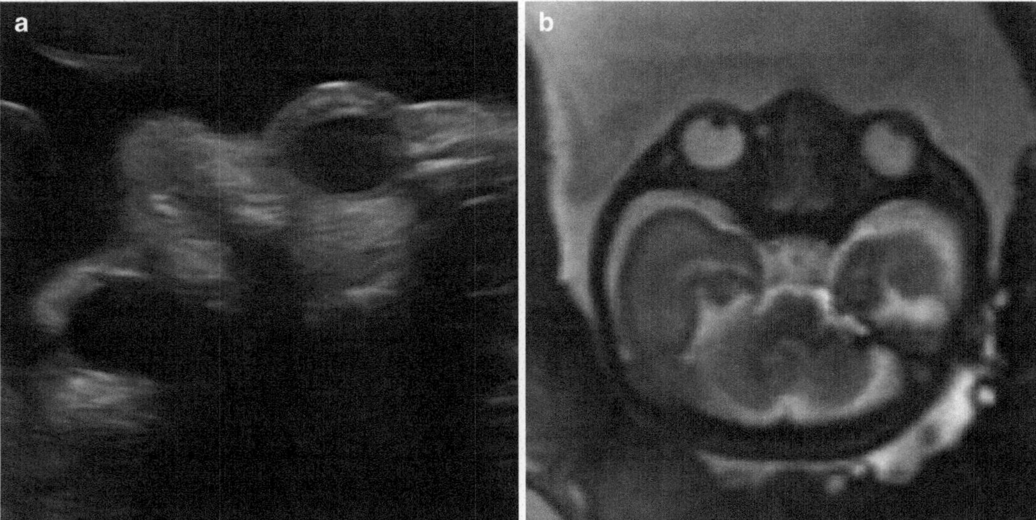

Fig. 6.3 Ultrasound (**a**) and axial HASTE MRI (**b**) images of the orbits demonstrating exorbitism. Note hypertelorism and shallow appearance of the orbits

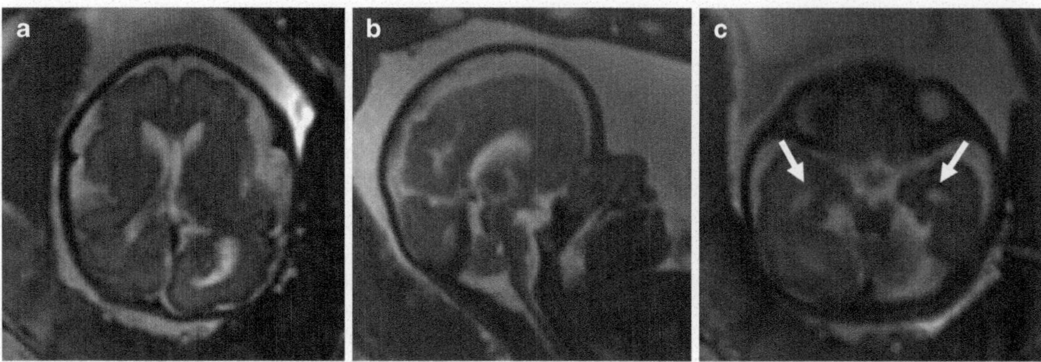

Fig. 6.4 Axial T2 HASTE image (**a**) with brachycephaly. Sagittal T2 HASTE image (**b**) demonstrating frontal bossing and maxillary hypoplasia. Axial T2 HASTE image (**c**) with over convolution of the temporal lobes (white arrow)

Musculoskeletal Imaging

Spinal Findings

Cervical spine abnormalities are a frequent yet underrecognized feature of Apert syndrome. In a cohort of 57 patients who underwent cervical spine imaging, approximately half of the cases reportedly had abnormalities affecting the cervical spine [13]. The most common abnormalities encountered in this cohort were congenital fusion anomalies, which were more evident in the posterior elements than the vertebral bodies. The overall prevalence of congenital spinal fusion is higher if non-osseous fusion anomalies are also considered [13, 14]. These typically manifest as reduced intervertebral disc spaces and/or small vertebral bodies in the anterior spinal column (Fig. 6.5a, b). The cervical levels most affected in Apert syndrome are the C5–C6 and C3–C4 levels, respectively. In contrast, with Crouzon syndrome, another FGFR-related syndrome, involvement of the C2–C3 level is more common [14]. Spinal fusion anomalies can also rarely be encountered in the thoracolumbar spine (Fig. 6.5c, d) [15].

In addition, osseous dysraphic defects (Fig. 6.5e, f) and formation anomalies (e.g., hemivertebra) have been described in Apert syndrome albeit less commonly compared with the fusion anomalies. Scoliotic and kyphotic spine deformities have also been observed in association with the congenital spinal anomalies [15].

Extremity Findings

Syndactyly of the hands, involving soft tissue and osseous fusion, is one of the hallmark features of Apert syndrome. Radiographs are the primary tool for assessing the extent of syndactyly and the degree of fusion between the bony structures.

Hand syndactyly in Apert syndrome commonly presents with a radially-deviated short thumb, complex osseous fusion of the second to fourth digits, simple syndactyly across the fourth interdigital webspace and symbrachyphalangism. The severity and pattern of hand syndactyly vary between patients but are typically classified into three types [16]:

1. *Type 1 Syndactyly ("spade hand")*: Fusion of the middle three digits along with partial to near-complete soft tissue fusion of the fifth digit. The thumb remains short and broad with radial clinodactyly. The palm is flat. This type is the most frequent form of syndactyly in Apert syndrome (Fig. 6.6).
2. *Type 2 Syndactyly ("mitten hand")*: More severe form of fusion with partial or complete simple (soft tissue) syndactyly of the radially

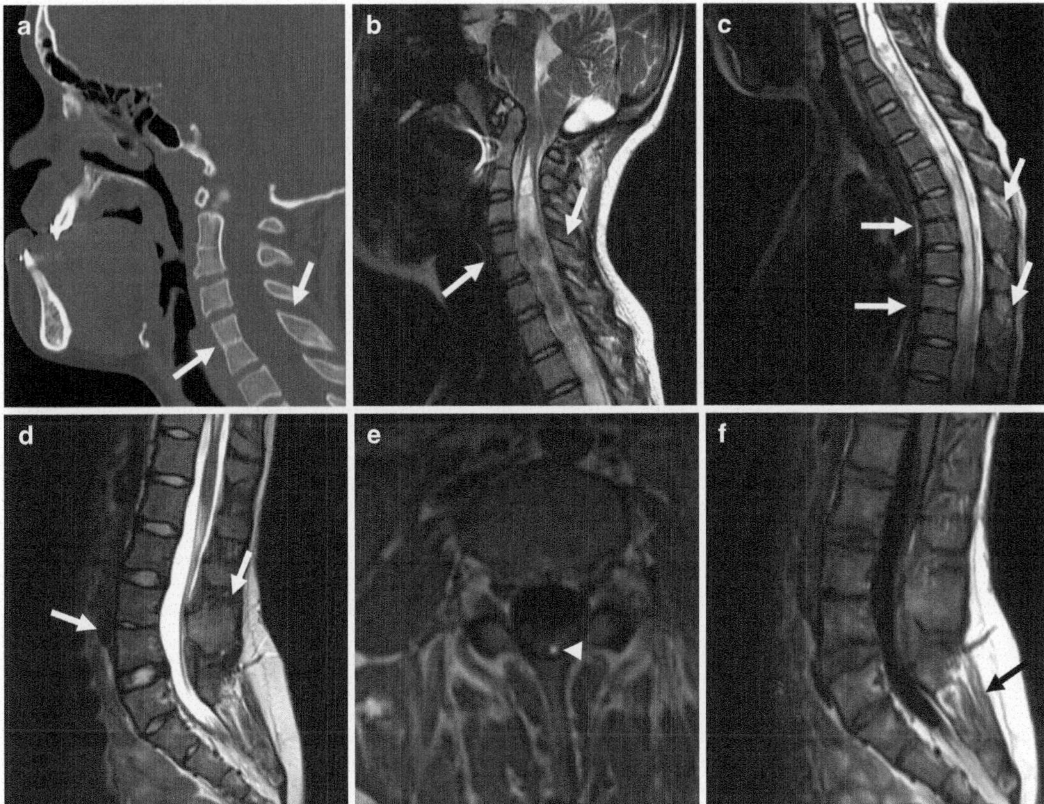

Fig. 6.5 A 14-year-old patient with Apert syndrome. Sagittal CT (**a**) and sagittal T2-weighted MR images (**b**) demonstrate osseous fusion (posterior > anterior) of C4–C5 vertebrae of the cervical spine (white arrows). Other craniofacial features typical of Apert syndrome can also be noted, including maxillary hypoplasia, anomaly of the craniocervical junction, Chiari deformity and syringohydromyelia of the spinal cord. Sagittal T2-weighted MR images of the cervicothoracic (**c**) and thoracolumbar (**d**) spine in the same patient reveal additional sites of vertebral fusion anomalies (white arrows) within the mid-thoracic spine and lumbar spine characterized by diminutive intervertebral discs and fusion of the posterior elements. Axial (**e**) and sagittal (**f**) T1-weighted MR images of the lumbosacral spine also show fatty infiltration of the terminal filum (white arrowhead) and osseous deficiency of the posterior elements at the lumbosacral junction (black arrow), respectively

deviated, deformed thumb to the mid digital hand mass. The complex (osseous) fusion of the digits is associated with splaying of the metacarpals resulting in the palmar concavity (Fig. 6.7).

3. *Type 3 Syndactyly ("rosebud hand")*: Complete fusion of all five digits. The palm is deeply concave and cup-shaped. It is the least common form of syndactyly (Fig. 6.8).

Elsewhere in the hand, metacarpal synostoses involving the fourth and fifth rays as well as carpal coalitions, often between the capitate and hamate, have been described [16]. Longitudinal radiographic studies of the hands also reveal progressive osseous fusion of various bony structures, which have been shown to be preceded by cartilaginous coalitions histologically [16, 17]. Surgical separation of the digits is commonly performed in stages, and postoperative radiographs are crucial for assessing bone remodeling and growth [18]. CT angiography may be obtained preoperatively to assess the pattern of vascular supply to the hand and digits for surgical planning [19].

In addition to the hands, patients with Apert syndrome often exhibit significant joint dysplasia in the shoulder and elbow joints of the upper

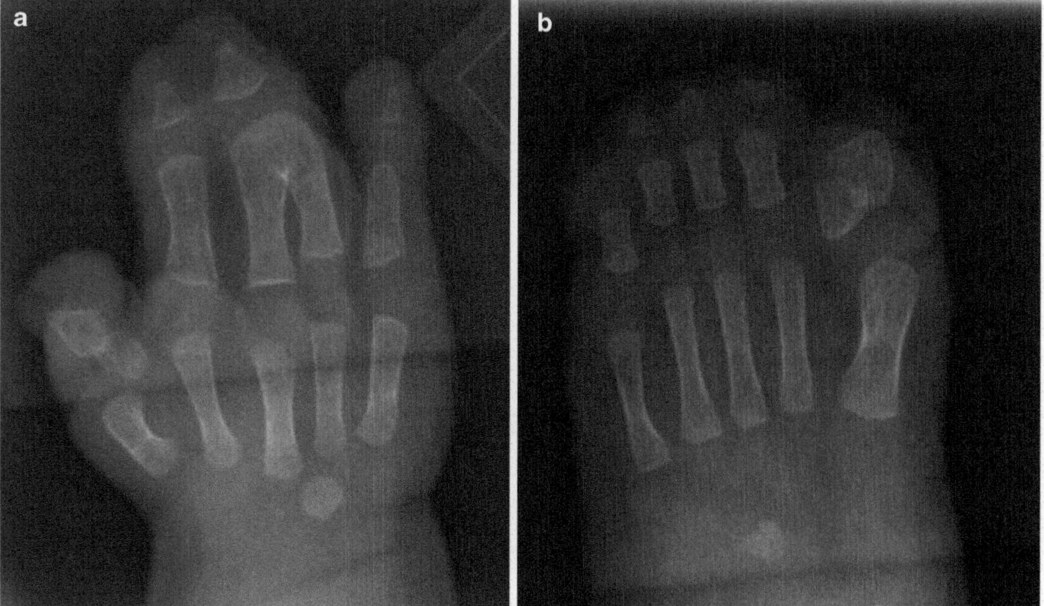

Fig. 6.6 A 2-month-old male infant with Apert syndrome and type I deformities of the hands and feet. (**a**) AP view of the hand shows a short, radially deviated thumb, complex syndactyly of the second, third and fourth digits and partial simple syndactyly of the fourth and fifth digits. (**b**) AP view of the foot reveals a short and dysmorphic great toe characterized by a wedge-shaped proximal phalanx articulating along the lateral side of the first metatarsal head with medial deviation of the distal hallux. The distal phalanx in the great toe is broad. The middle phalanges are missing in the remaining toes

extremities. While less commonly discussed than syndactyly, shoulder and elbow deformities can also lead to significant functional impairment [20].

The shoulder joint may initially appear radiographically normal at birth [16]. However, with growth, inferior-predominant glenoid hypoplasia and abnormal inclination with relative prominence of the acromion become increasingly evident. Additionally, the humeral head typically appears hypoplastic medially with relative overgrowth of the greater tuberosity [15, 16, 20, 21]. As a result, the proximal humerus loses the usual sphericity of the head and distinction of the head/neck junction, and both the glenoid fossa and humeral head become flattened and elongated (Fig. 6.9) [20, 21]. Overall, the combination of the developmental abnormalities leads to limitations in abduction, forward flexion and external rotation, and simulates anterior glenohumeral subluxation clinically [15, 16]. Glenohumeral joint arthropathy, and rarely, ankylosis can occur in this setting [20, 21]. Apart from the glenohumeral joint abnormalities, the humeral shaft is characteristically short in Apert syndrome (Fig. 6.10) [15].

The radiographic findings of the elbow joint are more variable, but tend to involve the radiocapitellar joint and spare the ulnotrochlear joint [15]. Flattening of the radial head and capitellum is the most reported abnormality, which may be associated with radial head subluxation or dislocation (Fig. 6.11) [17, 20]. Some patients may exhibit an angular appearance of the proximal radius or, more rarely, radiohumeral synostosis where the radius and humerus are fused, leading to reduced elbow mobility [15, 16].

In the lower extremities, the most frequently involved and well-studied site is the foot. Unlike the hands, the lateral four toes of the feet may demonstrate simple syndactyly without associated bony fusion [16]. The most observed radiographic abnormality in the feet is absence of the middle phalanx of the toes

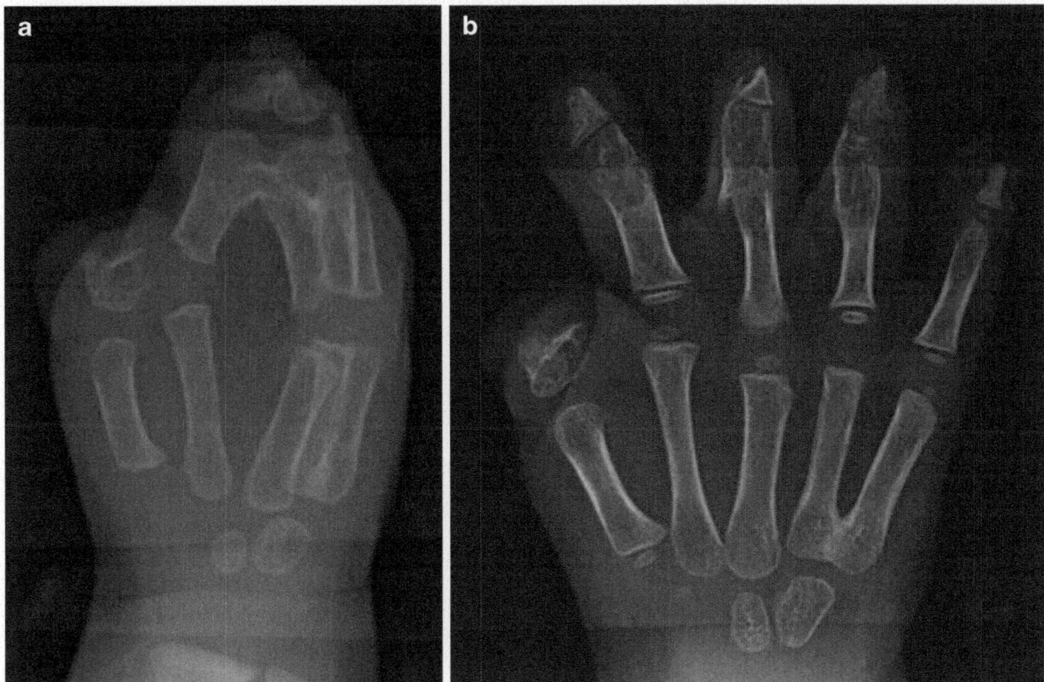

Fig. 6.7 A 16-month-old patient with Apert syndrome and type 2 hands. (**a**) Frontal radiograph of the hand reveals complex osseous syndactyly of the second-fourth digits with near-complete soft tissue syndactyly in the fourth interdigital web space with associated metacarpal splaying as seen with type 2 hand deformities. Partial soft tissue syndactyly is also present between the thumb and index fingers along with classic radial deviation of the thumb distally. (**b**) Frontal radiograph of the same hand is shown status post syndactyly releases and reconstructive osteotomies 2 years later. Of note, synostosis of the proximal fourth and fifth metacarpals becomes more evident compared to earlier radiographs

that is frequently associated with osseous fusion of the phalanges with growth [17, 22]. In the great toe, the triangular appearance of the proximal phalanx is seen nearly universally, which tends to be laterally positioned and hypoplastic with a bracketed epiphysis along the medial side of the phalanx (Fig. 6.6b) [16, 22]. This is associated with hallux varus angulation and deviation, which becomes increasingly more evident with growth [16, 17]. The distal phalanx of the great toe is typically wide, and phalangeal fusion across the first interphalangeal joint is commonly observed on radiographs with age [22].

Elsewhere in the foot, partial duplication of the proximal first metatarsal is commonly seen (Fig. 6.12a) and has been noted in about half the cases in one study cohort [22]. This observation is used to classify the feet in Apert syndrome into two types where the presence of the first metatarsal duplication constitutes the type 2 pattern [16, 17]. With growth, the feet become progressively more distorted due to variable osseous fusion between the tarsals and metatarsals (Fig. 6.12b). The secondary skeletal deformities tend to be more severe in the type 2 pattern than type 1 where five intact metatarsals are present at birth [16, 17].

No consistent radiographic abnormality has been reported in the hips and knees, and functional impairments related to deformities of those joints are uncommon [15, 16].

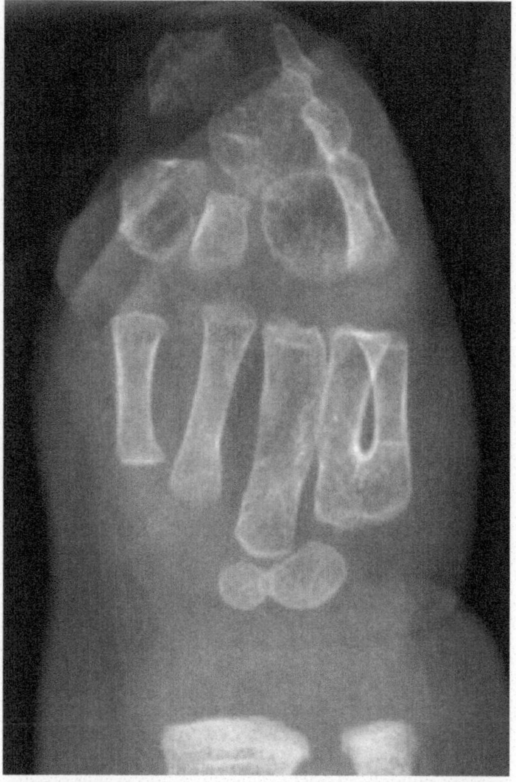

Fig. 6.8 A 9-month-old infant with Apert syndrome and type 3 hands. Frontal radiograph of the hand shows complex syndactyly involving all 5 digits with associated metacarpal synostosis of the fourth and fifth rays and early fusion of the capitate and hamate

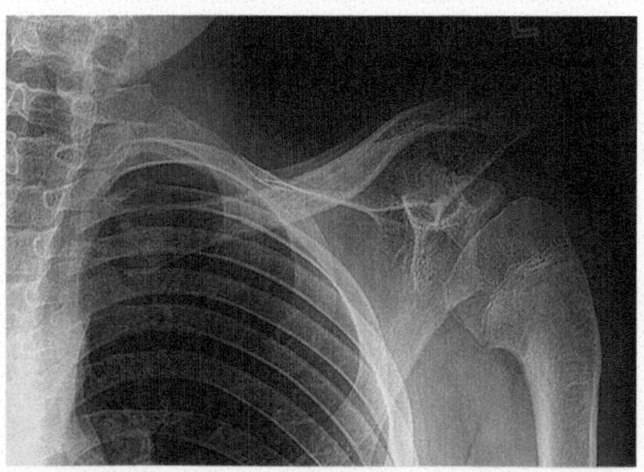

Fig. 6.9 A 14-year-old patient with Apert syndrome and left shoulder pain. AP view of the shoulder in external rotation demonstrates inferior-predominant glenoid hypoplasia and inferior inclination with dysplasia and loss of the sphericity of the humeral head

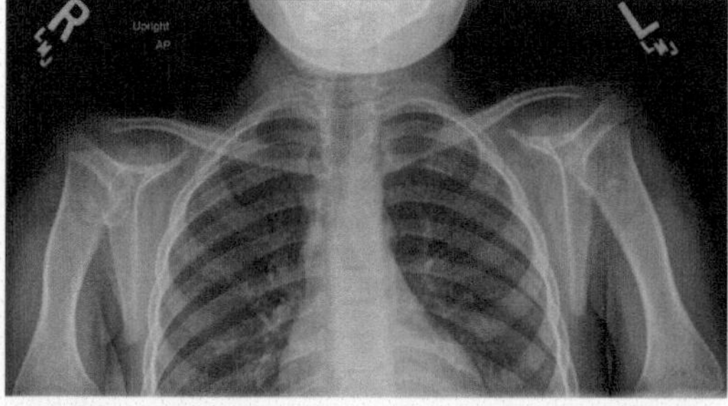

Fig. 6.10 A 3-year-old patient with Apert syndrome and limited shoulder movement. AP radiograph of both shoulders show bilateral glenohumeral synostosis and abnormally short humeral shafts

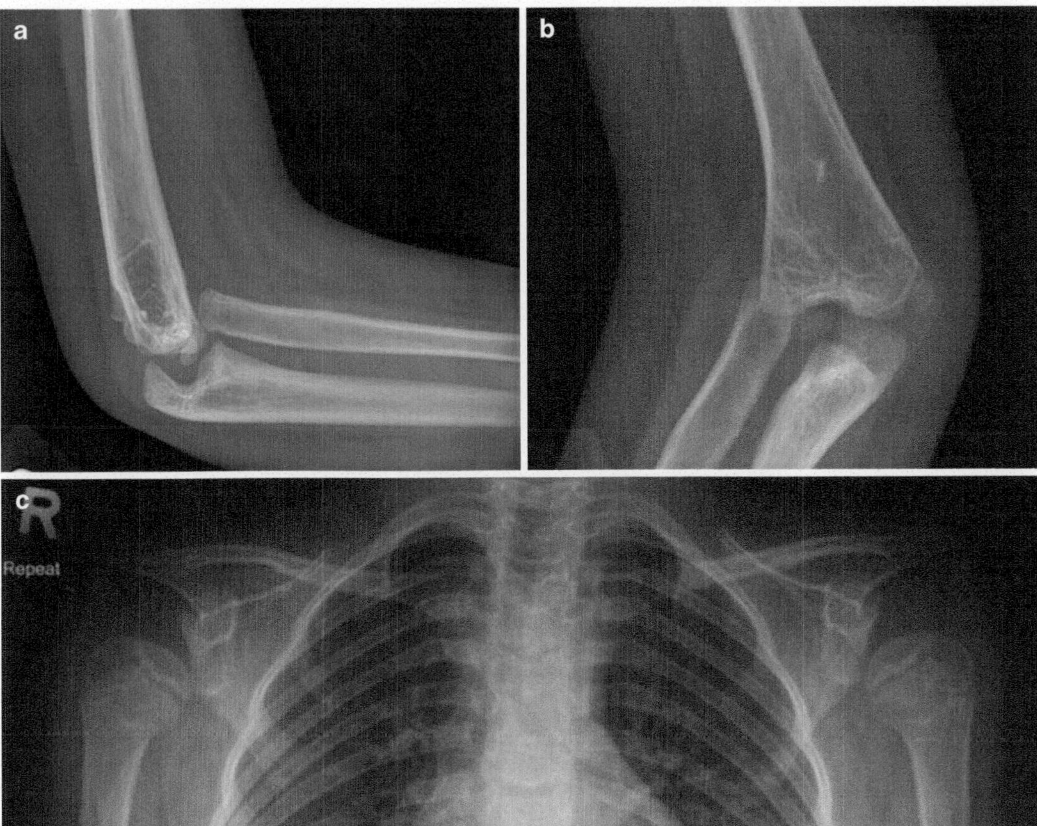

Fig. 6.11 A 4-year-old patient with Apert syndrome and limited elbow function. Oblique (**a**) and lateral (**b**) radiographs of the elbow show dysplastic radiocapitellar and ulnotrochlear joints with hypoplasia and anterior subluxation of the radial head relative to the hypoplastic capitellum. (**c**) AP radiograph of the shoulders in the same patient demonstrates bilateral (left greater than right) glenohumeral dysplasia as typically seen in Apert syndrome with apparent anterior-inferior subluxation of the left more than right humeral heads relative to the glenoids

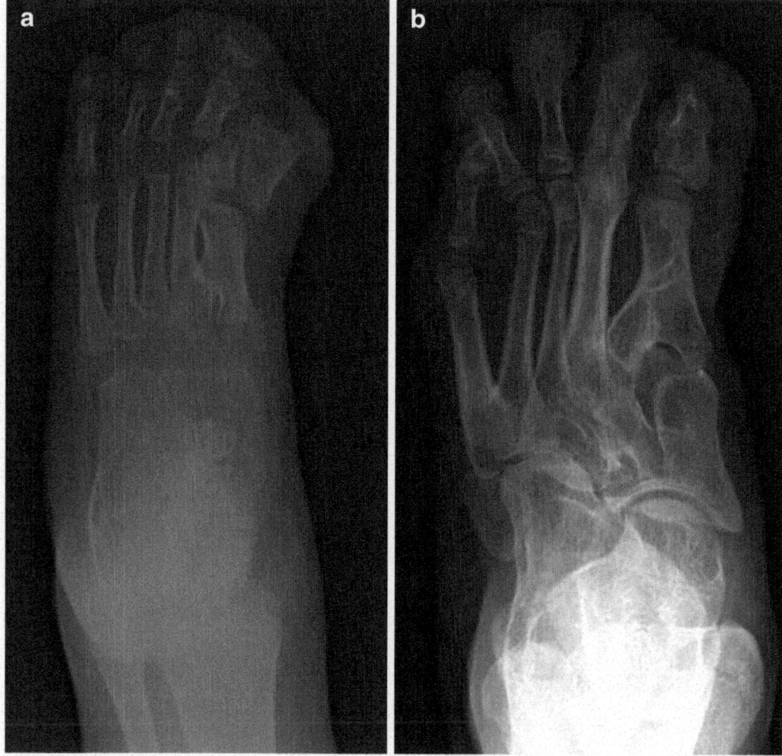

Fig. 6.12 A 3-year-old female with Apert syndrome and type II deformity of the feet. (**a**) Frontal radiograph of the foot shows the classic bifid appearance of the first metatarsal proximally. The radiograph also illustrates soft tissue syndactyly of the forefoot, medial deviation of the short and dysmorphic great toe, and calcaneocuboid fusion. (**b**) Frontal radiograph nearly a decade later shows the extent of osseous deformities that typically become more evident with age, including various sites of osseous fusions involving the navicular, cuneiforms and metatarsals

Craniofacial

Radiographs

In cases of low-risk craniosynostosis, a four-view radiograph is usually obtained as an initial imaging study to assess patency of cranial sutures [3]. In these low-risk cases, if radiographic evaluation is inconclusive, a CT with 3D reconstructions can be obtained for further evaluation. In cases of syndromic craniosynostosis, such as Apert syndrome, CT is obtained as the first line of choice for preoperative planning and evaluation of additional craniofacial features.

CT

CT imaging with 3D reconstruction is imperative for preoperative planning and evaluation of craniofacial morphology. CT imaging allows for the highest sensitivity evaluation of craniosynostosis with images acquired at 0.6 mm with 3 mm reconstructions in axial, sagittal, and coronal planes in bone and soft tissue windows.

In evaluation of the calvarial sutures, most commonly in Apert syndrome, the coronal sutures will be prematurely fused with resultant foreshortening of the anterior cranial fossa and brachycephaly; however, there is variability in the severity of fusion of additional sutures (Fig. 6.13a). A typical feature of Apert syndrome is pronounced widening of the anterior fontanelle and metopic and sagittal sutures often with delayed fusion up to the age of 4 [23]. In comparison with other syndromic craniosynostosis, Apert syndrome often demonstrates progressive fusion of sutures over time. Most often, at the time of imaging, patients will be imaged with the diagnosis of Apert syndrome, and the role of imaging is to determine the extent of abnormalities and assess for any features that might contribute to operative complications.

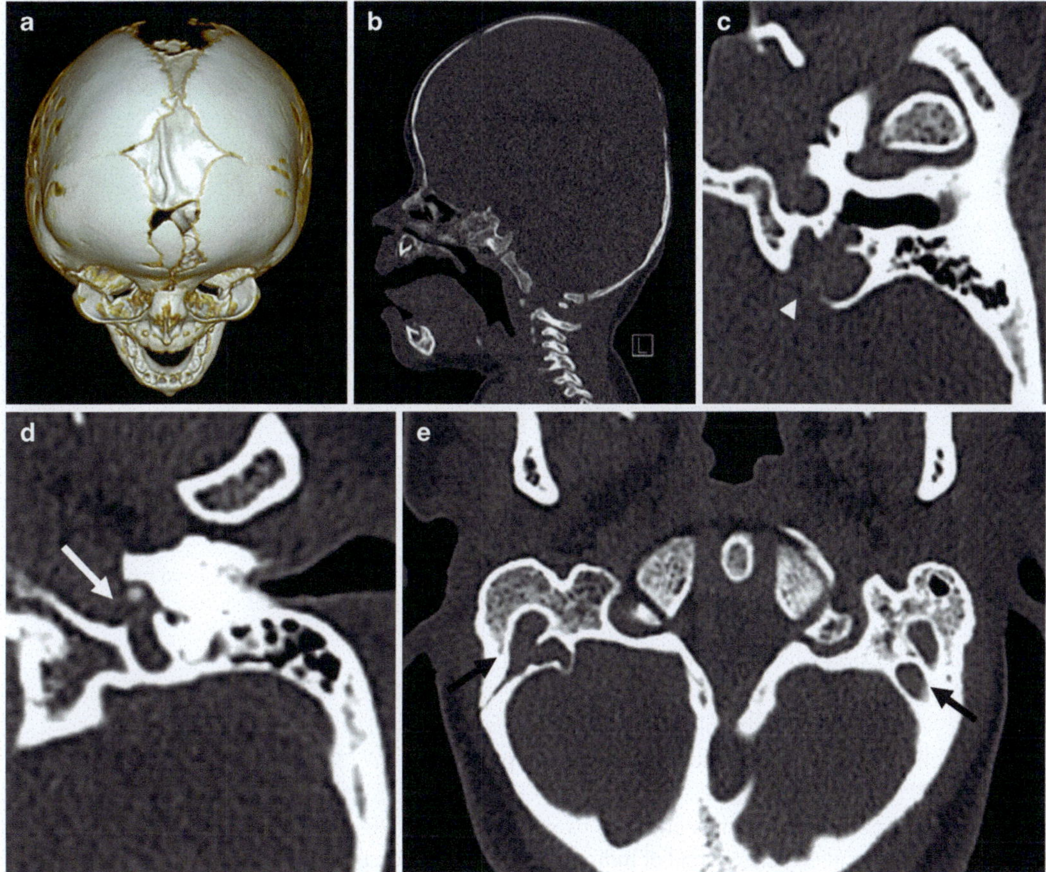

Fig. 6.13 3D-CT reconstruction (**a**) demonstrating premature fusion of the coronal sutures resulting in brachycephaly. Notice that the anterior fontanelle, metopic and sagittal sutures appear widened. Sagittal CT (**b**) reveals a sloping anterior cranial fossa in addition to midface hypoplasia. Axial CT images (**c–e**) through the temporal bone and posterior fossa with stenosis of the jugular fossa at the skull base (white arrow), jugular bulb dehiscence (white arrowhead) and prominent emissary veins (black arrows)

When evaluating the calvarium of patients with Apert syndrome, it is important to evaluate the skull base for preoperative planning. The anterior cranial fossa demonstrates a foreshortened and often a "sagging" configuration (Fig. 6.13b), increasing the risk of dural tear and meningoencephalocele during midface osteotomy and distraction osteogenesis [24]. In addition, careful evaluation of the jugular foramina may reveal that the combined cross-sectional area of both jugular foramina at the skull base is small with associated hypoplasia or atresia of the internal jugular veins and sometimes sigmoid sinuses with compensatory enlargement of the mastoid and central occipital emissary veins (Fig. 6.13c–e) [25]. It is imperative to identify these prominent emissary veins and other distended scalp veins to avoid inadvertent injury during surgery.

In addition to premature fusion of sutures, craniofacial CT allows for optimal detection of craniofacial morphology. Premature closure of the facial sutures can result in midface hypoplasia. In Apert syndrome, premature fusion of the spheno-occipital synchondrosis has been reported [26]. Findings include midface hypoplasia with resultant Class III malocclusion with anteroposterior dimensions of the maxilla being narrowed and posterior rotation of the pterygoid plates [27]. Altered maxillary development also produces a

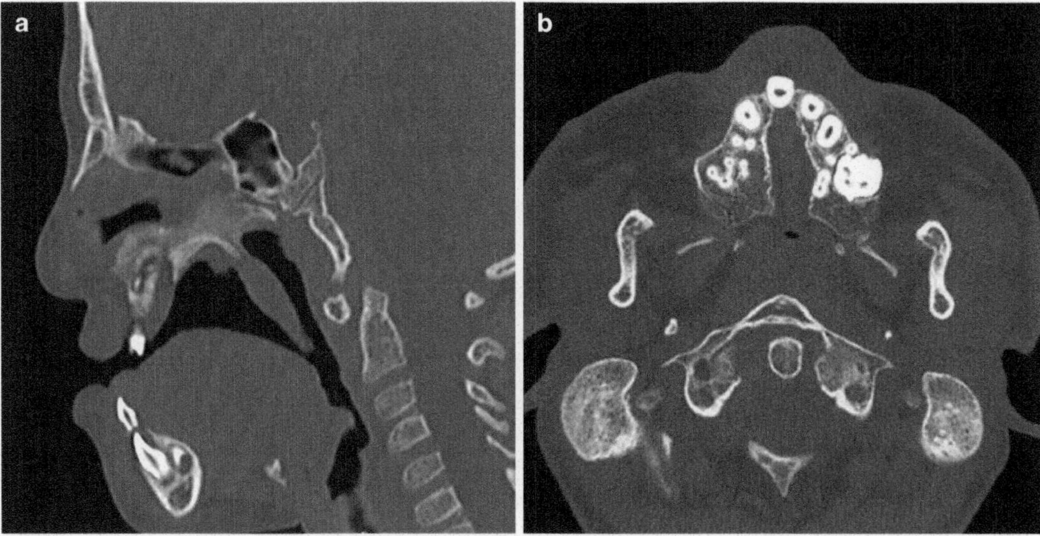

Fig. 6.14 Sagittal CT (**a**) image of the face demonstrating class III malocclusion and a high arched palate. Axial CT (**b**) demonstrates dental crowding within the maxilla and narrowed transverse dimension of the maxilla

high arched palate and dental crowding (Fig. 6.14a, b) [26]. Mandibular length may be small. Additional findings can include congenital bony nasal stenosis in association with midface hypoplasia [28, 29].

Children with Apert syndrome have a high incidence of inner ear malformations, with studies reporting up to 67–90% involvement of inner ear structures [30, 31]. High-resolution CT imaging of the temporal bones offers superior anatomic evaluation of inner and middle ear malformations. The most commonly encountered anomaly in Apert syndrome is an absent bone island of the lateral semicircular canal with an enlarged lateral semicircular canal that is continuous with the vestibule (Fig. 6.15) [31]. Anomalies of the vestibule can be variable, ranging from a bulbous appearance to fusion with the horizontal semicircular canal [31]. Additional identified features include cochlear hypoplasia, dehiscence of the posterior semicircular canal, high riding and sometimes dehiscent jugular bulb, and enlargement of the superior semicircular canal [30]. Heavily weighted T2 MR imaging such as T2 SPACE (Sampling Perfection with Application optimized Contrasts using different flip-angle Evolution) or FIESTA (Fast Imaging Employing Steady-State Acquisition) can also be used to identify the above anomalies. However, CT offers the added benefit of visualization of the inner ear structures as fusion of the ossicles has been described [31]. Eustachian tube dysfunction with chronic otitis media is also common with resultant mastoid air cell under-pneumatization and surrounding sclerosis with mastoid and tympanic cavity opacification.

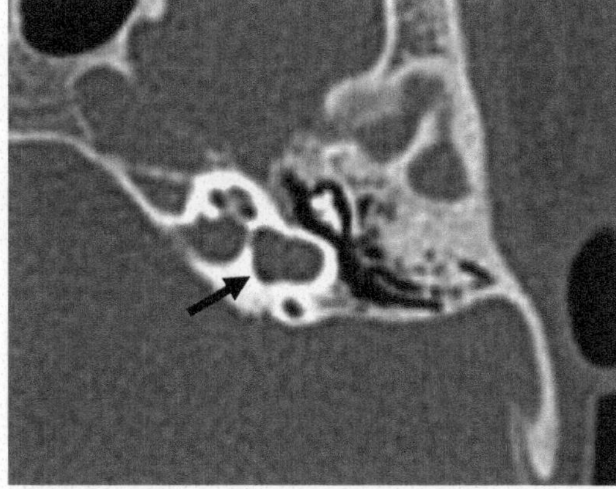

Fig. 6.15 Axial CT of the temporal bone reveals enlargement of the vestibule which is continuous with the horizontal semicircular canal in the setting of an absent bone island (black arrow)

MRI

With Apert syndrome, intracranial anomalies are best assessed on MR examination, with certain features reflecting a primary brain malformation and others being a secondary cause of craniosynostosis. Ventriculomegaly is a common finding in Apert syndrome with the majority of cases being non-progressive and an incidence of up to 60% (Fig. 6.16a) [32]. There are several underlying hypotheses as to the cause of ventriculomegaly. Some postulate that the finding is related to venous hypertension in craniosynostosis. Prior studies have shown that jugular vein atresia or stenosis can occur in syndromic synostosis, leading to prominent emissary veins [25], likely in elevated venous pressures. Venous hypertension results in higher cerebrospinal fluid (CSF) pressure and intracranial hypertension. When evaluating patients with syndromic craniosynostosis, it is important to evaluate the venous foramina for the presence of enlarged emissary veins. At surgery, these veins pose a risk for large hemorrhage. In comparison with other types of syndromic craniosynostosis, jugular foraminal stenosis is less common in Apert syndrome. In addition, although the coronal sutures fuse early, fusion of the lambdoid and sagittal sutures is usually later [33]. These differences likely account for a lower incidence of progressive hydrocephalus in patients with Apert syndrome. An alternative theory for ventriculomegaly is that the ventricular promi-

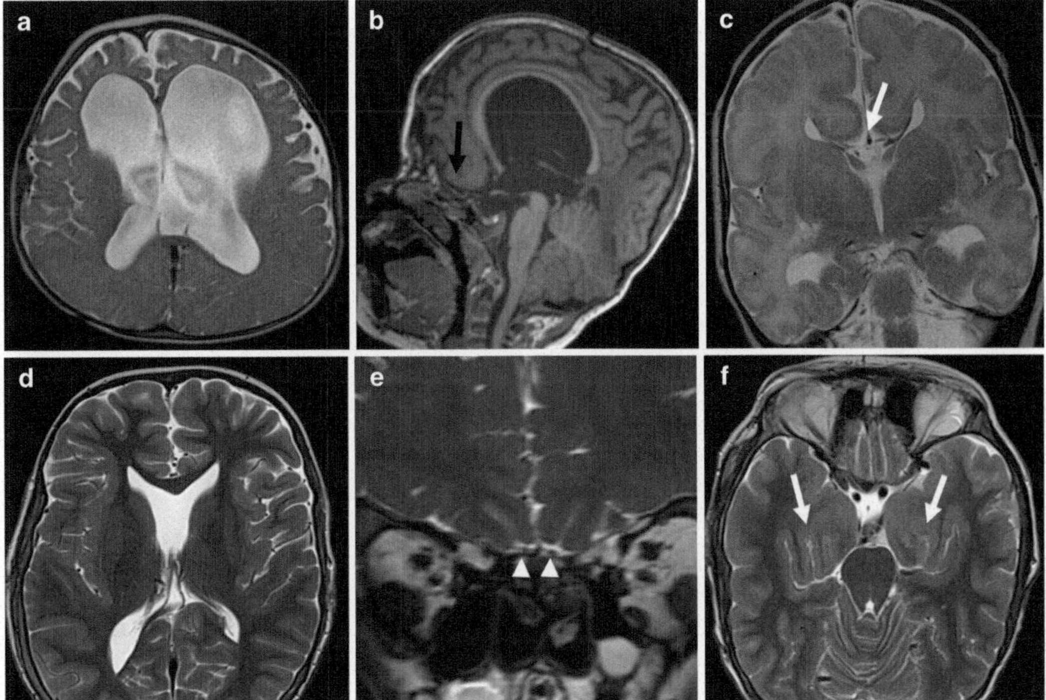

Fig. 6.16 Axial T2 HASTE (**a**) imaging demonstrates ventriculomegaly with characteristic enlargement of the frontal horns. Sagittal T1 MPRAGE (**b**) imaging revealed low lying cerebellar tonsils and Chiari I deformity. Notice addition craniofacial features such as midface hypoplasia and down sloping of the anterior cranial fossa (black arrow). There is also bowing of the corpus callosum in the setting of ventriculomegaly. Coronal T2 (**c**) and Axial T2 weighted images (**d**) demonstrate midline anomalies such as absence of the corpus callosum (white arrow) and septum pellucidum. There is a classic bull-horn configuration of the ventricles in the setting of callosal agenesis. Coronal CISS image (**e**) demonstrates shallow olfactory grooves and hypoplasia olfactory bulbs (white arrowheads). Axial T2 weighted images (**f**) at the level of the temporal lobes with over-convolution and a transverse fold (white arrows)

nence is related to depressed parenchymal white matter volume [34]. Generalized reduction in white matter is proposed in the setting of FGFR mutation and the inability of L1 cell adhesion molecule (L1CAM1) to interact with FGFR2 leading to maldevelopment of white matter. Tokumaru postulated that the ventriculomegaly could be secondary to abnormal calvarial morphology, given that the frontal horns are often more prominent [35]. Although most cases are non-progressive, progressive hydrocephalus can occur and may be an indication for surgery.

Chiari I malformation deformity, similar to hydrocephalus, is not as common in Apert syndrome compared with other syndromic craniosynostoses (such as Crouzon syndrome), with a reported incidence as low as 1.9% in the Apert population [33], and occasionally iatrogenically induced. Most children with Apert have a large head size, which is generally beneficial for brain growth. In cases where the ventriculomegaly has been shunted, an abnormally small head size can result, leading to herniation of the cerebellum through the foramen magnum. Chiari I malformation can also result from premature fusion of the lambdoid sutures resulting in a small posterior fossa; however, this is rare, more likely to occur in children with shunts, and occurs later in Apert syndrome compared to other syndromic synostoses, accounting for the lower incidence of Chiari I deformity. Although a Chiari I deformity may not be present, there is more commonly crowding of the foramen magnum (36%) [32]. It should be noted that asymptomatic Chiari I does not require surgical treatment.

Midline anomalies may include absence of the septum pellucidum and corpus callosum agenesis or dysgenesis (Fig. 6.16c, d) [36, 37]. Anomalies of the olfactory complex have also been described in Apert syndrome, including absence of the olfactory bulbs and tracts, fusion of the olfactory tubercles, and incomplete development [38]. Malformations of cortical development, including polymicrogyria and gray matter heterotopia, have been reported [37], although the finding is rare. Previous studies have shown that calvarial synostosis in a rat model led to morphometrical and cytoarchitectural changes in the maturing brain, including areas of gray matter heterotopia and differences in cell density [39]. These malformations are distinct from temporal lobe abnormalities reported in Apert syndrome, because temporal lobe abnormalities are hypothesized to be related to abnormal calvarial morphology. Temporal lobe findings include overexpansion of the temporal lobe, over-convolution, and a transverse fold that occurs in the mid-hippocampal body [11]. It is important to note that these temporal lobe findings are seen in other FGFR-related craniosynostosis syndrome. Fused thalami, vermian hypoplasia, pyramidal tract abnormalities, and megalencephaly have also been previously reported in Apert syndrome.

Finally, encephaloceles, or protrusion of brain and its covering meninges through an osseous defect have been reported in patients with Apert syndrome, including occipital, temporal, and frontonasal encephaloceles [32].

In addition to using MR for parenchymal assessment, in recent years black bone MR imaging has shown promise as an alternative to CT for evaluation of craniosynostosis. This sequence optimizes contrast between soft tissues and the calvarium, allowing for the evaluation of the calvarial sutures [40, 41]. Black Bone imaging has also shown promise in the evaluation of temporal bone findings [42].

Potential for Artificial Intelligence

Recent advancements in artificial intelligence (AI) medical applications hold promise for transforming diagnostic approaches to Apert syndrome. Currently, dysmorphologists rely on their expertise and the scientific literature to correlate specific facial features with diagnostic cues and identify target genes, such as *FGFR2*. However, various research teams are now developing AI-driven methods to automatically detect characteristic features of Apert syndrome, including hypertelorism, maxillary hypoplasia, brachycephaly, and a beaked nose. The ultimate goal is to reduce diagnostic delay, or "diagnostic wandering," which refers to the interval between a patient's initial consultation and the identification of the underlying causative gene.

Several AI methodologies have been explored to enhance diagnostic precision. In 2019, Gurovich and colleagues [43] utilized deep learning algorithms applied to facial photographs to identify hundreds of genetic syndromes characterized by facial dysmorphia. Their model achieved a top-10 accuracy rate of 91%, outperforming expert clinicians and leading to the development of the Face2Gene tool, which is accessible on smartphones for clinical use. More recently, in 2022, Hsieh and colleagues [44] introduced the GestaltMatcher tool, which also employs deep learning techniques for facial photograph analysis.

An alternative approach, known as feature engineering, focuses on strategically selecting features for syndromic diagnosis. For instance, Hennocq and colleagues [45, 46] developed a novel tool that extracts landmarks, shapes, and textures from frontal and profile facial photographs. This tool enables diagnostic orientation toward Apert syndrome, achieving 90.7% accuracy, and aids in characterizing the syndrome's typical facial phenotype. Additionally, this methodology allowed the team to investigate phenotypic differences between the two primary genetic variants associated with Apert syndrome, *FGFR2* p.Pro253Arg and *FGFR2* p.Ser252Trp, finding no significant facial phenotype differences between these variants. As Apert syndrome has highly specific extra-cranial features (hand and feet syndactyly), adding simple targeted yes/no questions to facial analysis tools will greatly improve their efficiency in many syndromes. The applicability of these tools to low-resolution images [47] further opens doors to their use in telemedicine.

These innovative tools, collectively part of the emerging field of next-generation phenotyping, are anticipated to become integral to routine medical practice and enhance diagnostic accuracy in the near future.

Conclusion

In this chapter, we reviewed essential radiologic features of Apert syndrome. Each imaging modality contributes valuable diagnostic information. Beginning in fetal life, ultrasound and MRI provide complimentary diagnostic information that is paramount for initial diagnosis. Radiographs remain the primary modality in detecting musculoskeletal anomalies in the hands, feet, cranium, and spine. Low-dose CT can be used for the evaluation of craniofacial abnormalities and synostosis. Finally, MRI is the gold standard for evaluating intracranial pathology. Multimodality imaging plays a key role in diagnosis and management of Apert syndrome from initial stages of diagnosis through treatment.

References

1. Montoya JC, Eckel LJ, DeLone DR, Kotsenas AL, Diehn FE, Yu L, et al. Low-dose CT for craniosynostosis: preserving diagnostic benefit with substantial radiation dose reduction. AJNR Am J Neuroradiol. 2017;38(4):672–7.
2. Patel DM, Tubbs RS, Pate G, Johnston JM, Blount JP. Fast-sequence MRI studies for surveillance imaging in pediatric hydrocephalus. J Neurosurg Pediatr. 2014;13(4):440–7.
3. Mathijssen IMJ. Guideline for care of patients with the diagnoses of craniosynostosis: working group on craniosynostosis. J Craniofac Surg. 2015;26(6):1735–807.
4. Fjørtoft MI, Sevely A, Boetto S, Kessler S, Sarramon MF, Rolland M. Prenatal diagnosis of craniosynostosis: value of MR imaging. Neuroradiology. 2007;49(6):515–21.
5. Cater SW, Boyd BK, Ghate SV. Abnormalities of the fetal central nervous system: prenatal US diagnosis with postnatal correlation. Radiographics. 2020;40(5):1458–72.
6. Rubio EI, Blask A, Bulas DI. Ultrasound and MR imaging findings in prenatal diagnosis of craniosynostosis syndromes. Pediatr Radiol. 2016;46(5):709–18.
7. Varlas VN, Epistatu D, Varlas RG. Emphasis on early prenatal diagnosis and perinatal outcomes

analysis of Apert syndrome. Diagnostics (Basel). 2024;14(14):1480.
8. Werner H, Castro P, Daltro P, Lopes J, Ribeiro G, Araujo JE. Prenatal diagnosis of Apert syndrome using ultrasound, magnetic resonance imaging, and three-dimensional virtual/physical models: three case series and literature review. Childs Nerv Syst. 2018;34(8):1563–71.
9. Shekdar K, Feygin T. Fetal neuroimaging. Neuroimaging Clin N Am. 2011;21(3):677–703, ix.
10. Ketwaroo PD, Robson CD, Estroff JA. Prenatal imaging of craniosynostosis syndromes. Semin Ultrasound CT MR. 2015;36(6):453–64.
11. Stark Z, McGillivray G, Sampson A, Palma-Dias R, Edwards A, Said JM, et al. Apert syndrome: temporal lobe abnormalities on fetal brain imaging. Prenat Diagn. 2015;35(2):179–82.
12. Quintas-Neves M, Soares-Fernandes JP. Fetal brain MRI in Apert syndrome: early in vivo detection of temporal lobe malformation. Childs Nerv Syst. 2018;34(9):1617–8.
13. Thompson DN, Slaney SF, Hall CM, Shaw D, Jones BM, Hayward RD. Congenital cervical spinal fusion: a study in Apert syndrome. Pediatr Neurosurg. 1996;25(1):20–7.
14. Kreiborg S, Barr M, Cohen MM. Cervical spine in the Apert syndrome. Am J Med Genet. 1992;43(4):704–8.
15. Cohen MM, Kreiborg S. Skeletal abnormalities in the Apert syndrome. Am J Med Genet. 1993;47(5):624–32.
16. Upton J. Apert syndrome. Classification and pathologic anatomy of limb anomalies. Clin Plast Surg. 1991;18(2):321–55.
17. Cohen MM, Kreiborg S. Hands and feet in the Apert syndrome. Am J Med Genet. 1995;57(1):82–96.
18. Kim JH, Rhee SH, Gong HS, Lee HJ, Kwon ST, Baek GH. Characteristic radiographic features of the central ray in Apert syndrome. J Hand Surg Eur. 2013;38(3):257–64.
19. Harvey I, Brown S, Ayres O, Proudman T. The Apert hand--angiographic planning of a single-stage, 5-digit release for all classes of deformity. J Hand Surg Am. 2012;37(1):152–8.
20. Wood VE, Sauser DD, O'Hara RC. The shoulder and elbow in Apert syndrome. J Pediatr Orthop. 1995;15(5):648–51.
21. Murnaghan LM, Thurgur CH, Forster BB, Sawatzky BJ, Hawkins R, Tredwell SJ. A clinicoradiologic study of the shoulder in Apert syndrome. J Pediatr Orthop. 2007;27(7):838–43.
22. Anderson PJ, Hall CM, Evans RD, Hayward RD, Jones BM. The feet in Apert syndrome. J Pediatr Orthop. 1999;19(4):504–7.
23. Lowe LH, Booth TN, Joglar JM, Rollins NK. Midface anomalies in children. Radiographics. 2000;20(4):907–22.
24. Ridgway EB, Robson CD, Padwa BL, Goumnerova LC, Mulliken JB. Meningoencephalocele and other dural disruptions: complications of Le Fort III Midfacial osteotomies and distraction. J Craniofac Surg. 2011;22(1):182–6.
25. Robson CD, Mulliken JB, Robertson RL, Proctor MR, Steinberger D, Barnes PD, et al. Prominent basal emissary foramina in syndromic craniosynostosis: correlation with phenotypic and molecular diagnoses. AJNR Am J Neuroradiol. 2000;21(9):1707–17.
26. Han JT, Egbert MA, Ettinger RE, Kapadia HP, Susarla SM. Orthognathic surgery in patients with syndromic craniosynostosis. Oral Maxillofac Surg Clin North Am. 2022;34(3):477–87.
27. Forte AJ, Alonso N, Persing JA, Pfaff MJ, Brooks ED, Steinbacher DM. Analysis of midface retrusion in Crouzon and Apert syndromes. Plast Reconstr Surg. 2014;134(2):285–93.
28. Sargar KM, Singh AK, Kao SC. Imaging of skeletal disorders caused by fibroblast growth factor receptor gene mutations. Radiographics. 2017;37(6):1813–30.
29. Xie C, De S, Selby A. Management of the airway in Apert syndrome. J Craniofac Surg. 2016;27(1):137–41.
30. Hogg ES, Turgut NF, McCann E, Avula S, De S, Sharma SD. Inner ear anomalies in children with Apert syndrome: a radiological and audiological analysis. J Craniofac Surg. 2022;33(5):1428–30.
31. Zhou G, Schwartz LT, Gopen Q. Inner ear anomalies and conductive hearing loss in children with Apert syndrome: an overlooked otologic aspect. Otol Neurotol. 2009;30(2):184–9.
32. Breik O, Mahindu A, Moore MH, Molloy CJ, Santoreneos S, David DJ. Central nervous system and cervical spine abnormalities in Apert syndrome. Childs Nerv Syst. 2016;32(5):833–8.
33. Cinalli G, Renier D, Sebag G, Sainte-Rose C, Arnaud E, Pierre-Kahn A. Chronic tonsillar herniation in Crouzon's and Apert syndromes: the role of premature synostosis of the lambdoid suture. J Neurosurg. 1995;83(4):575–82.
34. Raybaud C, Di Rocco C. Brain malformation in syndromic craniosynostoses, a primary disorder of white matter: a review. Childs Nerv Syst. 2007;23(12):1379–88.
35. Tokumaru AM, Barkovich AJ, Ciricillo SF, Edwards MS. Skull base and calvarial deformities: association with intracranial changes in craniofacial syndromes. AJNR Am J Neuroradiol. 1996;17(4):619–30.
36. Quintero-Rivera F, Robson CD, Reiss RE, Levine D, Benson CB, Mulliken JB, et al. Intracranial anomalies detected by imaging studies in 30 patients with Apert syndrome. Am J Med Genet A. 2006;140(12):1337–8.
37. Tan AP, Mankad K. Apert syndrome: magnetic resonance imaging (MRI) of associated intracranial anomalies. Childs Nerv Syst. 2018;34(2):205–16.
38. Maksem JA, Roessmann U. Apert syndrome with central nervous system anomalies. Acta Neuropathol. 1979;48(1):59–61.
39. Lam CH, Sethi KA, Low WC. A morphometric, neuroanatomical, and behavioral study on the effects of

geometric constraint on the growing brain: the methyl 2-cyanoacrylate craniosynostosis model. J Neurosurg. 2005;102(4 Suppl):396–402.
40. Saarikko A, Mellanen E, Kuusela L, Leikola J, Karppinen A, Autti T, et al. Comparison of black bone MRI and 3D-CT in the preoperative evaluation of patients with craniosynostosis. J Plast Reconstr Aesthet Surg. 2020;73(4):723–31.
41. Ganau M, Syrmos NC, Magdum SA. Imaging in craniofacial disorders with special emphasis on gradient echo black-bone and zero time echo MRI sequences. J Pediatr Neurosci. 2022;17(Suppl 1):S14–20.
42. Valeggia S, Dremmen MHG, Mathijssen IMJ, Gaillard L, Manara R, Ceccato R, et al. Black bone MRI vs. CT in temporal bone assessment in craniosynostosis: a radiation-free alternative. Neuroradiology. 2025;67(1):257–67.
43. Gurovich Y, Hanani Y, Bar O, Nadav G, Fleischer N, Gelbman D, et al. Identifying facial phenotypes of genetic disorders using deep learning. Nat Med. 2019;25(1):60–4.
44. Hsieh TC, Bar-Haim A, Moosa S, Ehmke N, Gripp KW, Pantel JT, et al. GestaltMatcher facilitates rare disease matching using facial phenotype descriptors. Nat Genet. 2022;54(3):349–57.
45. Hennocq Q, Bongibault T, Bizière M, Delassus O, Douillet M, Cormier-Daire V, et al. An automatic facial landmarking for children with rare diseases. Am J Med Genet A. 2023;191(5):1210–21.
46. Hennocq Q, Paternoster G, Collet C, Amiel J, Bongibault T, Bouygues T, et al. AI-based diagnosis and phenotype - genotype correlations in syndromic craniosynostoses. J Craniomaxillofac Surg. 2024;52(10):1172–87.
47. Hennocq Q, Bongibault T, Garcelon N, Khonsari RH. Humanitarian facial recognition for rare craniofacial malformations. Plast Reconstr Surg Glob Open. 2024;12(5):e5780.

Part II

Surgical Management

7 Perioperative and Anesthesia Management of the Pediatric Patient with Apert Syndrome

Marisol Zuluaga Giraldo, Luciano Brandao Machado, and Susan M. Goobie

Introduction

Apert syndrome is a congenital autosomal dominant disease with an incidence of 1 per 160,000 live births that affects all sexes equally. It is caused by a mutation in the fibroblast growth factor receptor 2 (FGFR2) gene, which has a role in tissue repair. The syndrome is evident at birth and accounts for 4.5% of all cases of craniosynostosis. Craniofacial abnormalities include hypertelorism, midface hypoplasia, and choanal stenosis [1, 2]. The other dominant clinical feature is symmetrical syndactyly of the fingers and toes (cutaneous and bony fusion), which generally affects the upper limbs more severely than the lower limbs. The synostotic presentation in these patients often involves the coronal sutures bilaterally, resulting in turribrachycephaly (high, steep, flat forehead, and occiput), short anterior cranial fossa, and orbital hypertelorism. A high-arched palate, often covered with excessive soft tissue, a collapsed maxillary arch, and an overt or sub mucous cleft palate can be found in approximately 30% of these patients [3]. Neurological and intracranial anomalies include ventriculomegaly, hydrocephalus, and developmental delays. Apert syndrome is often associated with neuropsychological problems, such as attention deficit hyperactivity disorder, and developmental delay [4]. Associated comorbidities include congenital cardiac disease (which occurs in approximately 10% of patients), polycystic kidneys, and pyloric stenosis. Heart issues include congenital cardiac defects (e.g., ventricular septal and atrial septal defects), overriding aorta, and pulmonary hypertension secondary to chronic hypoventilation [4].

Surgical and Procedural Types in Patients with Apert Syndrome

Pediatric patients with this syndrome require general anesthetics for surgeries and procedures of varying complexities. Procedures involving anesthesia care with either general anesthesia or sedation include diagnostic imaging (computed tomography [CT] and magnetic resonance imaging [MRI] scans) and otolaryngological (ORL) examination of the airway. If the patient needs an imaging diagnostic procedure before surgery, sedation should be used cautiously to produce safe and quality care [5]. We recommend general anesthesia with a supraglottic device (laryngeal

M. Z. Giraldo
Consultant Pediatric Anesthesia, King Abdullah Children's Hospital, Riyadh, Saudi Arabia

L. B. Machado
Division of Anesthesia, Hospital for Rehabilitation of Craniofacial Anomalies, Vila Nova Cidade Universitária, Bauru, São Paulo, Brazil

S. M. Goobie (✉)
Department of Anesthesiology, Critical Care and Pain Medicine, Boston Children's Hospital, Boston, MA, USA
Harvard Medical School, Boston, MA, USA
e-mail: Susan.Goobie@childrens.harvard.edu

J. G. Meara et al. (eds.), *Apert Syndrome*, https://doi.org/10.1007/978-3-032-12551-4_7

mask airway) and spontaneous breathing with either inhaled sevoflurane or total intravenous anesthesia for tomography or resonance images as this technique carries the smallest risk of complications while yielding the highest quality of images [6]

Surgical procedures that might be necessary include cleft lip and palate correction, syndactyly release, dental surgery, orthognathic procedures (such as infantile mandibular distraction device placement), tracheostomy and/or endoscopic assisted minimally invasive surgery (most commonly for bilateral coronal craniosynostosis release) (Fig. 7.1), posterior vault distraction (Fig. 7.2), frontal orbital advancement, and open cranial multiple suture total calvarial remodeling procedures (Fig. 7.3) [7, 8].

Major surgical management for craniosynostosis may involve calvarial vault reconstruction and/or midface advancement. Some general surgical intervention goals are as follows: (1) to prevent the progression of the abnormality, (2) to correct the abnormality, and (3) to reduce the risk of raised intracranial pressure (ICP) and subsequent neurological deterioration, which could occur if surgery is not performed.

Calvarial vault procedures include neuroendoscopically assisted release early in infancy or open cranial reconstruction in older infants or children, typically involving a combined procedure with a neurosurgeon and a plastic surgeon.

Children with midface hypoplasia may have associated upper airway obstruction and obstructive sleep apnea (OSA). Definite surgical management if indicated consists of midface advancement and includes Le Fort I maxillary advancement, Le Fort III midface advancement (often around 6–8 years old), and/or monobloc

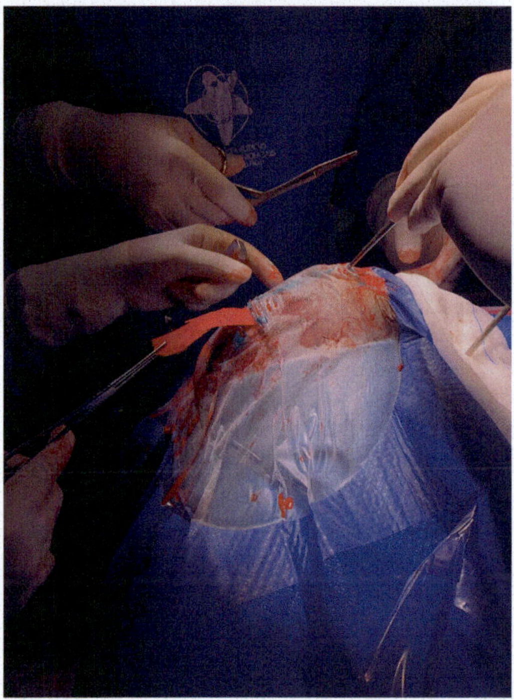

Fig. 7.1 Endoscopic strip craniectomy for sagittal synostosis

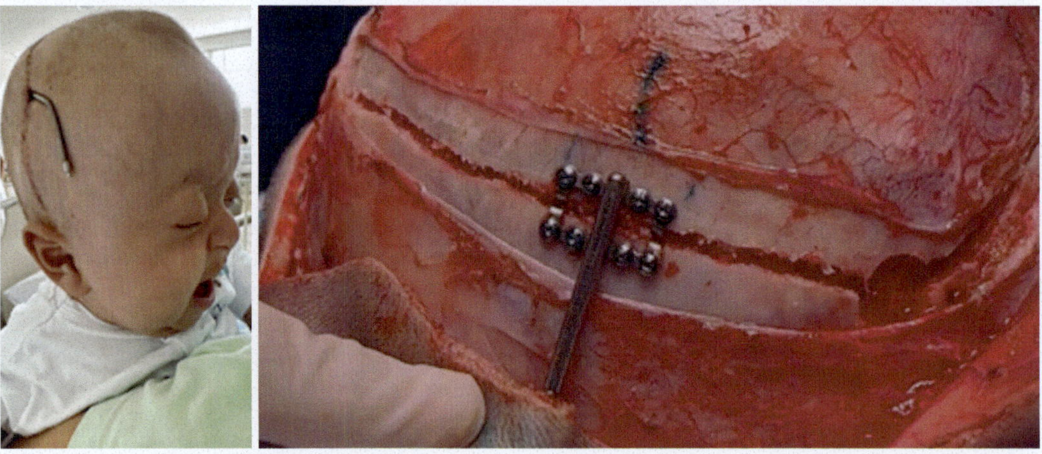

Fig. 7.2 Posterior cranial vault distraction

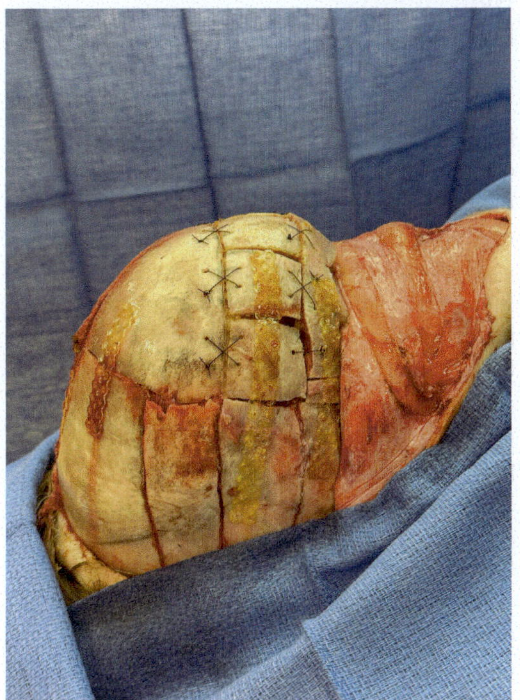

Fig. 7.3 Bilateral fronto-orbital advancement for multisuture synostosis

advancement, which involves the maxilla, upper face, orbits, and forehead. In severe cases, tracheostomy may be required in infancy, with the goal of future decannulation following midface advancement [9]

Perioperative Anesthetic Concerns in Patients with Apert Syndrome

General perioperative anesthesia considerations in patients with craniofacial syndromes such as Apert syndrome include difficult airway, difficult intravenous access, obstructive sleep apnea, bronchospasm, raised intracranial pressure, clinically significant blood loss, blood transfusion and its associated complications, as well as prolonged duration of surgery, intensive care stay, and hospital length of stay [10, 11]. Table 7.1 outlines the unique perioperative considerations for patients with Apert syndrome.

Preoperative Anesthetic Considerations

In addition to preoperative surgical planning, neonates, infants and children undergoing these procedures require comprehensive medical evaluation, laboratory testing, and appropriate diagnostic workup before surgery. General considerations include screening for preoperative anemia, and optimizing comorbidities such as airway, respiratory, cardiac, neurological, and hematologic conditions. Early preoperative evaluation and timely medical management of comorbidities before elective procedures is crucial to ensure the medically complex child is optimized for surgery. Elective surgery should be postponed until all modifiable risks are appropriately addressed and optimized. However, there are times when the surgery is more urgent, and the risks and benefits of rapid surgical intervention must be balanced. Multidisciplinary team-based consultations should be identified and initiated when appropriate, including anesthesiology, pediatrics, surgical services (otolaryngology, plastic, maxillofacial, neurosurgery), and ophthalmology. Age-appropriate and weight-based individualized physiological assessment and management are important.

Preoperative laboratory testing for all children should include a complete blood cell count (hemoglobin [Hgb], hematocrit [Hct], and platelet count). Many centers routinely order a coagulation profile (prothrombin time [PT]/international normalized ratio [INR], partial thromboplastin time [PTT]) and fibrinogen level for major surgery.

Diagnostic testing should be ordered and reviewed preoperatively when indicated based on the child's comorbidities and include a workups with X-rays, CT and MRI studies, sleep studies, pulmonary functions test, and echocardiography (ECHO) when indicated.

Preoperative fasting considerations for the child with Apert syndrome include avoiding dehydration. Pediatric international consensus fasting guidelines recommend following rules before surgery; healthy patients should fast for 8 hours after heavy meals; 6 hours after a light,

Table 7.1 Perioperative considerations and management strategies for patients with Apert syndrome

Apert syndrome characteristic	Anesthetic concern	Perioperative management strategies
Midface hypoplasia—choanal stenosis	Difficult bag-mask ventilation	Consider insertion of oral or nasopharyngeal airway (if patent nares) Use a supraglottic airway device Consider options for optimization and management of difficult airway
Midface hypoplasia High incidence of obstructive sleep apnea Cleft palate	Increased risk for upper airway obstruction Potential difficult intubation	Consider continuous positive airway pressure Employ difficult airway management protocol including video-assisted laryngoscopy with supplemental oxygen Use sedation cautiously
Tracheobronchial secretions Tracheal anomalies (bamboo trachea)	Increased oropharyngeal secretions Increased risk of bronchospasm	Airway, oropharyngeal, and tracheal suctioning Preemptive antisialagogue medication Limited airway instrumentation Deepening of anesthesia and paralysis Bronchodilator therapy
Limb deformities Syndactyly	Difficult venous access Increased risk of peripheral intravenous infiltration or extravasation	Improve success by utilizing local warming, transillumination, and/or ultrasonography. Consider alternatives to peripheral access such as central venous access, intraosseous placement, and venous cutdown
Craniosynostosis	Intracranial hypertension Clinically significant bleeding during open surgery	Avoidance medications and maneuvers that increase intracranial pressure (ICP). Employment of techniques to reduce ICP (maintain hemodynamics, hyperventilation) Multimodal goal-directed patient blood management strategies (Table 7.2)
Exophthalmos	Risk for orbital injury	Ensure eyes well-lubricated, taping/suturing eyes closed and careful padding eyes to avoid pressure, tarsorrhaphies
Cardiac anomalies	Hemodynamical instability risk Increased risk of venous air embolis (VAE)	Consider cardiology consult and echocardiography if required Optimize fluid management Consider vasopressors Prevent and monitor for VAE
Temperature dysregualtion	Hyperpyrexia risk Hypothermia risk	Continuous temperature monitoring Active cooling or warming techniques to maintain normothermia: forced air convectionblankets, circulating warming techniques to maintain normothermia: forced air convection blankets, circulating warm water mattresses, overhead radiant lights, and fluid warmers.
Severe obstructive sleep apnea Chronic hypoventilation	Pulmonary hypertension	Management depends on severity. Avoid hypoxemia, hypercapnia
Oculocardiac reflex (trigeminovagal reflex)	Bradycardia	Decrease surgical stimulus /avoid pressure on eyes Atropine

nonfatty meal or non-human milk; 4 hours after breastmilk, 2 hours after clear liquids for adolescents and adults; and 1 hour after clear liquids for infants and children [12].

Anemia

The global prevalence of anemia reported by the World Health Organization (WHO) is >40% in children and >25% of preschool-aged children in industrialized countries and up to 75% in lower-income environments. Iron deficiency (ID) is the largest contributing factor to anemia across all pediatric age groups.

Preoperative anemia in neonates and children is independently associated with over a twofold increased morbidity compared to matched cohorts undergoing non-cardiac surgery in US hospitals—this is independent of exposure to a blood transfusion [13]. Preoperative anemia has also been reported to be independently associated with an increased risk of any postoperative complication inlcuding a higher risk of surgical site infections [14]. Preoperative anemia is an independent predictor of intraoperative blood transfusion. As a comorbidity in pediatric surgical patients, anemia is associated with adverse outcomes including increased morbidity, mortality, longer length of stay in hospital and in the intensive care unit (ICU), and an overall diminished quality of life [15].

Expert consensus suggests that elective surgery be postponed to optimize unless the surgery is urgent or must be performed sooner. The Society for the Advancement of Patient Blood Management: Pediatric and Neonatal Medicine recommends for preoperative anemia: *Don't proceed with non-emergent major surgery until anemia is evaluated and treated.* Expert consensus guidelines recommend screening 3–6 weeks before major elective surgery [16]. Targeted preventative and therapeutic strategies include oral iron supplementation, to improve the hematologic status of anemic patients prior to surgery and could reduce blood transfusions, improve outcomes and safety, and decrease costs. Treatment must be based on non-transfusion modalities (due to the risks of blood transfusions) and harness the child's own hematopoiesis capacity.

Anemia should be either be diagnosed, corrected, or mitigated prior to the day of surgery. Anemia screening should begin during surgery. Since iron deficiency anemia (IDA) is the most commonly encountered etiology of preoperative anemia, targeted preventative and therapeutic strategies, including iron supplementation (oral or intravenous), to improve the hematologic status of anemic patients prior to surgery with a first-line treatment for patients who have at least 4–6 weeks prior to surgery. In addition, to expedite effect, intravenous iron is an option. Generally given in combination with iron, the use of erythropoietic stimulation agents to improve preoperative anemia can also be considered in certain high-risk situations, weighing the risk/benefit ratio.

Obstructive Sleep Apnea

Almost 50% of patients with Apert syndrome develop OSA [17, 18] attributed to the nasopharyngeal malformation [9, 19]. The obstruction can occur at various levels, but midface hypoplasia, which distorts the nasopharyngeal anatomy, is a common feature. A timely intervention, such as the insertion of a nasopharyngeal airway (NPA) if the nares are patent, may be indicated early in infancy, and such airways have an established role in managing upper airway obstruction in these children. Patients sometimes require continuous positive airway pressure (CPAP) preoperatively. Postoperatively the OSA can be exacerbated due to a combination of airway compromise from prolonged intubation, swelling from surgical manipulation, and a depressed respiratory drive from sedative/narcotic medications. Airway support options, best utilized in an ICU or Operating Room setting, include intubation, a supraglottic airway device, or noninvasive ventilation strategies; such as CPAP, or BiPAP (Bilevel Positive Airway Presure) together with oxygen.

It is also important to consider the effect of chronic upper airway obstruction on the cardiovascular and central nervous systems. During sleep, respiratory obstruction can develop in children with complex craniosynostosis forming part of a vicious cycle with elevated ICP and increased cerebral perfusion pressure (CPP). During the active phases of sleep, research has shown an increase in ICP and a subsequent decrease in cerebral perfusion pressure (CPP). These changes have a temporal relationship with upper airway obstruction. Recurrent episodes of intermittent reduction in CPP have a negative effect on neurological and cognitive development in the long term.

Intracranial Hypertension

Untreated craniosynostosis can lead to elevated intracranial pressure (ICP), as well as intellectual and neurologic developmental delays [20]. Children may present with evidence of elevated ICP, (with clinical symptoms manifesting as nausea, vomiting, or headaches) which can be diagnosed by an ophthalmic examination (papilledema), or CT scan [21]. Elevated ICP is

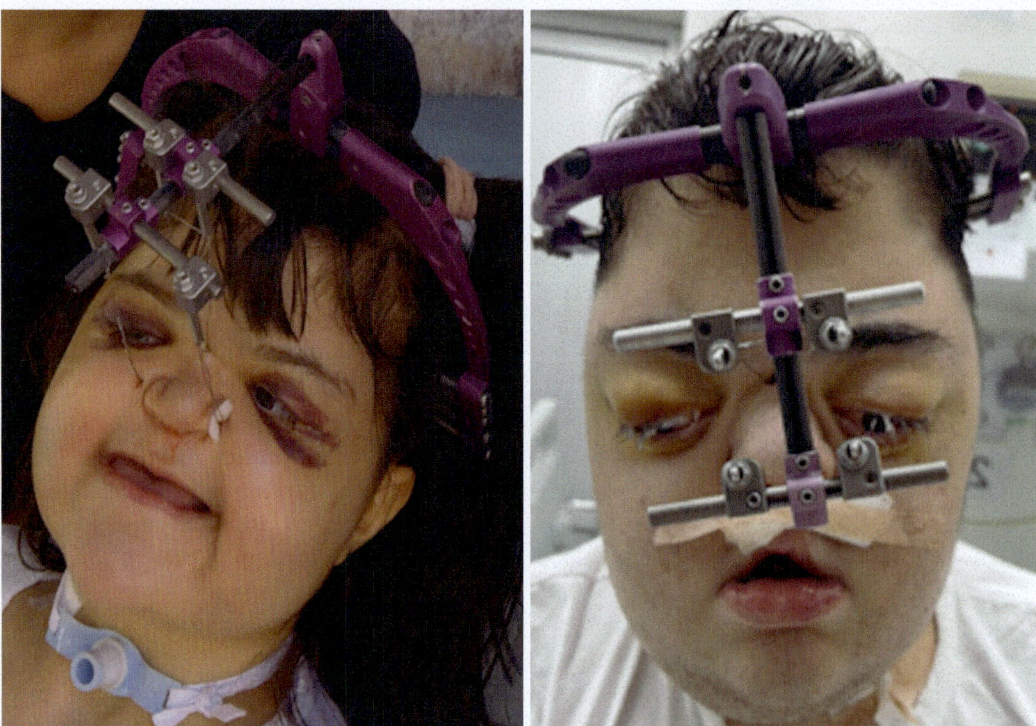

Fig. 7.4 External distractor in place

common in syndromic craniosynostosis with multiple sutures with an average incidence of 47% [2]. It can be associated with and accelerated by hydrocephalus, airway obstruction, craniocerebral disproportion, and/or abnormalities in the brain's venous drainage [2].

Airway Considerations

Infants and children undergoing craniofacial surgery may present with a wide range of diseases and conditions, posing an array of challenges to the anesthesiologist. Optimal perioperative care requires understanding these diseases and their impact on airway and anesthetic management [23, 24]. For children with anomalies affecting airway anatomy, soft tissues of the head and neck, or skeletal mobility, advanced airway management techniques (i.e., modalities other than direct laryngoscopy such as video laryngoscopy or fiberoptic intubation via a supraglottic airway) may be required to secure the airway [25]. Additionally, some craniofacial surgical procedures have direct implications on airway management, such as with Le Fort III midface advancement involving halo distractor application, where the distractor device precludes face-mask ventilation (Fig. 7.4) [26].

Midface hypoplasia and proptosis in children with Apert syndrome can make face mask ventilation difficult [27]. Small nares and a degree of choanal stenosis cause high resistance to airflow through the nasal route, so these patients are obligate mouth breathers. Face mask ventilation can be challenging, but simple airway maneuvers or adjuncts such as an oropharyngeal airway or nasopharyngeal airway along with continuous positive airway pressure (CPAP) are usually effective in relieving the obstruction. A significant proportion of children with Apert syndrome also have fused cervical vertebrae [2]. Cervical spine anomalies occur in 71% of these patients and mainly consist of a complex fusion of the spine at the C5–C6 level. This, however, is of little consequence in the intubation of these patients, as positioning for intubation involves the movement at upper cervical spine levels. As stated, achieving a

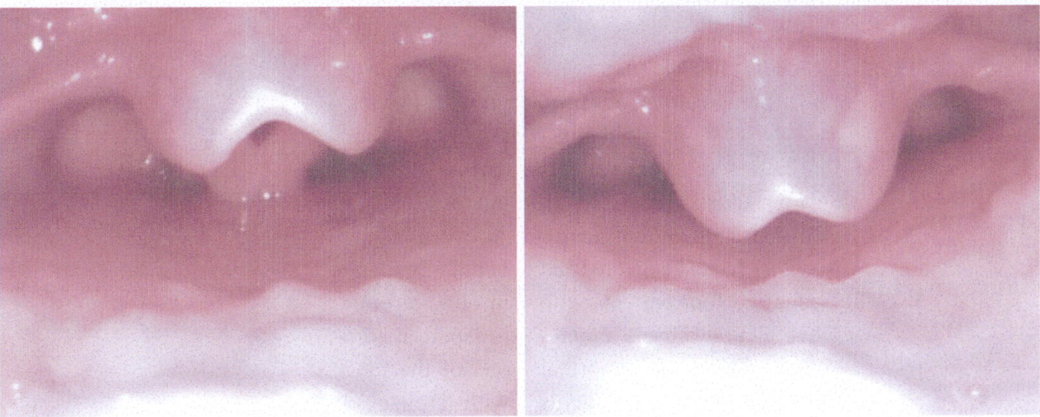

Fig. 7.5 Fiberoptic showing glossoptosis in a patient with Apert syndrome

good mask seal may be difficult; therefore, different sizes and types of masks should be available. Intubation via direct laryngoscopy is successful in the majority of cases; however, an indirect appraoch via video laryngoscope may be the best option. Continuous oxygen should be supplied via nasal canulae during intubation to avoid hypoxia. An important exception to this is children who have undergone front facial advancement. In these patients, intubation may be more difficult due to the altered relationships between the maxilla and mandible, along with reduced temporomandibular joint movement [9].

Patients with Apert syndrome may have "bamboo trachea," or a narrowing of their trachea with fused tracheal rings. A retrospective review of children with Apert syndrome undergoing anesthesia found that respiratory complications, primarily wheezing, were frequent. Complications were severe enough to lead to cancellation in several cases, with others resolving with bronchodilators and deepening of the anesthetic. The physiological mechanism for these complications is unknown, and laryngomalacia or tracheomalacia from a previous tracheostomy combined with increased tracheobronchial secretions from limited airway clearance may be contributing factors (Fig. 7.5). This information may be useful in formulating anesthetic plans for these children.

Barnett et al., in a series of 509 anesthetics administered to 61 patients with Apert syndrome over 14 years, reported that although the incidence of respiratory complications was low in this group of patients (6.1%), a significant proportion of complications arose from supraglottic airway obstruction at the time of induction and the emergence from anesthesia [28].

Bronchospasm is also more common in these patients than the rest of the population. The higher incidence of airway complications in this population could be related to the fact that these children suffer from tracheal anomalies in the form of complete or partial cartilage sleeve abnormalities, which may cause an accumulation of secretions that lead to bronchospasm. Wheezing is the most common respiratory symptom; in some cases, this is sufficiently severe to result in the abandonment of the operation. One proposed explanation for wheezing in this patient group is the lower airway compromise caused by stiff or vertically fused tracheal rings and the accumulation of secretions, which results in monophonic wheezing. This may respond to treatment with tracheal suctioning, deepening of anesthesia, and bronchodilator therapy.

On emergence, the presence of an internal or external device combined with postoperative swelling of the upper airway are the main anesthesia airway management consideratiosn immediately following midface advancement surgery in children with Apert syndrome [29].

Intraoperative Management Considerations in Patients with Apert Syndrome

Induction and Maintenance of Anesthesia

The method of inducing anesthesia will likely depend upon the individual anesthetist's expertise, preference and, to some extent, the patient's condition.

Specific issues that should be considered include the possibility that intravenous access may be difficult generally because of young age and because of anatomical differences in the limbs of a patient with Apert syndrome. Therefore, oral premedication followed by inhalation induction may be preferred to optimize conditions for securing intravenous access. The risk of airway obstruction may be increased with syndromic craniosynostosis. Table 7.1 outlines specific management strategies.

Current recommendations aim to achieve a balanced technique that provides hemodynamic cardiovascular stability and include using hypnotic agents, opioids, non-opioid analgesics, dexmedetomidine, muscle relaxants, and volatile agents.

Positioning

Careful positioning is required for optimal surgical access during craniosynostosis surgery and to minimize the risk of complications. The potential for prolonged duration of surgery means greater attention should be paid to areas at risk of neurovascular compromise caused by prolonged pressure effects. This includes ensuring adequate padding over invasive lines or monitoring leads in direct contact with the skin.

During cranial vault reconstruction procedures in the supine position, surgeons may prefer that the patient's eyes not be taped closed because they are within the surgical field. An ophthalmic ointment should instead be applied, the eyelids may be sutured shut, and all team members should pay careful attention to the patient's eyes, as they are a vulnerable area. Children with syndromic forms of craniosynostosis can have proptosis so severe that full eyelid closure is difficult. In these cases, the surgeons may perform tarsorrhaphies. Infants undergoing procedures in the prone position are placed on a horseshoe headrest. The head must be positioned and the headrest configured to ensure no pressure on the orbits when prone or other pressure points. Special concerns about satisfactory positioning should be periodically reassessed throughout the operation, as there are reports of severe visual disturbances after prone transcranial surgery [30].

Invasive Monitoring

Craniofacial surgery may be associated with hemodynamic and cardiovascular instability due to ongoing and rapid blood loss. Invasive arterial pressure monitoring is generally recommended for intracranial procedures because it allows for immediate hypotension detection and frequent blood sampling. Intravascular volume status is assessed most commonly through invasive arterial pressure measurement and invasive arterial pressure waveform assessment. There is a body of evidence supporting the efficacy of using changes in variability in pulse pressure/systolic pressure with positive pressure ventilation as a tool to direct fluid management. While central venous catheters (CVC) are useful to continuously measure central venous pressure to guide fluid and transfusion management, most centers reserve their use for high-risk children in whom adequate peripheral access is difficult to obtain. The indication for the CVC line must weighed with the risks such as the incidence of catheter-related thrombosis is higher in children with a CVC. CVC access via femoral vein cannulation is an option in children as it avoids pneumothorax and does not compromise cerebral venous return [31]. One study reported an increase in thrombosis related to central catheterization in children under 12 months of age, duration of catheterization longer than 15 days, catheter length greater than 9 cm, and associated coagulopathies, suggesting a preference for peripheral catheterization in some cases [32].

Peripheral Venous Access

All infants should have at least two peripheral intravenous (PIV) lines, preferably 22 gauge or

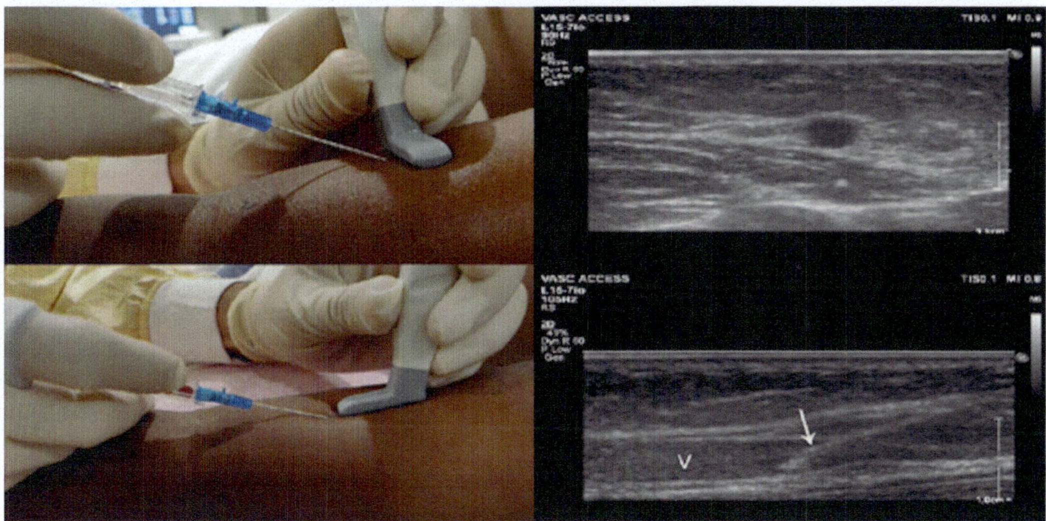

Fig. 7.6 Ultrasound-guided techniques for peripheral intravenous placement catheter over the needle

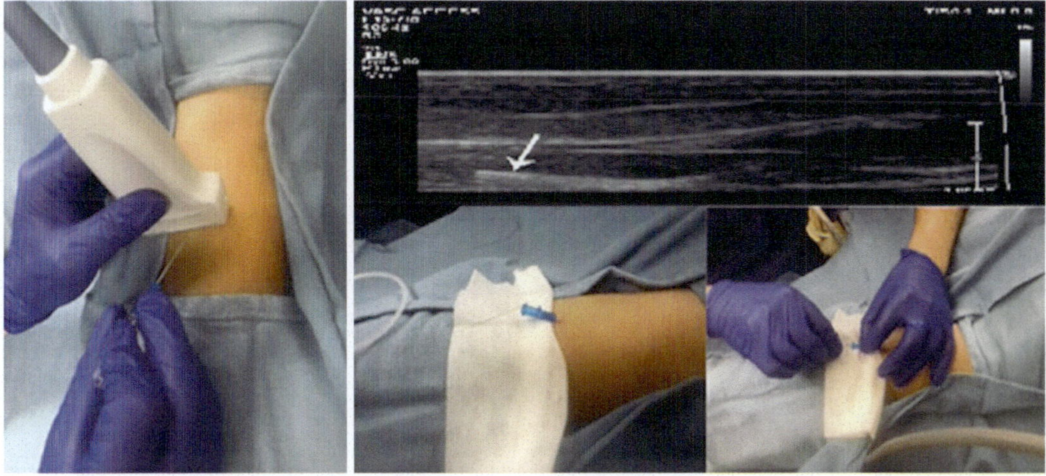

Fig. 7.7 Ultrasound-guided techniques for peripheral intravenous placement catheter over wire

larger, when possible. Blood products should be administered through large-bore peripheral intravenous lines rather than a central line because peripheral administration allows potentially high potassium content and citrate to mix and be diluted before it returns to the heart. In endoscopic surgery, a less invasive and faster procedure, one reliable peripheral access line and non-invasive blood pressure monitoring may be safely recommended. Obtaining peripheral intravenous (PIV) access in children with Apert syndrome can be challenging wiht reports ranging from a 10–50% incidence of difficult venous access in these children [33]. Difficulty with the placement of PIVs following inhalational induction may lead to prolonged times during which children are vulnerable to adverse airway events. Different techniques have been used to improve first-pass success rates in children with a known history of difficult access, including surface landmarking, local warming, transillumination, ultrasonography, central venous access, intraosseous placement, and venous cutdown. Ultrasound (US) guidance has garnered the most success and should be a standard of care if available (Figs. 7.6 and 7.7) [33, 34].

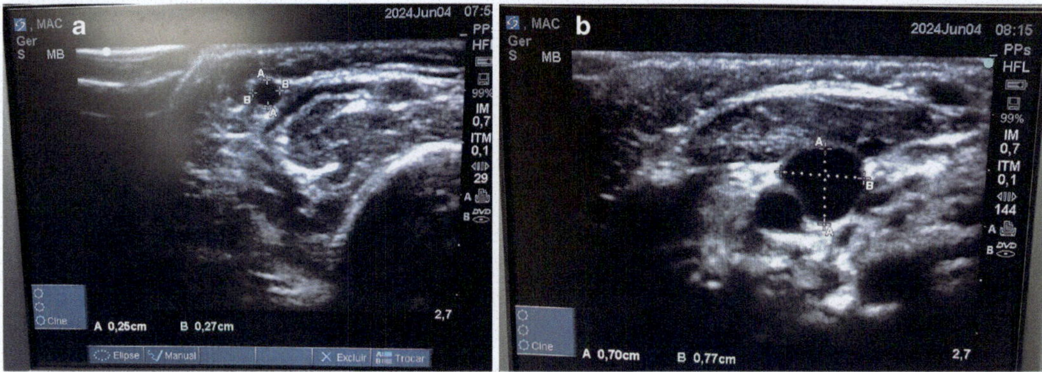

Fig. 7.8 Basilic vein (**a**) and internal jugular vein (**b**) in a 10 month old child. Observe the small diameter of the veins

The technical description of US-guided PIV placement, including the short axis out of plane (SA-OOP) and long axis in plane approaches, has been well reported. The SA-OOP approach is more commonly used in children, particularly infants, due to the smaller diameter of peripheral veins. Appropriate vein selection is an important, often overlooked, consideration to avoid vessel damage during US-guided PIV placement in children (Fig. 7.8). Many children with known difficult PIV access may need future venous access for bloodwork, procedures, or Peripherally Inserted Central Catheter (PICC) placement. The preferred veins for US-guided PIV placement are the forearm's superficial veins, the usual tributaries to the cephalic vein. The greater (or internal) saphenous vein is a common alternative when the forearm's veins are inaccessible. The basilic and brachial veins are deep veins of the arm that should only be accessed if no other options exist. Accessing the brachial vein requires a high level of expertise as there is a significant risk of brachial artery and median nerve injury. Midline catheters, shorter than a PICC line but longer than a peripheral cannula, are a safe potential alternative when attempting access of deeper veins [33, 35].

All PIV lines should be regularly checked intraoperatively to detect and prevent infiltration or extravasation (PIVIE) in a timely manner, which can be limb-threatening if unnoticed. Risk factors for PIVIE include medically complex patients (ASA level III or IV), prolonged surgery, ultrasound placement, and difficult IV placement. Any concern for intravenous catheter infiltration (i.e., difficulty flushing, intravenous fluids not readily dripping, decrease in pulsatility index (PI) of saturation monitor placed on same limb) should prompt inspection and assessment of the intravenous catheter site. The following are recommended PIVIE prevention and monitoring strategies:

1. When possible, intravenous catheters should be placed in areas that will be accessible for inspection during the case (non-tucked sites, sites not draped into field).
2. When clinically feasible, intravenous catheters that are accessible for inspection should be prioritized for use.
3. Consider long intravenous catheters if feasible when using ultrasound for placement.
4. Consider hourly intravenous catheter site checks when sites are accessible.
5. Consider periodic inspection of non-immediately accessible intravenous catheter sites (arms tucked, placement close to surgeons) if clinically feasible and appropriate (appropriate time of surgery, will not contaminate field).

Temperature

Patients with Apert syndrome may not need active warming when undergoing peripheral

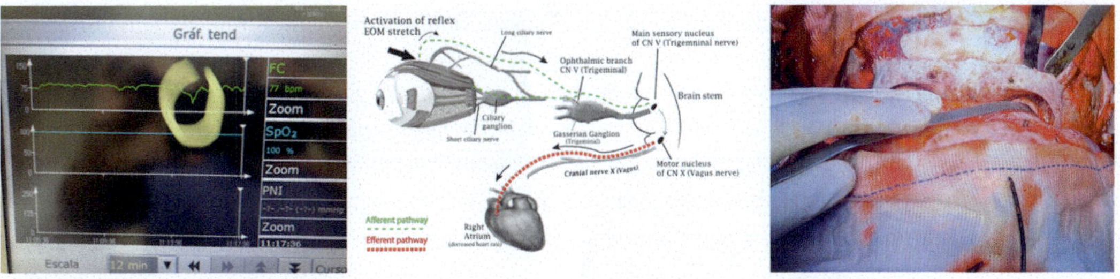

Fig. 7.9 Oculocardiac reflex during craniofacial surgery

surgery due to their inherent temperature dysregulation. If they are actively warmed there is a potential risk of pyrexia, therefore internal body temperature should consistently be monitored.

In craniosynostosis surgery, a large surface area is exposed to the atmosphere, which may result in excessive heat loss. Intraoperatively, the large surface area and high perfusion of an infant's head, coupled with anesthetic effects and the administration of large volumes of cool intravenous fluids, can result in hypothermia. With the proper measures in place, hypothermia can be prevented, but it requires attention by the team. Active warming techniques include a warm operating room, forced air convection blankets, circulating warm water mattresses, overhead radiant lights, and fluid warmers. Even mild hypothermia (less than 36 °C) impairs coagulation enzyme function and is associated with increased bleeding; therefore, management must be directed to prevent it [10, 36].

Oculocardiac Reflex

The oculocardiac reflex (OCR), also known as the Aschner reflex or trigeminovagal reflex, was first described as a bradycardia when direct pressure is placed on the eyeball. A heart rate decrease >20%, is followed by arterial pressure reduction, and may progress to arrhythmia, asystole, and even cardiac arrest [37]. The pediatric population faces a higher risk of OCR, and attention is crucial when manipulating the orbital bandeau during face osteotomies (Fig. 7.9) [38]. Anesthetists must immediately alert the surgeon to ease off the physical stimulus. In most cases, the heart rate returns to normal values spontaneously. Atropine is indicated in cases of persistent bradycardia, as the tachycardia effect of atropine may cause excessive bleeding.

Assessment of Intravascular Volume Status

One of the greatest challenges of complex cranial vault reconstruction and open craniectomy procedures is accurate measurement of blood loss and optimal hemodynamic resuscitation. It is often impossible to estimate ongoing losses accurately because blood seeps into and underneath surgical drapes, mixes with irrigation fluid, or is otherwise difficult to account for in surgical sponges. Therefore, there is no one accurate method for calculating blood loss intraoperatively, and it is common to underestimate or overestimate it. Underestimating blood loss has been identified as a cause of hypovolemic intraoperative cardiac arrest in children.

Many indicators and parameters may be used, including weighing swaps, measuring volume in suction bottles, visual inspection of the drapes, surgical field, and floor to estimate blood loss volumes. Estimation of blood loss may also be evaluated by assessing the patient's physiology and biochemistry through cardiovascular parameters such as heart rate, capillary refill time, blood pressure arterial waveform analysis, central venous pressure, surrogate measures of cardiac output, and biochemical levels such as lactate and base deficit. Serial hourly hemoglobin measurements are recommented to guide management during active bleeding and volume resusitation.

Calculating the allowable blood loss (ABL) may also help identify a point at which to consider blood transfusion, particularly in children where a small volume may be clinically significant. In conjunction with other parameters, ABL can help in appreciating the point at which transfusion may be required.

A typical ABL formulae is as follows:

$$ABL = \left[\text{weight}(\text{kg}) \times \text{estimated blood volume}\right] \times \left[\text{Hb}_{\text{initial}}(\text{g/dL}) - \text{Hb}_{\text{final}}(\text{g/dL})\right] \text{Hb}_{\text{initial}}(\text{g/dL})$$

Where for each age group the estimated blood volume (EBV) is as follows:

Full-term neonate 90 mL/kg, infant 80 mL/kg, child 75 mL/kg, and teenager 70 mL/kg

And $\text{Hb}_{\text{initial}}$ = starting Hemoglobin (Hb) and Hb_{final} = desired final Hb

Constant surgical and anesthetic hemovigilance remain the best tools for successfully assessing intravascular volume and blood status and preventing hypovolemia caused by blood loss. In practice, all available clinical data are combined to guide fluid administration. This includes direct observation of the surgical field and directing close attention to the invasive blood pressure and waveform, central venous pressure (if monitored), response to fluid challenges, urine output, hemoglobin measurements, and blood gas assessments.

Perioperative Management of Fluids

Balanced fluid administration is a key component in perioperative care. Maintaining the physiological state with normal hydration status for adequate tissue perfusion and normal metabolic function is one of our main goals in perioperative anesthetic care. Avoidance of under and overhydration (hemodilution) is paramount. Fluid and electrolyte management is a component of the care provided to every child undergoing craniosynostosis surgery. The anesthesiologist aims to assess and compensate for any perturbations to fluid homeostasis to maintain end-organ tissue perfusion, cellular metabolism, and acid–base status in physiological limits and avoid tissue edema.

The goal of giving fluid during surgery is to provide hydration for basal metabolism and to maintain circulating volume and electrolyte homeostasis. Balanced isotonic crystalloids (e.g., Ringer Lactate™ or Plasmalyte™) are the first-line fluids for intraoperative maintenance and volume replacement. In infants and children, fluid responsiveness describes the ability of intravenous fluids to improve cardiovascular function, tissue perfusion, and metabolic physiology. Infused fluids aim to increase preload, improve cardiac output, reduce peripheral vasoconstriction, and optimize blood rheology [39].

Large volume infusion of crystalloids during surgery (>40–60 mL kg) may induce endothelial dysfunction, increased transfer of fluid to the interstitial space, and fluid overload. Glucose supplementation is not usually necessary for healthy children undergoing surgery who have followed conservative fasting guidelines. Beyond the neonatal period, children have sufficient metabolic and energy reserves to maintain normoglycemia for most surgeries. Exceptions to this include children with malnutrition, hypermetabolism, liver failure, hypothermia, mitochondrial disorders, beta-blocker therapy, or critical illness. Blood sugar concentrations should be monitored closely in long surgery where glucose is not infused [40].

Bleeding and Transfusion Management

Craniosynostosis surgery has been associated with clinically significant surgical blood loss due to the proximity of many sutures to the brain's venous sinuses, the rich blood supply of the scalp and cranium, and the relatively small size and blood volume of the patients undergoing this extensive surgery. Approximately 80% or more of vault remodeling operations historically require intraoperative allogeneic blood product transfusion [41]. Blood loss in craniosynostosis may be slow and insidious or sudden and acute. The successful management of clinically significant hemorrhage requires careful preparation, anticipation, knowledge of the surgical technique and plan, and hemovigilance [42, 43]. The percentage of total body blood volume lost increases with small children due to both their young age and lower weight. This is because the relatively large head creates an increased surface area for blood loss, and because the head has a proportionally greater percentage of blood volume [44].

Meticulous surgical technique is the first critical step in reducing perioperative blood loss and includes infiltration of the tissues with epinephrine and liberal cautery hemostasis remain core principles in conserving blood loss. Prolonged surgery of more than 5 hours increases blood volume loss. Surgical time can be rendered more efficient and decreased with preoperative planning involving three-dimensional models. There are surgical stages where sudden and extensive blood loss may occur. Knowledge of these stages and the surgeon's technique enables the anesthetist to predict and prepare for hemorrhage. The first stage is during initial scalp dissection and raising the periosteum. The second involves the bony work, less in the frontal–orbital advance-

Table 7.2 Multimodal perioperative pediatric patient blood conservation strategies

Preoperative	Intraoperative	Postoperative
Diagnosis and treat anemia at least 3–6 weeks before elective surgery (ideally within an anemia clinic setting). Consider cancelling elective major surgery to optimize hemoglobin in high-risk patients.	Careful blood pressure and fluid management (avoid hemodilution)	Tolerate anemia and consider non-transfusion methods to management
Stimulate erythropoiesis to maximize red blood cell mass	Restrictive transfusion strategy[a] guided by physiological parameters[b]	Restrictive transfusion strategy guided by physiological parameters
Implementation of PBM program	Goal-directed transfusion algorithms[c] with point of care testing[d]	Goal-directed transfusion algorithms with point of care testing
	Optimize hemostatic surgical technique[e]	Tolerate coagulopathy especially if patient not bleeding
	Antifibrinolytics	Antifibrinolytics
	Consider topical hemostatic agents[f]	Minimize iatrogenic blood loss and limit routine blood draws
	Consider recombinant coagulation products[g]	
	Autologous cell salvage	
	Consider normovolemic hemodilution	
	Maintain normothermia[h]	

[a]Restrictive transfusion strategy: In the majority of pediatric patients who are hemodynamically stable with Hgb > 7.0 g/dL, erythrocyte transfusion is advised against (1B). The exceptions are premature babies and cyanotic newborns [3, 8, 12]

[b]Physiological parameters include measures of oxygen delivery, consumption, end-organ perfusion such as serial/continuous measurements of oxygen delivery (DO_2), mixed venous oxygen saturation (SVO_2), lactate levels, cerebral and somatic regional oximetry (rSO_2) and NIRS (Near-infrared spectroscopy)and end-organ function/demand such as hemodynamic status non-invasive blood pressure (NIBP), pulse pressure variation (PPV), arterial blood pressure (ABP) respiratory support, severity of illness, nutritional status [8]

[c]Goal-directed transfusion protocols such as massive hemorrhage management pathways (Fig. 7.10) [3]

[d]Point-of-care testing includes viscoelastic testing such as thromboelastography (TEG) or thromboelastometry (ROTEM) [29]

[e]Optimizing surgical technique can include hemovigilance, local vasoconstrictors, meticulous surgical technique, cautery, minimally invasive surgery, preoperative surgical planning with 3D models, and preoperative embolization

[f]Topical coagulation products include gelatin sponges (*Gelfoam*), *Surgicel, Avitene*, topical thrombin preparations, fibrin glue/fibrin sealant (products that combine thrombin and fibrinogen, such as Crosseal, which contains fibrinogen, thrombin, and TXA, Floseal, and Evicel), and topical antifibrinolytics

[g]Recombinant coagulation products include fibrinogen concentrate and prothrombin complex concentrates

[h]For each decrease in temperature below 36 °C, there is a 10% increase in coagulopathy

ment procedures and more in the total calvarial remodeling ones.

In addition to the key stages associated with acute blood loss, the capacity for gradual but significant blood loss exists throughout the whole surgical procedure. It extends into the postoperative period [45]. Communication between the surgeon and anesthetist is vital, and a verbal warning as the key stages are approached ensures prompt management and close proximity of packed red blood cells (PRBCs).

During the intraoperative period, direct assessment of blood volume loss is difficult. The amount of blood collected in the suction is often minimal, with most blood lost to surgical drapes and the surrounding area. Therefore, calculating blood volume loss often depends upon assessing the volume of fluid resuscitation required and blood products transfused [46, 47]. Implementation of a well-structured multimodal anesthetic plan incorporating blood conservation techniques described herein is essential for the effective management of intraoperative bleeding during craniofacial surgeries in patients with Apert syndrome. Such an approach is pivotal to ensuring optimal outcomes and minimizing complications associated with these complex procedures (Table 7.2).

Management of Massive Hemorrhage

Massive blood loss is defined as:

1. The loss of one blood volume in 24 hours,
2. 50% loss of one blood volume in 3 hours,
3. Losses over 1.5 mL/kg/min for 20 minutes
4. A blood transfusion of over 40 mL/kg of red cells in 3 hours or
5. A blood transfusion at a rate of 10% of total blood volume every 10 minutes [48].

Major blood loss should be acknowledged early, and the shock and its consequences, such as coagulopathy, must be treated promptly. Massive transfusion is associated with coagulopathy secondary to tissue trauma, hypoperfusion, dilution and coagulation factors, and platelets consumption [49].

Dilution of coagulation factors and platelets is an important cause of coagulopathy in massively transfused patients [50]. Hemodilution induces interstitial edema, disruption of microcirculation, and oxygenation, resulting in acidosis [51].

Hypothermia-induced coagulopathy is attributed to platelet dysfunction, reduced coagulation factors activity, and induction of fibrinolysis [52]. Hypothermia induces platelet morphological changes and disrupts activation, adhesion, and aggregation. The enzyme cascade for coagulation factors is efficient if the temperature is above 35 °C; there is a 10% decrease in the coagulation factors activity per every one degree of temperature decrease. The effect of hypothermia on in vivo coagulation is usually underestimated because the evaluations of the conventional coagulation tests are done at 37 °C. In massively transfused patients, hypoperfusion and saline overdosing during resuscitation often induce acidosis [53]. Acidosis alters coagulation through various pathways: platelets change their structure and shape and become spherical and deprived of their pseudopods at a pH below 7.4. Factor VII bonding to tissue factor is decreased, and the coagulation factors' activity diminishes, resulting in lower thrombin generation, the main cause of coagulopathic bleeding. Moreover, acidosis leads to increased fibrin degradation, further worsening the coagulopathy. Anemia contributes to coagulopathy because the red blood cells induce the marginalization of platelets by enabling their binding to the endothelium. Moreover, the red blood cells modulate the biochemical and functional responses within the activated platelets. They support the generation of thrombin through the exposure of membrane pro-coagulating phospholipids, stimulate the release of alpha granules, and the platelet production of cyclooxygenase [54].

Optimal massive bleeding management in major surgery involving pediatric patients requires a comprehensive knowledge of their hemostatic system and of the disruptions in the coagulation system during the specific surgical procedure. Early intervention is a must to avoid any coagulopathy-triggering factors such as hypothermia, acidosis, and hemodilution.

Adequate blood loss replacement is essential to reduce morbidity and mortality in pediatric surgical patients with craniosynostosis. Readiness is of the essence in situations where massive bleeding is expected.

Complications of massive hemorrhage not only relate to the immediate concerns of hypovolemia but also the sequelae of incorrect replacement with crystalloids, colloids, and blood components. These sequelae include metabolic acidosis, dilutional coagulopathy, thrombocytopenia, hyperkalemia (from high potassium content of stored packed red blood cells), hypocalcemia (citrate toxicity), and hypothermia [55, 56].

Rapid administration of packed red blood cells with prolonged storage, particularly in the setting of hypovolemia, can result in hyperkalemic cardiac arrest [55–57].

The potassium concentration in a unit of packed red blood cells increases linearly with time. Blood irradiation drastically accelerates the transmembrane leakage of potassium from stored red blood cells. In an advisory statement, the Wake-up Safe group recommends using RBCs less than 7 days from collection or packed red blood cells that have been washed and resuspended in saline to minimize the risk of hyperkalemia in scenarios where massive hemorrhage is anticipated [57, 59].

Patient Blood Management

Allogeneic blood transfusion is associated with significant and well-known risks (https://www.shotuk.org/shot-reports). These include acute hemolytic reactions, transfusion-related acute lung injury, infection, along with the complications of massive transfusions, such as coagulopathy and electrolyte and acid-base disturbance. It has been reported that transfusion with all types of blood products was one of the independent predictors of adverse postoperative outcomes in terms of morbidity and length of hospital stay. Hospitalization costs were increased in transfused patients compared with non-transfused patients [59–61]. Transfusion-related acute lung injury (TRALI) has been the leading case of transfusion-related mortality in the US for the last decade, according to the US Food and Drug Administration. A previous report presented a case of TRALI in a pediatric spine surgical patient who received transfused leukoreduced red blood cells [63].

For these reasons, many strategies have been developed to decrease blood transfusion.

Patient blood management (PBM) is a personalized, evidence-based, multidisciplinary strategy to improve patient outcomes and reduce unnecessary exposure to blood and blood products [64, 65].

PBM can be defined in many ways and may consist of hundreds of single measures to improve patient safety. Traditionally, PBM is based on three pillars and is defined as:

1. The optimization of the endogenous red blood cell mass through the targeted management of anemia, stimulation of erythropoiesis, and the treatment of modifiable underlying disorders,
2. The minimization of diagnostic, interventional, and surgical blood loss to preserve the patient's own blood, and
3. The optimization of the patient-specific tolerance to anemia and coagulopathy through adherence to physiological transfusion thresholds.

PBM should be considered in all patients presenting for surgery, particularly those with a high potential for blood loss [39, 61, 62]. Implementing PBM strategies has been shown to decrease blood transfusion, morbidity and mortality, and hospital costs [66]. The World Health Organization has advocated for PBM implementation as a standard of care.

Hemoglobin and Transfusion Triggers

Anemia is a known predictor of higher transfusion needs and in-hospital mortality in pediatric surgery patients; thus, strategies to improve preoperative hemoglobin may significantly improve the patient outcome and reduce transfusion requirements [67]. Nearly 20% of children are reported to have anemia in industrialized countries, as compared to nearly 40–60% of children in low- and middle-income countries (LMICs) [68]. Iron deficiency is one of the most common causes of anemia in children. Iron deficiency is associated with adverse psychomotor, cognitive, and socio-emotional development in young children. Anemia in neonates and children is independently associated with a twofold increase in morbidity compared to matched cohorts undergoing non-cardiac surgery in the United States, independent of blood transfusions.

Furthermore, preoperative anemia is an independent predictor of intraoperative blood transfusion and is associated with postoperative complications, including increased mortality, increased length of stay in hospital and intensive care units, surgical site infections, and diminished quality of life. Expert consensus guidelines recommend screening for anemia at least 3–6 weeks before major elective surgery [69]. This allows time for targeted therapeutic strategies, such as iron supplementation (either oral or intravenous) and/or erythropoietin administration, to increase the child's own hematopoietic capacity before surgery. Australian National Health and Medical Research Council, in their Neonatal and Pediatrics PBM Guideline, recommends not to proceed with non-emergent major surgery until anemia is evaluated and treated [69].

The optimization of hematocrit (Hct) preoperatively includes diagnosing and treating preexisting anemia, iron supplementation, and erythropoietin. Recombinant human erythropoietin Alpha (EPO) can be administered before surgery to increase red blood cell production and theoretically reduce the need for allogenic transfusion. EPO is one of the most widely studied approaches to blood conservation in craniofacial surgery [70]. Drawbacks of EPO include considerations regarding cost, as well as the need for multiple preoperative visits that require bloodwork and parenteral administration of the medication.

Several studies have reported improved outcomes with preoperative EPO administration; however, dosing varied in amount and frequency from 300 to 600 U/kg subcutaneously weekly, typically for 3–8 weeks [71]. Some of these studies included adjunctive ferrous sulfate supplementation (2–6 mg/kg/d), B12 vitamin, E vitamin, and folic acid as part of their EPO protocol. Thus, strong evidence supports the utilization of preoperative EPO with elemental iron supplementation in children undergoing craniosynostosis surgery. EPO given subcutaneously weekly for 3–8 weeks before the surgery, along with supplemental iron, folic acid, B12 vitamin, and E vitamin, can markedly increase the preoperative Hct by 28–56% and decrease transfusion requirements [70–72].

Blood transfusion is a precious resource and can be life and limb saving. PBM strategies include managing blood transfusion toward the "right component, in the right dose, to the right patient, at the right time, for the right reason." Lacroix and colleagues published a landmark multicenter randomized control trial in pediatric intensive care patients (TRIPICU) that compared a restrictive (Hgb < 7.0 g/dL) versus a liberal (Hgb < 9.5 g/dL) transfusion strategy in critically ill children with the primary outcome designated as new or progressive multiorgan failure [74]. This trial demonstrated that the restrictive transfusion strategy was as safe as the liberal transfusion strategy, but red blood cell transfusions were halved in the restrictive transfusion group.

It must be remembered that a restrictive transfusion threshold must be maintained throughout the perioperative period. There is no evidence that transfusion benefits a hemodynamically stable patient unless the hemoglobin is less than 7 g/dL [75]. The evidence is less clear for unstable patients, bleeding patients, and patients with cyanotic heart disease; some clinical judgment is required.

So then, when should we transfuse? A threshold of 7 g/dL should be used in a stable child undergoing craniofacial surgery without major comorbidity or ongoing blood loss. This restrictive transfusion practice has no association with increased adverse outcomes and is associated with reduced blood use [76]. Decisions to transfuse should also anticipate any further drop in hemoglobin, especially if frequent monitoring is not possible.

The hemoglobin concentration is not the only consideration in whether a blood transfusion is required. During active blood loss, it is helpful to calculate the point at which blood transfusion is required. This includes an appreciation of how blood volume varies with age: a neonate has a circulating volume of 90 mL/kg, an infant 75–80 mL/kg, and a child 70–75 mL/kg. This allows a calculation of the volume at which a patient has lost a certain percentage of their circulating volume and to appreciate how small volumes may mean significant blood loss.

Goal-Directed Massive Hemorrhage and Massive Transfusion Protocols

Blood is an indispensable resource, yet it is becoming increasingly scarce. At the same time, the transfusion of foreign blood is associated with risks for recipients if there is inadequate indication for its use. For this reason, a rational approach to the use of allogeneic blood transfusions is recommended in all areas of medicine and encouraged by the World Health Organization (WHO).

Implementation of standardized transfusion protocols is a simple, inexpensive, and effective strategy to minimize transfusion safely. Moreover, there is a body of scientific evidence demonstrating efficacy. Standardized transfusion thresholds have been shown to reduce red blood cell transfusion without an increased incidence of adverse events in adult patients, critically ill children, and pediatric postoperative patients. Transfusion protocols have been recommended for pediatric craniofacial surgery. Restrictive transfusion strategies are alternatives to liberal practices to reduce transfusion rates (Fig. 7.10) [74–76].

The European Society of Anesthesiology and Intensive Care's (ESAIC) guidelines for severe perioperative bleeding, revised in 2022, advise against transfusion if the child is hemodynamically stable and the Hgb concentration is at least 7 g/dL [76, 78]. The decision to transfuse red blood cell concentrates should not only be based on laboratory results but should also depend on the child's clinical condition and take the risks and advantages of transfusion into account.

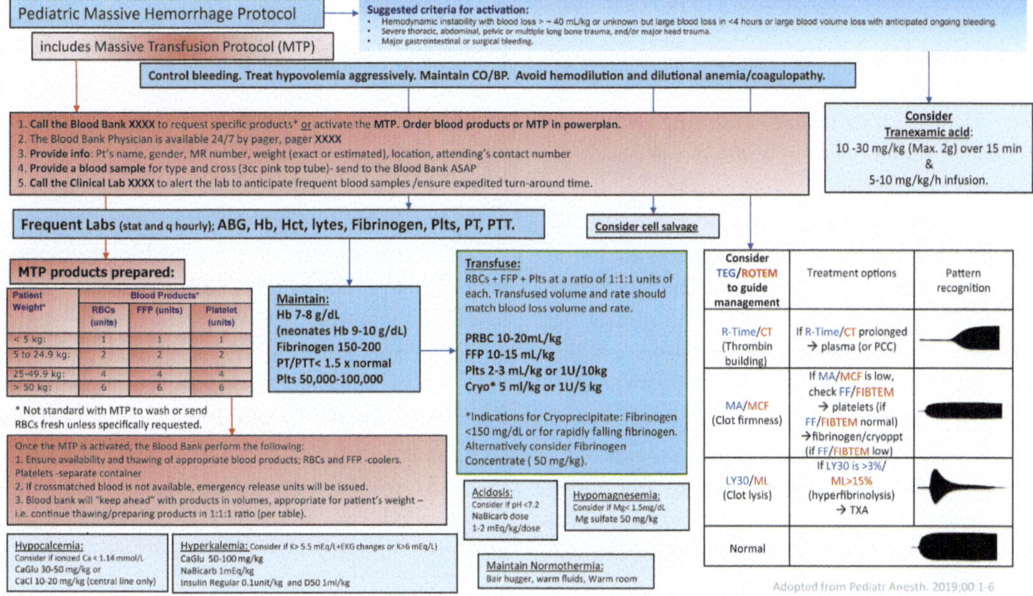

Fig. 7.10 Boston Children's Hospital Massive Hemorrhage Protocol

Identification of "safe" hemoglobin thresholds for children is extremely important in practical anesthesia and perioperative medicine. A transfusion decision should never be made solely based on the Hgb value, and this is especially true for pediatric patients. Oxygen supply and demand, lactate levels, regional oxygen saturation, and hemodynamic and respiratory status should, together with other parameters, be considered as part of the decision-making process.

In children with hemorrhagic shock, it is recommended to transfuse red blood cells, plasma, and platelets empirically in ratios between 2:1:1 and 1:1:1 until the bleeding is no longer life-threatening.

Therapeutic plasma administration is indicated for active bleeding with coagulopathy, along with abnormal point-of-care viscoelastic testing (VET) and a perioperative increase in activated partial thromboplastin time (aPTT and PT). Plasma is an essential component of massive transfusion in massive bleeding. Regardless of age and laboratory parameters, therapeutic plasma should not be administered as protection against bleeding except before major surgery and for severe coagulation imbalance. Its prophylactic administration, such as correcting laboratory abnormalities, is contraindicated. Plasma should not be used for volume replacement.

The decision to transfuse platelets should be based on the platelet count and function in point-of-care VET, as well as the patient's clinical status. Platelet transfusion volume should be calculated based on weight and desired increase in platelet increment.

Hypofibrinogenemia is a significant risk factor for bleeding in clinical settings, including pediatric surgery. Fibrinogen reference ranges are 150–300 mg/dL in infants and newborns, and some studies recommend keeping levels at least around 150–200 mg/dL for craniofacial surgeries [79, 80].

The decision to supplement fibrinogen firstly relies on adequate measurement of fibrinogen. There are many pitfalls around the optimal fibrinogen measurement in children. Cryoprecipitate and fibrinogen concentrate both effectively restore fibrinogen levels, but each product has its own set of advantages and constraints specific to its use in children. In children, dosing for therapeutic cryoprecipitate indications should be calculated considering the child's weight. Most pediatric transfusion guidelines dose cryoprecipitate based on the child's weight as a single variable. Many advise doses of 5–10 mL/kg, with exceptions of 20 mL/kg, for treating congenital fibrinogen deficiency with pathogen-reduced cryoprecipitate. Fibrinogen concentrate is dosed by most clinical guidelines from 50 to 70 mg/kg. There remains considerable uncertainty in children of all ages around optimal fibrinogen levels and the best fibrinogen replacement strategies [49, 81, 82].

Pediatric patients with massive hemorrhage or active critical bleeding should be managed with a goal-directed massive hemorrhage protocol, which may include a ratio-driven, balanced resuscitation strategy until the child is stabilized and the bleeding is controlled [83]. These recommendations exclude patients with acute brain injury, oncologic disease, stem cell transplantation, sickle cell anemia, severe acute respiratory distress syndrome, mechanical support, or cardiac disease, all of whom may require a higher hemoglobin level.

Evidence for the use of prothrombin complex concentrate (PCC) in pediatrics is weak. PCC contains factors II, VII, IX, and X, the vitamin K-dependent factors, and can be given to pediatric patients undergoing invasive surgery who are receiving vitamin K antagonists. There is no evidence of efficacy, safety, or dosing of PCCs in pediatric patients [84]. The use of PCCs is reported in cardiac surgery with cardiopulmonary bypass.

Transfusion guidelines for all blood components should be weight and age-appropriate, based on laboratory and physiologic/clinical criteria. When supported by published evidence and expert consensus, restrictive transfusion thresholds should be used for allogeneic red blood cell transfusion. The decision to transfuse fresh frozen plasma, platelets, and cryoprecipitate should be based on the etiology of the coagulopathy, clinical bleeding, and point-of-care VET [85].

Viscoelastic Testing

Viscoelastic hemostatic assays, such as thromboelastography (TEG) and rotational thromboelastometry (ROTEM), have undergone renewed interest and use since their initial description in the 1950s. Viscoelastic testing (VET) assays analyze the viscoelastic properties of clot formation and fibrinolysis in real-time, including the contribution of platelets and fibrinogen platelets to coagulation.

Point-of-care VET allows the anesthesia team to track hemostatic derangements, guiding the point of care, goal-directed management of coagulation, and targeted transfusion of the hemostatic blood components (fresh frozen plasma, cryoprecipitate, and/ recombinant products such as fibrinogen concentrate or prothrombin complex concentrates) [86]. Goal-directed bleeding management protocols based on VET benefit hemostatic management of the bleeding pedaitric patient.. The use of a VET-based transfusion algorithm should be considered for surgical procedures associated with a high bleeding risk (e.g., liver transplant, neuro craniofacial, spine, and cardiac surgeries) as well as in pediatric trauma. VET guided management for major craniofacial surgeries within a perioperative bleeding management protocol has been reported to be associated with a reduction/elminication in the transfusion of platelets and plasma (as no deterioration in MCF and CT), while hypofibrinogenemia (as assessed by low FIBTEM™ results) was the only consistently reported abnormal finding being effectively treated by administering fibrinogen concentrate. Employing a goal directed VET protocol has also been reported to be associated with a reduction in total costs for perioperative bleeding management in this patient population [87].

Cell Salvage

Intraoperative blood salvage (IOBS) allows blood lost from a surgical procedure to be transfused back to the patient perioperatively. This technique is alternatively known in the literature as autologous blood transfusion, cell salvage, or autotransfusion, and has become widely used in large-volume blood loss procedures [88]. The goal of IOBS is to mitigate the need for allogeneic (homologous) blood transfusions, which are well-known to be associated with adverse effects. The Association of Anesthetists consensus statement recommends that IOBS be considered if the anticipated blood loss is >8 mL/kg in children weighing >10 kg. IOBS has been shown to reduce allogeneic transfusions in pediatric surgery for craniosynostosis, scoliosis, and congenital cardiac disease.

The use of IOBS appears to be a safe option during the surgical management of craniosynostosis. With pediatric-specific parameters and smaller collection bowls, homologous transfusions can be minimized, avoiding associated risks [89].

IOBS is a technique that may reduce transfusions in infant craniofacial surgery. The machines used require small initial volumes for processing and can subsequently process blood as it is recovered. In prospective randomized controlled trials, IOBS has significantly reduced red blood cell transfusions in cardiac and non-cardiac surgeries in infants and children [88].

Antifibrinolytics

Inhibition of fibrinolysis is imperative to minimize perioperative blood loss and avoid unnecessary allogeneic blood component transfusion. Tranexamic acid (TXA) is the most common antifibrinolytic used worldwide, and it has proven efficacy [90]. Major pediatric surgeries are recommended to decrease blood loss as part of a comprehensive perioperative blood management protocol. Prophylactic administration of TXA is essential to an effective perioperative PBM strategy and expert consensus guidelines [47, 91].

Antifibrinolytic drugs such as TXA are synthetic lysine analogs that competitively inhibit plasminogen activation to plasmin, thus preventing fibrinolysis [92]. TXA may also have anti-inflammatory effects by reducing vasoactive peptide release [93]. At higher doses, TXA is a direct inhibitor of plasmin and, consequently, an indirect inhibitor of all pathways activated by plasmin (e.g., platelets, complement, inflammation) [94]. It is excreted in the urine largely unchanged, with filtration inversely proportional to plasma creatinine. Large doses of TXA have the potential to promote thrombosis and, due to its ability to pass the blood-brain barrier, can cause central nervous system hyperexcitability (seizures) by blocking the action of the inhibitory neurotransmitters gamma-aminobutyric acid and glycine [95, 96].

A multicenter observational study from the Pediatric Craniofacial Collaborative Group reviewed 1814 patients from 33 institutions across the US and Canada and found that TXA was associated with a 50% reduction in the odds of requiring blood transfusion and a 37% reduction in the odds of a major postoperative complication. TXA is effective across all craniosynostosis procedures but is particularly important in open vault remodeling operations, as it reduces hematological complications, transfusion incidence and volume, and overall complications [97].

The use of antifibrinolytics has emerged as a safe and effective prophylactic method of minimizing perioperative blood loss and transfusion requirements in pediatric patients undergoing craniosynostosis surgery [98]. Recent studies have shown that a low-dose TXA regimen is equally effective and safe [99]. Based on pharmacokinetic studies, a TXA dose between 10–30 mg/kg loading dose and 5–10 mg/kg/h maintenance infusion rate to maintain plasma concentrations between the 20 and 70 mg/mL range may be considered as a target for pediatric trauma and surgery [90, 98–100].

Absolute contraindications for antifibrinolytics include known hypersensitivity, active thromboembolic disease, and fibrinolytic conditions with consumption coagulopathy [94]. Relative contraindications include renal impairment (dose adjustment), disorders of thrombosis, preexisting coagulopathy, or the use of oral anticoagulants. TXA is not contraindicated in children with a seizure disorder, given the growing evidence supporting the safety profile of therapeutic dosing regimens. TXA-associated seizures have been reported in high-risk pediatric cardiac surgery patients with high doses (e.g., 100 mg/kg) [95]. The reported TXA-associated seizure incidence for non-cardiac pediatric surgery is extremely low. In pediatric craniofacial surgery, the incidence of seizures with antifibrinolytics is comparable to the incidence reported in children not exposed to TXA.

Acute Normovolemic Hemodilution

Acute normovolemic hemodilution (ANH) is an operative blood conservation technique involving the removal and storage of patient blood after the induction of anesthesia, with the maintenance of normovolemia by crystalloid and/or colloid replacement. ANH has also been reported in pediatric cardiac, scoliosis, craniofacial, maxillofacial, and liver transplant surgeries, in which high blood loss is anticipated [101–104].

While there is no standardized approach to pediatric ANH, generally, blood is removed in proportion to the patient's starting Hct and replaced with crystalloid or colloid to achieve a goal Hct of 20–25%. Exact recommendations for hemodilution targets and fluid replacement ratios should consider individual patient and surgical characteristics and vary widely between patients and surgeries.

ANH could be considered when high blood loss is anticipated or when other PBM strategies cannot reasonably be pursued due to patient issues (such as a difficult cross-match) or institutional barriers.

A known limitation of ANH is the requirement to have a robust starting red blood cell mass and the need to anticipate high blood loss, which makes it not conducive to surgical emergencies. Furthermore, this strategy may be inappropriate for patients who are intolerant of rapid fluid shifts or have low oxygen-carrying capacity. ANH may be unsafe in severely dehydrated patients, patients with significant baseline anemia or other hematologic disorders such as sickle cell anemia, infants with small blood volumes, and patients with cardiac or pulmonary disease. Finally, ANH is more labor-intensive for the anesthesia team than traditional transfusion and requires additional expertise, equipment, and preparation.

Because ANH has fallen out of vogue over the past decades, a now common barrier to the utilization of ANH in appropriate patients is a lack of institutional experience and guidelines. A pediatric-specific ANH protocol should be developed within institutions to help guide clinicians, which has been based on and extrapolated from published guidelines from the Association for the Advancement of Blood and Biotherapies [106]. While overall transfusion goals can be borrowed from established protocols, each institution must address its own specific strategy, which includes standardized blood storage equipment and methodology, transfusion goals, and ongoing quality improvement surveillance. This process is likely best navigated via multidisciplinary conversations between anesthesiologists, surgeons, and hematologists with expertise in blood banking or conservation.

Postoperative Blood Conservation

Many intraoperative PBM strategies can also be applied to the postoperative period depending on the etiology of the patient's anemia, bleeding diathesis, and/or hemostatic imbalance. Postoperative blood conservation measures include minimizing blood loss, using TXA, using small-volume phlebotomy tubes, point-of-care devices, closed sampling systems, and eliminating "standing daily" laboratory orders.

Anemia should be managed first by non-transfusion therapeutic preventive and treatment modalities, including limiting further blood loss and providing the substrates needed for hematopoiesis and clotting factor production such as Iron, EPO, and vitamins and minerals (B12 and K) and folate. The goal is to harness and maximize the patient's physiological tolerance of anemia and coagulopathy by promoting optimal pulmonary and cardiac function while considering restrictive transfusion thresholds. While there are many trials supporting the idea that restrictive Hgb thresholds (Hgb >7 g/dL in the absence of comorbidities) are non-inferior or superior to liberal thresholds (Hgb >9 g/dL) across a wide variety of clinical scenarios, strategies should move away from a Hgb threshold. Instead, the physiological status of the individual patient should guide decision-making.

Besides minimizing loss, adapting restrictive thresholds for both hemoglobin and coagulation derangements would be very effective in minimizing transfusion without increasing adverse events. This practice is further supported by the published decision trees recommended by The Pediatric Critical Care Transfusion and Anemia Expertise Initiative Consensus (TAXI) and the TAXI-Control Avoidance of Bleeding (TAXI-CAB) [107].

Furthermore, iatrogenic or hospital-induced anemia in the postoperative period is an area that has the most opportunity for improvement and best practice quality improvement initiatives. Routine phlebotomy is a common and preventable cause of hospital-acquired anemia and a modifiable blood transfusion risk factor. The importance of iatrogenic anemia is even more relevant in the pediatric population when adult-size tubes are often used, despite the availability of microtubes that would allow for a smaller volume of blood. Unnecessary phlebotomy reduces hemoglobin levels and may unnecessarily trigger red blood cell transfusions based on a numeric threshold despite adequate oxygen-carrying capacity. Routine frequent blood draws should be avoided, and if necessary, laboratory investigations should be consolidated when appropriate, using minimal volume withdrawal and closed loop collecting systems.

Metabolic Disturbance

The metabolic disturbance that occurs during the perioperative period for pediatric craniofacial surgery in terms of acid–base and electrolyte derangement is primarily related to significant blood loss and the resultant transfusion of crystalloid and colloid (including blood products).

Mannitol 20% should not be a strategy in Apert craniofacial surgeries despite routine clinical use in lowering ICP for states of traumatic brain injury [108, 109]. Cerebral salt wasting syndrome (CSW) is common in craniosynostosis surgery, a condition that presents with hyponatremia due to renal loss of sodium and has not been defined clearly yet [110]. Mannitol may worsen hyponatremia as well as hemodilution, resulting in an altered coagulation state.

In summary, careful attention should be paid to postoperative electrolyte disturbances, particularly hyponatremia [111]. This may be related partly to the use of crystalloid infusions intraoperatively and also to inappropriate antidiuretic hormone release (SIADH) as a result of the surgical insult or raised intracranial pressure [112]. A retrospective record review of patients developing hyponatremia post-craniosynostosis surgery suggested that patients at increased risk of this complication included those with preoperative raised ICP, increased volume blood transfusion, and female sex (regardless of ICP). The use of hyponatremic fluids or mannitol intraoperatively further increases the risk. It is important to differentiate hyponatremia due to SIADH or CSW because treatment is the opposite for each of them; SIADH needs fluid restriction, whereas CSW needs fluid and electrolyte resuscitation [113, 114].

Venous Air Embolism

A surgical osteotomy at a level above the heart creates a potential risk of venous air embolism. A VAE begins with the entrainment of air/air bubbles into the patient's venous system (usually via surgically exposed venous sinuses), traveling to the right side of the heart, essentially preventing the normal circulation of blood due to "mechanical" obstruction. The blood can enter either through veins or venous channels in the bones, but not on the arterial side where the pressures are much higher. Risk factors for this phenomenon include operating in regions of the body that are elevated above the heart, operating in the setting of blood loss and hypovolemia where central venous pressures are low, and operating around enlarged exposed area of bone. In order of clinical severity: Grade 1 VAE is defined as a subjective *millwheel murmur* heard on precordial Doppler as turbulent flow detected during systole. Grade 2 VAE is defined as a decrease/loss of the expired end-tidal carbon dioxide measurement due to obstruction of flow in the pulmonary vasculature and failure of the lungs to clear CO_2. Grade 3 VAE is defined as tachycardia and hypotension. Grade 4 VAE is the most serious with complete cardiovascular collapse.

Many centers routinely monitor for a VEA in high-risk cases by using a precordial Doppler placed on the chest over the right side of the heart. The incidence of venous air embolism during cranial vault reconstruction has historically been as high as 83%. However, most episodes are clinically silent and not associated with hemodynamic compromise. Venous air embolism can also occur during endoscopic procedures; however, the reported incidence is much lower (8%) and is infrequently associated with hemodynamic instability [109, 115]. Prevention and early detection are key. The use of precordial Doppler is routine in most centers. Controlled hypotension should be avoided, as decreased venous pressures make air entry into the venous system more likely to occur. Providing good surgical hemostasis, avoiding hypovolemia, knowledge of emergency responses including flooding the surgical field with saline, and, in the most extreme cases, providing cardiovascular support are management strategies every anesthesiologist should be aware of.

Anesthetic Considerations for Postoperative Care

All children who have had a craniotomy as part of their procedure are typically admitted to the ICU postoperatively [45]. Infants who may require postoperative intubation and mechanical ventilation include those in the prone position for lengthy procedures with significant facial swelling and infants with syndromic craniosynostosis who have significant preoperative obstructive sleep apnea. Otherwise, immediate extubation can be considered the standard of care with the potential need for oxygen supplementation and/or CPAP for obstructive sleep apnea management. Attention to serum biochemistry and hematology is imperative during the initial postoperative period. Blood conservation techniques should be considered including non-transfusion management of anemia (po or iv Iron), following restrictive transfusion strategies, continuing tranexamic acid postoperatively and goal-directed transfusion management. Of particular importance is the risk of hyponatremia, which is present after any major pediatric surgery but may be increased after craniofacial surgery. The cause of hyponatremia is likely to be related to anti-diuretic syndrome secretion or administration of hypotonic intravenous fluids. The risks of hyponatremia include cerebral edema, seizures, and death; low sodium-containing intravenous fluids should be avoided [116].

The patient should be monitored postoperatively for signs of airway obstruction. A nasopharyngeal airway may be required to alleviate supraglottic obstruction in the postoperative period, although it may be difficult to place due to the reduced nasopharyngeal volume.

Implementing an ambulatory protocol for minor procedures such as cleft lip and palate surgery is considered adequate [117]. Nowadays, with the endoscopic treatment of craniosynostosis, the in-hospital period is typically one day [118, 119].

Perioperative Pain Management

Craniosynostosis can be corrected through craniotomies and cranioplasties, which are invasive and painful procedures due to the extensive handling of the scalp and periosteum. Postoperative analgesia following open craniosynostosis repair is considered a challenge among plastic and reconstructive surgeons. There is a persistent problem with pediatric patients suffering from acute post-surgical pain that is poorly treated. Although numerous studies describe the etiology, evaluation, and treatment of craniosynostosis, few describe its pain management, even though some studies indicate a high prevalence of moderate-to-severe pain postoperatively [120].

Currently, there is no standard protocol for managing perioperative pain associated with craniosynostosis repair. Several studies have shown that steroids can be used preoperatively to reduce postoperative pain as a secondary benefit, along with other benefits such as reducing facial edema, reducing postoperative ecchymosis, and improving nausea and vomiting.

Craniotomy-related pain is mainly caused by skin incisions and muscle breaks rather than the operation on the brain parenchyma. The scalp is mainly innervated by the trigeminal nerve and the second and third cervical nerve roots. The sensory nerves in the head that are more commonly chosen for clinical block include the supraorbital nerve, supratrochlear nerve, auriculotemporal nerve, greater occipital nerve, and lesser occipital nerve. Therefore, using scalp nerve blocks in pediatric craniotomy can reduce intraoperative stress while providing some postoperative analgesia and helping speed up postoperative recovery. Scalp nerve blocks have been reported to be adjuncts to traditional postoperative analgesia and as interventions for reducing intraoperative blood loss.

Scalp nerve blocks may suppress the conduction of peripheral pain signals to the central nervous system and reduce the amount of perioperative opioids with no adverse effects (such as nausea or drowsiness). Since cranial suture reconstruction requires a long incision and may induce severe pain, ultrasound-guided scalp nerve block with general anesthesia may be employed in children with craniosynostosis who are receiving cranial suture reconstruction. A preoperative scalp nerve block may also attenuate hemodynamic fluctuation and is more effective for postoperative analgesia, which promotes postoperative recovery [121].

An infraorbital nerve block is recommended for lip surgery [120, 122] (Fig. 7.11). It is possible to perform the ultrasound-guided suprazygomatic maxillary nerve block for cleft palate and major craniofacial procedures with

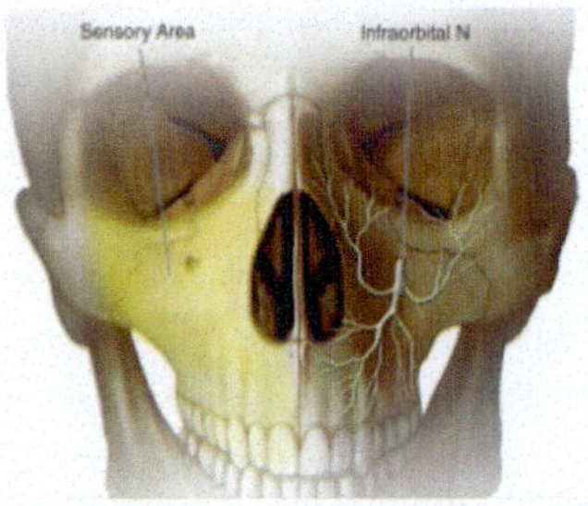

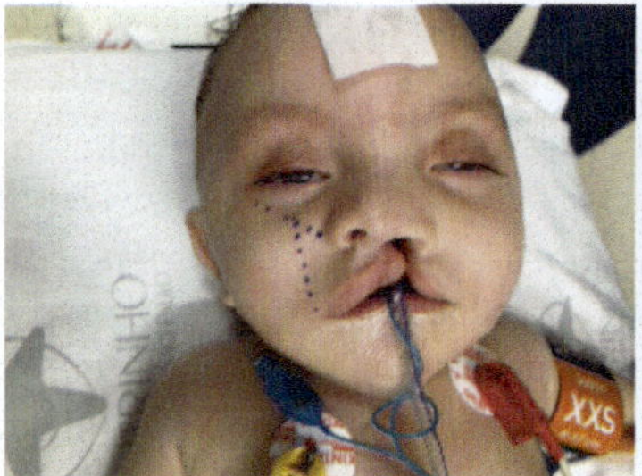

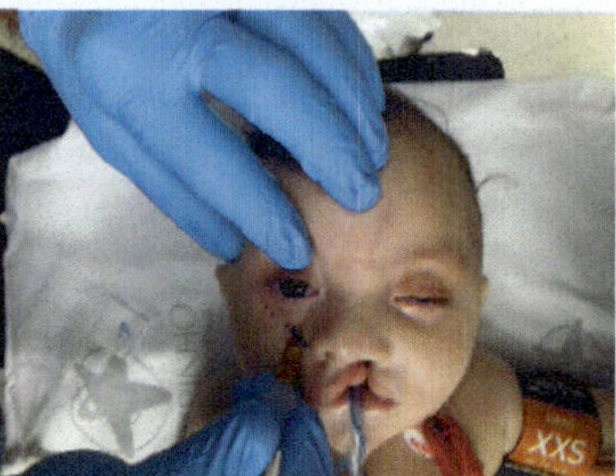

Fig. 7.11 Infraorbital nerve block

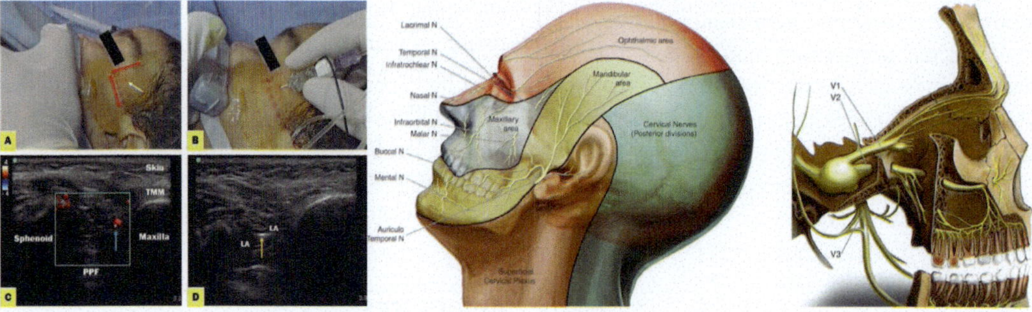

Fig. 7.12 Ultrasound-guided suprazygomatic maxillary nerve block. (Left figure from Mansour and Abdelghany [124], middle and right figures from: "Nysora.com", NYSORA, Inc (The New York School of Regional Anesthesia), 2585 Broadway, Suite 183, New York, NY 10025, USA)

satisfactory postoperative analgesia [121–124] (Fig. 7.12). Some other techniques, such as transversus abdominal plane block (TAP Block) and erector spine plane block, are effective for analgesia of donation areas in case of intercostal or iliac bone grafts [126]. In Apert syndactyly surgery, it is possible to perform an ultrasound-guided infraclavicular brachial plexus block for pain control [127, 128].

As for postoperative analgesia, most studies used multimodal analgesia, with opioids (e.g., Morphine, Tramadol) and acetaminophen, nonsteroidal anti-inflammatory drugs (NSAIDs), and gabapentin. Morphine is the most commonly used opioid as a single treatment, in combination with NSAIDs or acetaminophen. According to the results of this systematic review, the authors suggest the following: first, the use of opioids in combination with ketorolac, as it is found to have the shortest length of hospitalization and the lowest dose of opioids to control the pain. Second, scalp nerve blocks should be added to the intraoperative regimen as it is found to limit narcotic use postoperatively [129].

The known side effects of opioids range from nausea, vomiting, and urinary retention to more serious adverse effects such as respiratory depression, oversedation, and hypotension. Dexmedetomidine has been used in some studies with good results as a substitute for opioids to minimize these effects [129].

Conclusion

Children with Apert syndrome undergoing diagnostic and surgical procedures of varied complexity present unique perioperative and anesthetic management challenges. Preoperative optimization is imperative and includes timely management of modifiable risk factors such as anemia and comorbidities before elective procedures. Intraoperative considerations include airway management, difficult intravenous access, managing respiratory comorbidities, and using hemostatic measures to decrease blood loss. Employing optimal hemodynamic and blood conservation strategies to minimize blood transfusion and preserve vital organ function is paramount. Herein contemporary perioperative evidence-based management strategies are outlined for the high-risk patient with Apert syndrome. Ultimately patent care benefits from the mastery of teamwork; consisting of familiar and solid anesthesia, surgical and nursing teams working together to deliver compassionate, effective, and safe care.

References

1. Das S, Munshi A. Research advances in Apert syndrome. J Oral Biol Craniofac Res. 2018;8:194–9.
2. Breik O, Mahindu A, Moore MH, Molloy CJ, Santoreneos S, David DJ. Central nervous system and cervical spine abnormalities in Apert syndrome. Childs Nerv Syst. 2016;32:833–8.
3. Willie D, Holmes G, Jabs EW, Wu M. Cleft palate in Apert syndrome. J Dev Biol. 2022; https://doi.org/10.3390/jdb10030033.
4. Wenger TL, Hing AV, Evans KN, Adam MP, Feldman J, Mirzaa GM. Apert syndrome. In: Gene reviews. Seattle: University of Washington; 2019. p. 1993–2024.
5. González DG, Giraldo MZ. Sedation in pediatrics. Revista Chilena de Anestesia. 2023;52:244–50.
6. Wadod MA, Aboelazm OM, El Rawas MM. Effect of laryngeal mask airway on image quality in pediatric patients undergoing brain magnetic resonance imaging: a randomized controlled trial. Anesth Pain Med. 2023;13(2):e129532. https://doi.org/10.5812/aapm-129532.
7. Raposo-Amaral CE, Denadai R, de Oliveira YM, Ghizoni E, Raposo-Amaral CA. Apert syndrome management: changing treatment algorithm. J Craniofac Surg. 2020;31:648–52.
8. Fadda M, Ierardo G, Ladniak B, et al. Treatment timing and multidisciplinary approach in Apert syndrome. Ann Stomatol. 2015;6:58–63.
9. Garcia-Marcinkiewicz AG, Stricker PA. Craniofacial surgery and specific airway problems. Paediatr Anaesth. 2020;30:296–303.
10. Kumar N, Arora S, Bindra A, Goyal K. Anesthetic management of craniosynostosis repair in patient with Apert syndrome. Saudi J Anaesth. 2014;8:399–401.
11. Mangal H, Santlani P. Anesthetic management of craniosynostosis repair in a 13-month-old boy with Apert syndrome. Indian J Case Rep. 2021;7:214–6.
12. Dobson G, Chau A, Denomme J, et al. Guidelines to the practice of anesthesia: revised edition 2023. Can J Anesth. 2023;70:16–55.
13. Faraoni D, Dinardo JA, Goobie SM. Relationship between preoperative anemia and in-hospital mortality in children undergoing noncardiac surgery. Anesth Analg. 2016;123:1582–7.
14. Meyer HM, Torborg A, Cronje L, et al. The association between preoperative anemia and postoperative morbidity in pediatric surgical patients: a secondary analysis of a prospective observational cohort study. Paediatr Anaesth. 2020;30:759–65.
15. Stricker PA, Goobie SM, Cladis FP, Haberkern CM, Meier PM, Reddy SK, Nguyen TT, Cai L, Polansky M, Szmuk P. Perioperative outcomes and management in pediatric complex cranial vault reconstruction: a multicenter study from the Pediatric Craniofacial Collaborative Group. Anesthesiology. 2017;126:276–87.
16. Karnik P, Dave NM, Sayed M. Anesthesia management in craniosynostosis surgery: a retrospective, single-center experience. J Res Innov Anesth. 2021;6:27–30.
17. Bansal T, Jaiswal R, Hooda S, Mangla P. Apert syndrome: anaesthetic concerns and challenges. Egypt J Anaesth. 2015;31:85–7.
18. Purwoko P, Azhar A, Permana SA. Difficult airway management in Apert syndrome for maxillofacial reconstruction: a case report. Anaesth Pain Intensive Care. 2022;26:119–22.
19. Sinha S, Kadni RR, Chakravarthy J, Zachariah V. Anaesthetic management and literature review of syndromic craniosynostosis in infants-a case series. J Clin Diagn Res. 2022; https://doi.org/10.7860/jcdr/2022/50287.16236.
20. Brandao MM, Tonello C, Parizotto I, Machado LB, Alonso N. Analysis of intracranial pressure waveform using a non-invasive method in individuals with craniosynostosis. Childs Nerv Syst. 2024;40:145–52.
21. Brandao Machado L, Brandao MM, Ferro A, Minei TSS, Gualberto IJN, Alonso N. Anesthesia for preoperative non-invasive intracranial pressure measurement in a child with Apert syndrome: a case report. Arch Pediatr Neurosurg. 2024; https://doi.org/10.46900/apn.v5i3.190.
22. Raj D, Luginbuehl I. Managing the difficult airway in the syndromic child. CEACCP. 2015;15:7–13.
23. Apfelbaum JL, Hagberg CA, Connis RT, et al. 2022 American Society of Anesthesiologists Practice Guidelines for management of the difficult airway. Anesthesiology. 2022;136:31–81.
24. Nargozian C. The airway in patients with craniofacial abnormalities. Paediatr Anaesth. 2004:53–9.
25. Forte AJ, Lu X, Hashim PW, Steinbacher DM, Alperovich M, Persing JA, Alonso N. Airway analysis in Apert syndrome. Plast Reconstr Surg. 2019;144:704–9.
26. Barnett S, Moloney C, Bingham R. Perioperative complications in children with Apert syndrome:

a review of 509 anesthetics. Paediatr Anaesth. 2011;21:72–7.
27. Glover CD, Fernandez AM, Huang H, et al. Perioperative outcomes and management in midface advancement surgery: a multicenter observational descriptive study from the Pediatric Craniofacial Collaborative Group. Paediatr Anaesth. 2018;28:710–8.
28. Roumeliotis G, Campbell S, Das S, Hildebrand GD, Charbel Issa P, Jayamohan J, Lawrence T, Magdum S, Wall S, Johnson D. Central retinal artery occlusion following prone transcranial surgery for craniosynostosis and discussion of risk factors. J Craniofac Surg. 2020;31:1597–601.
29. Soriano SG, Eldredge EA, Rockoff MA. Pediatric neuroanesthesia. Anesthesiol Clin North Am. 2002;20:389–404.
30. Li S, Luo Y, Deng J, Zeng J, Fan M, Wang T, Xia Q. Risk factors for central venous catheter-related thrombosis in hospitalized children: a single-center a retrospective cohort study. Transl Pediatr. 2022;11:1840–51.
31. Munshey F, Parra DA, McDonnell C, Matava C. Ultrasound-guided techniques for peripheral intravenous placement in children with difficult venous access. Paediatr Anaesth. 2020;30:108–15.
32. Heinrichs J, Fritze Z, Vandermeer B, Klassen T, Curtis S. Ultrasonographically guided peripheral intravenous cannulation of children and adults: a systematic review and meta-analysis. Ann Emerg Med. 2013; https://doi.org/10.1016/j.annemergmed.2012.11.014.
33. Samoya SW. Real time ultrasound guided peripheral vascular access in pediatric patients. Anesth Analg. 2010;111:823–5.
34. Thomas K, Hughes C, Johnson D, Das S. Anesthesia for surgery related to craniosynostosis: a review. Part 1. Paediatr Anaesth. 2012;22:1033–41.
35. Arnold RW. The oculocardiac reflex: a review. Clin Ophthalmol. 2021;15:2693–725.
36. Patel S, Barnacle A, Mailli L, Osborne S, Vahdani K, Ratnam L. The oculocardiac reflex: a rare but significant cardiovascular complication during percutaneous sclerotherapy of a retro-bulbar low flow venolymphatic malformation. Cardiovasc Intervent Radiol. 2023;46:411–3.
37. Beels M, Stevens S, Saldien V. Perioperative fluid management in children: an updated review. Acta Anaesth Bel. 2022;73(3):179–89.
38. Eaddy N, Watene C. Perioperative management of fluids and electrolytes in children. BJA Educ. 2023;23:273–8.
39. Pearson A, Matava CT. Anaesthetic management for craniosynostosis repair in children. BJA Educ. 2016;16:410–6.
40. Giraldo MZ. Pediatric perioperative bleeding -basic considerations. Rev Colomb Anestesiol. 2013;41:44–9.
41. Yuki K, Dinardo JA, Koutsogiannaki S. The role of anesthetic selection in perioperative bleeding. Biomed Res Int. 2021; https://doi.org/10.1155/2021/5510634.
42. Beethe AB, Spitznagel RA, Kugler JA, Goeller JK, Franzen MH, Hamlin RJ, Lockhart TJ, Lyden ER, Glogowski KR, Leriger MM. The road to transfusion-free craniosynostosis repair in children less than 24 months old: a quality improvement initiative. Pediatr Qual Saf. 2020; https://doi.org/10.1097/pq9.0000000000000331.
43. Goobie SM, Zurakowski D, Proctor MR, Meara JG, Meier PM, Young VJ, Rogers GF. Predictors of clinically significant postoperative events after open craniosynostosis surgery. Anesthesiology. 2015;122:1021–32.
44. Bonfield CM, Sharma J, Cochrane DD, Singhal A, Steinbok P. Minimizing blood transfusions in the surgical correction of craniosynostosis: a 10-year single-center experience. Childs Nerv Syst. 2016;32:143–51.
45. Goobie SM, Haas T. Bleeding management for pediatric craniotomies and craniofacial surgery. Paediatr Anaesth. 2014;24:678–89.
46. Wojciechowski PJ, Samol N, Walker J. Coagulopathy in massive transfusion. Int Anesthesiol Clin. 2005;43:01–20.
47. Giraldo MZ. Management of perioperative bleeding in children. Step by step review. Rev Colomb Anestesiol. 2013;41:50–6.
48. Maw G, Furyk C. Pediatric massive transfusion a systematic review. Pedriatic Emerg Care. 2018;34:594–8.
49. Warner DS, Bolliger D, Gö K, Tanaka KA. Pathophysiology and treatment of coagulopathy in massive hemorrhage and hemodilution. Anesthesiology. 2010;113(5):1205–19.
50. Pötzsch B, Ivaskevicius V. Haemostasis management of massive bleeding. Hamostaseologie. 2011;31:15–20.
51. Johansson PI, Ostrowski SR, Secher NH. Management of major blood loss: an update. Acta Anaesthesiol Scand. 2010;54:1039–49.
52. Thomas D, Wee M, Clyburn P, Walker I, Brohi K, Collins P, Doughty H, Isaac J, Mahoney PF, Shewry L. Blood transfusion and the anaesthetist: management of massive haemorrhage. In: Anaesthesia; 2010. p. 1153–61.
53. Lee AC, Reduque LL, Luban NLC, Ness PM, Anton B, Heitmiller ES. Transfusion-associated hyperkalemic cardiac arrest in pediatric patients receiving massive transfusion. Transfusion (Paris). 2014;54:244–54.
54. Sesok-Pizzini D, Pizzini MA. Hyperkalemic cardiac arrest in pediatric patients undergoing massive transfusion: unplanned emergencies. Transfusion (Paris). 2014;54:4–7.
55. Lee AC, Heitmiller ES. Preventing pediatric transfusion-associated incidents of hyperkalemic cardiac arrest a wake up safe quality improvement initiative; 2014.

56. Bhananker SM, Ramamoorthy C, Geiduschek JM, Posner KL, Domino KB, Haberkern CM, Campos JS, Morray JP. Anesthesia-related cardiac arrest in children: update from the pediatric perioperative cardiac arrest registry. Anesth Analg. 2007;105:344–50.
57. Strauss RG. Red blood cell storage and avoiding hyperkalemia from transfusions to neonates and infants. Transfusion (Paris). 2010;50:1862–5.
58. Kumba C, Cresci F, Picard C, Thiry C, Albinni S, Orliaguet G. Transfusion and Morbi-mortality factors: an observational descriptive retrospective pediatric cohort study. J Anesth Crit Care. 2017; https://doi.org/10.15406/jaccoa.2017.08.00315.
59. Kumba C. Transfusion in pediatric surgical settings: economic aspects and hospitalization costs. Acta Sci Paediatr. 2021;4:3–6.
60. Hicks K, Perez M, Ryan S, Spotts A. Neonatal sepsis in the emergency department. Curr Pediatr Res. 2019;23:20.
61. Goobie SM. A blood transfusion can save a child's life or threaten it. Paediatr Anaesth. 2015;25:1182–3.
62. Sullivan HC, Roback JD. The pillars of patient blood management: key to successful implementation (Article, p. 2840). Transfusion (Paris). 2019;59:2763–7.
63. Zacharowski K, Spahn DR. Patient blood management equals patient safety. Best Pract Res Clin Anaesthesiol. 2016;30:159–69.
64. Al-Mozain N, Arora S, Goel R, Pavenski K, So-Osman C. Patient blood management in adults and children: what have we achieved, and what still needs to be addressed? Transfus Clin Biol. 2023;30:355–9.
65. Evans S, Klein A, Pearce L, Boyd-Carson H, Anaemia Guideline Working Group. Guideline for the management of anaemia in the perioperative pathway; 2022.
66. Tan GM, Murto K, Downey LA, Wilder MS, Goobie SM. Error traps in pediatric patient blood management in the perioperative period. Paediatr Anaesth. 2023;33:609–19.
67. National Blood Authority. Patient blood management guidelines. Module 6. Neonatal and paediatrics; 2016.
68. Coombs DM, Knackstedt R, Patel N. Optimizing blood loss and management in craniosynostosis surgery: a systematic review of outcomes over the last 40 years. Cleft Palate Craniofac J. 2023;60:1632–44.
69. Aljaaly HA, Aldekhayel SA, Diaz-Abele J, Karunanayka M, Gilardino MS. Effect of erythropoietin on transfusion requirements for craniosynostosis surgery in children. J Craniofac Surg. 2017;28:1315–9.
70. Kurlander DE, Ascha M, Marshall DC, et al. Impact of multidisciplinary engagement in a quality improvement blood conservation protocol for craniosynostosis. J Neurosurg Pediatr. 2020;26:406–14.
71. dos Santos AA, de Castro AJM, Soriano S. Tratamento de anemia e diretrizes para terapia com eritropoietina. World Health Organization (WHO); 2021. p. 01–9.
72. Lacroix J, Hébert PC, Hutchison JS, et al. Transfusion strategies for patients in pediatric intensive care units. N Engl J Med. 2007;356:1609–19.
73. Goobie SM, Gallagher T, Gross I, Shander A. Society for the advancement of blood management administrative and clinical standards for patient blood management programs. 4th edition (pediatric version). Paediatr Anaesth. 2019;29:231–6.
74. Downey LA, Goobie SM. Perioperative pediatric erythrocyte transfusions: incorporating hemoglobin thresholds and physiologic parameters in decision-making. Anesthesiology. 2022;137:604–19.
75. Stricker PA, Fiadjoe JE, Kilbaugh TJ, Pruitt EY, Taylor JA, Bartlett SP, McCloskey JJ. Effect of transfusion guidelines on postoperative transfusion in children undergoing craniofacial reconstruction surgery. Pediatr Crit Care Med. 2012; https://doi.org/10.1097/PCC.0b013e31825b561b.
76. Kietaibl S, Ahmed A, Afshari A, et al. Management of severe peri-operative bleeding: guidelines from the European Society of Anaesthesiology and Intensive Care: second update 2022. Eur J Anaesthesiol. 2023;40:226–304.
77. Haas T, Spielmann N, Restin T, Seifert B, Henze G, Obwegeser J, Min K, Jeszenszky D, Weiss M, Schmugge M. Higher fibrinogen concentrations for reduction of transfusion requirements during major paediatric surgery: a prospective randomised controlled trial. Br J Anaesth. 2015;115:234–43.
78. Tavares C, Sazaki S, Murata KN, Joaquim AF, Tedeschi H. Evaluation of the safety of fibrinogen concentrate administration for bleeding control in neurosurgery. Braz J Neurosurg. 2014;25:343–8.
79. Huisman EJ, Crighton GL. Pediatric fibrinogen PART I—pitfalls in fibrinogen evaluation and use of fibrinogen replacement products in children. Front Pediatr. 2021; https://doi.org/10.3389/fped.2021.617500.
80. Crighton GL, Huisman EJ. Pediatric fibrinogen PART II—overview of indications for fibrinogen use in critically ill children. Front Pediatr. 2021; https://doi.org/10.3389/fped.2021.647680.
81. Valentine SL, Cholette JM, Goobie SM. Transfusion strategies for hemostatic blood products in critically ill children: a narrative review and update on expert consensus guidelines. Anesth Analg. 2022;135:545–57.
82. Munlemvo DM, Tobias JD, Chenault KM, Naguib A. Prothrombin complex concentrates to treat coagulation disturbances: an overview with a focus on use in infants and children. Cardiol Res. 2022;13:18–26.
83. Wittenmeier E, Piekarski F, Steinbicker AU. Blood product transfusions for children in the perioperative period and for critically ill children. Dtsch Arztebl Int. 2024;121:58–65.
84. Haas T, Goobie S, Spielmann N, Weiss M, Schmugge M. Improvements in patient blood management for pediatric craniosynostosis surgery using

a ROTEM®-assisted strategy - feasibility and costs. Paediatr Anaesth. 2014;24:774–80.
85. Haas T, Faraoni D. Viscoelastic testing in pediatric patients. Transfusion (Paris). 2020;60:S75–85.
86. Klein AA, Bailey CR, Charlton AJ, et al. Association of Anaesthetists guidelines: cell salvage for perioperative blood conservation 2018. Anaesthesia. 2018;73:1141–50.
87. Nathan S, Shang M, Reid R. Systematic review of intraoperative blood salvage in the surgical management of craniosynostosis. Face. 2022;3:53–8.
88. King MR, Staffa SJ, Stricker PA, et al. Safety of antifibrinolytics in 6583 pediatric patients having craniosynostosis surgery: a decade of data reported from the multicenter Pediatric Craniofacial Collaborative Group. Paediatr Anaesth. 2022;32:1339–46.
89. Goobie SM, Zurakowski D, Glotzbecker MP, McCann ME, Hedequist D, Brustowicz RM, Sethna NF, Karlin LI, Emans JB, Hresko MT. Tranexamic acid is efficacious at decreasing the rate of blood loss in adolescent scoliosis surgery. J Bone Joint Surg. 2018;100:2024–32.
90. Wang JT, Seshadri SC, Butler CG, Staffa SJ, Kordun AS, Lukovits KE, Goobie SM. Tranexamic acid use in pediatric craniotomies at a large tertiary care pediatric hospital: a five year retrospective study. J Clin Med. 2023; https://doi.org/10.3390/jcm12134403.
91. Fenger-Eriksen C, D'Amore Lindholm A, Nørholt SE, von Oettingen G, Tarpgaard M, Krogh L, Juul N, Hvas AM, Rasmussen M. Reduced perioperative blood loss in children undergoing craniosynostosis surgery using prolonged tranexamic acid infusion: a randomised trial. Br J Anaesth. 2019;122:760–6.
92. Varidel AD, Meara JG, Proctor MR, Goobie SM. Antifibrinolytics as a patient blood management modality in craniosynostosis surgery: current concepts and a view to the future. Curr Anesthesiol Rep. 2023;13:148–58.
93. Lecker I, Wang DS, Whissell PD, Avramescu S, Mazer CD, Orser BA. Tranexamic acid-associated seizures: causes and treatment. Ann Neurol. 2016;79:18–26.
94. Patel PA, Wyrobek JA, Butwick AJ, Pivalizza EG, Hare GMT, Mazer CD, Goobie SM. Update on applications and limitations of perioperative tranexamic acid. Anesth Analg. 2022;135:460–73.
95. Goobie SM, Cladis FP, Glover CD, et al. Safety of antifibrinolytics in cranial vault reconstructive surgery: a report from the pediatric craniofacial collaborative group. Paediatr Anaesth. 2017;27:271–81.
96. Rossaint R, Afshari A, Bouillon B, et al. The European guideline on management of major bleeding and coagulopathy following trauma: sixth edition. Crit Care. 2023; https://doi.org/10.1186/s13054-023-04327-7.
97. Goobie SM, Staffa SJ, Meara JG, Proctor MR, Tumolo M, Cangemi G, Disma N. High-dose versus low-dose tranexamic acid for paediatric craniosynostosis surgery: a double-blind randomised controlled non-inferiority trial. Br J Anaesth. 2020;125:336–45.
98. Kumba C. Patient blood management in craniosynostosis surgery. Open J Modern Neurosurg. 2021;11:211–22.
99. Goobie SM, Faraoni D. Tranexamic acid and perioperative bleeding in children: what do we still need to know? Curr Opin Anaesthesiol. 2019;32:343–52.
100. Longacre MM, Seshadri SC, Adil E, Baird LC, Goobie SM. Perioperative management of pediatric patients undergoing juvenile angiofibroma resection. A case series and educational review highlighting patient blood management. Paediatr Anaesth. 2023;33:510–9.
101. Haberkern M, Dangel P. Normovolaemic haemodilution and intraoperative autotransfusion in children: experience with 30 cases of spinal fusion. Eur J Pediatr Surg. 1991;1:30–5.
102. Jabbour N, Gagandeep S, Mateo R, Sher L, Genyk Y, Selby R. Transfusion free surgery: single institution experience of 27 consecutive liver transplants in Jehovah's witnesses. J Am Coll Surg. 2005;201:412–7.
103. Jawan B, de Villa V, Luk H-N, et al. Perioperative normovolemic anemia is safe in pediatric living-donor liver transplantation. Transplantation. 2004;77:1394–8.
104. Association for the Advancement of Blood & Biotherapies. Standards for perioperative autologous blood collection and administration. American Association of Blood Banks; 2021. p. 01–67.
105. Valentine SL, Bembea MM, Muszynski JA, et al. Consensus recommendations for rbc transfusion practice in critically ill children from the pediatric critical care transfusion and anemia expertise initiative. Pediatr Crit Care Med. 2018;19:884–98.
106. Bernhardt K, McClune W, Rowland MJ, Shah A. Hypertonic saline versus other intracranial-pressure-lowering agents for patients with acute traumatic brain injury: a systematic review and meta-analysis. Neurocrit Care. 2024;40:769–84.
107. Stopa BM, Dolmans RGF, Broekman MLD, Gormley WB, Mannix R, Izzy S. Hyperosmolar therapy in pediatric severe traumatic brain injury - a systematic review. Crit Care Med. 2019;47:e1022–31.
108. Gencay I. Apert syndrome: intraoperative and postoperative hyponatremia. J Craniofac Surg. 2019;30:508–9.
109. Hosking J, Dowling K, Costi D. Intraoperative and postoperative hyponatremia with craniosynostosis surgery. Paediatr Anaesth. 2012;22:654–60.
110. Cladis FP, Bykowski M, Schmitt E, Naran S, Moritz ML, Cray J, Grunwaldt L, Losee J. Postoperative hyponatremia following calvarial vault remodeling in craniosynostosis. Paediatr Anaesth. 2011;21:1020–5.
111. Levine JP, Stelnicki E, Weiner HL, Bradley JP, McCarthy JG. Hyponatremia in the postoperative craniofacial pediatric patient population: a connection to cerebral salt wasting syndrome and management of the disorder. Plast Reconstr Surg. 2001;108:1501–8.

112. Ju Lee S, Ju Huh E, Hee Byeon J. Two cases of cerebral salt wasting syndrome developing after cranial vault remodeling in craniosynostosis children. J Korean Med Sci. 2004;19:627–30.
113. Stricker PA, Fiadjoe JE. Anesthesia for craniofacial surgery in infancy. Anesthesiol Clin. 2014;32:215–35.
114. Hughes C, Thomas K, Johnson D, Das S. Anesthesia for surgery related to craniosynostosis: a review. Part 2. Paediatr Anaesth. 2013;23:22–7.
115. Park JJ, Colon RR, Chaya BF, Rochlin DH, Chibarro PD, Shetye PR, Staffenberg DA, Flores RL. Implementation of an ambulatory cleft lip repair protocol: surgical outcomes. Cleft Palate Craniofac J. 2023;60:1220–9.
116. Riordan CP, Zurakowski D, Meier PM, Alexopoulos G, Meara JG, Proctor MR, Goobie SM. Minimally invasive endoscopic surgery for infantile craniosynostosis: a longitudinal cohort study. In: Journal of Pediatrics. Mosby Inc; 2020. p. 142–149.e2.
117. Arts S, Delye H, van Lindert EJ, Blok L, Borstlap W, Driessen J. Evaluation of anesthesia in endoscopic strip craniectomy: a review of 121 patients. Paediatr Anaesth. 2018;28:647–53.
118. Morzycki A, Nickel K, Newton D, Ng MC, Guilfoyle R. In search of the optimal pain management strategy for children undergoing cleft lip and palate repair: a systematic review and meta-analysis. J Plast Reconstr Aesthet Surg. 2022;75:4221–32.
119. Zou T, Yu S, Ding G, Wei R. Ultrasound-guided scalp nerve block in anesthesia of children receiving cranial suture reconstruction. BMC Anesthesiol. 2023; https://doi.org/10.1186/s12871-023-02223-9.
120. Hadzic A, Vloka JD. Nysora.com, Nerve blocks of the face. Nysora.com; 2024.
121. Echaniz G, Chan V, Maynes JT, Jozaghi Y, Agur A. Ultrasound-guided maxillary nerve block: an anatomical study using the suprazygomatic approach. Can J Anesth. 2020;67:186–93.
122. Esquerré T, Mure M, Minville V, Prevost A, Lauwers F, Ferré F. Bilateral ultrasound-guided maxillary and mandibular combined nerves block reduces morphine consumption after double-jaw orthognathic surgery: a randomized controlled trial. Reg Anesth Pain Med. 2024; https://doi.org/10.1136/rapm-2024-105497.
123. Mansour RF, Abdelghany MS. Ultrasound-guided suprazygomatic maxillary nerve block in cleft palate surgery: the efficacy of adding dexmedetomidine to bupivacaine. Egypt J Anaesth. 2021;37:329–36.
124. Forero M, Adhikary SD, Lopez H, Tsui C, Chin KJ. The erector spinae plane block a novel analgesic technique in thoracic neuropathic pain. Reg Anesth Pain Med. 2016;41:621–7.
125. Sandhu NS, Capan LM. Ultrasound-guided infraclavicular brachial plexus block. Br J Anaesth. 2002;89:254–9.
126. Chen L, Shen Y, Liu S, Cao Y. Minimum effective volume of 0.2% ropivacaine for ultrasound-guided axillary brachial plexus block in preschool-age children. Sci Rep. 2021; https://doi.org/10.1038/s41598-021-96582-3.
127. Mortada H, AlKhashan R, Alhindi N, AlWaily HB, Alsadhan GA, Alrobaiea S, Arab K. The management of perioperative pain in craniosynostosis repair: a systematic literature review of the current practices and guidelines for the future. Maxillofac Plast Reconstr Surg. 2022; https://doi.org/10.1186/s40902-022-00363-5.
128. Ghaly RF. Do neurosurgeons need neuroanesthesiologists? Should every neurosurgical case be done by a neuroanesthesiologist? Surg Neurol Int. 2014; https://doi.org/10.4103/2152-7806.133106.

8 Ophthalmic Evaluation

Linda R. Dagi, Yoon-Hee Chang, Matthieu Robert, Romain Touzé,
Isabella de Oliveira Lima Parizotto Paula,
and Raul Gonçalves de Paula

Ophthalmic evaluation is critical as a part of a multidisciplinary approach that includes early detection of vision-threatening conditions associated with craniosynostosis more generally, and Apert syndrome, in particular. Expeditious diagnosis and management of exposure keratopathy, eyelid deformities, refractive errors, amblyopia, and strabismus in addition to surveillance for papilledema as an indicator of elevated intracranial pressure can optimize outcomes. This chapter will focus on common ophthalmic disorders associated with Apert syndrome and review their non-surgical management. Surgical intervention for these problems will be detailed in the chapter on ophthalmic surgery.

L. R. Dagi (✉) · Y.-H. Chang
Department of Ophthalmology, Boston Children's Hospital, Boston, MA, USA
e-mail: Linda.Dagi@childrens.harvard.edu

M. Robert · R. Touzé
Department of Pediatric Ophthalmology, Hôpital Necker–Enfants malades, Paris, France

I. de O. L. P. Paula
Department of Craniofacial Surgery, Hospital for Rehabilitation of Craniofacial Anomalies, University of São Paulo, Bauru, São Paulo, Brazil

Bauru Eye Hospital, Bauru, São Paulo, Brazil

R. G. de Paula
Department of Craniofacial Surgery, Hospital for Rehabilitation of Craniofacial Anomalies, University of São Paulo, São Paulo, Brazil

Anisometropia and Amblyopia

Astigmatism and hypermetropia are very common refractive errors in both non-syndromic and syndromic craniosynostosis. Amblyopia secondary to strabismus and refractive errors has a prevalence of 14–70% in populations with craniosynostosis [1].

Anisometropia (50%) and, in particular, oblique astigmatism (34%) are very common in Apert syndrome. The presence of oblique astigmatism during childhood is associated with the development of amblyopia. In addition, anisometropia (a significant difference in the refractive error between the two eyes) can exacerbate visual deprivation and amblyopia [2]. In patients with significant oblique astigmatism, anisometropia, or high hyperopia, the use of optical correction in the form of glasses or other refractive correction may be very important. Finding comfortable spectacle correction that will stably rest on the nose, and will not touch the corneas (given globe protrusion) can be challenging. Although highly flexible soft frames often prove sufficient, there is more recent experience with facial scans that facilitate the production of three-dimensional (3D)-printed glasses to better meet this population's needs [3]. In addition to proper optical correction, treating amblyopia by occlusion therapy of the "better" eye with patching or pharmacological penalization with atropine eye drops can reverse suppression of the unfavored eye. In some cases, atropine penalization is preferable as the

J. G. Meara et al. (eds.), *Apert Syndrome*, https://doi.org/10.1007/978-3-032-12551-4_8

child can readily remove an occlusive patch. If there are other causes of diminished vision in one eye (exposure keratopathy, more significant ptosis), evaluating and managing these contributing factors should not be overlooked [4].

In population studies, the prevalence of visual impairment equal to or worse than 6/12 in school-age children ranges from 1.8% to 7.4%. In patients with Apert syndrome this level of visual impairment is common, occurring in 54% of patients in at least one eye. Usually, visual acuity limitation is unilateral and not primarily due to optic neuropathy from elevated intracranial pressure, but due to unrecognized or insufficiently addressed amblyopia due to strabismus or refractive errors. The prevalence of amblyopia is 35% compared with only 3.9–6.5% in population studies of school-age children. Thus, in addition to surveillance for papilledema or optic atrophy, equal attention should be paid to providing ideal refractive correction, treating amblyopia and strabismus, and preventing and treating exposure keratopathy [2, 5].

Hypertelorism Due to Orbital Dysmorphology

The Apert orbit is typically characterized by hypertelorism, proptosis, and shortening of the orbital roof and floor. The mean height is increased, and the greater wing of the sphenoid may protrude (Fig. 8.1).

Hypertelorism is always present (Fig. 8.2). Inner and outer canthal distances measured in patients with Apert syndrome are typically above the 97th and 75th percentiles, respectively [6].

Early fusion of the sphenoparietal and sphenofrontal sutures results in a shortened orbital plate, and marked retrusion and elevation of the supraorbital margin, most pronounced laterally. An interruption of the eyebrow corresponds to this defect [6, 7].

These orbital malformations alter the position of the eyes and eyelids, which can result in secondary ophthalmic disorders including ptosis, oblique astigmatism, exposure keratopathy, and strabismus.

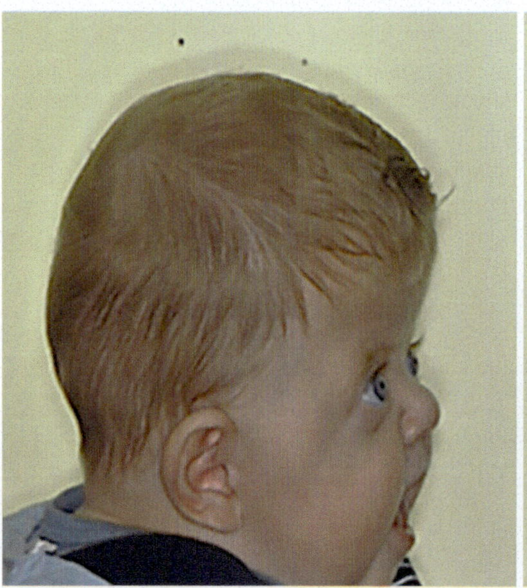
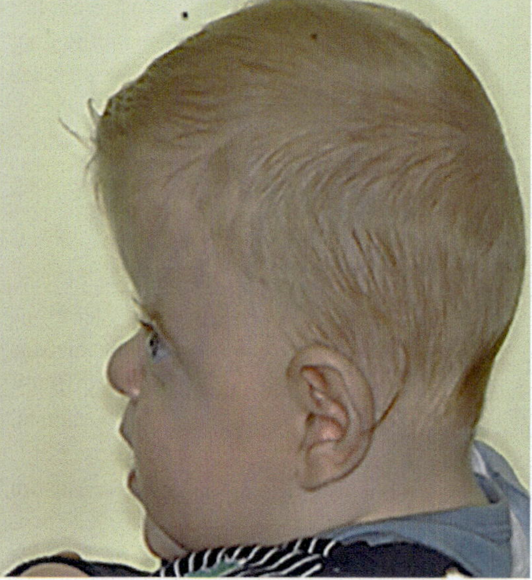

Fig. 8.1 Retrusion of the upper and lower margin of the orbital rim. The orbital retrusion in Apert syndrome extends to the midface, causing maxillary hypoplasia

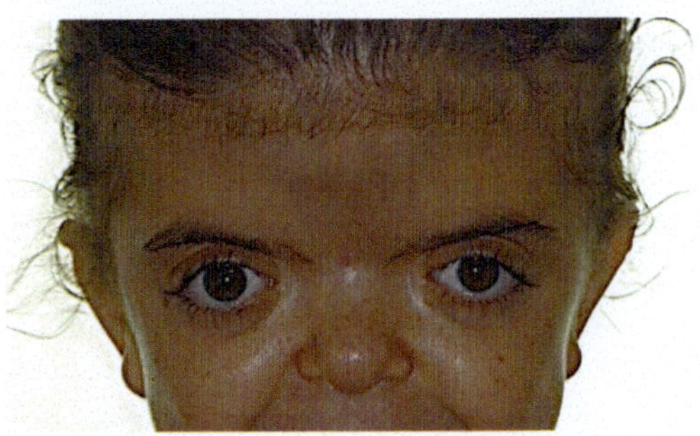

Fig. 8.2 Hypertelorism in Apert syndrome

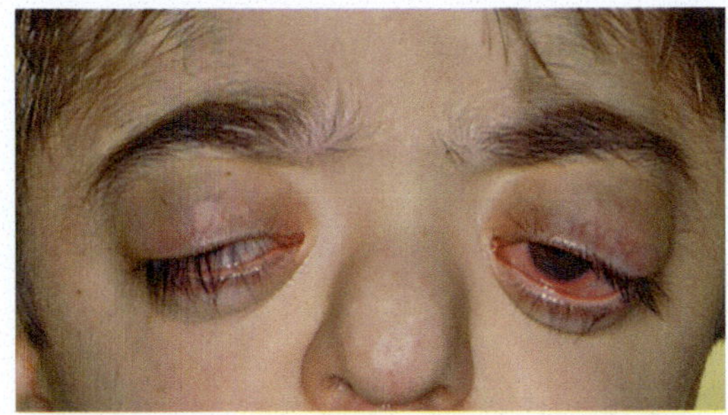

Fig. 8.3 Lagophthalmos due to protrusion of the eyeball associated with conjunctival inflammation

Proptosis and Exposure Keratopathy

Retrusion of the upper and lower orbital margins and shallowing of the orbit causes relative proptosis or protrusion of the globe outside the safe confines of the orbital rim. Exposure keratopathy may occur and there is a risk of traumatic globe rupture. Parents should be asked if eyelid closure is complete when their child is asleep. With incomplete closure, potentially exacerbated by a poor Bell's phenomenon, exposure will occur and the child will be photophobic, and tearful upon awakening. There is risk of developing inferior corneal scarring.

If significant exposure keratopathy is present, ocular lubricating gels and ointment must be used with great frequency and early lateral tarsorrhaphy considered. Exposure keratopathy may result in a permanent reduction in acuity due to conjunctival infection, acute and chronic keratitis, and, ultimately, corneal ulceration and scarring [8] (Fig. 8.3). The associated discomfort reduces quality of life, hampers normal childhood development and visual prognosis, and impairs the ability to examine the optic nerves of the child. Surgical intervention by tarsorrhaphy will be discussed in Chap. 9—Surgery on the Eyes and Eyelids.

Eyelid Disorders

The orbital characteristics of patients with Apert syndrome result in palpebral fissure downslanting and telecanthus (Fig. 8.4).

Ptosis can be present in children with Apert syndrome (Fig. 8.5). Because of the downslanting of the eyelids, ptosis is worse laterally. If the ptosis covers the visual axis, functional superior visual deficits and a chin up posture may result. Some children will recruit the frontalis muscle of the forehead to help elevate the lids, reducing the functional severity of the ptosis. Clinical evaluation and consideration of surgery require quantifying the levator function while eliminating frontalis support, and assessing the quality of the Bell's response.

In some cases of ptosis, proptosis is helpful as the upper lid is relatively retracted along the superior surface of the protuberant globe. For this reason, in cases of asymmetric proptosis, a greater degree of ptosis may be apparent on the side with less proptosis, even when there is no asymmetry in levator function.

The value of surgical correction of ptosis depends on the balance between the risk of amblyopia from ptosis and the benefit that ptosis provides in preventing exposure keratopathy (see Chap. 9, Surgery on the Eyes and Eyelids).

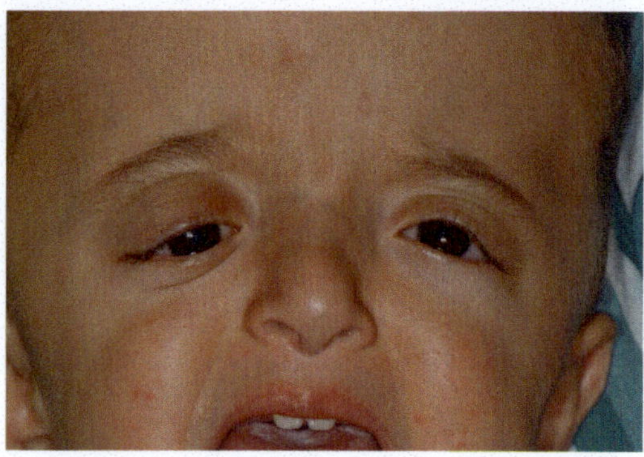

Fig. 8.4 Palpebral fissure downslanting

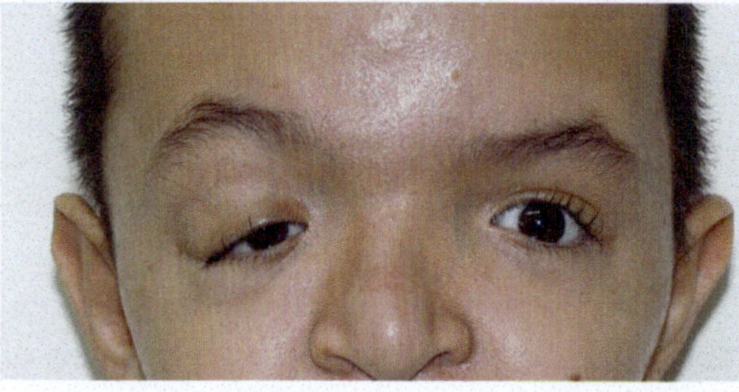

Fig. 8.5 Unilateral ptosis with poor function of the levator muscle of the right eyelid. Note that the child is recruiting the frontalis muscle of the forehead (see the elevation of the eyebrow) to try to open the right eye as much as possible. The weak or underdeveloped levator muscle of the right upper eyelid results in the lack of a formed eyelid crease

Strabismus

Prevalence

Strabismus is present in 50–93% of patients with Apert syndrome [1, 2, 9–12], and has been identified as a significant amblyogenic risk factor [9]. Primary position alignment varies as some studies report exotropia to be most common [9, 10], some note an equal prevalence of esotropia and exotropia [11, 13], and others report more frequent esotropia [2, 14]. Some report a shift from exotropia to esotropia during follow-up [2, 9], and Khong et al. describe the notable shift towards esotropia after craniofacial surgery [2, 10]. Regardless of the alignment in true primary position, V-pattern strabismus due to true or "pseudo" superior oblique palsy and accompanied by esotropia in downgaze and exotropia in upgaze is reported in 28–79% of patients with Apert syndrome [2, 6, 11, 13].

Genetics and Strabismus

Apert syndrome frequently results from fibroblast growth factor receptor 2 (FGFR2) mutations with autosomal dominant inheritance. It is most commonly seen with Ser252Trp (S252W) or Pro253Arg (P253R) mutations of FGFR2. Compared to P253R mutation, S252W is more common, and the prevalence of strabismus is possibly higher, although the difference reported is not statistically significant [15, 16]. Jadico et al. have compared ocular phenotypes and found that strabismus is a common finding in both mutations: 91% in S252W mutation and 85% in P253R [15]. They noted, however, that the number of patients treated surgically for their strabismus was significantly higher among those with S252W mutation, consistent with the reports of greater severity and more frequent apparent superior oblique underaction with this mutation.

Mechanism and Clinical Manifestation of Strabismus

Several mechanisms of strabismus, in particular of V-pattern strabismus, have been proposed in this population. These include abnormal origins and insertions of the extraocular muscles on the globe, extraocular muscle dysgenesis, displacement of the trochlea, and excyclorotation of the rectus muscles due to the shallow orbits [17–20] (Fig. 8.6). A quantitative appraisal by Dagi et al. revealed a highly significant association between severity of V-pattern strabismus and Apert syndrome [17]. They found that patients with Apert syndrome were more likely to have moderate-to-severe or seesaw V-pattern, while patients with Crouzon or Pfeiffer syndromes were more likely to have mild or moderate V-patterns. The magnitude of excyclorotation of the rectus muscles was highly associated with more severe V-pattern. In addition, excyclorotation of the rectus muscles was present not only at the insertion of these muscles on the globe, but as far posteriorly as

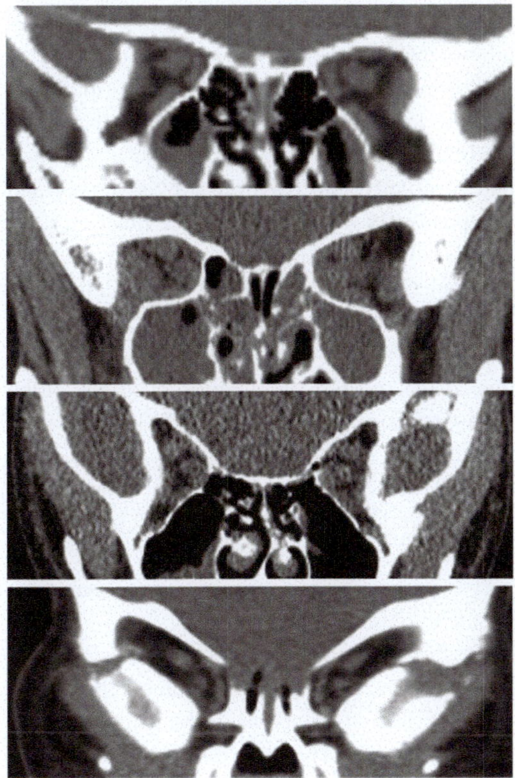

Fig. 8.6 CT coronal views. From the top: Mild; moderate; moderate to severe; and seesaw V-pattern. In patients with mild and moderate V-pattern strabismus, the orbital walls encase typically oriented rectus muscles. In patients with moderate-to-severe V-pattern strabismus, medial bowing of sphenoid greater wing infra-places the lateral rectus. In the most severe or "seesaw" V-pattern strabismus, the latter is exacerbated by temporal expansion of orbital roof with resultant lateral displacement of the superior rectus. This most severe V-pattern is most common in patients with Apert syndrome [17]

their origins at the orbital apex [17]. The unique feature of seesaw V-pattern characterized by inability to elevate the abducted eye above midline and the resultant "seesaw" ductional movements was more common in the Apert population (Fig. 8.7). This is consistent with early reports of apparent superior rectus underaction [17]. Touzé et al. used geometric morphometrics with 3D orbital magnetic resonance imaging (MRI) to evaluate the extraocular muscle positions in unicoronal synostosis [18]. By demonstrating excyclorotation of the rectus muscles as well as lateral, superior, and posterior displacement of the trochlea of the superior oblique muscle, they provided a quantitative proof of two mechanisms of V-pattern in this population. Posterior displacement of the trochlea results in superior oblique tendon laxity with superior oblique underaction and subsequent inferior oblique overaction. Consequently, the imbalance between superior and inferior oblique tone plays a significant role in developing V-pattern strabismus in addition to excyclorotation of the extraocular muscles [19]. Another potential cause of V-pattern is displacement of the trochlea after fronto-orbital advancement (FOA). Dalmas et al. demonstrated another biomechanical impact of FOA on the orbital anatomy and extraocular muscles in patients with unicoronal synostosis [21]. They showed that supraorbital advancement can aggravate the excyclotorsion of the orbit, potentially contributing to the V-pattern strabismus in these patients. Lee et al. [22] associated the wide shal-

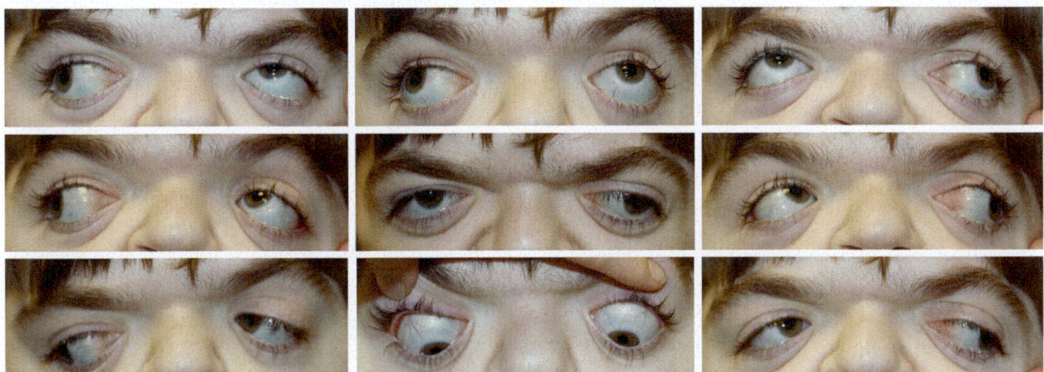

Fig. 8.7 Seesaw V-pattern strabismus in Apert syndrome

low orbits and inward bowing of the medial orbital wall with the associated strabismus.

Other reported extraocular muscle anomalies include dysgenesis, filmy diaphanous muscles, bifid muscles, inelastic muscles, fibrosed muscles, and abnormal muscle insertions in patients with syndromic craniosynostosis [23, 24]. In Apert syndrome, absent extraocular muscles or abnormal muscle insertions have been reported [15, 25]. Jadico et al. reported four patients with Apert syndrome with extraocular muscle anomalies: three patients with absence or abnormal insertion of the superior oblique/superior rectus muscle complex and one patient with bilateral absence of the medial rectus muscle [15]. Most of these extraocular muscle anomalies were not apparent on preoperative computed tomographic (CT) imaging but were discovered intraoperatively. They also noted that all four patients had the S252W mutation of the FGFR2 gene and that this mutation may alter extraocular muscle development. A histological analysis showed atypical inferior oblique muscles in patients with Apert syndrome and controls [26].

Surgical interventions for strabismus are discussed in detail in Chap. 9—Surgery on the Eyes and Eyelids.

Optic Neuropathy

Neuro-ophthalmological assessment in patients with Apert syndrome is critically important as analysis of the optic disc structure and function can help determine whether there is raised intracranial pressure (ICP); in addition, if severe papilledema or secondary optic atrophy are present, this information may provide insight on visual prognosis. Around 65% of children with syndromic craniosynostosis have at least one eye with a visual acuity less than or equal to 20/40, including 40% with a visual acuity less than, or equal to 20/40 in the best eye [14]. Although amblyopia is the most common cause of vision loss, optic neuropathy is the second most common cause in children with craniosynostosis [13]. Optic neuropathy is more likely to impact the visual acuity of both eyes.

Several mechanisms can lead to optic neuropathy in this population. The premature closure of one or more sutures can result in abnormal skull growth, leaving insufficient space for the growing brain. In addition, venous outflow obstruction and obstructive sleep apnea may adversely and independently impact optic nerve function [27]. Above all, chronically elevated ICP will cause papilledema and, if significant, ultimately result in optic atrophy. The prevalence of papilledema in Apert syndrome is estimated to be 9–11%—one of the most at-risk craniosynostoses, along with Crouzon and oxycephaly [28]. Optic neuropathy with papilledema is, however, most prevalent in Crouzon syndrome (34%) followed by Apert syndrome (9–11%) [1, 13, 28–30]. Compression or chronic elongation of the optic nerves within the orbit or optic canal may contribute to optic atrophy.

In this context, the name "papilledema" is believed to be a complex phenomenon that starts with swelling of the axons of the ganglion fibers in the optic disc. The optic disc is the most anterior, intraocular portion of the optic nerve, also called the prelaminar region because it is located anterior to the *lamina cribrosa*, a sheet of collagen pierced with numerous orifices that allow retinal axons and vessels to pass [31]. The role of the *lamina cribrosa* is to protect nerve structures from pressure gradients between the intra- and extraocular compartments of the optic nerve. Prelaminar axonal lesions, whatever the mechanism, can slow down cytoplasmic transport, accumulating toxic substances responsible for axonal swelling [31]. In papilledema, elevated ICP is transmitted to the sheath of the optic nerves, leading to their tortuosity and dilation with cerebrospinal fluid. An imbalance is created between intraocular and extraocular pressure (also called translaminar pressure gradient). It may result in injury or compression of venules in that region, with secondary venous stasis and fluid leakage that leads to the accumulation of extracellular fluid [32, 33]. Significant papilledema may result in an apparent elevation of the optic nerve head "into" the globe on MRI or CT imaging.

Any papilledema should be graded according to two classifications: the quantitative Frisén staging [34] (Table 8.1) and the evolutive Hoyt & Beesten staging (early, fully developed, chronic, atrophic). At best and as soon as it is feasible, the papilledema should also be documented by pictures and quantified using retinal nerve fiber layer (RNFL), and optic nerve height and volume by optical coherence tomography (OCT). To note, RNFL is mostly reproducible and useful in Frisén grade 1 and 2 papilledema, while OCT measures of optic nerve height and volume and infrared and/or conventional retinal photography are better ways to assess more severe papilledema. In papilledema, the risk of atrophy depends on two criteria: on the one hand the severity of the papilledema and on the other hand its duration: thus, a minimal papilledema, Frisén grade 1 or 2, can often be tolerated with no functional consequence for several months or even years. Conversely, an untreated Frisén grade 5 papilledema can result in irreversible destruction of the optic nerve fibers within a few days. Lowering the ICP is then a true emergency. For papilledema of intermediate severity, the prognosis mostly depends on its duration (Fig. 8.8). The presence of mild through more severe optic atrophy can be assessed as well as monitored by surveillance of the ganglion cell layer by OCT [35]. Post-papilledema RNFL may map within the "normal' range" in cases of mild optic atrophy but diagnosed by a reduced ganglion cell layer. In such cases it is likely that the RNFL prior to papilledema hovered at the upper end of normal, and post-papilledema has diminished to the "lower end of normal; the reduction in RNFL is consistent with mid atrophy. In the presence of an optic atrophy, the absence of papilledema has much less value in excluding elevated ICP. Destroyed ganglion fibers cannot swell anymore and those that remain may swell, but the swelling localized within the confines of the lamina cribrosa and thus difficult to detect even with the help of OCT.

Table 8.1 Papilledema grading system (Frisén scale)

Stage 0—Normal Optic Disc. Blurring of nasal, superior and inferior poles in inverse proportion to disc diameter. Radial nerve fiber layer (NFL) without NFL tortuosity. Rare obscuration of a major blood vessel, usually on the upper pole.
Stage 1—Very early papilledema. Obscuration of the nasal border of the disc. No elevation of the disc borders. Disruption of the normal radial NFL arrangement with greyish opacity accentuating nerve fiber layer bundles. Normal temporal disc margin. Subtle greyish halo with temporal gap (best seen with indirect ophthalmoscopy). Concentric or radial retro choroidal folds.
Stage 2—Early papilledema. Obscuration of all borders. Elevation of the nasal border. Complete peripapillary halo.
Stage 3—Moderate papilledema. Obscuration of all borders. Increased diameter of optic nerve head. Obscuration of one or more segments of major blood vessels leaving the disc. Peripapillary halo irregular outer fringe with finger like extensions.
Stage 4—Marked papilledema. Elevation of the entire nerve head. Obscuration of all borders. Peripapillary halo. Total obscuration on the disc of a segment of a major blood vessel.
Stage 5—Severe papilledema. Dome shaped protrusions representing anterior expansion of the optic nerve head. Peripapillary halo is narrow and smoothly demarcated. Total obscuration of a segment of a major blood vessel may or may not be present. Obliteration of the optic cup.

The question of the sensitivity of papilledema in the diagnosis of raised ICP is complex and highly debated. Papilledema is, by definition, specific for raised ICP: once the differential diagnoses of optic disc swelling have been eliminated (which is easy in the presence of important papilledema or of a recent papilledema with previously documented normal discs, but often difficult in case of moderate edema, see Box 8.1), its presence indicates elevated ICP. However, papilledema is not always a reliable way to detect elevated ICP, particularly in patients with syndromic craniosynostosis. Some studies have reported a sensitivity not exceeding 17–40% [36, 37]. Recent data suggest that sensitivity is lower in young patients, or those below 8 years of age [36, 38]. The absence of papilledema in these patients therefore does not allow formal exclusion of elevated ICP [30, 39]. Apert syndrome results from specific mutations in *FGFR2*. As FGFR2 is expressed during the development of the fetal orbit within the muscular, cartilaginous structures, and in the sheath of the optic nerves [40], mutations in *FGFR2* may lead to structural abnormalities of the *lamina cribrosa*, which

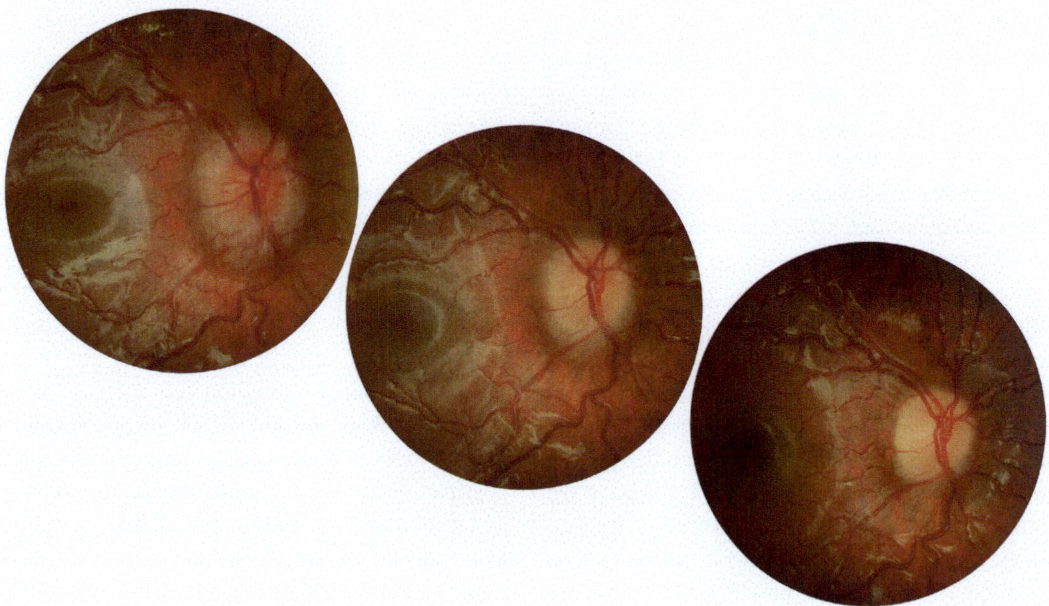

Fig. 8.8 Natural history of papilledema, from a long-lasting moderate optic disc swelling to a moderate optic atrophy (notice that disc pallor typically predominates temporally)

could alter the relation between translaminar pressure gradient and papilledema, and explain this poor sensitivity [39].

Several teams have use visual evoked potentials (VEPs) to detect raised ICP. The VEPs should be performed and analyzed according to the International Society for Clinical Electrophysiology of Vision (ISCEV) standard [41]. Rufai et al. found a sensitivity around 60% with specificity of 83% in the detection of raised ICP in children with craniosynostosis [38]. In comparison, they found a sensitivity of 30% of fundoscopy to detect raised ICP.

Another helpful diagnostic option within the realm of OCT is monitoring for the presence of peripapillary hyperreflective ovoid mass-like structures (PHOMS), a more novel OCT characteristic first described in 2018. PHOMS are highly associated with papilledema and axoplasmic stasis in disorders such as idiopathic intracranial hypertension, but are also present (less frequently) in the normal population, and, for example, in cases of pseudopapilledema, and in association with drusen [42, 43]. In patients with craniosynostosis, they are reliably associated with papilledema, odds ratio 40:1 95% confidence interval [CI]: 6.6–248.0, $P < 0.001$) with a positive predictive value of *86% and negative predictive value of 77%* [43].

Patients with Apert syndrome may also present with pseudopapilledema. The differential diagnosis is often difficult and requires expert assessment. Whenever possible, the use of multimodal imaging of the optic nerve, combining conventional fundus photography, fluorescein angiography, RNFL but also raster and radial OCT, helps distinguish papilledema (due to raised ICP) from pseudopapilledema caused by constitutive anatomical alteration of the optic nerve head in these patients. Importantly, none of these complementary exams have a very high sensitivity and specificity, so their combination and the evolution of disc characteristics, clinical signs and symptoms, and cerebral imaging, are key in determining whether there is raised ICP. In cases where the age and behavior of the children do not allow for any optic disc imaging, exam under sedation or general anesthesia can be performed. The goal of this assessment is, on the one hand, to avoid overlooking cases of raised ICP, and on the other hand, to avoid unnecessary direct measurements of the ICP.

In the presence of papilledema, once ICP is normalized, papilledema will resolve within a variable amount of time, depending on the grade of papilledema and on individual factors. While improvement may be noted within weeks, in some cases it can take up to 3 months before complete normalization.

Although papilledema is a relatively specific but not always sensitive sign of elevated ICP in cases of syndromic craniosynostosis, it is nonetheless a key element for follow-up monitoring for these children. It is critical to note that papilledema associated with elevation in intracranial pressure may not be accompanied by other clinical signs and symptoms of raised ICP in these children [44].

Respiratory disorders are also involved in the pathogenesis of optic neuropathy in patients with syndromic craniosynostosis. Facial and respiratory malformations can lead to severe obstructive apnea aggravating elevated ICP and optic neuropathy. Patients with Apert syndrome have the highest prevalence with 80% demonstrating obstructive sleep apnea. Nguyen et al. found that obstructive sleep apnea increases the risk of optic neuropathy, especially when associated with elevated ICP [27].

Considering these data, we recommend an ophthalmological assessment with fundus examination at the time of diagnosis, and then several months after the primary craniofacial surgery. Some recommend follow up every 6 months through 9 years and every year thereafter [45]. Patients with active treatment of amblyopia, strabismus, and exposure keratopathy may require more frequent monitoring, and others with apparently well-controlled ICP and absent other ophthalmic concerns may be followed with annual evaluation at an earlier age. Conventional fundus photography and OCT should be performed systematically, as soon as possible. Even if the disc appears clinically normal, having a clear baseline facilitates appreciation of change over time.

Box 8.1 Diagnosing Papilledema

It is difficult to distinguish between optic disc swelling due to raised ICP (called papilledema) and elevated optic disc from other causes, grouped under the generic term "pseudo-papilledema," most often related to the presence of buried optic disc *drusen, and sometimes seen in association with high hypermetropia* (Fig. 8.9). Optic disc drusen are accumulations of cytoplasmic material associated with peculiar constitutional features of the optic disc. They increase very slowly in size, become more superficial and apparent with age, and thus are easier to appreciate in adulthood. In children, optic disc *drusen* are more commonly buried; it is not always possible to visualize them ophthalmoscopically; enhanced depth OCT may help distinguish drusen from PHOMS and from true papilledema; drusen are often calcified and the diagnosis may be confirmed by OCT. To note, pseudopapilledema due to optic disc drusen can also lead to progressive optic neuropathy; however, this is more common in an adult population. There is no treatment, per se, for drusen-associated optic neuropathy, unlike papilledema, which will resolve with ICP normalization.

Visual impairment in Apert syndrome may be due to amblyopia due to uncorrected refractive error, strabismus and ptosis, exposure keratopathy, optic neuropathy, or any combination. Scheduled periodic ophthalmic evaluations based on the patients' age, cooperation, and ophthalmic manifestations are critical to optimizing outcomes. PHOMS in patients with papilledema and craniosynostosis typically resolve after surgical reduction in ICP [46].

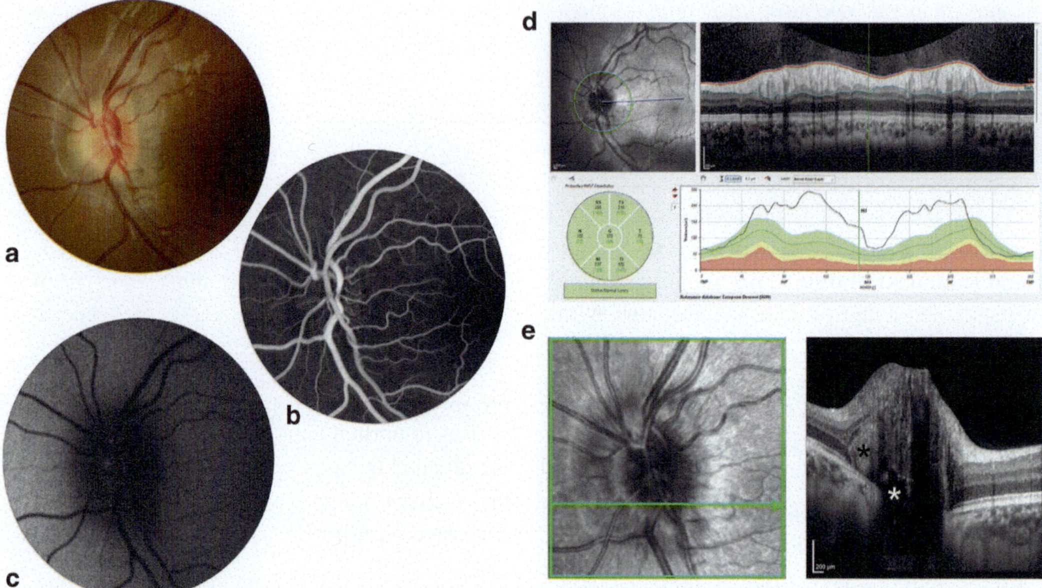

Fig. 8.9 Optic disc swelling due to buried drusen in an eight-year-old girl. (**a**) Fundus photography shows optic disc swelling, predominating nasally; (**b**) Absence of diffusion at late stage of fluoresceine angiography; (**c**) Hyper-autofluorescence is hardly visible since the drusen are buried; (**d**) Increased thickness of the retinal nerve fiber layer (RNFL) on optical coherence tomography (OCT); (**e**) Association of peripapillary hyperreflective ovoid mass-like structure (PHOMS; black star) and deep hyporeflective buried drusen (white star) with hyperreflective boundaries

References

1. Rostamzad P, Arslan ZF, Mathijssen IMJ, Koudstaal MJ, Pleumeekers MM, Versnel SL, et al. Prevalence of ocular anomalies in craniosynostosis: a systematic review and meta-analysis. J Clin Med. 2022;11(4)
2. Khong JJ, Anderson P, Gray TL, Hammerton M, Selva D, David D. Ophthalmic findings in Apert's syndrome after craniofacial surgery: twenty-nine years' experience. Ophthalmology. 2006;113(2):347–52.
3. de Alba Campomanes AG, Meer E, Clarke M, Brodie FL. Using a smartphone 3-dimensional surface imaging technique to manufacture custom 3-dimensional-printed eyeglasses. JAMA Ophthalmol. 2022;140(10):966–73.
4. Ganesh A, Edmond J, Forbes B, Katowitz WR, Nischal KK, Miller M, et al. An update of ophthalmic management in craniosynostosis. J AAPOS. 2019;23(2):66–76.
5. Preslan MW, Novak A. Baltimore vision screening project. Ophthalmology. 1996;103(1):105–9.
6. Kreiborg S, Cohen MM Jr. Ocular manifestations of Apert and Crouzon syndromes: qualitative and quantitative findings. J Craniofac Surg. 2010;21(5):1354–7.
7. Fadda MT, Ierardo G, Ladniak B, Di Giorgio G, Caporlingua A, Raponi I, et al. Treatment timing and multidisciplinary approach in Apert syndrome. Ann Stomatol (Roma). 2015;6(2):58–63.
8. Chauvel-Picard J, Allavena J, Beuriat PA, Di Rocco F, Gleizal A, Paulus C. Lipofilling of the lower eyelids: a craniofacial tool to postpone the facial advancement in craniofacial syndromes. J Stomatol Oral Maxillofac Surg. 2022;123(4):448–51.
9. Hinds AM, Thompson DA, Rufai SR, Weston K, Schwiebert K, Panteli V, et al. Visual outcomes in children with syndromic craniosynostosis: a review of 165 cases. Eye (Lond). 2022;36(5):1005–11.
10. Khong JJ, Anderson P, Gray TL, Hammerton M, Selva D, David D. Ophthalmic findings in apert syndrome prior to craniofacial surgery. Am J Ophthalmol. 2006;142(2):328–30.
11. Nelson LB, Ingoglia S, Breinin GM. Sensorimotor disturbances in craniostenosis. J Pediatr Ophthalmol Strabismus. 1981;18(5):32–41.
12. Rosenberg JB, Tepper OM, Medow NB. Strabismus in craniosynostosis. J Pediatr Ophthalmol Strabismus. 2013;50(3):140–8.
13. Tay T, Martin F, Rowe N, Johnson K, Poole M, Tan K, et al. Prevalence and causes of visual impairment in craniosynostotic syndromes. Clin Experiment Ophthalmol. 2006;34(5):434–40.
14. Khan SH, Nischal KK, Dean F, Hayward RD, Walker J. Visual outcomes and amblyogenic risk factors in

craniosynostotic syndromes: a review of 141 cases. Br J Ophthalmol. 2003;87(8):999–1003.
15. Jadico SK, Young DA, Huebner A, Edmond JC, Pollock AN, McDonald-McGinn DM, et al. Ocular abnormalities in Apert syndrome: genotype/phenotype correlations with fibroblast growth factor receptor type 2 mutations. J AAPOS. 2006;10(6):521–7.
16. Khong JJ, Anderson PJ, Hammerton M, Roscioli T, Selva D, David DJ. Differential effects of FGFR2 mutation in ophthalmic findings in Apert syndrome. J Craniofac Surg. 2007;18(1):39–42.
17. Dagi LR, MacKinnon S, Zurakowski D, Prabhu SP. Rectus muscle excyclorotation and V-pattern strabismus: a quantitative appraisal of clinical relevance in syndromic craniosynostosis. Br J Ophthalmol. 2017;101(11):1560–5.
18. Touzé R, Heuze Y, Robert MP, Bremond-Gignac D, Roux CJ, James S, et al. Extraocular muscle positions in anterior plagiocephaly: V-pattern strabismus explained using geometric mophometrics. Br J Ophthalmol. 2020;104(8):1156–60.
19. Ron Y, Dagi LR. The etiology of V pattern strabismus in patients with craniosynostosis. Int Ophthalmol Clin. 2008;48(2):215–23.
20. Velez FG, Thacker N, Britt MT, Rosenbaum AL. Cause of V pattern strabismus in craniosynostosis: a case report. Br J Ophthalmol. 2004;88(12):1598–9.
21. Dalmas F, Thollon L, Beylerian M, Godio Raboutet Y, David T, Scavarda D, et al. Impact of the craniofacial surgery simulation in anterior plagiocephaly on orbits and oculomotor muscles: biomechanical analysis with a finite element model. J Craniofac Surg. 2021;32(7):2344–8.
22. Lee TC, Walker E, Ting MA, Bolar DS, Koning J, Korn BS, et al. The influence of orbital architecture on strabismus in craniosynostosis. J AAPOS. 2024;28(1):103812.
23. Diamond GR, Katowitz JA, Whitaker LA, Quinn GE, Schaffer DB. Variations in extraocular muscle number and structure in craniofacial dysostosis. Am J Ophthalmol. 1980;90(3):416–8.
24. Lueder GT. Anomalous orbital structures resulting in unusual strabismus. Surv Ophthalmol. 2002;47(1):27–35.
25. Bustos DE, Donahue SP. Absence of all cyclovertical extraocular muscles in a child who has Apert syndrome. J AAPOS. 2007;11(4):408–9.
26. Rudell JC, Stager D Jr, Felius J, McLoon LK. Morphological differences in the inferior oblique muscles from subjects with over-elevation in adduction. Invest Ophthalmol Vis Sci. 2020;61(6):33.
27. Nguyen JQN, Resnick CM, Chang YH, Hansen RM, Fulton AB, Moskowitz A, et al. Impact of obstructive sleep apnea on optic nerve function in patients with craniosynostosis and recurrent intracranial hypertension. Am J Ophthalmol. 2019;207:356–62.
28. Renier D, Lajeunie É, Catala M, Arnaud É, Marchac D. Craniosténoses. EMC - Pédiatrie. 2008;43(2):1–19.
29. Gupta S, Ghose S, Rohatgi M, Kumar A, Das A. The optic nerve in children with craniosynostosis. A pre and post surgical evaluation. Doc Ophthalmol. 1993;83(4):271–8.
30. Bannink N, Joosten KF, van Veelen ML, Bartels MC, Tasker RC, van Adrichem LN, et al. Papilledema in patients with Apert, Crouzon, and Pfeiffer syndrome: prevalence, efficacy of treatment, and risk factors. J Craniofac Surg. 2008;19(1):121–7.
31. Héran F, Koskas P, Vignal C. Nerf optique. EMC - Ophtalmol. 2010;7(1):1–9.
32. Hayreh SS. Optic disc edema in raised intracranial pressure. V. Pathogenesis. Arch Ophthalmol. 1977;95(9):1553–65.
33. Hayreh SS. Pathogenesis of optic disc edema in raised intracranial pressure. Prog Retin Eye Res. 2016;50:108–44.
34. Frisen L. Swelling of the optic nerve head: a staging scheme. J Neurol Neurosurg Psychiatry. 1982;45(1):13–8.
35. Chang YH, Staffa SJ, Yavuz Saricay L, Zurakowski D, Gise R, Dagi LR. Sensitivity, specificity, and cutoff identifying optic atrophy by macular ganglion cell layer volume in syndromic craniosynostosis. Ophthalmology. 2024;131(3):341–8.
36. Tuite GF, Chong WK, Evanson J, Narita A, Taylor D, Harkness WF, et al. The effectiveness of papilledema as an indicator of raised intracranial pressure in children with craniosynostosis. Neurosurgery. 1996;38(2):272–8.
37. Judy BF, Swanson JW, Yang W, Storm PB, Bartlett SP, Taylor JA, et al. Intraoperative intracranial pressure monitoring in the pediatric craniosynostosis population. J Neurosurg Pediatr. 2018;22(5):475–80.
38. Rufai SR, Marmoy OR, Thompson DA, van de Lande LS, Breakey RW, Bunce C, et al. Electrophysiological and fundoscopic detection of intracranial hypertension in craniosynostosis. Eye (Lond). 2023;37(1):139–45.
39. Nischal KK. Visual surveillance in craniosynostoses. Am Orthopt J. 2014;64:24–31.
40. Khan SH, Britto JA, Evans RD, Nischal KK. Expression of FGFR-2 and FGFR-3 in the normal human fetal orbit. Br J Ophthalmol. 2005;89(12):1643–5.
41. Constable PA, Bach M, Frishman LJ, Jeffrey BG, Robson AG. International Society for Clinical Electrophysiology of V. ISCEV standard for clinical electro-oculography (2017 update). Doc Ophthalmol. 2017;134(1):1–9.
42. Maalej R, Bouassida M, Picard H, Clermont CV, Hage R. Are peripapillary hyperreflective ovoid mass-like structures with an elevated optic disc still a diagnosis dilemma? Ophthalmology. 2025;132(3):309–16.
43. Jeon-Chapman JG, Estrela T, Zurakowski D, Chang YH, Dagi LR, Gise RA. Prevalence and clinical associations of peripapillary hyperreflective ovoid mass-like structures in craniosynostosis. J Neuroophthalmol. 2025. Online ahead of print; https://doi.org/10.1097/WNO.0000000000002315.
44. Bartels MC, Vaandrager JM, de Jong TH, Simonsz HJ. Visual loss in syndromic craniosynostosis with papilledema but without other symptoms

of intracranial hypertension. J Craniofac Surg. 2004;15(6):1019–22; discussion 23–4.
45. Touzé R, Bremond-Gignac D, Robert MP. Ophthalmological management in craniosynostosis. Neurochirurgie. 2019;65(5):310–7.
46. Chang YH, Gise R, Estrela T, Zurakowski D, Staffa SJ, Jeon-Chapman J, Dagi LR. Peripapillary Hyperreflective Ovoid Mass-like Structures before and after Intracranial Decompression: A Longitudinal Cohort Study. Ophthalmology. 2025;132(12):1402–10. https://doi.org/10.1016/j.ophtha.2025.07.025. Epub 2025 Jul 28. PMID: 40738333.

Surgery on the Eyes and Eyelids

9

Linda R. Dagi, Yoon-Hee Chang, Eric Arnaud, Roman H. Khonsari, Isabella de Oliveira Lima Parizotto Paula, Raul Gonçalves de Paula, Matthieu Robert, and Romain Touzé

We have discussed common ophthalmic manifestations of Apert syndrome and their non-surgical management. Some of these ophthalmologic conditions are best managed with surgical intervention in addition to conservative measures. In this chapter, we will discuss surgical management of relevant ophthalmic conditions previously covered.

Exposure Keratopathy

The shallow orbits, globe luxation, eyelid malformations, or eyelid malposition may cause exposure keratopathy with resultant astigmatism, exposure keratitis, photophobia, and corneal scarring. Corneal perforation, globe rupture, and endophthalmitis may ensue in rare cases. Although lubricating eye drops during the day and ointment at bedtime can help, sometimes lateral tarsorrhaphy is necessary to protect the ocular surface.

A tarsorrhaphy can be temporary or permanent, partial or complete, and mechanical or pharmacological. The type and timing of tarsorrhaphy depend on treatment goals. The most effective tarsorrhaphy is accomplished by suturing the lateral eyelids together [1]. This procedure involves splitting the upper and lower lid margins with removal of the distal posterior lamella. The anterior lamellae of the upper and lower lids are sutured together, and the raw edges of the posterior lamella form a bond by scarring to each other [2]. Permanent tarsorrhaphies are usually performed laterally as this location is less likely to block the pupil, and does not impair lacrimal function, a risk associated with medial tarsorrhaphy [1] (Fig. 9.1). If indicated, successful lateral tarsorrhaphy may provide corneal protection and reduce photophobia, enhancing the ability to examine a child with Apert syndrome.

Other options, in addition to temporary tarsorrhaphy, include injection of botulinum toxin in the upper eyelid. This pharmacologic technique inhibits the action of the levator palpebral muscle, thus generating ptosis that usually last up to 6 weeks [3]. One notable drawback is that secondary amblyopia that can result from blocking the central pupillary axis. In addition, if the botu-

L. R. Dagi (✉) · Y.-H. Chang
Department of Ophthalmology, Boston Children's Hospital, Boston, MA, USA
e-mail: Linda.Dagi@childrens.harvard.edu

E. Arnaud · R. H. Khonsari
Craniofacial Unit, Hôpital Necker–Enfants malades, Paris, France

I. de O. L. P. Paula
Department of Craniofacial Surgery, Hospital for Rehabilitation of Craniofacial Anomalies, University of São Paulo, Bauru, São Paulo, Brazil

Bauru Eye Hospital, Bauru, São Paulo, Brazil

R. G. de Paula
Bauru Eye Hospital, Bauru, São Paulo, Brazil

M. Robert · R. Touzé
Department of Pediatric Ophthalmology, Hôpital Necker–Enfants malades, Paris, France

J. G. Meara et al. (eds.), *Apert Syndrome*, https://doi.org/10.1007/978-3-032-12551-4_9

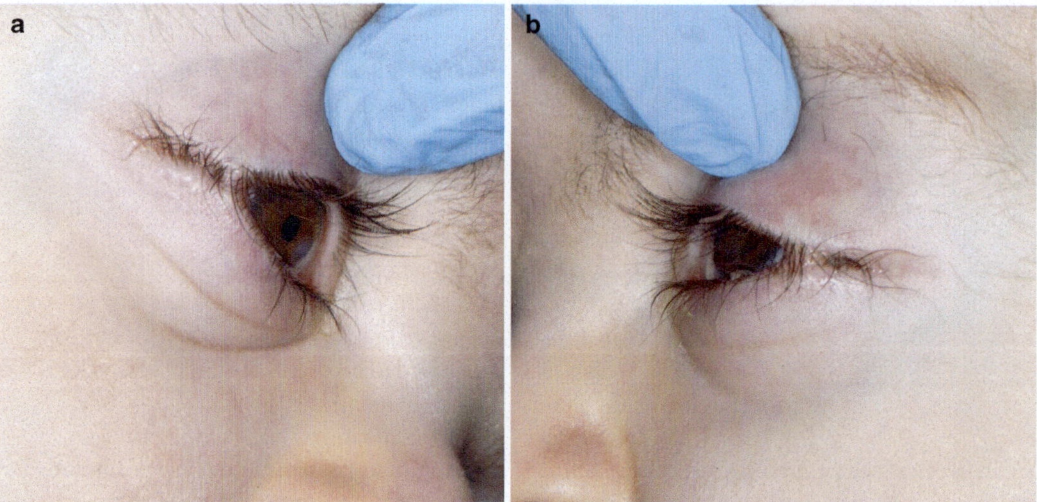

Fig. 9.1 Final aspect of lateral tarsorrhaphy. (**a**) Right eye; (**b**) Left eye

linum toxin extravasates and spreads to surrounding muscles such as the adjacent superior rectus muscle, secondary strabismus may occur.

It is important to appreciate that while both lateral tarsorrhaphy and pharmacologically induced ptosis provide substantial relief from exposure keratopathy, neither of these two techniques protect a globe that is significantly proptotic from the risk of globe rupture associated with accidental trauma. This protection is usually afforded by a combination of fronto-orbital advancement and later midface advancement, which provides protection for the globe by advancing the orbital rim.

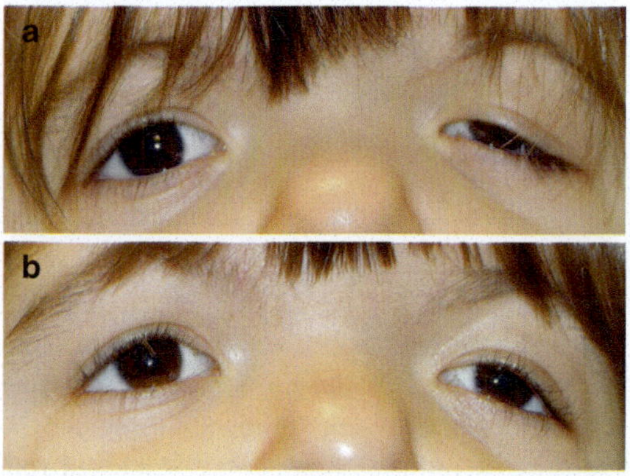

Eyelid Ptosis

Depending on the severity of ptosis, surgical intervention may be indicated to reduce this and prevent amblyopia. In these cases, poor function of the upper eyelid levator muscle is the rule, and thus, a frontalis muscle suspension technique using fascia lata or silicone thread or direct frontalis flap may be considered among other techniques [4] (Fig. 9.2). Procedures need to be conservative to prevent secondary exposure keratopathy.

Fig. 9.2 Three-year-old with Apert syndrome before (**a**) and after (**b**) levator frontalis sling with silicone rod left eye to reduce amblyogenic ptosis

Strabismus

Strabismus management plays an important role in maintaining or enhancing the potential for normal binocular function and can help reduce the burden of amblyopia. Nevertheless, the optimal timing of strabismus surgery and the potential impact of craniofacial procedures remains somewhat controversial [1, 5–10]. The current trend toward earlier craniofacial intervention (by 4 months of age for endoscopic procedures and about a year of age for primary cranial vault expansion) makes delay until completion of the primary craniofacial repair both reasonable and typical. Although secondary craniofacial surgery may prove necessary in later years, it is rarely advisable to delay strabismus surgery, if it is indicated, until late in childhood as the opportunity for binocular function may be lost [1, 6]. It has been our experience, however, that surgical fatigue on the part of Apert families, often related to the number of early childhood procedures to address syndactyly, may result in a parental desire to delay strabismus surgery. This is an important consideration. In children with Apert syndrome who appear to lack binocular potential, early childhood surgical intervention for the associated strabismus can be delayed.

Management of strabismus in Apert syndrome is a therapeutic challenge. While standard surgical procedures for horizontal strabismus are generally effective, the outcomes may be less satisfactory and unpredictable given the degree of incomitance, even in the absence of anomalous extraocular muscles [1]. Preoperative imaging with CT, or more favorably with MRI, may provide helpful information on the position of the extraocular muscles [5, 7, 11–14]. In particular, imaging may determine whether excyclorotation of the rectus muscles significantly contributes to V-pattern [6]. Occasionally, extraocular muscles present on imaging may not be readily "found" at the time of surgery [1]. These extraocular muscles may be morphologically atypical, or their insertions unusually placed; some reports of "absent" extraocular muscles may simply describe situations where the muscle insertions were not easily identified [15].

In patients with significant ocular torticollis, the preoperative monocular patch test helps predict whether the strabismus surgery is likely to remedy torticollis and strabismus. Although there are exceptions, if the placement of a patch over one eye does *not* significantly reduce torticollis (i.e., the atypical head position is *not* being used to enhance binocular fusion) eye muscle surgery, while reducing the strabismus, is unlikely to resolve the problem of torticollis.

In patients with mild V-pattern and evident of fusion, inferior oblique weakening procedures, such as myectomy and recession, reduce V-pattern and excyclotorsion, just as these procedures do in patients without craniosynostosis. If inferior oblique weakening proves to be insufficient, superior oblique tuck or combination of procedures designed to reduce inferior oblique function (recession, myectomy, antero-nasal transposition) and enhance superior oblique function (advancement or tuck) may be considered (Fig. 9.3). Generally, significant superior oblique underaction indicates treatment by tuck, which may in some cases effectively reverse V pattern and fundus excyclotorsion [16]. However, in the presence of an extremely lax superior oblique, hypoplastic superior oblique, or aberrant trajectory of the superior oblique, tucking is less successful resulting in a more modest reduction in V-pattern and fundus torsion [6]. This is common when the tendonous notch of the superior oblique has been displaced posteriorly, sometimes in conjunction with fronto-orbital advancement.

In cases with severe excyclorotation and V-pattern, success has been demonstrated with anterior and nasal transposition of the inferior oblique muscle [17] (Fig. 9.4). This is a very powerful procedure and best preserved for extremely severe V-pattern, as it markedly reduces elevation in adduction and excyclotorsion, though not reducing esotropia in downgaze. If excyclorotated rectus muscles are notable, correcting the path by, for example, infraplacement of the medial rectus and supraplacement of the lateral rectus can effectively reduce hyper-elevation in adduction (Fig. 9.3). More than one procedure is often indicated in many such patients to optimize ocular alignment [1, 5, 6]. The challenge is even greater in cases with absent or aberrant muscles; as their insertions may be thin and atypically placed, care should be taken during initial exposure and exploration of the extraocular muscles.

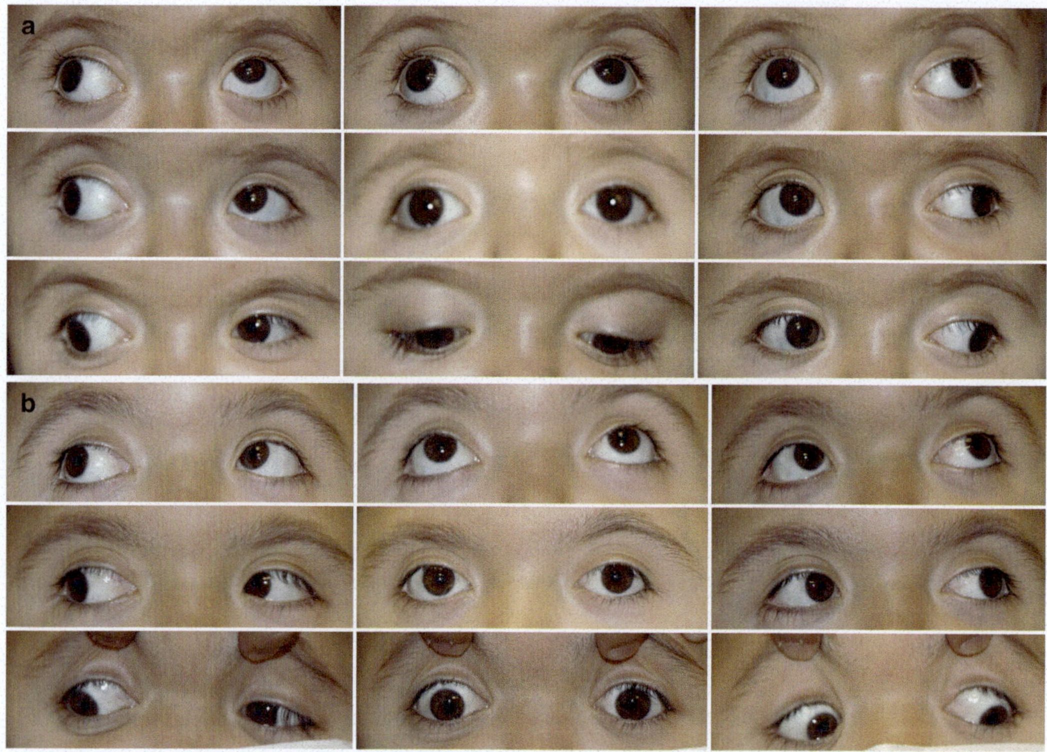

Fig. 9.3 Patients with Apert syndrome and severe V-pattern strabismus. This patient underwent bilateral lateral rectus recessions with a half tendon-width supraplacement and bilateral inferior oblique myectomies, which effectively reduced V-pattern. (**a**) Preoperative photos; (**b**) Postoperative photos

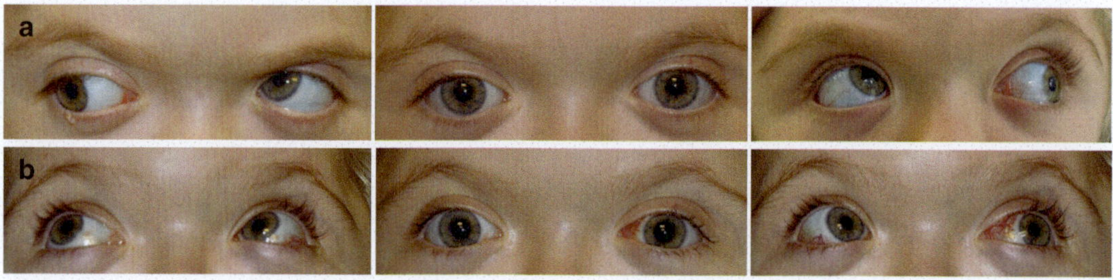

Fig. 9.4 Patient with Apert syndrome and extreme V-pattern before and after anterior nasal transposition of the inferior oblique muscle. (**a**) Preoperative photos; (**b**) Postoperative photos, 4 days after surgery

V-pattern strabismus is common finding in Apert syndrome. Careful review of orbital imaging for possible aberrancy and excyclorotation of extraocular muscles, and consideration of the superior and inferior oblique tone, forced ductions more generally, as well as evidence of binocular fusion and fusional potential help guide a reasonable course of treatment.

The Orbit and Craniofacial Surgery

Patients with Apert syndrome demonstrate orbital dysmorphology, including a short anteroposterior orbit, downslanting of the orbital floor, a shallow lateral orbital wall, decreased orbital soft-tissue volume and excyclorotation or extraocular muscle insertions with resultant in changes in eyelid positioning, and eye alignment [11].

In Apert syndrome, the extreme protrusion of the lateral orbital wall (thereby narrowing the orbit capacity) and the shallow posterior orbit are thought to account for abnormal protrusion of the globe. Comparing the position of the eyeball in patients with normal orbits, the projection in Apert syndrome is 1.56 versus 0.78 cm in typical patients [18].

The first major craniofacial surgery, fronto-orbital advancement (FOA), is traditionally performed close to a year of age. Endoscopic strip craniectomy (ESC) is a less-invasive alternative recently reintroduced as an option for this population if patients present by about 4 months of age or younger. This procedure consists of endoscopically opening the fused sutures and orthosis promoted by helmeting until 1 year of age. Mackinnon et al. reported that children with unicoronal synostosis treated by early ESC developed less severe V-pattern strabismus, excyclotorsion, and range of aniso-astigmatism than those treated by later FOA [19–21]. Due to the success of this early endoscopic intervention, some patients with multi-suture syndromic synostosis and associated bicoronal synostosis, such as patients with Apert syndrome, are being offered early endoscopic repair for their initial craniofacial repair.

It has been reported that eyelid downslanting in patients with Apert syndrome whose primary intervention was FOA remains more severe than those treated with early ESC and orthosis. At about one year of age, patients treated with either intervention had similar angles of palpebral fissure downslanting. By 3 years of age and continuing through 5 years of age, a statistically significant difference in angle of downslanting was present, with more severe downslanting noted in the FOA-treated group. However, a small number of patients, treated initially with ESC, ultimately required FOA or other intervention to improve control of intracranial pressure [22] (Fig. 9.5).

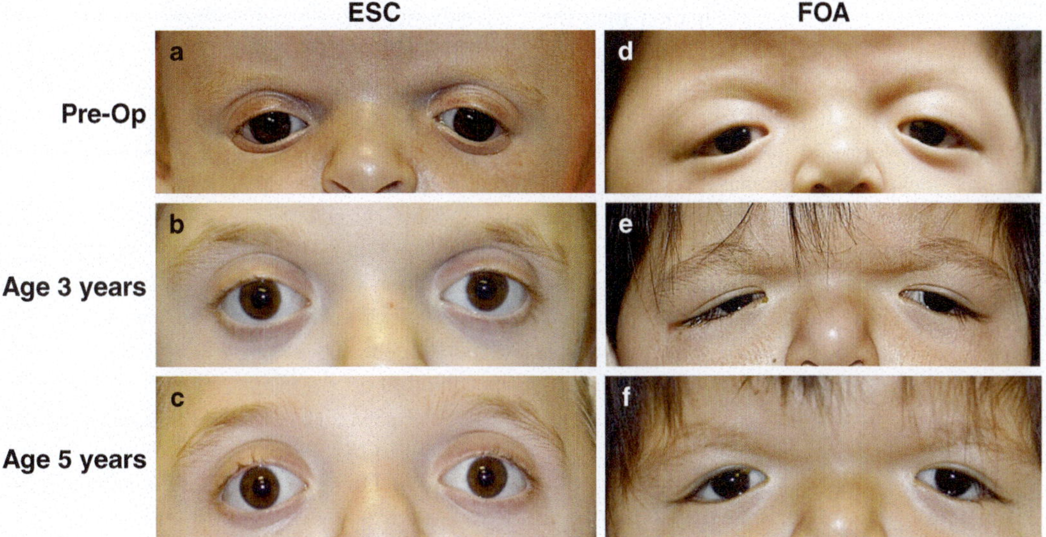

Fig. 9.5 Preoperative and early and late postoperative photographs of patients treated by ESC (**a**–**c**) and FOA (**d**–**f**). Both patients have the SER 252 TRP mutation of FGFR2. ESC: Endoscopic strip craniectomy; FOA: fronto-orbital advancement; FGFR2: fibroblast growth factor receptor 2

FOA results in an anterior translation of the upper orbit and orbital rim only. Later in childhood, Lefort III osteotomy with or without distraction is typically performed, successfully advancing the midface. Both help "replace" the globe back into the orbit very successfully resolving exposure keratopathy, and providing needed protection of the globe [23].

Imai et al. identified that preoperative orbital volumes in patients with Apert syndrome ranged from 7.2 to 10.8 cm^3 (mean, 9.1 cm^3). After FOA there was a significant orbital expansion to 11.6 to 13.2 cm^3 (mean 12.4 cm^3). The average of orbital volume relative to the normal volume was 69% (56–81%) preoperatively and 88% (81–95%) postoperatively. In most cases, alleviation of preoperative symptoms (exophthalmos/eyeball prolapse, corneal keratopathy, conjunctivitis) occurred after surgery, suggesting that the orbit was sufficiently expanded. However, some complications such as entropion were reported [24].

Lateral Canthopexies in Apert

The phenotype of the patient with Apert syndrome is characterized by downslanting of the palpebral fissure wherein the lateral canthus is lower than the medial canthus. This aspect is corrected by a facial osteotomy which involves a medialization of both hemifaces after a medial facial split or a zygomatic repositioning.

Therefore, the lateral canthopexy can be performed through a coronal approach when a Le Fort III or a Monobloc is performed, or through a lateral upper eyelid incision if a coronal approach is not necessary [25, 26].

(a) *Lateral canthopexy through coronal approach*

External canthopexies are performed using surgical stainless-steel sutures and fixed to the fronto-zygomatic plates with moderate over-correction (Figs. 9.6 and 9.7).

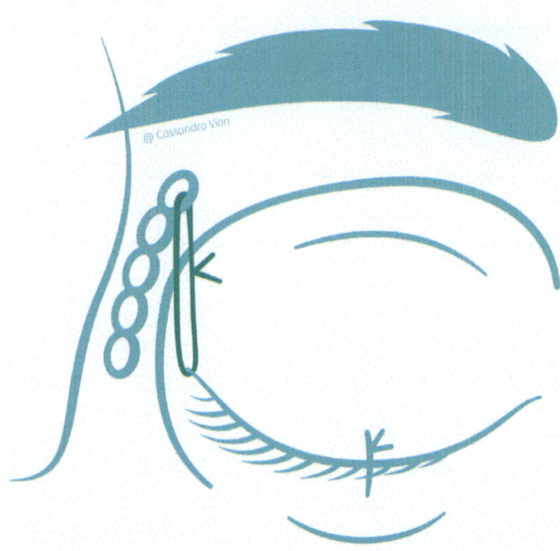

Fig. 9.6 External canthopexy using stainless steel sutures

(b) *Lateral canthopexy through upper eyelid lateral incision*

As an ancillary procedure during aesthetic refinement, a lateral canthopexy can be performed through a small eyelid incision, in its external part above the lateral rim. This aims at correcting the antimongoloid axis of eyelids, whenever present, and creates a normal, slight mongoloid, canthus.

After skin incision, the orbicularis muscle is dissected, allowing an approach to the bony rim. The periosteum is incised vertically and elevated with a small subperiosteal elevator both internally and externally. Then a small hole is drilled in the bone. A colorless Prolene 4/0 is passed through the hole and then toward the lateral canthus, grabbing the lateral part of the cartilaginous tarsus of the inferior eyelid. Then the retaining ligaments of the lateral canthus are released from the deep attachments to allow freedom of movement upward. The tension is adapted to the proper angulation. Suture is performed layer by layer (Fig. 9.8).

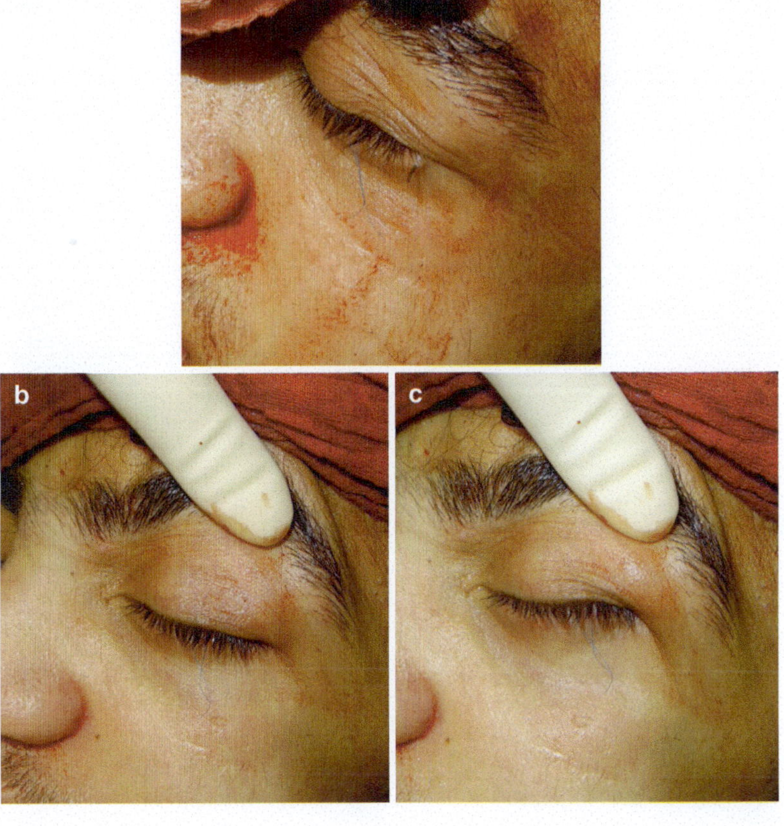

Fig. 9.7 Direction of the suture in external canthopexies. (**a**) Exit point of the stainless-steel suture when performing an external canthopexy; (**b**) Position of the external canthus before suturing the canthopexy to the fronto-zygomatic plate; (**c**) Position of the external canthus after the suture of the canthopexy

(c) *Limits of lateral canthopexies*

The lateral canthopexies, internal or external, are limited by the importance of remaining exorbitism: if the eye is still exophthalmic, the lateral canthopexy will not act properly, and will tend to sling the eyelid under the globe, creating a very inappropriate look. Therefore, the rule is to correct the exorbitism by enlarging the orbit, before any adjustment on the eyelids.

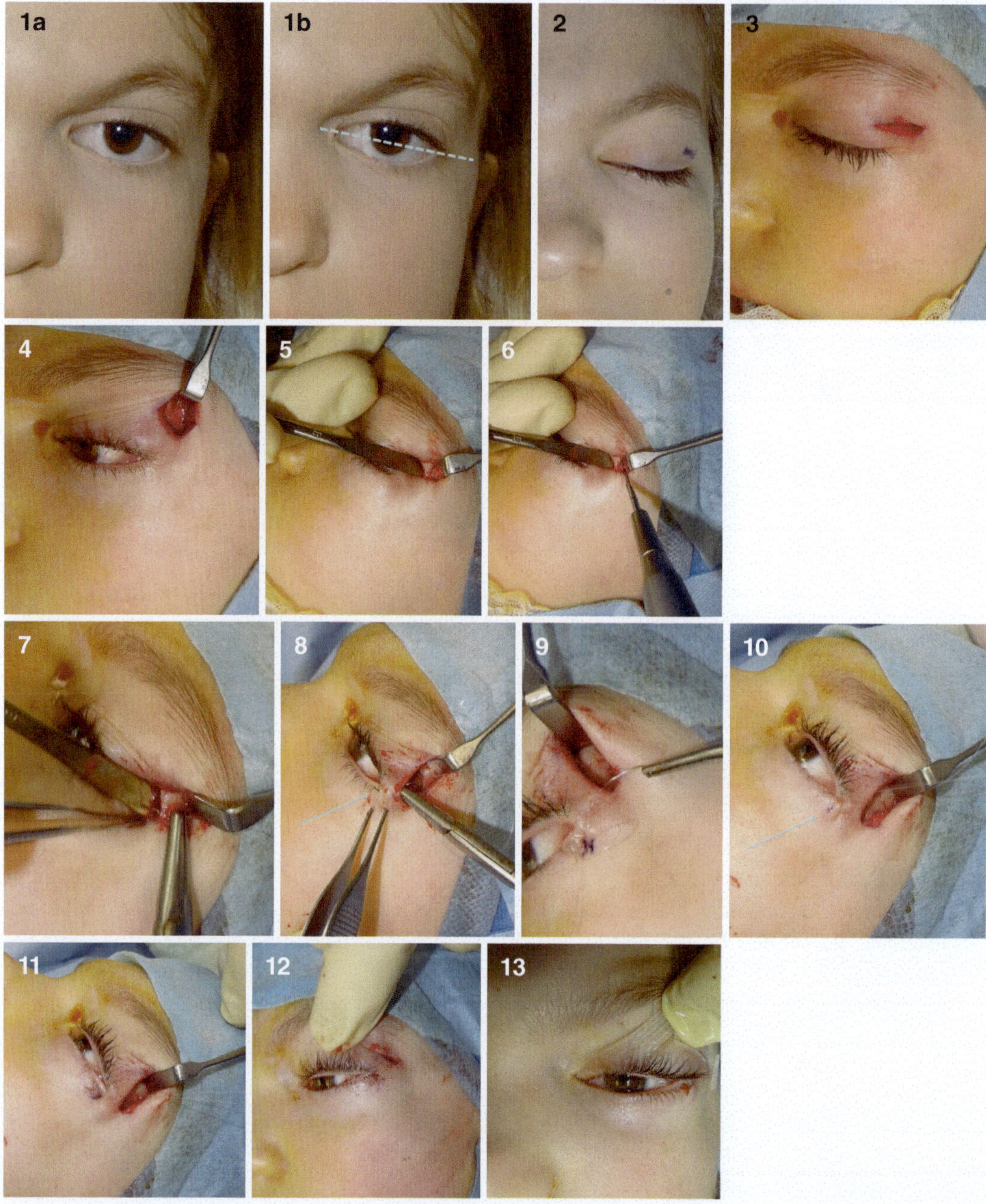

Fig. 9.8 Lateral canthopexy by eyelid approach. 1A: Downslanting palpebral fissure; 1B: Dotted line showing the inverted angle; 2: Lateral incision of upper eyelid above the lateral rim of the orbit; 3: Dissection of the orbicularis muscle; 4: Periosteal incision at the border of the rim; 5: Subperiosteal dissection in the medial and lateral aspect of the lateral rim; 6: Drilling of the bone with a1.2mm drill; 7: Passage of the needle through the bone (Prolene4/0); 8: Perforation of the tarsus of the inferior eyelid medially to the lateral canthus; 9: The needle is exteriorized through a tunnel; 10: Verification of the catch of the lateral canthus; 11: Release of retaining ligaments if necessary; 12: The effect of the canthopexy should be discretely excessive; 13: Suture in layers and Steri-Strips

Surgery to Address Papilledema and Risk of Optic Atrophy

Elevated intracranial pressure with secondary papilledema and the risk of subsequent optic atrophy require consideration of surgical intervention; intracranial pressure can sometimes be temporarily medically controlled with the use of a carbonic anhydrase inhibitor such as acetazolamide. Options for surgically controlling intracranial pressure include the various forms of cranial vault expansion, ventriculoperitoneal shunt, and endoscopic third ventriculostomy [27]. These options are covered in Chaps. 14–19. Finally, checking for the presence of obstructive sleep apnea, commonly seen in children with Apert syndrome, is critical since chronic obstructive sleep apnea is an independent risk factor for the development of optic atrophy in patients with syndromic craniosynostosis [28–30]. Surgical interventions to remedy obstructive sleep apnea are covered in Chap. 13.

References

1. Ganesh A, Edmond J, Forbes B, Katowitz WR, Nischal KK, Miller M, et al. An update of ophthalmic management in craniosynostosis. J AAPOS. 2019;23(2):66–76.
2. de Silva DJ, Ramkissoon YD, Ismail AR, Beaconsfield M. Surgical technique: modified lateral tarsorrhaphy. Ophthalmic Plast Reconstr Surg. 2011;27(3):216–8.
3. Ellis MF, Daniell M. An evaluation of the safety and efficacy of botulinum toxin type A (BOTOX) when used to produce a protective ptosis. Clin Experiment Ophthalmol. 2001;29(6):394–9.
4. SooHoo JR, Davies BW, Allard FD, Durairaj VD. Congenital ptosis. Surv Ophthalmol. 2014;59(5):483–92.
5. Touzé R, Bremond-Gignac D, Robert MP. Ophthalmological management in craniosynostosis. Neurochirurgie. 2019;65(5):310–7.
6. Elhusseiny AM, Huynh EM, Dagi LR. Evaluation and Management of V pattern strabismus in Craniosynostosis. J Binocul Vis Ocul Motil. 2020;70(1):40–5.
7. Rosenberg JB, Tepper OM, Medow NB. Strabismus in craniosynostosis. J Pediatr Ophthalmol Strabismus. 2013;50(3):140–8.
8. Diamond GR, Katowitz JA, Whitaker LH, Quinn GE, Schaffer DB. Ocular alignment after craniofacial reconstruction. Am J Ophthalmol. 1980;90(2):248–50.
9. Diamond GR, Whitaker L. Ocular motility in craniofacial reconstruction. Plast Reconstr Surg. 1984;73(1):31–7.
10. Morax S. Change in eye position after cranio-facial surgery. J Maxillofac Surg. 1984;12(2):47–55.
11. Dagi LR, MacKinnon S, Zurakowski D, Prabhu SP. Rectus muscle excyclorotation and V-pattern strabismus: a quantitative appraisal of clinical relevance in syndromic craniosynostosis. Br J Ophthalmol. 2017;101(11):1560–5.
12. Touzé R, Heuze Y, Robert MP, Bremond-Gignac D, Roux CJ, James S, et al. Extraocular muscle positions in anterior plagiocephaly: V-pattern strabismus explained using geometric mophometrics. Br J Ophthalmol. 2020;104(8):1156–60.
13. Jadico SK, Young DA, Huebner A, Edmond JC, Pollock AN, DM MD-MG, et al. Ocular abnormalities in Apert syndrome: genotype/phenotype correlations with fibroblast growth factor receptor type 2 mutations. J AAPOS. 2006;10(6):521–7.
14. Romano PE. Absent or hypoplastic extraocular muscles? J Med Genet. 1989;26(3):216.
15. Ron Y, Dagi LR. The etiology of V pattern strabismus in patients with craniosynostosis. Int Ophthalmol Clin. 2008;48(2):215–23.
16. Holmes JM, Hatt SR, Leske DA. Superior oblique tucks for apparent inferior oblique overaction and V-pattern strabismus associated with craniosynostosis. Strabismus. 2010;18(3):111–5.
17. Hussein MA, Stager DR Sr, Beauchamp GR, Stager DR Jr, Felius J. Anterior and nasal transposition of the inferior oblique muscles in patients with missing superior oblique tendons. J AAPOS. 2007;11(1):29–33.
18. Forte AJ, Steinbacher DM, Persing JA, Brooks ED, Andrew TW, Alonso N. Orbital Dysmorphology in untreated children with Crouzon and Apert syndromes. Plast Reconstr Surg. 2015;136(5):1054–62.
19. MacKinnon S, Rogers GF, Gregas M, Proctor MR, Mulliken JB, Dagi LR. Treatment of unilateral coronal synostosis by endoscopic strip craniectomy or fronto-orbital advancement: ophthalmologic findings. J AAPOS. 2009;13(2):155–60.
20. MacKinnon S, Proctor MR, Rogers GF, Meara JG, Whitecross S, Dagi LR. Improving ophthalmic outcomes in children with unilateral coronal synostosis by treatment with endoscopic strip craniectomy and helmet therapy rather than fronto-orbital advancement. J AAPOS. 2013;17(3):259–65.
21. Elhusseiny AM, MacKinnon S, Zurakowski D, Huynh E, Dagi LR. Long-term ophthalmic outcomes in 120 children with unilateral coronal synostosis: a 20-year retrospective analysis. J AAPOS. 2021;25(2):76 e1–e5.
22. Dohlman JC, Prabhu SP, Staffa SJ, Kanack MD, Mackinnon S, Warkad VU, et al. Orbital and eyelid characteristics, strabismus, and intracranial pressure control in Apert children treated by endoscopic strip Craniectomy versus Fronto-orbital advancement. Plast Reconstr Surg Glob Open. 2023;11(5):e4937.

23. Holmes AD, Wright GW, Meara JG, Heggie AA, Probert TC. LeFort III internal distraction in syndromic craniosynostosis. J Craniofac Surg. 2002;13(2):262–72.
24. Imai K, Fujimoto T, Takahashi M, Maruyama Y, Yamaguchi K. Preoperative and postoperative orbital volume in patients with Crouzon and Apert syndrome. J Craniofac Surg. 2013;24(1):191–4.
25. Chetty V, Haber SE, Khonsari RH, Arnaud E. Improvement of periorbital appearance in Apert syndrome after subcranial Le fort III with bipartition and distraction. J Craniofac Surg. 2020;31(3):711–5.
26. Cruz A, Akaishi P, Arnaud E, Marchac D, Renier D. Palpebral fissure changes after monobloc frontofacial advancement in faciocraniosynostosis. J Craniofac Surg. 2008;9(1):1–4.
27. Bonfield CM, Shannon CN, Reeder RW, Browd S, Drake J, Hauptman JS, et al. Hydrocephalus treatment in patients with craniosynostosis: an analysis from the Hydrocephalus Clinical Research Network prospective registry. Neurosurg Focus. 2021;50(4):E11.
28. Nguyen JQN, Resnick CM, Chang YH, Hansen RM, Fulton AB, Moskowitz A, et al. Impact of obstructive sleep apnea on optic nerve function in patients with Craniosynostosis and recurrent intracranial hypertension. Am J Ophthalmol. 2019;207:356–62.
29. Chang YH, Staffa SJ, Yavuz Saricay L, Zurakowski D, Gise R, Dagi LR. Sensitivity, specificity, and cutoff identifying optic atrophy by macular ganglion cell layer volume in syndromic Craniosynostosis. Ophthalmology. 2024;131(3):341–8.
30. Estrela T, Dagi LR. Optic neuropathy in craniosynostosis. Front Ophthalmol (Lausanne). 2023;3:1303723.

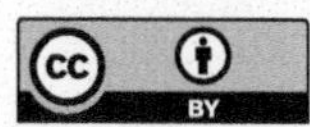

10 Otologic Disorders

Romain Luscan, Alice Briozzo, Charlotte Celerier, Vincent Couloigner, and Marine Parodi

Introduction

Hearing impairment is common in patients with Apert syndrome [1–4]. A large retrospective study analyzing audiologic and otologic findings in 125 patients with Apert syndrome found hearing loss in 80% of patients [2]. Hearing impairment is classically divided into three groups: conductive, sensorineural, and mixed hearing loss. Conductive hearing loss (CHL) is due to external or middle ear pathology that alters sound conduction to the inner ear. Sensorineural hearing loss (SNHL) is linked to a malformation or a functional disorder of the inner ear or the auditory nerve. Mixed hearing loss (MHL) involves a combination of CHL and SNHL, affecting both sound transmission and inner ear function.

In most cases, hearing impairment in patients with Apert syndrome is conductive, occurring in with 93% of patients ($n = 93/100$) in the aforementioned review, but SNHL has also been described [2]. Several factors contribute to the frequent association between Apert syndrome and hearing loss. First, cranial base malformations are associated with a narrowing of the Eustachian tube, predisposing to chronic otitis media and its numerous complications. Additionally, fibroblast growth factor receptor 2 (*FGFR2*), the gene implicated in the pathogenesis of Apert syndrome, is implicated in the embryonic development of the external and middle ear, leading to various malformations of these structures. Lastly, *FGFR2* also plays a critical role in developing inner ear structures, further contributing to auditory impairments.

This chapter provides a comprehensive overview of the various otologic disorders encountered in Apert syndrome and outlines the diagnostic approach and treatment options.

R. Luscan (✉) · A. Briozzo · C. Celerier
V. Couloigner · M. Parodi
Pediatric Otorhinolaryngology and Head and Neck Department, AP-HP, Hôpital Necker–Enfants malades, Paris, France
e-mail: romain.luscan@aphp.fr

Brief Overview of the Anatomy of the Ear and the Auditory Physiology

Anatomy of the Ear

The ear is anatomically divided into three main parts: the external ear, the middle ear, and the inner ear (Fig. 10.1a, b). The external ear includes the auricle and the external auditory canal. Its primary function is to collect sound waves and direct them toward the tympanic membrane. The shape of the auricle and binaural hearing help localize sound, while the external auditory canal amplifies it. The tympanic membrane separates the external ear and the middle ear. A thin membrane, its integrity is mandatory for sound wave transmission to the ossicles. The middle ear is an air-filled cavity containing the

J. G. Meara et al. (eds.), *Apert Syndrome*, https://doi.org/10.1007/978-3-032-12551-4_10

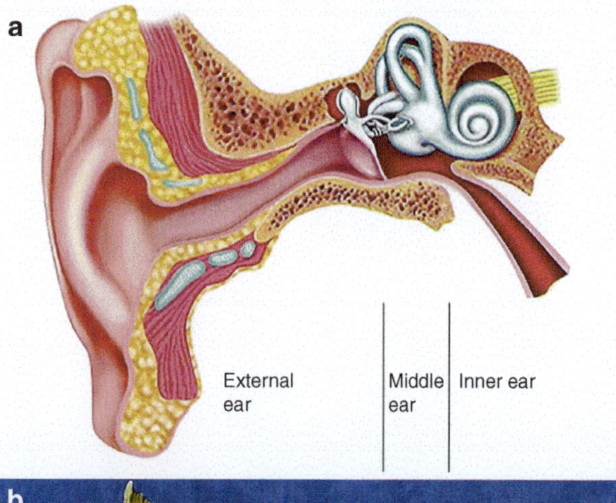

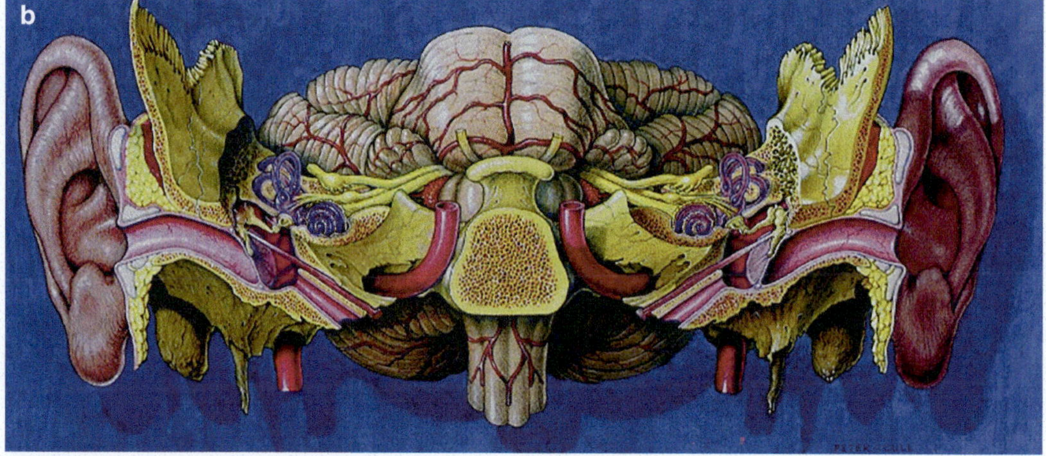

Fig. 10.1 Anatomy of the Ear: (**a**) Anatomy of the inner, middle and external ears. (**b**) The organs of hearing and the cerebellum

three ossicles: the malleus, incus, and stapes. These bones form a chain that amplifies and transmits sound vibrations from the tympanic membrane to the oval window, a membrane separating the middle ear and the cochlea. The Eustachian tube connects the middle ear to the nasopharynx, ensuring the ventilation of the middle ear and helping to equalize pressure on either side of the tympanic membrane. The inner ear—localized in the petrous part of the temporal bone—comprises the cochlea and the vestibule. The cochlea, involved in hearing, is a spiral-shaped structure filled with fluid and lined with sensory cells (i.e., hair cells) that detect sound vibrations. The vestibule, involved in balance, comprises the semicircular canals oriented along the three planes of space, as well as the utricle and saccule, which perceive vertical and horizontal acceleration movements.

Auditory Physiology

Hearing involves a complex, multi-step process to convert sound waves into an electrical signal that the brain can interpret. The sound waves are initially captured by the auricle and funneled down the external auditory canal, causing the tympanic membrane to vibrate. Then, the vibrations are transmitted through the ossicles in the middle ear. The small size of the stapes footplate relative to the tympanic membrane, along with the lever action of the ossicles, amplifies the sound pressure. The stapes pushes against the oval window, generating waves in the fluid-filled cochlea. Within the cochlea, the basilar membrane vibrates at specific points depending on the sound frequency. This vibration excites hair cells in the organ of Corti, leading to the release of neurotransmitters and the generation of electrical impulses in the auditory nerve. Finally, the auditory nerve carries the signals to the brainstem and auditory cortex, where the signals are processed and interpreted as sound.

Brief Overview of the Embryology of the Ear

The development of the ear is a complex process that begins early in embryogenesis, involving contributions from all three germ layers: ectoderm, mesoderm, and endoderm [5]. These structures arise from distinct embryological origins and develop in a coordinated manner to form the functional organ of hearing and balance. The external and middle ears arise from structures of the first and second pharyngeal arches and the intervening pharyngeal cleft and pouch. The inner ear develops from an epidermal otic placode (Fig. 10.2).

Development of the External Ear

The development of the auricle begins at 5–6 weeks of gestation. Six auricular hillocks develop on the facing edges of the first and second arches, around the first pharyngeal cleft. These hillocks enlarge, differentiate, and fuse to produce the mature auricle by the 20th week of gestation. The external auditory canal develops by deepening the first pharyngeal cleft during the sixth week. Its epithelial lining is of ectodermal origin.

Development of the Middle Ear

The tympanic membrane is derived from the pharyngeal membrane that separates the first pharyngeal pouch (forming the middle ear) and cleft (at the origin of the external auditory canal). It is a three-layered structure composed of an external layer of ectoderm, a mesodermal fibrous stratum, and an inner endoderm layer.

By the fourth week of development, the first pharyngeal pouch elongates to form a tubotympanic recess, which gives rise to the tympanic cavity and Eustachian tube. The ossicles develop from the condensations of cartilaginous precursors in the mesenchyme of the first and second pharyngeal arches. Specifically, the malleus and incus arise from the cartilage of the first arch, while the stapes are formed from the cartilage of the second arch. The ossicles are initially embedded in the mesenchyme adjacent to the tympanic cavity and become surrounded by the expanding tympanic cavity during the late fetal period (around the eighth month of gestation). The associated middle ear muscles—the tensor tympani and stapedius—also develop from mesenchyme associated with the first and second arches, respectively.

Development of the Inner Ear

In the third week of gestation, the inner ear begins to form with the appearance of a thickening of ectoderm, the otic placode, next to the developing hindbrain. By the fourth week, the otic placode invaginates and then pinches off to form the otic vesicle. The otic vesicle rapidly differentiates into three structures: the dorsal endolymphatic duct and sac; a central utricle, giving rise to the semicircular canals and utricle; and the ventral saccule, which forms the saccule and cochlea. By the eighth week, the cochlear duct elongates and spirals to form the definitive cochlea. Specialized sensory structures, such as the organ of Corti, develop within the cochlear duct, while the vestibular sensory organs differentiate in the utricle and semicircular canals. Surrounding mesenchyme condenses to form the bony labyrinth, while the perilymphatic space emerges between the membranous and bony labyrinths.

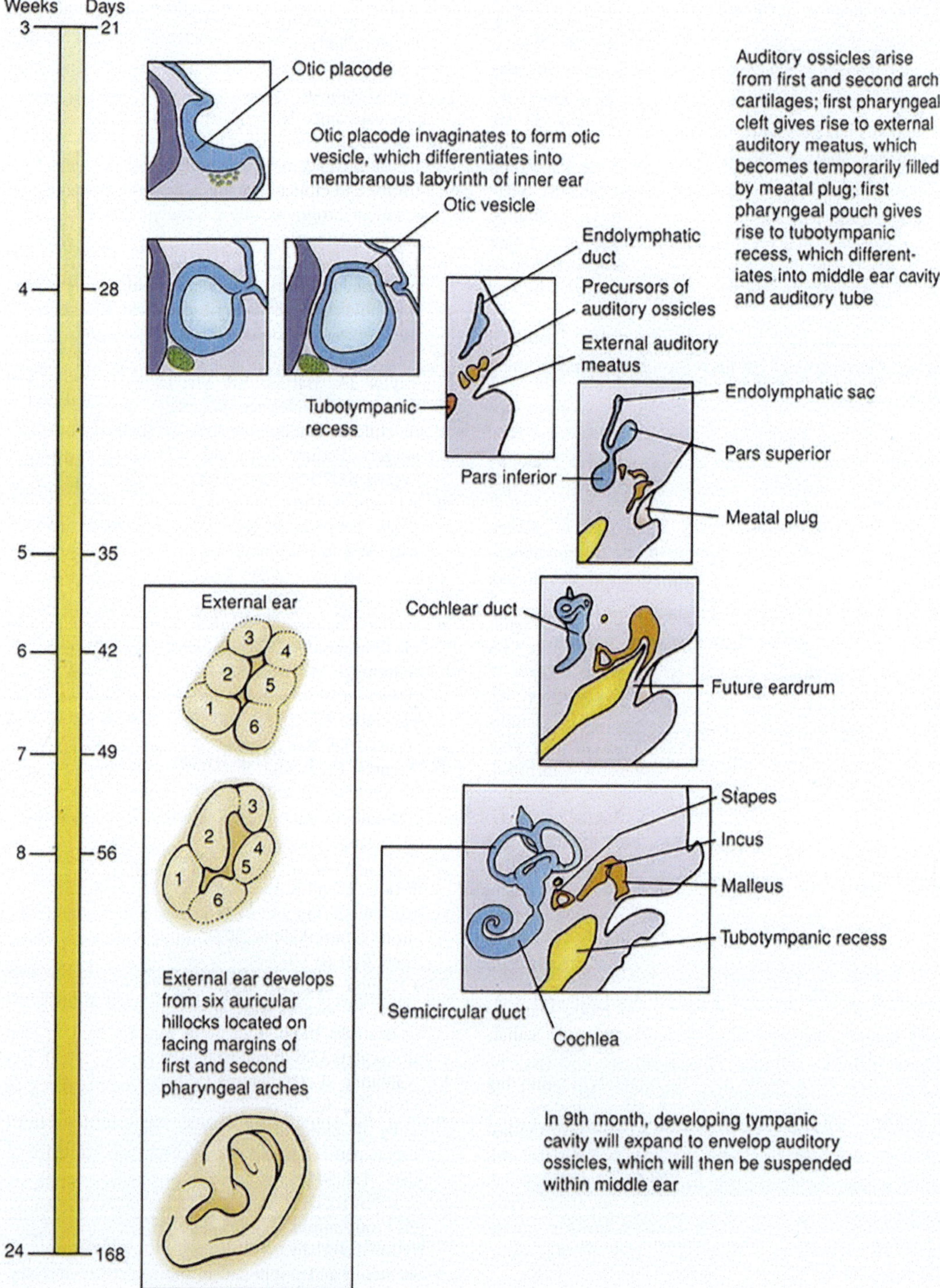

Fig. 10.2 Embryology of the Ear: timeline of development of the inner, middle and external ears

Implication of FGFR2 in Otologic Development

Two adjacent mutations in the *FGFR2* gene on chromosome 10q are responsible for Apert syndrome. *FGFR2* signaling is essential for the proper morphogenesis of the external and middle ear structures. *FGF* signaling is also crucial for otic development and functions at multiple stages. Indeed, *FGF* cascades from the endoderm, mesoderm, and hindbrain are required for otic placode induction [6]. *FGFR2* also plays a vital role in inner ear development and hair cell differentiation. Urness et al. demonstrated the importance of *FGFR2*b ligands *fgf3* and *fgf10* in the development of the inner ear in mouse models [6]. Indeed, the alteration of *fgf3* and *fgf10* expression induces various morphological variations in the inner ear structure, and mice double null mutants (i.e., *F3KO; F10KO*) have no inner ear [6].

FGFR Craniosynostosis (CS) and Otologic Findings

Hearing Loss in Non-syndromic and Syndromic CS

Determining the precise incidence of hearing loss in patients with craniosynostosis (CS) is difficult. Indeed, the incidence varies in the literature depending on whether the criteria studied include congenital hearing loss only, congenital and acquired hearing loss, or hearing loss that includes impairment that is transient and/or related to otitis media with effusion. Regardless of these variations, evidence indicates that hearing loss is a common condition in patients with CS, particularly in those with syndromic craniosynostosis. In a study including 31 patients with CS (9 non-syndromic and 22 syndromic), Goh et al. reported that 18 out of 22 patients with syndromic CS (82%) had hearing loss, compared to only 2 out of 9 (22%) with non-syndromic CS ($p < 0.001$) [4]. Similarly, Biamino et al. found hearing loss in 7 of 11 patients (64%) with syndromic CS [3]. Other studies also report high rates of hearing loss in Apert syndrome and other types of syndromic CS [7–9]. Conversely, Rajenderkumar et al. and Tovetjärn et al. observed lower rates of hearing loss in their series on Apert syndrome, further underscoring the difficulty of estimating the true incidence (Table 10.1) [10, 11].

Regarding the type of hearing loss, the majority of cases reported in the literature presented CHL, followed by MHL and, in a few cases, SNHL. In the study by Goh et al., CHL in syndromic CS was more likely to be associated with a SNHL when compared to non-syndromic CS ($p < 0.01$) [4]. Rajenderkumar et al. report that most patients with Apert syndrome present with acquired hearing loss, despite the frequency of congenital malformations [10]. The level of hearing loss is primarily mild to moderate (Table 10.1).

Comparing hearing loss across different CS syndromes, a literature review by Agochukwu et al. revealed the following incidences of hearing loss in *FGFR* craniosynostoses: 61% in Muenke syndrome, 80% in Apert syndrome, 92% in Pfeiffer syndrome, 74% in Crouzon syndrome, 68% in Jackson Weiss syndrome, 4% in Beare Stevenson syndrome, and 14% in Crouzon syndrome with Acanthosis Nigricans. The majority of the hearing loss was conductive, with the exception of Muenke syndrome—which was associated with a majority of SNHL—and Crouzon syndrome, where almost half of the patients have a pure SNHL or a MHL [2, 12]. Table 10.1 presents an overview of the types and levels of hearing loss observed in different series.

Focus on Otologic Findings in Apert Syndrome

A literature review revealed that 100 of 125 patients with Apert syndrome (80%) had transient or permanent hearing loss [2]. As with the majority of syndromic CS, hearing loss in Apert

Table 10.1 Otologic findings in patients with craniosynostosis

Article	Type of craniosynostosis	n (patient)	Degree of hearing loss[a]	n (ear)	Type of hearing loss[a]	n (ear)
Goh et al. [4]	Apert	9	Normal	10	CHL	26
	Crouzon	7	Mild	14	SHL	0
	Pfeiffer	5	Moderate	16	MHL	14
	Saethre–Chotzen	1	Severe + profound	12		
	Non-syndromic	18				
Huang et al. [18]	Apert	1	Moderate	1	CHL	1
David et al. [22]	Apert	28	Normal	26	CHL	7
			Mild	6		
			Severe	1		
			Missing data	30		
Desai et al. [23]	Pfeiffer	20	Normal	3	CHL	23
			Mild	21	SHL	2
			Moderate	10	MHL	6
			Severe	2	Missing data	6
			Missing data	4		
De Jong et al. [24]	Apert	25	Normal	14		
			Mild	6		
			Moderate	5		
	Crouzon	42	Normal	30		
			Mild	8		
			Moderate	4		
	Muenke syndrome	29	Normal	11		
			Mild	14		
			Moderate	4		
	Saethre–Chotzen syndrome	21	Normal	15		
			Mild	6		
			Moderate	0		
Rajenderkumar et al. [10]	Apert	70	Normal	n (patient) 57	Congenital CHL	2
			Mild	11	Congenital SNHL	2
			Moderate	8	Acquired CHL	19
			Missing data	4		
Tovetjärn et al. [11]	Apert	28	Normal	15		
			« hearing problems »	9		
Barber et al. [25]	Pfeiffer	1	Profound	1	SNHL	1
Phillips et al. [8]	Apert	3	Normal	2	CHL	2
			Mild	1	MHL	2
			Moderate	3		
Gould et al. [9]	Apert	17	Normal	4	CHL	30
			Mild	16		
			Moderate	14		
Orvidas et al. [26]	Crouzon		Normal	11	CHL	8
			Moderate	1	SNHL	8

(continued)

Table 10.1 (continued)

Article	Type of craniosynostosis	*n* (patient)	Degree of hearing loss[a]	*n* (ear)	Type of hearing loss[a]	*n* (ear)
			Unknown level of hearing loss	18	MHL	3
Kilcoyne et al. [27]	Crouzon with acanthosis nigricans	6	Mild	*n* (patient) 2	CHL	*n* (patient) 5
			Moderate	3	SNHL	1
			Missing data	1		
Zhou et al. [7]	Apert	20	Normal	7	CHL	*n* (patient) 16
			« Mild—moderate hearing loss »	33	MHL	2
Hogg et al. [20]	Apert	19	Normal	*n* (patient) 2	CHL	*n* (patient) 9
			« hearing loss »	9		7
			Unknown	8		
Bergstrom et al. [28]	Apert		Moderate	7	CHL	7
			Severe	1		
Gopen et al. [29]	Apert	1	Normal	1	MHL	1
			Moderate	1		
Biamino et al. [3]	Apert	4	Normal	1	CHL	5
			Mild	2	MHL	2
			Moderate	5	SNH	0
	Crouzon	1	Mild	1	CHL	2
			Moderate	1		
	Pfeiffer	1	Normal	2		
	Saethre-Chotzen	3	Normal	2	CHL	4
			Mild	4		
	Muenke	2	Normal	4		

Mild hearing loss: AC 21–40 dB, Moderate hearing loss: AC 41–70 dB, Severe hearing loss: AC 71–90 dB, Severe hearing loss: 91–110 dB

CHL conductive hearing loss, *MHL* mixed hearing loss, *SNHL* sensorineural hearing loss

[a]The degree and type of hearing loss are most often reported as the number of ears (*n* = ear), but occasionally, they are expressed as the number of patients. In such cases, the notation "*n* = patient" is provided alongside the data

is mainly conductive, but MHL and SNHL are also described (Table 10.1) [2]. In most cases, patients had mild-to-moderate hearing loss. The most frequent condition was otitis media with effusion (OME) and its associated complications. The insertion of ventilation tubes in patients with Apert syndrome is frequent [10]. The key role of *FGFR2* signaling in the development of external, middle, and inner ear is associated with the broad number of different malformations in patients with Apert syndrome reported in the literature (Table 10.2).

Table 10.2 Type of ear malformations encountered in patients with Apert syndrome

Article	Type of malformation	*n*
Huang et al. [18]	Abnormal vestibules Enlarged LSCC Slight dilatation of IACs Dehiscent fallopian canal Overhanging facial nerve in the oval window	1 1 1 1 1
de Jong et al. [24]	Atelectasis or retraction	19
Phillips et al. [8]	Low set ears Congenitally fixed stapes Thickened footplate Abnormally thick posterior stapedial crus Constricted ear canal Dehiscent jugular bulb Fixed incus	1 2 1 1 1 2 1
Farkas et al. [17]	Short and narrow ear Wide ears Long and wide ears Disproportionally wide ear Disproportionally long ear	1 2 1 2 1
Gould et al. [9]	Grade 1 microtia Posteriorly rotated ears Tympanic membrane perforation Tympanic membrane atelectasis Cholesteatoma Incus erosion due to chronic infection Fused incus mallear mass Large diameter to the LSCC Exhibited bilateral canting of the temporal bone Exhibited unilateral canting of the temporal bone Congenitally fixed footplate Dehiscent jugular bulb	7 9 2 2 1 1 1 1 2 1 1 2
Zhou et al. [7]	Bilateral inner ear abnormalities Dilation / enlargement of the vestibule Bulbous vestibule Hypoplastic cochlea High riding jugular bulb Dehiscent PSCC Malformed / fused middle ear ossicles, calcification of ligaments	18 11 9 18 12 4 8
Hogg et al. [20]	No anomaly	6
	Absent bony window of the LSCC Enlarged lateral SCC that is continuous with the vestibule Near dehiscence of the PSCC High riding jugular bulb Slightly enlarged SSCC	12 12 6 4 1
	Absent bony island and enlarged LSCC = rectangular vestibular cavity	12

(continued)

Table 10.2 (continued)

Article	Type of malformation	*n*
Rajenderkumar et al. [10]	Low-set ears Microtia, macrotia Abnormal surface configuration of pinna Posteriorly rotated external ears Eustachian tube dysfunction Constricted external canal Conductive hearing loss Ossicular fixation (stapes footplate fixation) Wide cochlear aqueduct Otitis media with effusion Atelectasis/retraction Perforation of the eardrum	NA NA NA NA NA NA NA NA NA 65 8 4
Bergstrom et al. [28]	Congenital fixation of the stapes footplate Perilymph leak, and abnormally wide cochlear aqueduct Enlarged internal auditory meatus Absence of stapedius reflex, ossicular fixation	1 1 1 1
Gopen et al. [29]	PSCC dehiscence	1
Biamino et al. [3]	Recurrent otitis media[a] Cholesteatoma[a] Tympanic atelectasis[a]	7 1 1
Lindsay et al. [30]	Cartilaginous fixation of the stapes footplate Large fissula ante fenestram, filled with cartilage Incompletely developed annular ligament Absent otoconia and hair cells over the lower anterior saccular macula	1 1 1 1

Only series were included, literature review were excluded

LSCC lateral semicircular canal, *PSCC* posterior semicircular canal, *SSCC* superior semicircular canal, *IAC* internal auditory canal

[a]Mixed data of patients with Apert, Crouzon, Muenken, Pfeiffer or Saethre–Chotzen syndrome

Hearing Assessment

The incidence of congenital hearing loss in patients with Apert syndrome is estimated to be 3–6%, which is higher than that in the general population [10, 13] and underscores the essential need for systematic neonatal hearing screening. In most high-income countries, universal hearing screening is conducted in all newborns. Given that craniofacial malformations are a known risk factor for hearing loss, neonatal hearing screenings are all the more important in patients with Apert syndrome [14]. In the event of normal screening results at birth, the risk of congenital moderate-to-profound SNHL can be ruled out. Hearing follow-up care should be performed regularly, with particular attention given to the possible repercussions of chronic otitis, including transient mild-to-moderate deafness that typically regresses with otitis treatment. Given the risk of repercussions on auditory perception and speech development, management of hearing issues is particularly important in patients with a syndrome associated with neurodevelopmental disorders. Moderate-to-severe intellectual disability and variable developmental delay occur in more than half of Apert syndrome cases.

Children with Apert syndrome require multidisciplinary monitoring for issues including sleep apnea, airway problems, and hearing loss. An ear, nose, and throat (ENT) specialist can monitor and, when appropriate, provide early diagnosis of hearing issues via careful tympanic examination. Tympanometry is a helpful tool for the diagnosing of serous otitis. The ENT specialist will also perform a hearing test if indicated based on parental impressions and language level. Depending on the child's age, hearing tests can be subjective and/or objective. For example, age-appropriate behavioral audiometry is subjective, whereas the auditory evoked potentials, auditory steady state response, and otoacoustic emissions assessments are objective. International guidelines on the frequency of hearing monitoring in children with Apert syndrome have not been established, but Wenger et al. and Mathijssen et al. recommend annual assessment [12, 15].

Later in childhood, the prevalence of developing a hearing impairment is estimated to be 0.3–0.5% in the general population and is influenced by various medical and environmental factors [16]. However, the incidence of hearing impairment is higher in patients with Apert syndrome. In a series including 34 patients with Apert syndrome aged 10–20 years, 19 (56%) developed a CHL [13]. A study including 28 adults with Apert syndrome reported that adult patients had significantly more otologic problems than the general population, emphasizing the importance of lifelong otologic follow-up [11]. At Necker Enfants Malades Hospital, all patients with CS have annual otologic examinations and regular hearing tests, with the otologic aspect and presence of any ear malformation informing the frequency of hearing assessment.

Conductive Hearing Loss

Chronic Otitis Media

An early cause of CHL in Apert syndrome is OME, a common condition in children. Patients with Apert syndrome are particularly prone to OME due to the narrowness of the Eustachian tube caused by cranial base malformation. OME can lead to mild-to-moderate CHL and recurrent acute otitis media.

The first-line treatment of chronic OME is ventilation tube placement and, if necessary, an adenoidectomy. A short video presenting the procedure of ventilation tube placement is available on our department's YouTube otologic channel.[1] This procedure relieves hearing loss and prevents subsequent complications. Ventilation tubes are often kept in place for at least 2 years in patients with Apert syndrome—longer than in the general population—because craniofacial anomalies increase both the risk and persistence of tubal dysfunction and nasal obstruction. Of note, adenoidectomy is contraindicated if velar insufficiency, bifid uvula, or adenoid hypertrophy is present due to the risk of increased nasal emission during speech that decreases speech intelligibility. Given the narrowness of the Eustachian tube, untreatable otorrhea sometimes appears after ventilation tube placement. In these rare instances, ventilation tubes are removed, and hearing aids are indicated to treat the CHL in case of OME recurrency.

Chronic OME, if not properly diagnosed and treated, can lead to different forms of chronic otitis—such as tympanic perforation, tympanic membrane retraction pocket, atelectasis or cholesteatoma, and tympanosclerosis (Fig. 10.3)—resulting in CHL or MHL. The treatment of such pathologies is primarily surgical. After performing a surgical retraction pocket or cholesteatoma

[1] Video is available at https://www.youtube.com/watch?v=onww_yRPgMw&t=3s (accessed June 10, 2025).

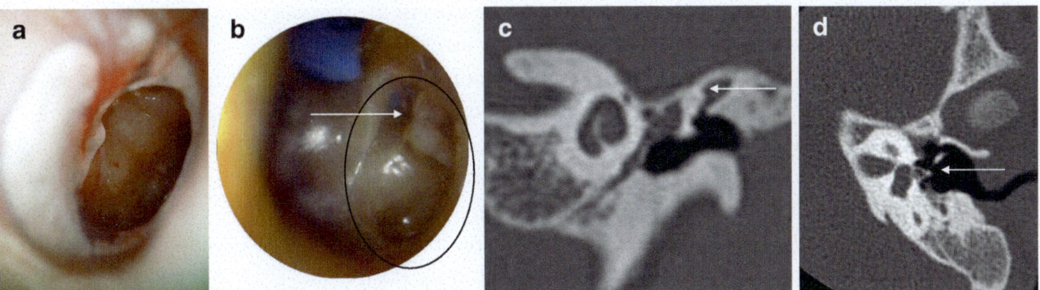

Fig. 10.3 Different pathologies of the middle ear encountered in patients with Apert syndrome. (**a**) Tympanic membrane perforation of the anterior quadrant associated with myringosclerosis. (**b**) Retraction pocket of a left tympanic membrane with a lysis of the incus and a ventilation tube. (**c**) Computed tomography (CT) scan, coronal view of epitympanic fixation of the malleus (arrow). (**d**) CT scan, axial view of lysis of the long process of the incus (arrow)

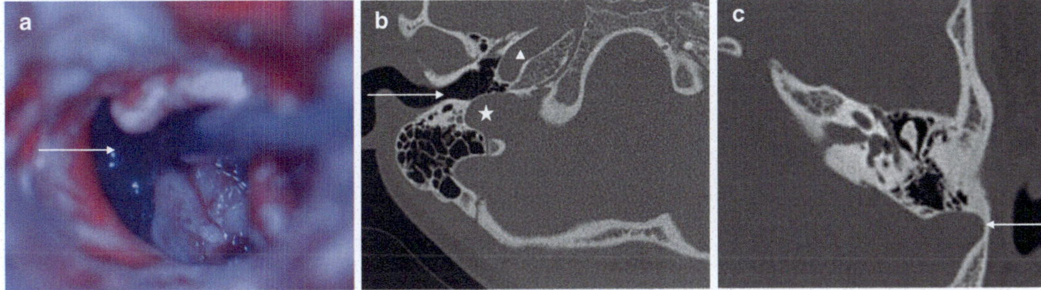

Fig. 10.4 Different vascular malformations encountered in patients with Apert syndrome. (**a**) Operative view of a left high riding jugular bulb (arrow). (**b**) Computed tomography (CT) scan, axial view of right narrow external ear canal (arrow), high riding jugular bulb (star), and inner carotid protrusion (triangle). (**c**) CT scan, axial view of left lateral sinus protrusion (arrow)

treatment, a tympanic cartilage graft is placed to close the tympanic perforation or to reinforce the tympanic membrane. Anatomical findings observed in patients with Apert syndrome include a narrow external ear canal and high-riding jugular bulb, which pose challenges to middle ear access during surgery (Fig. 10.4) [9].

External Ear Malformations

Other rare causes of CHL in Apert syndrome include external ear malformations such as microtia and external ear canal stenosis) (Fig. 10.5) [2]. In these cases, hearing aids are prescribed to treat hearing impairment. The indication of surgical canaloplasty is under debate. Although it is recommended in cases of cholesteatoma due to skin retention in the external canal, the auditory benefit of this surgery is not proven. In a series including 11 patients with Apert syndrome, Farkas et al. observed different external ear particularities in four patients (Table 10.2) [17]. These morphological variations are not associated with any hearing impairment.

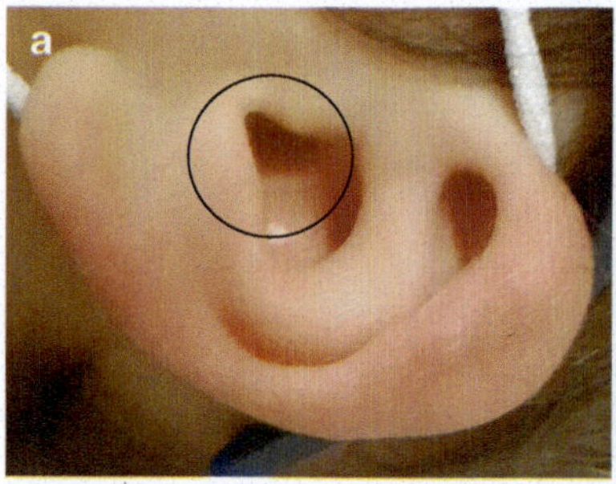

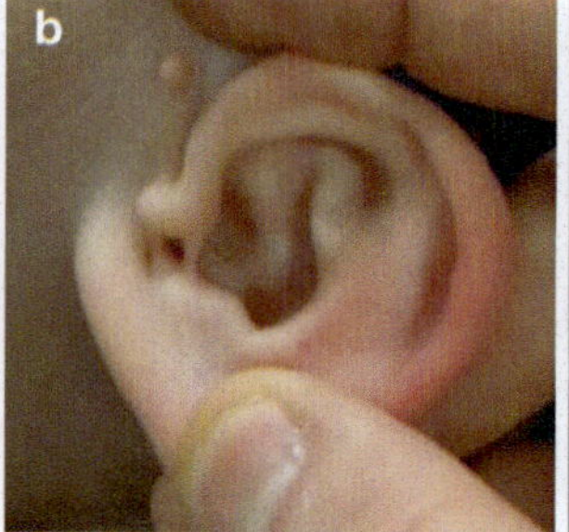

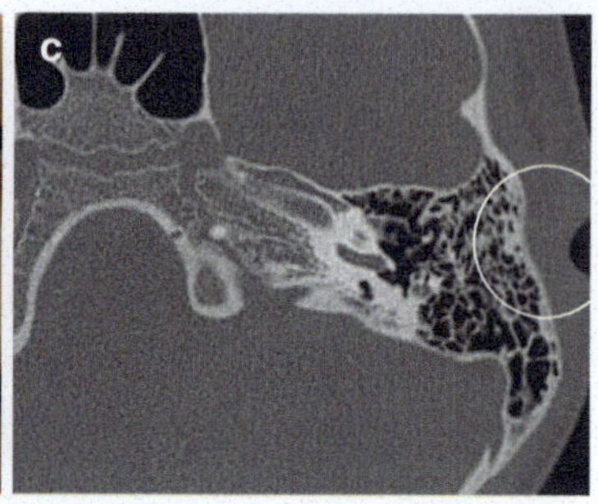

Fig. 10.5 Different malformations of the external ear encountered in patients with Apert syndrome. (**a**) Left external auditory canal atresia. (**b**) Left external auditory canal atresia. (**c**) Computed tomography (CT) scan, axial view of left external auditory canal atresia

Ossicular Malformations

Ossicular malformations or fixation have been described in patients with Apert syndrome (Fig. 10.3) [18]. The most frequently encountered ossicular malformation is the stapes and footplate fixation, both of which originate from the second branchial arch and otic capsule [18]. This rare malformation is responsible for mild-to-severe CHL, and the first line of treatment is hearing aids. Surgical ossiculoplasty is only proposed if the child is unsatisfied with the hearing aids and motivated for surgery. Depending on the encountered anomalies, surgical treatment consists of a stapes mobilization, a stapedotomy (i.e., footplate trephination and piston placement) that can be performed independently or in conjunction with the stapes mobilization, or a stapedectomy. Patients must be informed that surgery for ossicular malformations carries the risk of total hearing loss. Given this risk, surgical treatment is only proposed in adolescents or adults. Additionally, stapes fixation can be associated with "stapes gusher," a rare phenomenon in which perilymphatic fluid suddenly exits during surgical stapedotomy or stapedectomy. This complication is caused by a congenital malformation that results in abnormal communication between the perilymphatic and subarachnoid spaces. Computed tomography (CT) scan images with variable findings—small cochlea, dilated inner auditory canal, incomplete partition of the cochlear coils, dilatation of the semicircular canals, vestibulum, or vestibular and/or cochlear aqueduct—can inform suspicion of stapes gusher [18]. Surgery is contraindicated in this context due to the risk of total hearing loss secondary to the opening of the inner ear.

Vascular Anomalies

A high-riding or dehiscent jugular bulb has been described in several cases of patients with Apert syndrome (Table 10.2) (Fig. 10.4). These anatomical particularities have no impact on hearing or balance, but can lead to difficult access to the middle ear during tympanoplasty. No surgical treatment is recommended to modify the route or cover the jugular bulb. To date, no malformation of the internal carotid in the otologic area is described in the literature.

Sensorineural Hearing Loss

Less than 5% patients with Apert syndrome have SNHL [2]. Various inner malformations have been reported in this patient group, including dilated vestibule, malformed lateral semicircular canal, and cochlear dysplasia (Table 10.2) [5]. In a series including 20 patients with Apert syndrome, Zhou et al. found that all the patients had some form of inner ear anomaly [7]. Although this finding is likely an overestimation, it underscores the importance of systematic CT imaging of the ears and a precise expert analysis. In most cases, SNHL in patients with Apert syndrome is congenital, primarily due to the role of *FGFR2* in the development of the otic placode and the differentiation of hair cells. However, acquired SNHL resulting from various factors has also been documented. Factors include auditory nerve compression secondary to inner auditory canal malformation, prolonged hospital stays for airway or intracranial complications, exposure to ototoxic medications, mechanical ventilation, and recurrent infections. These factors are well-known contributors to inner ear damage and auditory neuropathies [19]. Sometimes, inner ear malformations are not associated with hearing impairment and are incidentally discovered during routine CT scans performed in children with Apert syndrome.

Vestibular Anomalies

In a series including 19 patients with Apert syndrome, the most commonly observed anomalies were an absent bony window of the lateral semicircular canal and an enlarged lateral semicircular canal (Fig. 10.6) [20]. Anomalies of the posterior semicircular canal have also been described. Patients with Apert syndrome can present dilation or enlargement of the vestibule or a bulbous vestibule (Table 10.2). Vestibular or semicircular canal malformations can be responsible for SNHL but are also associated with CHL or MHL by creating a "third mobile window."

Balance Issues in Patients with CS

Many inner ear anomalies described above can be associated with balance issues. However, only one series in the literature reports disequilibrium and vertigo in a patient with a "congenital unilateral craniosynostosis" [21]. Given that vestibular assessments in children are a recent pediatric ENT offering available in only a limited number of centers, balance issues may be undiagnosed. Moreover, vestibular exploration is not routinely performed in patients with CS. Further investigation into this area would undoubtedly be of value.

Cochlear and Windows Malformations

Several cochlear abnormalities, such as hypoplastic cochlea, have been described in patients with CS, and may or may not be associated with vestibular malformations. Dilation of the cochlear aqueduct—a small canal that connects the cochlea to the subarachnoid space and plays a role in fluid regulation and pressure balance—has been observed. This last malformation can be associated with the stapes gusher phenomenon described in this chapter.

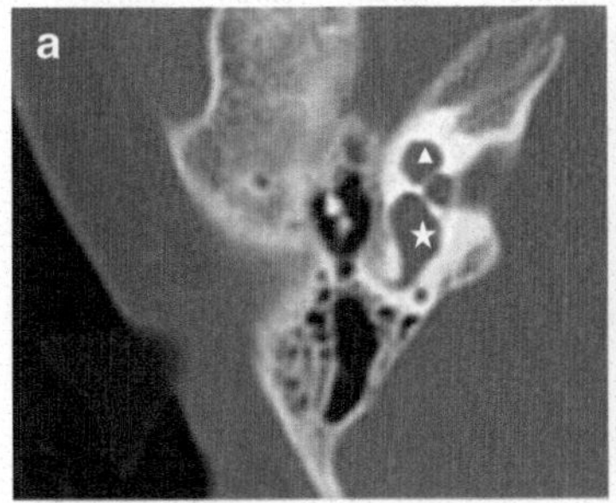

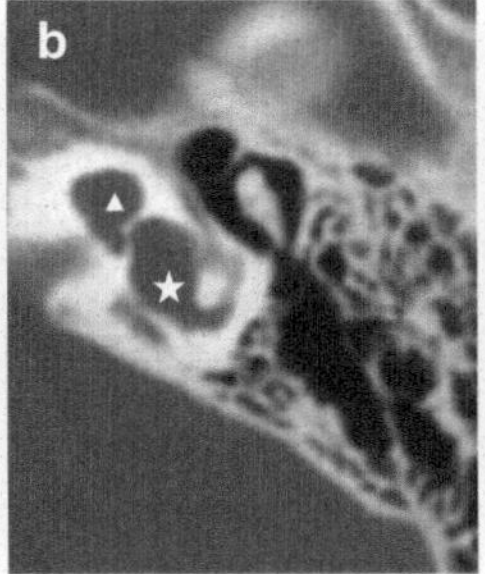

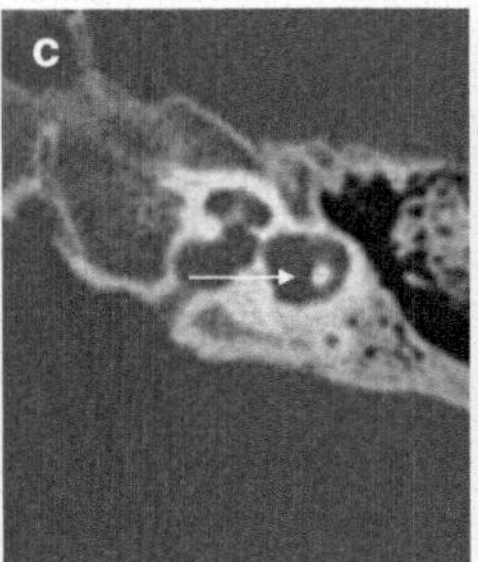

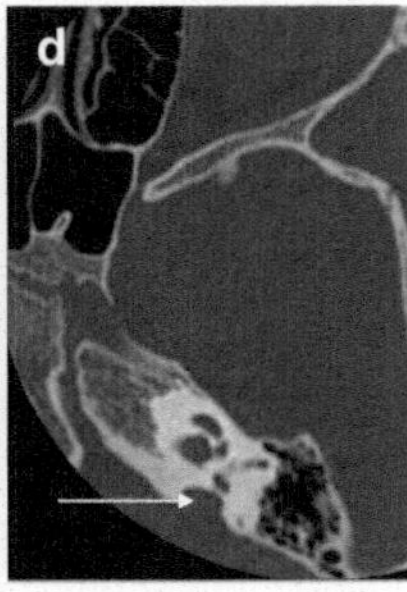

Fig. 10.6 Different malformations of the inner ear encountered in patients with Apert syndrome. (**a**) Computed tomography (CT) scan, axial view of vestibular dilation (star) and cochlear hypoplasia (triangle). (**b**) CT scan of vestibular dilation (star) and cochlear hypoplasia (triangle). (**c**) CT scan of vestibular malformation; small-sized central bony island and enlarged lateral semicircular canal (arrow). (**d**) CT scan of abnormally wide vestibular aqueduct (arrow)

Additionally, anatomical anomalies of the oval and round windows, leading to CHL or SNHL, have been described (Table 10.2).

Conclusion

Although the otolaryngology management of children with Apert syndrome mainly focuses on nasal obstruction and obstructive sleep apnea, close otologic follow-up, consisting of otoscopic examination and radiologic investigation, is essential. OME, the most frequent otologic pathology in patients with Apert syndrome, requires appropriate diagnosis and treatment to address hearing loss and avoid complications such as retraction pocket or cholesteatoma. In addition, many various malformations of the external, middle, and inner ear have been described in the literature as responsible for CHL, MHL, or SNHL. Although hearing loss in patients with Apert syndrome can be congenital, it is primarily acquired, highlighting the importance of lifelong otologic follow-up.

References

1. Couloigner V, Ayari Khalfallah S. Craniosynostosis and ENT. Neurochirurgie. 2019;65(5):318–21.
2. Agochukwu NB, Solomon BD, Muenke M. Hearing loss in syndromic craniosynostoses: otologic manifestations and clinical findings. Int J Pediatr Otorhinolaryngol. 2014;78(12):2037–47.
3. Biamino E, Canale A, Lacilla M, Marinosci A, Dagna F, Genitori L, et al. Prevention and management of hearing loss in syndromic craniosynostosis: a case series. Int J Pediatr Otorhinolaryngol. 2016;85:95–8.
4. Goh LC, Azman A, Siti HBK, Khoo WV, Muthukumarasamy PA, Thong MK, et al. An audiological evaluation of syndromic and non-syndromic craniosynostosis in pre-school going children. Int J Pediatr Otorhinolaryngol. 2018;109:50–3.
5. Larsen's Human Embryology, 6th Edition. 2020.
6. Urness LD, Wang X, Doan H, Shumway N, Noyes CA, Gutierrez-Magana E, et al. Spatial and temporal inhibition of FGFR2b ligands reveals continuous requirements and novel targets in mouse inner ear morphogenesis. Dev Camb Engl. 2018;145(24):dev170142.
7. Zhou G, Schwartz LT, Gopen Q. Inner ear anomalies and conductive hearing loss in children with Apert syndrome: an overlooked otologic aspect. Otol Neurotol. 2009;30(2):184–9.
8. Phillips SG, Miyamoto RT. Congenital conductive hearing loss in Apert syndrome. Otolaryngol Head Neck Surg. 1986;95(4):429–33.
9. Gould HJ, Caldarelli DD. Hearing and otopathology in Apert syndrome. Arch Otolaryngol Chic Ill 1960. 1982;108(6):347–9.
10. Rajenderkumar D, Bamiou DE, Sirimanna T. Audiological profile in Apert syndrome. Arch Dis Child. 2005;90(6):592–3.
11. Tovetjärn R, Tarnow P, Maltese G, Fischer S, Sahlin PE, Kölby L. Children with Apert syndrome as adults: a follow-up study of 28 Scandinavian patients. Plast Reconstr Surg. 2012;130(4):572e–6e.
12. Wenger T, Miller D, Evans K. FGFR Craniosynostosis syndromes overview. In: GeneReviews®. Seattle: University of Washington; 1993.
13. Rajenderkumar D, Bamiou D, Sirimanna T. Management of hearing loss in Apert syndrome. J Laryngol Otol. 2005;119(5):385–90.
14. Year 2019 Position Statement: Principles and Guidelines for Early Hearing Detection and Intervention Programs. J Early Hear Detect Interv. 9(1):1–53, 4(2), 1–44. https://doi.org/10.15142/fptk-b748.
15. Mathijssen IMJ. Working group guideline Craniosynostosis. Updated guideline on treatment and management of craniosynostosis. J Craniofac Surg. 2021;32(1):371–450.
16. Lieu JEC, Kenna M, Anne S, Davidson L. Hearing loss in children: a review. JAMA. 2020;324(21):2195–205.
17. Farkas LG. Ear morphology in Treacher Collins', Apert's, and Crouzon's syndromes. Arch Otorhinolaryngol. 1978;220(1–2):153–7.
18. Huang F, Sweet R, Tewfik TL. Apert syndrome and hearing loss with ear anomalies: a case report and literature review. Int J Pediatr Otorhinolaryngol. 2004;68(4):495–501.
19. Church MW, Parent-Jenkins L, Rozzelle AA, Eldis FE, Kazzi SNJ. Auditory brainstem response abnormalities and hearing loss in children with craniosynostosis. Pediatrics. 2007;119(6):e1351–60.
20. Hogg ES, Turgut NF, McCann E, Avula S, De S, Sharma SD. Inner ear anomalies in children with Apert syndrome: a radiological and Audiological analysis. J Craniofac Surg. 2022;33(5):1428–30.
21. Grundfast KM, Bluestone CD. Sudden or fluctuating hearing loss and vertigo in children due to perilymph fistula. Ann Otol Rhinol Laryngol. 1978;87(6 Pt 1):761–71.
22. David DJ, Anderson P, Flapper W, Syme-Grant J, Santoreneos S, Moore M. Apert syndrome: outcomes from the Australian craniofacial unit's birth to maturity management protocol. J Craniofac Surg. 2016;27(5):1125–34.
23. Desai U, Rosen H, Mulliken JB, Gopen Q, Meara JG, Rogers GF. Audiologic findings in Pfeiffer syndrome. J Craniofac Surg. 2010;21(5):1411–8.

24. de Jong T, Toll MS, de Gier HHW, Mathijssen IMJ. Audiological profile of children and young adults with syndromic and complex craniosynostosis. Arch Otolaryngol Head Neck Surg. 2011;137(8):775–8.
25. Barber SR, Remenschneider AK, Kozin ED, Cunnane ME, Nahed BV, Leslie-Mazwi T, et al. Cochlear implantation in a patient with Pfeiffer syndrome and temporal bone vascular anomalies. Otol Neurotol. 2016;37(3):241–3.
26. Orvidas LJ, Fabry LB, Diacova S, McDonald TJ. Hearing and otopathology in Crouzon syndrome. Laryngoscope. 1999;109(9):1372–5.
27. Kilcoyne S, Scully P, Overton S, Brockbank S, Thomas GPL, Ching RC, et al. Speech and language development, hearing, and feeding in patients with genetically confirmed Crouzon syndrome with acanthosis Nigricans: a 36-year longitudinal retrospective review of patients at the Oxford craniofacial unit. J Craniofac Surg. 2024.
28. Bergstrom L, Neblett LM, Hemenway WG. Otologic manifestations of acrocephalosyndactyly. Arch Otolaryngol Chic Ill 1960. 1972;96(2):117–23.
29. Gopen Q, Zhou G, Poe D, Kenna M, Jones D. Posterior semicircular canal dehiscence: first reported case series. Otol Neurotol. 2010;31(2):339–44.
30. Lindsay JR, Black FO, Donnelly WH. Acrocephalosyndactly (Apert's syndrome): temporal bone findings. Ann Otol Rhinol Laryngol. 1975;84(2 PART 1):174–8.

11 Cleft Palate

Ingrid M. Ganske, Melissa Zattoni Antonelli, and Nivaldo Alonso

Take Home Messages

- High arched palate with progressively enlarging bilateral flanking tissue prominences gives Apert syndrome a "pseudocleft" appearance.
- Overt and submucosal clefting is more common in this syndrome than in other craniofacial synostosis.
- The goals of palate repair include improved oral feeding (prevention of nasal regurgitation) and speech.
- The palate should be addressed secondarily to treatment of the cranium to minimize risks of prolonged elevation of intracranial pressure and at a slightly older age than typical palate repair to minimize risks of post-operative airway obstruction.
- Concurrent facial differences, particularly maxillary hypoplasia, possible facial asymmetry/deviated septum, and choanal atresia, may increase the child's risk of worsened obstructive breathing after palate repair.
- Midfacial hypoplasia often causes hyponasal speech outcomes; once midfacial advancement is performed, velopharyngeal insufficiency is often noted, at least temporarily.
- Comprehensive speech therapy addresses resonance, velopharyngeal function, articulation challenges attributable to malocclusion, and general speech-language skills related to concurrent developmental delay.
- Cognitive function can affect speech evaluation and outcomes in individuals with Apert syndrome.

I. M. Ganske (✉)
Department of Plastic and Oral Surgery, Boston Children's Hospital, Boston, MA, USA

Harvard Medical School, Boston, MA, USA
e-mail: Ingrid.ganske@childrens.harvard.edu

M. Z. Antonelli
Speech and Hearing Department, Hospital for Rehabilitation of Craniofacial Anomalies and University of São Paulo, Sao Paulo, Brazil

N. Alonso
Department of Plastic Surgery, Faculdade de Medicina da Universidade de São Paulo, São Paulo, São Paulo, Brazil

Craniofacial Division, Hospital for Rehabilitation of Craniofacial Anomalies and University of São Paulo, São Paulo, São Paulo, Brazil

Introduction

Cleft palate is a common finding in Apert syndrome. It is also one of the most common congenital craniofacial anomalies in isolation, occurring in approximately 6 per 10,000 infants [24]. The standard techniques, timing, and outcomes of cleft palate repair are well established; specific considerations in other craniofacial conditions, such as Robin Sequence [48], hemifacial microsomia [8], and syndromes such as 22q [4] have also been described. In Apert syndrome, the features of palatal anatomy are well described; however, this population's outcomes of palate

J. G. Meara et al. (eds.), *Apert Syndrome*, https://doi.org/10.1007/978-3-032-12551-4_11

repair and technical considerations are not. We attempt to summarize the available literature and the experiences of our two institutions (HRCA and BCH).

Palatal Findings in Apert Syndrome

In Apert syndrome, the palate demonstrates soft tissue mounds over the hard palate separated by a narrow, high arch centrally. Pruzansky and Lis [35] noted that this "pseudocleft" phenomenon becomes progressively more pronounced with age. Gorlin et al. [14] referred to the palatal configuration as a "Byzantine arch palate" with an incomplete fusion of the palatine processes of the maxilla with the nasal spine. Indeed, this configuration has been documented in nearly all individuals with Apert syndrome [20]. Solomon et al. [39] found a possible explanation for gingival hypertrophy in patients with Apert syndrome: a high deposit of acid mucopolysaccharides in hard palate mucosa and palatal bone hyperplasia with age (Fig. 11.1). The maxillary sutures have been shown to fuse earlier than in unaffected children, preventing circummaxillary growth [28]. With increasing age, the narrowness of the palate becomes more pronounced. Additionally, the hard palate is shorter than it is in unaffected individuals, whereas the soft palate is longer than normal [33]. Computed tomographic scans of children with Apert syndrome have demonstrated that, compared to controls, there is normal nasal length and width (similar nasal airway volume to controls); however, there is a limited airway dimension posterior to the palate and small overall pharyngeal airway size that leads to obstructed breathing often seen in this condition [10, 17, 22] (Fig. 11.2).

Apert syndrome may or may not include a cleft palate (Fig. 11.3). In a series of 119 patients with Apert syndrome, Kreiborg and Cohen Jr [20] found cleft palate or bifid uvula in 75%. Previous reports had documented bifid uvula in 66.7% and true cleft at only 10.5% [32]. A smaller study of 17 cases of Apert syndrome by Arroyo Carrera et al. [3] identified cleft palate in 23.5%. Variation in the incidence of clefting evident in other studies may be attributable to whether bifid uvula and submucous forms are included in the tally and potential misdiagnosis of the severely high and narrowly arched "pseudocleft."

There is a well-established difference in the risk of cleft palate occurring between the two different mutations within FGFR2 (fibroblast growth factor receptor 2) responsible for Apert syndrome—Ser252Trp and Pro253Arg. Park et al. [30] found that cleft palate occurred with much higher frequency in the S252W genotype than in the P253R genotype. Slaney et al. [38] found that individuals with the S252W variant

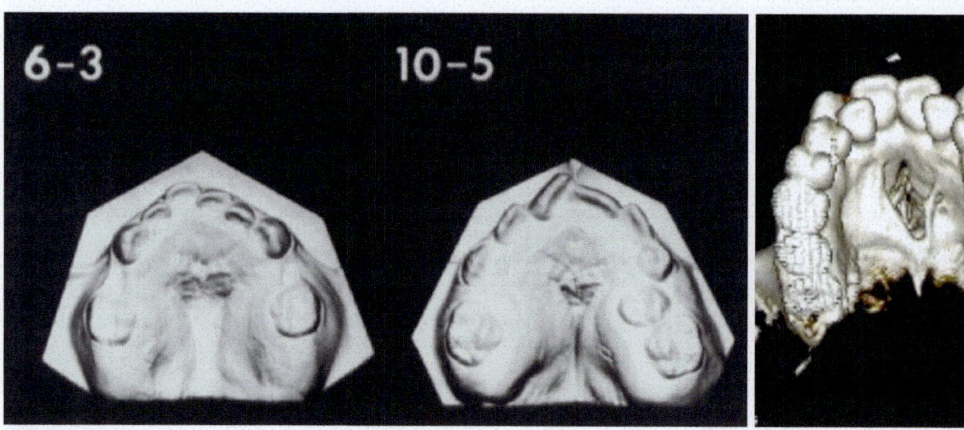

Fig. 11.1 Evolution of hard palate deformity with age. Left: Hard palate model at age 6 years and at 10 years with progressive thickening of mucopolysaccharide deposition (Solomon et al. [39]). Right: Similar accumulations seen on CT scan in another patient with Apert syndrome at 23 years

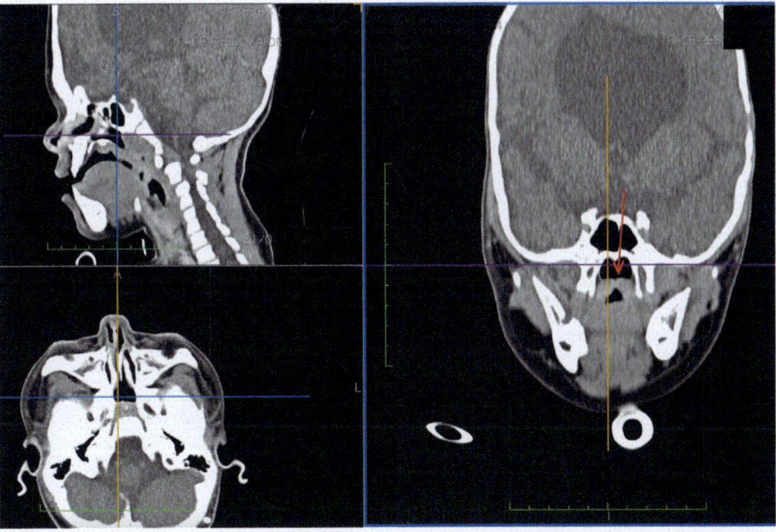

Fig. 11.2 CT imaging in unoperated patient with Apert syndrome. Left above: Sagittal section showing a short posterior airway and soft palate touching the posterior pharyngeal wall. Left below: Axial section showing a transversely narrow posterior airway. Right: Coronal section showing submucous cleft palate (arrow)

also had more severe facial findings based on supraorbital ridging, marked maxillary hypoplasia, ocular proptosis, down-slanting palpebral fissures, and facial asymmetry. In their series, cleft palate occurred more often in this subtype (58.5%) than in those with the P253R variation (17.4%), and there was a higher prevalence of choanal atresia with S252W as well. A more severe craniofacial phenotype in S252W has been supported by several other subsequent studies, which report cleft palate in approximately 60% of those with the S252W variant and only 15% of those with P253R [18, 21, 36, 46, 49]. In a review of 44 patients with Apert, Wagner et al. [47] found significantly smaller nasopharyngeal airway cross-sectional volumes, shorter maxillae, and increased incidence of obstructive sleep apnea in those with Ser252Trp mutations than those with Pro253Arg [47].

Mouse models provide the opportunity to investigate the role of FGF (fibroblast growth factor) signaling in palatal defects in Apert syndrome. The pathogenic variants in FGFR2 potentially alter a complex signaling network in epithelial–mesenchymal interactions during palatogenesis, resulting in cleft palate [49]. The difference in phenotypes resulting from the two mutations has been linked to variably enhanced binding to FGF2 and other fibroblast growth factors expressed in cranial sutures, with a greater increase in affinity for the S252W mutation than the P253R mutation [1, 16]. Studies on the activating FGFR2 mutation of S252W have led to speculation that it confers a specific functional effect on KGFR signaling that interferes with human palatal shelf fusion by disrupting epithelial-mesenchymal differentiation disruption of apoptosis, or both [6, 51]. In mouse models [25] demonstrated that the S252W palatal development is characterized by aberrant cellular behaviors that cause premature fusion of the anterior transverse sutures (right and left maxillary-palatine sutures) as well as failure of closure of the midline inter-premaxillary and inter-palatine sutures, resulting in clefting.

As with complex syndactyly, cleft palate is often described as a unique finding in Apert compared to other forms of syndromic craniosynostosis, but there are reports of frequently high-arched palates and occasional clefting in Pfeiffer and, to a lesser extent, in Saethre-Chotzen syndrome [41, 42]. Submucous cleft palate, while certainly more common in Apert syndrome, has also been described to occur somewhat more frequently in non-syndromic craniosynostosis (8%) than in the general population (between 1% and 4%) [29].

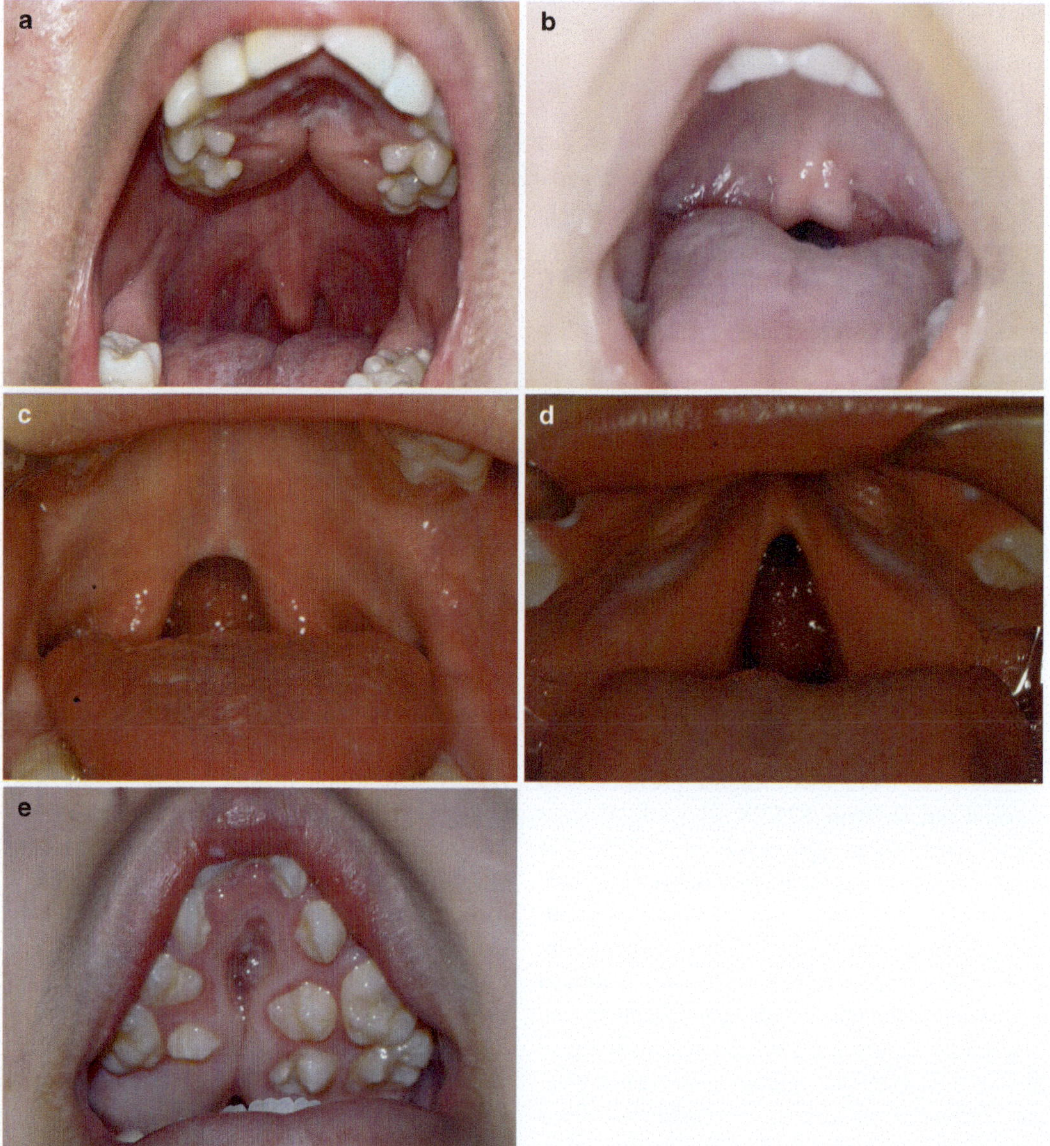

Fig. 11.3 Spectrum of palate anatomy in Apert syndrome. (**a**) Pseudocleft of the hard palate with long soft palate. (**b**) Bifid uvula. (**c**) Veau I cleft of soft palate, with pseudo cleft of hard palate flanked by soft tissue prominences. (**d**) Veau II cleft of the soft and hard palate. (**e**) Teenager with unrepaired, high-arched cleft palate with narrow maxilla and dental crowding. Note more pronounced flanking soft tissue accumulations at this older age

Goals of Palate Repair

Cleft palate results in incomplete closure of the oropharynx and nasopharynx. In normal palate anatomy, an intact muscular velar sling controls oronasal airflow during speech, prevents nasal regurgitation during feeding, and plays a role in proper Eustachian tube function. The goals of cleft palate repair are to reposition the aberrant soft tissue musculature into a functional velopharyngeal sling for speech and to provide an intact division between the mouth and nose to facilitate eating.

Management of Cleft Palate in Apert

Little has been published that may specifically guide management in caring for patients with Apert syndrome who have a cleft palate. General principles described for the more substantial population of infants with cleft palate and other syndromic diagnoses or causes for medical complexity are applicable.

Feeding

Feeding challenges in Apert syndrome are multifactorial. When a cleft is present, there is an inability to create negative intraoral pressure, resulting in inefficient suction and allowing feeds to be readily regurgitated nasally. This compounds the feeding challenges already inherent in Apert syndrome and attributable to malocclusion from midfacial hypoplasia, baseline respiratory obstruction that can contribute to fatigue with oral feeding, breathing-suction-swallowing incoordination, and possible dyscoordination stemming from abnormalities of the central nervous system [13, 31]. For infants with Apert syndrome, simply positioning the bottle nipple in the infant's mouth can hinder or prevent any necessary mouth breathing. Bottle feeding in Apert syndrome is typically prolonged with increased noisy breathing as the feed progresses [34, 44] and frequent coughing or even choking during feeding, indicative of aspiration [45]. Increased respiratory effort during feeding often results in failure to thrive and inadequate weight gain [31]. Pereira et al. [31] used video fluoroscopy to assess swallow function in infants with Apert and noted that even when obstructive breathing was managed with a tracheostomy, the dysphagia often persisted and likely reflected central nervous system dyscoordination of swallow.

When a cleft palate is present, non-suction types of bottles are necessary (Fig. 11.4). Most of these utilize maxillomandibular compression to express liquid from the nipple. When midfacial hypoplasia is severe, infant-driven compression of the bottle nipples may be challenging, and parent-assisted squirt-bottle systems (Haberman™ or syringes) may enable better liquid delivery with less energy expenditure by the infant. In low and middle-income countries where specialty bottle systems are unavailable, very soft-tip silicone nipples can enable successful oral feeding without suction (Fig. 11.5). If there are concerns about uncoordinated feeding and aspiration, video fluoroscopy is indicated, and thickened liquids may be helpful. Formula concentration provides additional caloric content to address failure to thrive from feeding-related energy expenditures. Using a nasogastric tube or placing a percutaneous gastrostomy tube may be necessary; however, the goal is for children to become orally competent without the need for any such ongoing support, which is nearly always achievable. During the tube feeding period, if required, it is important to provide oral stimulation; for example, using an adapted pacifier that allows both oral stimulation and mouth breathing. An interdisciplinary approach to the management of issues with feeding and swallowing is necessary, especially in the first months of life.

Timing of Palate Repair

Children presenting with isolated cleft palate typically undergo palate repair within the first year of life to optimize speech outcomes. For children with Apert syndrome, cleft palate repair may exacerbate airway obstruction and evalua-

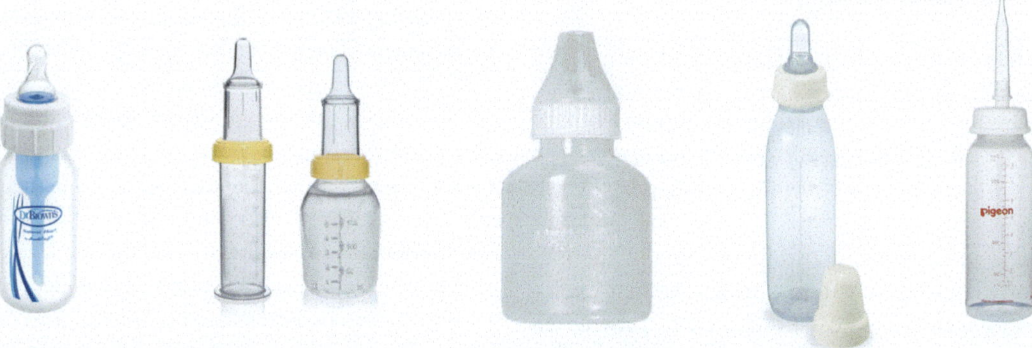

Fig. 11.4 Various options of cleft feeders. From left to right: Dr. Brown's® Specialty feeder, Medela Special Needs Haberman feeder™, Mead Johnson Cleft Palate Nurser™, Pigeon® Cleft Palate bottle with round and syringe nipples

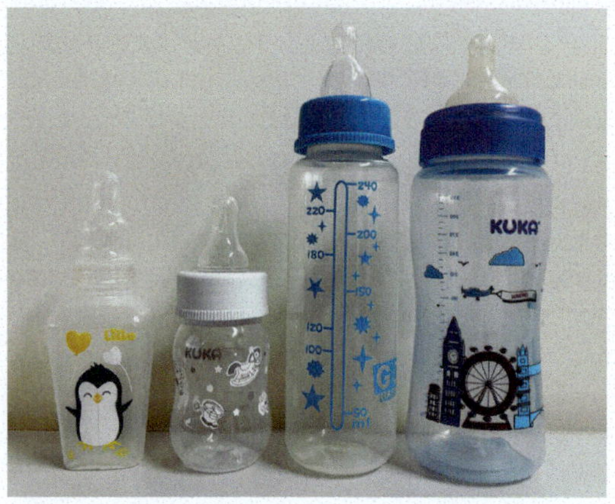

Fig. 11.5 Examples of very soft silicone nipples that may be used instead of cleft feeders

tion of tonsilectomy should be considered before any procedure [50]. Pre-operative polysomnography (PSG), where available, can help identify infants who may be at higher risk due to baseline respiratory physiology [17]. Andiné et al. [2] retrospectively reviewed 14 patients with Apert syndrome following cleft palate repair. Although the study was too small to find statistically significant predictors of postoperative respiratory complications, the authors noted that those who experienced complications or required ICU care had palate repair at a younger age (less than 20 months). Notably, preoperative PSG results were not available for risk stratification. They also found that patients who had post-operative respiratory issues all had palate repair in conjunction with other procedures, suggesting the potential risk factors of longer anesthesia time, surgical stress, or baseline health conditions necessitating the coordinated procedures (such as gastrostomy tube placement) [2]. Careful consideration should be given to whether palate repair should be done at a later age than in the non-Apert population. Rather than attempting to coordinate procedures, other interventions often done in the first year, including correction of craniosynostosis and syndactyly [43], may be prioritized. When repairing the palate at an older age, removing tonsils and adenoids first may help reduce the risk of post-operative airway compromise.

Thus, the ideal timing of cleft palate repair must account for other planned procedures and the extent and type of cleft, balanced with the severity of breathing concerns. Peterson-Falzone et al. [33] raised the possibility that an overt cleft palate may be an unexpected benefit for patients with Apert syndrome, providing additional nasopharyngeal airway patency [33]. Awaiting further orofacial growth before repair may help decrease the obstructing effect of repairing the open cleft airway. Midfacial retrusion may partially minimize air escape through a soft palatal cleft. Although no studies evaluate speech and resonance in children with Apert syndrome who have unrepaired cleft palate, it is feasible that the outcomes are less hypernasal than would otherwise occur in isolated unrepaired cleft palate without craniofacial synostosis. This could result in fewer negative consequences to the child regarding compensatory speech error development, thus mitigating the worst speech outcomes resulting from repair later in childhood in non-Apert populations.

Techniques of Palate Repair

Well-established techniques of palate repair include either uni-pedicled or bi-pedicled repair of the hard palate, coupled with closure of the soft palate using straight line closure with intravelar veloplasty [40], Furlow double opposing Z-plasty [11], and possible inclusion of buccal fat or myomucosal flaps [27]. These are described elsewhere in detail [12, 15, 23, 26]. Considering the specific, unique anatomy of Apert syndrome, including the long soft palate in conjunction with the already heightened concern for sleep apnea from midfacial hypoplasia, further lengthening the soft palate with a Furlow repair would not be advisable. The authors recommend straight-line closure with intravelar veloplasty. Visualization and dissection of the hard palatal flaps can be more challenging than the typical cleft palate due to the high-arched configuration, but are typically achievable with standard intraoral retractors and loupe magnification. Additional surgical maneuvers may be necessary, particularly when the palate is repaired later in childhood after the gingival protuberances have become more pronounced (Fig. 11.6).

Postoperative Care

Airway monitoring is critical immediately following cleft palate repair. Postoperative palatal swelling from the repair, compounded by possible tongue swelling from the intraoperative retraction, exacerbates baseline obstructive tendencies from the midfacial hypoplasia. Consideration may be given to extended intubation through the period of peak swelling, 48 h postoperatively. If immediate extubation is performed, a short-term nasopharyngeal tube may be placed to bypass the palatal swelling. Postoperative steroids may be used to minimize swelling. Intensive care capabilities should be available, if not preemptively arranged, for monitoring overnight.

Patients are allowed to resume oral feeding as they are able. A liquid and soft puree consistency is followed for the first 4–6 weeks until the palate is healed.

Speech and Language Development and the Role of Speech Therapy

Palatal components to speech include velar closure to generate adequate pressure for oral sounds

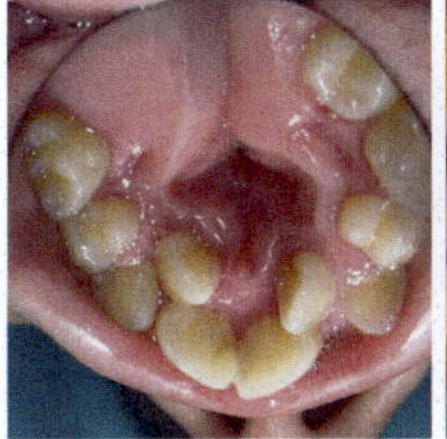
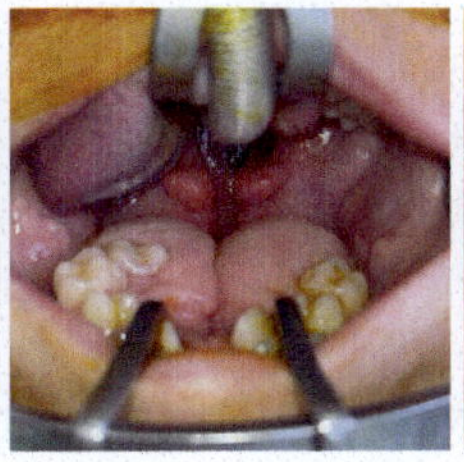
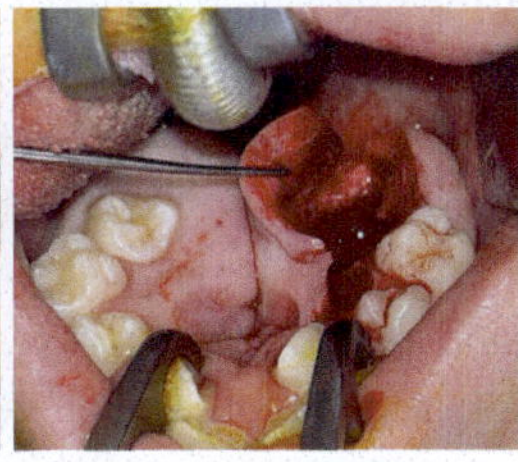
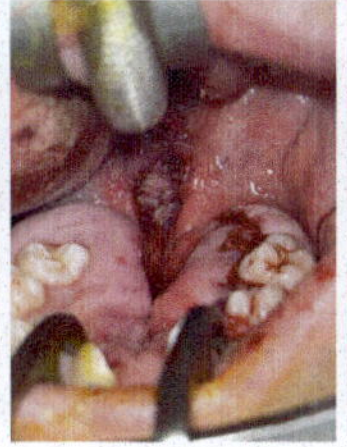
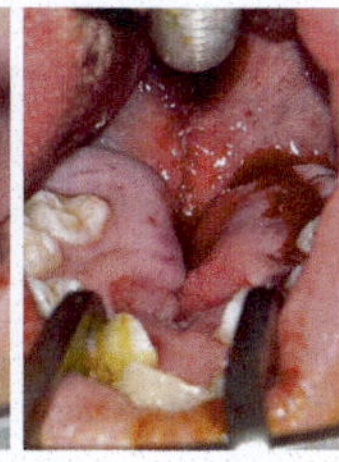

Fig. 11.6 Soft palate cleft repair requiring reduction of hard palate gingiva for access and visualization. (**a**) Pseudocleft of the hard palate. (**b**) Cleft soft palate with prominent hard palate mucosa obscuring access. (**c**) Exposure and resection of redundant hard palate mucosa, as well as removal of impacted molars. (**d**) Improved visualization of the soft palate to facilitate repair. (**e**) Following intravelar-veloplasty and oral closure

and resonance of the voice. Communication skills in Apert syndrome may be impacted by more than speech sound disorders stemming from cleft palate. Language disorders, hearing loss, and its associated communication difficulties, social communication difficulties, and any associated cognitive impairment all contribute to the overall intelligibility of speech [18, 37].

Cognitive abilities are pertinent to language development and engaging productively in speech therapy. Lajeunie et al. [21] assessed IQ in 24 patients with Apert syndrome and found IQ less than 70 (normal) in over half. Of the eleven patients in their series with cleft palate and neurocognitive testing results, seven (63%) had low IQ. Still, others had IQs ranging from 70 to 114, indicating variable prognosis regarding developmental delay that may impact speech and communication skills.

In a review of hearing, speech, and communication in 55 children with Apert syndrome, Kilcoyne et al. [18] found that almost all had speech sound disorders in both FGFR2 genotype variants. Patients with S252W mutation were more likely to have moderate to severe difficulties with communication participation than the P253R group [18]. In the majority of all individuals, this was attributable to structural anomalies such as dental crowding, anterior open bite, and high arched palate, and not to cleft-type speech characteristics. In fact, hyponasal resonance was found in 75% of both subtypes; however, the study did not indicate the age of speech assessments or the temporal relationship of the assessment to any mid-facial advancement operations performed. A nearly pervasive need for speech and language therapy has been noted in both genotypes [18].

Outcomes of Palate Repair in Apert Syndrome

Following palate repair, the primary outcomes of concern include avoidance of worsened airway obstruction, avoidance of fistula, and establishment of velopharyngeal competency. There is only a single study to date reporting the outcomes of any of these variables. Andiné et al. [2] presented the short-term results of 14 patients with Apert syndrome and cleft palate who had repair at an average age of 22 months. In their cohort, 29% had worsened airway obstruction post-operatively, and 36% required ICU-level care for one night. One patient required CPAP after the palate repair; none required a tracheostomy [2].

Andiné et al. also reported one reoperation for palatal fistula (7%) [2]. The development of a palatal fistula is of immediate post-operative concern with any palate repair. In Apert syndrome, the repaired cleft palate is again at risk of injury during subsequent procedures, with potential for fistula formation during monobloc and Le Fort advancement. Care must be taken to fully release the tissues before advancement with Rowe retractors; otherwise, tear of the palatal tissue may ensue.

Assessment of speech outcomes following palate repair in Apert syndrome is challenging because of the confounding developmental and communication issues involved and the variability of results in relation to the midfacial correction. In early childhood, before maxillary advancement, there is rarely concern about velopharyngeal insufficiency; in fact, more commonly, the speech is hyponasal. Any type of facial advancement theoretically could lead to loss of velar contact with the posterior pharyngeal wall and development of hypernasality; this is well established in the non-syndromic cleft palate population following Le Fort I advancement with or without distraction [19]. (Fig. 11.7) In Apert syndrome, when midfacial advancement is performed, the hyponasality improves, and speech often becomes hypernasal at least temporarily. Cedars et al. [7] described finding transient borderline to overt velopharyngeal insufficiency in nearly half of patients with craniofacial synostosis (Apert and Crouzon syndromes) undergoing midface distraction techniques, even in the absence of cleft palate. Others have found nearly universal transient velopharyngeal insufficiency (VPI) in children with Apert syndrome, including those with and without cleft palate, after midfacial advancement [52]. Fearon [9] noted that the temporary VPI in patients following Halo dis-

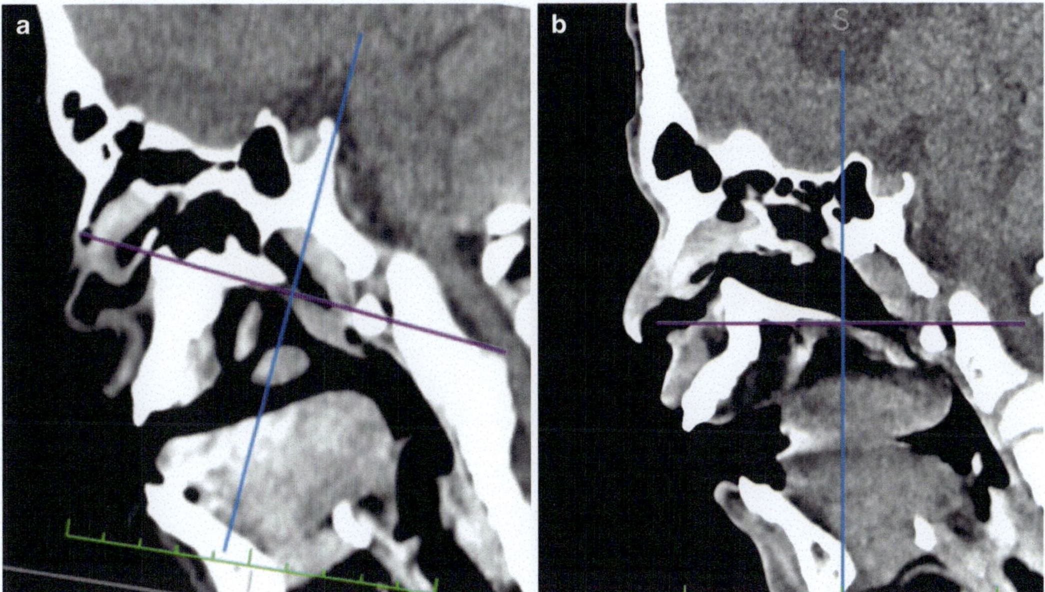

Fig. 11.7 Sagittal CT sections showing changes in the soft palate position and posterior pharyngeal dimension before (left) and after (right) frontofacial monobloc advancement in a patient with Apert syndrome

traction of Le Fort III in syndromic craniosynostosis typically completely resolved by 6 weeks postoperatively. Meanwhile, others have found a need for speech surgery after midfacial advancement in Apert syndrome. Bordbar et al. [5] reported that 75% with cleft palate needed speech surgery after advancement, and 25% without cleft palate had worse hypernasality and needed intervention as well; however, the follow-up duration at the time of the assessment was heterogeneous, and in some cases as early as 2 months post-operative [5]. Speech and resonance should be reevaluated before and after mid-facial advancement.

The authors report the experience of our combined centers. Of 152 patients with Apert syndrome seen in São Paulo and Bauru from 1987 to the present, 49 patients were treated by the senior surgeon (NA). Of those, 22 (45%) had an abnormal palate, including four with overt submucous cleft palate and bifid uvula, two with Veau II cleft palate, and the majority (16, 73%) with Veau I. Of the 22 patients with cleft palate who had palate repair, there was one postoperative palatal fistula after palatoplasty (Fig. 11.8) and a second fistula after frontofacial monobloc advancement during the facial mobilization with Rowe forceps. Most patients had palatoplasty done after 24 months, and five underwent repair later than 4 years of age. One patient had primary palatoplasty at 13 years old, not because of velopharyngeal insufficiency but exclusively due to concerns of nasal regurgitation. In this patient, the surgery was technically very difficult because of the gingival hypertrophy of the hard palate, including many impacted teeth (see Fig. 11.5 above).

At Boston Children's Hospital, 62 patients with Apert syndrome were treated over a 12-year period from 2008 to 2020. Some form of palatal clefting was found in 17 (22.5%). Seven (41%) had submucosal clefts, none of whom required repair. Of those with Veau I (4, 23.5%), Veau II (3, 17.5%), or unspecified overt clefting (3, 17.5%), all but two had repair, which was performed at an average age of 13.5 months. Two patients had true clefts that were not repaired. In both instances, repair was deferred in infancy due to severe airway obstruction; later repair was not done in one child due to lack of language development, and in the other because of lack of symptoms from the unrepaired cleft palate (no velopharyngeal insufficiency or nasal regurgita-

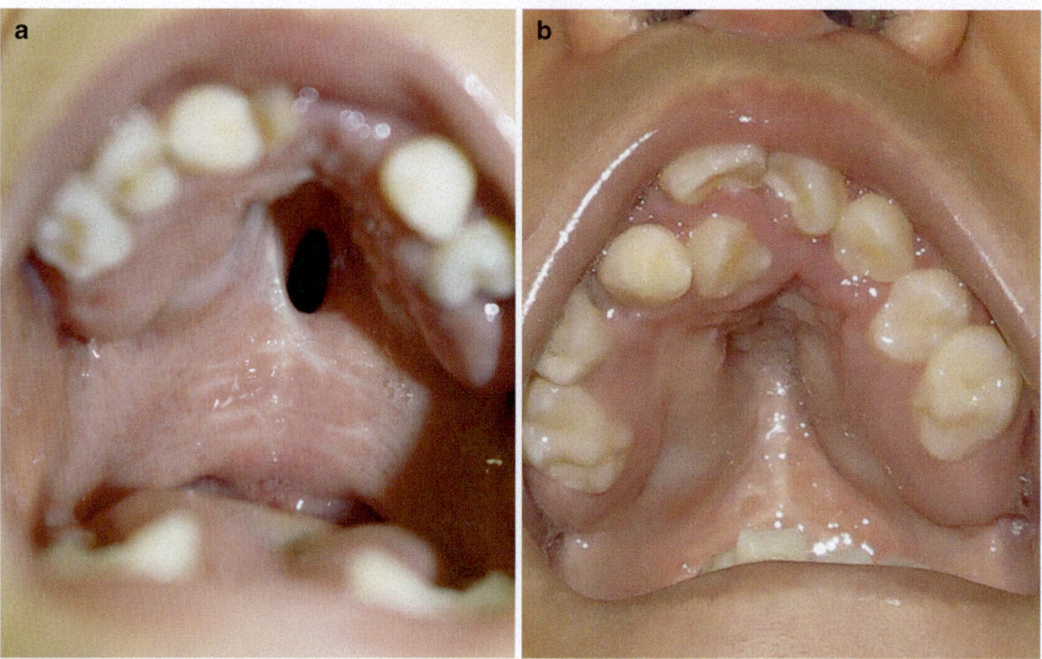

Fig. 11.8 (**a**) Repaired Cleft palate in Apert patient with a fistula in the junction of hard and soft palate. (**b**) Following fistula closure, note maxillary dentition crowding

tion). Of those who had repairs, there was one instance of postoperative airway obstruction; this occurred in an 11-month old who subsequently required continuous positive airway pressure (CPAP) throughout childhood that was eventually found attributable, at least in part, to a severely deviated septum. There were no palatal fistulae and no instances of VPI; however, the speech results are incomplete as many of the children had yet to undergo Le Fort III advancement at the time of review.

Conclusions

Individuals with Apert syndrome have multiple problems related to the genetic disorder, all of which can directly impact the functional and psychosocial outcomes of their multidisciplinary treatment. In São Paulo, an ongoing unpublished study about the quality of life in Apert syndrome utilizes the questionnaire HUI 3 (Health Utilities Index) to assess patients who have undergone the full institutional treatment protocol to date (early cranial decompression, monobloc advancement, palate repair if cleft, and Le Fort and orthognathic surgery as needed). Eight attributes are evaluated and correlated with the time of surgical treatment, speech among them. Of the 20 patients evaluated to date, common negative contributors to quality of life have been speech, emotion, and knowledge. In this preliminary review, all patients with Apert syndrome had decreased quality of life affected by speech, even when the evaluator deemed their speech to be good. This underscores the need for speech and language support for all those with Apert syndrome, independent of cleft palate, as satisfaction with speech and language skills is critical to holistic care.

Our review of the topic and institutional experiences shows that palatoplasty can safely be performed in Apert syndrome but is best delayed until approximately 24 months of age. Preoperative efforts should be directed at identifying and mitigating the risk of airway obstruction. Postoperatively, speech and language outcomes typically reflect broader cognitive and communication challenges than palatal contributions to speech intelligibility. Following patients through the completion of facial growth and final orthognathic procedures is critical, as VPI can occur due to these later anatomic changes.

Acknowledgment The authors thank Brent Whiting, of Harvard Dental School, and Stephen Stearns, of Harvard Medical School, for their assistance with data collection, which made this review possible.

References

1. Anderson J, Burns HD, Enriquez-Harris P, Wilkie AO, Heath JK. Apert syndrome mutations in fibroblast growth factor receptor 2 exhibit increased affinity for FGF ligand. Hum Mol Genet. 1998;7:1475–83.
2. Andiné A, Tarnow P, Boivie P. Cleft palate in Apert syndrome: a descriptive study of incidence and surgical outcome. Cleft Palate Craniofac J. 2023:10556656231194445. Epub ahead of print.
3. Arroyo Carrera I, Martínez-Frías ML, Marco Pérez JJ, Paisán Grisolía L, Cárdenes Rodríguez A, Nieto Conde C, Félix Rodríguez V, Egüés Jimeno JJ, Morales Fernández MC, Gómez-Ullate Vergara J, Pardo Romero M, Peñas Valiente A. Oliván del Cacho MJ, Lara Palma A. Síndrome de Apert: análisis clínico-epidemiológico de una serie consecutiva de casos en España [Apert syndrome: Clinico-epidemiological analysis of a series of consecutive cases in Spain]. An Esp Pediatr. 1999;51:667–72.
4. Bezuhly M, Fischbach S, Klaiman P, Fisher DM. Impact of 22q deletion syndrome on speech outcomes following primary surgery for submucous cleft palate. Plast Reconstr Surg. 2012;129:502e–10e.
5. Bordbar P, Blumenow W, Duncan C, Richardson D. Resonance and speech articulation after midface advancement in craniofacial dysostosis. J Craniofac Surg. 2012;23:e100–3.
6. Britto JA, Evans RD, Hayward RD, Jones BM. Toward pathogenesis of Apert cleft palate: FGF, FGFR, and TGF beta genes are differentially expressed in sequential stages of human palatal shelf fusion. Cleft Palate Craniofac J. 2002;39:332–40.
7. Cedars MG, Linck DL 2nd, Chin M, Toth BA. Advancement of the midface using distraction techniques. Plast Reconstr Surg. 1999;103:429–41.
8. Dentino KM, Valstar A, Padwa BL. Cleft characteristics and treatment outcomes in hemifacial microsomia compared to non-syndromic cleft lip/palate. Int J Oral Maxillofac Surg. 2016;45:679–82.
9. Fearon JA. Halo distraction of the Le Fort III in syndromic craniosynostosis: a long-term assessment. Plast Reconstr Surg. 2005;115:1524–36.
10. Forte AJ, Lu X, Hashim PW, Steinbacher DM, Alperovich M, Persing JA, Alonso N. Airway analysis in Apert syndrome. Plast Reconstr Surg. 2019;144:704–9.
11. Furlow LT Jr. Cleft palate repair by double opposing Z-plasty. Plast Reconstr Surg. 1986;78:724–38.
12. Ganske IM, Rogers-Vizena CR. Cleft lip and palate: principles and management. In: Chung KC, editor. Grabb and smith's plastic surgery. 9th ed. Wolters Kluwer; 2025.
13. Gonsalez SL, Thompson D, Hayward R, Lane R. Breathing patterns in children with craniofacial dysostosis and hindbrain herniation. Eur Respir J. 1998;11:866–72.
14. Gorlin RJ, Cervenka J, Pruzansky S. Facial clefting and its syndromes. Birth Defects Orig Art Ser. 1971;7:3–49.
15. Hamdan US, Rogers-Vizena CR, Vyas RM, Sommerlad BC, Low DW. Interdisciplinary cleft care: global perspectives. Plural Publishing; 2023.
16. Ibrahimi OA, Zhang F, Eliseenkova AV, Itoh N, Linhardt RJ, Mohammadi M. Biochemical analysis of pathogenic ligand-dependent FGFR2 mutations suggests distinct pathophysiological mechanisms for craniofacial and limb abnormalities. Hum Mol Genet. 2004;13:2313–24.
17. Inverso G, Brustowicz KA, Katz E, Padwa BL. The prevalence of obstructive sleep apnea in symptomatic patients with syndromic craniosynostosis. Int J Oral Maxillofac Surg. 2016;45:167–9.
18. Kilcoyne S, Luscombe C, Scull P, Overton S, Brockbank S, Swan MC, Johnson D, Wall S, Wilkie AOM. Hearing, speech, language, and communicative participation in patients with Apert syndrome: analysis of correlation with fibroblast growth factor receptor 2 mutation. J Craniofac Surg. 2022;33:243–50.
19. Kinter S, Susarla S, Delaney JC, Chapman K, Kapadia H, Weiss N. Does distraction lower risk of VPI compared to conventional maxillary advancement? A retrospective cohort study of adolescents with cleft palate. Cleft Palate Craniofac J. 2024;61:422–32.
20. Kreiborg S, Cohen MM Jr. The oral manifestations of Apert syndrome. J Craniofac Genet Dev Biol. 1992;12:41–8.
21. Lajeunie E, Cameron R, El Ghouzzi V, et al. Clinical variability in patients with Apert's syndrome. J Neurosurg. 1999;90:443.
22. Lu X, Sawh-Martinez R, Forte AJ, Wu R, Cabrejo R, Wilson A, Steinbacher DM, Alperovich M, Alonso N, Persing JA. Mandibular spatial reorientation and morphological alteration of Crouzon and Apert syndrome. Ann Plast Surg. 2019b;83:568–82.
23. Lossee JE, Kirshner R. Comprehensive cleft care. 2nd ed. Thieme; 2016.
24. Mai CT, Cassell CH, Meyer RE, Isenburg J, Canfield MA, Rickard R, Olney RS, Stallings EB, Beck M, Hashmi SS, Cho SJ, Kirby RS, National Birth Defects Prevention Network. Birth defects data from

population-based birth defects surveillance programs in the United States, 2007 to 2011: highlighting orofacial clefts. Birth Defects Res A Clin Mol Teratol. 2014;100:895–904.
25. Martínez-Abadías N, Holmes G, Pankratz T, Wang Y, Zhou X, Jabs EW, Richtsmeier JT. From shape to cells: mouse models reveal mechanisms altering palate development in Apert syndrome. Dis Model Mech. 2013;6(3):768–79.
26. Millard RDJ. Cleft Craft. Little, Brown, and Company; 1976.
27. Mann RJ, Neaman KC, Armstrong SD, Ebner B, Bajnrauh R, Naum S. The double-opposing buccal flap procedure for palatal lengthening. Plast Reconstr Surg. 2011;127:2413–8.
28. Meazzini MC, Corradi F, Mazzoleni F, De Ponti E, Maccagni M, Novelli G, Bozzetti A. Circummaxillary sutures in patients with Apert, Crouzon, and Pfeiffer syndromes compared to nonsyndromic children: growth, orthodontic, and surgical implications. Cleft Palate Craniofac J. 2021;58:299–305.
29. Naran S, Miller M, Shakir S, Ware B, Camison L, Ford M, Goldstein J, Losee J. Nonsyndromic craniosynostosis and associated abnormal speech and language development. Plast Reconstr Surg. 2017;140:62e.
30. Park WJ, Theda C, Maestri NE, et al. Analysis of phenotypic features and FGFR2 mutations in Apert syndrome. Am J Hum Genet. 1995;57:321.
31. Pereira V, Sacher P, Ryan M, Hayward R. Dysphagia and nutrition problems in infants with Apert syndrome. Cleft Palate Craniofac J. 2009;46:285–91.
32. Peterson SJ, Pruzansky S. Palatal anomalies in the syndromes of Apert and Crouzon. Cleft Palate J. 1974;11:394–403.
33. Peterson-Falzone SJ, Pruzansky S, Parris PJ, Laffer JL. Nasopharyngeal dysmorphology in the syndromes of Apert and Crouzon. Cleft Palate J. 1981;18:237–50.
34. Posnick JC. Craniofacial dysostosis syndromes: a staged reconstructive approach. In: Tuvey TA, Vig KW, Fonseca RJ, editors. Facial clefts and craniosynostosis: principles and management. London: WB Saunders; 1996.
35. Pruzansky W, Lis EF. Cephalometric roentgenography of infants: sedation, instrumentation and research. Am J Orthod. 1958;44:159–86.
36. Sakai N, Tokunaga K, Yamazaki Y, Shida H, Sakata Y, Susami T, Nakakita N, Takato T, Uchinuma E. Sequence analysis of fibroblast growth factor receptor 2 (FGFR2) in Japanese patients with craniosynostosis. J Craniofac Surg. 2001;12:580–5.
37. Shipster C, Hearst D, Dockrell JE, Kilby E, Hayward R. Speech and language skills and cognitive functioning in children with Apert syndrome: a pilot study. Int J Lang Commun Disord. 2002;37:325–43.
38. Slaney SF, Oldridge M, Hurst JA, Morriss-Kay GM, Hall CM, Poole MD, Wilkie AOM. Differential effects of FGFR2 mutations on syndactyly and cleft palate in Apert syndrome. Am J Hum Genet. 1996;58:923–32.
39. Solomon LM, Medenica M, Pruzansky S, Kreiborg S. Apert syndrome and palatal mucopolysaccharides. Teratology. 1973;8:287–91.
40. Sommerlad BC. A technique for cleft palate repair. Plast Reconstr Surg. 2003;112:1542–8.
41. Stoler JM, Rosen H, Desai U, Mulliken JB, Meara JG, Rogers GF. Cleft palate in Pfeiffer syndrome. J Craniofac Surg. 2009a;20:1375–7.
42. Stoler JM, Rogers GF, Mulliken JB. The frequency of palatal anomalies in Saethre-Chotzen syndrome. Cleft Palate Craniofac J. 2009b;46:280–4.
43. Theman TA, Upton J, Taghinia AH, Firriolo JM, Nuzzi LC, Labow BI. Central coalition osteotomy of phalangeal synostoses in the management of the Type III Apert hand. J Hand Surg Am. 2018;43:1042.e1–8.
44. Thompson D, Jones B, Hayward R, Harkness W. Assessment and treatment of craniosynostosis. Acta Neurochir. 1994;120:123–5.
45. Tuchman DN, Walter RS. Disorders of feeding and swallowing in infants and children. Pathophysiology, diagnosis, and treatment. San Diego: Singular Publishing; 1994.
46. Von Gernet S, Golla A, Ehrenfels Y, Schuffenhauer S, Fairley JD. Genotype-phenotype analysis in Apert syndrome suggests opposite effects of the two recurrent mutations on syndactyly and outcome of craniofacial surgery. Clin Genet. 2000;57:137.
47. Wagner CS, Wietlisbach LE, Kota A, Villavisanis DF, Pontell ME, Barrero CE, Salinero LK, Swanson JW, Taylor JA, Bartlett SP. Genetic subtypes of Apert syndrome are associated with differences in airway morphology and early upper airway obstruction. J Craniofac Surg. 2023;34:1999–2003.
48. Wang C, Shi B, Li J. Management of cleft palate among patients with Pierre Robin sequence. Br J Oral Maxillofac Surg. 2023;61:475–81.
49. Willie D, Holmes G, Jabs EW, Wu M. Cleft palate in Apert syndrome. J Dev Biol. 2022;10:33.
50. Willington AJ, Ramsden JD. Adenotonsillectomy for the management of obstructive sleep apnea in children with congenital craniosynostosis syndromes. J Craniofac Surg. 2012;23:1020–2.
51. Yeh E, Fanganiello RD, Sunaga DY, Zhou X, Holmes G, Rocha KM, Alonso N, Matushita H, Wang Y, Jabs EW, Passos-Bueno MR. Novel molecular pathways elicited by mutant FGFR2 may account for brain abnormalities in Apert syndrome. PLoS One. 2013;8:e60439.
52. Zimmerman CE, Sun J, Wes AM, Vu GH, Kalmar CL, Humphries LS, Bartlett SP, Cohen MA, Swanson JW, Taylor JA. Long term speech outcomes following midface advancement in syndromic craniosynostosis. J Craniofac Surg. 2020;31:1775–9.

Orthodontic Care

12

Marielle Pillon, Brigitte Vi-Fane, Thomas Bondi, Roman H. Khonsari, Eric Arnaud, and Catherine Tomat

Introduction

Orthodontic intervention typically begins around the age of six, coinciding with the eruption of the first molars into the dental arch. An early orthodontic consultation facilitates a comprehensive diagnosis and allows for an initial discussion with the family regarding the complementary roles of orthodontic treatment and maxillofacial surgical procedures.

The primary goal of the initial treatment phase is to expand the transverse dimension of the maxilla by acting on the mid-palatal suture. If the suture remains patent, an orthodontic appliance is applied to induce expansion. In cases where the mid-palatal suture is fused, and / or orthopedic expansion proves unsuccessful, a surgically-assisted intermaxillary disjunction becomes necessary [1].

Following a period of collaborative monitoring with the maxillofacial surgeon, orthodontic treatment is typically delayed until late adolescence, often around the age of fourteen, unless there is a need to reposition impacted or ectopic teeth into the dental arches before this time. In cases of severe midface hypoplasia or significant obstructive sleep apnea syndrome, patients may require a Le Fort III osteotomy. This procedure is ideally performed between the ages of twelve and fourteen, without prior orthodontic preparation, except in cases where a facial bipartition is necessary. Here, orthodontic preparation may involve placing a palatal plate to prevent overcorrection of the maxillary transverse dimension and/or to modify the angles of the incisor roots to avoid injuries during the inter-maxillary osteotomy. The final surgical intervention in occlusal management typically involves a maxillomandibular osteotomy performed at skeletal maturity (around age eighteen).

Notably, early craniofacial interventions such as frontofacial monobloc advancement (FFMBA) lead to significant dental damage, complicating the orthodontic treatment and indicating implant placement to rehabilitate the posterior maxilla [2].

Orthodontic treatment aligns impacted teeth and coordinates the dental arches in preparation for orthognathic surgery at the end of growth. Its primary objective is to correct dentoalveolar compensations in three dimensions, while orthognathic surgery addresses the underlying skeletal anomalies. The orthodontist plays a critical role both in the pre-surgical preparation and in the postoperative finishing and retention phases [1, 3–7].

M. Pillon · B. Vi-Fane · T. Bondi · R. H. Khonsari
E. Arnaud · C. Tomat (✉)
Department of Maxillofacial Surgery and Plastic Surgery, and Craniofacial Unit, Hôpital Necker–Enfants malades, Assistance publique–Hôpitaux de Paris, Paris, France

J. G. Meara et al. (eds.), *Apert Syndrome*, https://doi.org/10.1007/978-3-032-12551-4_12

Initial Orthodontic Evaluation

Diagnosis

During the initial consultation, a comprehensive clinical examination is performed. The diagnosis is established through an assessment of facial aesthetics, analysis of static and dynamic occlusal relationships, evaluation of functional aspects, and review of supplementary diagnostic tools such as dental casts and radiographic imaging.

Extraoral Examination

Facial observation is conducted from both frontal and lateral views. In the frontal view, facial harmony is assessed based on the degree of symmetry on either side of the mid-vertical axis and the proportionality of the three horizontal facial thirds.

Intraoral Examination

The overall dental health, along with the condition of the oral mucosa, is evaluated. Skeletal and alveolar orthodontic anomalies are also diagnosed. A dynamic occlusal analysis evaluates Planas' functional masticatory angles (AFMP). This assessment of masticatory dynamics enables the identification of whether the patient exhibits normal or imbalanced mastication, aiding in the detection of prematurity, functional abnormalities, and their potential effects on the temporomandibular joint (TMJ), occlusal plane rotation, overbite, and open bite, as well as the assessment of the transverse dimension and any midline deviations. Static occlusion is analyzed directly from the study models.

Function Assessment

A functional assessment is also performed, as dysfunctions—particularly lingual—are frequently observed [8]. These dysfunctions contribute to respiratory disorders, including mouth breathing, obstructive sleep apnea syndrome (OSAS), and snoring without OSAS during sleep, in addition to speech and masticatory difficulties resulting from the misalignment of skeletal structures, dental impactions, and dental dystopias [3]. Collaboration with a speech therapist may be advantageous for correcting and managing these functional impairments. This multidisciplinary approach helps to maintain the stability of treatment outcomes and reduces the risk of recurrence [9].

Study of Complementary Examinations

Photographs

Standard frontal, lateral, and intraoral photographs are essential for monitoring treatment progress and evaluating ongoing clinical changes.

Study Models and Setup

Dental casts are employed to analyze the dental arches and confirm the clinical diagnosis. They provide additional insights that may not be readily apparent during the initial clinical examination, including canine and molar classifications, ectopias, rotations, the degree of crowding, arch form, symmetry, and the extent of dentoalveolar compensations. They are relevant in Apert syndrome as most patients present with maxillary retrusion. A setup, created either from study models mounted on an articulator or a digital workflow, is an invaluable tool for communication between the surgeon and orthodontist. It also aids in the simulation of the surgical procedure [10].

Orthopantomogram (OTP)

This radiograph enables the counting of teeth, facilitating the identification of dental anomalies such as damaged tooth germs from prior craniofacial surgeries (Fig. 12.1), and the localization of impacted teeth. A preliminary assessment of the temporomandibular joints (TMJs) can also be performed.

Frontal and Lateral Cephalometric Radiographs

The lateral cephalometric radiograph is utilized for cephalometric analysis, which is crucial for quantifying skeletal dysmorphia and assessing its impact on the dental arches. It plays a key role in defining treatment objectives and identifying alveolar compensations that require correction during orthodontic preparation. Additionally, this

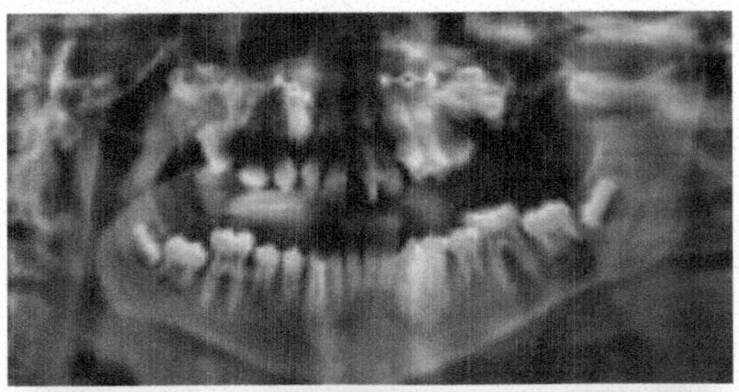

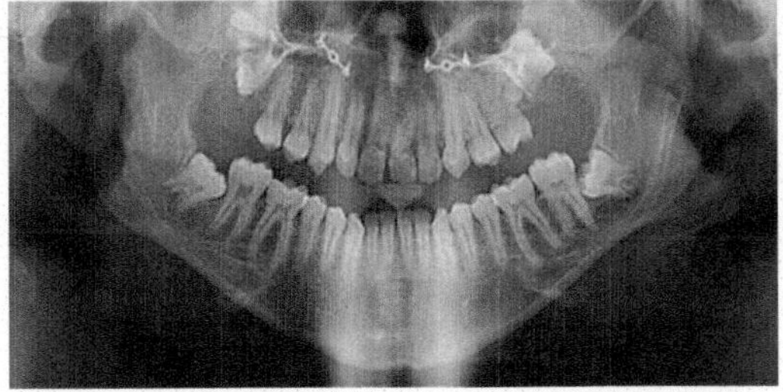

Fig. 12.1 Dental X-rays between 10 and 15 years of age, before and after orthodontic management in a patient with Apert syndrome. Posterior edentulism secondary to early fronto-facial monobloc advancement led to anchoring difficulties. The orthodontic appliance allowed the placement of included teeth on the arch and the coordination of the arches before orthognathic surgery

radiograph is invaluable for conducting longitudinal studies on facial growth and development. The frontal cephalometric radiograph aids in confirming the diagnosis of maxillary retrognathism and detecting facial or mandibular asymmetry.

Cone Beam Computed Tomography (CBCT)

A cone beam computed tomography (CBCT) scan is essential for evaluating the degree of craniofacial asymmetry, facilitating the planning of surgical correction, and is used for fabricating 3D-printed surgical splints in digital workflows. CBCT also allows for precise visualization of the position of impacted teeth and is useful for assessing the maturation stage of the mid-palatal suture before undertaking orthopedic disjunction. The assessment of the intermaxillary suture maturation in orthodontics is based on works by Melsen [11]. Maturation progresses through three stages: infantile (Y-shaped), juvenile (T-shaped), and adult (complex interdigitated suture). Conventional X-rays present limitations in interpretation primarily due to superimposition artifacts. CBCT is thus recommended for the 3D visualization of the midpalatal suture [12].

A new classification system by Angelieri et al. [13] identifies five stages of suture maturation, ranging from Stage A (nearly straight suture) to Stage E (complete fusion). Additionally, cervical vertebral maturation stages, as described by Baccetti [14], are correlated with suture maturation [15, 16].

Principles of Orthodontic Management in Apert Syndrome

Following the initial consultation, the orthodontist formulates a diagnosis and emphasizes to the family the importance of a multidisciplinary follow-up. A comprehensive therapeutic strategy is then developed in collaboration with the maxillofacial surgeon. Before initiating any orthodontic treatment, ensuring optimal oral hygiene and dental health is essential. When necessary, the patient should be referred to their general dentist for any required treatments, as orthodontic intervention must be conducted on a healthy dental and periodontal foundation. Additionally, since orthodontic appliances can interfere with magnetic resonance imaging (MRI), the orthodontist must validate the treatment plan with the multidisciplinary team before proceeding, especially in cases where repeated brain or spinal imaging may be required. It is crucial to understand that orthodontics may be optional within the broader treatment framework for these patients [17]. Nevertheless, despite the data on midpalatal suture fusion, maxillary expansion is always the first option to manage the transverse dimension, and surgery is considered only after the failure of orthopedic methods.

Children with Apert syndrome face a significantly increased risk of intellectual disability, making orthodontic treatment more difficult. Parents of children with syndromic conditions report greater social challenges, attention deficits, and internalizing behaviors compared to parents of children without such conditions. There is a strong correlation between social, emotional, and behavioral difficulties and cognitive development. Additionally, parents of affected children often report a lower quality of life for their child in comparison to the control population [18].

Treating children with special healthcare needs, particularly those with craniofacial anomalies, typically requires more frequent clinical appointments, which may lead to less favorable outcomes. However, overall treatment duration, behavior score, and dental health and aesthetic component scores are comparable to children without special healthcare needs [19].

The Transverse Dimension

When the diagnosis reveals a deficiency in the transverse dimension, the orthodontist should initiate treatment by expanding the maxilla. Orthopedic rapid maxillary expansion (RME) is typically achieved using an intraoral expander, as demonstrated in our observational study at Necker Hospital, where treatment is initiated around the age of 10 [20]. The success of this approach depends mainly on the degree of suture fusion. The appliance facilitates ultra-rapid maxillary expansion, achieving a daily expansion rate of 0.75 mm with an activation screw, which is adjusted by the parents twice daily for approximately 15 days. The degree of activation is determined based on the extent of the transverse discrepancy. In syndromic cases, sagittal skeletal discrepancies are often pronounced; future maxillary advancement must be considered to adapt the relative width of maxillary and mandibular dental arches at the end of treatment and the excessive correction of the transverse dimension.

A follow-up appointment should be scheduled after 1 week to assess expansion progress, verified by the presence of an inter-incisal diastema and the absence of molar tipping or confirmed via occlusal X-rays. Intermaxillary suture maturation varies considerably among individuals, and in the general population, the suture remains largely unossified throughout life, justifying the initial orthopedic approach, even though patients with Apert syndrome most probably present with a higher rate of fused sutures at early ages [21].

Once the targeted expansion is reached, the appliance is locked in position, allowing for suture healing and adaptation of the surrounding soft tissues and perioral musculature, typically over 6 months.

A significant challenge in transverse maxillary expansion for patients with Apert syndrome is the lack of retention in supporting teeth. These patients often exhibit delayed dental eruption and have primary teeth with nonretentive morphology. Ideally, the anchorage is dental, utilizing bands on the first molars [16, 26] or sealed retainers in cases of retention issues. While retainers may enhance appliance retention, they introduce hygiene difficulties, particularly in patients with restricted mouth opening. Additionally, many patients present with intellectual disabilities or limited mouth opening, further complicating dental hygiene (see above).

In cases of severe maxillary retrognathism, bone support can be achieved using bone anchors, like miniscrews [1, 21]. Generally, this method poses few complications, aside from issues related to gingival health due to the difficulty of maintaining hygiene around appliances bonded to retainers or in bone anchorage situations. In syndromic patients, the thick gingival mucosa can contribute to complications such as mucositis or inflammation around the bone anchorage sites [22] (Fig. 12.2).

If the mid-palatal suture has fused and orthopedic expansion is unsuccessful, surgically-assisted rapid maxillary expansion (SARME) is required [1, 23]. This technique combines surgical and orthodontic approaches to create additional space in the maxillary arch, facilitating proper dental alignment; the same device can be employed for various methods of jaw expansion, including RME and SARME. As noted in our observational study, SARME is typically indicated in cases where the orthopedic expansion method has failed, beginning around the age of 10 [8, 20].

SARME also significantly increases the maxillary apical (dentoalveolar) base and expands the

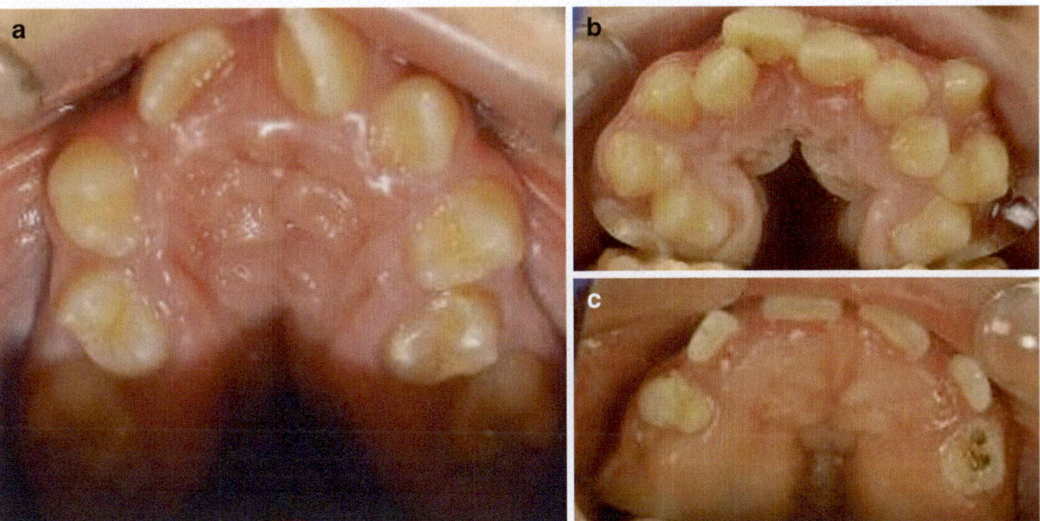

Fig. 12.2 Mucosal thickening in a 10-year-old patient (**a** and **b**) and iatrogenic posterior edentulism in 8-year-old patient with only teeth 11, 12, 14, 21, 22, and 64 on the arch (**c**)

palatal arch, enhancing tongue movement during swallowing. Furthermore, SARME often results in subjective improvements in nasal breathing due to widening the narrowest section of the nasal cavity and increasing its overall volume, even though this point requires further investigations in cases of Apert syndrome [8, 9, 24].

An additional complication arises in patients with an associated cleft palate. In many cases, particularly at advanced ages (8–10 years), the hard palate portion of the cleft may not have been closed due to technical constraints or the cumulative burden of care. Technical difficulties are often related to the unique palatal anatomy in Apert syndrome, which involves a deep midline and thick palatal mucosa. In these cases, the decision to close the palate either before or after maxillary expansion must be made individually, considering the patient's specific anatomical and clinical circumstances.

Placement of Teeth in the Dental Arch

Orthodontic preparation is influenced by patient compliance and, more critically, by the timing of arch preparation and its specific objectives, such as creating adequate space for the eruption and alignment of impacted teeth to avoid extractions (Fig. 12.3). Impacted teeth must be integrated into the dental arch, but in some instances, extractions may be necessary. The selection of teeth for extraction, typically related to space constraints, is determined by local anatomical factors and the patient's motivation and preferences—particularly regarding their satisfaction with facial morphology or their desire for a more harmonious profile. While first premolars are often the primary candidates for extraction, second premolars and even canines may be considered in some cases.

In addition, the risk of obstructive sleep apnea syndrome (OSAS) and the space required for proper tongue function must be carefully evaluated, particularly when considering mandibular premolar extractions.

In cases with a mildly expressed phenotype, guided extractions and exclusive orthodontic treatment with dentoalveolar compensation may be sufficient to address dental arch discrepancies and minor sagittal intermaxillary discrepancies. However, most cases necessitate orthognathic surgery once growth is complete [24].

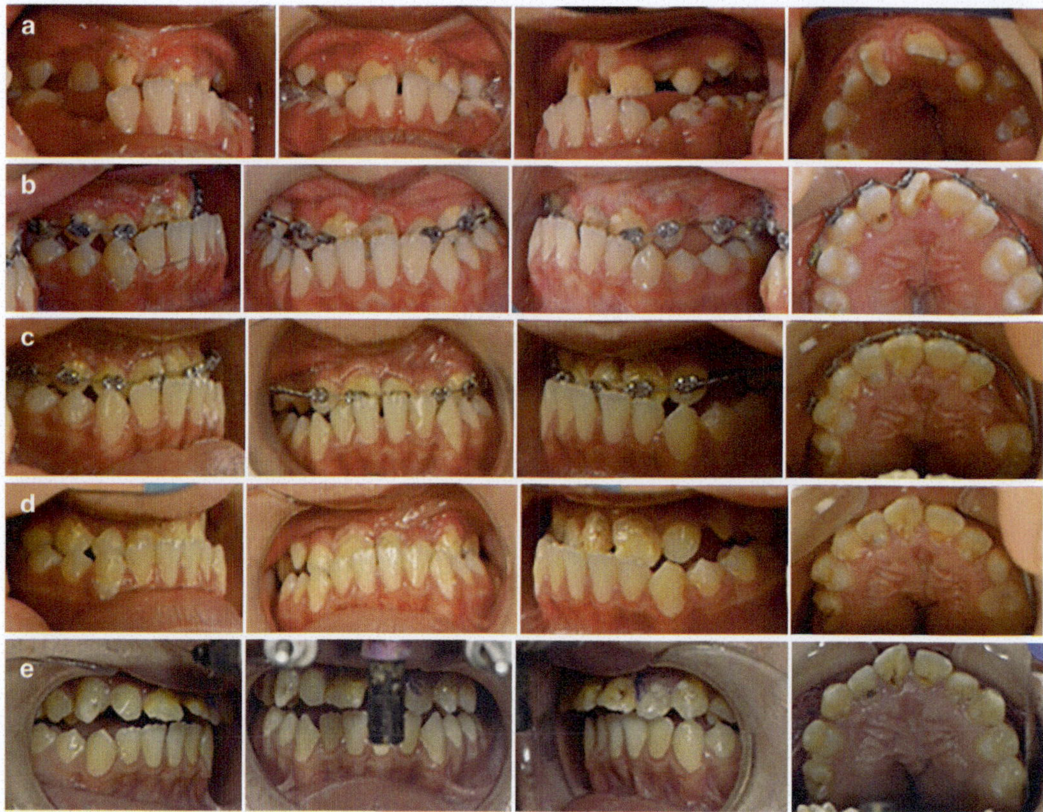

Fig. 12.3 Before, during and after orthodontic treatment in a patient with Apert syndrome. (**a**) Initial situation with dental crowding and 13 included at 10 years of age. (**b**) Orthodontic management to align teeth and create space for tooth 13 at 12 years of age. (**c**) orthodontic management to position tooth 13 on the arch at 13 years of age. (**d**) Coordinated arch before surgery at 14 years of age. (**e**) After Le Fort III osteotomy at 15 years of age

According to an observational study at Necker–Enfants malades Hospital, the average age for placing a multi-bracket appliance for arch preparation is 14 years; however, it is advisable to address impacted teeth earlier. The timing of bracket placement for impacted teeth is determined through a multidisciplinary approach, customized to each case of syndromic craniosynostosis [20].

Preparation for Surgery

Orthodontic preparation in syndromic cases necessitates a collaborative, multidisciplinary approach. Close communication between the orthodontist and the surgeon is essential to ensure a mutual understanding of each other's limitations and to tailor treatments accordingly. In certain situations, it is critical to accept therapeutic compromises to achieve optimal outcomes.

Le Fort III Osteotomy

Le Fort III osteotomy effectively addresses midface retrusion, reduces exophthalmos, and alleviates respiratory issues, yielding significant psychological and social benefits. If necessary, the procedure can be repeated to achieve full correction. Advancing the midface increases orbital volume and enhances the oronasal-pharyngeal airway while improving intermaxillary relationships. However, the procedure does not primarily aim to close open bites or achieve Class I occlusion, as the final position of the maxilla cannot be controlled [8, 25]. Furthermore, the specific technique used in our institution with internal and external distraction leads to a counterclockwise maxillary rotation during advancement, leading to a severe open bite to be corrected secondarily during the maxillomandibular osteotomy at the end of growth (Fig. 12.4).

Considerable controversy surrounds the optimal timing of midface advancement. Currently, the timing is determined based on each patient's individual needs, whether early intervention is required to ameliorate obstructive sleep apnea and avoid tracheostomy or for ophthalmological reasons, such as globe protection. It is generally recommended that midface advancement be performed as late as possible to minimize the need for repeat surgeries [3].

Orthodontic preparation in mixed or permanent dentition may be necessary in some cases. Occasionally, a brief phase of orthodontic treatment is recommended in the maxillary arch to align and level the arch in preparation for maxillary advancement (Fig. 12.3). This limited orthodontic phase should aim to facilitate the proper eruption of permanent teeth and address any

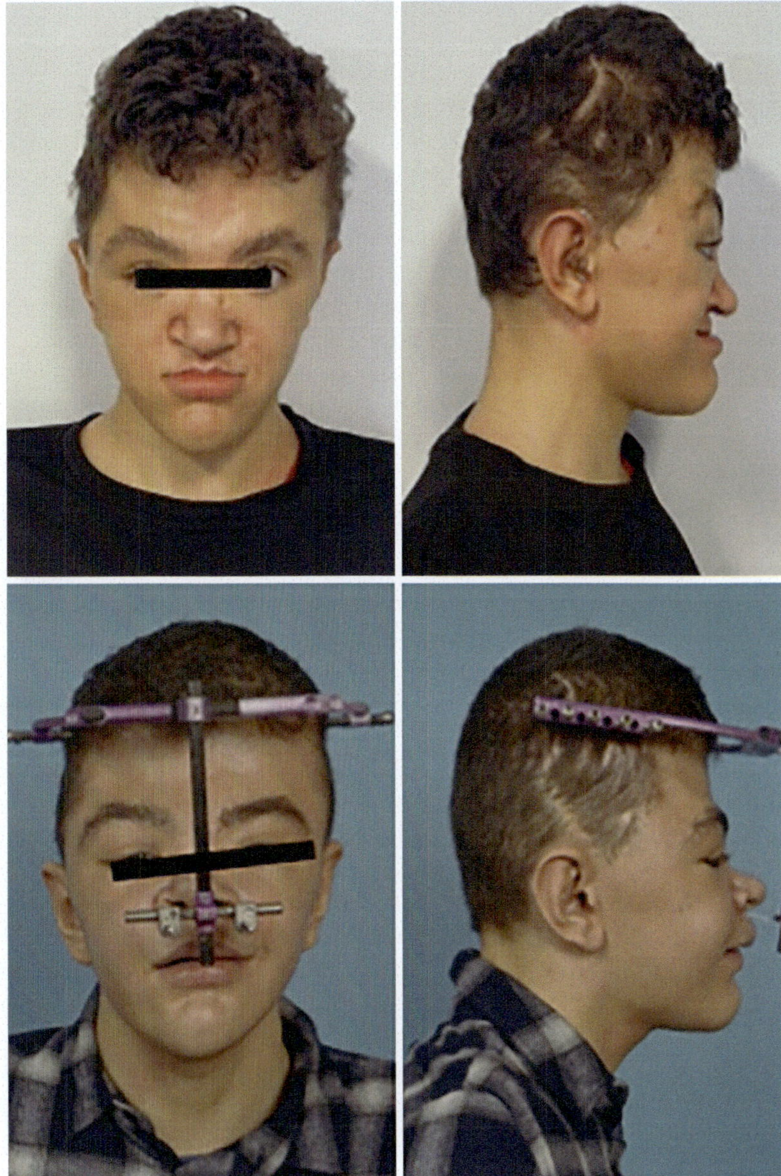

Fig. 12.4 Before and after Le Fort III osteotomy with internal and external distraction in a 13-year-old patient with Apert syndrome

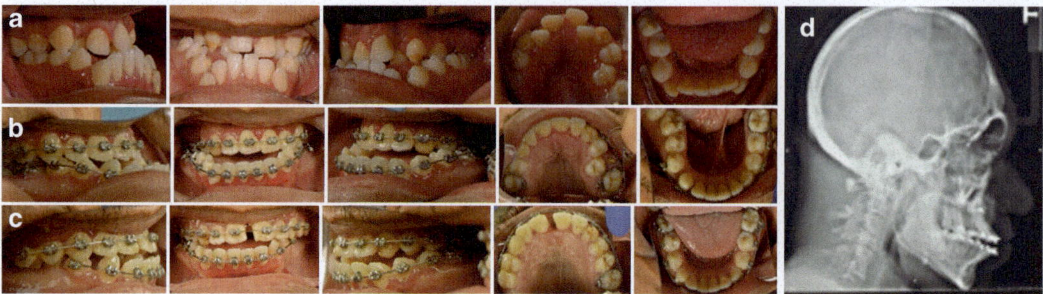

Fig. 12.5 Orthodontic and surgical management in a patient with Apert syndrome. (**a**) Initial situation with dental crowding and retrusive maxilla at 14 years of age. (**b**) Orthodontic management to align teeth after the first orthodontic phase of RME at 15 years of age. (**c**) After transverse expansion at 18 years of age. (**d**) After orthodontic and before surgical treatment

impactions. To avoid overburdening the patient, the duration of this phase should be kept within 6–9 months [3, 4].

In cases where a Le Fort III osteotomy with facial bipartition is planned, the orthodontist may be asked to position an expansion device to control intraoperative maxillary expansion, regardless of whether such a device was previously used in the patient's management. Action on the axes of the central incisors to avoid injuries during the intermaxillary osteotomy may also be necessary.

Controlling hypercorrection of the transverse dimension in cases of associated facial bipartition is critical. Furthermore, slight overcorrection of the midface advancement is preferable, as a small degree of relapse is generally expected, mainly at the maxillary level rather than at the orbital level (Fig. 12.5).

Orthognathic Surgery

During the permanent dentition phase, orthodontic preparation involves utilizing fixed appliances to prepare the dental arches in anticipation of orthognathic surgery, with the extraction of impacted teeth as necessary (Fig. 12.5). Treatment should be coordinated with the surgical timeline, with the bonding of fixed appliances occurring either at the end of growth (approximately 15–16 years of age) or earlier if impacted teeth need to be removed. Orthodontic preparation for presurgical cases in syndromic patients requires a departure from traditional orthodontic principles. Presurgical orthodontics aims to accentuate inter-arch discrepancies that have arisen to compensate for underlying skeletal dysmorphia. This preparation involves three main objectives:

- Correction of dento-maxillary disharmony and alignment of the arches,
- Elimination of dental compensations for skeletal discrepancies,
- Creation of arch forms that will facilitate optimal interdigitation at the time of surgical fixation.

Orthodontic correction of dental rotations, individual tooth dystopias, and achieving parallelism of the dental axes are critical to ensuring proper inter-arch occlusion at surgery. Arch leveling is completed to establish the occlusion, ensuring adequate incisal overlap for stability. Any spaces created through extractions are closed orthodontically before surgery [6]. Thus, presurgical orthodontics focuses on aligning and repositioning teeth within their skeletal bases without targeting ideal occlusal relationships, as the skeletal discrepancies are yet to be corrected.

In the anteroposterior dimension, orthodontic treatment often exacerbates existing issues. In Class III malocclusions, the maxillary incisors may be retroclined (palatoversion) while the mandibular incisors are proclined (vestibuloversion) using Class II elastics. Vertically, if an open bite is present and an osteotomy is planned, it is preferable not to close the open bite, as dental relapse is more common than skeletal relapse post-surgery (Fig. 12.6).

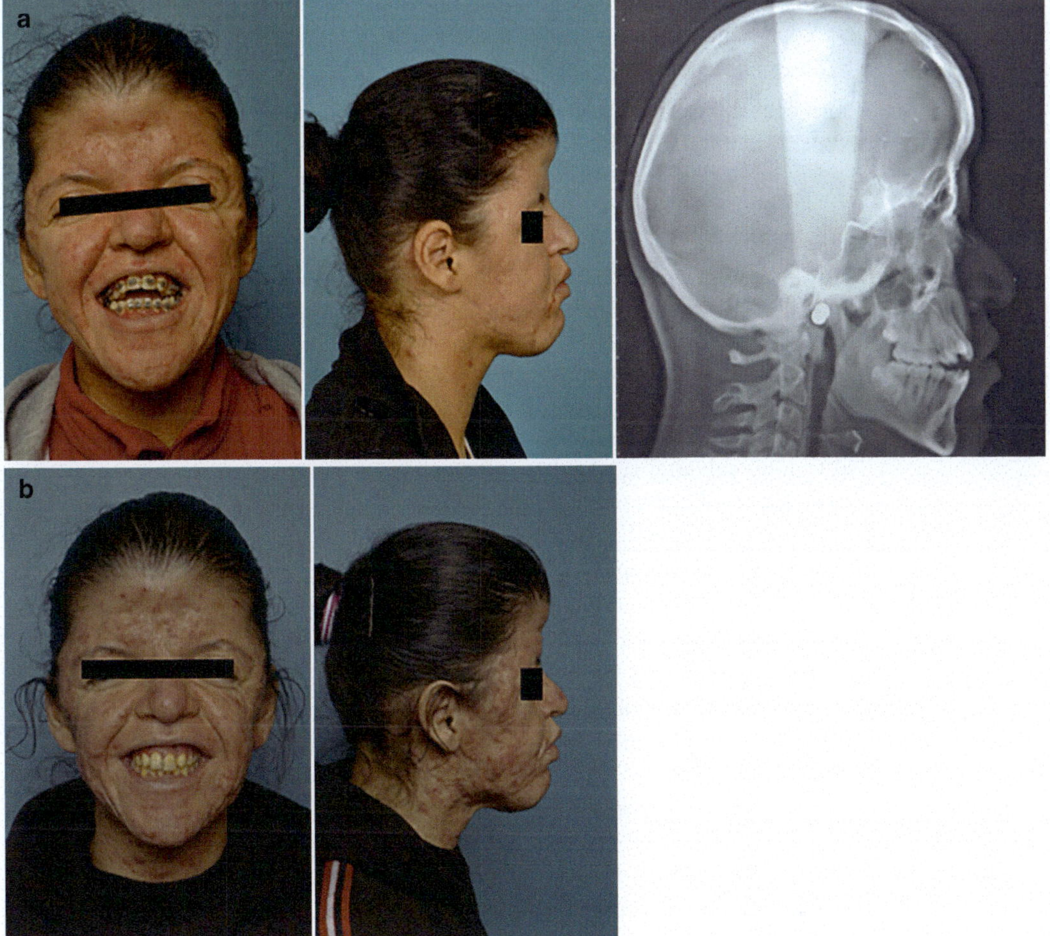

Fig. 12.6 Before (**a**) and after (**b**) orthognathic surgery at 21 years of age

Orthodontic preparation is accomplished using fixed appliances and intermaxillary elastics. Once orthodontic preparation is complete, surgical intervention should proceed promptly, as the dentoalveolar arches are in an unstable state due to untreated skeletal anomalies and uncorrected muscle attachments [3]. Pre-surgical impressions and setup are essential for verifying arch congruence, form, and symmetry, especially in Class III cases. These preparations allow the surgeon to visualize the movements required and the desired interdigitation.

At the end of the orthodontic preparation, patients are referred for surgery to discuss the surgical procedure. An inter-occlusal splint, fabricated from pre-surgical impressions mounted on a physiological articulator, is essential for post-surgical retention. This acrylic splint features imprints of the occlusal surfaces of both arches and is free from resin overhangs on the buccal surfaces, facilitating the use of intermaxillary elastics.

The splint serves two key functions. First, it provides an accurate guide for the surgeon during the repositioning of the skeletal segments. Second, it stabilizes the maxillomandibular fixation after surgery. In some cases, Le Fort III osteotomy may result in molar infra-occlusion due to segmental movement of the maxilla or mandible, though this is not systematic and depends on surgical planning. This cannot be mitigated during orthodontic preparation, as the molar groups remain in occlusion preoperatively. The interocclusal splint functions as a wedge to maintain stable fixation of the bony segments, and any resulting molar infra-occlusion is corrected orthodontically once the osteotomized segments have consolidated.

In the frequent cases of combined maxillary and mandibular surgery, two splints are fabricated: the first for maxillary positioning and the second for final mandibular positioning relative to the repositioned maxilla, ensuring maxillomandibular fixation. Intermaxillary fixation may be achieved using various methods, with traction elastics being the most employed. These elastics not only stabilize the arches but also minimize relapse depending on their positioning.

After postoperative edema subsides and normal mouth opening is restored, orthodontic treatment can resume. Typically, this occurs 3–6 months post-surgery, beginning with a classical finishing phase. During the first 3 months following surgery, patients experience enhanced cellular turnover due to the healing response, facilitating orthodontic movement [26].

In some cases, early midface advancement can negatively affect the development of the maxillary molar germs, leading to posterior edentulism (see above). There is currently no consensus on the optimal timing of such interventions. Prosthetic options should be considered to restore missing molars in affected patients.

Before surgery, it is advisable to assess the position of the molars and work with the surgical team to mitigate potential risks to undrilled teeth. FFMBA involves pterygomaxillary disjunction (PMD), which risks injuring the developing germs of the permanent molars. The lack of maxillary molars can hinder orthopedic maxillary expansion. To improve the management protocol for these patients, additional research is necessary to compare dental results according to the different techniques for performing PMD (intra-oral, infratemporal, or with endoscopic guidance) [27].

Complications such as pulp necrosis of the central incisors have been reported in cases involving facial bipartition, requiring endodontic treatment or, in severe cases, prosthetic replacement with implants or bridges. For this reason, the axes of the roots of the central incisors should be assessed when a bipartition is considered and modified using orthodontics in cases with major convergence interfering with intermaxillary osteotomy. Additionally, separation of the palate between the incisors during surgery may lead to gingival recession, necessitating periodontal care. Patients must receive appropriate dental referrals postorthodontic treatment for replacement of missing teeth and long-term dental care after their transition to adult units [1].

The final phase of orthodontic treatment is retention, designed to prevent relapse due to the natural tendency of teeth to return to their original positions. Treatment success depends on long-term stability, making this phase both essential and challenging. There is no consensus on the most effective retention method, and retention plans must be individualized based on the patient's initial malocclusion [10].

Common retention methods include:

- Removable devices:
  - Passive: Hawley retainers, night-time lingual wraps, thermoformed splints,
  - Active: Positioners,
- Fixed devices: Bonded retainers using mesh or wire (braided or round) attached to the lingual surfaces of the teeth.

Relapse can be dental, alveolar, or skeletal in origin. Common causes of relapse include:

- Unfavorable post-treatment growth, which can be mitigated by performing surgery after growth has ceased,
- Poorly balanced static and dynamic occlusal relationships, causing periodontal tension, which should be avoided through precise surgical planning,
- Muscular imbalances and functional disorders, particularly in patients with long-term tracheostomies, which can be minimized through physical and speech therapy, though these remain challenging issues,
- 'Wire syndrome' related to the use of fixed retainers, corresponding to dental movements described as unexplained or undesirable in the

presence of an intact orthodontic retainer, without detachment or fracture [28].

Proposal for a Care Protocol for Orthodontic Management in Apert Syndrome

Orthodontic management of Apert syndrome presents numerous challenges, requiring a comprehensive, multidisciplinary approach. Collaboration with a rare disease center and timely communication with all healthcare professionals involved in the patient's care is recommended immediately following the first consultation. The orthodontist plays a critical role within the craniofacial team. Orthodontic interventions are categorized into three key phases: primary dentition, mixed dentition, and permanent dentition.

I. Orthodontic Management in Primary Dentition

During early childhood, the primary goal of managing patients with Apert syndrome is to support normal brain development, avoiding complications from intracranial hypertension, while promoting cranial and facial growth to prevent ocular and respiratory issues. In the primary dentition phase, orthodontic intervention is typically limited to cases of obstructive sleep apnea syndrome (OSAS), where early intermaxillary orthopedic disjunction (RME type) may be indicated to increase the volume of the nasal airways, with potential complex retention issues [9, 24].

II. Orthodontic Management in Mixed Dentition

In mixed dentition, the orthodontist's primary challenge is to facilitate the eruption of all teeth within the dental arch and to normalize the transverse dimension when necessary. If a narrow maxillary arch is diagnosed, RME should be initiated. If orthopedic expansion fails, SARME may be required, utilizing the same device.

III. Orthodontic Management in Permanent Dentition

In the permanent dentition phase, orthodontic preparation involves the use of fixed appliances to prepare the dental arches in anticipation of orthognathic surgery, with the extraction of impacted teeth when necessary. Treatment should be timed to align with the surgical schedule, with bonding of the fixed appliance occurring either at the end of growth (around 15–16 years of age) or earlier if impacted teeth require extraction.

Orthodontic treatment for craniosynostosis requires the involvement of a multidisciplinary team. It is important to recognize that orthodontics may be optional in the broader treatment pathway for these patients.

Main Messages

- Orthodontic management starts around the age of 6 with discussions on the indications for transversal maxillary expansion.
- Orthopedic rapid maxillary expansion is indicated initially, while surgically-assisted rapid maxillary expansion is required in case of failure of orthopedic devices due to a fused mid-palatal suture.
- Orthodontic management is complicated by frequent iatrogenic damage to maxillary molars due to early pterygo-zygomatic disjunctions associated with frontofacial monobloc advancement, and cognitive issues may interfere with compliance.
- Le Fort III osteotomy does not require orthodontic preparation except for the design of palatal plates to avoid excessive correction of the narrow palatal width during the subcranial bipartition and action on the direction of the incisor roots to avoid damage during the intermaxillary osteotomy.

- Orthodontics should be delayed until the age of 14–15, except for the traction of impacted teeth to avoid prolonged treatment, as all patients will require orthognathic surgery with pre-surgical preparation of dental arches.

References

1. Vargervik K, Rubin MS, Grayson BH, Figueroa AA, Kreiborg S, Shirley JC, et al. Parameters of care for craniosynostosis: dental and orthodontic perspectives. Am J Orthod Dentofacial Orthop. 2012;141(4):S68–73.
2. Sicard L, Hounkpevi M, Tomat C, James S, Paternoster G, Khonsari RH, et al. Dental consequences of pterygomaxillary dysjunction during fronto-facial monobloc advancement with internal distraction for Crouzon syndrome. J Craniofac Surg. 2018;46(9):1476–9.
3. Azoulay-Avinoam S, Bruun R, MacLaine J, Allareddy V, Resnick CM, Padwa BL. An overview of Craniosynostosis craniofacial syndromes for combined orthodontic and surgical management. Oral Maxillofac Surg Clin N Am. 2020;32(2):233–47.
4. Yamamoto S, Kurosaka H, Mihara K, Onoda M, Haraguchi S, Yamashiro T. Long-term follow-up of a patient diagnosed with Crouzon syndrome who underwent Le Fort I and III distraction osteogenesis using a rigid external distractor system. Angle Orthod. 2023;93(6):736–46.
5. Ghesquiere E. Prise en charge chirurgico-orthodontique de patients porteurs d'une craniofaciosténose. La distraction: une alternative au traitement chirurgico- orthodontique conventionnel? Lille: Université du droit et de la santé; 2008. 228 p.
6. Nurko C, Quinones R. Dental and orthodontic management of patients with Apert and Crouzon syndromes. Oral Maxillofac Surg Clin N Am. 2004;16(4):541–53.
7. Kahnberg KE, Hagberg C. Orthognathic surgery in patients with craniofacial syndrome. I. A 5-year overview of combined orthodontic and surgical correction. J Plast Surg Hand Surg. 2010;44(6):282–8.
8. Meazzini MC, Brusati R, Bozzetti A, Mazzoleni F, Felisati G, Garattini G, et al. Craniofacial anomalies: surgical-orthodontic management. Kindle 2014.
9. Garg RK, Afifi AM, Garland CB, Sanchez R, Mount DL. Pediatric obstructive sleep apnea: consensus, controversy, and craniofacial considerations. Plast Reconstr Surg. 2017;140(5):987–97.
10. Pinto RDO, Tonello C, Peixoto AP, De Jesus AS, Santos-Pinto AD, Raveli DB. Three-dimensional evaluation of dental arches in individuals with syndromic craniosynostosis. Khalaf K, editor. Int J Dent. 2023;2023:1–8.
11. Melsen B. Palatal growth studied on human autopsy material. Am J Orthod. 1975;68(1):42–54.
12. Soufflet E, Moison R, Sergent JF, Khenafi H, Veyssiere A, Benateau H. Étude rétrospective sur l'intérêt de l'imagerie 3D dans l'évaluation de la suture mésio-palatine. Soyer Y, editor. Rev Orthop Dento-Faciale. 2023;57(3):237–44.
13. Angelieri F, Cevidanes LHS, Franchi L, Gonçalves JR, Benavides E, McNamara JA Jr. Midpalatal suture maturation: classification method for individual assessment before rapid maxillary expansion. Am J Orthod Dentofacial Orthop. 2013;144(5):759–69.
14. Baccetti T, Franchi L, Cameron CG, McNamara JA. Treatment timing for rapid maxillary expansion. Angle Orthod. 2001;71(5):343–50.
15. Kwak KH, Kim SS, Kim YI, Kim YD. Quantitative evaluation of midpalatal suture maturation via fractal analysis. Korean J Orthod. 2016;46(5):323.
16. Isfeld D, Lagravere M, Leon-Salazar V, Flores-Mir C. Novel methodologies and technologies to assess mid-palatal suture maturation: a systematic review. Head Face Med. 2017;13(1):13.
17. Shetye PR. Orthodontic management in syndromic craniosynostosis. In: Shetye PR, Gibson TL, editors. Cleft and craniofacial orthodontics [Internet]. 1st ed. Wiley; 2023 [cited 2024 Jul 24]. p. 678–89. Available from: https://onlinelibrary.wiley.com/doi/10.1002/9781119778387.ch52.
18. Mathijssen IMJ. Updated guideline on treatment and management of craniosynostosis. J Craniofac Surg. 2021 Jan;32(1):371–450.
19. Taddei M, D'Alessandro G, Amunni F, Piana G. Orthodontic treatment of a particular subgroup of children with special health care needs, children with craniofacial anomalies: an analysis of treatment length and clinical outcome. Angle Orthod. 2016;86(1):115–20.
20. Pillon M, Bondi T, Khonsari RH. Orthodontic and surgical management of FGFR-related craniosynostoses: observation study on 136 patients. 2024
21. Garrec P, Vi-Fane B, Jordan L. L'expansion rapide maxillaire (ERM) Est-ce toujours une question d'âge? Rev Orthopédie Dento-Faciale. 2017;51(4):531–9.
22. Dalben GDS, Neves LTD, Gomide MR. Oral findings in patients with Apert syndrome. J Appl Oral Sci. 2006;14(6):465–9.
23. Arnaud E, Paternoster G, James S, Morisseau-Durand MP, Couloigner V, Diner P, et al. Stratégie cranio-faciale pour les faciocraniosténoses. Ann Chir Plast Esthét. 2016;61(5):408–19.

24. Fauroux B, Amaddeo A. Cas particulier des troubles respiratoires du sommeil des patients syndromiques. Rev Orthopédie Dento-Faciale. 2015;49(2):127–32.
25. Mathijssen I, Arnaud E, Marchac D, Mireau E, Morisseau-Durand MP, Guérin P, et al. Respiratory outcome of mid-face advancement with distraction: a comparison between Le Fort III and Frontofacial Monobloc. J Craniofac Surg. 2006;17(5):880–2.
26. Moncayo Pinos JS, Pezantes Solano SM. Osteotomía y Corticotomía en la aceleración del movimiento dental: revisión de la literatura. Religación. 2023;9(39):e2401125.
27. Arnaud E, Paternoster G, Khonsari RH, Haber SE. Dental consequences of FFMBA. In: Arnaud E, Paternoster G, Khonsari RH, Haber SE, editors. Frontofacial Monobloc advancement with internal distraction: tactics and strategy in Faciocraniosynostosis [Internet]. Cham: Springer International Publishing; 2023. p. 171–5. Available from: https://doi.org/10.1007/978-3-031-07574-2_8.
28. Charavet C, Vives F, Aroca S, Dridi SM. "Wire syndrome" following bonded orthodontic retainers: a systematic review of the literature. Healthc Basel Switz. 2022;10(2):379.

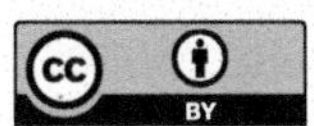

13 Airway Assessment and Management

Brigitte Fauroux, Briac Thierry, Sonia Khirani, Vincent Couloigner, and Romain Luscan

Introduction

Patients with Apert syndrome have mid-face hypoplasia associated with mandibular hypoplasia or other airway anomalies. Indeed, a temporal analysis of craniofacial 3-dimensional cephalometries showed that facial deformity of Apert syndrome begins with the midface and affects the orbit and mandible later in life [1]. These anatomical anomalies put these patients at high risk of obstructive sleep apnea (OSA), which is defined as repeated periods of total (apnea) or partial (hypopnea) closure of the upper airway during sleep. OSA is associated with neurocognitive dysfunction, memory, attention, and executive function impairment, and behavioral disorders with various degrees of hyperactivity or aggressiveness, which may result in deterioration in learning abilities and school performance [2]. OSA may cause feeding difficulties, leading to insufficient weight gain and growth retardation. OSA may also increase intracranial pressure and contribute to or aggravate intracranial hypertension. Finally, OSA may be associated with metabolic syndrome, cardiovascular stress, and, in particular, arterial hypertension. OSA screening and treatment are thus essential in patients with Apert syndrome. This chapter aims to comprehensively overview airway issues in patients with Apert syndrome, including screening, management, and follow-up.

B. Fauroux (✉)
Pediatric Noninvasive Ventilation and Sleep Unit, AP-HP, Hôpital Necker–Enfants malades, Paris, France

EA 7330 VIFASOM (Vigilance Fatigue Sommeil et Santé Publique), Paris University, Paris, France
e-mail: brigitte.fauroux@aphp.fr

B. Thierry · V. Couloigner · R. Luscan
Pediatric Otorhinolaryngology and Head and Neck Department, AP-HP, Hôpital Necker–Enfants malades, Paris, France

S. Khirani
Pediatric Noninvasive Ventilation and Sleep Unit, AP-HP, Hôpital Necker–Enfants malades, Paris, France

ASV Santé, Gennevilliers, France

Breathing Issues in Patients with Apert Syndrome

Sleep-Disordered Breathing in Apert Syndrome

The most common breathing issue in patients with Apert syndrome is OSA. As shown in imaging studies, OSA is caused by reduced airway caliber and patency. Fifty children with syndromic craniosynostosis, with 19 children having Apert syndrome, had a lateral cephalogram between the ages of 6–18 years [3]. Patients with prior midfacial advancement were excluded. Patients were classified as having OSA, documented on polysomnography (PSG), or no OSA on a PSG or the absence of sleep-disordered

J. G. Meara et al. (eds.), *Apert Syndrome*, https://doi.org/10.1007/978-3-032-12551-4_13

breathing symptoms. According to the apnea-hypopnea index (AHI), all the patients with OSA had severe OSA with a mean AHI of 24 ± 5 events/h. When comparing the cephalometric parameters between the OSA and non-OSA groups, the upper airway length was longer, and the posterior airway space was smaller in the patients with OSA. Upper airway length was the primary predictor for OSA. OSA severity correlated negatively with age, and none of the cephalometric parameters correlated with clinical severity or the AHI. In another study, 24 out of 153 children with syndromic craniosynostosis had a PSG, with 16 patients having OSA and 8 having no OSA [4]. Compared to patients without OSA, those with OSA had significantly smaller upper airway volume, nasal cavity volume, nasopharyngeal volume, retropalatal cross-sectional airway, and a longer retropalatal length. Again, no correlation was observed between the airway measurements and the AHI, which may be explained by the fact that imaging techniques cannot assess the dynamic collapse of the upper airways or the glossoptosis during sleep and the different sleep stages. In another Fibroblast Growth Factor Receptor (FGFR) syndrome, Pfeiffer syndrome, a prospective study compared the pre-operative skull computed tomography in 30 infants with Pfeiffer syndrome, at a mean age of 0.6 ± 0.9 years, to 42 age-matched healthy controls [5]. Compared to healthy controls, infants with Pfeiffer syndrome had a 50% reduction in nasal airway volume and a 44% reduction in pharyngeal airway volume. The nasal airway was reduced in length, height, and width with choanal stenosis. The authors concluded that mediolateral maxillary expansion and maxillo-mandibular advancement may benefit these children by increasing the upper airway volume and thus reducing the risk of OSA.

These severe anatomical abnormalities of the upper airway explain the high prevalence and severity of OSA in patients with Apert syndrome. Indeed, a 70% prevalence of OSA was reported in a cohort of 20 patients aged 0.2–21.6 years [6]. In our own experience, the mean pre-operative monobloc AHI of 109 children with syndromic craniosynostosis, of whom 20 had Apert syndrome, was as high as 19 ± 17 events/h [7]. Similar data were reported in a study of 18 children with syndromic craniosynostosis [8]. The six patients with Apert syndrome had an AHI ranging from 7 to 62 events/h, with two patients requiring a non-invasive continuous positive airway pressure (CPAP) treatment. Again, the AHI did not correlate with symptoms and clinical findings, underlining the need for a systematic screening of OSA in patients with Apert syndrome. In children with Apert syndrome, OSA is usually severe. In a retrospective review of 47 children with syndromic craniosynostosis (Apert 66%, Crouzon 15%, and Pfeiffer syndromes 19%) seen at Boston Children's Hospital from January 2001 through April 2011, 83% of the patients had OSA, with 42% severe, 19% moderate, and 22% mild OSA [9]. In another study of 25 infants with craniofacial synostosis, the pre-operative AHI of the six children with Apert syndrome ranged between 7 and 66 events/h, with four children having an AHI >18 events/h [8]. Importantly, OSA has been shown to be more severe in the first months of life [3]. Also, OSA may occur at any age and relapse after treatment, requiring a follow-up until the end of the pubertal growth spurt. In our own experience, in a cohort of 108 patients with craniosynostosis who had an early fronto-facial monobloc, 17 (15.7%) patients, three had Apert syndrome, required a secondary Le Fort III for residual OSA [10]. Of note, this secondary Le Fort III normalized the AHI in 15 (88%) patients, and two of the four patients with a tracheotomy could be decannulated.

Central sleep apnea (CSA) represents the other breathing abnormality that may be theoretically observed in patients with syndromic craniosynostosis. A cervico-occipital compression may cause an injury of the brain stem with a consequent dysfunction of the central breathing drive. This may cause central apneas, characterized by a cessation of airflow, due to the lack of contraction of the inspiratory muscles, without any reduction in the airway caliber. But in practice, this type of sleep-disordered breathing has not been observed in a study of 138 patients with syndromic craniosynostosis, of whom 20 had Apert syndrome [11].

Diagnosis of Sleep-Disordered Breathing

Sleep-disordered breathing should be diagnosed and treated in children, as OSA is associated with neurocognitive dysfunction and abnormal behavior. This applies to typically developing children without any associated disorder, but also to children with an underlying anomaly of the upper airways, as children with Apert syndrome. Indeed, OSA may favor or aggravate neurocognitive impairment, abnormal behavior, working memory, and quality of life in these children [12]. OSA has also been shown to be associated with a significantly lower weight-for-height standard deviation score in children with complex or syndromic craniosynostosis [13].

Symptoms, clinical examination, and sleep questionnaires are insufficiently sensitive and specific as screening tools to document OSA and its severity in patients with any upper airway anomaly [14–17]. This lack of correlation has also been observed in children with syndromic craniosynostosis [3, 4, 8], underlining the need for systematic sleep studies in these patients.

PSG remains the gold standard for the diagnosis of OSA and includes electroencephalography (EEG), electrooculogram, submental and leg electromyogram, oronasal airflow, abdominal and chest wall movements, pulse oximetry (SpO_2), partial pressure or end-tidal or transcutaneous carbon dioxide ($PtcCO_2$), and a video recording [18]. There are standardized indications for PSG in children aged 1–18 years and for younger children (<2 years of age), which include children with an upper airway anomaly [19, 20]. However, access, availability, and costs remain obstacles to the widespread utilization of PSG. Respiratory polygraphy (PG), a limited-channel overnight recording, has been demonstrated to be a feasible and practical alternative to PSG [21, 22]. PG, also referred to as a cardio-respiratory sleep study, is a scaled-down PSG with fewer leads that has been used in the hospital or home setting. There are no electro-ocular graphs or EEG leads, so sleep staging and arousal scoring are not possible. Nasal airflow is measured with a nasal cannula pressure transducer, and respiratory effort is assessed using combined thoracic and abdominal respiratory inductance plethysmography (RIP) belts. Electrocardiography and body position may also be recorded. Notably, a pediatric sleep expert should perform a PSG or PG scoring manually, ideally having craniosynostosis competency. The European Respiratory Society (ERS) has included PG in the diagnostic algorithms for sleep-disordered breathing in infants and young children [19, 20]. PG has been shown to be safe and feasible for many children in the home setting [21], comprising children with syndromic craniosynostosis. Indeed, in a large cohort of 123 patients, who had 149 PSG and 108 ambulatory PG, no significant difference was found between the two types of sleep studies regarding sleep study parameters [23].

The standard parameter derived from PSG and PG is the AHI, which is the frequency of significant respiratory events (apneas and hypopneas). The OSA threshold for diagnosis in children is lower than required in adulthood. An AHI > 1 event/h is most used for diagnosing OSA in children [24, 25], with an AHI between 1 and 5 events/h indicating mild OSA, between 5 and 10 events/h, moderate OSA, and ≥10 events/h, severe OSA.

Overnight recordings of SpO_2 and $PtcCO_2$ may show clusters of desaturation, which may or may not be associated with concomitant increases in $PtcCO_2$ levels [26]. These abnormalities reflect the consequences of OSA on the nocturnal gas exchange. These abnormalities should prompt an effective treatment of OSA, but they do not give any information on the precise type of sleep-disordered breathing or on the objective severity of OSA. This type of investigation is thus insufficient for the optimal therapeutic management of OSA in a patient with Apert syndrome.

Treatment of Sleep-Disordered Breathing

OSA treatment requires a multidisciplinary team comprising a pediatric neurosurgeon, ENT surgeon, maxillofacial surgeon and orthodontist, sleep specialist, pulmonologist, ophthalmologist, radiologist, geneticist, and psychologist. OSA management follows a stepwise approach, taking into account the patient's age, clinical status (intracranial hypertension, sleep-disordered breathing symptoms, nutrition, and growth), and PSG or PG data (Fig. 13.1).

The first step consists of a complete clinical evaluation of the upper airways, associating buccal and oropharyngeal exam, anterior rhinoscopy, and flexible scope. This last exam can be impossible due to the very narrow nasal cavities. The aim of a complete evaluation of the upper airway is to identify all potential obstructive sites responsible for OSA, such as congenital nasal pyriform aperture stenosis, inferior turbinal hypertrophy/midface stenosis, septal deviation, choanal atresia, narrow nasopharynx, adenoid hypertrophy, tonsil hypertrophy, pharyngomalacia, glossoptosis, tongue base hypertrophy, and laryngomalacia.

To evaluate precisely the role of each obstructive site during sleep, drug-induced sleep endoscopy (DISE) has been developed in the last decade in children. DISE consists of a complete evaluation of the upper airway, using a flexible scope, during an "artificial sleep," mimicking natural sleep in the operating room. During the procedure, a complete scoring of each site is performed, allowing an understanding of all the different collapsing sites during sleep [27, 28].

Nasal obstruction can be treated by saline nasal instillation. In case of severe symptoms, topical steroid treatment [29] or nasal instillations of epinephrine (in a hospital setting) may be useful. If laryngeal examination with a flexible scope shows suggestive signs of gastro-esophageal reflux, pH monitoring may be performed with the prescription of proton pump inhibitors in case of gastro-esophageal reflux.

In the more severe cases, surgical treatment is indicated. Depending on the obstructive site(s), different surgical procedures may be proposed, such as [6, 9, 30–34] (Table 13.1):

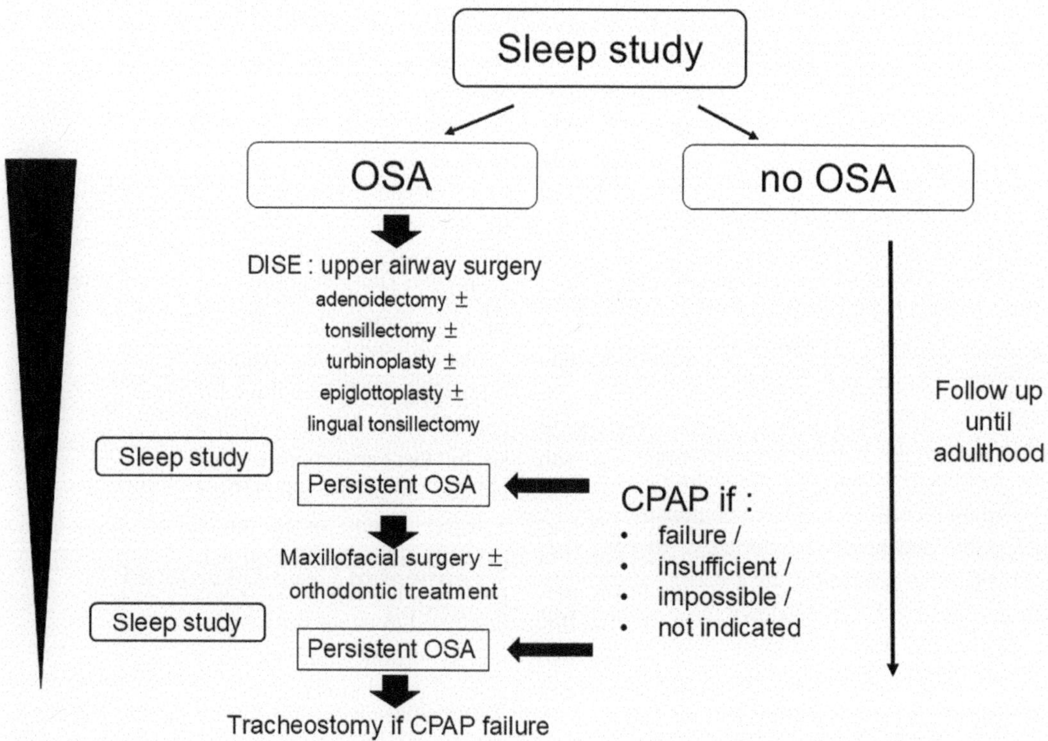

Fig. 13.1 Stepwise algorithm for the management of OSA

Table 13.1 Necker's technical surgical notes

(a) Congenital piriform aperture dilatation
A sublabial approach is performed to enlarge the piriform aperture with a bur. In order to boost the surgical result at the end of the procedure, an endonasal ballon dilatation can be proposed
(b) Inferior turbinectomy/turbinoplasty
Given the narrowness of the nasal cavity due to midface stenosis, we recommend a full-length removal of the inferior half of the inferior turbinate to improve nasal patency at the end of the operation
(c) Resection of the posterior part of the vomer to widen the nasopharynx
In order to widen the nasopharynx, we perform a resection of the posterior third part of the vomer with cold instrument
(d) Partial or total tonsillectomy
Partial tonsillectomy can be performed using cold instruments /bipolar, the Ellman® (Ellman, Hicksville, New York), Coblator device® (Smith & Nephew, London, UK) or another device. Around 80% of the tonsils is removed and the residual tissue can be cauterized with a bipolar coagulation in order to decrease the risk of regrowth
In case of total tonsillectomy, the dissection is performed lateral to the tonsil in the plane between the tonsillar capsule and the pharyngeal musculature
(e) Pharyngeal expansion
Pharyngoplasty consisted in the reduction of the length of the soft palate by removing a half-moon part of velar mucosa, associating with the isolation and rotation of the two palatopharyngeus muscles supero-anterolaterally
(f) Tongue base reduction
We perform the reduction of the lingual tonsils using the Coblator device®. The objective is to obtain a clear vallecular space. Hemostasis was performed using the same device. We don't perform any posterior midline glossectomy
(g) Supraglottoplasty
Depending on the obstructive site, different procedure can be proposed:
Section of the aryepiglottic folds with cold instruments
Epiglottoplasty: Cauterization of the lingual face of the epiglottis using thulium LASER RevoLix® fiber (laser in surgery®, Epinay-sous-Sénart, France) or a bipolar
Arytenoidoplasty: Partial resection or vaporization of floppy supra-arytenoid mucosal tissue

- Congenital piriform aperture dilatation
- Inferior turbinectomy/turbinoplasty
- Septoplasty
- Resection of the posterior part of the vomer to widen the nasopharynx
- Adenoidectomy
- Partial or total tonsillectomy
- Pharyngeal expansion
- Tongue base reduction
- Supraglottoplasty

The classical surgical procedure to treat OSA in children consists of an adenotonsillectomy. However, in patients with Apert syndrome, this procedure is rarely sufficient to cure OSA, even in the case of significant hypertrophy of the adenoids and tonsils. Indeed, in a meta-analysis including three studies, Saengthong et al. observed no statistically significant reduction in the postoperative AHI despite an average decrease in the AHI of 5 events/h [31]. This shows the high prevalence of multi-level airway obstruction in Apert syndrome [35].

In neonates and infants, the lymphoid tissue of the upper airways is still virtual or poorly developed. At this young age, the most frequent obstructive sites are the nasal fossa due to the anteroposterior and lateral midface stenosis (Fig. 13.2). The functional impact is significant as newborns only breathe through the nose. The first surgical intervention consists of a permeabilization/dilatation/enlargement of the nasal airways and the nasopharynx. Depending on the obstructive sites, it can include congenital piriform aperture dilation, turbinoplasty/turbinectomy, choanal atresia treatment, or anteriorization of the vomer to widen the nasopharynx (Fig. 13.3). Laryngomalacia is frequently encountered in young patients with Apert syndrome and is significantly more symptomatic than in non-syndromic patients [36].

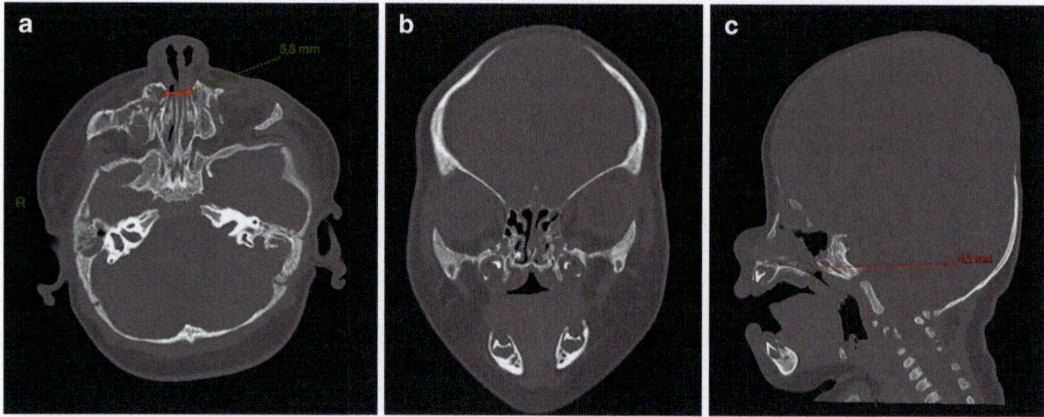

Fig. 13.2 CT-scan of a 2-month-old girl with Apert syndrome. On the axial slice (**a**), we can see the narrowness of the entire nasal cavity due to the midface stenosis (transversal diameter = 8.8 mm). On the coronal slice (**b**), we appreciate the relatively inferior turbinate hypertrophy (white star) due to the narrowness of the nasal fossa. On the sagittal section (**c**), we can visualize the narrowness of the nasopharynx (4.2 mm)

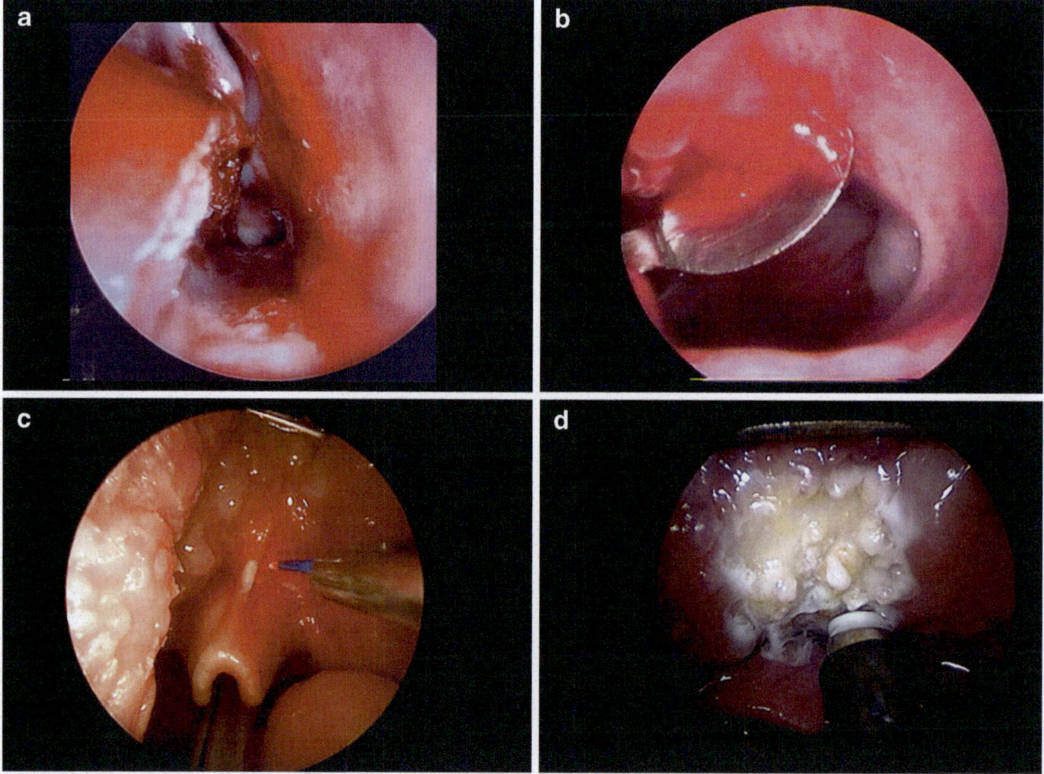

Fig. 13.3 Peroperative registration of different surgical procedures to relieve upper airway obstruction. (**a**) Postoperative view after right inferior turbinectomy. (**b**) Resection of the posterior part of the vomer to widen the nasopharynx. (**c**) Epiglottoplasty with LASER. (**d**) Tongue base reduction using a coblation device

Hypertrophy of the adenoids and tonsils occurs later in life due to recurrent viral infections of the upper airways. Adeno-tonsillectomy is frequently indicated in the case of OSA around the age of 2–5 years. Partial tonsillectomy (also called intracapsular tonsillectomy or tonsillotomy) is nowadays preferred to total tonsillectomy because it reduces the risk of postoperative hemorrhage and pain and facilitates a quicker return to a normal diet and activity [37, 38]. Adenoidectomy is contraindicated in the case of cleft palate due to the risks of postoperative velar insufficiency.

In clinical practice, a wide range of surgical procedures may be necessary in patients with Apert syndrome. In a retrospective series of patients with Apert syndrome from 1990 to 2013, dilatation of nasal airways and choanal atresia repair, adenoidectomy, tonsillectomy, early midface advancement, and/or non-invasive ventilation were performed in those with OSA [33].

Patients with syndromic craniosynostosis present a high risk of residual OSA after upper airway surgery, underlining the need for a systematic clinical follow-up after surgery. Of the 47 children with syndromic craniosynostosis seen at Boston Children's Hospital from January 2001 through April 2011, 62% had an adenotonsillectomy, and 45% had a pre- and postoperative PSG [9]. After surgery, the mean AHI was not significantly different, and OSA persisted in 11 of 13 children. A small meta-analysis on three retrospective studies (24 patients) did not identify a statistically significant difference between preoperative and postoperative AHI despite an overall reduction of AHI of 5 events/h. However, there was a statistically significant decrease in the postoperative oxygen desaturation index (ODI) as compared to the preoperative ODI, with an overall reduction of 8.5 events/h [31].

Upper airway surgery also comprises maxillofacial and neurosurgical procedures detailed in the corresponding chapters. These additional or complementary orthodontic or surgical procedures should be discussed within a multidisciplinary team before proposing other treatments, such as continuous positive airway pressure (CPAP) or, ultimately, a tracheostomy.

Indeed, when the patient presents with persisting severe OSA, after failure of all other treatments, or when other treatments are not indicated or not feasible, a treatment with CPAP is indicated (Fig. 13.1) [11, 39]. CPAP consists of delivering air pressure into the upper airways (nose, mouth, pharynx, larynx, and trachea) to keep them open during the entire breathing cycle (inspiration and expiration). CPAP is used during sleep (overnight and during naps in infants) and at home to preserve the patient's and family's quality of life. The main advantage of CPAP is that it is a non-invasive treatment that can be used on demand at home. CPAP is also a multilevel treatment that may overcome multi-level upper airway obstruction [39].

The decision to treat with CPAP is based on a combination of criteria that may vary from one child to another and include the child's age, clinical status, and growth, OSA symptoms, and PSG or PG data.

CPAP equipment is made up of the following:

- CPAP *machine* that delivers air at a titrated pressure,
- *Circuit* (tube) that provides the air pressure from the machine to the child
- The interface (or mask) is positioned on the child's face and held in place by a headgear.

Different interfaces may be used:

- *Nasal mask* that covers the nose
- *Oronasal mask* covers the mouth and nose, and is used in children who breathe through their mouth whilst sleeping
- *Nasal pillows* (or nasal canula or nasal prongs) cover the nostrils and can be used in older children.
- *Facial mask* covers the whole face and is only used in exceptional circumstances in children.

The interface choice depends on the child's age, his way of breathing during the night (through the nose or mouth), the shape of the face and skull, and the comfort and preference of the child. Of note, in infants, only nasal masks are available.

The efficacy of CPAP should be checked by analyzing the built-in software data of the CPAP device, together with an overnight recording of SpO_2 and $PtcCO_2$ [39]. A control PSG or PG with

CPAP is reserved for patients who fail this standard follow-up.

The primary limitations and side effects of CPAP are the risk of skin injury and facial deformity due to the pressure exerted by the interface [40]. Indeed, in young children, the long-term use of CPAP may induce a maxillary retrusion, which may aggravate the midface hypoplasia and retrusion in children who have intrinsically an anatomical facial deformity. For this reason, the decision to initiate CPAP should be made by a multidisciplinary team, with a systematic maxillary assessment during follow-up.

Treatment adherence is a significant issue. In children, the aim is to achieve CPAP use during normal, physiological sleep duration for age [39]. Therapeutic education has been shown to be essential to achieve this goal [41]. During follow-up, the correction or persistence of OSA should be checked by a PSG or PG after any procedure that may improve OSA, such as any upper airway surgery, to wean the patient from CPAP as early as possible [39, 42]. And finally, CPAP is a temporary treatment used to normalize breathing and sleep while waiting for the optimal timing of definitive curative surgical procedures. Indeed, the aim is to wean the patient from CPAP at the end of puberty, before adulthood.

In a national French survey, 1449 children were treated with long-term (>3 months) CPAP or non-invasive ventilation at home in June 2019 [43]. Among these 1449 children, 48 were treated with long-term CPAP for craniosynostosis.

At least, when CPAP fails because OSA is too severe or when CPAP is required for more than 16/24 h, the ultimate solution is a tracheostomy. This procedure can be challenging due to the frequent association of Apert syndrome and a "cartilaginous sleeve trachea," a rare tracheal malformation consisting of a fusion of the tracheal cartilage rings [44]. In a series including patients with major craniofacial anomalies, craniofacial synostosis patients had the highest rate of tracheotomy (48% [28/59]) [45].

Tracheostomy is a 100% efficient procedure to treat OSA, but in children, it is associated with significant morbidity (up to 20%) and mortality (0.5–1% per year). Consequently, a tracheostomy should remain the ultimate therapeutic option [46].

Nasopharyngeal airway tube placement has also been reported to reduce the need for CPAP or a tracheostomy [47, 48]. To bypass the rhinopharyngeal narrowing, a tube is placed up to the supraglottic space and can be maintained for several weeks. In a series of 27 patients with craniosynostosis, 26 (96%) improved AHI with this technique.

Recently, we analyzed the upper airway and craniofacial management of 28 patients with Apert syndrome followed at our national reference center during a period of 25 years (personal data). Mean age at baseline PG was 3.9 ± 5.4 years with a mean AHI of 5.7 ± 10.2 events/h. Ten (36%) patients had mild-to-severe OSA, with 3 (11%) patients having severe OSA. No patient had central apneas. Among the three patients with severe OSA, one patient had upper airway surgery, one patient was started on CPAP, and one patient continued CPAP. During follow-up, 22/28 (79%) patients had repeated PG. Among the four patients with mild OSA at baseline PG, two patients had persistent mild OSA and one patient developed severe OSA. Among the three patients with moderate OSA at baseline PG, none of the patients developed severe OSA during follow-up. Among the three patients with severe OSA, one patient continued CPAP and the two others improved. At the same time, patients had also undergone numerous surgical interventions. All patients but one patient, aged 0.7 years, had at least one craniofacial procedure. In total, 17/28 (61%) patients had a posterior cranial vault decompression, 16/28 (57%) patients had a fronto-orbital advancement, among which two patients had a repeated procedure. Nine (32%) patients had a frontofacial monobloc advancement, and 7/28 (25%) patients had a Le Fort three distraction, among which one patient had a repeated procedure. Among these patients, one patient had a frontofacial monobloc advancement to treat severe OSA, and three patients had a Le Fort three distraction to allow CPAP weaning. In conclusion, multiple surgeries, combining upper airway, craniofacial, and maxillofacial surgeries, were necessary to treat upper airway obstruction. Moreover, CPAP was also necessary in case of persistent OSA, and was effective in delaying craniofacial surgeries.

In conclusion, OSA is highly prevalent in patients with Apert syndrome and peaks in the first months of life. Diagnosis can only be made on a PSG or PG. OSA is usually severe and may relapse during childhood, underlining the need for a long-term follow-up. Treatment strategies should be personalized and developed by a multidisciplinary team of pediatric experts. CPAP is an effective, non-invasive treatment of severe OSA while waiting for curative surgery. A systematic assessment of sleep and neurocognitive function is mandatory for these children to diagnose and treat OSA and sleep-disordered breathing as early and efficiently as possible. Indeed, we should not miss a potential therapeutic window for improvement in these severely affected children.

Take-Home Messages—Necker Protocol

- Patients with Apert syndrome have midface hypoplasia associated with mandibular hypoplasia or other airway anomalies, which puts them at risk of obstructive sleep apnea (OSA).
- OSA is highly prevalent in patients with Apert syndrome and peaks in the first months of life.
- Diagnosis of OSA can only be made on a polysomnography or respiratory polygraphy.
- OSA is usually severe and may relapse during childhood, underlining the need for a long-term follow-up.
- Treatment strategy should be personalized and made by a pediatric expert multidisciplinary team and associates with upper airway surgery, maxillofacial surgery, and/or neurosurgery.
- Continuous positive airway pressure (CPAP) is an effective non-invasive treatment of severe OSA while waiting for curative surgery.
- A systematic assessment of sleep and neurocognitive function is mandatory in patients with Apert syndrome to diagnose and treat OSA as early and as efficiently as possible.

References

1. Lu X, Forte AJ, Sawh-Martinez R, Wu R, Cabrejo R, Gabrick K, et al. Temporal evaluation of craniofacial relationships in Apert syndrome. J Craniofac Surg. 2019;30(2):317–25.
2. Menzies B, Teng A, Burns M, Lah S. Neurocognitive outcomes of children with sleep disordered breathing: a systematic review with meta-analysis. Sleep Med Rev. 2022;63:101629.
3. Dentino K, Ganjawalla K, Inverso G, Mulliken JB, Padwa BL. Upper airway length is predictive of obstructive sleep apnea in syndromic Craniosynostosis. J Oral Maxillofac Surg Off J Am Assoc Oral Maxillofac Surg. 2015;73(12 Suppl):S20–5.
4. Resnick CM, Middleton JK, Calabrese CE, Ganjawalla K, Padwa BL. Retropalatal cross-sectional area is predictive of obstructive sleep apnea in patients with syndromic Craniosynostosis. Cleft Palate-Craniofacial J Off Publ Am Cleft Palate-Craniofacial Assoc. 2020;57(5):560–5.
5. Lu X, Forte AJ, Allam O, Park KE, Junn A, Alperovich M, et al. Nasopharyngeal airway and subcranial space analysis in Pfeiffer syndrome. Br J Oral Maxillofac Surg. 2021;59(5):592–8.
6. Driessen C, Joosten KFM, Bannink N, Bredero-Boelhouwer HH, Hoeve HLJ, Wolvius EB, et al. How does obstructive sleep apnoea evolve in syndromic craniosynostosis? A prospective cohort study. Arch Dis Child. 2013;98(7):538–43.
7. Khonsari RH, Haber S, Paternoster G, Fauroux B, Morisseau-Durand MP, Cormier-Daire V, et al. The influence of fronto-facial monobloc advancement on obstructive sleep apnea: an assessment of 109 syndromic craniosynostoses cases. J Cranio-Maxillo-fac Surg Off Publ Eur Assoc Cranio-Maxillo-fac Surg. 2020;48(6):536–47.
8. Mannelli G, Arcuri F, Spacca B, Genitori L, Spinelli G. Respiratory and volumetric changes of the upper airways in craniofacial synostosis patients. J Cranio-Maxillo-fac Surg Off Publ Eur Assoc Cranio-Maxillo-fac Surg. 2019;47(4):548–55.
9. Zandieh SO, Padwa BL, Katz ES. Adenotonsillectomy for obstructive sleep apnea in children with syndromic craniosynostosis. Plast Reconstr Surg. 2013;131(4):847–52.
10. Haber SE, Leikola J, Nowinski D, Fauroux B, Morisseau-Durand MP, Paternoster G, Khonsari RH, Arnaud E. Secondary Le Fort III after early fronto-facial monobloc normalizes sleep apnea in faciocraniosynostosis: a cohort study. J Plast Reconstr Aesthet Surg. 2022;75:2706–18.
11. Driessen C, Mathijssen IMJ, De Groot MR, Joosten KFM. Does central sleep apnea occur in children with syndromic craniosynostosis? Respir Physiol Neurobiol. 2012;181(3):321–5.
12. Bannink N, Maliepaard M, Raat H, Joosten KFM, Mathijssen IMJ. Obstructive sleep apnea-specific

quality of life and behavioral problems in children with syndromic craniosynostosis. J Dev Behav Pediatr JDBP. 2011;32(3):233–8.
13. Yang S, Mathijssen IMJ, Joosten KFM. The impact of obstructive sleep apnea on growth in patients with syndromic and complex craniosynostosis: a retrospective study. Eur J Pediatr. 2022;181(12):4191–7.
14. Kalyoncu M, Namlı N, Yegit CY, Yanaz M, Gulieva A, Ergenekon AP, et al. Is the pediatric sleep questionnaire sensitive for sleep-disordered breathing in children with complex chronic disease? Sleep Breath Schlaf Atm. 2024;28(1):331–7.
15. Julliand S, Boulé M, Baujat G, Ramirez A, Couloigner V, Beydon N, et al. Lung function, diagnosis, and treatment of sleep-disordered breathing in children with achondroplasia. Am J Med Genet A. 2012;158A(8):1987–93.
16. Breslin J, Spanò G, Bootzin R, Anand P, Nadel L, Edgin J. Obstructive sleep apnea syndrome and cognition in down syndrome. Dev Med Child Neurol. 2014;56(7):657–64.
17. Maris M, Verhulst S, Wojciechowski M, Van de Heyning P, Boudewyns A. Prevalence of obstructive sleep apnea in children with down syndrome. Sleep. 2016;39(3):699–704.
18. Berry RB, Budhiraja R, Gottlieb DJ, Gozal D, Iber C, Kapur VK, et al. Rules for scoring respiratory events in sleep: update of the 2007 AASM manual for the scoring of sleep and associated events. Deliberations of the sleep apnea definitions task force of the American Academy of Sleep Medicine. J Clin Sleep Med JCSM Off Publ Am Acad Sleep Med. 2012;8(5):597–619.
19. Kaditis AG, Alonso Alvarez ML, Boudewyns A, Abel F, Alexopoulos EI, Ersu R, et al. ERS statement on obstructive sleep disordered breathing in 1- to 23-month-old children. Eur Respir J. 2017;50(6):1700985.
20. Kaditis AG, Alonso Alvarez ML, Boudewyns A, Alexopoulos EI, Ersu R, Joosten K, et al. Obstructive sleep disordered breathing in 2- to 18-year-old children: diagnosis and management. Eur Respir J. 2016;47(1):69–94.
21. Alonso-Álvarez ML, Terán-Santos J, Ordax Carbajo E, Cordero-Guevara JA, Navazo-Egüia AI, Kheirandish-Gozal L, et al. Reliability of home respiratory polygraphy for the diagnosis of sleep apnea in children. Chest. 2015;147(4):1020–8.
22. Parakh A, Dhingra D, Abel F. Sleep Studies in Children. Indian Pediatr. 2021;58(11):1085–90.
23. Yang S, de Goederen R, Bredero-Boelhouwer H, Joosten KFM, Mathijssen IMJ. Accuracy of detecting obstructive sleep apnea using ambulatory sleep studies in patients with syndromic Craniosynostosis. J Craniofac Surg. 2022;33(8):2538–42.
24. Marcus CL, Omlin KJ, Basinki DJ, Bailey SL, Rachal AB, Von Pechmann WS, et al. Normal polysomnographic values for children and adolescents. Am Rev Respir Dis. 1992;146(5 Pt 1):1235–9.
25. Montgomery-Downs HE, O'Brien LM, Gulliver TE, Gozal D. Polysomnographic characteristics in normal preschool and early school-aged children. Pediatrics. 2006;117(3):741–53.
26. Amaddeo A, Moreau J, Frapin A, Khirani S, Felix O, Fernandez-Bolanos M, et al. Long term continuous positive airway pressure (CPAP) and noninvasive ventilation (NIV) in children: initiation criteria in real life. Pediatr Pulmonol. 2016;51(9):968–74.
27. Baldassari CM, Lam DJ, Ishman SL, Chernobilsky B, Friedman NR, Giordano T, et al. Expert consensus statement: pediatric drug-induced sleep endoscopy. Otolaryngol Head Neck Surg. 2021;165(4):578–91.
28. Parikh SR, Boudewyns A, Friedman NR, Schwartz SR, Baldassari CM, Benedek P, et al. International pediatric otolaryngology group (IPOG) consensus on scoring of pediatric drug induced sleep endoscopy (DISE). Int J Pediatr Otorhinolaryngol. 2023;171:111627.
29. Adil E, Huntley C, Choudhary A, Carr M. Congenital nasal obstruction: clinical and radiologic review. Eur J Pediatr. 2012;171(4):641–50.
30. Tan HL, Kheirandish-Gozal L, Abel F, Gozal D. Craniofacial syndromes and sleep-related breathing disorders. Sleep Med Rev. 2016;27:74–88.
31. Saengthong P, Chaitusaney B, Hirunwiwatkul P, Charakorn N. Adenotonsillectomy in children with syndromic craniosynostosis: a systematic review and meta-analysis. European Archives of Oto-Rhino-Laryngology. 2019;276(6):1555–60.
32. Moraleda-Cibrián M, Edwards SP, Kasten SJ, Buchman SR, Berger M, O'Brien LM. Obstructive sleep apnea pretreatment and posttreatment in symptomatic children with congenital craniofacial malformations. J Clin Sleep Med JCSM. 2015;11(1):37–43.
33. Xie C, De S, Selby A. Management of the airway in Apert syndrome. J Craniofac Surg. 2016;27(1):137–41.
34. Raghavan U, Fuad F, Gibbin KP. Congenital midnasal stenosis in an infant. Int J Pediatr Otorhinolaryngol. 2004;68(6):823–5.
35. Doerga PN, Spruijt B, Mathijssen IMJ, Wolvius EB, Joosten KFM, van der Schroeff MP. Upper airway endoscopy to optimize obstructive sleep apnea treatment in Apert and Crouzon syndromes. J Cranio-Maxillo-fac Surg. 2016;44(2):191–6.
36. Mathews F, Shaffer AD, Georg MW, Ford MD, Jabbour N, Simons JP. Laryngomalacia in patients with craniosynostosis. Ann Otol Rhinol Laryngol. 2018;127(8):543–50.
37. Lee HS, Yoon HY, Jin HJ, Hwang SH. The safety and efficacy of powered intracapsular tonsillectomy in children: a meta-analysis. Laryngoscope. 2018;128(3):732–44.
38. Zhang LY, Zhong L, David M, Cervin A. Tonsillectomy or tonsillotomy? A systematic review for paediatric sleep-disordered breathing. Int J Pediatr Otorhinolaryngol. 2017;103:41–50.
39. Fauroux B, Abel F, Amaddeo A, Bignamini E, Chan E, Corel L, et al. ERS statement on paediatric long-term noninvasive respiratory support. Eur Respir J. 2022;59(6):2101404.

40. Fauroux B, Lavis JF, Nicot F, Picard A, Boelle PY, Clément A, et al. Facial side effects during noninvasive positive pressure ventilation in children. Intensive Care Med. 2005;31(7):965–9.
41. Edwards JD, Panitch HB, George M, Cirrilla AM, Grunstein E, Wolfe J, et al. Development and validation of a novel informational booklet for pediatric long-term ventilation decision support. Pediatr Pulmonol. 2021;56(5):1198–204.
42. Mastouri M, Amaddeo A, Griffon L, Frapin A, Touil S, Ramirez A, et al. Weaning from long term continuous positive airway pressure or noninvasive ventilation in children. Pediatr Pulmonol. 2017;52(10):1349–54.
43. Fauroux B, Khirani S, Amaddeo A, Massenavette B, Bierme P, Taytard J, et al. Paediatric long term continuous positive airway pressure and noninvasive ventilation in France: a cross-sectional study. Respir Med. 2021;181:106388.
44. Noble AR, Cunningham ML, Lam A, Wenger TL, Sie KC, Perkins JA, et al. Complex airway management in patients with tracheal cartilaginous sleeves. Laryngoscope. 2022;132(1):215–21.
45. Sculerati N, Gottlieb MD, Zimbler MS, Chibbaro PD, McCarthy JG. Airway management in children with major craniofacial anomalies. Laryngoscope. 1998;108(12):1806–12.
46. Wetmore RF, Marsh RR, Thompson ME, Tom LW. Pediatric tracheostomy: a changing procedure? Ann Otol Rhinol Laryngol. 1999;108(7 Pt 1):695–9.
47. Randhawa PS, Ahmed J, Nouraei SR, Wyatt ME. Impact of long-term nasopharyngeal airway on health-related quality of life of children with obstructive sleep apnea caused by syndromic craniosynostosis. J Craniofac Surg. 2011;22(1):125–8.
48. Ahmed J, Marucci D, Cochrane L, Heywood RL, Wyatt ME, Leighton SEJ. The role of the nasopharyngeal airway for obstructive sleep apnea in syndromic craniosynostosis. J Craniofac Surg. 2008;19(3):659–63.

Neurosurgical Considerations

14

Giovanna Paternoster, Tatiana Protzenko, Roman H. Khonsari, Syril James, and Eric Arnaud

Introduction

Apert syndrome is one of the most severe craniofacial disorders, caused by mutations in the fibroblast growth factor receptor 2 (FGFR2) gene, and characterized by craniosynostosis (premature fusion of skull bones), facial abnormalities, and syndactyly (fusion of fingers and toes).

Neurosurgical considerations in managing patients with Apert syndrome are critical due to the potential neurological and developmental challenges associated with the condition. Many specific findings differentiate patients with Apert syndrome from Crouzon and Pfeiffer.

Intracranial hypertension is a crucial problem in complex craniosynostosis and is related to:

- Brain compression (related to reduced skull growth due to craniosynostosis),
- Cerebrospinal fluid (CSF) circulation obstruction (related to Chiari malformation—CM).
- Venous hypertension (associated with venous sinus stenosis and collateral venous anomalies).
- Hydrocephalus (that can have obstructive and venous components).

In patients with Apert syndrome, the risk of intracranial hypertension is reduced compared to other syndromic forms of synostosis. Hydrocephalus and ventriculoperitoneal (VP) shunt insertion are hardly necessary. In addition, CM is rarely described, and venous anomalies are less frequent.

The resolution of the turri-brachycephaly of patients with Apert syndrome can be managed with posterior or anterior approaches that normally allow the complete resolution of intracranial pressure problems.

The number of surgical procedures is lower than in other syndromic conditions:

G. Paternoster
Craniofacial Unit of Necker Hospital, Paris, France

Pediatric Neurosurgical Department, French National Reference Center for Rare Disease (CRANIOST), and European Rare Disease Network member (ERN CRANIO), Paris, France

T. Protzenko
National Institute of Health for Women, Children and Adolescents Fernandes Figueira/Osvaldo Cruz Fondation, Rio de Janiero, Brazil

R. H. Khonsari · E. Arnaud (✉)
Craniofacial Unit, Hôpital Necker–Enfants malades, Paris, France

Pediatric Neurosurgical Department, French National Reference Center for Rare Disease (CRANIOST), and European Rare Disease Network member (ERN CRANIO), Paris, France

Clinique Marcel Sembat, Centre de Competence Maladies Rares CRANIOST, Ramsay-Generale de Santé, Boulogne Billancourt, France

S. James
Clinique Marcel Sembat, Centre de Competence Maladies Rares CRANIOST, Ramsay-Generale de Santé, Boulogne Billancourt, France

J. G. Meara et al. (eds.), *Apert Syndrome*, https://doi.org/10.1007/978-3-032-12551-4_14

- No VP shunt insertion (or Endoscopic Third Ventriculostomy (ETV)) is generally required,
- No cervical junction procedures for CM,
- Decreased risk of repeated cranial vault surgery for recurrence of elevated intracranial pressure (ICP).

The main issues in surgical decision-making for these patients relate to the management of airways difficulties and sleep obstructive apnea syndrome (SOAS) problems and the need to integrate cranial procedures into the schedule of ENT/ maxillofacial surgeries.

Similar to other forms of craniosynostosis, it is important to operate on patients with Apert syndrome before the age of one year. This is well demonstrated by the improved long-term cognitive outcome in patients operated on at a younger age [23].

Hydrocephalus and Ventricular Size

Some series report up to 60% ventriculomegaly in Apert syndrome [18], and Munarriz et al. presented as much as 51.3% [17]. However, nonprogressive ventriculomegaly is far more frequent than true hydrocephalus [2, 5, 7, 10, 19] (Fig. 14.1).

Tokumaru et al. stressed that true hydrocephalus is uncommon in Apert syndrome and could be differentiated from the more common non-progressive ventriculomegaly by the dilatation of the anterior third ventricle [31].

Considering the typical cranial deformity of patients with Apert syndrome, we can envision that the ventricular enlargement mostly affects the frontal horns and mirrors the misshaped and widened calvarium.

Real signs or symptoms of progressive hydrocephalus (clinical or radiological) are exceptional in Apert syndrome. This is why in 1971 Hogan and Bauman evoked the diagnosis of normal pressure hydrocephalus in Apert syndrome [14].

Unlike other forms of syndromic synostosis, the lower predominance of venous hypertension in patients with Apert syndrome due to normal jugular foramina leads to decreased brain pressures and normal CSF re-absorption. These children generally also have a normal posterior fossa with no obstruction of CSF circulation, reducing the incidence of hydrocephalus.

In literature, the incidence of VP shunt insertion in patients with Apert syndrome can vary

Article	*n* (total)	*n* (with CT or MRI images)	VP shunt	Tonsillar herniation	Corpus callosum anomalies*	Septum pellucidum anomalies†
Hanieh and David[17] (1993, North Adelaide, Australia)	33	13	0% (0/33)	-	-	-
Murovic *et al.*[26] (1993, Toronto, Canada)	44	25	23% (10/44)	-	12% (agenesis) (3/25)	-
Posnick *et al.*[28] (1994, Washington D.C., USA)	8	8	25% (2/8)	-	-	-
Cinalli *et al.*[6] (1995, Paris, France)‡	65	55	6.15% (4/65)	1.9% (1/55)	32.7% (18/55)	50.9% (28/55)
McCarthy *et al.*[24] (1995, New York, USA)	24	24	20.8% (5/24)	-	-	-
Renier *et al.*[30] (1996, Paris, France)‡	70	60	11.7% (7/60)	1.7% (1/60)	30% (18/60)	55% (33/60)
Cinalli *et al.*[7] (1998, Paris, France)‡	77	77	6.5% (5/77)	1.3% (1/77)	-	-
Yacubian-Fernandes *et al.*[37] (2004, Sao Paulo, Brazil)	18	18	0% (0/18)	-	27.8% (5/18)	38.9% (7/18))
Collmann *et al.*[11] (2005, Würzburg, Germany)	45	-	4.4% (2/45)	-	-	-
Marucci *et al.*[23] (2008, London, UK)	24	24	12.5% (3/24	-	-	-
Fearon and Podner[16] (2013, Dallas, USA)	135	135	18.5% (25/135)	29%	12%	24%
Breik *et al.*[4] (2016, North Adelaide, Australia)	94	94	7.45% (7/94)	4% (4/94)	11% (agenesis) (10/94)	13% (12/94)
Munarriz *et al.* (2020, Madrid, Spain)	37	37	24.3% (9/37)	21.6% (8/37)	43.2% (16/37)	59.5% (22/37)

*Corpus callosum anomalies include agenesis and hypoplasia. †Septum pellucidum anomalies include partial absence, complete absence, cavum vergae, or cystic septum. ‡Three papers from the same hospital; thus, they correspond to a series of patients that are very similar to each other

Fig. 14.1 Comparison of different series of patients with Apert syndrome—Munarriz et al. [17]

from 0 to 25%, with higher rates in the older series [17]. In the last reviews and in the centers with a large volume of patients, it is clear that there should be reluctance to consider CSF drainage, and that most children with Apert syndrome do not have pathological hydrocephalus [21, 30].

Chiari Malformation

Chiari I deformity is rare in Apert syndrome, estimated at <2% in most series [4, 24]. A convincing correlation has been found between chronic tonsillar herniation and the premature closure of the lambdoid suture (before 24 months), and this premature fusion is much less common in Apert syndrome than in Crouzon syndrome [3, 4].

This finding is consistent with normal embryology and development, as cerebellar growth is especially accelerated compared to the forebrain and brainstem during these first two years of age. Consequently, a patient with early lambdoid craniosynostosis (and of the synchondroses of the cranial base) would be at a higher risk of CM [3, 5, 6].

In a recent study about the role of posterior fossa volume in developing CM, Rijken et al. demonstrated that none of the individual syndromes was associated with a restricted Posterior Fossa Volume [27].

In only a few papers, Chiari has been found in a higher percentage of patients: in Munarriz et al. around 21% had CM and three patients required surgery (8.1%) [17]. Raposo et al. found that 14% of patients presented with CM, and were treated by posterior expansion or foramen magnum decompression.

It is likely that in these cases, a more severe phenotype, with a cloverleaf skull condition and evidence of increased intracranial hypertension, might, plays a major role in the development of CM.

Radiological Aspects

Skull

Patients with Apert syndrome present a more homogeneous phenotype, characterized by bilateral closure of the coronal sutures, although in rare cases, the synostosis is unilateral [24]. In addition, most infants have a wider-than-normal metopic and sagittal suture separation. In contrast with other syndromes, progressive suture closure over time has rarely been described.

The persistent opening of the lambdoid sutures in these patients allows for the development of a normal posterior fossa and a reduced risk of Chiari malformation (CM).

In the Apert syndrome, the spheno-occipital, petro-occipital, and occipital synchondrosis are never fused in the first year of life and begin to fuse between 12 and 48 months, with complete fusion after four years of age [15].

The sagittal suture is generally widely patent and larger than normal [22]. This wide sagittal suture separation is likely an adaptation of the interparietal diameter to the brachycephaly induced by the coronal synostosis, and may play a role in the architecture of the Apert posterior fossa, which is usually larger than normal [25, 26] and is rarely associated with CM [4, 6, 24].

There are several other stereotypic features of the skull base. The skull base angle in newborns with Apert syndrome is significantly smaller than controls. The foramen magnum area at birth is normal, but the growth is disturbed; The clivus length is significantly shorter at birth, with a significant growth retardation; the tonsillar position was significantly higher at birth compared to controls, and it lowered faster throughout life. The exact role of each parameter remains unclear [12] (Figs. 14.2 and 14.3).

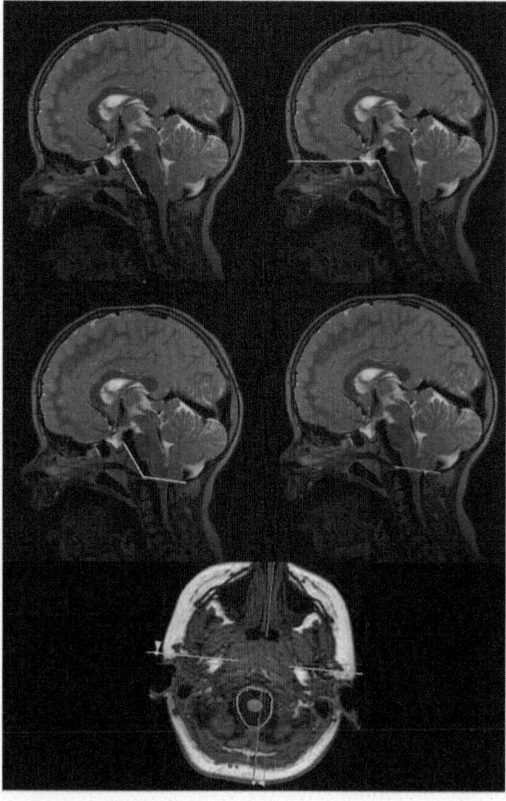

Fig. 14.2 Measured parameters in a patient with syndromic synostosis. Above, left: clivus length. Above, right: skull base angle. Middle, left: Boogard's angle. Middle, right: tonsillar position. Below: foramen magnum area [12]

Brain

Most brain malformations related to Apert syndrome correspond to abnormalities of midline development, specifically involving the olfactory-limbic-septal-callosal structures [2, 17]. The olfactory bulbs and tract were present in most case.

Hypoplasia of the Corpus Callosum (CC) was defined as a reduction in the extension or thickness of the CC, which is well seen in patients with Apert syndrome, along with abnormalities of the septum pellucidum.

Mesial temporal abnormalities are prominent: a redundant, over convoluted cortex (without polymicrogyria) in the anterior mesial temporal pole, with a poorly formed amygdala, a large temporal horn, and locally hypoplastic white matter. These findings are more likely to be real developmental abnormalities related to the skull deformity. No clear explanation has been identified regarding whether the cause of the temporal white matter anomalies is a cortical abnormality or if the white matter defect is secondary to the parenchymal disorganization.

There are several indicators of white matter abnormalities in addition to those found in the temporal lobe. There are other findings of global reduction of white matter volume with an abnormal corpus callosum, the defective interhemispheric commissural, the absence of septum pellucidum and the hypoplastic pyramidal tracts, as well as the non-progressive ventriculomegaly [22]. The role of white matter in the connectivity is well recognized; therefore, these diffuse white matter anomalies may influence the neurocognitive dysfunction often seen in patients with Apert syndrome. As such, developmental delay in patients with Apert syndrome may be a consequence of white matter maldevelopment rather than secondary to hydrocephalus or skull restriction [22, 29]. In some papers, the hypothesis of the role of gene mutation in white matter abnormalities associates to craniosynostosis has been promoted [22, 23] (Table. 14.1).

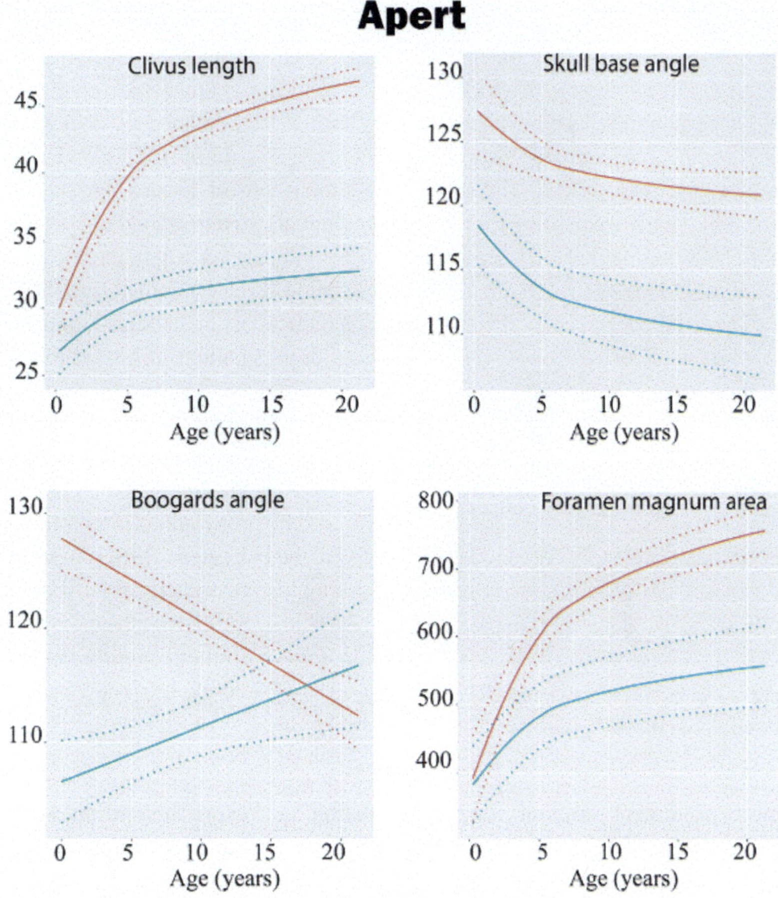

Fig. 14.3 Mean fitted values of the linear mixed models comparing skull base parameters between Apert craniosynostosis (blue line) and controls (red line) [12]

Table. 14.1 Cerebral abnormalities in Apert syndrome [22]

	Normal (%)	Abnormal (%)
Brain	28	72
Corpus callosum	70	thin 27, absent 3
Septum pellucidum	45	cavum 25, absent 30
Cerebellum	98	Chiari I 1.9

Venous System Abnormalities

Venous outflow anomalies are recognized in patients with complex craniosynostosis and have been the focus of recent studies [11, 13]. Venous sinus stenosis and associated venous collateral circulation are related to both intrinsic and extrinsic factors.

The origin of collateral venous circulation and its relationship with the morphology of the skull base is still controversial. Literature suggests that changes in the skull base would be responsible for stenosis of the dural venous sinuses, leading to the development of compensatory collateral circulation or persistence of fetal venous sinuses [28]. As the jugular foramen contains the sigmoid sinus and the jugular bulb, it would not be difficult to imagine that its stenosis could lead to stenosis of the drainage and collateral circulation pathways. However, somewhat contradictory data has also been reported. Coll and colleagues (2019) compared the area of the jugular foramen among patients with Crouzon, Pfeiffer, and Apert syndromes under two years of age. They found that the only group that showed truly reduced jugular foramina when compared to control was the Apert group. Therefore, it would be obvious that the extracranial venous circulation would be more exuberant in patients with Apert syndrome. However, this is not true, and many studies report

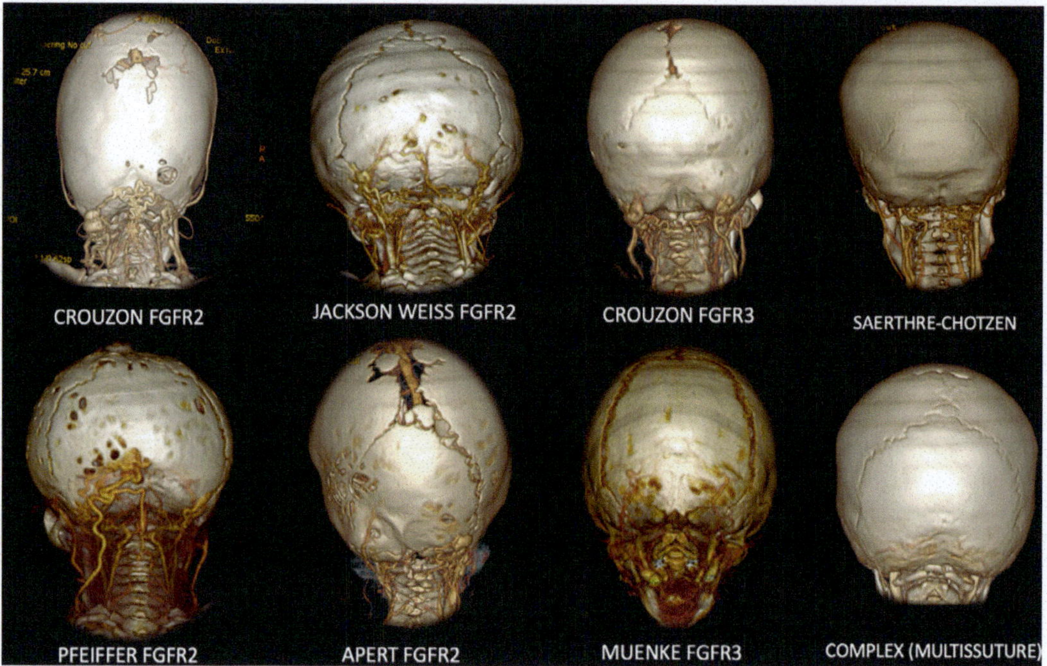

Fig. 14.4 Venous outflow differences between syndromes. Apert group shows less severe changes comparing to Crouzon and Pfeiffer groups

more prominent external venous circulation in patients with Pfeiffer syndrome (100%), followed by Crouzon (84%) and Apert syndromes (64%) (Copeland). This demonstrates, as suggested by Coll and colleagues [8], that bone measurements alone do not explain the changes of the cranial venous outflow tracts in syndromic patients [9].

Other authors reported that patients with enlarged emissary veins are more likely to have elevated ICP, ventriculomegaly or shunted hydrocephalus, Chiari I malformation, and obstructive sleep apnea (Copeland). In these cases, collateral circulation would be a compensatory mechanism for intracranial hypertension. However, we know neither CMI nor hydrocephalus is common in Apert syndrome, even though they can change venous outflow, mainly in the occipital region.

This suggests that the stenosis of the jugular foramen is not directly or uniquely related to the venous anomalies, and that additional intrinsic factors could be involved. A possible intrinsic theory is based on a primary vascular abnormality resulting from a similar dysplastic process that occurs in the bones of the skull. FGFR gene expression products have been detected in cranial vascular endothelium and in synostotic sutures in patients with syndromic craniosynostosis by immunohistochemical examination [16, 32]. Also, collaterals in newborn patients found in a retrospective series implies that collateral development could be an intrinsic disorder [1].

Regardless of the mechanism of abnormal venous outflow, these vessels are increasingly focused on in preoperative planning since the rupture of this circulation can have fatal consequences. Therefore, a venous study should be considered in all patients with syndromic craniosynostosis, although less severe changes are found in patients with Apert syndrome than in Crouzon and Pfeiffer patients (Fig. 14.4).

Developmental Impairments

Children with Apert syndrome often experience developmental delays, including cognitive, motor, and speech delays. Historically, neurocognitive deficiency is common, with less than half of the patients (48%) with an intelligence quotient above 70 and one fifth (21%) below 50 [20]. However, it should be stressed that much of this information might be related to older ages at surgery in the historical cohorts. In any case, neurosurgeons should collaborate with pediatric neurologists and developmental specialists to monitor neurological function and cognitive development. Early neurodevelopmental interventions are crucial, including speech, occupational, and physical therapy. The delays can be attributed to several factors, including craniosynostosis, structural brain differences, and early-life challenges related to physical disabilities such as syndactyly and facial deformities.

Cognitive and Intellectual Delays

Rener et al. in 1996 described which factors can be involved in the cognitive development of patients with Apert syndrome. Thirty-two percent of patients with significant follow-up review had an intelligence quotient (IQ) greater than 70. Age at operation appeared to be the main factor associated with changes in mental development: 50% of patients operated on before one year of age versus only 7.1% in patients operated on later in life ($p = 0.01$). Malformations of the corpus callosum and size of the ventricles played no role in the final IQ, whereas anomalies of the septum pellucidum had a significant effect. Quality of the family environment was the third factor involved in intellectual achievement: only 12.5% of institutionalized children reached a normal IQ level compared to 39.3% of children from a traditional family background [23].

Cognitive impairments in Apert syndrome can vary widely. Some children may have normal intelligence or only mild delays, while others may experience moderate-to-severe intellectual disabilities. Early developmental assessments can help determine the level of cognitive delay, allowing for early intervention programs to support cognitive growth. Children with Apert syndrome are often enrolled in special education programs and receive individualized educational support to help them progress at their own pace.

- *Motor Delays*

Due to syndactyly (fusion of fingers and toes) and other musculoskeletal abnormalities, children with Apert syndrome may have motor coordination issues and fine motor difficulties.

Early surgical correction of syndactyly (separating fused fingers and toes) is important to allow for normal hand and foot function, which in turn helps with fine motor skills development.

Physical therapy is crucial in helping children develop gross motor skills (such as walking, running, and balancing), while occupational therapy focuses on fine motor skills (like writing, grasping objects, and buttoning clothes).

- *Speech and Language Delays*

Many children with Apert syndrome experience delays in speech development, which can be attributed to facial abnormalities (such as a high-arched palate, clefting, or underdeveloped jaw) and hearing problems (such as middle ear dysfunction due to craniofacial malformations).

Speech therapy is essential in managing these delays. Therapists often work on articulation, language skills, and communication strategies. If speech development is significantly delayed, some children may require the use of alternative communication devices.

- *Social and Emotional Development*

As with other areas of development, social and emotional development can also be affected. Children with significant physical differences due to Apert syndrome may experience social challenges or low self-esteem due to their appearance.

Psychological support, such as counselling and social skills training, can help children build coping mechanisms, improve self-confidence, and develop social relationships with peers. As Renier stated in 1996, the quality of socio-familial environment is critical to obtain the best mental outcome in the child affected with Apert syndrome.

Surgical Procedures

The timing of neurosurgical interventions is believed to be an important factor in minimizing neurological deficits. Early surgery for craniosynostosis (around 6–12 months) improves outcomes by preventing developmental delays and alleviating the pressure on the brain.

Once surgery has been performed, regular follow-up is needed to assess cognitive and motor development, as delayed surgery, inadequate surgery, or the need for additional surgery can lead to significant neurodevelopmental impairments.

Early intervention (usually within the first year of life) is necessary to prevent intracranial pressure (ICP) buildup and to allow normal brain development. Surgical options may include:

- *Posterior cranial vault remodeling:* To reshape the skull and reduce the turricephaly.
- *Frontal-orbital advancement:* To reposition the forehead and eye sockets, correcting exorbitism and reducing brachycephaly.
- *Endoscopic strip craniectomies* performed very early.
- *Frontofacial monobloc advancement:* To manage in a single procedure the intracranial hypertension, exorbitism (+/− subluxation risk), and respiratory impairment, reducing the possible requirement for tracheostomy. This procedure can be performed even at an early age.

Important Messages

- Among faciocraniosynostoses syndromes, patients with Apert syndrome present more frequently with an associated brain malformation.
- Ventriculomegaly is often mistaken with hydrocephalus, but shunting is rarely necessary.
- Raised ICP in the infant patient with Apert syndrome is rare because the synostosis is limited to coronal sutures and associated with a wide median frontal dehiscence acting like a pressure release valve.
- Because of the absence of lambdoid synostosis, cerebellum tonsillar herniation (Chiari malformation) is extremely rare.
- Our data in Necker support the evidence that reinforced parental education, absence of brain malformation, and early surgical surgery before one year of age are associated with a better mental outcome [23].
- Early release of the skull may be carried out with a posterior distraction, an endoscopic strip craniectomy or fronto-orbital advancement before one year of age.
- The early management of impaired airways is critical to achieve the optimal prognosis. Tracheostomy should be restricted to life-threatening neonatal situations.
- Necessity for frontofacial monobloc in the patient with Apert syndrome is less frequent than in Crouzon or Pfeiffer, and should be reserved for patients with severe exorbitism and OSAS.
- In case a shunt is needed, it should be delayed until after skull expansions, as it impedes further skull growth and can lead to relative microcephaly and pansynostosis.

References

1. Armand T, Schaefer E, Di Rocco F, Edery P, Collet C, Rossi M. Genetic bases of craniosynostoses: an update. Neurochirurgie. 2019;65(5):196–201.
2. Breik O, Mahindu A, Moore MH, Molloy CJ, Santoreneos S, David DJ. Central nervous system and cervical spine abnormalities in Apert syndrome. Childs Nerv Syst. 2016;32:833–8.
3. Cinalli G, Chumas P, Arnaud E, Sainte-Rose C, Renier D. Occipital remodeling and suboccipital decompression in severe craniosynostosis associated with tonsillar herniation. Neurosurgery. 1998;42:66–73.
4. Cinalli G, Renier D, Sebag G, Sainte-Rose C, Arnaud E, Pierre-Kahn A. Chronic tonsillar herniation in Crouzon and Apert syndrome: the role of the premature synostosis of the lambdoid suture. J Neurosurg. 1995;83:575–82.
5. Cinalli G, Sainte-Rose C, Kollar EM, Zerah M, Brunelle F, Chumas P, et al. Hydrocephalus and craniosynostosis. J Neurosurg. 1998;88:209–14.

6. Cinalli G, Spennato P, Sainte-Rose C, Arnaud E, Aliberti F, Brunelle F, Cianciulli E, Renier D. Chiari malformation in craniosynostosis. Childs Nerv Syst. 2005;21(10):889–901.
7. Cohen MM Jr, Kreiborg S. The central nervous system in the Apert syndrome. Am J Med Genet. 1990;35:36–45.
8. Coll G, Abed Rabbo F, Jecko V, Sakka L, Di Rocco F, Delion M. The growth of the posterior cranial fossa in FGFR2-induced faciocraniosynostosis: a review. Neurochirurgie. 2019 Nov;65(5):221–7.
9. Coll G, Arnaud E, Collet C, Brunelle F, Sainte-Rose C, Di Rocco F. Skull Base morphology in fibroblast growth factor receptor type 2-related faciocraniosynostosis. Neurosurgery. 2015;76(5):571–83.
10. Collmann H, Sörensen N, Krauss J. Hydrocephalus in craniosynostosis: a review. Childs Nerv Syst. 2005;21:902–12.
11. Copeland AE, Hoffman CE, Tsitouras V, Jeevan DS, Ho ES, Drake JM, et al. Clinical significance of venous anomalies in syndromic craniosynostosis: plastic and reconstructive surgery. Global Open. 2018;6(1):e1613.
12. den Ottelander BK, Dremmen MHG, de Planque CA, van der Oest MJW, Mathijssen IMJ, van Veelen MC. Does the association between abnormal anatomy of the skull base and cerebellar tonsillar position also exist in syndromic craniosynostosis? J Plast Reconstr Aesthet Surg. 2022 Feb;75(2):797–805.
13. Florisson JMG, Barmpalios G, Lequin M, van Veelen MLC, Bannink N, Hayward RD, et al. Venous hypertension in syndromic and complex craniosynostosis: the abnormal anatomy of the jugular foramen and collaterals. J Craniofac Surg. 2015;43(3):312–8.
14. Hogan GR, Bauman ML. Hydrocephalus in Apert's syndrome. J Pediatr. 1971;79:782–7.
15. Kreiborg S, Marsh JL, Cohen MM Jr, Liversage M, Pedersen H, Skovby F, Børgesen SE, Vannier MW. Comparative three-dimensional analysis of CT-scans of the calvaria and cranial base in Apert and Crouzon syndromes. J Craniomaxillofac Surg. 21:181–8.
16. Lajeunie E, Le Merrer M, Bonaïti-Pellie C, Marchac D, Renier D. Genetic study of nonsyndromic coronal craniosynostosis. Am J Med Genet. 1995;55(4):500–4.
17. Munarriz PM, Pascual B, Castaño-Leon AM, García-Recuero I, Redondo M, de Aragón AM, Romance A. Apert syndrome: cranial procedures and brain malformations in a series of patients. Surg Neurol Int. 2020;29(11):361.
18. Murovic JA, Posnick JC, Drake JM, Humphreys RP, Hoffman HJ, Hendricks EB. Hydrocephalus in Apert syndrome: a retrospective review. Pediatr Neurosurg. 1993;19:151–5.
19. Noetzel MJ, Marsh JL, Palkes H, Gado M. Hydrocephalus and mental retardation in craniosynostosis. J Pediatr. 1985;107:885–92.
20. Patton MA, Goodship J, Hayward R, Lansdown R. Intellectual development in Apert's syndrome: a long term follow-up of 29 patients. J Med Genet. 1988;25:164–7.
21. Raposo-Amaral CE, Vincenzi-Lemes M, Medeiros ML, Raposo-Amaral CA, Ghizoni E. Apert syndrome: neurosurgical outcomes and complications following posterior vault distraction osteogenesis. Childs Nerv Syst. 2024 Aug;40(8):2557–63.
22. Raybaud C. Di Rocco C brain malformation in syndromic craniosynostoses, a primary disorder of white matter: a review. Childs Nerv Syst. 2007;23(12):1379–88.
23. Renier D, Arnaud E, Cinalli G, Sebag G, Zerah M, Marchac D. Prognosis for mental function in Apert's syndrome. J Neurosurg. 1996;85:66–72.
24. Renier D, Lajeunie E, Arnaud E, Marchac D. Management of craniosynostoses. Childs Nerv Syst. 2000;16(10–11):645–58.
25. Richtsmeier JT. Comparative study of normal, Crouzon and Apert craniofacial morphology using finite element scaling analysis. Am J Phys Anthropol. 1987;74:473–93.
26. Richtsmeier JT. Craniofacial growth in Apert syndrome as measured by finite-element scaling analysis. Acta Anat. 1988;133:50–6.
27. Rijken BF, Lequin MH, van der Lijn F, van Veelen-Vincent ML, de Rooi J, Hoogendam YY, Niessen WJ, Mathijssen IM. The role of the posterior fossa in developing Chiari I malformation in children with craniosynostosis syndromes. J Craniomaxillofac Surg. 2015 Jul;43(6):813–9.
28. Robson CD, Mulliken JB, Robertson RL, Proctor MR, Steinberger D, Barnes PD, et al. Prominent basal emissary foramina in syndromic craniosynostosis: correlation with phenotypic and molecular diagnoses. AJNR Am J Neuroradiol. 2000;21(9):1707–17.
29. Tan AP, Mankad K. Apert syndrome: magnetic resonance imaging (MRI) of associated intracranial anomalies. Childs Nerv Syst. 2018;34(2):205–16.
30. Tcherbbis Testa V, Jaimovich S, Argañaraz R, Mantese B. Management of ventriculomegaly in pediatric patients with syndromic craniosynostosis: a single center experience. Acta Neurochir. 2021;163(11):3083–91.
31. Tokumaru AM, Barkovich AJ, Ciricillo SF, Edwards MSB. Skull base and calvarial deformities: association with intracranial changes in craniofacial syndromes. Am J Neuroradiol. 1996;17:619–30.
32. Wang JC, Nagy L, Demke JC. Syndromic Craniosynostosis. Facial Plast Surg Clin North Am. 2016 Nov;24(4):531–43.

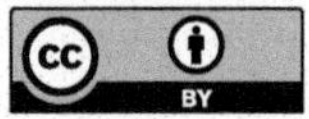

15 Early Surgery: Endoscopic Strip Craniectomy (ESC)

Mark R. Proctor and Emma K. Hartman

Introduction

Patients with Apert syndrome often suffer from associated multi-suture craniosynostosis, especially bilateral coronal synostosis (Fig. 15.1) [1, 2]. Craniosynostosis associated with Apert syndrome generally benefits from surgical intervention during infancy to prevent elevated intracranial pressure (ICP), visual impairment, and improve significant head-shape deformities such as turribrachycephaly [1]. The traditional approach has been cranial vault reconstruction towards the end of the first year, but the results regarding the height of the skull have been suboptimal. Turricephaly is a vexing problem that is difficult to repair in single-stage cranial vault reconstruction. As a result, many centers now offer an early operation during the first several months to prevent the progression of turricephaly, essentially staging the full repair of the cranial vault [3]. At many centers, this is accomplished by posterior cranial vault expansion, either in a single procedure or via distraction osteogenesis. Since the primary underlying issue is bilateral coronal synostosis, our center has developed a protocol for early endoscopic bilateral coronal strip craniectomy (ESC), which offers the possibility of a single-stage repair in many cases. In this chapter, we outline the technique and outcomes.

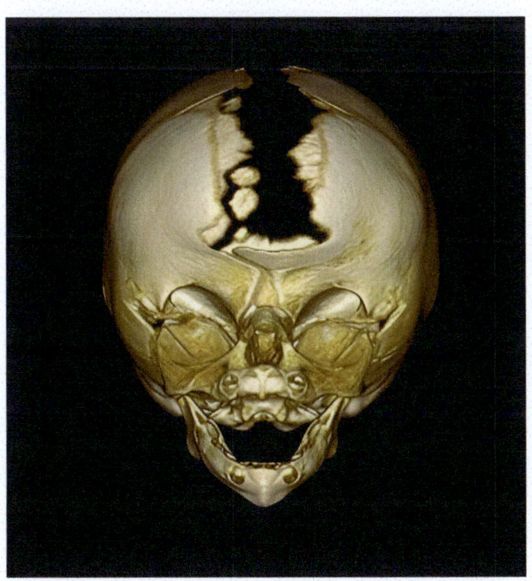

Fig. 15.1 3D reconstruction of the Apert skull seen from the anterior view with bilateral coronal synostosis

M. R. Proctor (✉) · E. K. Hartman
Department of Neurosurgery, Boston Children's Hospital, Boston, MA, USA
e-mail: Mark.Proctor@childrens.harvard.edu

History of ESC

Evidence of craniosynostosis can be traced back to the writings of Hippocrates, but the first viable treatment options were only developed in the last century. In the late 1800s, surgeons initially attempted to treat single-suture craniosynostosis with an open procedure known as the strip craniectomy, which entailed a large incision followed by surgical removal of the fused cranial suture

J. G. Meara et al. (eds.), *Apert Syndrome*, https://doi.org/10.1007/978-3-032-12551-4_15

[4]. Unfortunately, in these early surgeries patient selection was likely poor, and morbidity and mortality were high. Later on, when strip craniectomy became safer and the patients were appropriately selected, results were often not optimal because the operated suture refused too quickly, preventing adequate corrections. This led to an era of larger surgeries.

From the early 1960s to the mid-1990s, several larger open procedures were developed to address these limitations and treat multi-suture craniosynostosis, commonly found in syndromic patients. Fueled by significant advances in anesthesia and blood transfusion, innovations from Dr. Tessier led to total calvarial remodeling procedures (CVRs) that involve the removal and repositioning of segments of cranial bone to a more anatomical position [4, 5]. This approach produced improved cosmetic outcomes relative to the strip craniectomy, but it was associated with high rates of blood loss requiring significant transfusion volumes, as well as long operative and anesthesia times and postoperative stays. In addition, it became clear that while immediate results were excellent, long-term growth could lead to regression and inadequate outcomes [6, 7].

In the 1990s, Drs. Jimenez and Barone sought to address these drawbacks via the use of newly available technologies, including the endoscope and cranial orthoses. They developed an endoscopic approach to the traditional strip craniectomy technique, which they coupled with postoperative helmet therapy. The endoscope was used to perform the traditional strip craniectomy through small incisions. This approach allowed for minimal blood loss, with less local tissue disruption and the associated negative impact on bone growth, which is substantially influenced by the dura and periosteum. The postoperative use of orthosis ensured subsequent skull growth progressed in the desired direction, preventing the rapid refusion of the suture that had been seen historically. This groundbreaking advancement ushered in a new era of endoscopic surgery for craniosynostosis [8–12].

Endoscopic strip craniectomy with postoperative orthotics has now been shown effective for the treatment of both single-suture craniosynostosis and multi-suture or syndromic craniosynostosis, as either a single operation or part of a staged approach in these complex patients. Despite numerous peer-reviewed articles on endoscopic techniques for craniosynostosis correction published throughout the 1990s and early 2000s, many centers have been slower to adopt this technology than they were to adopt the larger cranial vault operations when they were initially introduced by Tessier. That notwithstanding, there is excellent evidence of the effectiveness of these endoscopic operations in the appropriate patients, and comprehensive craniofacial centers should be proficient in both open and endoscopic interventions, to offer the most modern and comprehensive care to their patients [4].

ESC Compared to Other Treatments

Traditionally, bicoronal craniosynostosis in syndromic and nonsyndromic patients has been treated with open procedures usually performed between 9 and 11 months of age. However, it has been challenging to correct turribrachycephaly effectively using these operations, which has led to early surgery as a well-adopted standard of care for children with Apert syndrome. As discussed, many centers have adopted an approach that addresses this by expanding the posterior calvarium early in life through a posterior cranial vault reconstruction or posterior cranial vault distraction. Jimenez was the first to publish on the use of endoscopic surgery addressing the fused coronal sutures to treat this condition and prevent the progression of turricephaly [12]. At our center, ESC between 2–4 months of age has become the preferred procedure in patients with Apert syndrome due to its effectiveness in correcting turricephaly, which is present at birth and progresses over the first year of life in the absence of intervention [1]. Similar to the posterior approaches that are commonly used, by preventing worsening turricephaly, early intervention with ESC promises better overall outcomes [2, 11–13]. In contrast to the posterior approaches, a substantial advantage of endoscopic surgery is that it addresses the primary problem. Therefore, there is the possibility of it being a single-stage treatment, unlike the three-stage treatment algorithms used when posterior distraction is the preferred intervention, which requires distraction placement, distraction removal, and ultimate frontal orbital advancement [14].

Endoscopic strip craniectomy has been well-studied in the treatment of children with Apert syndrome. Previously published data has shown improvement in many elements of turribrachycephaly based on computed tomography (CT) analysis of bilateral coronal synostosis patients treated with endoscopic release [2]. With regard to ophthalmologic outcomes, endoscopic release also results in less severe palpebral fissure downslanting and V-pattern strabismus in patients with Apert syndrome, similar to what has previously been found in unilateral coronal synostosis patients, thus helping to normalize appearance and ocular function [15, 16]. ESC has also been demonstrated to be equally effective in normalizing head growth and cephalic index (CI)—proxies for measuring intracranial volume and turribrachycephaly, respectively—by the time patients reach 2 years of age, with fewer complications relative to FOA/CVR [1, 2]. Moreover, while some critics argue that ESC may not achieve similar supraorbital rim advancement as is seen with fronto-orbital advancement (FOA), we know that reoperation rates for bilateral coronal synostosis are high even after open surgery. A series by Wong et al. documented a 100% reoperation rate in patients with Apert syndrome who were initially treated with an FOA [17]. This research indicates that even an FOA could require revision for improved supraorbital protection and contour, underscoring that reoperations in syndromic populations are common regardless of initial surgical intervention.

Reoperation after craniofacial surgery is, unfortunately, a common, well-known problem after all types of surgical repair [18–25]. Children with synostosis are immediately at risk for reclosure of the original sutures or other cranial sutures. Consistent with this, the associated mutation in the characteristic Apert FGFR2 gene is a gain-of-function mutation, prompting appropriate concerns about premature postoperative suture reossification. There is substantial literature that after both open and endoscopic surgery centers should closely follow patients over time, at least until the point at which full brain growth is substantially complete. Studies have shown this to be approximately 6 years of age [26, 27]. Despite our best treatments in either the open or minimally invasive realms, the genetics of synostosis are such that all of these patients need close follow-up until at least this point in time. At our center we routinely follow all synostosis patients until at least 6 years of age, and syndromic patients are followed until adulthood. This is true after open cranial vault repair and is certainly also true after endoscopic surgery. In our published experience, on average 30% of patients with Apert syndrome who undergo early endoscopic surgery experience premature reossification of the osteotomized sutures [1]. More extended data suggests that the rate of requiring additional surgery is as high as 44%, with the indication for surgery being either inadequate cosmetic result in the forehead or the need for additional intracranial space. The latter is often detected via the routine assessment of head circumference, ophthalmologic exams, and repeat imaging as necessary.

It is important to emphasize, as is well-known to any craniofacial surgeon, that there are many ways of achieving similar goals. In general it should be the goal of the craniofacial team to achieve the best results regarding both form and function in a way that require the least morbidity and fewest interventions for the child. In this regard, ESC offers advantages over other procedures such as posterior vault distraction osteogenesis (PVDO) or reconstruction as an initial approach to Apert syndrome. PVDO involves a three-surgery treatment plan (posterior craniotomy with distractor placement, removal of distractors, and FOA). In contrast, ESC offers a chance at resolution with a single surgery in over 50% of patients [11–14, 28, 29]. Additionally, ESC addresses the pathologic sutures directly, rather than involving a nonpathologic area of the skull, as PVDO does. It is common knowledge in craniofacial surgery that when intervening on normal sutures, you often terminally interrupt their anatomy. Indeed, postoperative CT scans after cranial vault reconstruction often show a complete absence of cranial sutures in the operated portions of the skull (Fig. 15.2).

Endoscopic surgery, which only involves surgery on the affected suture and does not interrupt the normal sutures avoids a direct surgical insult that places the functioning sutures at risk for premature fusion. Indeed, there is excellent evidence in syndromic and nonsyndromic patients that after minimally invasive surgery they can develop a neosuture which leads to more normalized skull growth over time (Fig. 15.3) [30].

In summary, since studies have shown that morphological improvement in patients with bilateral coronal craniosynostosis who undergo ESC is at least equivalent to posterior cranial vault distraction, along with lower morbidity and the possibility of a single-stage treatment algorithm for the correction of cranial dysmorphology, we feel that endoscopic surgery has several potential advantages and should be part of a routine treatment algorithm [2].

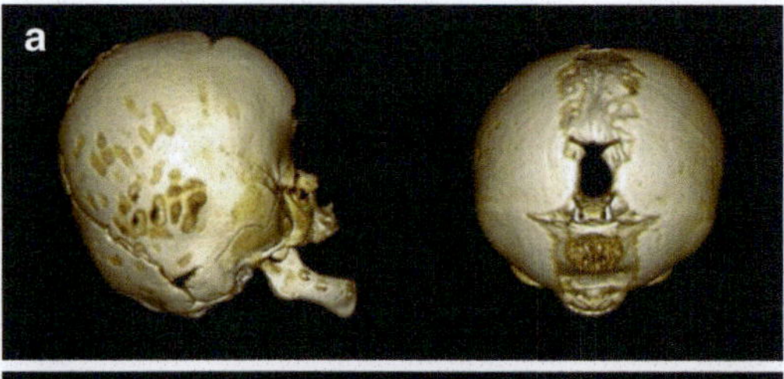

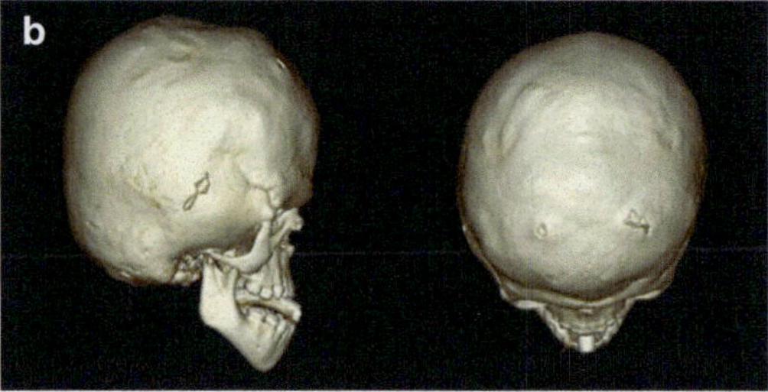

Fig. 15.2 (**a**) Preoperative lateral and superior view of infant with Apert syndrome showing bilateral coronal synostosis with patency of all other sutures. (**b**) Postoperative CT at 3 years of age in same patient after open calvarial vault remodeling surgery showing loss of all normal sutures

Patient Selection and Preoperative Care

Patients with Apert syndrome should have an evaluation for craniosynostosis with a craniofacial surgeon between the ages of 1 and 3 months. Most patients with Apert syndrome present with bilateral coronal synostosis, although some may have variations that include unilateral coronal synostosis or additional fused sutures. As discussed previously, because of the progressive deformity over time, along with the risks to bring growth and development that might be mitigated by early surgery, early diagnosis and intervention are believed important in the treatment algorithm.

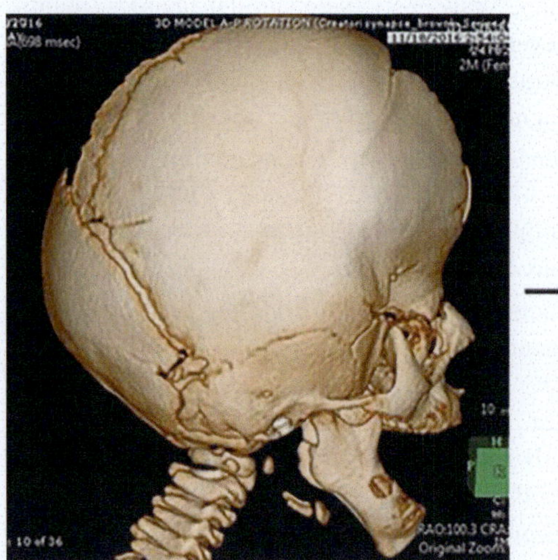

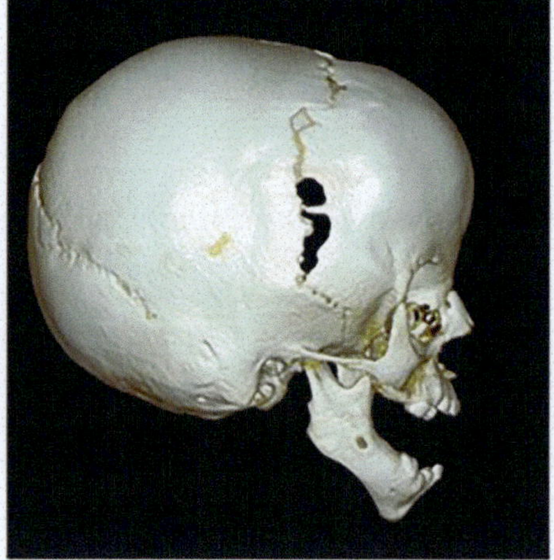

Fig. 15.3 Postoperative neosuture formation in an patient with Apert syndrome

Craniosynostosis can be diagnosed clinically in patients with Apert syndrome through manual palpitation of the cranial sutures, although magnetic resonance imaging (MRI), X-ray, or computed tomography (CT) can be used to further evaluate, manage, or confirm the diagnosis.

In most cases of nonsyndromic craniosynostosis at our institution, an endoscopic strip craniectomy—also known as an endoscopic suturectomy or endoscopic suture release—is performed when the child is between 2 and 4 months old. Since ESC seeks to restore normal anatomy, as opposed to open procedures which entail reconstructing the skull surgically, it relies on subsequent brain and skull growth to sustain the endoscopic correction [1]. Consequently, endoscopic surgery should be performed early as the brain grows rapidly over the first 3–6 months of life and the profound turricephaly found in children with Apert syndrome will likely not respond to endoscopic techniques at older ages [5]. An interesting approach, that we do not have experience with, could be the addition of adjuvant devices such as distractors or springs to slowly push the frontal and parietal skull bones apart after an endoscopic release. Endoscopic surgery by the age of 3 months is ideal, but minor variations in timing are acceptable up to the age of 6 months given general infant health or weight. In our experience infants should weigh >5 kg to be considered suitable candidates for ESC. This was based on early data from our first 100 patients, where infants having reached this threshold were much better surgical and anesthetic risks with lower rates of blood transfusion [31]. For surgeons unfamiliar with this type of surgery, endoscopic techniques are feasible and straightforward due to the ease of separation of the dura from the bone at a fused suture. Therefore, we consider it a very safe operation with low risk of dural injury, although cerebrospinal fluid (CSF) leak should be avoided assiduously when making the burr hole. Finally, minimally invasive surgery is part of a complex treatment algorithm and should be performed only by surgeons with expertise in open and endoscopic techniques [32].

Compared to nonsyndromic patients, patients with Apert syndrome who undergo endoscopic suturectomy are at increased risk of requiring a blood transfusion, longer hospital stay, or secondary operation. However, these rates remain very low, and the average hospital stay is 1 day [33]. Yet these concerns also exist with open procedures, which are inherently higher risk than ESC for all patient populations, including patients with Apert syndrome [1, 17, 34, 35]. Extended discussion on the potential challenges and benefits of open and endoscopic approaches must be undertaken with the family. Early endoscopic intervention is performed with the expectation that another open procedure may still be required in the future to fully correct the condition, as sutures may fuse again, and inadequate cosmetic result could be a problem even if the sutures remain open [2, 36]. Unlike nonsyndromic patients, we recommend that patients with Apert syndrome undergo a preoperative CT scan for surgical planning and to understand any underlying anatomic abnormalities of the brain. In addition, we generally obtain a postoperative scan between 12 and 24 months of age to assess the status of the sutures and the brain.

All craniosynostosis patients at our institution undergo a preoperative anesthesia clinic visit involving a comprehensive evaluation. They have routine laboratory samples drawn at this time so that blood can be crossmatched and readily available in the operating room (OR) at the start of the case [5]. Patients are admitted postoperatively to the neurosurgical floor, with the intensive care unit (ICU) reserved for the rare subset of patients with significant respiratory compromise due to midface hypoplasia.

Surgical Technique

The patient is prepared for surgery with general endotracheal anesthesia and two intravenous catheter lines. No arterial line or central line is used. Precordial Doppler ultrasonography is employed in all cases to assess for air embolism. Patients with Apert syndrome with bicoronal synostosis are positioned supine and the head is placed on a horseshoe headholder. After the hair is shaved in the appropriate area, the scalp is prepared with a povidone-iodine solution (see Fig. 15.4 for steps to surgery).

Two 2-cm incisions are made perpendicularly to each coronal suture. *It is important to obtain bone removal as far inferior as the lateral canthus and as far midline as the fontanelle.* A single dose of preoperative antibiotics is administered. After sterile prep and drape, the incisions are infused with local anesthesia (Marcaine 0.25% and epinephrine 1/200,000). We then open using a Colorado needle to do this as bloodlessly as possible. Once the incisions are made, we identify the underlying bone and place a burr hole over the fused suture. Often this area can be identified from a ridge, but occasionally it is not externally visible. Care is taken to avoid tearing the dura, and a curette is used to expand the burr hole locally. Kerrison Rongeurs are then employed. The goal is to get an approximate 1- to 2-cm width of bone, with the ultimate objec-

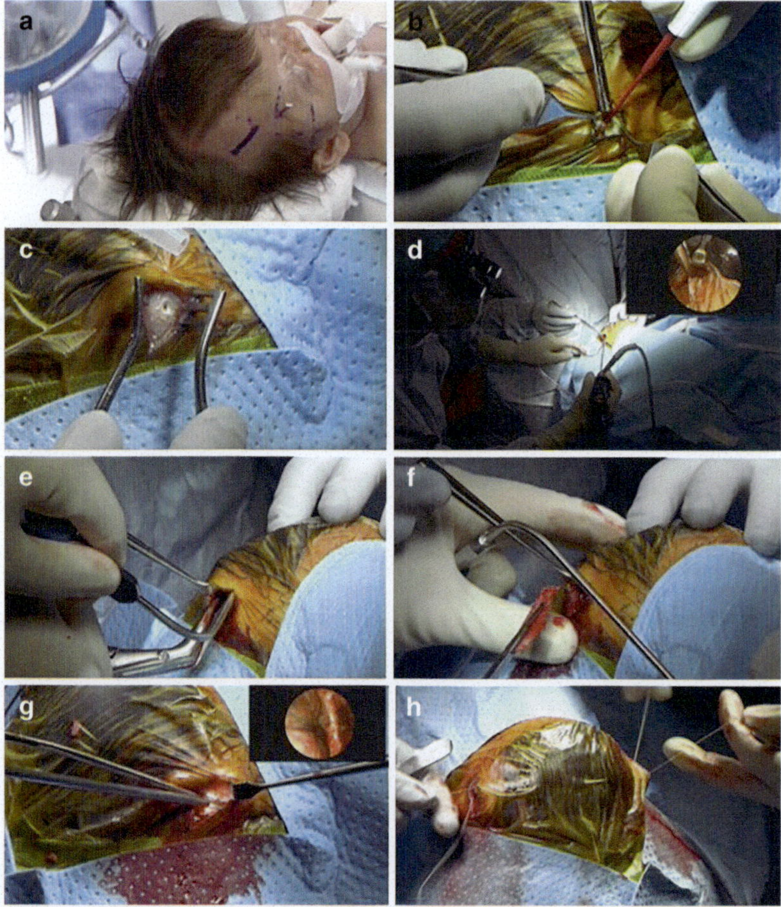

Fig. 15.4 (**a**) This is the planned location of the incision on the right side of the patient, with a mirror image incision on the left. The "angle" markings represent the presumed course of the sphenoid ridge. (**b**) The incision is opened with a Colorado needle monopolar cautery to avoid blood loss on the exposure. (**c**) A single bur hole is placed with a high-speed drill, which allows a 1 cm gap to be created using rongeurs. (**d**) Once the bur hole has been created the endoscope is introduced to safely dissect the dura off of the bone, first moving superiorly and then repeating this process towards the floor of the temporal fossa, shown in figure 7. (**e**) Tessier bone cutting scissors are used to separate the strip once the dura has been safely dissected off of the bone. (**f**) After the bone cuts have been made, the strip is removed. (**g**) The endoscope is now used to dissect inferiorly. In the inset, the endoscopic view shows the instruments passing the sphenoid wing, the point of greatest adherence to the dura, and greatest thickness of the bone. (**h**) In this figure, one can see the relative position of each incision as they are being closed with absorbable sutures

tive of the operation being to unlock the bones, not necessarily to create a wide gap. Once the burr hole and gap are created, the site is locally expanded with more Kerrisons, and we move superiorly toward the fontanelle. Bone-cutting scissors are then used to complete the craniectomy to midline. Once the two cuts have been made, the bone can be withdrawn. It is often connected to soft tissues, and a gentle twist of the bones allows it to be excised in one large piece. The medial portion along the fontanelle should be visible on the removed bone specimen.

After the medial portion has been removed, attention is turned inferiorly. This step is often the most problematic part of the operation, as the dura can be invaginated in this region by the anteriorly rotated sphenoid wing. If a dural tear is to occur, it is likely in this area, so we are quite careful. Once the dura has been dissected, we again use instruments including bone-cutting scissors and pituitary rongeurs to remove the bone all the way down to the lateral canthus. Note that it is not technically viable or necessary to continue to follow the sphenoid, which continues anteriorly to the orbital roof. Once the sphenoid is crossed, the bony separation is angled more posteriorly to the squamosal suture. At completion, the bony region under the inferior temporal lobe is visible, allowing us to confirm that the frontal and parietal bones are separated and mobile. This procedure is repeated on the contralateral side. Once separation is complete, the bony edges are lined with Gelfoam, and we rigorously ensure all the bones are mobile. We have found that moist Gelfoam alone, without thrombin, is adequate for hemostasis. We do not routinely cauterize the bone edges and use bone wax selectively; however, our anesthesia team typically administers tranexamic acid (TXA) for patients with Apert syndrome and other syndromic diagnoses. The incision is irrigated with povidine and closed in two layers using 4-0 Vicryls in the galea, followed by 4-0 Vicryl Rapide in the skin as a running suture. The closure is sterilely dressed. Average time in the OR is 72 min. Postoperative hematocrit is checked before leaving the operating room. If postoperative hematocrit was greater than 20% and no significant intraoperative bleeding occurred, hematocrit is not checked again unless there is clinical concern for hypovolemia. If hematocrit was 18–20%, it is rechecked later that day or the following morning, but a further drop is rarely seen. If it was less than 18%, a transfusion of 15 mL of red blood cells/kg is generally administered. The transfusion rate for patients with Apert syndrome undergoing ESC at our institution is 26%.

Postoperative Care

Most nonsyndromic patients can be admitted to the floor postoperatively for 23-h monitoring, but patients with Apert syndrome may require intensive care unit supervision if they have respiratory comorbidities (e.g., airway obstruction, which is often associated with the disorder) or experience intraoperative complications that require additional observation or intervention. Immediate routine postoperative imaging is not performed on ESC unless there is a postoperative concern.

Potential postoperative complications from ESC include bone defect, CSF leak, respiratory problems, wound infections, and transfusion-related complications. Overall, complications are rare. No patients with Apert syndrome who underwent ESC at our institution have had clinically significant cranial defects following their procedure or required revision cranioplasty to repair non-healing bone defects. Of the patients with Apert syndrome treated with ESC at our center, two patients experienced a postoperative CSF leak requiring a lumbar drain, and one required additional revision surgery for the leak. No other patients returned to the OR within 30 days, and we will discuss the long-term need for reoperations later in the chapter. Recovery after endoscopic strip craniectomy is quick: patients typically are discharged from the hospital without restrictions on postoperative day 1, although syndromic patients with airway issues might require additional observation.

Cranial Remolding Helmets and Follow-Up Care

After discharge and within 1 week of the procedure, patients undergo three-dimensional (3D) laser imaging and are fitted with a helmet custom-made by an experienced certified orthotist. Each helmet is designed with contours to contact all areas of the patient's cranium, except for the sites where growth is desirable; for Apert syndrome this means restrictions in height and width, but unrestricted anterior posterior growth. The helmet treatment period typically lasts 6–9 months until the patient reaches one year of age, or until the desired phenotype (normocephaly) is obtained and sustained upon serial clinical examination [5]. Patients initially wear the helmet 23 h a day, but the duration often decreases over time. The average cost of orthosis is $2200/helmet; most patients only require one or two helmets over the treatment period [5]. Previous literature from our center and others has shown substantial cost reduction from open surgery [37, 38]. Helmets are advantageous over other technologies, such as springs and distractors for their ability to modify skull growth in three dimensions and to be adjusted in all dimensions in response to skull growth [5].

An experienced orthotist is crucial for the postoperative care and outcomes of craniosynostosis patients with Apert syndrome. However, we do not restrict our patients to stay in our local region for helmet therapy, as many orthotists have gained experience in treatment with a cranial orthotic therapy. Proper orthotic fitting requires a detailed conceptualization of how cranial growth in specified areas will correct the deformity. The orthotist must understand which areas of the skull are to be contained to limit growth and which areas must be allowed to grow freely [5]. Since shape changes of the skull are most pronounced early in treatment, careful assessment and thoughtful adjustments planned jointly by an orthotist and the craniofacial team are necessary during the first 3–4 months, and we do have close follow-up of our patients during this time. In the early stages of our program's development, we routinely saw patients every 2–3 weeks postoperatively to ensure that the orthotic helmet was fitted and contoured appropriately. As our orthotist partners became more experienced, the frequency relaxed accordingly. A lack of attention to postoperative orthotics—whether it be poor compliance or insufficient duration of helmet therapy—can be a significant driver of suboptimal outcomes following endoscopic suture release [5].

Follow-Up Care

At our institution, patients are followed postoperatively in the outpatient craniofacial clinic for 5–6 years for non-syndromic patients, when brain growth is substantially complete [26, 27]. Syndromic patients are followed until adulthood [32]. During the first year, patients attend follow-ups every 3 months and then annually to assess how well the skull is reshaping and the brain is developing. In each clinic visit, patients have head circumference measurements taken, and dilated funduscopic examinations are performed annually, along with clinical evaluation. All patients with Apert syndrome undergo standard CT imaging at 18 months postoperatively to ensure suture patency (Fig. 15.5). Over time, following ESC with postoperative orthotic therapy, patients with Apert syndrome usually develop similar head circumference relative to nonsyndromic age- and gender-matched peers (Fig. 15.6) [1]. Our center also uses routine neuropsychological evaluations.

Our clinical follow-up data has shown that head growth in patients with Apert syndrome grows along their curve. At 28.5 months post-ESC, patients with Apert syndrome on average had head circumferences at or above the 85th percentile [1]. In our morphological studies, median preoperative CI was 0.95 but decreased to 0.85 postoperatively [1]. Neither the surgeons nor the family expressed complaints of asymmetry in these patients. ESC with subsequent orthotic therapy also improves anterior turricephaly and corrects frontal bossing and brachycephaly in patients with bilateral coronal craniosynostosis by stabilizing anterior cranial height and lengthening anterior cranial

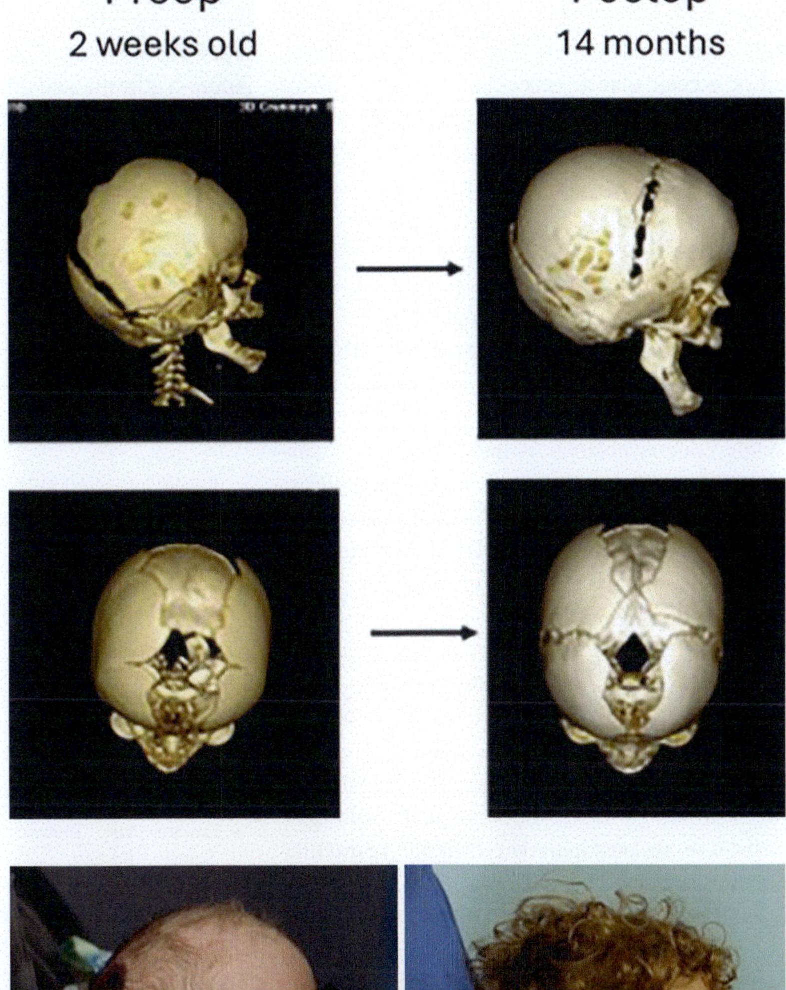

Fig. 15.5 Successful single-stage ESC

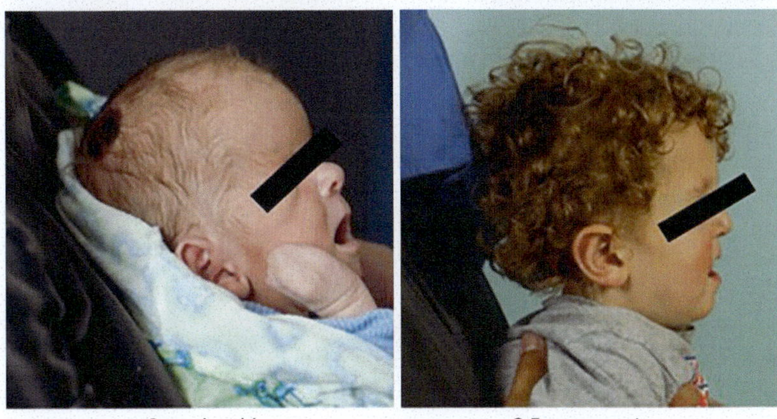

Fig. 15.6 Before and after pictures for an patient with Apert syndrome who underwent successful single-stage ESC

base length [2]. Interestingly, many patients had persistent gaps with formation of a neosuture which correlated with phenotypic improvement that continued to improve over time [30].

Throughout the follow-up period, concerning clinical symptoms, papilledema, and diminished cranial growth are seen as indications for further workup, often with computerized tomography (CT). The need for subsequent FOA procedures depends on multiple clinical parameters observed during the follow-up period, such as the presence of intracranial hypertension, or significant frontal retrusion leading to poor eye protection. In our program's clinical experience, 44% of patients with Apert syndrome with mean clinical follow-up of greater than 6 years required a follow-up FOA due to elevated ICP concerns or frontal retrusion. The average time to follow-up FOA was 3.53 years and the average age at follow-up surgery was 4 years.

Advantages to Endoscopic Management in Lower- and Middle-Income Countries

While craniosynostosis is understood and managed effectively in most high-income countries, care and research disparities persist in low- and middle-income countries (LMICs), especially in the treatment of syndromic patients, who constitute 25% of craniosynostosis cases globally [39]. As we have discussed in this chapter, compared to delayed open surgical approaches, early endoscopic management of bicoronal synostosis in patients with Apert syndrome reduces operative time, length of stay, ICU stay, and transfusion rates. Although ESC patients incur additional costs due to postoperative orthotic helmeting needs, previous financial analyses in nonsyndromic cohorts have found open repair to be 73% more expensive than endoscopic repair [40]. Moreover, at our institution, relative to cranial vault remodeling patients, ESC patients were found to save an average of $31,744 in costs during postoperative year one [37]. Ultimately, the lower resource burden and cost to both families and the healthcare system relative to delayed open surgical repair make early endoscopic suturectomy a feasible and valuable treatment option for patients with Apert syndrome in LMICs or low-resource centers.

Conclusion

Early endoscopic strip craniectomy of the bilateral coronal sutures for patients with Apert syndrome and craniosynostosis offers a safe and effective alternative to other treatment options, including early posterior expansion operations or later open frontal advancements. Ongoing research into the genetic and molecular origins of Apert syndrome and craniosynostosis, as well as the development of AI for surgical planning and execution, will no doubt influence the future of endoscopic suture craniectomy, continuing its evolution and improving outcomes for patients.

References

1. Riesel JN, Riordan CP, Hughes CD, et al. Endoscopic strip craniectomy with orthotic helmeting for safe improvement of head growth in children with Apert syndrome. J Neurosurg Pediatr. 2022;29(6):659–66. https://doi.org/10.3171/2022.2.PEDS21340.
2. Rottgers SA, Syed HR, Jodeh DS, et al. Craniometric analysis of endoscopic suturectomy for bilateral coronal Craniosynostosis. Plast Reconstr Surg. 2019;143(1):183–96. https://doi.org/10.1097/PRS.0000000000005118.
3. Raposo-Amaral CE, Vincenzi-Lemes M, Medeiros ML, Raposo-Amaral CA, Ghizoni E. Apert syndrome: neurosurgical outcomes and complications following posterior vault distraction osteogenesis. Childs Nerv Syst ChNS Off J Int Soc Pediatr Neurosurg. 2024;40(8):2557–63. https://doi.org/10.1007/s00381-024-06436-2.
4. Proctor MR. Endoscopic craniosynostosis repair. Transl Pediatr. 2014;3(3):247–58. https://doi.org/10.3978/j.issn.2224-4336.2014.07.03.
5. Berry-Candelario J, Ridgway EB, Grondin RT, Rogers GF, Proctor MR. Endoscope-assisted strip craniectomy and postoperative helmet therapy for treatment of craniosynostosis. Neurosurg Focus. 2011;31(2):E5. https://doi.org/10.3171/2011.6.FOCUS1198.
6. Wu M, Massenburg BB, Villavisanis DF, et al. The evolution of unicoronal synostosis correction: long-term aesthetic outcomes of Fronto-orbital distraction versus traditional advancement. Plast Reconstr Surg. Published online March 24, 2021. https://doi.org/10.1097/PRS.0000000000011844.
7. Taylor JA, Paliga JT, Wes AM, et al. A critical evaluation of long-term aesthetic outcomes of fronto-orbital advancement and cranial vault remodeling in nonsyndromic unicoronal craniosynostosis. Plast Reconstr Surg. 2015;135(1):220–31. https://doi.org/10.1097/PRS.0000000000000829.
8. Jimenez DF, Barone CM. Endoscopic craniectomy for early surgical correction of sagittal craniosynostosis. J Neurosurg. 1998;88(1):77–81. https://doi.org/10.3171/jns.1998.88.1.0077.
9. Barone CM, Jimenez DF. Endoscopic craniectomy for early correction of craniosynostosis. Plast Reconstr Surg. 1999;104(7):1965–73; discussion 1974–1975. https://doi.org/10.1097/00006534-199912000-00003.

10. Jimenez DF, Barone CM, Cartwright CC, Baker L. Early management of craniosynostosis using endoscopic-assisted strip craniectomies and cranial orthotic molding therapy. Pediatrics. 2002;110(1 Pt 1):97–104. https://doi.org/10.1542/peds.110.1.97.
11. Jimenez DF, Barone CM. Multiple-suture nonsyndromic craniosynostosis: early and effective management using endoscopic techniques. J Neurosurg Pediatr. 2010;5(3):223–31. https://doi.org/10.3171/2009.10.PEDS09216.
12. Jimenez DF, Barone CM. Bilateral endoscopic craniectomies in the treatment of an infant with Apert syndrome. J Neurosurg Pediatr. 2012;10(4):310–4. https://doi.org/10.3171/2012.7.PEDS11281.
13. Rivero-Garvía M, Marquez-Rivas J, Rueda-Torres AB, Ollero-Ortiz A. Early endoscopy-assisted treatment of multiple-suture craniosynostosis. Childs Nerv Syst ChNS Off J Int Soc Pediatr Neurosurg. 2012;28(3):427–31. https://doi.org/10.1007/s00381-011-1621-8.
14. Wiberg A, Magdum S, Richards PG, Jayamohan J, Wall SA, Johnson D. Posterior calvarial distraction in craniosynostosis - an evolving technique. J Cranio-Maxillo-fac Surg Off Publ Eur Assoc Cranio-Maxillo-fac Surg. 2012;40(8):799–806. https://doi.org/10.1016/j.jcms.2012.02.018.
15. Dohlman JC, Prabhu SP, Staffa SJ, et al. Orbital and eyelid characteristics, strabismus, and intracranial pressure control in Apert children treated by endoscopic strip craniectomy versus Fronto-orbital advancement. Plast Reconstr Surg Glob Open. 2023;11(5):e4937. https://doi.org/10.1097/GOX.0000000000004937.
16. Tan SPK, Proctor MR, Mulliken JB, Rogers GF. Early frontofacial symmetry after correction of unilateral coronal synostosis: frontoorbital advancement vs endoscopic strip craniectomy and helmet therapy. J Craniofac Surg. 2013;24(4):1190–4. https://doi.org/10.1097/SCS.0b013e318299742e.
17. Wong GB, Kakulis EG, Mulliken JB. Analysis of fronto-orbital advancement for Apert, Crouzon, Pfeiffer, and Saethre-Chotzen syndromes. Plast Reconstr Surg. 2000;105(7):2314–23. https://doi.org/10.1097/00006534-200006000-00002.
18. Wu RT, Menard RM. Persistent cranial defects after endoscopic sagittal synostosis surgery. J Craniofac Surg. 2023;34(1):368–73. https://doi.org/10.1097/SCS.0000000000009044.
19. Klement KA, Adamson KA, Horriat NL, Denny AD. Surgical treatment of nonsyndromic craniosynostosis. J Craniofac Surg. 2017;28(7):1752–6. https://doi.org/10.1097/SCS.0000000000003950.
20. Goyal A, Lu VM, Yolcu YU, Elminawy M, Daniels DJ. Endoscopic versus open approach in craniosynostosis repair: a systematic review and meta-analysis of perioperative outcomes. Childs Nerv Syst. 2018;34(9):1627–37. https://doi.org/10.1007/s00381-018-3852-4.
21. Chiang SN, Skolnick GB, Naidoo SD, Smyth MD, Patel KB. Outcomes after endoscope-assisted strip craniectomy and orthotic therapy for syndromic craniosynostosis. Plast Reconstr Surg. 2023;151(4):832–42. https://doi.org/10.1097/PRS.0000000000010006.
22. Kanth A, Ditthakasem K, Herbert M, Fearon JA. Secondary corrections for single-suture craniosynostosis: perioperative outcomes and predisposing factors. Plast Reconstr Surg. 2023;152(2):397–404. https://doi.org/10.1097/PRS.0000000000010332.
23. Akai T, Yamashita M, Shiro T, et al. Long-term outcomes of non-syndromic and syndromic craniosynostosis: analysis of demographic, morphologic, and surgical factors. Neurol Med Chir (Tokyo). 2022;62(2):57–64. https://doi.org/10.2176/nmc.oa.2021-0101.
24. Morrison KA, Lee JC, Souweidane MM, Feldstein NA, Ascherman JA. Twenty-year outcome experience with open craniosynostosis repairs: an analysis of reoperation and complication rates. Ann Plast Surg. 2018;80(4 Suppl 4):S158–63. https://doi.org/10.1097/SAP.0000000000001365.
25. Belza CC, Modi RN, Kamel GN, et al. Perioperative comparison between open cranial vault remodeling and distraction osteogenesis for unilateral lambdoid craniosynostosis. J Craniofac Surg. 2023;34(4):1222–5. https://doi.org/10.1097/SCS.0000000000009227.
26. Lenroot RK, Giedd JN. Brain development in children and adolescents: insights from anatomical magnetic resonance imaging. Neurosci Biobehav Rev. 2006;30(6):718–29. https://doi.org/10.1016/j.neubiorev.2006.06.001.
27. Dekaban AS. Changes in brain weights during the span of human life: relation of brain weights to body heights and body weights. Ann Neurol. 1978;4(4):345–56. https://doi.org/10.1002/ana.410040410.
28. Goldstein JA, Paliga JT, Wink JD, Low DW, Bartlett SP, Taylor JA. A craniometric analysis of posterior cranial vault distraction osteogenesis. Plast Reconstr Surg. 2013;131(6):1367–75. https://doi.org/10.1097/PRS.0b013e31828bd541.
29. Davis C, MacFarlane MR, Wickremesekera A. Occipital expansion without osteotomies in Apert syndrome. Childs Nerv Syst ChNS Off J Int Soc Pediatr Neurosurg. 2010;26(11):1543–8. https://doi.org/10.1007/s00381-010-1144-8.
30. Sauerhammer TM, Seruya M, Ropper AE, Oh AK, Proctor MR, Rogers GF. Craniectomy gap patency and neosuture formation following endoscopic suturectomy for unilateral coronal craniosynostosis. Plast Reconstr Surg. 2014;134(1):81e–91e. https://doi.org/10.1097/PRS.0000000000000285.
31. Meier PM, Goobie SM, DiNardo JA, Proctor MR, Zurakowski D, Soriano SG. Endoscopic strip craniectomy in early infancy: the initial five years of anesthesia experience. Anesth Analg. 2011;112(2):407–14. https://doi.org/10.1213/ANE.0b013e31820471e4.
32. McCarthy JG, Warren SM, Bernstein J, et al. Parameters of care for craniosynostosis. Cleft Palate

Craniofacial J. 2012;49(1_suppl):1–24. https://doi.org/10.1597/11-138.

33. Rottgers SA, Lohani S, Proctor MR. Outcomes of endoscopic suturectomy with postoperative helmet therapy in bilateral coronal craniosynostosis. J Neurosurg Pediatr. 2016;18(3):281–6. https://doi.org/10.3171/2016.2.PEDS15693.
34. Kurnik NM, Bristol R, Maneri C, Singhal R, Singh DJ. Open craniosynostosis surgery: effect of early intraoperative blood transfusion on postoperative course. J Craniofac Surg. 2017;28(5):e505–10. https://doi.org/10.1097/SCS.0000000000003803.
35. Isaac KV, Meara JG, Proctor MR. Analysis of clinical outcomes for treatment of sagittal craniosynostosis: a comparison of endoscopic suturectomy and cranial vault remodeling. J Neurosurg Pediatr. 2018;22(5):467–74. https://doi.org/10.3171/2018.5.PEDS1846.
36. Hopper RA, Lee A. Discussion: craniometric analysis of endoscopic suturectomy for bilateral coronal craniosynostosis. Plast Reconstr Surg. 2019;143(1):199–201. https://doi.org/10.1097/PRS.0000000000005119.
37. Abbott MM, Rogers GF, Proctor MR, Busa K, Meara JG. Cost of treating sagittal synostosis in the first year of life. J Craniofac Surg. 2012;23(1):88–93. https://doi.org/10.1097/SCS.0b013e318240f965.
38. Vogel TW, Woo AS, Kane AA, Patel KB, Naidoo SD, Smyth MD. A comparison of costs associated with endoscope-assisted craniectomy versus open cranial vault repair for infants with sagittal synostosis. J Neurosurg Pediatr. 2014;13(3):324–31. https://doi.org/10.3171/2013.12.PEDS13320.
39. Insights into craniosynostosis management in low- and middle-income countries: A narrative review of outcomes, shortcomings and paediatric neurosurgery capacity – PMC. https://www.ncbi.nlm.nih.gov/pmc/articles/PMC10798110/. Accessed 13 Sep 2024.
40. Liles C, Dallas J, Hale AT, et al. The economic impact of open versus endoscope-assisted craniosynostosis surgery. J Neurosurg Pediatr. 2019;24(2):145–52. https://doi.org/10.3171/2019.4.PEDS18586.

Management of the Posterior Vault

16

Irene M. J. Mathijssen, Marie-Lise C. van Veelen, Jesse A. Taylor, Allison C. Hu, Jordan W. Swanson, Ben B. Massenburg, and Hamilton Matushita

Introduction

Patients with Apert syndrome require coordinated, multidisciplinary care from a specialized craniofacial team to address their complex needs. Classically, patients with Apert syndrome present with bicoronal suture synostosis, but other sutures can be involved. Incidental cases of genetically proven Apert syndrome without craniosynostosis are known, and vault surgery is not indicated in these individuals [1].

Premature fusing of cranial sutures results in a cranial vault unable to accommodate brain growth, leading to cephalocranial disproportion and increased intracranial pressure. Historically, surgical protocols for the cephalocranial disproportion associated with Apert syndrome were often based on those for single-suture non-syndromic cases, leading to suboptimal outcomes that frequently required additional surgeries [2]. Traditionally, Apert syndrome had been treated with a fronto-orbital advancement (FOA). Some centers performed FOA prophylactically in infancy for all patients with Apert syndrome, while other centers preferred expectant management and only performed FOA in the event of increased intracranial pressure (ICP) [3–5]. However, most teams found that early frontal surgery was associated with high rates of relapse and reoperation [6].

Over the past few decades, initial cranial vault expansion for patients with Apert syndrome has shifted from FOA to posterior vault expansion or posterior vault distraction osteogenesis (PVDO) [7]. These posterior surgeries allow the frontal surgery to be delayed to a point more likely to yield a stable result, and this creates the possibility of combining frontal surgery with midface surgery as a transcranial fronto-facial advancement, thereby reducing the overall surgical burden of these patients [8]. More recent approaches have adapted to the specific needs and natural history of syndromic craniosynostosis, significantly improving outcomes [9, 10]. These protocols emphasize the critical timing of staged surgeries and the integration of treatments for associated conditions such as Chiari malformation, hydrocephalus, and sleep-disordered breathing.

A large systematic review of surgical protocols for syndromic craniosynostosis was

I. M. J. Mathijssen (✉)
Department of Plastic and Reconstructive Surgery and Hand Surgery, Erasmus Medical Center, Rotterdam, the Netherlands
e-mail: i.mathijssen@erasmusmc.nl

M.-L. C. van Veelen
Department of Neurosurgery, Erasmus Medical Center, Rotterdam, the Netherlands

J. A. Taylor · A. C. Hu · J. W. Swanson
B. B. Massenburg
Division of Plastic, Reconstructive, and Oral Surgery, Children's Hospital of Philadelphia, Philadelphia, PA, USA

H. Matushita
Department of Neurosurgery, Division of Pediatric Neurosurgery, University of São Paulo, São Paulo, São Paulo, Brazil

J. G. Meara et al. (eds.), *Apert Syndrome*, https://doi.org/10.1007/978-3-032-12551-4_16

performed to update the guidelines for the treatment of these patients [11]. The review found that after more than five years of follow-up, PVDO results in a greater increase in intracranial volume and a significantly lower prevalence of tonsillar herniation and papilledema when compared to FOA or conventional posterior vault expansion without distraction [6, 12–15]. Some centers are exploring posterior expansion as the primary intervention for concurrent Chiari malformations in multisuture synostosis [16]. Early posterior expansion has also been shown to delay or halt progression of turricephaly and passively improve frontal morphology [7, 17, 18]. Several techniques for posterior cranial vault expansion have been described, including conventional open posterior cranial vault expansion [19, 20], PVDO [21, 22], and spring-assisted posterior vault expansion [23].

The evolution of posterior vault management in Apert syndrome reflects the broader progress in craniofacial surgery. From the initial focus on FOA to the incorporation of posterior vault expansion and the transformative impact of PVDO and springs, our field has made remarkable strides. This chapter will focus on the adapted protocols of three large craniofacial centers—in Philadelphia (USA), Rotterdam (Netherlands), and San Paolo (Brazil)—with significant experience in managing the posterior vault for patients with Apert syndrome.

Timing of Surgery and Preoperative Preparation

Occipital expansion, using either distractors or springs, is typically scheduled at about six months of age. This timing optimizes bone stock maturity, allowing for stable hardware fixation of the distractors and reducing the risk of hardware migration or loosening issues. However, surgery may be performed earlier if signs of raised ICP are present, including papilledema, a bulging fontanel, or a severe copper-beaten appearance on imaging. These findings are relatively uncommon in the first months of life in infants with Apert syndrome.

Before surgery is scheduled, the following examinations are undertaken:

- Fundoscopy to screen for papilledema as a sign of raised ICP.
- Three-dimensional computed tomography angiogram of the head to diagnose which sutures are affected, to check for the presence of both transverse sinuses, and to identify and locate occipital collateral veins. This aids in determining whether occipital collateral veins need to be preserved during the development of the occipital skin flap.
- Magnetic resonance imaging of the brain as reference for the size of the ventricles, position of the cerebellar tonsils, and other intracranial anomalies.
- Sleep study to diagnose the presence and severity of sleep-disturbed breathing. If signs of obstructed breathing are present, the patient is seen by the ear, nose, and throat surgeon, who will perform an upper airway endoscopy in combination with the posterior vault expansion. With the endoscopy, the various levels of obstruction can be visualized.

Parents are advised to position the child's head to the side during sleep. This allows better breathing by preventing both backward positioning of the tongue and flattening of the occiput. In cases where springs are used for the occipital expansion, the child can become accustomed to this position, as it is required postoperatively to allow expansion of the springs.

Distraction Versus Classic Expansion

Prior to the development of PVDO, FOA was the traditional initial cranial treatment for Apert syndrome. However, significant research has shown that early frontal surgery had higher rates of relapse and reoperation, and a posterior expansion could offer twice the intracranial volume when compared to FOA [6, 15]. PVDO also keeps the bone pedicled on the dura, allowing for slower, vascularized expansion. This, in addition to the soft tissue stretch that occurs with PVDO, confers significant advantage to distraction over classic expansion.

Type of Distraction Device: Springs Versus Distractors

The teams from Philadelphia and San Paolo favor using distractors, while the team from Rotterdam prefers springs. Both techniques appear to achieve the same goal, and these preferences are mainly based on the personal experience of the surgeons.

The Philadelphia team utilizes semi-buried, internal cranial distractors. This group believes that distractors offer several advantages over springs, including controlled expansion, versatility in vector selection, and predictable and stable outcomes. Typically, the distractors are placed in an anterior–posterior dimension on a flat aspect of the lateral skull. Both distractors must have a co-linear vector to avoid binding during activation. Occasionally, in the context of severe turribrachycephaly, the vector can also aim slightly inferior in attempts to decrease the skull height; the group has shown that posterior vault distraction has some ability to improve frontal morphology [17, 24, 25]. Additionally, distractors provide a stable framework throughout the distraction period, minimizing the risk of unintended shifts in bone segments. This stability reduces the chance of relapse or uneven expansion, which can be more challenging to control with springs that rely on recoil forces that vary over time.

The Rotterdam team performs posterior vault expansion in children with Apert syndrome with springs [23]. Springs offer the advantage of application in very thin bone with multiple defects. The bone of the posterior vault is tilted upwards by the springs, which allows correction of the flattened vertex. Thus, the largest volume expansion is created at the site of the posterior fossa. Moreover, the springs are covered by the skin, thereby lowering the risk of infection and trauma compared to distractors. In procedures performed in children older than 1.5–2 years of age, distractors are used to ensure good ossification.

Design of the Surgical Technique

The patient is in prone position, ensuring no pressure is exerted on the eyes.

A routine coronal incision is used, which allows this scar to be used in future frontal and midface advancement as needed. With the dissection of the skin flap, the venous collaterals are preserved whenever possible. This is most relevant if one or both transverse sinuses are aplastic or hypoplastic, a relatively common finding [26].

The posterior osteotomy is performed below the transverse sinus and the torcula [23, 27]. Alternatively, an osteotomy can be performed just above this level, visualizing and releasing the transverse sinuses and removing additional bone to expose them. In many cases, this approach appears to improve or mitigate Chiari malformation. The vertical part of the bilateral osteotomy is adapted according to the location of the fused coronal sutures, the remaining open portion of the posterior fontanel, and the shape of the vertex.

Distractors

The vertical aspect of the osteotomy may include a short, interdigitating, tongue-in-groove segment that may enhance the mechanical strength of the regenerate (Fig. 16.1). The segment must be placed in the correct distraction vector and the length must not cause bony interference during the activation phase. Distractors are usually positioned at the middle distance between the coronal and lambdoid suture parallel to the contralateral side. The group in Philadelphia most commonly places distractors in an anterior-posterior direction, although they may be aimed slightly inferior to reduce turricephaly. Additionally, barrel stave osteotomies are performed at the inferior occipital bone, below the low transverse osteotomy, to reduce the amount of bony step-offs that exist in this area at the end of distraction. Open lambdoid sutures may be rigidly fixated with resorbable plates and screws to prevent excursion across the open suture (i.e., “gull winging”). While this maneuver allows for the parietal and occipital

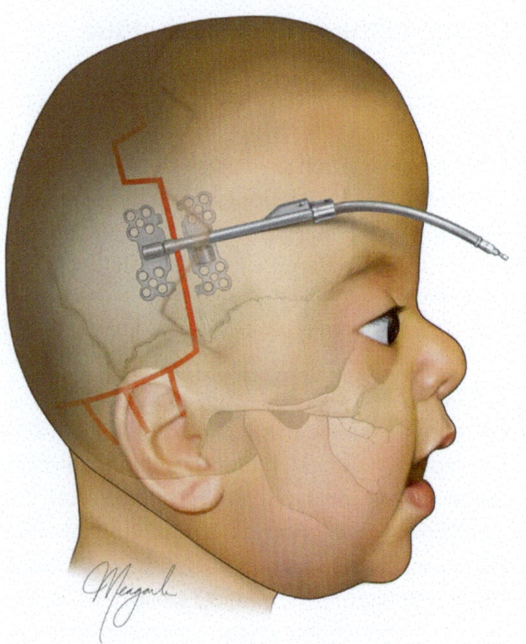

Fig. 16.1 Illustration of the interdigitating osteotomies for posterior vault distraction osteogenesis with the use of two distractors. (Illustration published in Wu et al. [8])

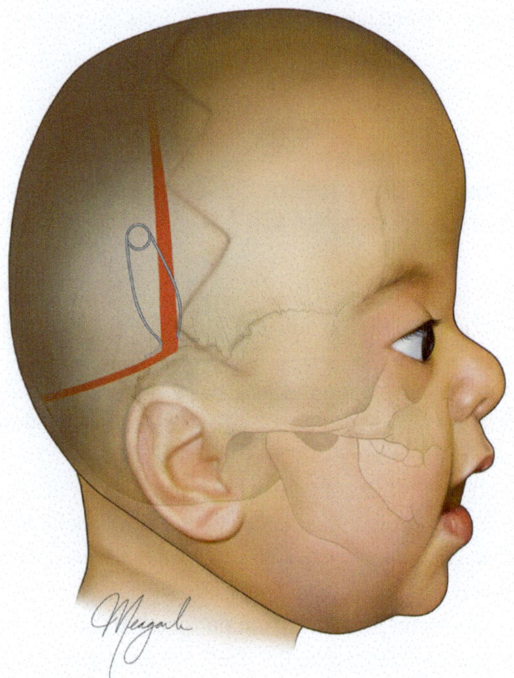

Fig. 16.2 Illustration of the osteotomies for posterior vault distraction osteogenesis with the use of two springs. (Illustration designed by Meagan Wu [8])

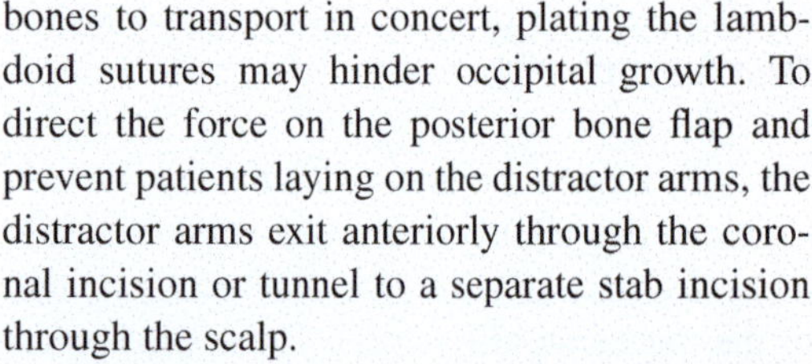

bones to transport in concert, plating the lambdoid sutures may hinder occipital growth. To direct the force on the posterior bone flap and prevent patients laying on the distractor arms, the distractor arms exit anteriorly through the coronal incision or tunnel to a separate stab incision through the scalp.

Distraction typically begins after an average latency of 4.0 days. Active distraction occurs at a rate of 0.5 mm twice daily or 1 mm once daily until the desired distraction length is achieved. The mean active phase lasts 26 days with a mean consolidation period of 63 days. On average, distractions are removed after an 11-week consolidation period.

Springs

One spring is inserted on each side. The springs are either 7 or 9 Newton (N), achieving 6–8 cm of expansion, respectively. The selection of spring strength and positioning is adapted to the pattern of lambdoid closure. If the lambdoid sutures are closed, one of the 7 N spring footplates is inserted at the osteotomy line and the other in a burr hole near the free edge of the occipital bone (Fig. 16.2). When the lambdoid sutures are open, this procedure could result in gull winging: the parietal bone edge lifts and the lambdoid sutures serve as hinges, preventing expansion of the posterior vault. In that event, we position a 9 N spring with one footplate at the osteotomy and the other footplate in a burr hole just next to the lambdoid suture. Given that the footplates are placed a few centimeters apart from one another, the total amount of distraction is approximately 6 cm.

At the top of the skull, a hinge is left intact and consists of either a bony bridge of 1–1.5 cm or the periosteum attached to the dura. The hinge adds to a more selective opening of the posterior fossa by pulling the bone upward.

Following surgery, the patient is positioned on the side to allow the springs to expand the posterior vault. Springs are removed 10–12 weeks after insertion.

Foramen Magnum Decompression

Simultaneous foramen magnum decompression is only performed in select cases, and these are rare in Apert syndrome. Indications include the presence of Chiari malformation, although the prevalence in Apert syndrome is rather low [28].

Outcome of Surgery and Follow-Up Schedule After Posterior Expansion

Over the past decade, PVDO has become an essential technique for cranial expansion, especially in patients with syndromic and multisuture craniosynostosis. Since 2009, the centers Philadelphia, San Paolo, and Rotterdam have adopted PVDO as the preferred initial cranial vault expansion method for syndromic patients due to its (1) low complication rate, (2) substantial volumetric expansion, (3) enhancement of both frontal and occipital contour, (4) potential to resolve Chiari malformation, (5) ability to delay the need for frontal surgery, and (6) potential to reduce the total surgical burden [6–8, 17, 24, 25, 29–31].

Since implementing the PVDO-first approach to syndromic craniosynostosis, these teams have found that PVDO delays the need for FOA. When looking at the subgroup of patients with Apert syndrome who had follow-up beyond the age of six years, only 50% of those treated with PVDO required an FOA, compared to 100% of those treated with conventional methods, 29% of whom needed a repeat FOA [8]. A comparable proportion of patients underwent midface procedures in each group; 50% of PVDO patients and 57% of conventional treatment patients had transcranial procedures, and 33% of PVDO patients and 43% of conventional treatment patients had subcranial procedures. A previous FOA significantly increases the risk profile when considering a transcranial frontofacial advancement, underscoring the importance of this finding [32, 33].

The timeline for follow-up after the occipital expansion is provided in Fig. 16.3. Follow-up care includes checks on skull growth and fundoscopy every three months in the first year, every six months in the second year, and then yearly. A second vault expansion is only indicated if symptoms of raised ICP are detected. Annual checks on sleep-disturbed breathing are performed with sleep studies.

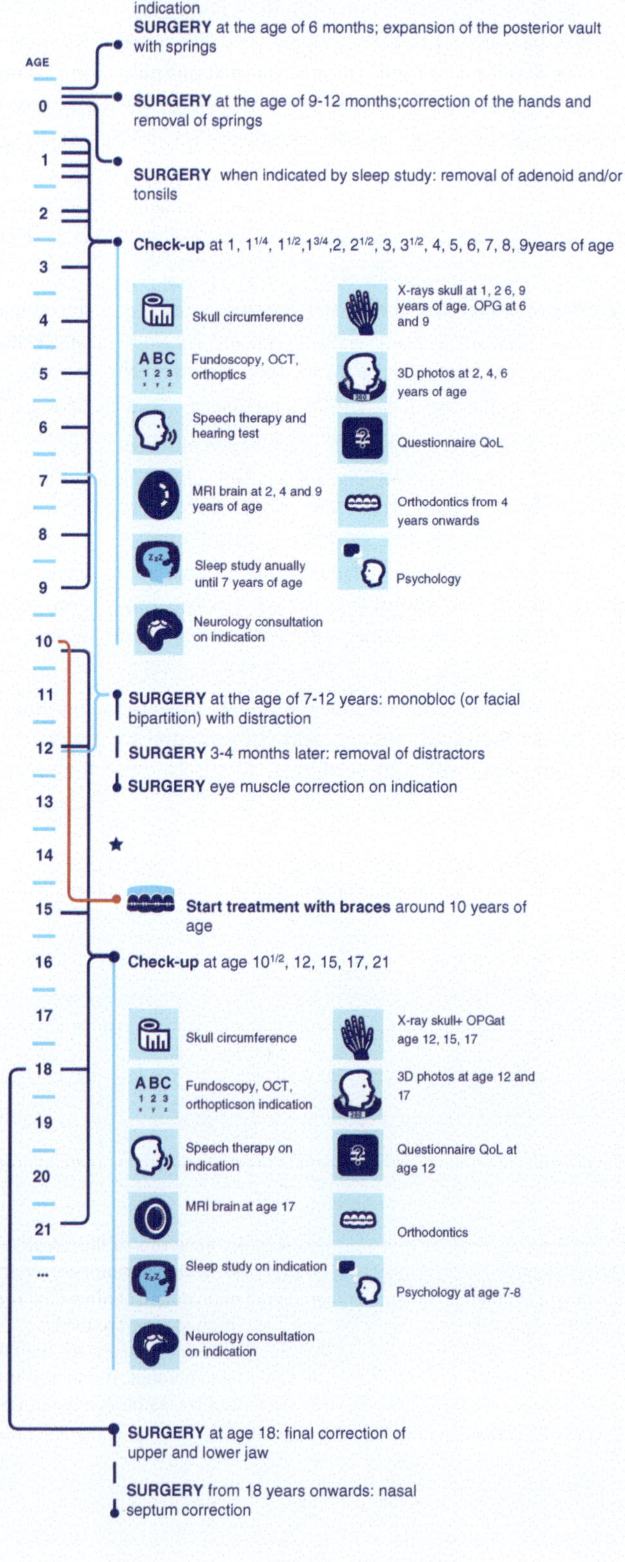

Fig. 16.3 Treatment timeline for patients with Apert syndrome

Conclusions

Posterior vault distraction with either distractors or springs is considered the best treatment for most patients with Apert syndrome when compared with FOA alone. PVDO outcomes are significantly better than an initial FOA or a posterior vault expansion without distraction. Given the low prevalence of raised ICP after PVDO, routine FOA as secondary vault expansion has been removed from the protocol. There is no evidence-based preference for either the use of distractors or springs in PVDO.

References

1. De Ângelis RD, Matushita H, Cardeal DD, Nascimento CNG, Teixeira MJ. Apert syndrome without craniosynostosis. Childs Nerv Syst. 2019;35(3):565–7.
2. McCarthy JG, Glasberg SB, Cutting CB, et al. Twenty-year experience with early surgery for craniosynostosis: II. The craniofacial synostosis syndromes and pansynostosis—results and unsolved problems. Plast Reconstr Surg. 1995;96(2):284–98. https://doi.org/10.1097/00006534-199508000-00005.
3. Bruce DA. Consensus: craniofacial synostoses. Apert and Crouzon syndromes. Childs Nerv Syst. 1996;12(11):734–6. https://doi.org/10.1007/BF00366159.
4. Sgouros S, Goldin JH, Hockley AD, Wake MJ. Posterior skull surgery in craniosynostosis. Childs Nerv Syst. 1996;12(11):727–33. https://doi.org/10.1007/BF00366158.
5. Marucci DD, Dunaway DJ, Jones BM, Hayward RD. Raised intracranial pressure in Apert syndrome. Plast Reconstr Surg. 2008;122:1162.
6. Derderian CA, Wink JD, McGrath JL, Collinsworth ARS, Bartlett SP, Taylor JA. Volumetric changes in cranial vault expansion: comparison of fronto-orbital advancement and posterior cranial vault distraction osteogenesis. Plast Reconstr Surg. 2015;135(6):1665–72. https://doi.org/10.1097/PRS.0000000000001294.
7. Swanson JW, Samra F, Bauder A, Mitchell BT, Taylor JA, Bartlett SP. An algorithm for managing syndromic craniosynostosis using posterior vault distraction osteogenesis. Plast Reconstr Surg. 2016;137(5):829e–41e. https://doi.org/10.1097/PRS.0000000000002127.
8. Wu M, Barnett SL, Massenburg BB, Ng JJ, Romeo DJ, Taylor JA, Bartlett SP, Swanson JW. Early posterior vault distraction osteogenesis changes the syndromic craniosynostosis treatment paradigm: long-term outcomes of a 23-year cohort study. ChNS. 2024;40(9):2811–23. https://doi.org/10.1007/s00381-024-06465-x.
9. Taylor JA, Bartlett SP. What's new in syndromic craniosynostosis surgery? Plast Reconstr Surg. 2017;140(1):82e–93e. https://doi.org/10.1097/PRS.0000000000003524.
10. Forrest CR, Hopper RA. Craniofacial syndromes and surgery. Plast Reconstr Surg. 2013;131(1):86–109.
11. Mathijssen IMJ, Working Group Guideline Craniosynostosis. Updated guideline on treatment and management of craniosynostosis. J Craniofac Surg. 2021;32(1):371–450. https://doi.org/10.1097/SCS.0000000000007035. PMID: 33156164; PMCID: PMC7769187
12. De Jong T, Van Veelen MLC, Mathijssen IMJ. Springs-assisted posterior vault expansion in multisuture craniosynostosis. Childs Nerv Syst. 2013;29:815–20.
13. Thomas GPL, Wall SA, Jayamohan J, et al. Lessons learned in posterior cranial vault distraction. J Craniofac Surg. 2014;25:1721–7.
14. Mundinger GS, Rehim SA, Johnson IIIO, et al. Distraction osteogenesis for surgical treatment of craniosynostosis: a systematic review. Plast Reconstr Surg. 2016;138:657–69.
15. Spruijt B, Rijken BFM, Den Ottelander BK, et al. First vault expansion in Apert and Crouzon-Pfeiffer syndromes: front or back? Plast Reconstr Surg. 2016;137:112e–21e.
16. Lo WB, Thant KZ, Kaderbhai J, et al. Posterior calvarial distraction for complex craniosynostosis and cerebellar tonsillar herniation. J Neurosurg Pediatr. 2020;26(4):421–30. https://doi.org/10.3171/2020.4.PEDS19742.
17. Ter Maaten NS, Mazzaferro DM, Wes AM, Naran S, Bartlett SP, Taylor JA. Craniometric analysis of frontal cranial morphology following posterior vault distraction. J Craniofac Surg. 2018;29(5):1169–73. https://doi.org/10.1097/SCS.0000000000004473.
18. Taylor JA, Derderian CA, Bartlett SP, Fiadjoe JE, Sussman EM, Stricker PA. Perioperative morbidity in posterior cranial vault expansion: distraction osteogenesis versus conventional osteotomy. Plast Reconstr Surg. 2012;129(4):1–3. https://doi.org/10.1097/PRS.0b013e3182443164.
19. Scott WW, Fearon JA, Swift DM, Sacco DJ. Suboccipital decompression during posterior cranial vault remodeling for selected cases of Chiari malformations associated with craniosynostosis: clinical article. J Neurosurg Pediatr. 2013;12(2):166–70. https://doi.org/10.3171/2013.4.PEDS12463.
20. Cinalli G, Chumas P, Arnaud E, Sainte-Rose C, Renier D. Occipital remodeling and suboccipital decompression in severe craniosynostosis associated with tonsillar herniation. Neurosurgery. 1998;42(1):66–73. https://doi.org/10.1097/00006123-199801000-00013.
21. White N, Evans M, Dover S, Noons P, Solanki G, Nishikawa H. Posterior calvarial vault expansion using distraction osteogenesis. Childs Nerv Syst. 2009;25(2):231–6. https://doi.org/10.1007/s00381-008-0758-6.

22. Steinbacher DMM, Skirpan J, Puchała J, Bartlett SPP. Expansion of the posterior cranial vault using distraction osteogenesis. Plast Reconstr Surg. 2011;127(2):792–801. https://doi.org/10.1097/PRS.0b013e318200ab83.
23. Mathijssen IMJ, Driessen C, Versnel SL, Dremmen MHG, van Veelen MLC. Posterior distraction using springs in syndromic and multisuture craniosynostosis: improving the technique. J Craniofac Surg. 2020;31(7):2095–6. https://doi.org/10.1097/SCS.0000000000006882.
24. Samra F, Swanson JW, Mitchell B, et al. Posterior vault distraction osteogenesis conveys anterior benefit in apert syndrome. Plast Reconstr Surg. 2015;136:51.
25. Goldstein JA, Paliga JT, Wink JD, et al. A craniometric analysis of posterior cranial vault distraction osteogenesis. Plast Reconstr Surg. 2013;131:1367–75.
26. Florisson JM, Barmpalios G, Lequin M, van Veelen ML, Bannink N, Hayward RD, Mathijssen IM. Venous hypertension in syndromic and complex craniosynostosis: the abnormal anatomy of the jugular foramen and collaterals. J Craniomaxillofac Surg. 2015;43(3):312–8. https://doi.org/10.1016/j.jcms.2014.11.023. Epub 2014 Dec 12.PMID: 25604402
27. Zapatero ZD, Kosyk MS, Kalmar CL, Cheung L, Carlson AR, Heuer GG, Bartlett SP, Taylor JA, Lang SS, Swanson JW. How low should we go? safety and craniometric impact of the low occipital osteotomy in posterior vault remodeling. Plast Reconstr Surg. 2022;150(5):1037e–48e. https://doi.org/10.1097/PRS.0000000000009626. Epub 2022 Aug 24. PMID: 35998141
28. Rijken BF, Lequin MH, Van Veelen ML, de Rooi J, Mathijssen IM. The formation of the foramen magnum and its role in developing ventriculomegaly and Chiari I malformation in children with craniosynostosis syndromes. J Craniomaxillofac Surg. 2015;43(7):1042–8. https://doi.org/10.1016/j.jcms.2015.04.025.
29. Greives MR, Ware BW, Tian AG, et al. Complications in posterior cranial vault distraction. Ann Plast Surg. 2016;76:211–5.
30. de Jong T, van Veelen ML, Mathijssen IM. Spring-assisted posterior vault expansion in multisuture craniosynostosis. Childs Nerv Syst. 2013;29(5):815–20. https://doi.org/10.1007/s00381-013-2033-8. Epub 2013 Jan 26
31. Mathijssen IMJ, Wolvius EB, Spoor JKH, van Veelen MC, Versnel SL. Secondary vault reconstruction after open or minimal invasive correction for unisutural, multisutural or syndromic craniosynostosis: a cohort study on the impact of diagnosis and type of initial surgical technique. J Plast Reconstr Aesthet Surg. 2021;74(5):1087–92. https://doi.org/10.1016/j.bjps.2020.10.049.
32. Wagner CS, Pontell ME, Hitchner MK, Barrero CE, Salinero LK, Swanson JW, Bartlett SP, Taylor JA. Prior fronto-orbital advancement associated with complications from transcranial midface surgery in patients with syndromic craniosynostosis. Childs Nerv Syst. 2023;39(6):1619–26. https://doi.org/10.1007/s00381-023-05879-3. Epub 2023 Feb 15. PMID: 36790494
33. Frontofacial Monobloc Advancement with Internal Distraction. Arnaud E, Paternoster G, Khonsari RH, Haber SE, editors. Tactics and strategy in faciocraniosynostosis. Springer. ISBN 978-3-031-07573-5

17 Two-Stage Strategy: FOA and Le Fort III

Natalie M. Plana, Pradip R. Shetye, and Roberto L. Flores

Apert syndrome manifests through a broad range of phenotypic presentations with the common treatment goals of normalizing intracranial pressure, eliminating upper airway obstruction, protecting the orbital contents, and improving facial dysmorphology. This autosomal dominant and possibly sporadic genetic mutation of fibroblast growth factor receptor (FGFR2) produces a spectrum of craniofacial anomalies commonly including multi-suture dysostosis with turribrachycephaly, shallow orbits with ocular proptosis and hypertelorism, midface hypoplasia commonly causing airway obstruction and dental malocclusion. Midface hypoplasia is multidimensional, including retrusion and midline hypoplasia resulting in a concave facial feature, foreshortened nose, and downward slanting of the palpebral fissures resulting from superior displacement of the medial canthus. Treatment pathways begin at birth and can continue well into adulthood representing a lifelong commitment to care. Algorithmic treatment patterns continue to evolve, and treatment protocols can be center- and surgeon-specific. We describe the protocol used selectively by our unit for midface advancement, which involves a two-staged strategy: fronto-orbital advancement followed by Le Fort III advancement.

NYU Institutional Protocol

The institutional protocol followed by the senior authors employs a three-tiered approach to addressing functional needs throughout childhood. The three generalized stages follow a top-down flow, first addressing cerebral constriction, second focusing on orbital hypoplasia with additional cranial expansion, and a third phase concentrating on alleviating respiratory function. The three general areas of craniofacial treatment can be addressed concurrently, but as a principle of care, they should each be assessed separately, and the care plan should be informed by the findings. Critical to these goals is protocol-driven interdisciplinary care including neurosurgery, ophthalmology, otolaryngology, dentistry, genetics, speech and feeding specialists, and psychologists to personalize care to the child's developmental needs. Ophthalmologic exams focus on corneal health in cases with exorbitism, but also garner insight into ocular pressures as a surrogate for possible intracranial pressure elevation. Dental assessment emphasizes appropriate oral hygiene in the younger ages, an important detail that can compromise future reconstruction if not followed. During midface reconstruction, a skilled craniofacial orthodontist will serve as a

N. M. Plana (✉)
Hansjorg Wyss Department of Plastic Surgery, NYU Langone Health, New York, NY, USA

Hanna Face and Jaw, New York, NY, USA

P. R. Shetye · R. L. Flores
Hansjorg Wyss Department of Plastic Surgery, NYU Langone Health, New York, NY, USA

J. G. Meara et al. (eds.), *Apert Syndrome*, https://doi.org/10.1007/978-3-032-12551-4_17

critical treatment partner. Airway management is performed in conjunction with otolaryngology specialists who can assist in informing the indication for midface advancement and offer more conservative interventions to alleviate obstructive sleep apnea to ensure appropriate timing of surgery. Speech and language pathologists play a pivotal role improving articulation in the background of a constricted upper and lower arch, anterior crossbite, and a cleft palate (when present). An important and at times overlooked team member is a clinical psychologist who can help patients and families mediate the psychosocial elements of their diagnosis and provide support during their surgical journey.

Within the first year of life, elevated intracranial pressures may be an indication for posterior vault distraction osteogenesis (PVDO). This initial intervention is focused solely on alleviating intracranial pressures and generating volumetric increases for the constricted brain. In persistent hydrocephalus, neurosurgery may elect to place a ventriculoperitoneal shunt for pressure alleviation before cranial expansion. If cranial constriction is mild to moderate, a fronto-orbital advancement (FOA) can be performed as an initial cranial intervention. In cases where PVDO is performed first, a FOA can be performed as a secondary operation during the PVDO device removal or as a separate procedure. This permits another operative opportunity to further correct craniocerebral disproportion with concurrent improvement in forehead retrusion and first-time orbital reconstruction. While the orbital skeleton is far from reaching skeletal maturity at this age, some lessened constraint can allow the ocular globe to better accommodate into the orbital space and help protect the cornea with eyelid closure. Temporary or permanent tarsorrhaphy can be performed concurrently or prior to cranial surgery to protect the globes until greater orbital expansion is performed at an older age. When the child reaches seven to nine years of age, the midface is addressed with a subcranial Le Fort III advancement procedure. This age range is selected to follow full physiologic maturity of the orbits and ossification of the anterior cranial vault. Furthermore, midface advancement performed at this age or later can avoid a secondary Le Fort III surgery prior to or at the time of facial maturity. In cases of severe midface retrusion causing severe upper airway obstruction, Le Fort III advancement may be considered at an earlier age to avoid tracheostomy. Overcorrection of the sagittal midface position should be pursued as anterior growth of the midface is limited after midface distraction. At the age of facial maturity, an orthognathic surgery can be pursued to restore occlusion definitively. In cases where the midface distraction is performed at an earlier age, there is a higher likelihood that a repeat distraction would be required before facial maturity. In these cases, the osteotomy is commonly more difficult to perform, there may be bony loss at the osteotomy sites due to incomplete bone generation, and there is typically more soft tissue scarring. These combined variables can affect the predictability of secondary and tertiary midface distraction and therefore it is better avoided, if possible, by performing this procedure at the age of mixed dentition. The patient's specific operative timeline is primarily driven by functional needs at presentation and during the child's development. For example, midface advancement has been performed at this institution as early as three years old for a patient with recalcitrant obstructive sleep apnea necessitating a tracheostomy. Younger age of intervention also poses greater risks to be considered including injury of deciduous dentition and higher relapse rates, which must be outweighed by the functional benefits to the airway.

Surgical Technique

The fronto-orbital advancement with cranial vault remodeling surgery will be described elsewhere in this textbook. Therefore, this chapter will only describe the surgical technique for the subcranial Le Fort III. Surgical approach to the Le Fort III advancement begins with a bicoronal incision following the existing scar pattern from previous intracranial procedures. Care is taken to radiographically identify any cranial defects before surgery to control the risks of dural violation during dissection. The scalp is ideally elevated in a subgaleal plane until the supraorbital bar is reached, at which point a subperiosteal plane is entered. Dissection continues anteriorly to the root of the nose and the supraorbital rims. Although maintenance of a subgaleal plane is preferred over the cranial portion of the dissection to limit bone bleeding, this may not be feasible in the setting of previous anterior cranial vault reconstruction. Blunt dissection is preferred when elevating the scalp tissue over a cranial defect to protect the underlying dura. The temporalis muscle remains in continuity with the overlying scalp. Once the supraorbital bar is reached, wide subperiosteal dissection is performed to expose the following structures: nasal radix and superior nasal bones, medial orbital wall including the superior aspects of the anterior and posterior lacrimal crests, superior orbital rim, lateral orbital rim, inferior orbital rim and orbital floor, inferior orbital fissure, and lateral aspect of the zygomatic body including the junction with the anterior zygomatic arch. Of note, the medical canthal tendon is preserved in its periosteal attachment and the temporalis muscle is detached from the lateral aspect of the lateral orbital rim. The zygomatic arch should be entirely free of periosteal and masseteric attachments at the anterior aspect to allow for the zygomatic osteotomy. If an intraoral approach for pterygomaxillary disjunction is desired, an upper gingivobuccal sulcus incision is required and subperiosteal dissection will follow up the maxilla and wrapping posteriorly towards the pterygoid process. The senior authors prefer performing the pterygomaxillary disjunction using the coronal incision only; however, the use of the intraoral sulcus incision will simplify the complete separation of the maxilla from the skull base.

Osteotomies are performed next. All osteotomies must be performed to completion and with appropriate irrigation (when mechanical saws are used) to limit thermal damage. Considering the limited visualization, certain critical osteotomies are not directly visualized. Rather, the pathway of the osteotomy is visualized in the "mind's eye." This reality can be difficult for the novice surgeon to adapt. In these cases, careful study of skulls and physical and digital models is strongly recommended for surgeons with less experience with these procedures. In this chapter, mechanical saws are used; however, ultrasonic saws can be substituted as per surgeon's preference. Only one side of the skeleton will be described.

A reciprocating saw is used to make an osteotomy at the junction of the zygomatic arch and body. It is important to perform this osteotomy anteriorly, within the lateral border of the zygomatic body, to create a wide area of bone-to-bone contact; this will improve the quality of the bone generate induced by distraction osteogenesis. The same saw is used to complete an osteotomy through the lateral orbital rim at the area of the frontozygomatic suture. The next osteotomy is vertically oriented, starting from the inferior orbital fissure and directed superiorly to the meet the osteotomy made at the frontozygomatic suture. The bony cut is started at the superior aspect of the lateral wall of the maxillary sinus which facilitates pterygomaxillary separation later in the surgery. Protection of the intraorbital contents is achieved with a malleable retractor and the tip of the saw blade within the orbit should be directly visualized at all times. A 3 mm osteotome is then employed to complete the osteotomy of the orbital floor towards the medial orbital wall, a much thinner bone than the lateral portion. This cut should remain about 6–10 mm posterior to the orbital rim. It is critical to directly visualize the inferior orbital rim during the completion of this osteotomy; blind osteotomy creates risk of a pathological fracture resulting in a separation of the zygoma from the Le Fort III segment. It is commonly not possible to reach the medial limit of the orbital floor with the osteotome and the remainder of the bone of the medial orbital floor is separated during down fracture. It is the senior author's preference that the pterygopalatine and posterior maxillary osteotomy is performed through the coronal incision approach, as opposed to through an intraoral approach. The pterygopalatine osteotomy is achieved with a curved Kawamoto osteotome and the opposing hand palpating transorally behind the maxillary tuberosity to confirm separation is made and the palatal mucosa is not injured. The osteotomy is continued superiorly and then anteriorly along the lateral wall of the maxillary sinus to meet the osteotomy made at the superior aspect of the lateral wall of the maxillary sinus. A straight osteotome is then used to separate any remaining bony connections within the osteotomies between the intraorbital fissure and pterygomaxillary suture. These remaining bony connections are more common in patients with a hypoplastic maxillary sinus.

The nasofrontal osteotomy is performed last. As intraorbital visualization can be limited, a 3 mm is first used to complete a vertical osteotomy, behind the posterior lacrimal crest, starting from the horizontal position of the anterior ethmoid artery, towards the orbital floor. A malleable retractor is used to gently translate the orbital contents laterally. It is usually not possible to reach the orbital floor with the osteotome and the remainder of the bony connections is separated during down fracture. A reciprocating saw is then used in an oblique orientation to connect the superior aspect of the osteotomy formed at the medial orbital wall with the nasal radix. This midline osteotomy must be below the level of the cribriform plate to maintain a subcranial separation. Patients with Apert syndrome commonly have an inferiorly located cribriform plate and the anterior cranial fossa is foreshortened. Therefore, careful preoperative study of the cranial base is important to inform the location of the osteotomy and avoid unintentional extension of the nasofrontal osteotomy into the intracranial space. The midline osteotomy is completed with a Tessier curved osteotomy directed towards the posterior nasal spine. This vector is best directed by placing a finger intraorally onto the posterior nasal spine to create a "target."

Complete craniofacial disjunction is achieved with firm, steady, downward pressure and use of Rowe maxillary disimpaction forceps. Any resistance should be respected and not forced to completion. Excessive force can result in a pathologic fracture. Rather, re-exploration of the osteotomy sites and confirmation of completeness with osteotomes should be performed. The maxillary sinus and pterygomaxillary suture are common areas for residual bony bridges. The curved osteotome can be used to section any remaining bony segments. Tessier straight osteotomes can also be used as levers to confirm appropriate separation in the nasofrontal junction and the pterygomaxillary suture. However, surgeons should avoid using excessive force when levering the Le Fort III segment. Full mobility should be confirmed before placing any distraction hardware.

The lateral canthal tendon can be resuspended to the lateral orbital rim in its new anterior position, as per the surgeon's preference. A small drill hole is made along the lateral orbital rim, slightly more superior than the position of the lateral canthal tendon. An Ethibond suture is used affix the lateral canthal tendon to the drill hole. Before securing this knot, the periorbital soft tissue flap is repositioned so the eyelid positioning can be directly visualized, and the suture is tied, resulting in a superior and lateral placement of the lateral canthus. The rate of relapse of lateral canthal tendon resuspension can be significant. The scalp wound is irrigated, and the coronal incision can be closed in a layered fashion over a closed suction drain.

In cases where a rigid external distraction (RED) device is used, surgeons may opt to cement a maxillary dental splint to the dentition which can be rigidly attached to the RED device (senior author's preference) or outriggers can be attached to the maxillary splint and steel wires then attached from the outriggers to the RED device. The external device is secured to the cranium with pins, carefully paying attention to a symmetric placement and avoid affixing of screws near cranial defects or thin bone. In young patients (3 years or younger), the cranial bone can be quite thin, significantly increasing the risk of intracranial violation. In these young age groups, an internal device is recommended. The vertical midline post of the external device is mounted, and vector is determined. There should be at least a 2 cm space between the external device and the forehead to account for postoperative swelling. The distraction vector can be adjusted to patient needs. Still, it should most commonly have an anterior transition to improve airway obstruction but also a clockwise rotation to lengthen the face and attempt at closing the anterior open bite. Considering the vertical deficiency in patients with Apert syndrome, a mild inferior vector is often used. Once the desired vector is reached, the vertical midline post is secured to the maxillary tooth-anchored splint with 26-gauge wires or through direct fixation to the RED device.

Patients are extubated at the end of surgery barring any intraoperative complications or pre-operative respiratory fragility. A five-day latency period is afforded followed by activation at a rate of 1–1.5 mm daily. Overcorrection is the goal in the growing face, resulting in significant class II occlusion, moderate enophthalmos, and exaggerated facial convexity. Typically, 16–26 mm advancement is performed, but these distances are ultimately patient-tailored. An eight-week consolidation phase is followed prior to removal of the RED device under general anesthesia.

Surgical Considerations and Rationale

In the described treatment algorithm, the forehead and midface are transposed through separate operations. There are several advantages to this approach. The restoration of the forehead and midface may require different vectors of translation and, therefore, are better performed separately to achieve a more complete aesthetic outcome. Functionally, the time to intervene for increased intracranial pressure (treated by cranial expansion) is commonly earlier than that for upper airway obstruction (treated by midface expansion). Furthermore, performing a subcranial Le Fort III is safer than a monobloc or facial bipartition distraction as the intracranial cavity is not violated.

Advancements beyond the apparent ideal is necessary to allow for facial growth and accommodate a degree of phenotypic relapse. It is important to note that the midface itself does not tend to relapse after an appropriately performed midface distraction. Rather, there is continued facial growth with limited anterior midface growth after distraction, causing the phenotype's recurrence as the rest of the face grows. Objective measurements to guide degree of overcorrection are patient-specific and thus generalized end-points are not typically followed. Instead, functional outcomes are followed while pushing the envelope as much as possible. Advancements as great as 26–29 mm have been reached with excellent patient tolerance. These distances may not be reasonable end-points when a monobloc is pursued.

Le Fort III procedure has some deferential effects on the soft tissue, namely when considering the degree of overcorrection targeted. Nasal lengthening and tip rotation are both exaggerated by overcorrecting to a class II occlusion, and in the Apert phenotype can be rather overt. Raposo et al. describe a "low Le Fort I" osteotomy design with a pivoting rotation centered on the nasoglabellar angle in an effort to minimize nasal lengthening while still achieving counterclockwise directionality of distraction [1]. However, any form of nasal reconstruction or rhinoplasty techniques should definitively be deferred to the teenage years and after all jaw and midface transpositions are complete. As the orbital construct is advanced uniformly, the medial and lateral canthi relationship is unchanged. Therefore, it is common and encouraged to perform a concurrent lateral canthotomy to resuspend the tendon and achieve a more aesthetic positive canthal tilt.

Review of Current Practices and Outcomes

Techniques to advance the Apert midface have evolved considerably in the past several decades. Monobloc advancement, for example, has been performed in early months of life for the most severe of patients with life-threatening sleep apnea or vision-threatening exorbitism [2]. Many variations in midface reconstruction have been informed by a more robust understanding of the facial dysmorphology associated with Apert syndrome. The Aperts phenotype is that of an abnormal midface in an abnormal position [3]. Hypoplasia of the orbits, zygoma, and maxilla exists in a multi-planar fashion with shortened height, width, and thickness. What results is a concavity of the face whereby the central face along the midline is more retrusive than lateral segments. Midfacial height from nasion to subnasale is shortened and the distance from subnasale to the upper dentition is increased. The nose itself is far more retruded than surrounding central features that leads to a concave appearance of the face both in the sagittal and coronal planes. Biconcavity of the face is a unique facial feature of Apert syndrome in addition to the hand and food syndactyly. The Apert midface is not one with a normal anatomy that is simply pushed back in the face, nor is it a presentation of isolated hypoplasia. It is in fact the combination of orbitozygomatic hypoplasia neighboring a both hypoplastic and retrusive maxilla. Therefore, advancing the forehead, orbits, zygomas, and maxilla wholly in a single forward vector simply displaces abnormal anatomy into a more anterior position.

Subcranial Versus Intracranial Osteotomy

Our institutional preference for subcranial Le Fort III distraction is predicated on the prior advancement of a frontal bandeau, which addresses the contour of the forehead and expands intracranial volume in early childhood. In this instance, subcranial Le Fort III as compared to intracranial monobloc can better focus on orbital correction and differential advancement of the midface and forehead. Le Fort III thus is most beneficial for the patient with isolated midface retrusion, whether that be due to a phenotypically less severe forehead retrusion or an adequately overcorrected frontal/brow position following front-orbital advancement [1]. Le Fort III more easily improves facial convexity due to the isolated facial advancement against a fixed frontal region. The contrasting monobloc procedure displaces the forehead anteriorly and lessens the sagittal discrepancy between the upper and middle thirds. Furthermore, the senior author's experience shows that the optimal degree of sagittal advancement is different in the forehead and midface in patients with Apert syndrome.

Early restoration of forehead shape and intracranial volume through FOA can preclude the need for a riskier intracranial operation once the patient reaches age of mixed dentition. A secondary anterior cranial expansion to address the supraorbital region remains an option for patients with recurrent forehead retrusion. Monobloc distraction is a common intervention at centers that rely on PVDO in infancy with demonstrated improvement in anterior contour owing to massive volumetric expansion [4]. Following this protocol, composite transposition with the monobloc can be easily relied upon to correct the small movement needed at the level of the frontal bone, concurrently with midface transposition. An untouched anterior cranial vault and midface is undoubtedly a major benefit in this treatment pathway. However, it is not clear if all patients undergoing monobloc distraction, following this treatment protocol, are indeed affected by elevated ICP.

Regarding the orbits, subcranial midface advancement focuses on the movement of the orbital–midface structures in isolation from the forehead, which inherently improves the convexity profile of the face instead of advancing an abnormal concave contour en bloc. This segmented concept is important as it anatomically divides abnormally developed structures that are in an abnormal relation to one another. Le Fort III osteotomy becomes most advantageous when this is considered, and movements are guided towards a dramatic anterior and downward vector directing clockwise rotation. This is limited in the monobloc as it would yield an unfavorable appearance of the upper face.

Segmentalizing the subcranial osteotomy is gaining popularity while inherently increasing surgical complexity. Le Fort II osteotomy with zygomatic repositioning differentially advances the central face independently of the lateral orbits and zygomas, each movement with varying rotation and advancement [5]. Obligatory use of distraction is seen with these segmentalized procedures to account for each subdivision's independent movements. A more recently described technique is that of zygomatic rotation with maxillary expansion whereby the medial orbital wall and nasal bones are excluded from the Le Fort III osteotomy and midline sagittal palatal split is performed [1]. This technique was designed for the patient with Apert syndrome with a long nasal span that should not be lengthened with midface advancement. In patient with a moderate-to-severe degree of hypertelorism, facial bipartition may be the more appropriate procedure to improve intradacryon distance. In this case, facial bipartition can be performed in combination with distraction osteogenesis. Several authors advocate for facial bipartition even in mild forms of hypertelorism as they cite medialization of the orbits is the only way to destigmatize the Apert appearance [6, 7].

Morbidity Profile

Morbidity risk is significant with any intracranial or midface procedure and these reconstructions should be performed in specialized centers with a significant volume of patients and a dedicated craniofacial and neurosurgical team. Major complications associated with FOA include intraoperative blood loss, intracranial venous hypertension, infection, wound breakdown hardware exposure, and injury to the intracranial and intraorbital contents. Major complications associated with Le Fort III distraction include infection, relapse, formation of poor bone generate, pathologic fracture of the Le Fort III segment, incomplete osteotomy resulting in limited midface translation, suboptimal vector of translation, hardware dislodgement, and damage to the globes. In experienced units, these complications tend to be limited. As surgical and postoperative experience has improved, the complication rate for Le Fort III advancement has decreased over time [8]. Distraction osteogenesis has improved patient safety while facilitating larger advancement distances, improved bony stability, management over vector control, and accommodation of the overlying soft tissue preventing relapse [9].

The limitations to understanding the true complication rate with these procedures is that these data are reported discretely by individual craniofacial groups with limited population numbers. Reported overall complications appear to be statistically similar between groups, ranging around 30–60% [10–13], when performed in adolescent ages.

Distractor Devices and Manipulation

Le Fort III distraction osteogenesis can follow one of two technical variations: a "push" method through use of internal distractor devices or a "pull" method which employ an external halo device. Both approaches can achieve similar surgical outcomes with differing complication profiles [14]. Proponents of interval devices note absence of transcutaneous scar creation, improved patient compliance, socially accepting appearance during the distraction and consolidation phases, and greater stability of the device with bony fixation [15]. Internal devices mandate precision during placement to ensure proper device alignment and vector selection, as the devices cannot be manipulated postoperatively. A second operation is also required for removal. Although this can be true for the external halo device as well, it is a simpler removal procedure. Infectious sequelae have been reported to be greater among buried distractor groups [13]. In contrast, advocates of external device assert the control of three-dimensional vector maneuvering and differential pull between segments as the primary advantage of these systems [16]. Patient-specific vector forces in multidimensional planes are better achieved by the external devices. Moreover, in the presence of fluid collection or infection, buried devices need be removed immediately and distraction stalled, while external distractors may not require removal as it can function as a temporary external fixation system. External devices can also be fixated with a dental attachment and therefore would not require a second operation for device removal. Pin site infections or migration, temporal bone fractures during from pin placement and bony pull, and patient compliance are referenced downfalls of the external distraction devices. In patients aged three year or younger, the bone stock may not be sufficient to withstand the fixation screws of the halo. The external device can also have significant psychosocial implications for the patient due to the effects on appearance.

Regardless of device employed, the desired vector for advancement should be one with a mild inferior vector. This direction is important to unfurl the central concavity for better projection and will achieve better nasal lengthening. Anterior maxillary growth is limited after frontofacial distraction [17–19] and sagittal overcorrection is necessary to compensate for the expected growth of the lower jaw into facial maturity. Patients who undergo midface distraction at the age of seven years or later and who have undergone appropriate sagittal overcorrection can commonly avoid the need of another Le Fort III procedure prior to or at the completion of facial growth. If any jaw surgery is required, it is usually in the form of a traditional orthognathic surgery.

Aesthetic Considerations

The decision tree followed to guide midface advancement techniques in Apert syndrome can have a variety of branching pathways and cognitive and airway function are central considerations to the timing and type of intervention. Although the functional and aesthetic changes associated with different interventions cannot typically be individually modified within each procedure, there are some variations to aesthetic changes when comparing different treatment protocols. Segmentalizing osteotomies affords surgeons greater degrees of freedom towards achieving their aesthetic goal through multipiece, multidimensional movement and are effective in correcting canthal relationship [20]. Facial bipartition can address hypertelorism and horizontal facial concavity. Le Fort III (with previous FOA) can precisely restore frontofacial sagittal relationships and is probably better suited for patients with mild-to-moderate expressions of Apert syndrome. Several authors report use of onlay prosthetic materials such as polyether ether ketone (PEEK) or porous polyethylene to augment the forehead and improve contour [1, 5]. This is to address not a relapse following FOA or a retrusive forehead, but rather a recession contour irregularity of 3–4 mm only. Advocates describe a presentation where the frontal bandeau maintains its advanced position and the middle to upper forehead fall into this recessed position, so this is where the thin implant is positioned.

Important soft tissue changes enacted by bony movement that are relevant to patients with Apert syndrome include nasal length, frontonasal angle, globe position relative to the orbits, and palpebral fissures. Conventional Le Fort III osteotomies can overlengthen the nose, cause notable step-offs at the lateral orbital walls and nasofrontal junction, and cause enophthalmos if the orbits are overcorrected. Definitive rhinoplasty is deferred until skeletal maturity, as is restoration of dental occlusion in orthognathic surgery.

Conclusion

The presented treatment plan for patients affected by Apert syndrome involves staging surgical management by (1) addressing intracranial hypertension through PVDO within the first year of life (if required), (2) returning to expand the anterior cranial vault and improve frontal contour with FOA at the age of two years, and (3) awaiting until the age of mixed dentition to advance the central face in the form of Le Fort III distraction. A variety of branching algorithms that differ from this approach are well described and justified by their functional outcomes, aesthetic outcomes, and safety profile. Ultimately, surgical decision-making should be focused on patient-specific needs dictated by the frontofacial dysmorphology and functional status.

References

1. Raposo-Amaral CE, Ghizoni E, Raposo-Amaral CA. Apert syndrome: selection rationale for midface advancement technique. Adv Tech Stand Neurosurg. 2023;46:245–66.
2. Ahmad F, Cobb ARM, Mills C, Jones BM, Hayward RD, Dunaway DJ. Frontofacial monobloc distraction in the very young: a review of 12 consecutive cases. Plast Reconstr Surg. 2012;129(3):488e–97e.
3. Hopper RA, Prucz RB, Iamphongsai S. Achieving differential facial changes with Le Fort III distraction osteogenesis: the use of nasal passenger grafts, cerclage hinges, and segmental movements. Plast Reconstr Surg. 2012;130(6):1281–8.
4. Swanson JW, Samra F, Bauder A, Mitchell BT, Taylor JA, Bartlett SP. An algorithm for managing syndromic craniosynostosis using posterior

vault distraction osteogenesis. Plast Reconstr Surg. 2016;137(5):829e–41e.
5. Hopper RA, Kapadia H, Susarla SM. Le Fort II distraction with zygomatic repositioning: a technique for differential correction of midface hypoplasia. J Oral Maxillofac Surg. 2018;76(9):2002.e1–2002.e14.
6. Raposo-Amaral CE, Denadai R, Oliveira YM, Ghizoni E, Raposo-Amaral CA. Apert syndrome management: changing treatment algorithm. J Craniofac Surg. 2020;31(3):648–52.
7. Allam KA, Wan DC, Khwanngern K, Kawamoto HK, Tanna N, Perry A, et al. Treatment of apert syndrome: a long-term follow-up study. Plast Reconstr Surg. 2011;127(4):1601–11.
8. Shetye PR, Boutros S, Grayson BH, McCarthy JG. Midterm follow-up of midface distraction for syndromic craniosynostosis: a clinical and cephalometric study. Plast Reconstr Surg. 2007;120(6):1621–32.
9. Fearon JA, Whitaker LA. Complications with facial advancement: a comparison between the Le Fort III and monobloc advancements. Plast Reconstr Surg. 1993;91(6):990–5.
10. Munabi NCO, Williams M, Nagengast ES, Fahradyan A, Goel P, Gould DJ, et al. Outcomes of intracranial versus subcranial approaches to the frontofacial skeleton. J Oral Maxillofac Surg. 2020;78(9):1609–16.
11. Zhang RS, Lin LO, Hoppe IC, Swanson JW, Bartlett SP, Taylor JA. Retrospective review of the complication profile associated with 71 subcranial and transcranial midface distraction procedures at a single institution. Plast Reconstr Surg. 2019;143(2):521–30.
12. Dunaway DJ, Britto JA, Abela C, Evans RD, Jeelani NU. Complications of frontofacial advancement. Childs Nerv Syst. 2012;28(9):1571–6.
13. Goldstein JA, Paliga JT, Taylor JA, Bartlett SP. Complications in 54 frontofacial distraction procedures in patients with syndromic craniosynostosis. J Craniofac Surg. 2015;26(1):124–8.
14. Meling TR, Høgevold HE, Due-Tønnessen BJ, Skjelbred P. Midface distraction osteogenesis: internal vs. external devices. Int J Oral Maxillofac Surg. 2011;40(2):139–45.
15. Chin M, Toth BA. Le Fort III advancement with gradual distraction using internal devices. Plast Reconstr Surg. 1997;100(4):819–30. discussion 31–2
16. Witherow H, Dunaway D, Evans R, Nischal KK, Shipster C, Pereira V, et al. Functional outcomes in monobloc advancement by distraction using the rigid external distractor device. Plast Reconstr Surg. 2008;121(4):1311–22.
17. Meazzini MC, Mazzoleni F, Caronni E, Bozzetti A. Le Fort III advancement osteotomy in the growing child affected by Crouzon's and Apert's syndromes: presurgical and postsurgical growth. J Craniofac Surg. 2005;16(3):369–77.
18. Fearon JA. Halo distraction of the Le Fort III in syndromic craniosynostosis: a long-term assessment. Plast Reconstr Surg. 2005;115(6):1524–36.
19. McCarthy JG, La Trenta GS, Breitbart AS, Grayson BH, Bookstein FL. The Le Fort III advancement osteotomy in the child under 7 years of age. Plast Reconstr Surg. 1990;86(4):633–46. discussion 47–9
20. Wu M, Massenburg BB, Ng JJ, Romeo DJ, Swanson JW, Bartlett SP, et al. The Kaleidoscope of midface management in apert syndrome: a 23-year single-institution experience. Plast Reconstr Surg. 2024;155:767e.

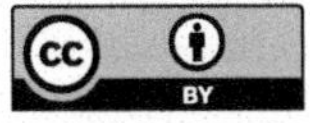

Monobloc Advancement with Internal Distraction

18

Eric Arnaud, Roman H. Khonsari, and Giovanna Paternoster

Introduction

Between 2000 and 2024, 210 Frontofacial Monobloc Advancements (FFMBA) have been performed for syndromic craniosynostoses in the Necker craniofacial unit. Among them 24 have been performed for patients with Apert syndrome. These represented a minority as most of them [35] underwent a classical two-stage anterior strategy, with a fronto-orbital advancement (FOA) followed by a Le Fort III advancement. The main difference between these two groups is the relatively less severe obstructive sleep apnea (OSA) in patients with Apert syndrome than other syndromes. The second reason is that some patients were treated initially in another center where an FOA had been the primary treatment without necessarily considering the OSA. Those patients treated with Le Fort III will be analyzed in chapters on Midface Advancement with Two Stage Strategy (variant of Le Fort 3 osteotomy with subcranial bi-partition).

The patients with Apert syndrome who underwent a FFMBA were at a mean of three years of age. Most had a prior posterior distraction before 18 months of age. The indication for FFMBA) includes the combination of exorbitism and obstructive sleep apnea syndrome (OSAS). At three years of age, the risk of raised ICP is minimal, especially if a preliminary skull expansion has been undertaken. As previously explained, the posterior distraction allows quicker closure of the common median frontal dehiscence. The mean Apnea–Hyponea Index (AHI) preoperatively was 15,3/h and post-operatively 6,5/h. At Necker, we try to avoid tracheostomy by any means, which implies a more frequent and earlier use of the FFMBA. Before FFMBA, continuous positive airway pressure (CPAP) is used whenever necessary to delay the FFMBA until the age of 2.5 years. As already observed, CPAP should not be used for a very long period as it worsens the facial retrusion. Several articles have described our initial techniques since 2001 and all the functional consequences with more than 20 years of follow-up [1–35].

The indication to FFMBA could be resumed in this simplified algorithm (see previous chapter introduction).

E. Arnaud (✉)
Craniofacial Unit, Hôpital Necker–Enfants malades, Reference Center for French Rare Disease Network CRANIOST, European Rare Disease Network ERN CRANIO, Paris, France

Competence Center for French Rare Disease Network CRANIOST, Clinique Marcel Sembat, Ramsay-Generale de santé, Boulogne Billancourt, France

R. H. Khonsari · G. Paternoster
Craniofacial Unit, Hôpital Necker–Enfants malades, Reference Center for French Rare Disease Network CRANIOST, European Rare Disease Network ERN CRANIO, Paris, France

J. G. Meara et al. (eds.), *Apert Syndrome*, https://doi.org/10.1007/978-3-032-12551-4_18

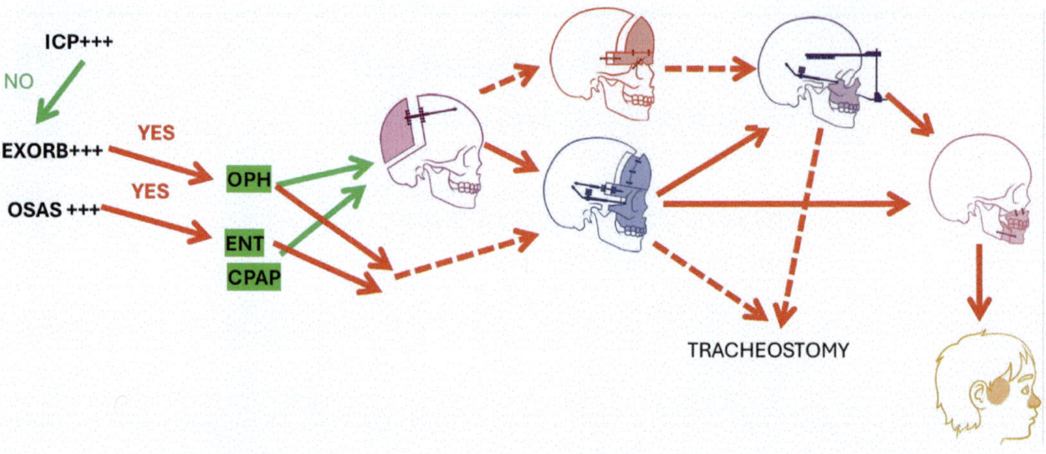

Standardized Technique of FFMBA[1]

Although slight modifications were introduced along the way, the technique was well standardized and can be summarized as follows and always included four internal distractors.

FFMBA is performed with the patient in a supine position with oral intubation (Figs. 18.1 and 18.2). The tube is sutured to the lower jaw using non-absorbable braided sutures (Fig. 18.3). Bilateral tarsorraphies are placed using non-absorbable monofilament sutures (Fig. 18.4). The child is positioned on a headrest and two chest rolls—one under the thighs and one under the shoulders—are taped to the operating table to prevent him from sliding down during the procedure (Fig. 18.2). An instrument table is fixed to the operating table at approximately 20–25 cm from the chin of the patient (Fig. 18.1).

[1] *Special note:* Some parts (text and images) of this chapter have been previously published by the same publisher (Springer) in the following release: Frontofacial Monobloc with distraction; Eric Arnaud, Giovanna Paternoster, Roman Hossein Khonsari, Samer Haber, Eds. Springer Nature Switzerland 1G 2023. Permission has been asked to reuse some of the materials. Original illustrations were produced by Cassandra Vion within a partnership with Ecole Estienne (Paris).

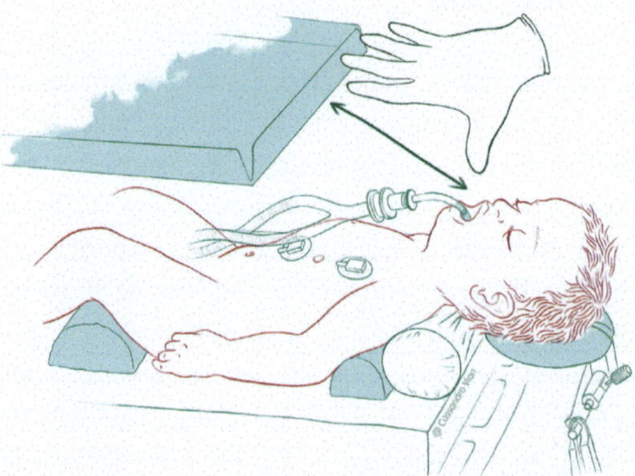

Fig. 18.1 Operating room setup and patient positioning

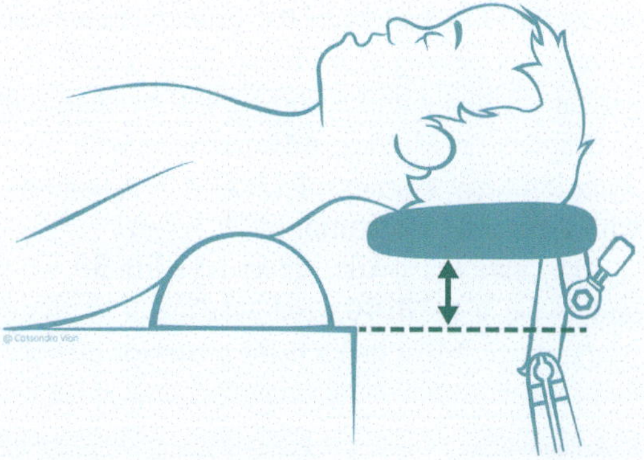

Fig. 18.2 Position of the headrest relative to the operating table

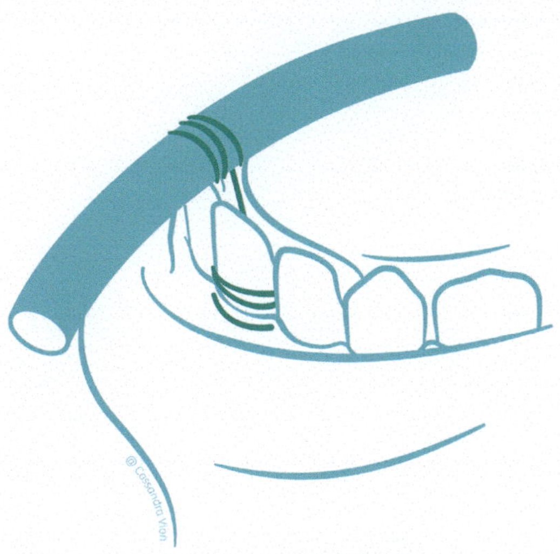

Fig. 18.3 Fixation of the tube to the lower jaw

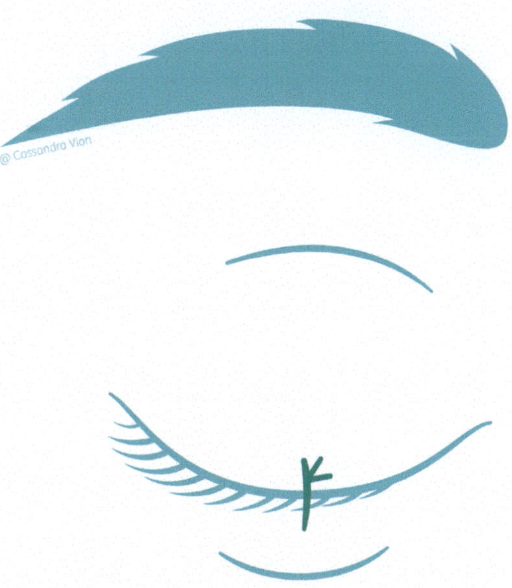

Fig. 18.4 Tarsorrhaphy

Skin markings are made for a zig-zag or undulated bi-coronal incision (Fig. 18.5). Usually, the scar from a previous posterior vault expansion is used. The hair is shaved over a 3 cm wide band around the incision line. Infiltration in subgaleal and subdermal planes using 1 mg/L adrenaline solution is performed along the incision line.

The subgaleal plane is undermined down to the superior orbital ridge and on the surface of the superficial layer of the deep temporal fascia,

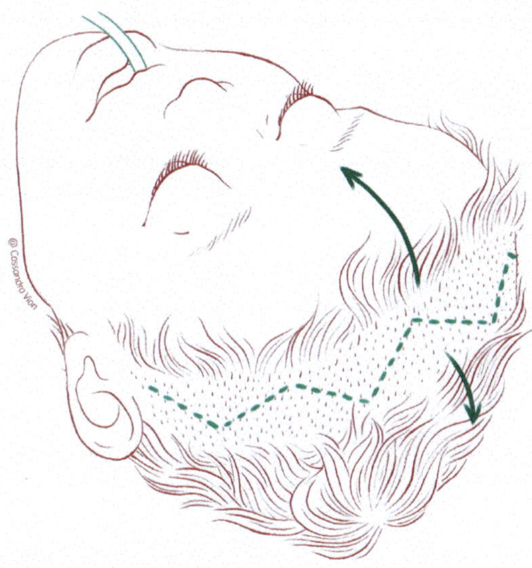

Fig. 18.5 Skin incision

to avoid facial nerve branch injuries. Two periosteal flaps are elevated containing the supra-orbital and supra-trochlear pedicles (Figs. 18.6 and 18.7). Small horizontal incisions of the superficial layer of the deep temporal fascia are performed in order to prepare the Tessier maneuver (Fig. 18.8a). The orbital roofs and the lateral orbital walls are dissected using a periosteal elevator. The bony vertex is exposed.

The surface of the zygoma and the zygomatic arch are exposed using the Tessier maneuver before raising the temporal muscles (Fig. 18.8a, c). The temporal muscles are then raised, exposing the lateral orbital wall (Fig. 18.8b).

Burr holes are performed lateral to the forehead in sufficient numbers to safely raise the forehead bone as a unit (Figs. 18.9, 18.10 and 18.11). The lower limit of the forehead is located 1 cm above the upper orbital rim. The forehead and two laterally adjacent coronal bony segments (Paternoster side-wings) are raised using a craniotome and/or piezosurgery (Fig. 18.12). The tongue and groove designs of the temporal osteotomies are illustrated in Fig. 18.13.

Deep tongue and groove designs are performed in the temporal regions with an antero-posterior length of 5 cm. An oscillating saw can be used for a cleaner cut of the vertical osteotomy at the edge of the tongue-and-groove (Figs. 18.11

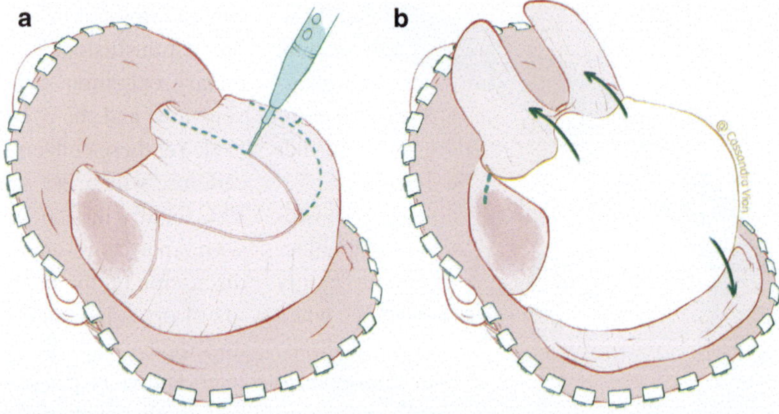

Fig. 18.6 (**a**, **b**) Elevation of the periosteal flaps and exposure of the skull vault

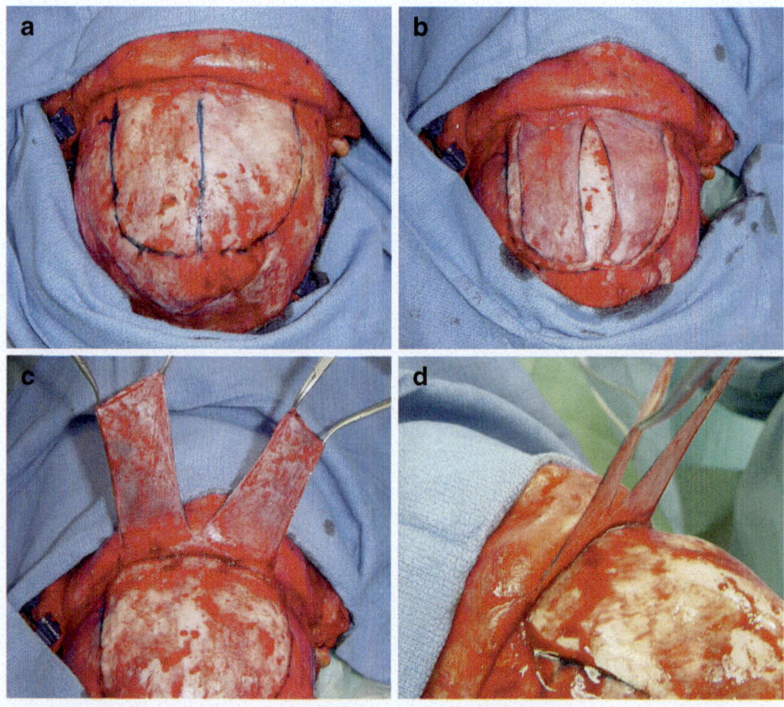

Fig. 18.7 (**a**–**d**) Elevation of the periosteal flaps, intraoperative view

and 18.12). Piezoelectric surgery can alternatively be used to perform all the previous steps. The zygomatic arches are sectioned using a reciprocating saw.

The lateral orbital wall is sectioned with the reciprocating saw directed upwards, until the osteotomy line meets the previous osteotomy at the lower border of the temporal tongue and groove design (Fig. 18.14). The reciprocating saw is then oriented downwards inside that same lateral orbital osteotomy line, to cut the body of the zygoma and the lateral part of the orbital floor.

The osteotomy of the orbital floor is performed using the reciprocating saw 2 mm anterior to the inferior orbital fissure. The osteotomy is extended towards the medial orbital wall using a curved osteotome oriented posteriorly, while applying extreme caution not to section the inferior orbital rim (Figs. 18.15 and 18.16). The orbits are very shallow in antero-posterior axis (AP), and the osteotomy line must be posterior enough to avoid anteriorly sectioning the inferior orbital rim. A critical instrument in this procedure step is a curved lighted retractor with built-

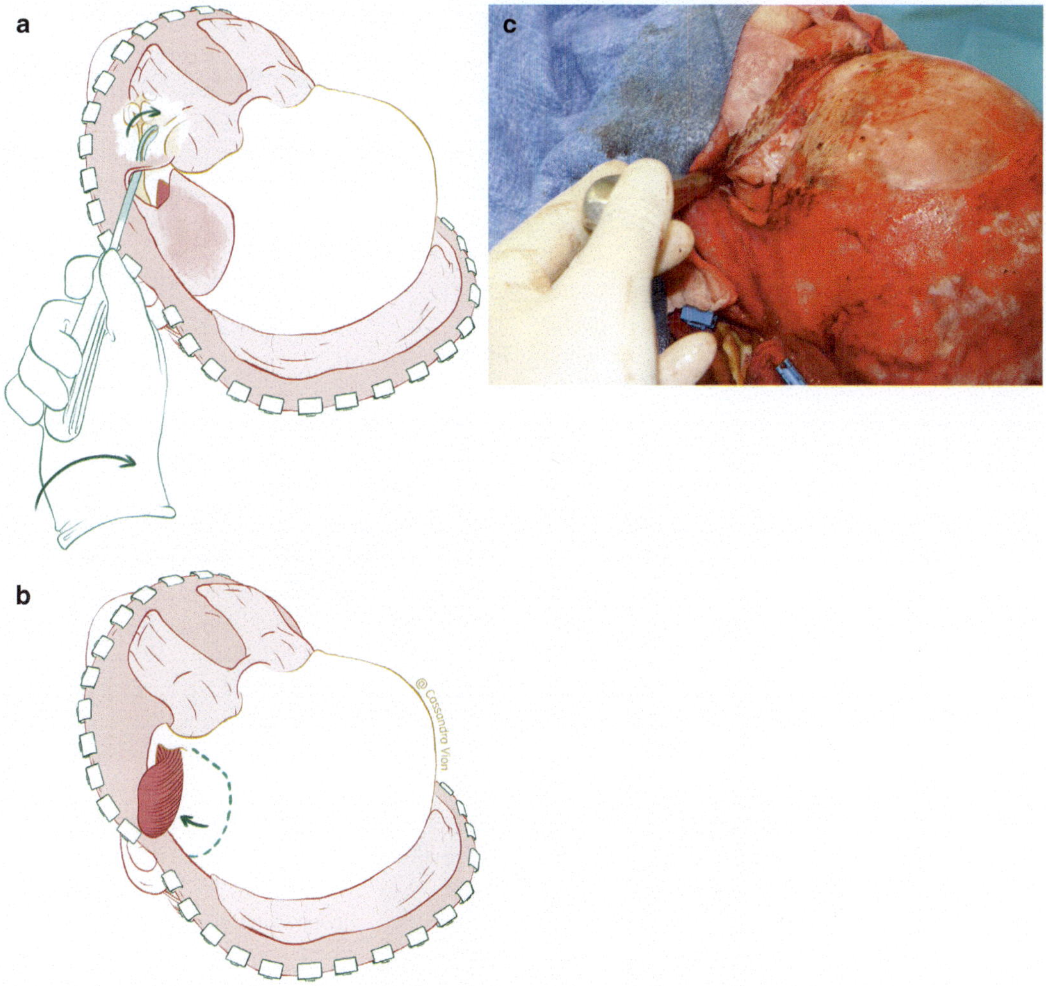

Fig. 18.8 (**a**) Tessier maneuver exposing the zygomatic surface and the zygomatic arch is performed before raising the temporal muscle but after dissecting the lateral orbital wall from the orbital contents. (**b**) Raising of the temporal muscle and exposure of the lateral orbital wall. (**c**) Intraoperative photograph demonstrating the Tessier maneuver

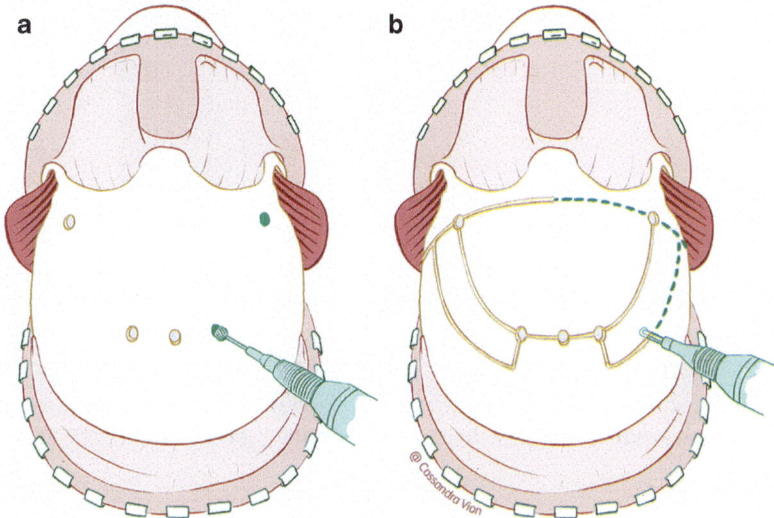

Fig. 18.9 (**a**) Burr holes lateral to the forehead, which is sectioned 1 cm above the upper orbital rim. (**b**) Two lateral coronal side-wings are raised on both sides of the forehead

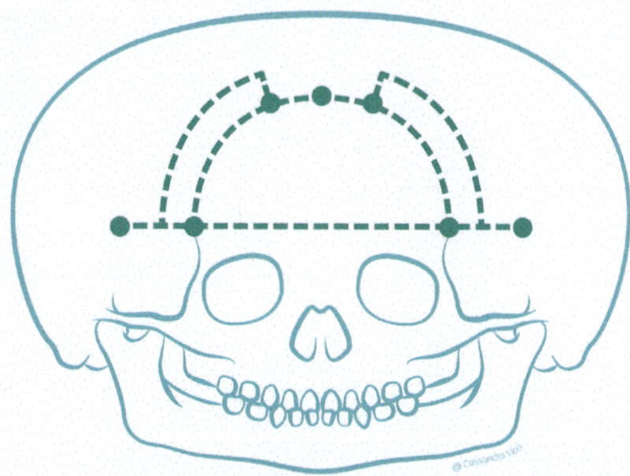

Fig. 18.10 Frontal osteotomy design

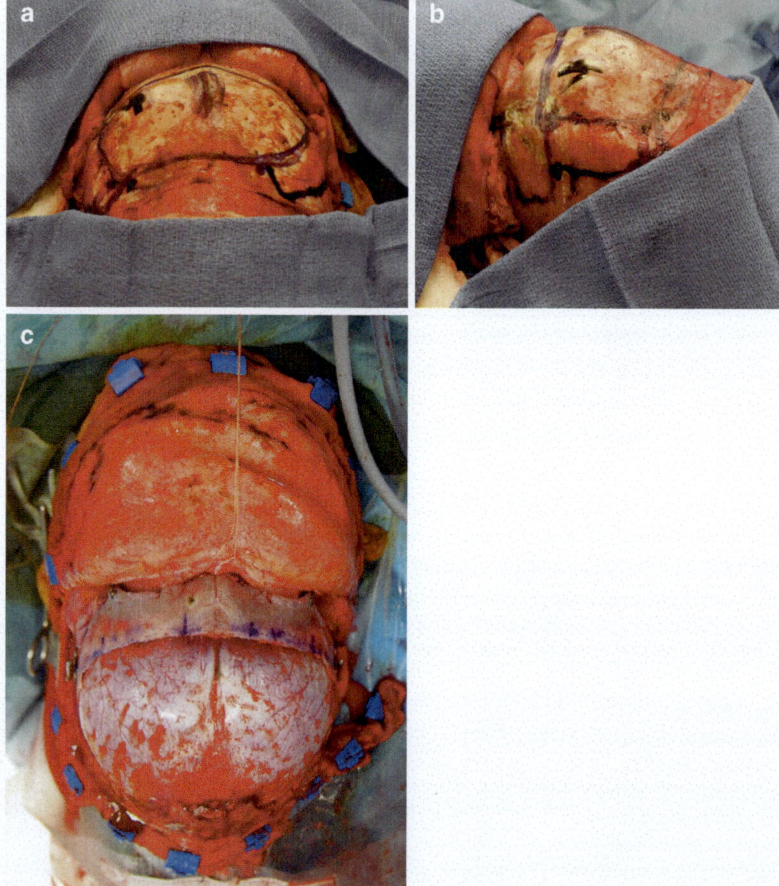

Fig. 18.11 (**a**, **b**) Lateral coronal bony side-wings. (**c**) Forehead raised 1 cm above the upper orbital rim

in suction. It allows for visualization of the orbital floor and protecting the orbital content while performing the osteotomy.

Three malleable retractor blades are then used to protect the temporal lobe under the lesser wing of the sphenoid bone, the eyeball, and the frontal lobe dura mater. The orbital roof osteotomy is then performed using a reciprocating saw starting at the posterior border of the lesser wing towards the midline (Fig. 18.17a). Piezoelectric surgery can also be used for this step of the procedure.

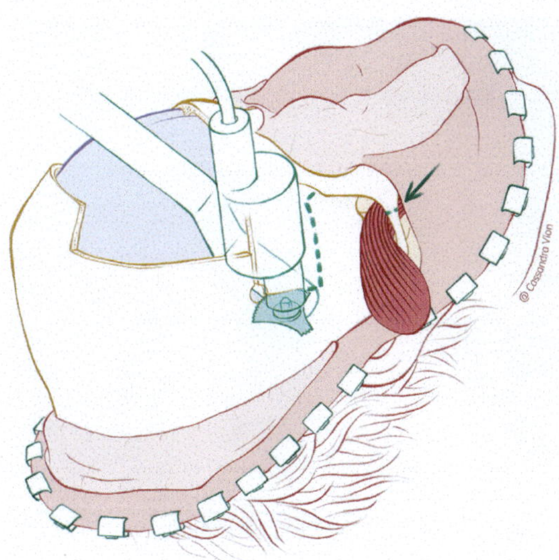

Fig. 18.12 Tongue and groove temporal osteotomies and section of the zygomatic arches

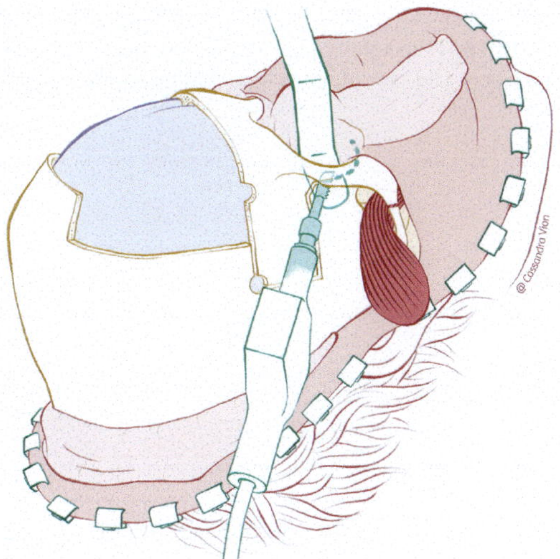

Fig. 18.14 Osteotomy of the lateral orbital wall

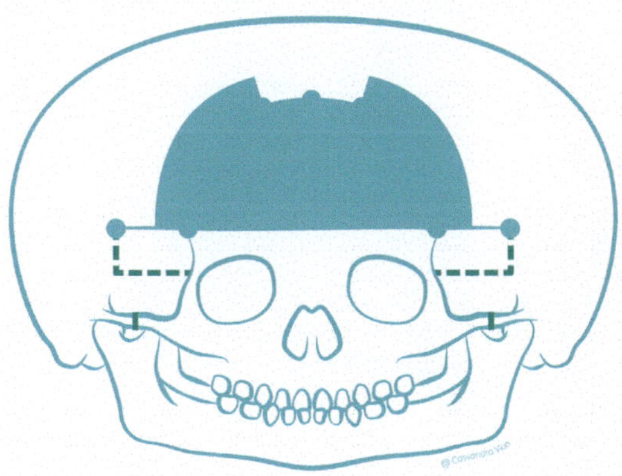

Fig. 18.13 Tongue and groove design after forehead elevation

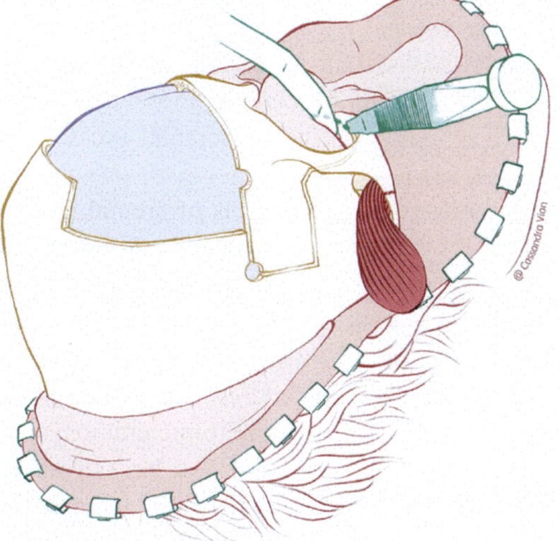

Fig. 18.15 Osteotomies of the orbital floor and medial orbital wall using a curved osteotome

On the midline, a small dural extension is a constant anatomic finding within the foramen cecum (Fig. 18.17b). It is dissected using bipolar electrocautery (Fig. 18.17c, d). The midline osteotomy of the ethmoid and the septum/vomer is performed using the reciprocating saw (and/or with the support of piezosurgery) (Fig. 18.17f). It is then completed with a curved osteotome all the way down to the vomer (Figs. 18.17e and 18.18).

Pterygomaxillary disjunction is performed using an infratemporal approach with an elevator or a curved osteotome. Intraoral digital control allows assessing the completeness of the disjunction (Fig. 18.19). Additional disjunction using an elevator rotated within the pterygopalatine junction is often necessary in younger patients (below 30 months of age) and in secondary cases due to consistent fibrosis of this anatomical region.

Craniofacial disjunction is performed using Rowe forceps without indentations protected intra-orally by silicon sleeves (Fig. 18.20 and 18.21). A counterclockwise movement (when the head of the patient is directed towards the right side) produces the disjunction, completed by careful lateral and clockwise movements to achieve posterior disjunctions in the nasal and oral areas. The two forceps must be handled

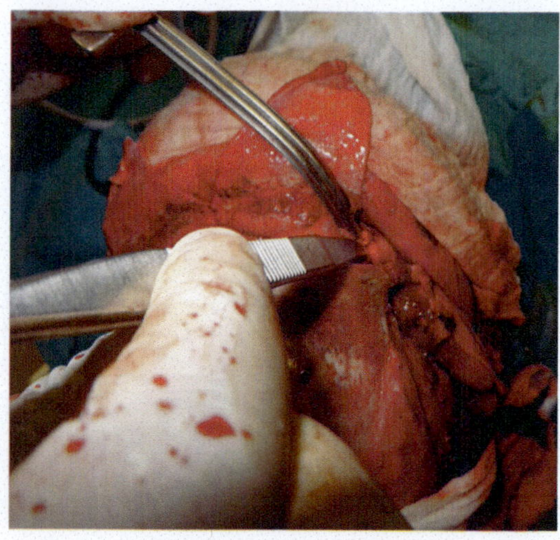

Fig. 18.16 Osteotomy of the orbital floor using a curved osteotome and an illuminated retractor with built-in suction

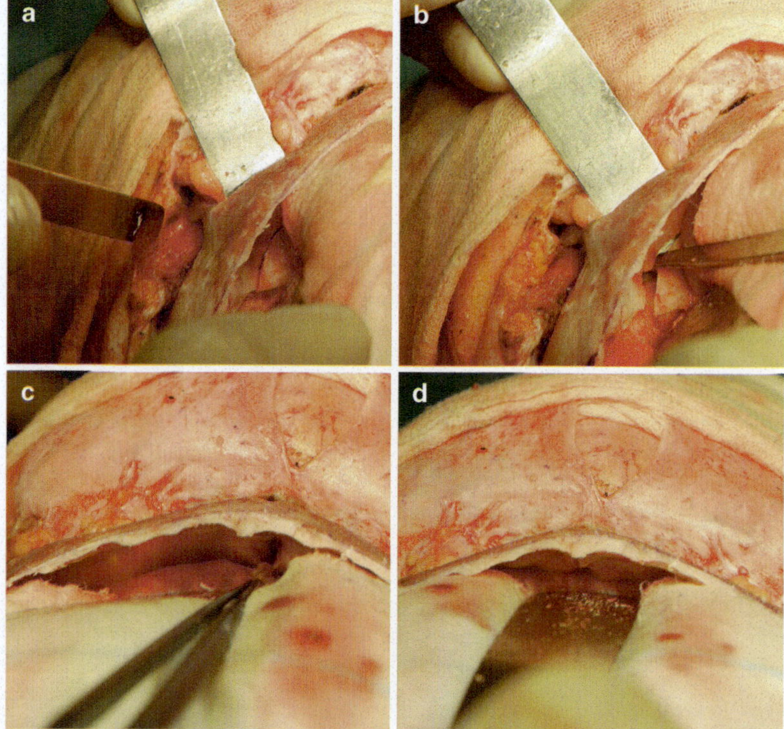

Fig. 18.17 (**a**) Osteotomy of the orbital roof starting at the lesser sphenoid wing. Malleable retractor blades protect the eyeball and the temporal lobe beneath the lesser sphenoid wing. (**b**) Complete release is verified at the convergence point of three osteotomies: lateral orbital, lesser wing, and inferior tenon. (**c**) Midline dural extension penetrating the foramen cecum. (**d**) Dissection of the foramen cecum using gentle bipolar electrocautery to retract the dura

together to avoid midline disjunction and palatal lacerations.

The anterior midline gap of the skull base is reconstructed using the two initially designed periosteal flaps, pulled through the orbital roof osteotomies (Figs. 18.22 and 18.23). One flap covers the midline gap and is sutured to the bandeau using two transosseous 5.0 non-absorbable nylon sutures and then glued. The other flap is used as a secondary cover, sutured to the bandeau and also glued. No sutures are performed to the dura to avoid tears during distraction.

The forehead is remodeled using barrel-stave osteotomies (Figs. 18.24, 18.25 and 18.26). Its inferior border is trimmed laterally to allow a posterior tilt after fixation. Forehead barrel-

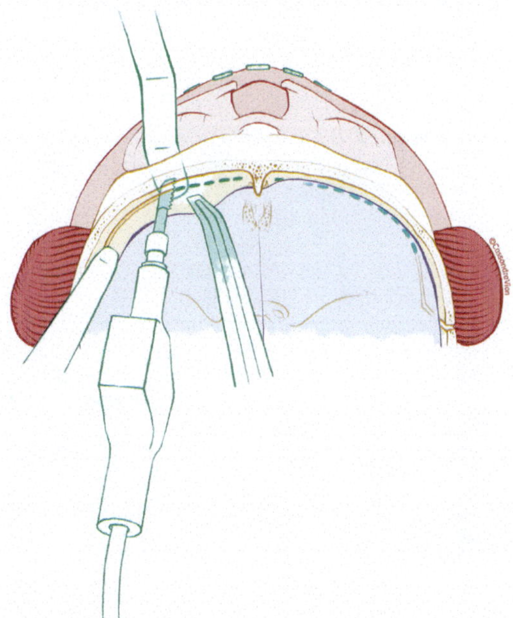

Fig. 18.17 (**e**) Skull base osteotomy using the reciprocating saw. Malleable blades are used to protect the dura mater and the orbital content

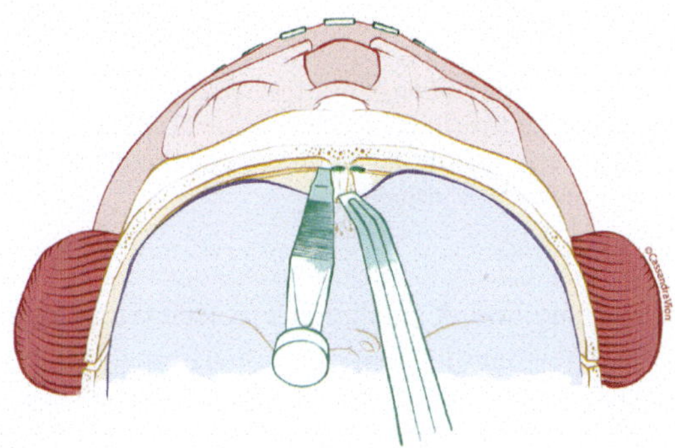

Fig. 18.17 (**f**) The skull base osteotomy is extended inferiorly at the medial wall of the orbit using a curved osteotome oriented posteriorly to the posterior lacrimal crest

staving is performed to control curvature and triangular lateral trimming allows inducing a posterior tilt after fixation. This tilt decreases the volume of the frontal dead space that will form secondary to the frontofacial advancement. Barrel-staving of the vault posterior to the fore-

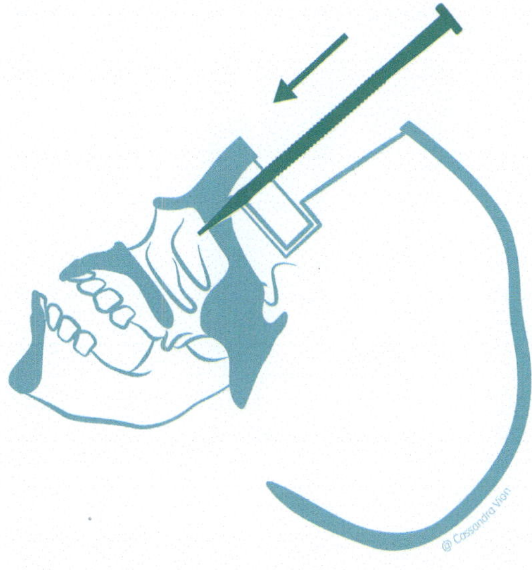

Fig. 18.18 Position of the osteotome when performing the midline osteotomy of the ethmoid and the vomer on a sagittal view

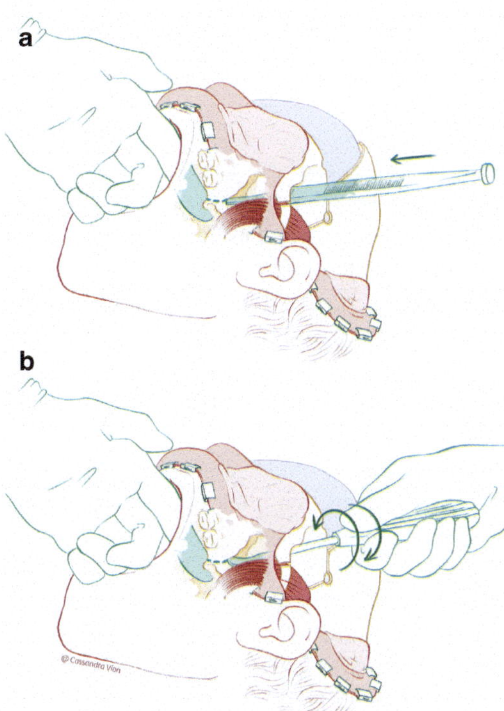

Fig. 18.19 (**a**) Pterygomaxillary disjunction using a curved osteotome. (**b**) Additional disjunction using an elevator

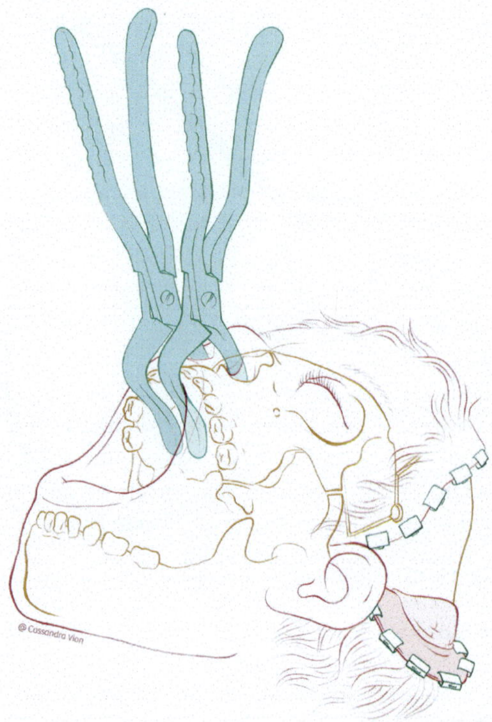

Fig. 18.20 Craniofacial disjunction using Rowe forceps

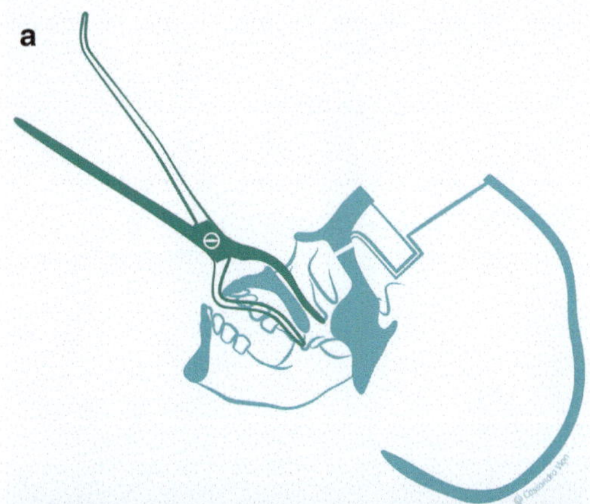

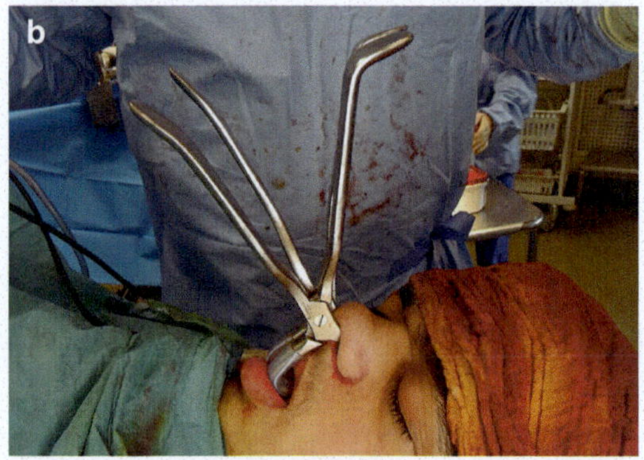

Fig. 18.21 (a) Position of the Rowe forceps on a sagittal section before performing craniofacial disjunction. (b) Intraoperative view of the position of the Rowe forceps before craniofacial disjunction

head osteotomy can also be performed to optimize the curvature of the skull (Fig. 18.27).

Fixation is performed using 2.0 monofilament absorbable sutures and stainless steel sutures (X3) (We try to avoid metallic or absorbable plates which are more prone to get infected). The coronal bony side-wings are used to cover the lateral defects and fixed laterally to the forehead using absorbable sutures.

Internal cranio-orbital distractors are placed and fixed using 4 mm blunt-tipped screws with potentially additional absorbable rivets (Sonicweld Rx®, KLS Martin Group). Intraoperative distraction of approximately 5 mm is performed. The activation arm pierces the skin posterior to the coronal incision line (Fig. 18.28a).

Internal temporo-zygomatic distractors are placed under the temporal muscle and fixed using the superior fixation zone only—the inferior fixation zone must be sectioned. The anterior arm of the temporo-zygomatic distractor is positioned low on the zygoma, close to the zygomatic arch osteotomy line. A small notch to secure the position of the anterior arm can be performed on the posterior aspect of the external orbital wall using gouge forceps. The activation arm is extruded posterior to the coronal incision line (Fig. 18.28b, 18.29 and 18.30).

Fronto-zygomatic osteosynthesis using a curved 1.5 mm titanium plate and 4 mm screws is performed to prevent frontozygomatic disjunction during distraction (Fig. 18.31).

When present, a vertex bulge can be remodeled using a sand dollar design and repositioned using fibrin glue (Fig. 18.32).

In younger patients (before 30 months of age), transfacial pinning using a 2.1 Kirschner wire through the bodies of the zygoma can be considered to avoid maxilla-zygomatic disjunction during distraction (Figs. 18.33 and 18.34).

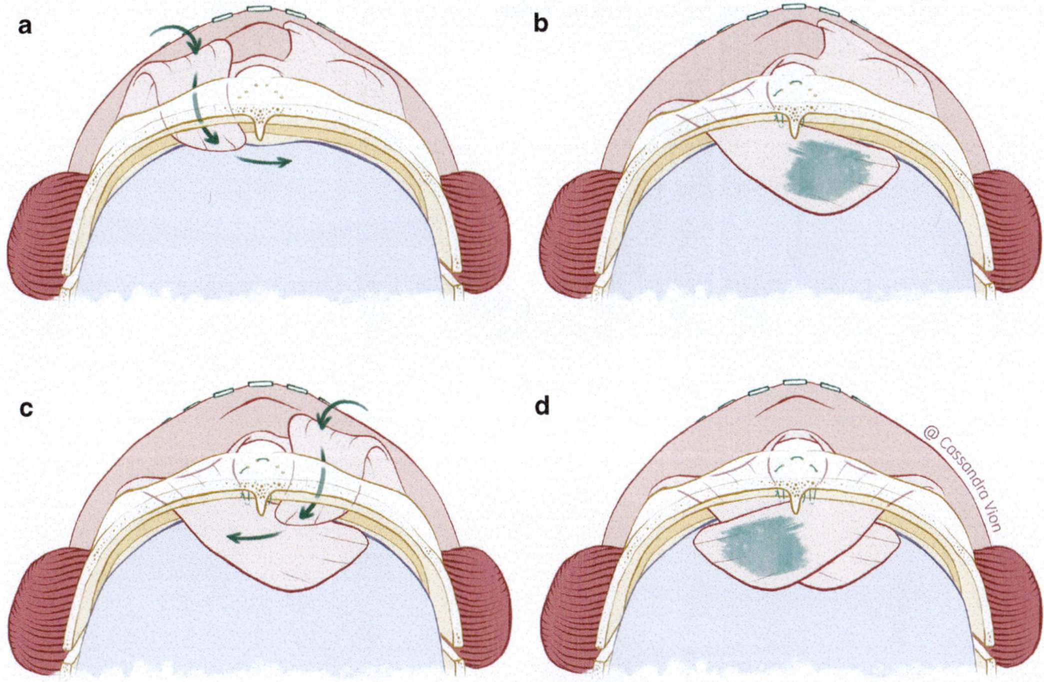

Fig. 18.22 (**a**) Anterior skull base transposition of transorbital periosteal flaps. (**b**) The left flap is sutured to the bandeau towards the right side and glued. (**c**) The same procedure is performed with the right flap towards the left side, creating a double layer on the midline (d) with sutures anteriorly and fibrin glue posteriorly

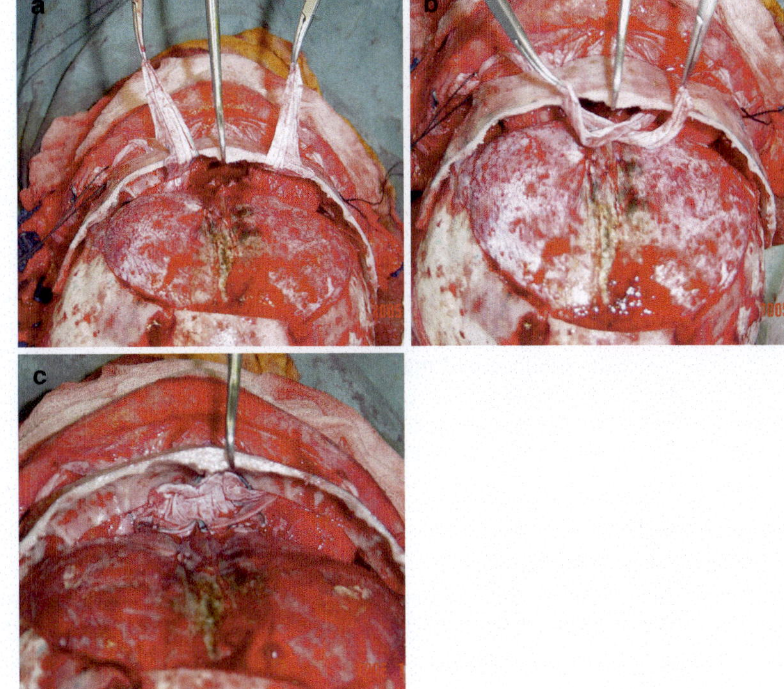

Fig. 18.23 Intraoperative views of anterior skull base reconstruction. (**a**) Transorbital periosteal flaps. (**b**) Crossing of the flaps and coverage of the anterior midline. (**c**) Final sealing using transosseous sutures and glue

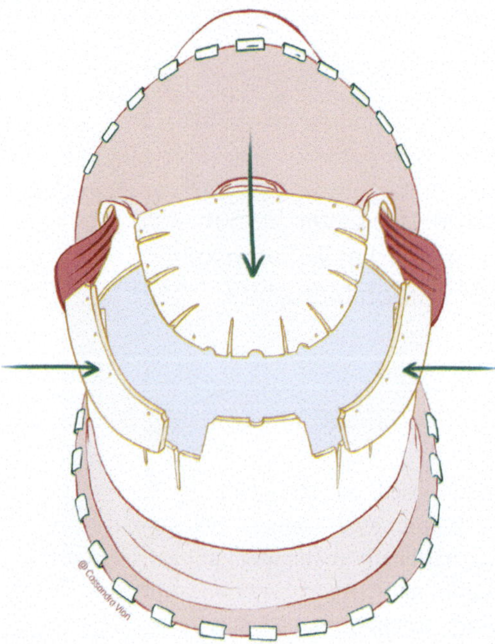

Fig. 18.24 Forehead reconstruction after lateral trimming and barrel-stave osteotomies. Positioning of the two lateral bony side wings

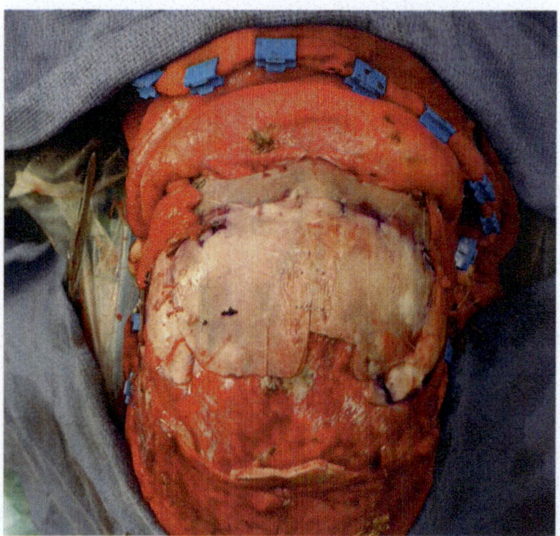

Fig. 18.25 Intraoperative view of a reconstructed forehead after lateral trimming, barrel-stave osteotomies, and fixation of the lateral bony side wings. Fixation is performed using a combination of monofilament absorbable sutures and absorbable osteosynthesis plates

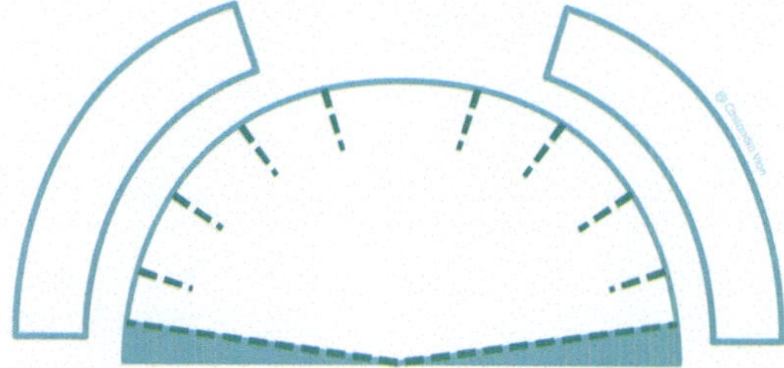

Fig. 18.26 Lateral triangular trimming of the inferior border of the forehead to induce a posterior tilt after firm fixation to the bandeau

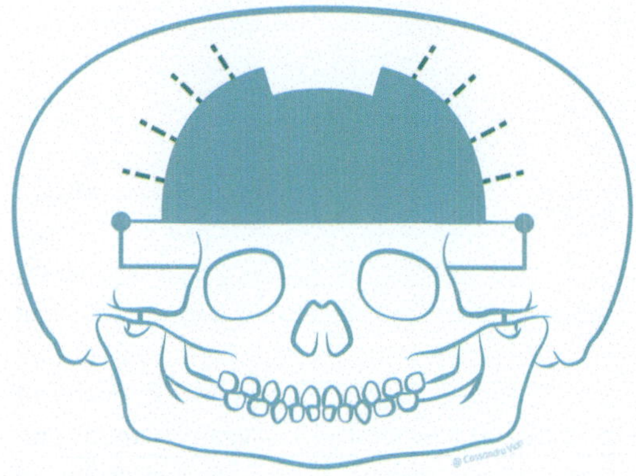

Fig. 18.27 Barrel-stave osteotomies of the skull vault posterior of the forehead osteotomy line

Transfacial pins are also used for external traction in very early FFMBA. Due to frequent severe facial retrusion in younger cases with small zygoma, the pinning can be difficult and lead to considerable damage of the tooth germs. Main justification of its use is the attempt of tracheostomy removal or the prevention of its insertion.

The temporal muscle is repositioned over the distractors and fixed using 3.0 monofilament absorbable sutures to prevent temporal hollowing (Fig. 18.35). A lower posterior backcut of the muscle can be required to allow adequate transposition anteriorly.

Residual bone gaps are filled using bone powder collected during the procedure. The powder is secured using fibrin glue (Fig. 18.36).

An external canthopexy using steel wires or non-adsorbable monofilament suture is performed and generally suspended to the frontozygomatic osteosynthesis plate (Fig. 18.37).

The posterior periosteum is redraped anteriorly to cover the bone fragments and glued (Fig. 18.38a). Suspension using absorbable 4.0 monofilament sutures can be used to drape the periosteum over the vault surface. Bilateral external drainage is used without aspiration in case of unnoticed cerebrospinal fluid leak (Fig. 18.38b).

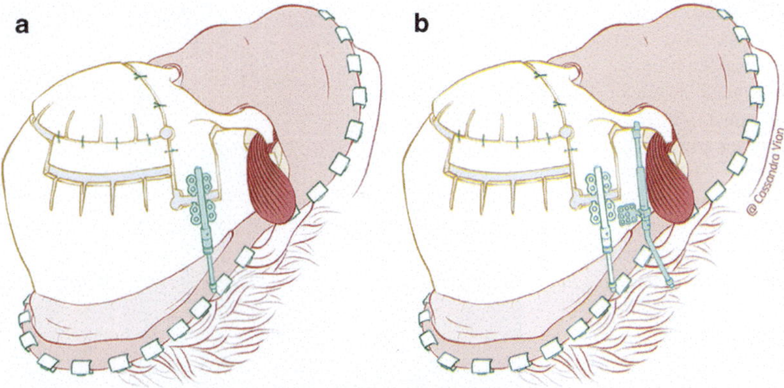

Fig. 18.28 (**a**) Internal cranio-orbital distraction. (**b**) Internal temporo-zygomatic distraction, placed under the temporal muscle

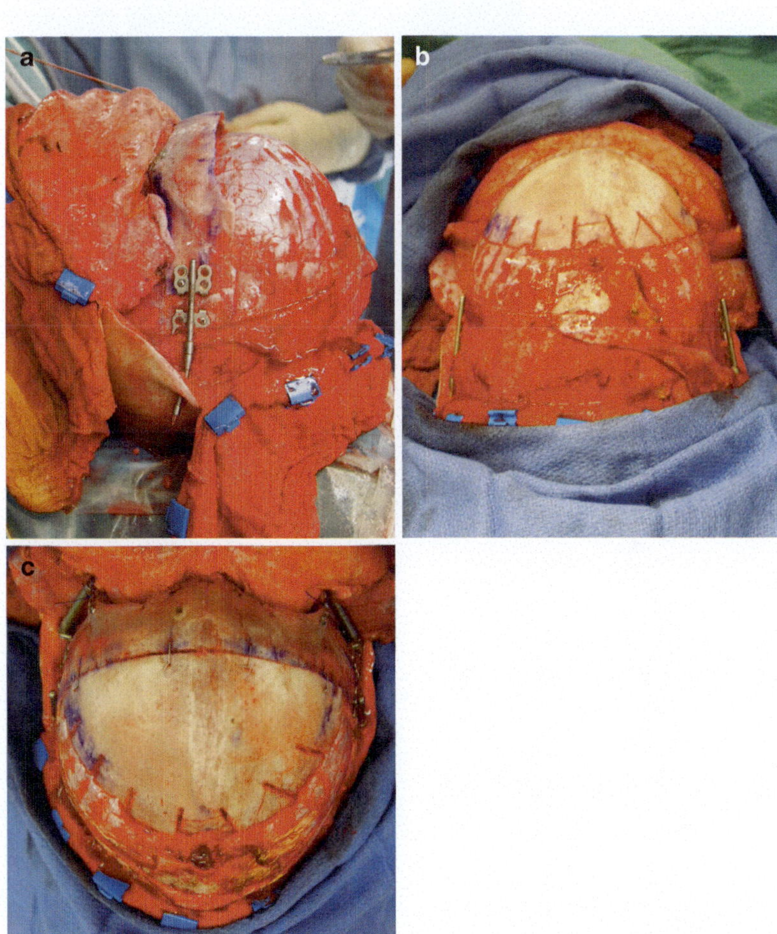

Fig. 18.29 (**a**–**c**) Intraoperative view of internal cranio-orbital activator placement through the skin

The skin is closed using 3.0 and 4.0 braided absorbable sutures with minimal subcutaneous points. Nasopharyngeal tubes with trans-septal fixation are used to maintain airway patency. The tips of the transfacial pin are protected using silicon tubes (Fig. 18.38c). A non-compressive dressing is made. All patients are managed in the pediatric intensive care unit after surgery. Extubation occurs on days 0–5, and nasopharyngeal tubes and tarsorrhaphies are removed according to edema decrease (generally day 3).

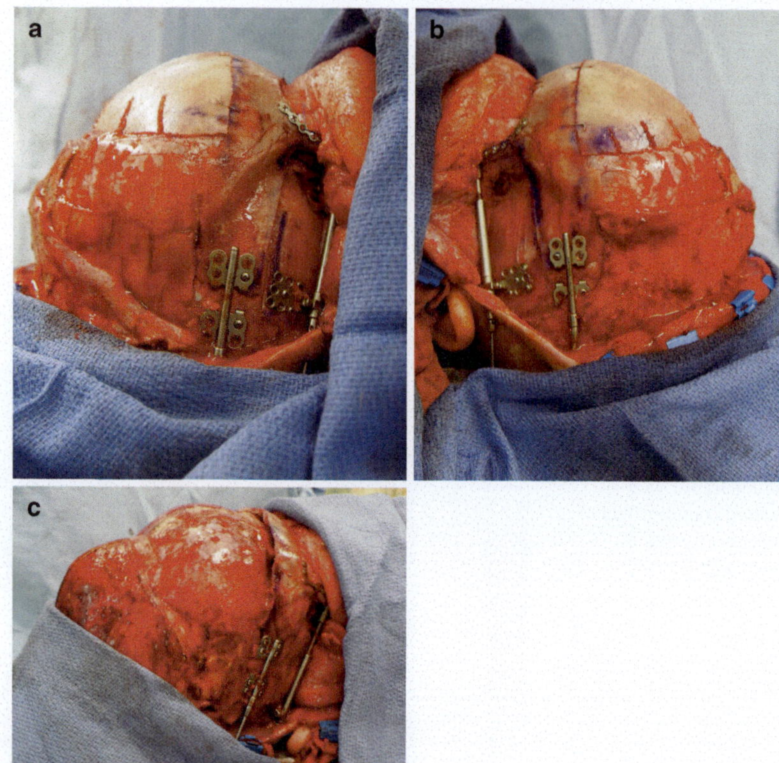

Fig. 18.30 (**a**, **b**) Intraoperative view of internal temporo-zygomatic distractor placement. (**c**) The anterior arm abuts against the lateral orbital rim. It is positioned low, at the level of the zygoma, and secured by performing a small notch on the external orbital rim

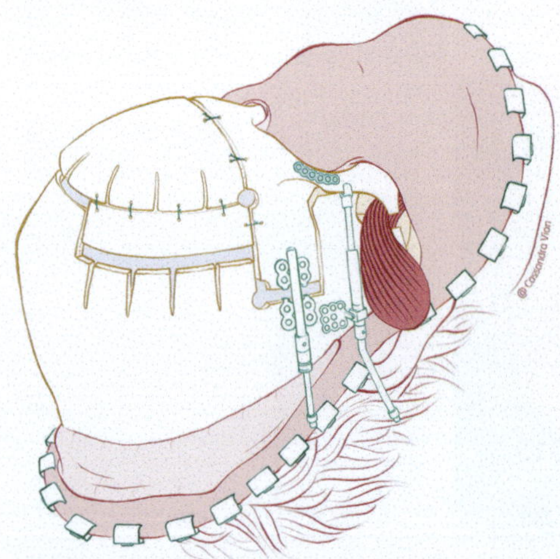

Fig. 18.31 Fronto-zygomatic osteosynthesis using a curved 1.5 mm titanium plate

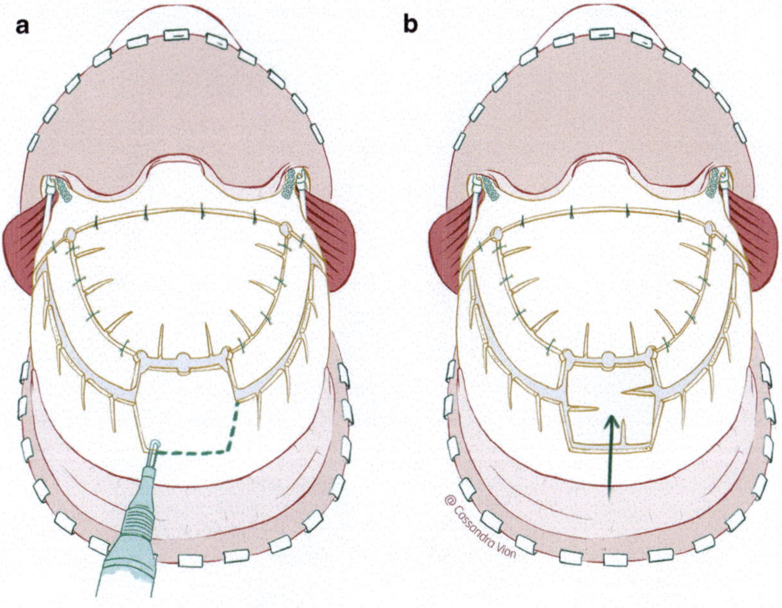

Fig. 18.32 (**a**) Vertex bulge osteotomy. (**b**) Vertex remodeling using a sand dollar design and repositioning using glue

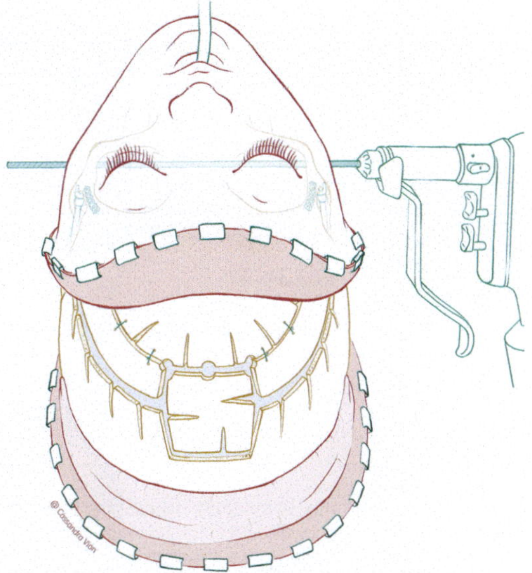

Fig. 18.33 Transfacial pinning using a 2.1 Kirschner wire

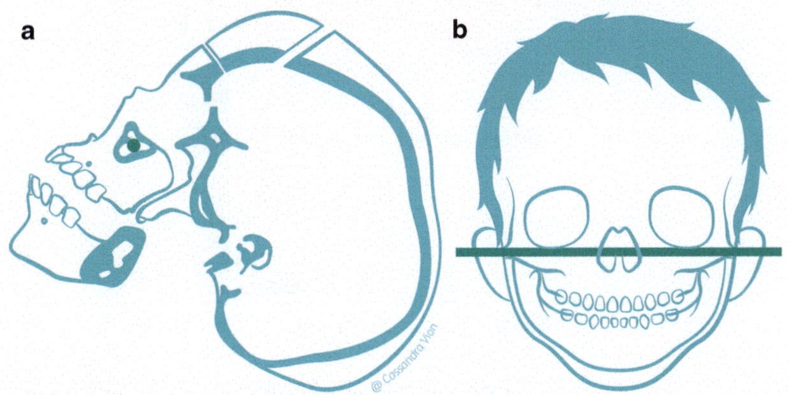

Fig. 18.34 (**a**) Sagittal section showing the transzygomatic position of the wire. (**b**) Frontal view showing the proximity of the pin with the orbital cavity

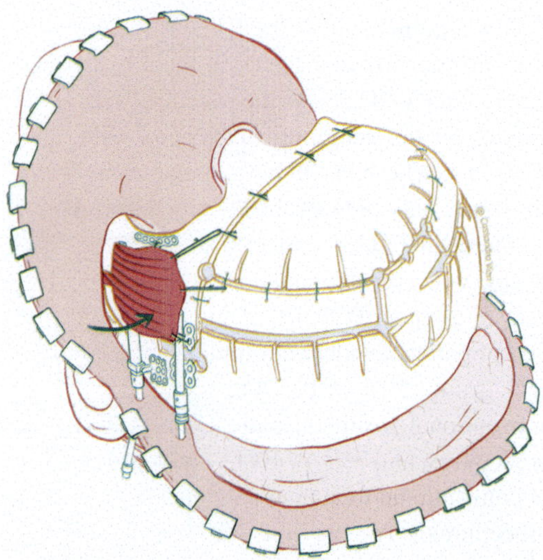

Fig. 18.35 Temporal muscle repositioning after anterior rotation assisted by a low backcut

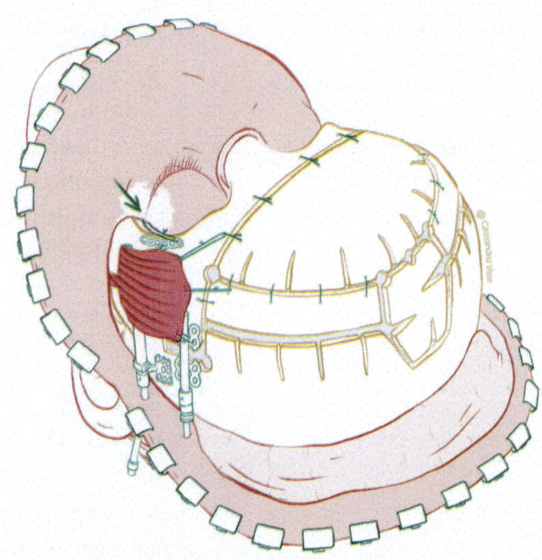

Fig. 18.37 External canthopexy with suspension to the fronto-zygomatic osteosynthesis plate

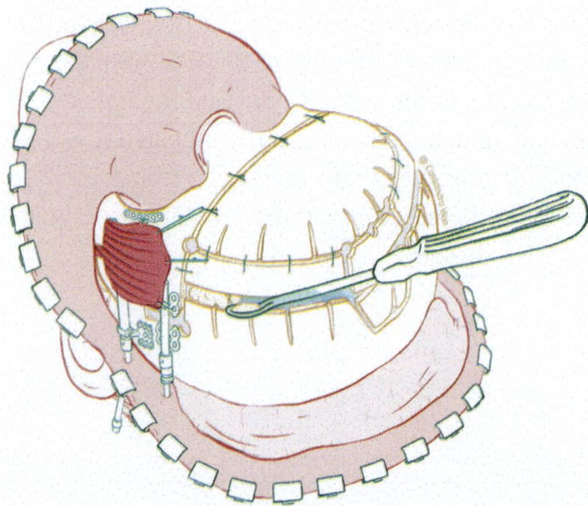

Fig. 18.36 Filling the bony gaps using glued bone powder

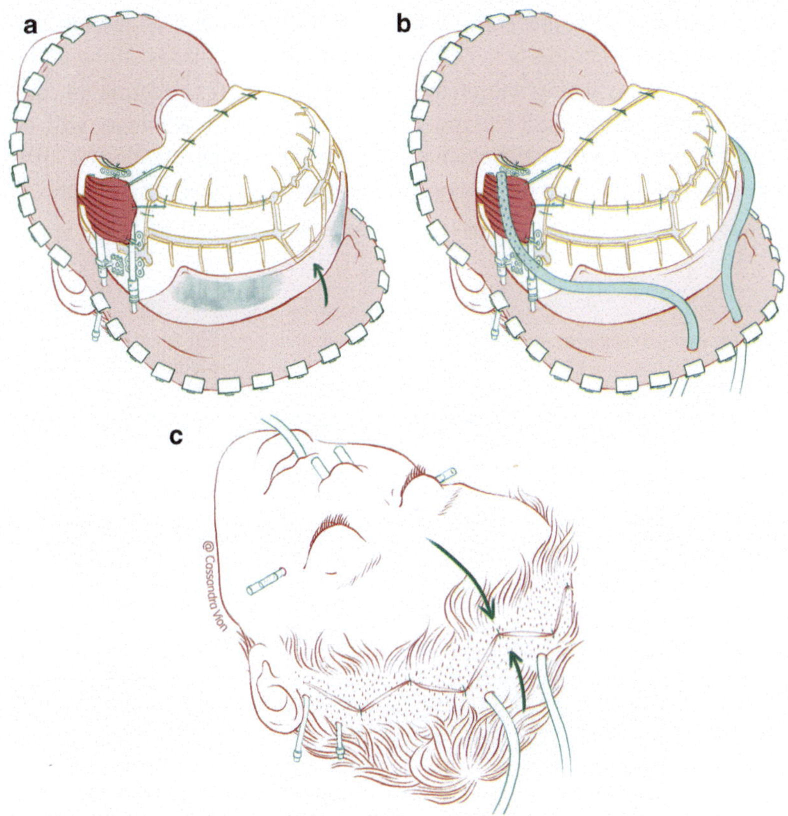

Fig. 18.38 (**a**) Periosteal draping over the skull vault surface. (**b**) External drainage without aspiration. (**c**) Skin closure using 4–0 running Vicryl Rapide (Ethicon) with eversion of the wound edges. Inverted sutures are avoided and reduced to a minimum to avoid suture extrusion. Nasopharyngeal tubes are inserted and the tips of an eventual transfacial pin are covered using silicon sleeves

The activation phase of distraction generally starts on day 2 after a control CT scan.

Results of FFMBA in the Patient with Apert Syndrome

The exorbitism was corrected in all cases. It is well known that FFMBA is the most powerful tool to enlarge an orbit. However, exorbitism in the patient with Apert syndrome is rarely extreme; therefore, the full correction was easily obtained.

The results of the correction of OSAS were less drastic: the mean AHI dropped from 15.2/h to 6.8 /h postoperatively. In the 24 patients with Apert syndrome, 17 of them underwent total correction of OSAS, but 7 were improved without attaining complete normalization. Those necessitated a secondary facial advancement with a Le Fort III with rotations of the hemi-faces. By splitting the cohort, it appears that the subgroup which were not quite corrected by FFMBA were more severe. As it appears in Table 18.1 the group who ended ip with both necessitating a FFMBA and a LF3 presented with a more severe OSAS.

Table 18.1 Effect of fronto-facial monobloc advancement (FFMBA) and Le Fort III osteotomy (LF3) on obstructive sleep apnea (quantified using Apnea–Hyponea Index (AHI) in Apert syndrome

APERT 16/24	All FFMBA	FFMBA alone	FFMBA and LF3
Age at surgery (year)	4.5	3	6
AHI pre-op.	15.8	11.3	24
AHI postop.	6.5	5.8	7.8

Adapted from Khonsari et al. [32], Haber et al. [34]

Considering those results, most patients with Apert syndrome treated by FFMBA could avoid an early secondary Le Fort III to reach a normal respiratory status. For the two patients who had a tracheostomy, the tracheostomy could be removed after Le Fort III advancement, but they were dependent on the need for a CPAP after surgery. In all cases, the preventive removal of tonsils and adenoids ensures better OSAS reduction, as it enlarges the airway and creates scar tissue, which reduces pharyngeal collapse.

In the subgroup of patients who did not need an early Le Fort III for respiratory reasons, there will be a time in the subsequent growth, at the latest at adolescent age, for a Le Fort III with split hemifaces allowing reduction in hypertelorism and correction of angulation of upper maxilla. This sequence will continue with orthognathic surgery followed by rhinoplasty and ancillary aesthetic procedures (See chapter on Aesthetic refinements).

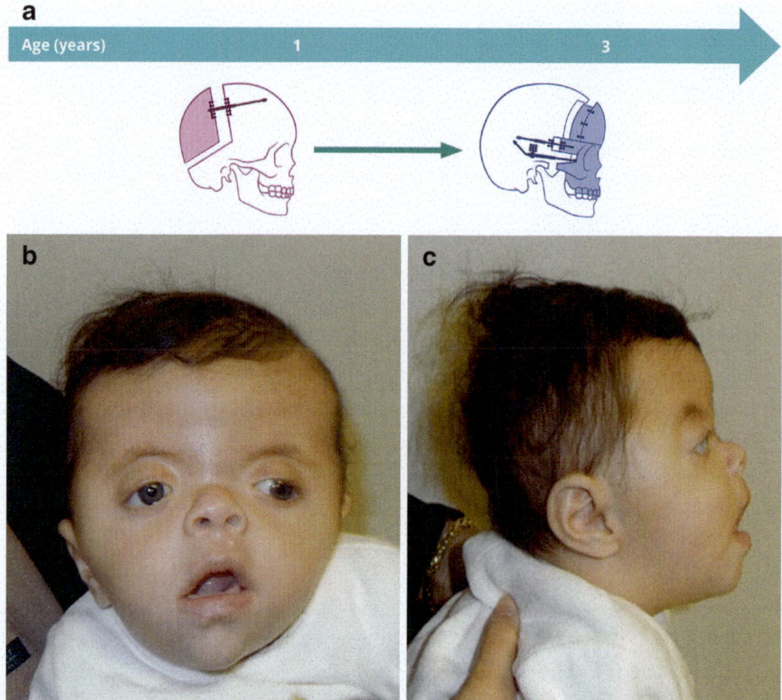

Fig. 18.39 In Fig 18.39, from a to b' there is a sequence from infancy to childhood, including posterior distraction and frontofacial monobloc

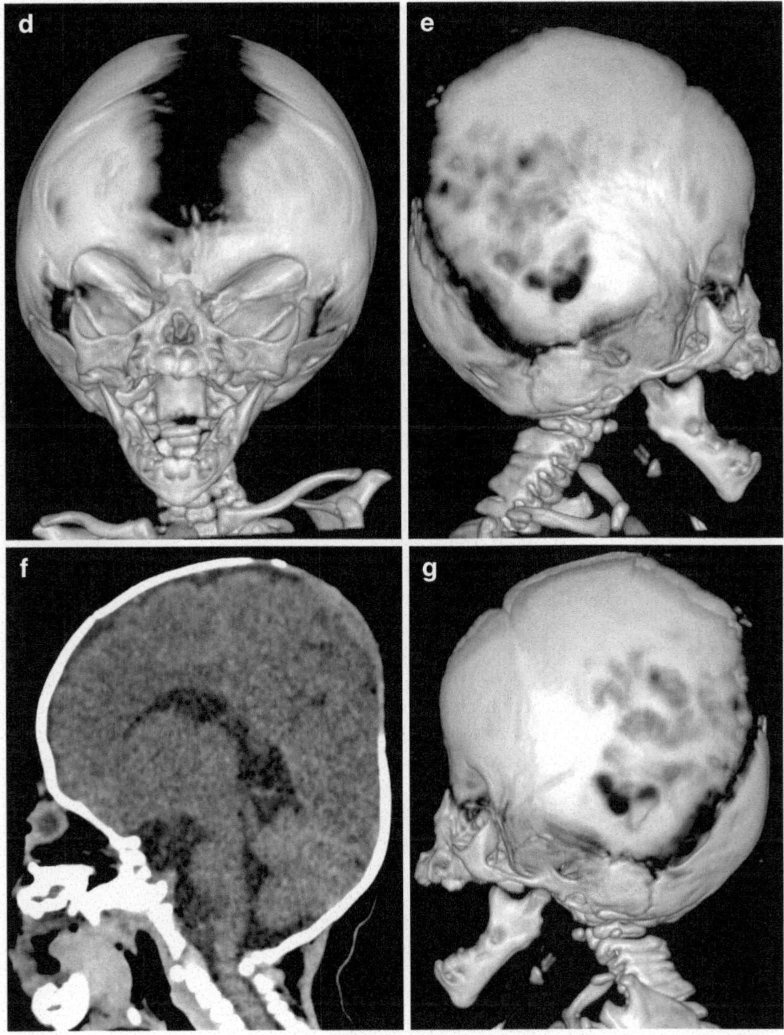

Fig. 18.39 (continued)

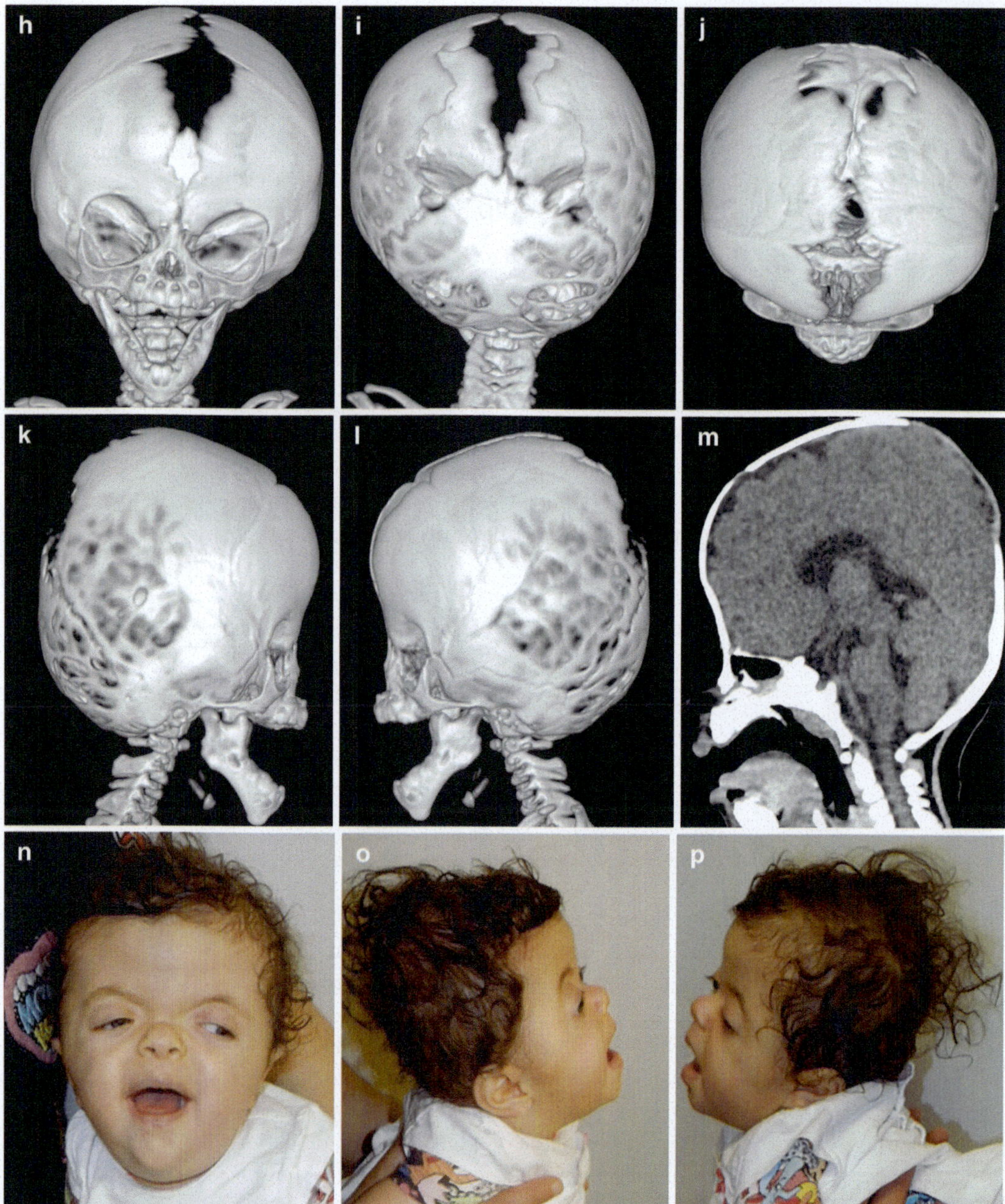

Fig. 18.39 (continued)

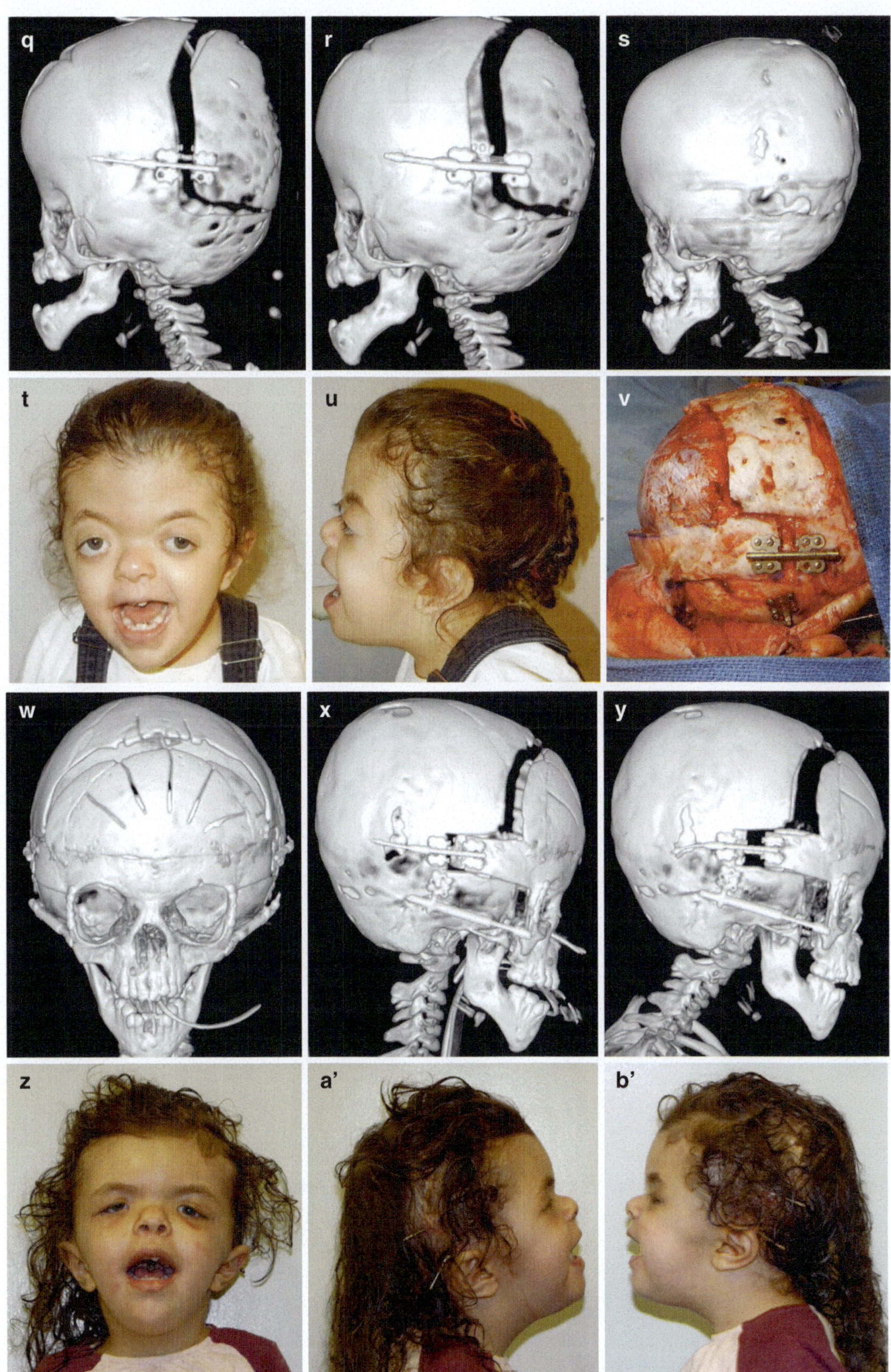

Fig. 18.39 (continued)

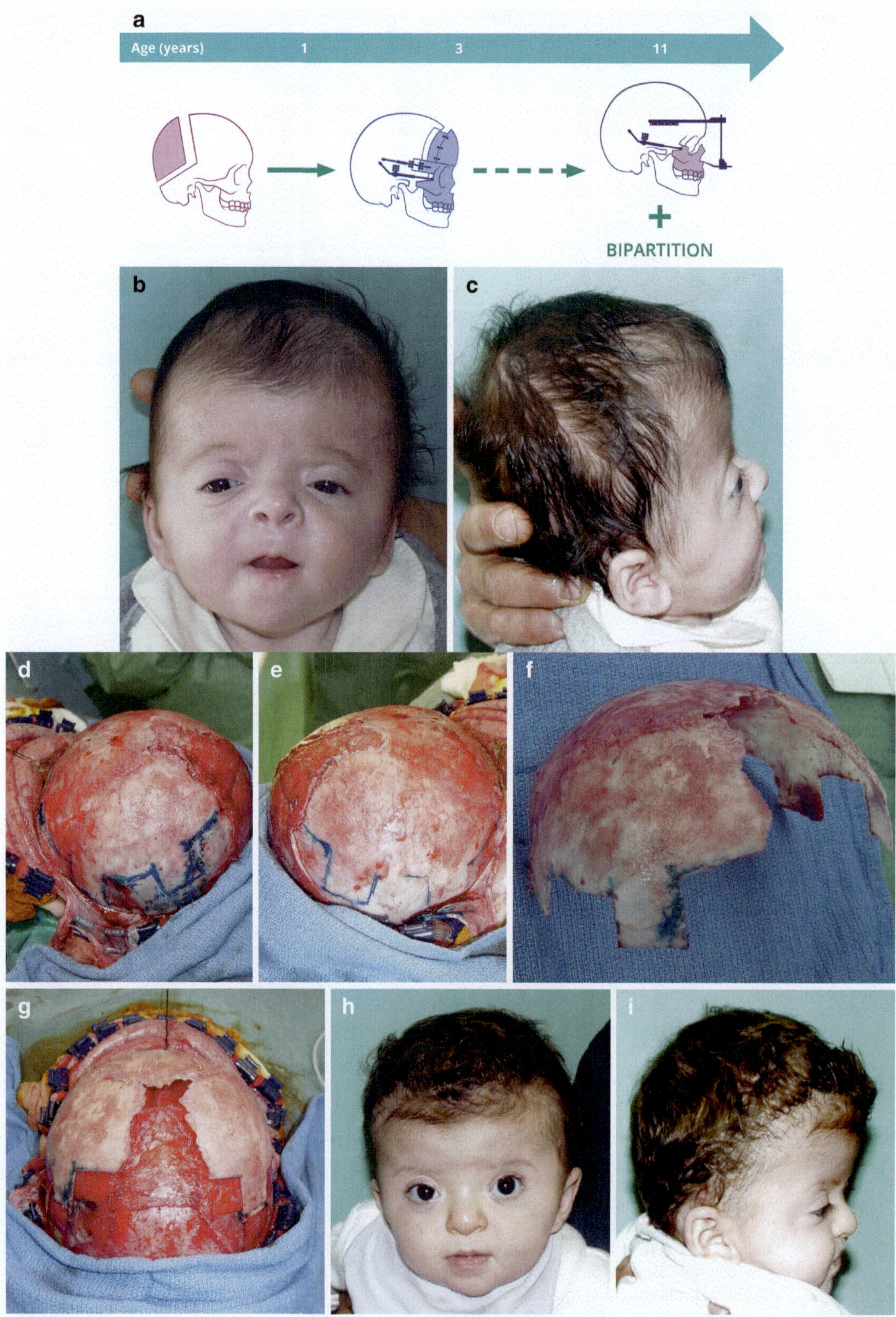

Fig. 18.40 In Fig 18.40, from a to g' there is a sequence from infancy to adolescence, including posterior expansion (without distraction), then frontofacial monobloc and LeFort 3 advancement

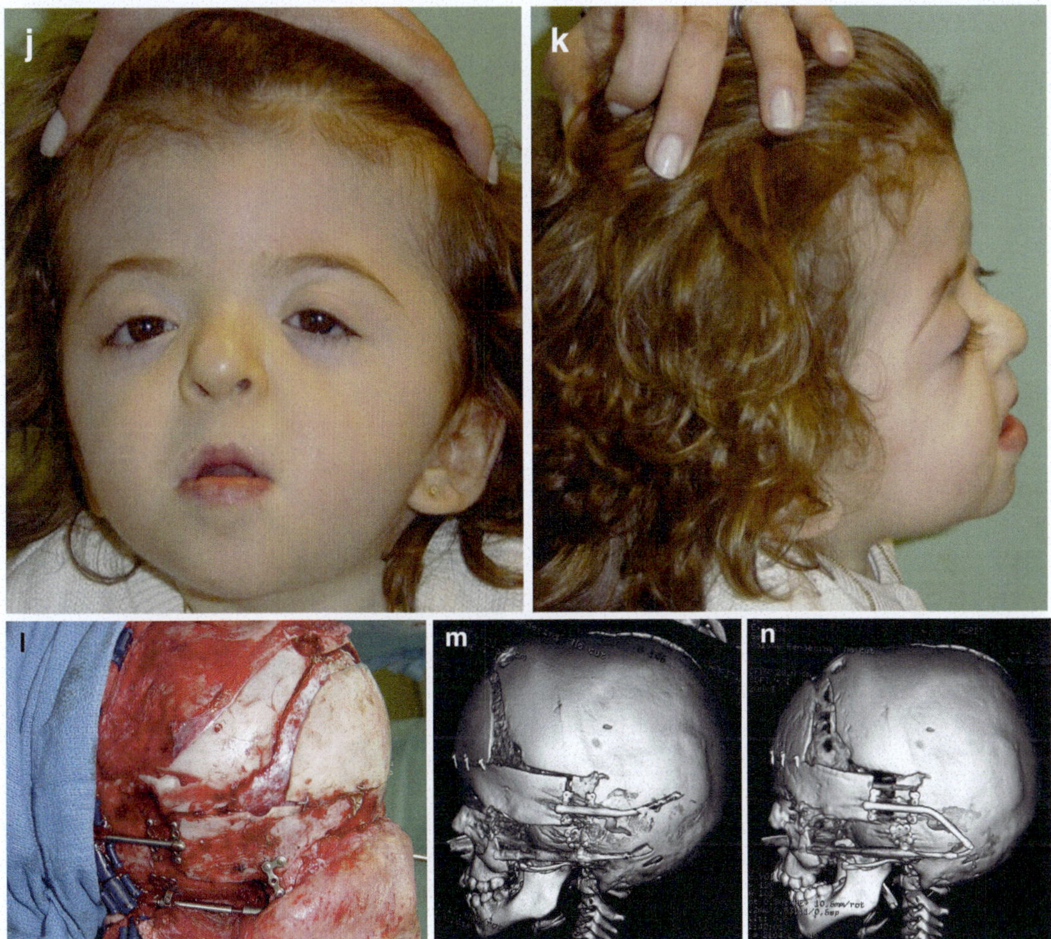

Fig. 18.40 (continued)

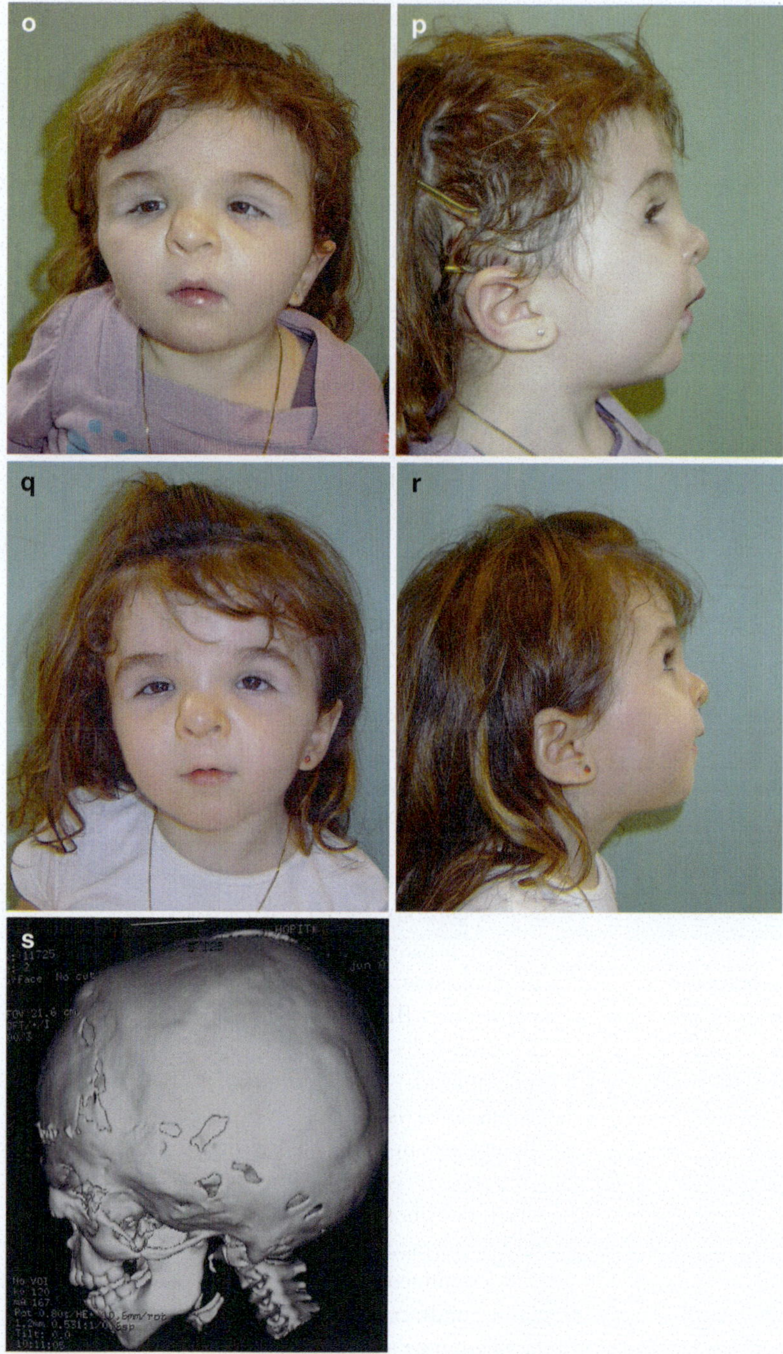

Fig. 18.40 (continued)

t u v w x y z

Fig. 18.40 (continued)

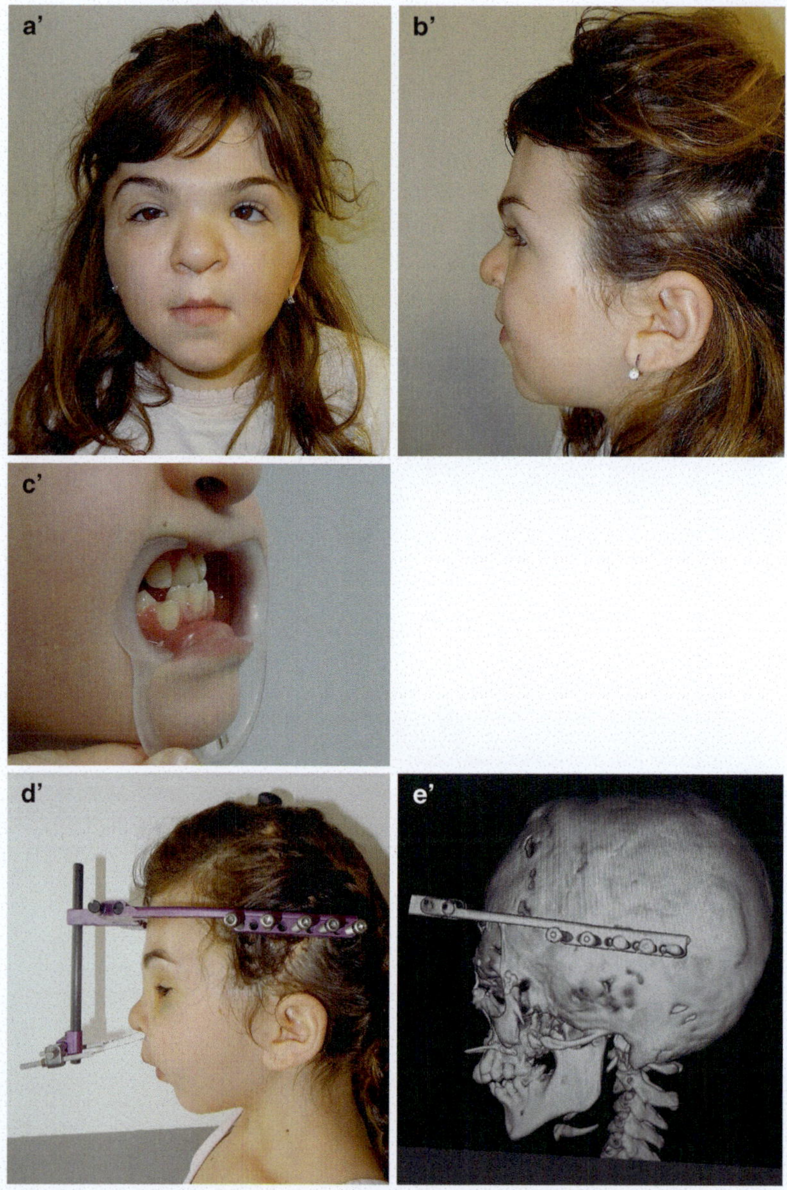

Fig. 18.40 (continued)

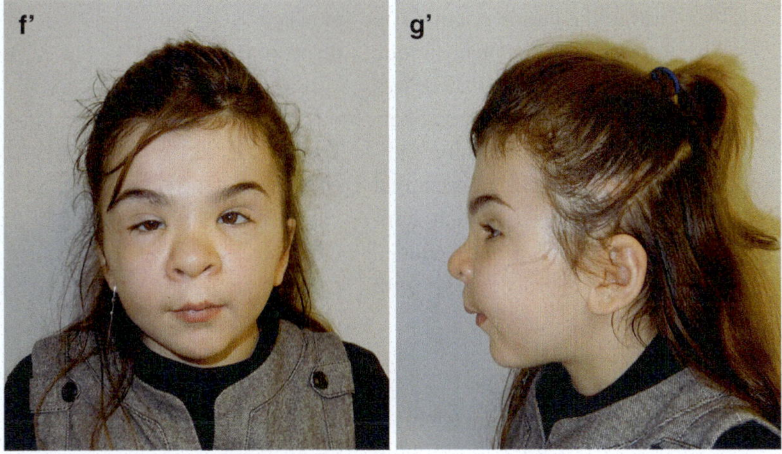

Fig. 18.40 (continued)

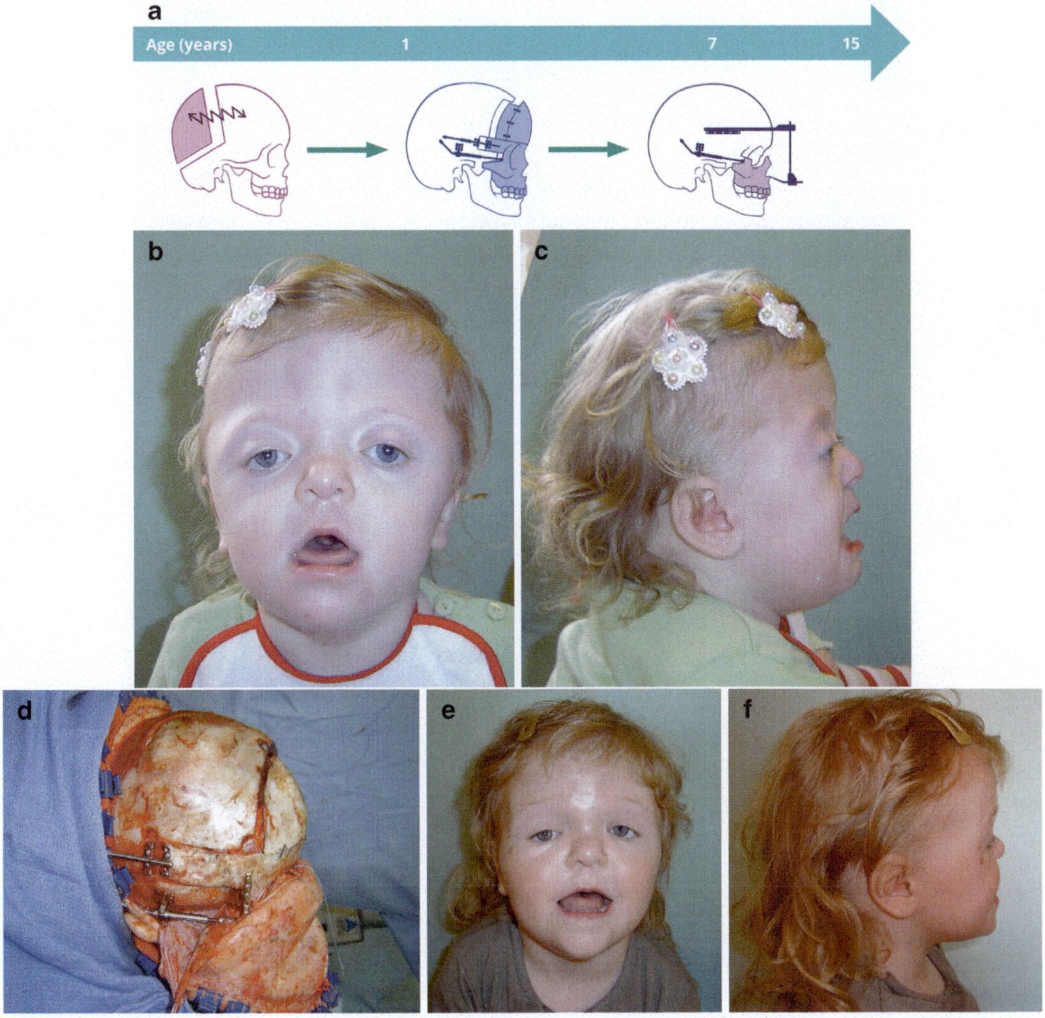

a

Age (years) 1 7 15

b c

d e f

Fig. 18.41 In Fig 18.41, from a to p there is a sequence from infancy to adolescence, including posterior distraction, frontofacial monobloc, and LeFort 3. Last pictures show patient before orthognatic surgery

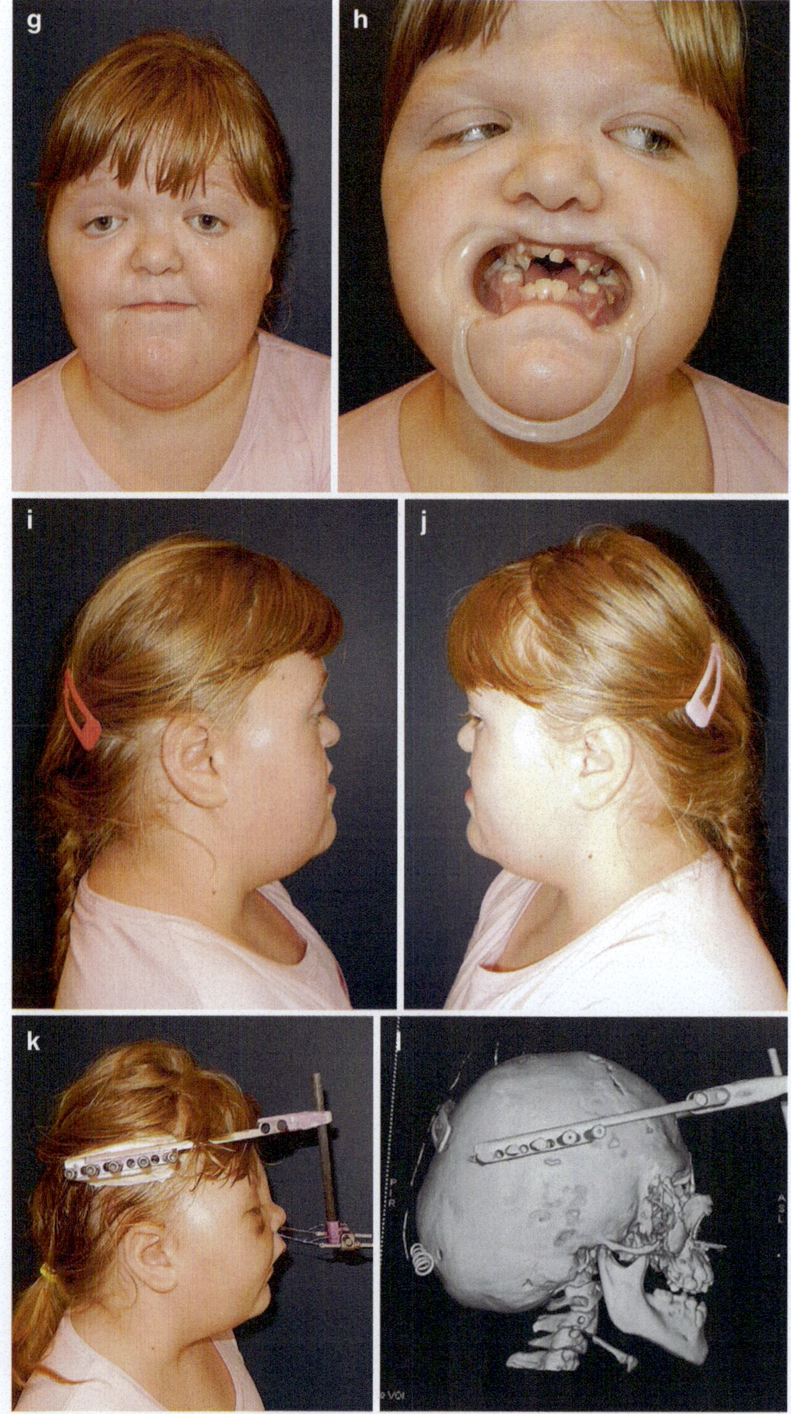

Fig. 18.41 (continued)

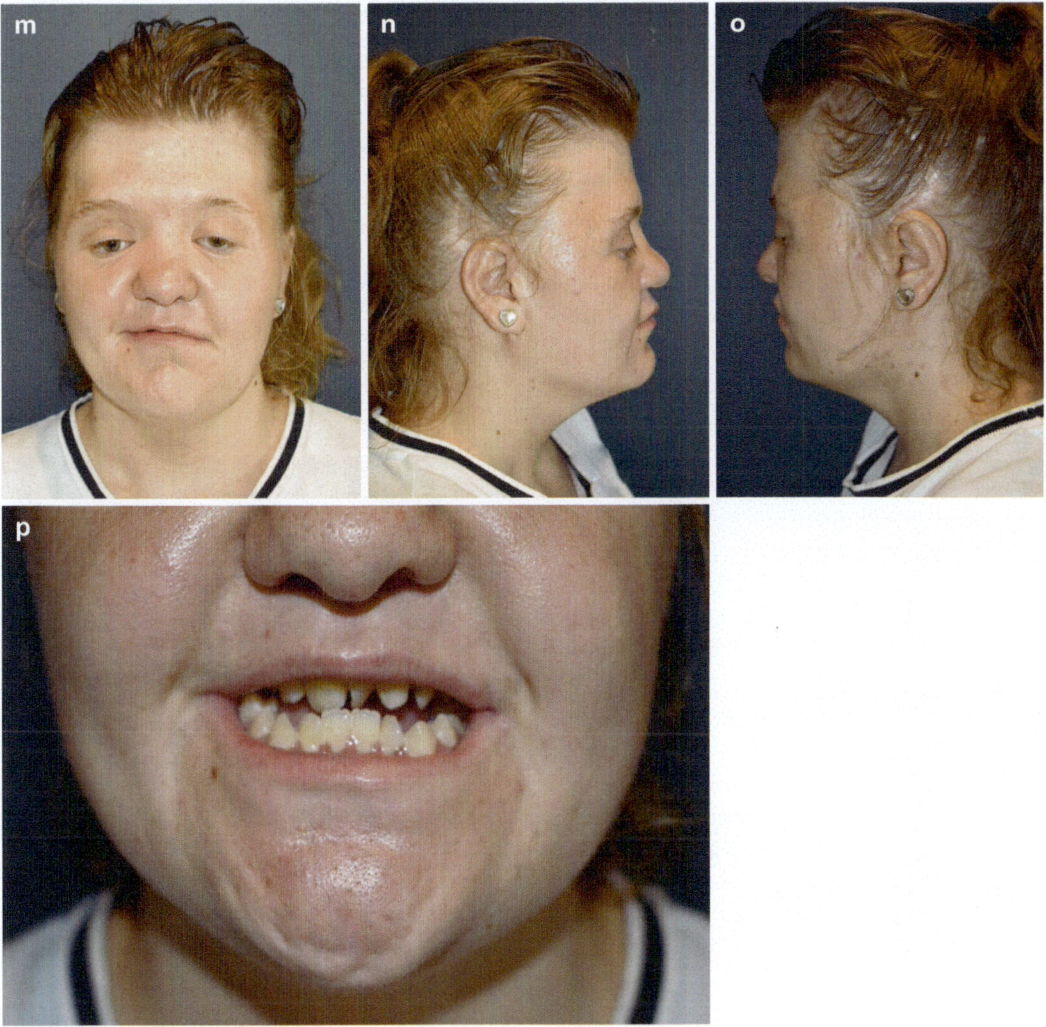

Fig. 18.41 (continued)

Examples of Patients with Apert Syndrome Who Underwent FFMBA (Figs. 18.39, 18.40 and 18.41)

Important Messages—Necker Protocol

- Most patients with Apert syndrome require a posterior distraction (PD), especially before FFMBA.
- Indication for FFMBA mainly relies on the association of significant exorbitism and OSAS.
- Internal distractors are preferred at a young age. The distraction rate might be slower (0.5 mm/day) and carefully monitored as brain

re-expansion is slower in patients with Apert syndrome.

- Exorbitism correction occurred in all patients.
- OSA correction occurred in 17/24 patients and 7/24 patients needed a secondary Le Fort III to treat the OSA, because of insufficient initial correction. OSA assessment by polysomnography should be performed at least six months after removal of internal distractors because the devices stimulate inflammation during the consolidation period, which will take time to disappear.
- FFMBA can provide 10 years free of symptoms and therefore delay secondary surgery.
- In patients with Apert syndrome, a Le Fort III with rotation of the hemifacial segments will be necessary at some point of the therapeutical sequences to address the triangular shape of the face, reduce the hypertelorism, and correct the palatal angulation.
- Tonsils and adenoids should be removed preventively before FFMBA to ensure a better respiratory status after FFMBA. CPAP is a useful tool whenever necessary before surgery or after FFMBA if a secondary Le Fort III is necessary to correct the OSAS.

References

1. Arnaud E, Marchac D, Renier D. Double internal distraction with monobloc advancement in infants. In E. Arnaud, P. A. Diner, Eds. Proceedings of the 3rd International Congress on cranial and facial bone distraction processes. Paris, France June 14–16, 2001: 455–460.
2. Arnaud E, Marchac D, Renier D. Evaluation of frontofacial monobloc advancement with quadruple internal distraction-abstract N° 20. Childs Nerv Syst. 2003;19:610.
3. Arnaud E, Marchac D, Renier D. Quadruple internal distraction with monobloc advancement: experience with 19 cases. Proceedings of the 3rd International Congress on cranial and facial bone distraction processes. Paris, France July 2–5, 2003:191–195.
4. Cinalli G, Renier D, Sebag G, et al. Chronic tonsillar herniation in Crouzon's and Apert's syndromes: the role of premature synostosis of the lambdoid suture. J Neurosurg. 1995;83(4):575–82.
5. Nowinski D, Di Rocco F, Renier D, et al. Posterior cranial vault expansion in the treatment of craniosynostosis. Comparison of current techniques. Childs Nerv Syst. 2012;28(9):1537–44.
6. Arnaud E, Marchac A, Jeblaoui Y, et al. Spring-assisted posterior skull expansion without osteotomies. Childs Nerv Syst. 2012;28(9):1545–9.
7. Swanson JW, Samra F, Bauder A, et al. An algorithm for managing syndromic craniosynostosis using posterior vault distraction osteogenesis. Plast Reconstr Surg. 2016;137(5):829e–41e.
8. Florisson JMG, Barmpalios G, Lequin M, et al. Venous hypertension in syndromic and complex craniosynostosis: the abnormal anatomy of the jugular foramen and collaterals. J Craniomaxillofac Surg. 2015;43(3):312–8.
9. Jeevan DS, Anlsow P, Jayamohan J. Abnormal venous drainage in syndromic craniosynostosis and the role of CT venography. Childs Nerv Syst. 2008;24(12):1413–20.
10. Cornelissen MJ, de Goederen R, Doerga P, et al. Pilot study of intracranial venous physiology in craniosynostosis. J Neurosurg Pediatr. 2018;21(6):626–31.
11. Ghali GZ, Zaki Ghali MG, Ghali EZ, et al. Intracranial venous hypertension in craniosynostosis: mechanistic underpinnings and therapeutic implications. World Neurosurg 2018 Aug 6
12. Arnaud E, Di Rocco F. Faciocraniosynostosis: monobloc frontofacial osteotomy replacing the two-stage strategy? Childs Nerv Syst. 2012;28(9):1557–64.
13. Arnaud E, Paternoster G, James S, et al. Craniofacial strategy for syndromic craniosynostosis. Ann Chir Plast Esthet. 2016;61(5):408–19.
14. Mathijssen I, Arnaud E, Marchac D, Morisseau-Durand MP, Mireau E, Guérin P, Renier D. Respiratory outcome of midface advancement with distraction: a comparison between Le Fort III and frontofacial monobloc. J Craniofac Surg. 2006;17(5):880–2.
15. Oyama A, Arnaud E, Marchac D, Renier D. Reossification of cranium and zygomatic arch after monobloc frontofacial distraction advancement for syndromic craniosynostosis. J Craniofac Surg. 2009;20(Suppl 2):1905–9.
16. Noordzij N, Brouwer R, van der Horst C. Incomplete reossification after craniosynostosis surgery. J Craniofac Surg. 2016;27(1):e105–8.
17. Thenier-Villa JL, Sanromán-Álvarez P, Miranda-Lloret P, et al. Incomplete reossification after craniosynostosis surgery-incidence and analysis of risk factors: a clinical-radiological assessment study. J Neurosurg Pediatr. 2018;22(2):120–7.
18. Bouaoud J, Hennocq Q, Paternoster G, et al. Excessive ossification of the bandeau in Crouzon and Apert syndromes. J Craniomaxillofac Surg. 2020;48(4):376–82.
19. Morice A, Paternoster G, Ostertag A, et al. Anterior skull base and pericranial flap ossification after frontofacial monobloc advancement. Plast Reconstr Surg. 2018;141(2):437–45.

20. Arnaud E, Paternoster G, James S, Meyer Ph. Prise en charge cranio-faciale du syndrome d'Apert. Gaz Soc F Orthop Ped. 2016, Mars-Avril; 45:10–11.
21. Arnaud E, Paternoster G, James S, Morisseau-Durand MP, Couloigner V, Diner P, Tomat C, Viot-Blanc V, Fauroux B, Cormier-Daire V, Baujat G, Robert M, Picard A, Antunez S, Khonsari H, Pamphile-Tabuteau L, Legros C, Zerah M, Meyer P. Stratégie craniofaciale pour les faciocraniosténoses. Ann Chir Plast. 2016;61:408–19.
22. Morice A, Paternoster G, Ostertag A, James S, Cohen-Solal M, Khonsari RH, Arnaud E. Anterior skull base and pericranial flap ossification after frontofacial monobloc advancement. Plast Reconstr Surg. 2018;141(2):437–45.
23. Sicard L, Hounkpevi M, Tomat C, James S, Paternoster G, Khonsari RH, Arnaud E. Dental consequences of pterygomaxillary dysjunction during fronto-facial monobloc advancement with internal distraction for Crouzon syndrome. J Craniomaxillofac Surg. 2018;46(9):1476–9.
24. Khonsari RH, Hennocq Q, Nysjö J, Sandy R, Haber S, James S, Britto JA, Paternoster G, Arnaud E. Defining critical ages for orbital shape changes after frontofacial advancement in Crouzon syndrome. Plast Reconstr Surg. 2019;144(5):841–52.
25. Khonsari H, Morice A, Paternoster G, James S, Sicard L, Morisseau-Durand MP, Fauroux B, Couloigner V, Diner P, Tomat C, Robert M, Arnaud E. Quantitative facial and orbital assessments of fronto-facial monobloc advancement with internal distraction in faciocraniosynostoses. ISCFS 2019 Paris Abstract Supplement. Plast Reconstr Surg -GO. 2019;7(8S-2):6–7.
26. Paternoster G, Dahiez X, Andre K, Pamphile-Tabuteau L, Angeard N, Khonsari H, James S, Zerah M, Arnaud E. Cognitive assessment in school age Crouzon and Pfeiffer after early frontofacial monobloc. ISCFS 2019 Paris Abstract Supplement. Plast Reconstr Surg -GO. 2019;7(8S-2):7–8.
27. Arnaud E, Paternoster G, Khonsari H, Haber S, Hennocq Q, James S, Morisseau-Durand MP, Fauroux B, Amaddeo A, Cormier-Daire V, Couloigner V, Diner P, Tomat C, Robert M, Meyer P. Necker experience of frontofacial monobloc advancement with distraction (FFMBA) about 145 cases in faciocraniosynostotic children. ISCFS 2019 Paris Abstract Supplement. Plast Reconstr Surg -GO. 2019;7(8S-2):8–9.
28. Arnaud E, Antunez S, Khonsari H, Haber S, Paternoster G, James S, Meyer P. Transfacial external traction and internal distraction for young and severe faciocraniosynostoses: the very early monobloc. ISCFS 2019 Paris Abstract Supplement. Plast Reconstr Surg -GO. 2019;7(8S-2):9.
29. Khonsari RH, Haber S, Paternoster G, Fauroux B, Morisseau-Durand MP, Cormier-Daire V, Legeai-Mallet L, James S, Hennocq Q, Arnaud E. The influence of fronto-facial monobloc advancement on obstructive sleep apnea: an assessment of 109 syndromic craniosynostoses cases. J Craniomaxillofac Surg. 2020;48(6):536–47.
30. Paternoster G, Haber SE, Khonsari RH, James S, Arnaud E. Craniosynostosis: Monobloc distraction with internal device and its variant for infants with severe craniosynostosis. Clin Plast Surg. 2021;48(3):497–506.
31. Haber SE, Leikola J, Nowinski D, Fauroux B, Morisseau-Durand MP, Paternoster G, Khonsari RH, Arnaud E. Secondary Le Fort III after early frontofacial monobloc normalizes sleep apnea in faciocraniosynostosis: a cohort study. J Plast Reconstr Aesthet Surg. 2022;1:S1748–6815(22)00123–1.
32. Rickart AJ, van de Lande LS, O' Sullivan E, Bloch K, Arnaud E, Schievano S, Jeelani NUO, Paternoster G, Khonsari R, Dunaway DJ. Comparison of internal and external distraction in frontofacial monobloc advancement: a three-dimensional quantification. Plast Reconstr Surg. 2023;152(3):612–22.
33. Landart M, Benichi S, James S, Arnaud É, Paternoster G, Khonsari RH. Frontal bone resorption after frontofacial monobloc advancement in FGFR-related craniosynostoses: predictive factors. Plast Reconstr Surg. 2024;11:1740. https://doi.org/10.1097/PRS.0000000000011740.
34. Guérin J, Hennocq Q, Paternoster G, Arnaud É, Khonsari RHJ. Distractor position and distraction amplitude in fronto-facial monobloc advancement: a case series. Stomatol Oral Maxillofac Surg. 2024;125(5S2):101942.
35. Kogane N, Hennocq Q, Collet C, Touzé R, Arnaud É, Paternoster G, Khonsari RH. Optic nerve elongation during fronto-facial surgery for Crouzon syndrome: 3D quantification and clinical implications. J Neurosurg Pediatr. 2024;34(4):414–22.

19 Monobloc Advancement with External Distraction

Nivaldo Alonso and Cristiano Tonello

Introduction

Apert syndrome is a complex autosomal dominant genetic disorder with early closure of cranial and facial sutures, midface retrusion, and limb anomalies. The syndrome is well known as acrocephalosyndactyly type I. The craniofacial findings include supraorbital ridging, marked maxillary hypoplasia, mild ocular proptosis, down slanting palpebral fissure, small nose, and convex face. In addition to these craniofacial phenotypic signs, findings include neurologic, cardiac, and intellectual abnormalities. Most patients with Apert syndrome have one of two mutations in the FGFR 2 gene. Many phenotypic variations in the skeleton and soft tissue are based on this genetic variation, such as the increased incidence of cleft palate found in patients with the Ser252Trp mutation and the complex syndactyly in the hands and feet found in patients with the Pro253Arg mutation [1]. Approximately 70% of patients with Apert syndrome carry the mutation Ser252Trp. This mutation induces abnormalities in the central nervous system in newborn Apert mouse models, indicating that patients with Apert syndrome could be similarly affected [2]. Yacubian-Fernandes et al. described more than 65% of brain malformations, with ventricular enlargement, septum pellucidum hypoplasia, and corpus callosum hypoplasia being the most prevalent [3]. Additionally, Chiari malformation and hydrocephalus could warrant early procedures, and choanal atresia is a clinical condition in some early intervention patients [4]. Despite these possibilities, our large series of patients with Apert syndrome only included three cases of hydrocephalus requiring a ventriculi-peritoneal shunt and one Chiari malformation.

Anatomic Considerations

Some anatomical issues—such as brain expansion, visual protection, and airway considerations—are crucial for surgical treatment. Forte et al. demonstrated that cranial and facial synostosis cause patients with Apert syndrome to have a shorter maxilla with a much more obtuse sphenoid divergence angle than normal controls at the same age. This explains a short anterior cranial fossa and the need for early cranial expansion, and here we could consider posterior vault distraction osteogenesis (PVDO) or frontal–orbital advancement (FOA) to expand the cranial vault [5]. Surgical options are based on the type of cra-

N. Alonso (✉)
Department of Plastic Surgery, Faculdade de Medicina da Universidade de São Paulo, São Paulo, São Paulo, Brazil

Craniofacial Division, Hospital for Rehabilitation of Craniofacial Anomalies and University of São Paulo, São Paulo, Brazil
e-mail: nivalonso@usp.br

C. Tonello
Craniofacial Unit HRAC Bauru USP Bauru, São Paulo, Brazil

J. G. Meara et al. (eds.), *Apert Syndrome*, https://doi.org/10.1007/978-3-032-12551-4_19

niosynostosis present. In cases with a wide fontanelle and only bi-coronal suture fusion, we prefer the option of late FOA at one year of age with multiple-suture fusion and PVDO. In a series of 31 patients with Apert syndrome who did not undergo surgery, Lu et al. observed that bi-coronal synostosis is the most common type of craniosynostosis; less common are pan synostosis and coronal with other sutures involved. In this study, the authors found important differences between the cranial fossa and the airway, with patients with bi-coronal synostosis more likely to require anterior expansion. However, airway obstruction is more severe in these patients because of the cranial base angle (Fig. 19.1) [6]. Due to the rapid evolution of cranial sutures in patients with Apert syndrome, observing those changes is important for identifying those that require immediate intervention (Fig. 19.2).

Patients with Apert syndrome have early closing of the sphenoidal sutures that result in shallow orbital floor and roof—causing short orbits—and retruded superior and inferior orbital margins. Additionally, the anterior cranial fossa enlarges lateral orbital walls, creating the need to expand the anterior cranial fossa (Fig. 19.3) [7, 8]. Enlarged temporal fossae can also cause problems with positioning internal distractors (ID) during future osteotomies, such as early frontofacial monobloc advancement (FFMBA). This makes it essential to expand the cranial vault before any facial advancement with ID.

Our previous studies analyzing the airways of patients with Apert syndrome demonstrated greater reductions in the laryngopharyngeal region than the nasopharyngeal region. Aside from the clinical appearance and short nose, the incidence of respiratory distress will always be significant from a surgical point of view (Fig. 19.4) [9]. In addition to facial osteotomies, other important steps to improve the airway include addressing septal deviation, tonsils, and

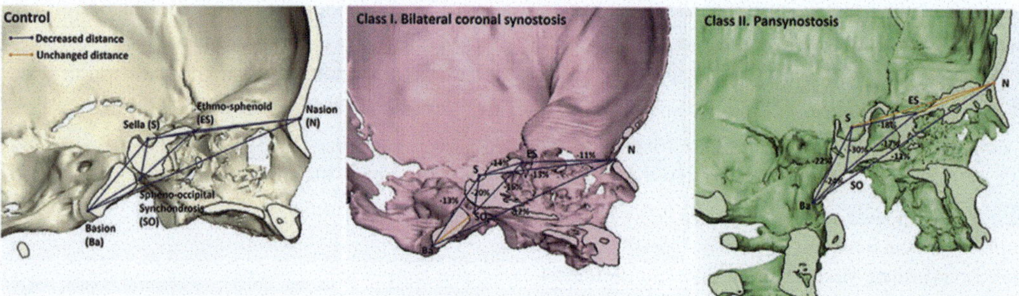

Fig. 19.1 Classification of Apert syndrome based on the type of cranial suture closed

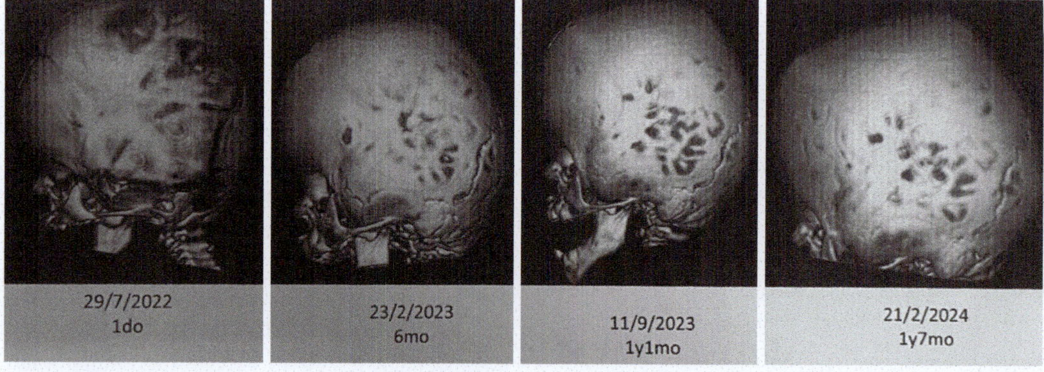

Fig. 19.2 Evolution of bi-coronal synostosis in patients with Apert syndrome from 1 day to 19 months, closing sagittal and lambdoid sutures, increased digital prints, and enlargement of the temporal fossa

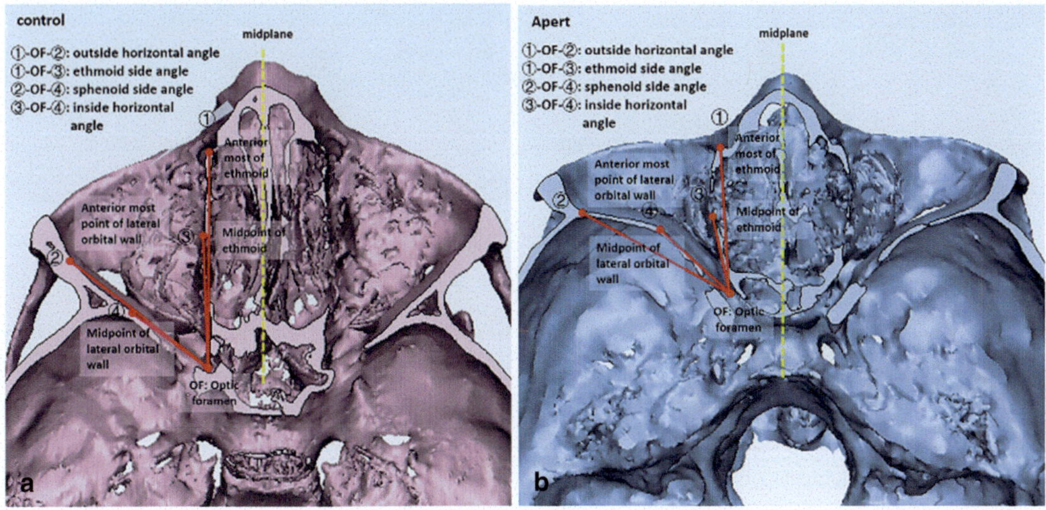

Fig. 19.3 The temporal enlargement and the convexity of the lateral wall produce a very short orbital cavity and medial wall by ethmoidal area

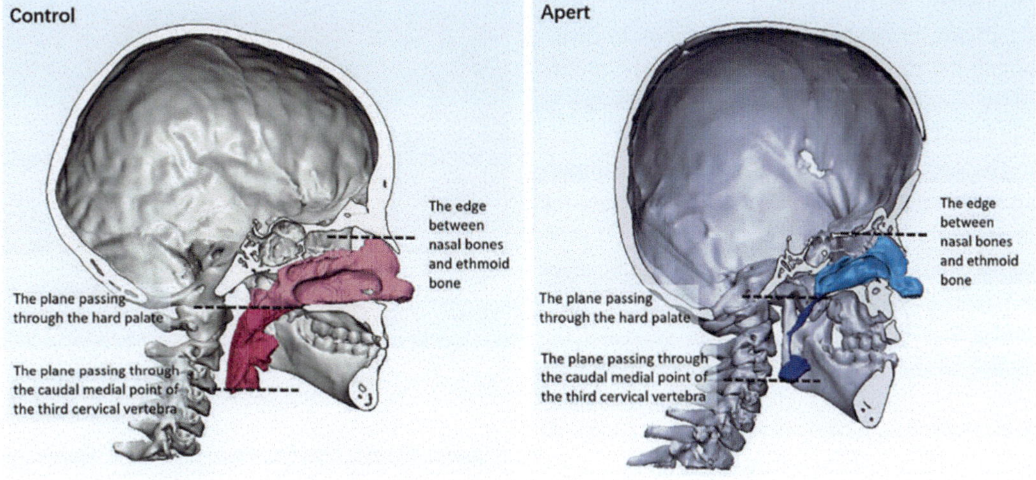

Fig. 19.4 Reduced pharyngeal airway in patient with Apert syndrome due to severe midface retrusion when compared to control

adenoids. Despite this airway obstruction in our series of 152 patients, only six patients had a tracheostomy—five of which were performed just after birth and one after surgeries including FOA and cranial decompression, performed in another service for high apnea index (Fig. 19.5). Two patients still have a tracheostomy in place after FFMBA was performed and are currently awaiting decannulation. In this series, we only found two patients with choanal atresia, who were operated on early upon diagnosis.

Previous studies of normal orbital development have shown that 77% of orbital volume growth and 85% of cranio-orbitozygomatic skeleton growth occur by the age of five years [11, 12]. The orbits of patients with Apert syndrome are hypoplastic and shallow, which can cause severe ocular complications stemming from globe exposure. The presence of intracranial hypertension can cause compression of the optic nerve, thereby jeopardizing vision and influencing the timing of surgery with respect to age.

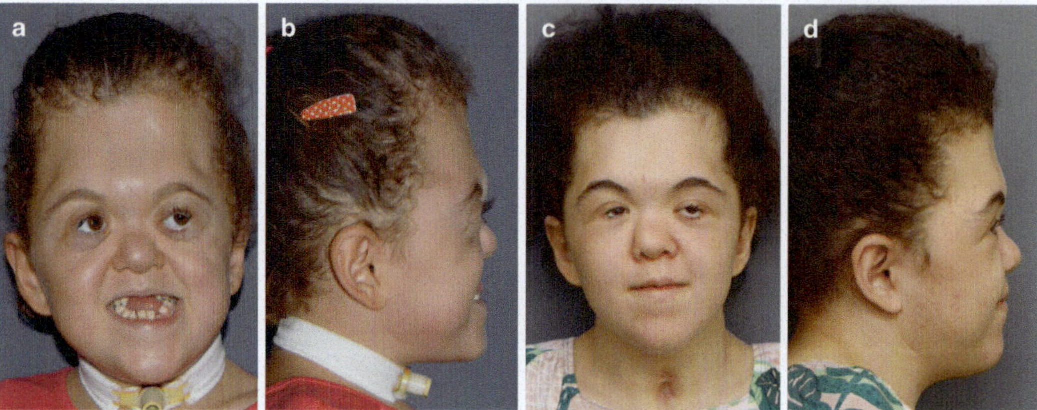

Fig. 19.5 Patient with Apert syndrome on tracheo and tarsorrhaphy since birth, frontal–orbital advancement and ventriculoperitoneal shunt at six months, and frontofacial monobloc advancement with distraction osteogenesis 14 mm at nine years

Fundoscopy and ultrasound of the optic nerve sheath are important pre-examinations in determining the timing for surgery. Presently, noninvasive measurement of intracranial pressure is being used in our unit [13].

The severity of the case is of crucial importance for selecting the procedure and timing the intervention. Both FFMBA and Le Fort III midface advancement procedures protect the eyes and increase the airway. Antunes et al. have shown that both procedures can increase the volume of the orbits in syndromic craniosynostosis. With these procedures, 1 mm advancement corresponds to a 0.719 mm^3 increase in orbital volume with FFMBA and 0.53 mm^3 with Le Fort III [14]. Due to the age at which patients presented, FFMBA was often our first procedure of choice. In these cases, FFMBA was able to correct orbit and midface retrusion at the same time. Our age limit for FFMBA was 14 years because of concerns regarding lack of brain expansion. Our first series used external devices (ED) with glabellar and dental traction. After some issues with dental traction, we pivoted to traction via pins fixed in the piriform aperture with an external skin incision. Although we prefer ID, particularly for young children, the ability to reuse ED influences device selection. This chapter does not reference any brand names because many different types of ED were used (Figs. 19.6a, 19.6b, and 19.6c).

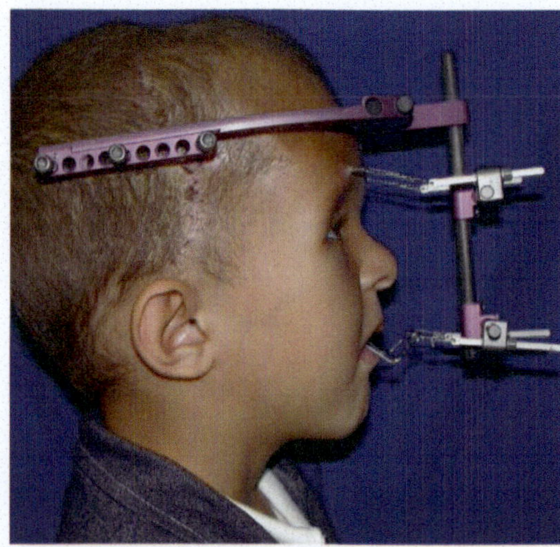

Fig. 19.6a Patient with Apert syndrome without previous surgery frontofacial monobloc advancement with frontal–external pins and dental traction

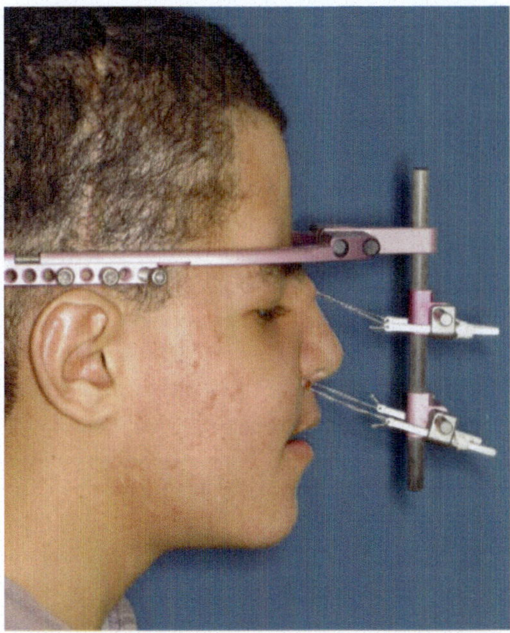

Fig. 19.6b Patient with Apert syndrome with previous frontal–orbital advancement and Le Fort III with nasal and maxillary traction

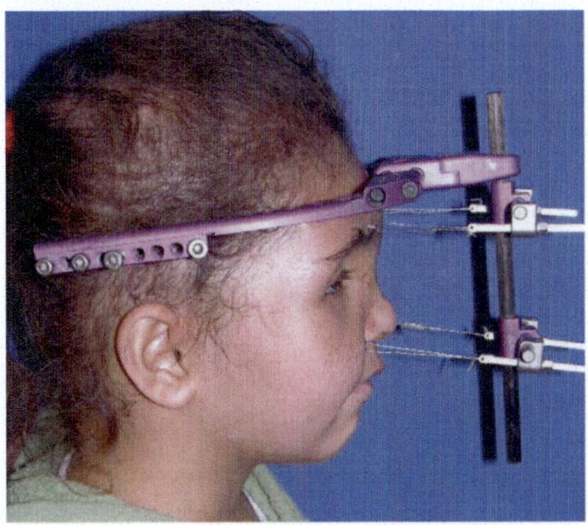

Fig. 19.6c Patient with Apert syndrome without previous surgery FFA with external distractors with frontal and maxillary traction

Authors Series

Previous procedures, such as FOA and PVDO, will be discussed in other chapters of this book. Our series of 152 patients with Apert syndrome from 1987 to the present includes 82 females and 70 males. Of these patients, 49 have had surgeries and long-term follow-up appointments with my team. This group includes 26 females and 23 males. FFMBA was performed in 32 patients, 12 of whom had ED and 22 had ID; two patients experienced problems with ID and were changed to ED. Of those 32 patients, FFMBA was associated with FOA in 11 cases and PVDO in 6 cases, while 14 patients had isolated FFMBA as the first operation. Another group of 18 patients had facial osteotomy type Le Fort III (Le Fort III) and FOA, 7 of which with ED devices. Additionally, 19 patients had FFMBA and FOA+ Le Fort III with the ED device. Our observations will focus on the 19 patients with Apert syndrome with FFMBA and Le Fort III procedures. Le Fort III was associated with FOA in 5 and 2, which were isolated.

Our protocol is FOA at the age of 1 year if only two coronal sutures are closed, posterior vault distraction (PVDO) between 3 and 6 months if more sutures are involved, and—depending on the brain development and other clinical signs present, such as severe exorbitism, respiratory distress, and presence of tracheostomy—FFMBA at the age of six years. In early cases, posterior vault decompression was performed with osteotomies without distractors. In only two cases, springs were not successful. Our current routine practice utilizes internal distractors. More recently, we had two patients who received endoscopic coronal sutures resection followed by helmet use for one year. This new protocol is currently being evaluated to determine whether it will allow FFMBA to be postponed (Fig. 19.7).

All our patients with Apert syndrome who have completed their facial growth require orthognathic surgery. From this series, we performed orthognathic surgeries on ten patients; not all patients met the indications for surgery, largely based on cognitive evaluation. Most shared the facial profile of a short face with anterior open bite and mandibular retrusion with clockwise rotation. Lu et al. described these clinical signs in 33 patients with Apert syndrome and mandible abnormalities in three dimensions: length, width, and height. This study showed that the narrowed angle between the mandible and cranial base reduced nasopharyngeal and oropharyngeal airway space [15].

Treatment Strategies (Fig. 19.7)

- Hand surgery starts at six months of age and involves two or three stages, depending on Upton's classification [16].
- The timing of FOA or PVDO is based on the type of sutures and clinical signs of cranial hypertension. FOA was performed on 21 patients aged 12 months and PVDO was performed on 7 patients aged 6 months. In this group of patients, 17 had FFMBA associated with FOA [9] or PVDO [7].
- A group of 14 patients had FFMBA as their first surgery due to their age at arrival and signs of intracranial hypertension, respiratory distress, and exorbitism. These patients ranged in age from 1 to 14 years old, with an average age of 8.28 years old. Five of these patients had ED and nine had ID.
- Early FFMBA was performed in three patients younger than four years of age. One of these patients had cranial hypertension, obstructive apnea, and no prior surgeries. The youngest patient (one year old) was an unusual case presenting other anomalies with severe proptosis. The third patient had hydrocephaly, obstructive apnea, and two previous craniectomies in another service. The majority of patients were operated on between five and nine years of age (18 patients).
- The determination to use ED versus ID was influenced by the ability to reuse ED within the unit. From 2000 to 2015, 12 patients had FFMBA operations and ED, and 7 patients had Le Fort III and ED.

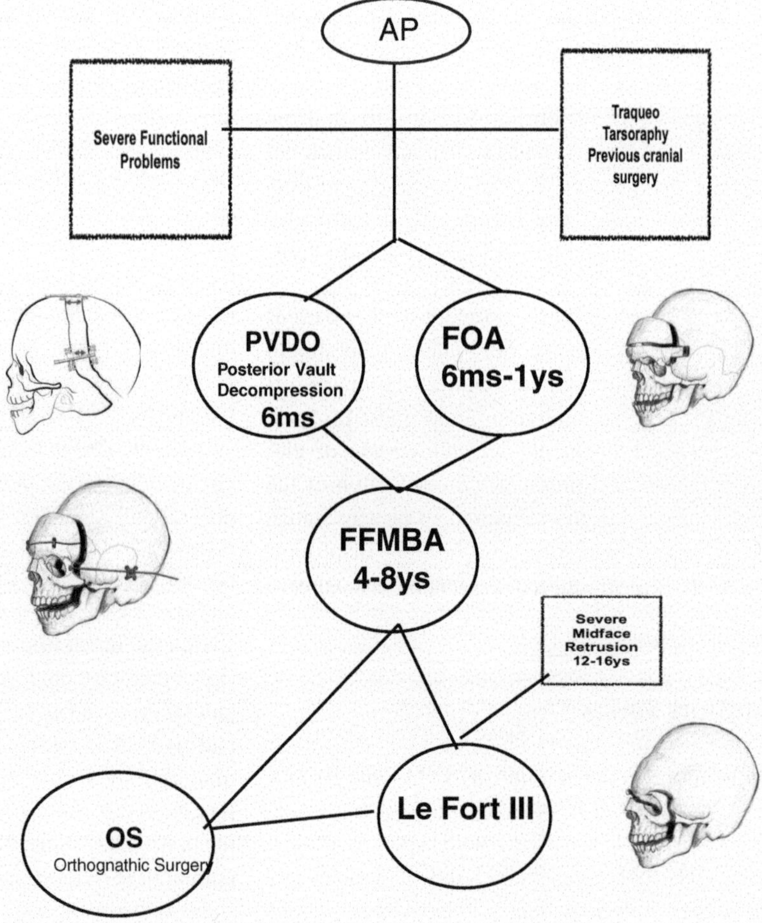

Fig. 19.7 Algorithm for Apert syndrome surgical treatment

Rescue surgery after FFMBA with ID was performed for two patients, both of whom had had an incomplete fracture in the maxillozygomatic suture and a unilateral pterygoid fracture. In these reoperations, ED was selected for FFMBA.

Surgical Technique

Surgical technique is the same for ED and ID, and important considerations include position on the table, temporary tarsorrhaphy, and oral intubation. A broken skin incision is made in the calvarium without any palpebral incision. Arnaud et al. describe this technique in detailed steps for FFMBA osteotomies with ID (Fig. 19.8) [17, 19].

Traditional osteotomy lines with small lateral bone extension begin with frontal craniotomy and orbital osteotomies, followed by pterygoid plate osteotomies done by coronal incision [18]. In a very small number of cases, an oral incision could help in the maxillary separation osteotomy. Bilateral galea flaps are used through the superior orbital osteotomy and attached to the dura with stitches and glue. Parallel lateral osteotomies are done in the cranium to expand the temporal region. When IDs are used, we position them with care so as not to have any space between the site of osteotomies. For ED, we mark the ED position points externally, place the plates and screws in the orbital margin, and then suture the bi-coronal incision. Positioning the ED device is one of the most important points for achieving good traction vectors. The ED has a horizontal part, which is fixed in the cranial bones, and a vertical part located in the facial midline with frontal and maxillary points of traction (Fig. 19.9).

The ED's external points of fixation in the face are (1) the superior margin of the orbit with plates and screws and (2) the piriform aperture and surrounding skin in the nasal alar implantation. We no longer use dental devices in patients with Apert syndrome because of dental crowding. For Le Fort III patients, we use a central traction point in the glabellar region. In contrast to ID, external traction starts as soon as the ED is in place without any activation. Even though the device is not activated, the position of the external device is sufficient for small forward traction (Fig. 19.10).

Our protocol entails device activation five days after placement and 0.5 mm expansion twice daily, totaling 1 mm a day. The criteria to stop are a clinical evaluation and always trying to overcorrection with the main concern in the orbital area. Distraction ranged from 14 to 26 mm for our patients. The average distraction time was 20 days and, once optimal distraction was

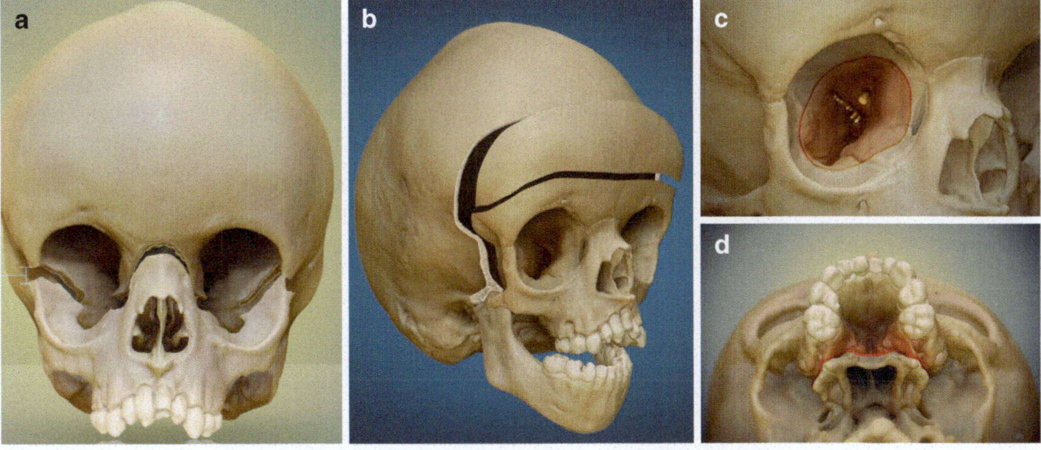

Fig. 19.8 Lines of osteotomies (**a**) Le Fort III, (**b**) frontofacial monobloc advancement, (**c**) landmarks for inner orbital osteotomie, and (**d**) pterygoid plates osteotomy

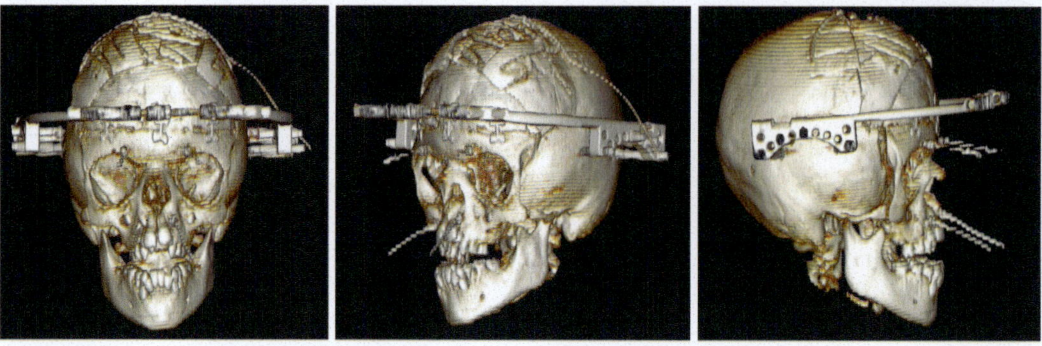

Fig. 19.9 Immediate postoperative just after external distractor (ED) three positions showing the frontal and maxillary fixation

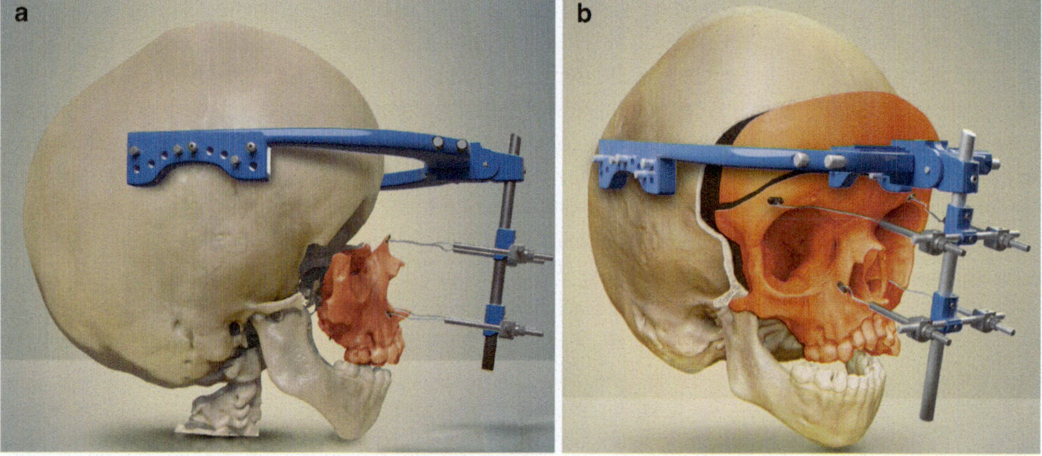

Fig. 19.10 External devices and its fixation points for Le Fort III and frontofacial monobloc advancement

attained, the RED remained in place for three months. In most patients with syndromic craniosynostosis, we did not observe relapse of the facial advancement. However, in patients with Apert syndrome, the midface and malar projection do not look like normal faces. Tonello et al. compared the preoperative and one-year-postoperative computed tomography (CT) scans of 16 patients with syndromic craniosynostosis—five of whom had Apert syndrome—with aged-matched control patients. Even though the results demonstrated desired change, the facial angle, maxillary dimensions, and facial growth were not similar to the control patients (Fig. 19.11) [20].

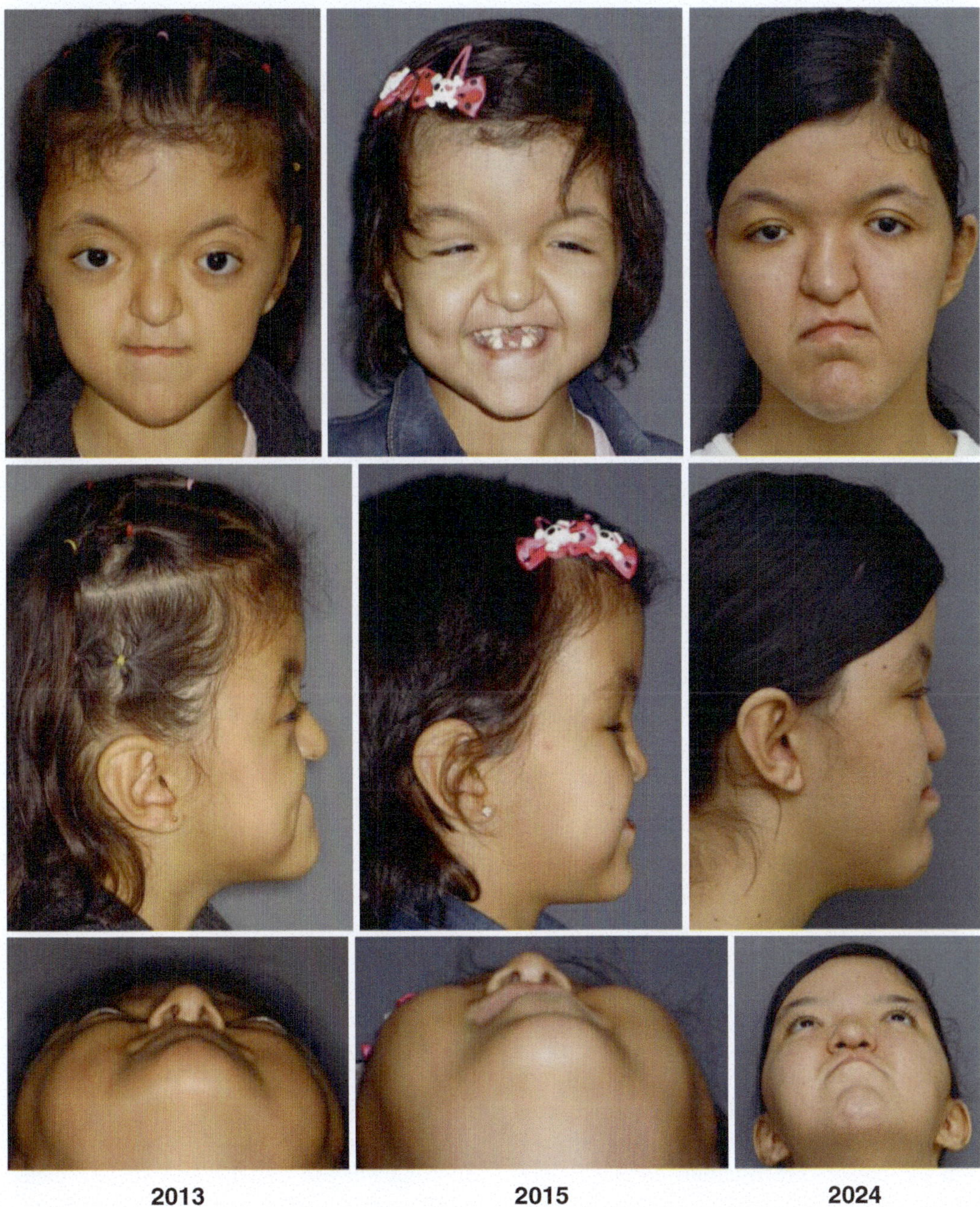

Fig. 19.11 Flatness of the midface persists even after FFMBA during facial growth. The transverse dimension of the face is broad, and maxillary retrusion is evident. Good superior orbital projection

Final Cognitive Evaluation of Patients with Apert Syndrome

Of the patients with Apert syndrome in this series, 20 were interviewed utilizing the Health Utilities Index 3 (HUI3), a quality of life questionnaire. This group comprised 14 females and 6 males; of these, 2 had completed college, 11 had not completed basic education, and only 9 could write and read. Of those, nine individuals had undergone cleft palate operations, six had cardiac diagnoses, and five reported seizures, with one patient indicating that seizures posed substantial challenges to daily living. The HUI3 indicated that 62% of participants had a very good global health evaluation. All 20 patients demonstrated some mental deficiency, ranging from mild to severe. One patient had his first surgery at 11 years old and presented with more severe mental deficiency. Twelve patients had hand surgery in the first year of life, and dexterity scores averaged 0.77 out of 1. Nine patients (45%) had appropriately timed surgeries—early cranial decompression, FFMBA, or Le Fort III—and three patients had no surgeries. The evaluation concluded that 12 patients (60%) had speech impairments, 10 (50%) had some level of mental deficiency, and 12 (60%) felt deeply affected by difficult emotions. Quality of life was profoundly affected for all patients with Apert syndrome we evaluated. In addition to the 20 patients interviewed, we documented one biomedical professional, one student applying for medical school, and one student attending a bilingual school. This study has not yet been published.

Complications

Upon analyzing our complications in FFMBA and comparing ID versus ED, ID were associated with more minor complications (e.g., disjunction of maxillary zygomatic suture or frontozygomatic fracture) because of the traction vector and type of ID. Other complications were not related to the type of distractor used. Two severe visual complications included temporary visual loss after FFMBA with ED that was recovered by stopping and reversing the distraction associated with the use of corticosteroids for seven days [21]. The other case involved ethmoidal encephalocele followed by a temporary visual loss after Le Fort III osteotomy with ED device, which was also reversed after surgical correction by intracranial access and skull base reconstruction. Other complications included five cases of cerebrospinal fistula, two cases of meningitis, one palatal fistula after FFMBA, two facial infections in the orbital area, and a complication related to the resorbable plates used. One patient with Apert syndrome using ED developed significant restriction in opening the mouth, and resolving the complication required surgery. Posterior calvarium alopecia occurred more often with ED than with ID after these procedures. In young patients, repositioning the ED was sometimes necessary. The use of ED in young, energetic patients carried risk of more severe complications, as seen in a patient with Crouzon syndrome with ED after FFMBA who had a broken cranial bone after a fall suit by fistula. This complication was an emergency requiring immediate reoperation. This could be prevented by recovering the cranial bone with non-resorbable mesh to support ED (Fig. 19.12).

Many clinical complications could be related to the procedure rather than the use of ED. Examples include a five-year-old patient with persistent and difficult-to-control seizures that were not present before surgery, one partial frontal resorption in a patient with ventriculoperitoneal shunt, and two patients who remain on tracheotomy. In this series, one patient had FOA at an early age, had Le Fort III with ED when she was 18 years old, and died at home at the age of 26 years. No information is available on the cause of death. Interestingly, this patient had attained a biomedical degree, and her final presentation before graduation was a publication about syndromic craniosynostosis [22] .

After comparing orbital volume evaluation following FFMBA and Le Fort III, we prefer FFMBA when exophthalmos and respiratory distress are present [14]. In long-term follow-up observations, no patients with Apert syndrome who received FFMBA operations required fur-

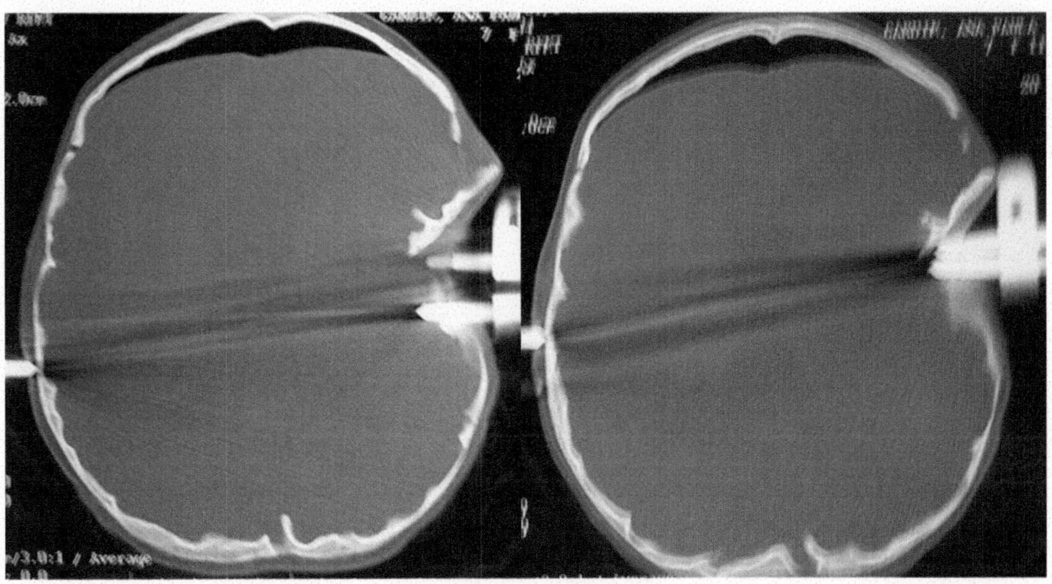

Fig. 19.12 Cerebrospinal fluid fistula after pin perforations in patient with Crouzon syndrome using external device

ther forehead or orbital surgery. However, all these patients needed midface advancement—either Le Fort III or orthognathic surgery—independent of ED or ID. In conclusion, our evaluation identified no major difference in complications between ED and ID and only minor differences in postoperative care and patient quality of life in this period. Additionally, we had opportunities to use two pairs of ID in four patients, but we did not observe any substantial differences. Ultimately, the benefits associated with ID did not justify the high expense for our service. Although there were no differences related to complications, it is worth highlighting that ID uses two different points of traction—one superior and another in the midface—that provide better midface forward traction than ED. Nonetheless, these patients nonetheless require Le Fort III or orthognathic surgery after facial growth is complete (Figs. 19.13, 19.14, and 19.15).

Published in 2009, our first series of syndromic craniosynostosis measured stability and facial growth (done with profile facial teleradiograph) in midface advancement with the use of ED. In this series, four patients had Apert syndrome. The average advancement for these patients was 12.31 mm, less than the actual series. Concluding that the vertical component of the ED vector was the most important, we found minimal horizontal relapse and clear vertical facial growth at the one-year evaluation [23]. This raises the question of whether to change to ID. Some challenges in utilizing ED should be noted, such as difficulty in keeping ED in position in young patients. Additionally, the bone fragility in secondary patients with previous cranial remodeling requires extra titanium mesh to support ED. An 8-year-old patient had numerous teeth buds in the piriform aperture, making it difficult to affix screws in this region, and more recently patients' information also have changed our mind about it. Despite these issues, we use the rigid ED and prefer it in cases where facial bones are thin and already osteotomized or when complications with ID arise.

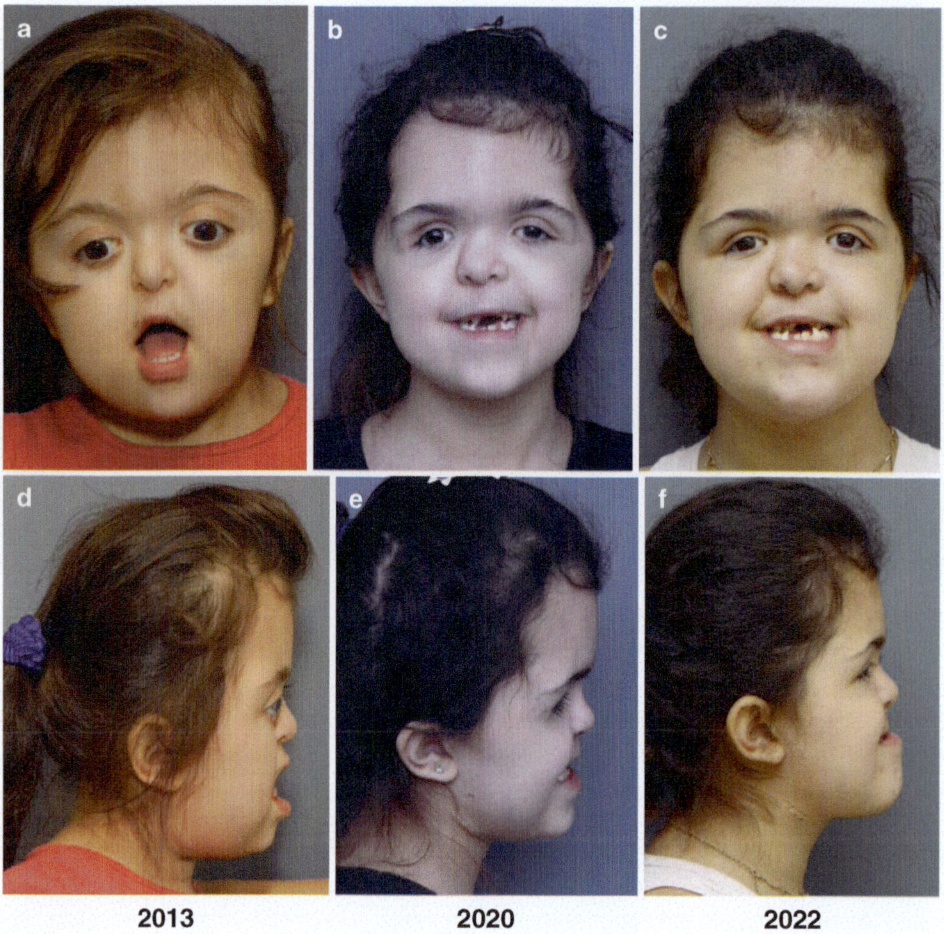

2013 2020 2022

Fig. 19.13 Long-term follow-up, 9 years, after FFMBA the nasal deviation is observed after the surgery and persist after facial growth

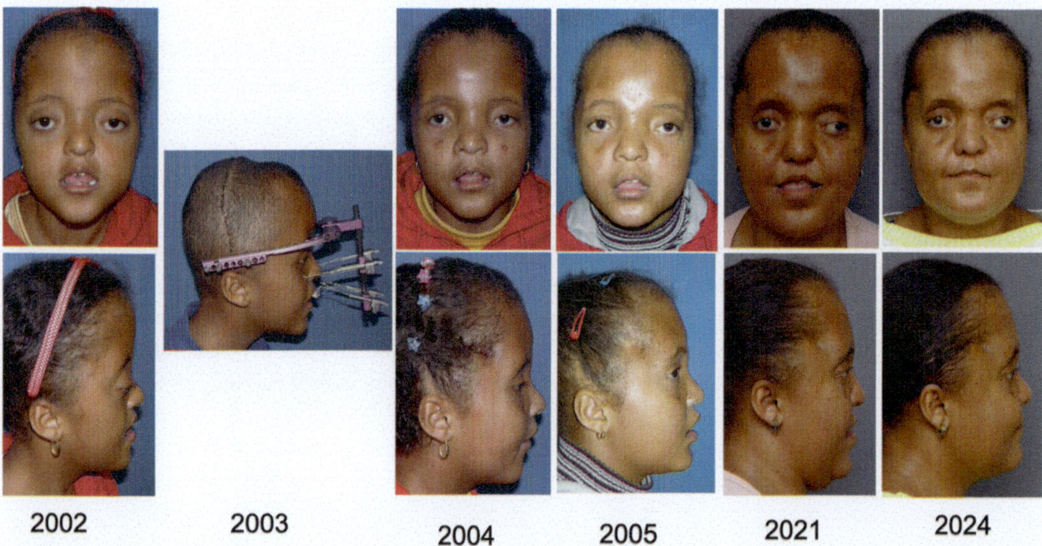

Fig. 19.14 Patient with Apert syndrome operated at 5 years old with 22 years follow-up after FFMBA, and orthognathic surgery

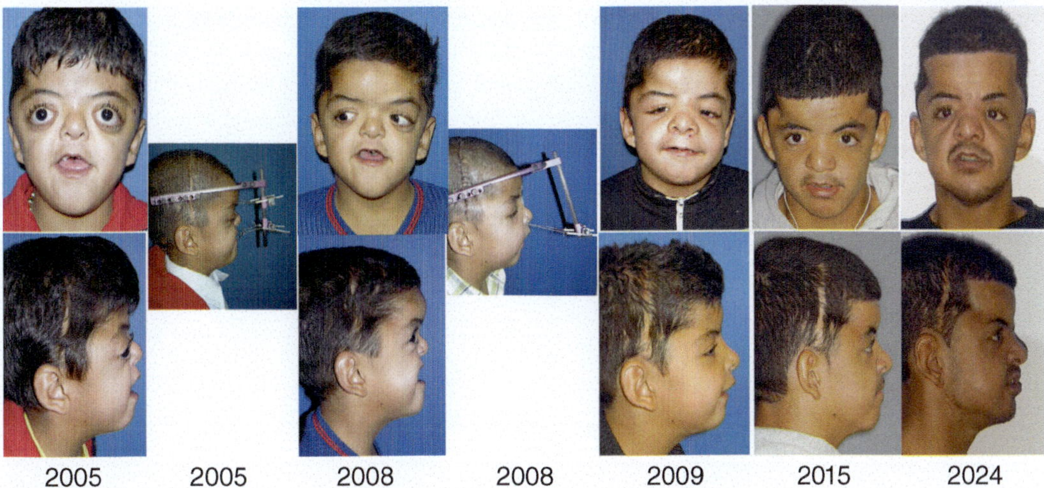

Fig. 19.15 AP with previous cranial surgery with exophthalmia, after FFMBA, three years late the patient still with obstructive sleep apnea (OSA) another early Le Fort III and after nine years follow-up without OSA

Pros and Cons of Device Types

An interesting paper by Rickart et al. compared radiological study results of ID and ED in patients with syndromic craniosynostosis from Crouzon syndrome and found that ED provide better midfacial advancement than ID, while ID provide more orbital movement forward [24]. This study was performed in two of the largest centers in the world that treat craniosynostosis. We observe that osteotomies should be performed completely and inspected at the end of the procedure using Rowe forceps. Whereas ID exert pressure on the orbital area, ED also offer traction in the piriform aperture by pulling forward. In addition to positioning, final facial appearance depends on facial growth, which is always abnormal in Apert syndrome, as demonstrated by Tonello et al. [20]. Our impression is that the point of traction in maxillary area appears beneficial in moving the maxilla forward. However, it is usually performed very early, and there is no normal facial growth in this area later because of the complete closing of the facial and skull base sutures. Thus, at the end of the facial growth, it still will not be normal and will need further surgeries for ED or ID.

The literature reflects many different protocols for treating complex cases of syndromic craniosynostosis, such as facial bipartition, Le Fort II with facial bipartition, and zygomatic Le Fort II osteotomies [24–26]. Long-term follow-up provides details regarding multiple facial osteotomies, the amount of facial bone resorption, and the quality of skin in patients with Apert syndrome; such factors could affect the facial appearance at the end of facial growth, regardless of the type of advancement performed (Figs. 19.16 and 19.17).

Facial bipartition in patients with Apert syndrome could be an interesting option for a few patients with Apert syndrome in our series. We found five patients with severe hypertelorism that could be corrected with FFMBA with facial bipartition. Conversely, at the end of facial growth, we see a high demand among our patients with Crouzon syndrome for cosmetic procedures such as rhinoplasty, chin advancement, or facelift. This is in contrast to our patients with Apert syndrome, and these unusual osteotomies are interesting to consider.

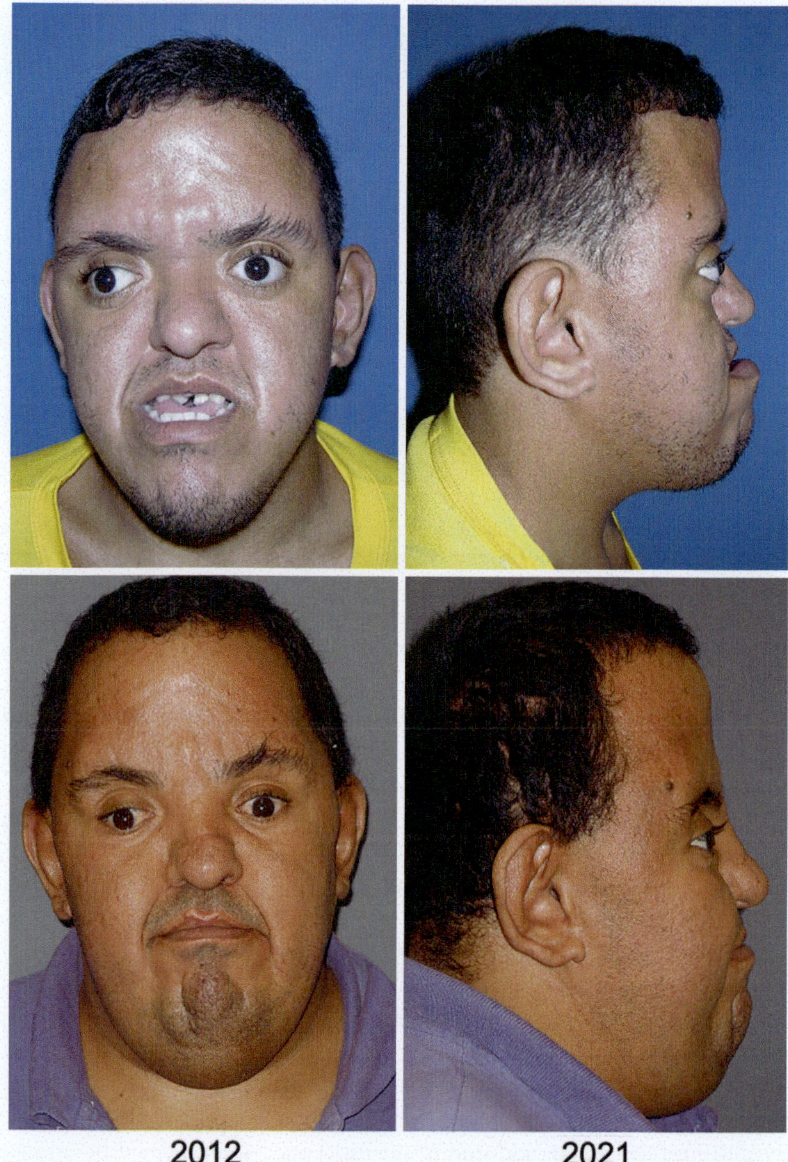

Fig. 19.16 AP without any surgery, 28 ys old with OSA submitted to Le Fort III with ED, picture after 9 years follow-up without any respiratory problem

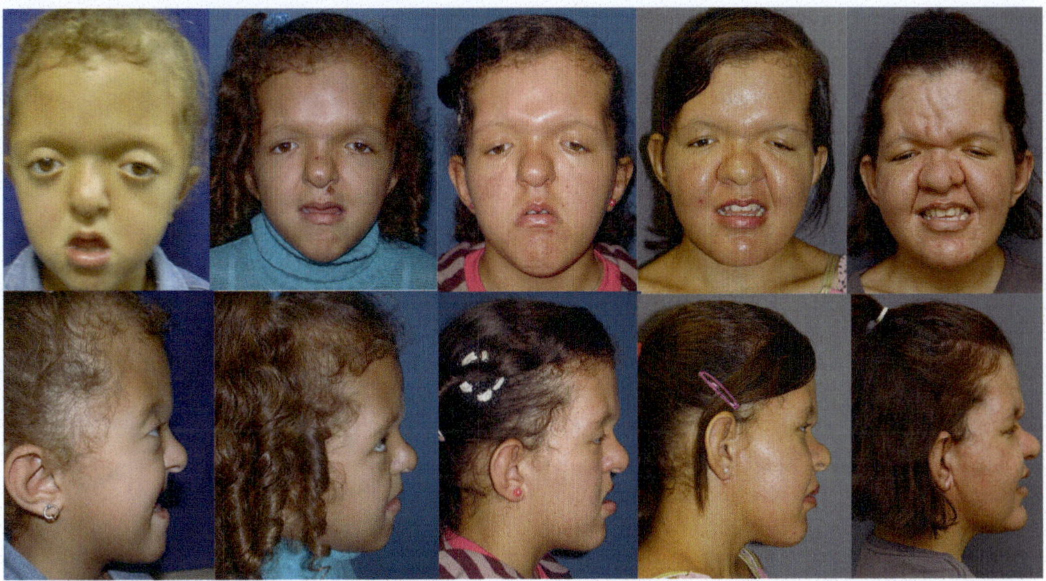

Fig. 19.17 Evolution of facial appearance in AP 23 years follow-up with only two procedures, FFMBA at 5 years old and orthognathic surgery at 18 years

Key Messages

- Frontofacial monobloc advancement osteotomy is an important tool for protecting the eyes and improving airway obstruction in patients with Apert syndrome.
- Internal distractors push the facial bones in the orbital area and force more frontozygomatic and maxillary zygomatic sutures than external distractors, which pull the frontal area and maxillary area without forcing sutures directly.
- External distractors have traction vectors for facial bone mobility in the orbital and maxillary regions and pull the facial bones from two external points of traction, one superior and another inferior.
- External distractors provide better traction in the maxillary region because the second point is located below the orbit in the maxilla.
- External distractors are important instruments for rescuing failure of internal distractors when there are limitations for facial bone advancement.
- The limitations of external distractors include the young age of surgical patients with Apert syndrome, the quality of cranial bone present, patient complaints, previous cranial remodeling, and the consolidation period with the external device.
- Another important limitation of external distractors is that they restrict patients' routine daily living activities like eating, sleeping, and working.

References

1. Wagner CS, Wietlisbach LE, Kota A, Villavisanis DF, Pontell ME, Barrero CE, et al. Genetic subtypes of Apert syndrome are associated with differences in airway morphology and early upper airway obstruction. J Craniofac Surg. 2023;34(7):1999–2003.
2. Yeh E, Fanganiello RD, Sunaga DY, Zhou X, Holmes G, Rocha KM, et al. Novel molecular pathways elicited by mutant FGFR2 may account for brain abnormalities in Apert syndrome. PLoS One. 2013;8(4):e60439.
3. Yacubian-Fernandes A, Palhares A, Giglio A, Gabarra RC, Zanini S, Portela L, et al. Apert syndrome: analysis of associated brain malformations and conformational changes determined by surgical treatment. J Neuroradiol [Internet] 2004 Mar [cited 2024 Oct

12];31(2):116–22. Available from: https://linkinghub.elsevier.com/retrieve/pii/S0150986104969787
4. Lesciotto KM, Heuzé Y, Jabs EW, Bernstein JM, Richtsmeier JT. Choanal atresia and craniosynostosis: development and disease. Plast Reconstr Surg [Internet]. 2018 Jan [cited 2024 Oct 12];141(1):156–68. Available from: https://journals.lww.com/00006534-201801000-00034
5. Forte AJ, Alonso N, Persing JA, Pfaff MJ, Brooks ED, Steinbacher DM. Analysis of midface retrusion in Crouzon and Apert syndromes. Plast Reconstr Surg. 2014;134(2):285–93.
6. Lu X, Sawh-Martinez R, Jorge Forte A, Wu R, Cabrejo R, Wilson A, et al. Classification of subtypes of Apert syndrome, based on the type of vault suture synostosis. Plast Reconstr Surg Glob Open. 2019;7(3):e2158.
7. Forte AJ, Steinbacher DM, Persing JA, Brooks ED, Andrew TW, Alonso N. Orbital dysmorphology in untreated children with Crouzon and Apert syndromes. Plast Reconstr Surg. 2015;136(5):1054–62.
8. Lu X, Forte AJ, Sawh-Martinez R, Wu R, Cabrejo R, Steinbacher DM, et al. Anterior convex lateral orbital wall: distinctive morphology in Apert syndrome. Br J Oral Maxillofac Surg [Internet]. 2018 Nov [cited 2024 Oct 12];56(9):864–9. Available from: https://linkinghub.elsevier.com/retrieve/pii/S0266435618303206
9. Forte AJ, Lu X, Hashim PW, Steinbacher DM, Alperovich M, Persing JA, et al. Airway analysis in Apert syndrome. Plast Reconstr Surg. 2019;144(3):704–9.
10. Bentley RP, Sgouros S, Natarajan K, Dover MS, Hockley AD. Changes in orbital volume during childhood in cases of craniosynostosis. J Neurosurg [Internet]. 2002 Apr [cited 2024 Oct 12];96(4):747–54. Available from: https://thejns.org/view/journals/j-neurosurg/96/4/article-p747.xml
11. Bentley RP, Sgouros S, Natarajan K, Dover MS, Hockley AD. Normal changes in orbital volume during childhood. J Neurosurg [Internet]. 2002 Apr [cited 2024 Oct 12];96(4):742–6. Available from: https://thejns.org/view/journals/j-neurosurg/96/4/article-p742.xml
12. Brandao MM, Tonello C, Parizotto I, Machado LB, Alonso N. Analysis of intracranial pressure waveform using a non-invasive method in individuals with craniosynostosis. Childs Nerv Syst [Internet]. 2024 Jan [cited 2024 Oct 12];40(1):145–52. Available from: https://link.springer.com/10.1007/s00381-023-06092-y
13. Antunes RB, Camilo AA, da Silva AM, da Silva JVL, Alonso N. Assessment of orbital volume in frontofacial advancements. J Craniofac Surg. 2015;26(3):843–8.
14. Lu X, Sawh-Martinez R, Forte AJ, Wu R, Cabrejo R, Wilson A, et al. Mandibular spatial reorientation and morphological alteration of Crouzon and Apert syndrome. Ann Plast Surg. 2019;83(5):568–82.
15. Raposo-Amaral CE, Denadai R, Furlan P, Raposo-Amaral CA. Treatment of Apert hand syndrome: strategies for achieving a five-digit hand. Plast Reconstr Surg [Internet] 2018 Oct [cited 2024 Oct 17];142(4):972–82. Available from: https://journals.lww.com/00006534-201810000-00025
16. Haber SE, Khonsari R, Paternoster G, Arnaud E. Frontofacial monobloc advancement with internal distraction tactics and strategy in faciocraniosynostosis [Internet]. Switzerland: Springer Nature; 2023 [cited 2024 Oct 20]. 319 p. https://doi.org/10.1007/978-3-031-07574-2.
17. Ferreira Junior TA, Fontoura RR, Marques do Nascimento L, Alcântara MT, Capuchinho-Júnior GA, Alonso N, et al. Frontofacial Monobloc advancement with internal distraction: surgical technique and osteotomy guide. Oper Neurosurg Hagerstown Md 2022;23(1):e33–e41.
18. Arnaud E, Marchac D, Renier D. Reduction of morbidity of the frontofacial monobloc advancement in children by the use of internal distraction: Plast Reconstr Surg [Internet] 2007 Sep [cited 2024 Oct 26];120(4):1009–26. Available from: http://journals.lww.com/00006534-200709150-00025
19. Tonello C, Cevidanes LHS, Ruellas ACO, Alonso N. Midface morphology and growth in syndromic craniosynostosis patients following Frontofacial Monobloc distraction. J Craniofac Surg. 2021;32(1):87–91.
20. Alonso N, Goldenberg D, Fonseca AS, Kanashiro E, Matsushita H, Freitas R d S, et al. Blindness as a complication of monobloc frontofacial advancement with distraction. J Craniofac Surg. 2008;19(4):1170–3.
21. Valezi KB, Quiezi RG. Correlação das mutações nos genes FGF e twist1 nas síndromes de apert, crouzon e pfeiffer—revisão de literatura. Rev Conex Saúde FIB [Internet]. 2018 Sep 8 [cited 2024 Oct 12];2(2). Available from: https://revistas.fibbauru.br/conexaosaude/article/view/310
22. Lima DSC, Alonso N, Câmara PRP, Goldenberg DC. Evaluation of cephalometric points in midface bone lengthening with the use of a rigid external device in syndromic craniosynostosis patients. Braz J Otorhinolaryngol. 2009;75(3):395–406.
23. Rickart AJ, Van De Lande LS, O' Sullivan E, Bloch K, Arnaud E, Schievano S, et al. Comparison of Internal and External Distraction in Frontofacial Monobloc Advancement: A Three-Dimensional Quantification. Plast Reconstr Surg [Internet]. 2023 Feb 28 [cited 2024 Oct 20]; Available from: https://journals.lww.com/10.1097/PRS.0000000000010331
24. Greig AVH, Britto JA, Abela C, Witherow H, Richards R, Evans RD, et al. Correcting the typical Apert face: combining bipartition with monobloc distraction. Plast Reconstr Surg [Internet]. 2013 Feb [cited 2024 Oct 12];131(2):219e–30e. Available from: http://journals.lww.com/00006534-201302000-00029

25. Purnell CA, Evans M, Massenburg BB, Kim S, Preston K, Kapadia H, et al. Lefort II distraction with zygomatic repositioning versus Lefort III distraction: a comparison of surgical outcomes and complications. J Cranio-Maxillofac Surg [Internet] 2021 Oct [cited 2024 Oct 20];49(10):905–13. Available from: https://linkinghub.elsevier.com/retrieve/pii/S1010518221001025
26. Chetty V, Haber SE, Khonsari RH, Arnaud E. Improvement of periorbital appearance in Apert syndrome after subcranial Le Fort III with bipartition and distraction. J Craniofac Surg [Internet] 2020 May [cited 2024 Oct 12];31(3):711–5. Available from: https://journals.lww.com/10.1097/SCS.0000000000006233

20 Midface Management: The CHOP Approach and the Role of Monobloc with Le Fort II Advancement

Allison C. Hu and Jesse A. Taylor

Introduction and Foundations of Midface Management in Apert Syndrome

The complex bi-concave midface with varying degrees of central versus peripheral hypoplasia, airway, ocular, and dental differences presents unique challenges to craniofacial surgeons [1]. Operative intervention during the mixed dentition period is often indicated to improve orbital protection, respiratory function, dental occlusion, and overall facial balance [2].

The craniofacial dysmorphology seen in Apert syndrome is defined by multidimensional skeletal deficiency. Midface hypoplasia spans the sagittal, vertical, and transverse planes, but disproportionately affects the nasomaxillary segment compared to the orbitozygomatic complex [3]. Clinically, this results in hallmark features: a depressed nasal bridge and "parrot-beak" nose, a retruded maxilla with counterclockwise rotation of the occlusal plane, and a low midface-to-orbital height ratio [4, 5]. Sagittal discrepancies between the maxilla and mandible contribute to class III malocclusion, anterior open bite, and an inverted "V" maxillary arch [6, 7]. Periorbital manifestations include shallow orbits, hypertelorism, down-slanting palpebral fissures, and pronounced globe protrusion [8]. As these features vary in severity and distribution, midface surgical planning must be individualized, with operative goals centered on airway improvement, globe protection, functional occlusion, and normalized facial proportions.

Historically, midface advancement in Apert syndrome was performed using monolithic osteotomies such as Le Fort III and monobloc procedures. These strategies sought to mobilize the midface or frontofacial skeleton en bloc, typically via acute advancement. The introduction of distraction osteogenesis marked a paradigm shift, offering gradual skeletal advancement with reduced soft tissue tension, better vascular preservation, and the potential for larger, safer movements [9]. Still, debate persists regarding the optimal technique, vector, and timing of advancement [5, 8, 10]. While Le Fort III and monobloc osteotomies remain widely utilized [11–15], evolving strategies now include multi-piece osteotomies such as the Le Fort II with zygomatic repositioning [5, 10, 16–20], facial bipartition, and hybrid constructs such as monobloc with Le Fort II or Le Fort III combined with Le Fort I [21–25]. Each carries tradeoffs in exposure, vector control, and risk profile.

A central consideration is whether cranial vault expansion and midface advancement should be performed in a single stage or as sequential procedures. Distraction-based frontofacial advancement reduces morbidity compared to acute advancement; however, it does not eliminate

A. C. Hu · J. A. Taylor (✉)
Division of Plastic, Reconstructive, and Oral Surgery, Children's Hospital of Philadelphia, Philadelphia, PA, USA

J. G. Meara et al. (eds.), *Apert Syndrome*, https://doi.org/10.1007/978-3-032-12551-4_20

the risk [25]. Transcranial approaches, such as monobloc or bipartition, address both orbital and cranial volume deficiencies but have been associated with higher complication rates, including cerebrospinal fluid (CSF) leaks and ascending infections [19, 26–29]. Subcranial approaches, though less invasive, may inadequately correct associated supraorbital deformities or cephalocranial disproportion, leading to persistent dysmorphology and the need for secondary cranioplasty [30].

At the Children's Hospital of Philadelphia (CHOP), our midface advancement algorithm for Apert syndrome has evolved over the past two decades, shaped by longitudinal experience and changing philosophical approaches to craniofacial reconstruction. Our treatment model emphasizes early posterior vault distraction osteogenesis (PVDO) as a first-line intervention in infants [31], which provides superior intracranial volume expansion compared to fronto-orbital advancement (FOA) [32] and often permits deferral or avoidance of transcranial surgery in infancy. In patients requiring further correction, frontal cranial surgery is typically delayed until orbital maturity, between five and eight years, when midface distraction can be safely combined with it. Surgical decisions at this stage are guided by morphologic analysis, occlusal pattern, airway status, globe position, and the presence of turribrachycephaly or elevated intracranial pressure.

Over time, our operative approach has transitioned from monolithic advancement to a segmentation-based strategy. We now employ modular osteotomies that allow for tailored vector control across craniofacial subunits. This reflects the recognition that the Apert face is not uniformly deficient; rather, it exhibits complex asymmetries across various dimensions. By segmenting the midface and upper facial skeleton into discrete units, we gain the flexibility to manipulate each independently, optimizing both function and aesthetics.

To this end, our institutional experience includes five primary distraction osteotomy constructs: Le Fort III, monobloc, Le Fort II with zygomatic repositioning, monobloc with facial bipartition, and monobloc with Le Fort II. Each is selected based on phenotypic characteristics and regional skeletal deficiency. In all cases, virtual surgical planning (VSP), computer-aided design/computer-aided manufacturing (CAD/CAM)-fabricated guides, and external halo distractors form the backbone of our workflow, facilitating submillimeter accuracy and multi-vector control.

In this chapter, we describe our evolution from traditional Le Fort III and monobloc techniques toward more refined, segmentation-based osteotomies. We review outcomes and complication profiles associated with each approach, emphasizing the rationale for technique selection based on individualized morphology. Particular attention is given to the Monobloc with Le Fort II advancement, an innovative dual-vector strategy developed at CHOP to address both vertical and sagittal midface deficiency in a single-stage procedure. We propose that this tailored, phenotype-guided approach represents a significant advancement in the surgical management of Apert midface dysmorphology.

The CHOP Strategy: Evolution to Segmental and Tailored Osteotomies

Over the past two decades, CHOP has developed a stepwise, phenotype-guided algorithm for midface management in Apert syndrome. Our approach to syndromic craniosynostosis begins with posterior vault distraction osteogenesis (PVDO) as the first-line strategy for cranial expansion [31]. PVDO generates greater intracranial volume than fronto-orbital advancement (FOA) [32], allowing us to defer frontal surgery until a later developmental stage. In some patients, FOA may be avoided entirely; in others, it is postponed until orbital maturity, typically between five and eight years of age, at which point transcranial midface advancement becomes less morbid. Patients without significant supraorbital or frontal bar involvement may instead undergo subcranial midface advancement. Osteotomy selection at this juncture is guided by individual phenotype, morphometric targets, and the relative morbidity of each approach (Fig. 20.1). Virtual surgical planning (VSP) is now fully integrated into our workflow, enabling precise osteotomy design and device placement. External halo-type distractors have become our standard due to their superior control of distraction vectors and adaptability for complex, multidimensional corrections.

Concurrently, our operative paradigm has shifted from monolithic to modular midface techniques. Before 2012, Le Fort III and monobloc osteotomies were predominant, reflecting a broader reliance on single-segment advancement. Since then, we have adopted multi-piece, segmental osteotomies that permit differential vector control across craniofacial subunits, which is better suited to the three-dimensional complexity of Apert morphology. From 2012 onward, five osteotomy types have emerged as our primary strategies: Le Fort III, monobloc, Le Fort II with zygomatic repositioning (LFII + ZR), monobloc with facial bipartition, and monobloc combined with Le Fort II. Each is chosen based on anatomical pattern and functional needs, allowing us to address the specific spatial patterns of dysmorphology with greater precision.

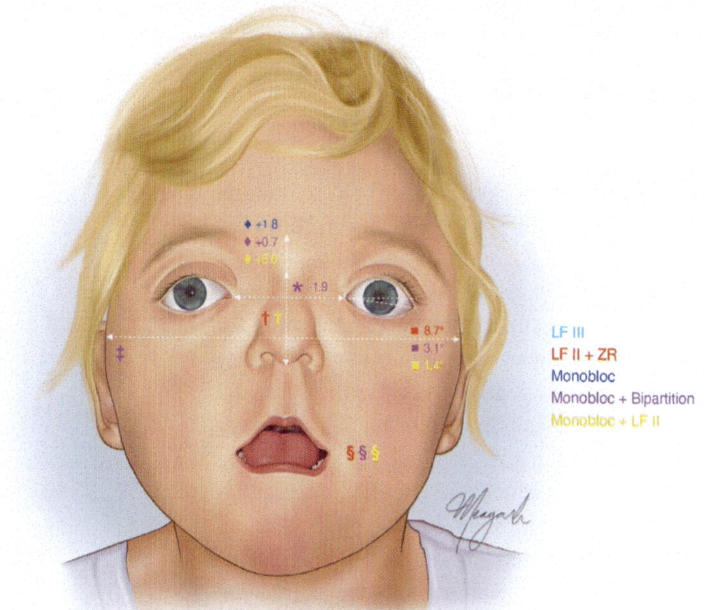

Fig. 20.1 Differential effects of midface osteotomy techniques on facial characteristics in Apert syndrome, with symbols denoting the specific morphometric corrections and colors representing the osteotomy techniques. Numbers represent median changes in middle facial third height and intercanthal distance (as percentages of facial height and width) as well as median changes in bilateral canthal tilt angle. A comparative risk-to-benefit assessment of the five osteotomy techniques is presented below the illustration

	Subcranial		Transcranial		
	LF III	LF II + ZR[a]	Monobloc	Monobloc + Bipartition[b]	Monobloc + LF II[a]
Differential advancement (central vs. peripheral)	-	+	-	+	+
Expands cranium	-	-	+	+	+
Lengthens midface ♦	-	+	-	+	+
Lengthens nose †	-	+	-	-	+
Decreases bizygomatic width ‡	-	-	-	+	-
Changes canthal tilt ■	-	+	-	+	+
Corrects hypertelorism*	-	-	-	+	-
Closes anterior open bite §	-	+ (level)	-	+ (V-shaped)	+
Morbidity profile	Lower	Lower	Higher	Higher	Higher

LF, Le Fort; ZR, zygomatic repositioning.
[a]Levels palpebral fissures by lowering the medial canthi.
[b]Levels palpebral fissures by raising the lateral canthi.

Selection Rationale by Phenotype

Our approach to midface osteotomy selection in Apert syndrome is phenotype-driven, based on the pattern and severity of skeletal involvement across sagittal, vertical, and axial dimensions (Fig. 20.1). Each technique offers unique advantages that align with specific craniofacial morphologies. All patients undergo a standardized distraction protocol, which includes a five-day latency phase followed by distraction at 1 mm/day. Consolidation is maintained for two to three months. As of 2010, we transitioned exclusively to external halo distraction systems, which allow for more precise intraoperative and postoperative vector control [26]. Over the past decade, the use of virtual surgical planning (VSP) has become central to our workflow, supported by advances in CAD/CAM technology [33, 34].

Le Fort III

Le Fort III advancement (Fig. 20.2), initially introduced by Gillies [35] and later refined by Tessier [36], mobilizes the midface as a single unit, including the zygomas, maxilla, and nasal bones [7]. This technique is most appropriate for patients with midface retrusion but normal brow projection and no signs of elevated intracranial pressure (ICP). It allows substantial improvement in upper airway volume, often resolving obstructive sleep apnea and enabling decannulation [2, 37, 38]. However, because the advancement vector is based on the bony orbital rims rather than globe projection, undercorrection can occur without intentional overadvancement [5, 7]. In our experience, Le Fort III produces greater sagittal improvement in facial profile than monobloc, with a median convexity change of 21.5° versus 17.5°. This likely reflects preservation of the nasion and glabellar architecture. Minor improvement in canthal tilt may result from lateral canthopexy routinely performed in these cases.

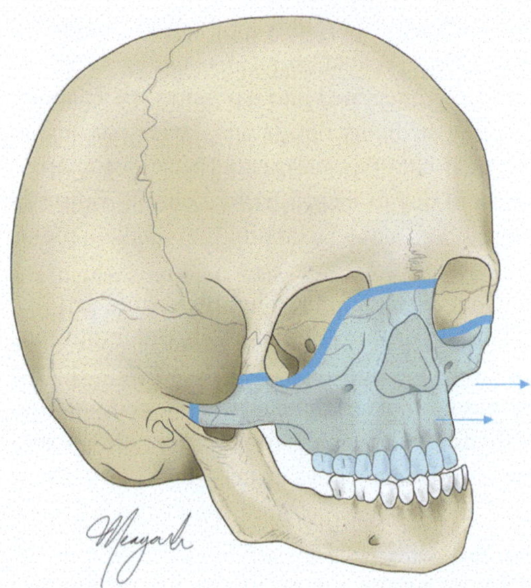

Fig. 20.2 Le Fort III osteotomy for midface advancement. The nasal, maxillary, and zygomatic complex is brought forward in one piece

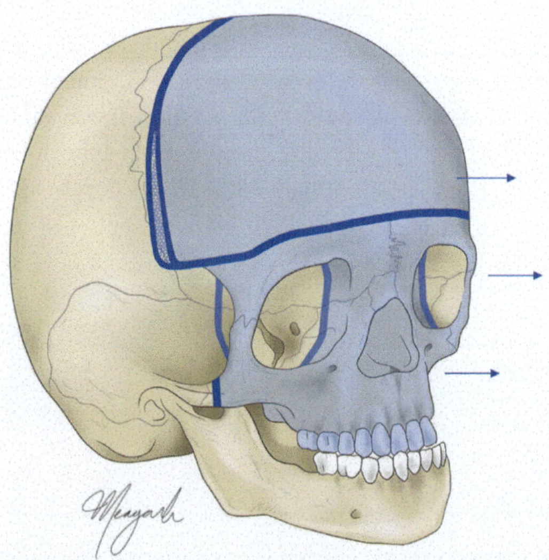

Fig. 20.3 Monobloc osteotomy for midface advancement. The orbital/forehead unit and midface are brought forward in one piece

Monobloc

For patients exhibiting retrusion of both the midface and supraorbital bar, often accompanied by exorbitism or signs of elevated ICP, we favor the monobloc osteotomy (Fig. 20.3) [18, 39]. This technique advances the forehead and midface en bloc, expanding both intracranial and orbital volume [40]. It can address multiple functional concerns in a single procedure, including airway obstruction and elevated ICP [41]. While monobloc is effective in the anteroposterior dimension, it does not significantly increase midface height, a common deficiency in Apert syndrome [24]. Nasal length and intercanthal width typically remain unchanged [42]. Because the approach is transcranial, it carries increased risk for intracranial complications, including meningitis from ascending infection [43].

Le Fort II with Zygomatic Repositioning (LF II + ZR)

Le Fort II osteotomy with zygomatic repositioning (Fig. 20.4), as detailed by Hopper et al. [5], is designed to address disproportionate central midface deficiency while preserving lateral orbital support. The zygomas are stabilized, enabling the central segment to be advanced independently in a clockwise arc [3]. This targeted movement addresses vertical and sagittal underdevelopment of the nasomaxillary complex while sparing the lateral orbit [5]. This strategy effectively levels the palpebral fissures by advancing and lowering the medial canthi while leaving the lateral canthi fixed [42]. In our cohort, it produced the largest improvement in canthal tilt (8.7° median change) and significant elongation of the midface (30.3° median increase in facial convexity). However, this method does not address hypertelorism or lateral facial width [8]. We apply LF II + ZR in cases with pronounced nasal shortening, reverse canthal tilt, and mild-to-moderate airway compromise. Compared to Le Fort III, it may offer improved nasopharyngeal airway expansion due to its more favorable rotational vector [44, 45]. Outcomes reported by Purnell et al. show comparable cephalometric correction and low relapse rates relative to Le Fort III [46].

Monobloc with Facial Bipartition

For patients with marked hypertelorism, biconcave midface profile, and axial facial widening, we utilize a combined monobloc and facial bipartition approach (Fig. 20.5), following the principles developed by Tessier [17] and later popularized by David Dunaway and the team at Great Ormond Street [10, 47]. This technique reshapes the central face by removing a midline bone wedge and rotating the lateral orbital segments medially [10]. Unlike techniques that lower the medial canthi, bipartition levels the

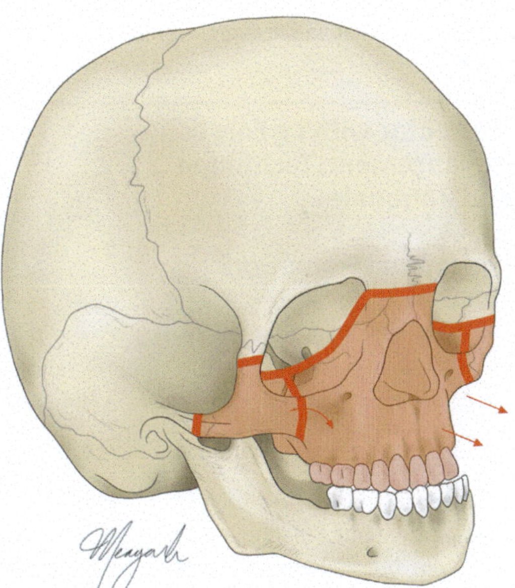

Fig. 20.4 Le Fort II with zygomatic repositioning osteotomy for midface advancement. The orbits and central midface are moved along different vectors

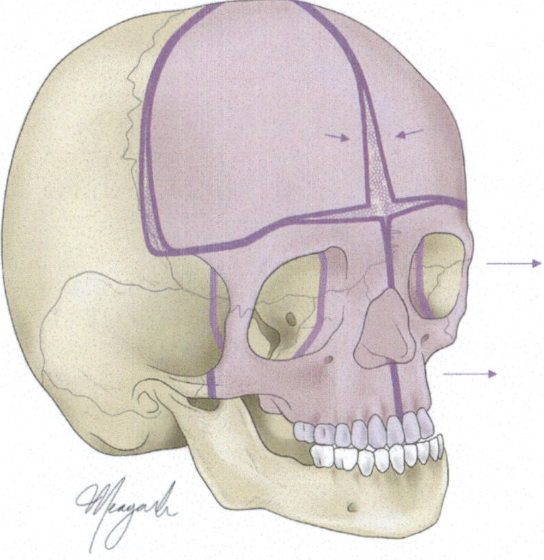

Fig. 20.5 Monobloc with facial bipartition osteotomy for midface advancement. The facial skeleton is separated then brought together via removal of a midline frontal bone segment, allowing for superomedial rotation of the lateral orbits

eyelid fissures by elevating the lateral canthi [10]. It also narrows the interorbital distance, unique among the methods we evaluated, and addresses bizygomatic width to improve overall facial harmony [27]. In our series, it was the only technique that significantly reduced intercanthal distance. Patients undergoing this approach demonstrated lower rates of exotropia and reduced need for ocular alignment procedures, with improved binocular function [48].

Monobloc with Le Fort II

We previously described a combined monobloc + Le Fort II strategy (Fig. 20.6) for patients with complex midface morphology involving both axial and vertical hypoplasia, often in the setting of turribrachycephaly, exorbitism, and airway compromise [24]. This technique enables independent vector control: monobloc distraction advances the fronto-orbital and zygomatic units, while Le Fort II distraction rotates and elongates the central midface and nasal pyramid.

This approach resulted in the largest improvement in facial projection in our cohort (median convexity increase of 35°) and reliably corrected class III malocclusion and open bite deformities [2]. Additionally, it facilitates decompression of elevated ICP in the face of cephalocranial disproportion.

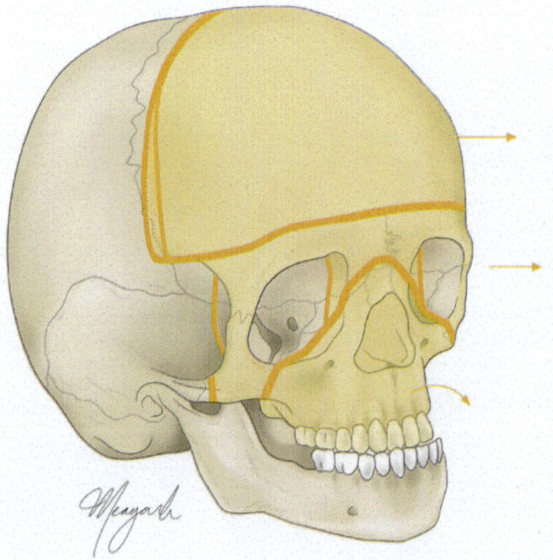

Fig. 20.6 Monobloc with Le Fort II osteotomy for midface advancement. The forehead and midface are advanced horizontally, while the Le Fort II segment follows an oblique vector and clockwise rotation

Toward Precision-Based, Segmental Midface Reconstruction

Our current philosophy emphasizes differential, rather than uniform, correction of the midface—recognizing that Apert syndrome rarely presents with symmetric or unidirectional skeletal deficiency. Segmental osteotomies enable targeted modification of distinct craniofacial subunits, improving the ability to address discordant vertical, sagittal, and axial dysmorphologies. This modular approach enhances facial proportionality, reduces the risk of overcorrection or undercorrection in any single region, and supports more stable occlusal and orbital outcomes. At CHOP, customized osteotomy planning using VSP allows us to simulate osteotomies, plan distraction vectors with sub-millimeter accuracy, and tailor operative sequences to the patient's specific anatomy. This precision-based strategy has become central to our management of Apert midface dysmorphology, enabling individualized, phenotype-specific correction with optimized functional and aesthetic results.

Monobloc with Le Fort II Advancement: Technique and Rationale

Conceptual Framework

The Monobloc with Le Fort II advancement represents a significant evolution in craniofacial distraction, introducing a two-vector osteotomy framework that targets the multidimensional deformities characteristic of Apert syndrome. Traditional approaches, such as Le Fort III or classic monobloc distraction, rely on a single vector en bloc advancement, which can inadequately address the regionally heterogeneous dysmorphology in syndromic patients. In contrast, the Monobloc with Le Fort II strategy enables independent mobilization of the cranial and midfacial segments along divergent trajectories.

In this approach, the monobloc component facilitates horizontal advancement of the forehead and orbital bandeau, effectively correcting frontal bar flattening, orbital retrusion, and increasing intracranial volume. The Le Fort II osteotomy simultaneously permits vertical elongation and clockwise rotation of the nasomaxillary unit, addressing occlusal plane canting, open bite deformities, nasal retrusion, and midface shortening. Clockwise rotational movement of the Le Fort II segment also allows for downward projection of the central midface while preserving lateral orbital position, thus optimizing palpebral fissure orientation and nasal projection.

Segmenting the craniofacial skeleton in this manner introduces surgical flexibility, allowing differential manipulation of each subunit in three planes of motion (e.g., pitch, yaw, and roll). This is particularly important in patients with Apert syndrome, where the composite facial morphology includes sagittal retrusion, vertical deficiency, axial concavity, and asymmetry. The ability to tailor correction to each axis results in a more harmonized facial profile, more durable functional outcomes, and potentially obviates the need for future staged procedures such as orthognathic surgery.

In essence, this technique departs from a uniform correction paradigm and instead supports phenotype-specific advancement strategies. It shifts the reconstructive philosophy from global translation to modular repositioning, enhancing surgical precision while addressing the structural and aesthetic goals of midface and orbital reconstruction.

Indications and Patient Selection

Monobloc with Le Fort II advancement is best suited for patients with severe, multi-planar Apert dysmorphology, particularly those demonstrating persistent panfacial deficiency despite prior cranial expansion. Indications include:

- Midface hypoplasia with sagittal and vertical deficiency.
- Nasal retrusion and flat midline profile.
- Class III malocclusion with anterior open bite and reverse occlusal cant.
- Orbital retrusion with pronounced exorbitism.
- Frontal bar flattening and reduced anterior cranial volume.
- Radiographic or clinical signs of elevated intracranial pressure (ICP).
- Residual deformities after posterior vault distraction osteogenesis (PVDO) or fronto-orbital advancement (FOA).

These patients frequently present during the mixed dentition phase with midfacial underprojection, poor ocular coverage, and airway compromise. The Monobloc + Le Fort II construct enables simultaneous correction of these features through dual-segment advancement. Importantly, the operation can be timed to reduce the burden of future orthognathic intervention by establishing functional occlusion early in development.

Patient selection is nuanced and benefits from a multidisciplinary assessment involving craniofacial surgeons, neurosurgeons, orthodontists, ophthalmologists, and speech-language pathologists. A thorough workup includes:

- High-resolution computed tomography (CT) with three-dimensional (3D) reconstruction to evaluate bone volume, sinus pneumatization, orbital depth, and plan distractor trajectories.
- Photographic analysis and 3D facial scanning to assess facial convexity and midfacial height.
- Dental impressions or digital occlusal scans for occlusal analysis and model surgery.
- Ophthalmologic evaluation for corneal protection, lagophthalmos, and globe position.
- Airway imaging or endoscopy as indicated.

Contraindications include active infection, unstable intracranial hypertension, insufficient bone stock for distractor fixation, and limited caregiver support to manage postoperative halo care. Informed consent must include counseling on the complexity of the procedure, halo care requirements, and potential risks.

Operative Technique

Operative planning for Monobloc with Le Fort II advancement begins with detailed virtual surgical planning (VSP), a cornerstone of our current workflow. Using high-resolution CT imaging, craniofacial and neurosurgical teams collaborate to simulate osteotomy patterns, define independent vector trajectories, and plan device placement. CAD/CAM technology is used to generate patient-specific cutting guides and distractor positioning jigs, based on two to three virtual planning sessions conducted jointly by surgical, orthodontic, and biomedical engineering teams.

Access is gained through a bicoronal incision combined with upper gingivobuccal sulcus incisions to expose the anterior cranial vault and midface. After fixation of the supraorbital cutting guide, bifrontal craniectomy is performed by the neurosurgical team. The monobloc osteotomy is performed in a standard fashion, mobilizing the frontal bone, orbital bandeau, and supraorbital bar as a single segment. Temporal bone tabs may be included to increase the low-vault contact area. Once the monobloc segment is released, attention is turned to the midface.

The Le Fort II osteotomy is initiated at the nasal radix, carried through the infraorbital rims, maxillary sinuses, and down to the pterygoid plates. Additional osteotomies are performed at the zygomaticomaxillary junction and nasion, fully separating the nasomaxillary segment from the monobloc to enable differential distraction. A pericranial flap is placed over the anterior cranial base to mitigate CSF leak risk and support dural integrity.

Distractor placement is guided by prepositioned CAD/CAM templates. Internal distractors are fixated bilaterally using 4-mm self-tapping screws to secure the temporal baseplates and zygomatic footplates. For the Le Fort II segment, a rigid external distraction device is mounted to the piriform rim using 27-mm transcutaneous pins secured to 1.5-mm plates. The frontal bone may be reshaped to reduce turricephaly and is then rigidly fixated to the monobloc to allow co-movement during distraction.

An external halo distractor is applied using bicortical pins across the bitemporal region to control monobloc vectoring. A latency phase of five days precedes distraction. The monobloc is advanced horizontally at a rate of 1 mm/day. Concurrently or in staggered fashion, the Le Fort II segment is distracted along an oblique vector to achieve anterior, inferior, and clockwise rotational movement. Total distraction typically spans two to three weeks.

Following distraction, an 8–12-week consolidation phase is observed. During this period, patients undergo weekly vector assessments and imaging to ensure fidelity of segment positioning. Serial clinical photographs and 3D facial scans are used to monitor progress. Caregiver education on halo care and vector adjustment may be instituted depending on stability and home resources.

Halo and hardware removal is performed under general anesthesia. This may coincide with secondary soft tissue procedures, such as canthopexy or minor contour refinements. Final assessment is made of bony union, soft tissue adaptation, and vector achievement. When performed with careful preoperative planning and multidisciplinary coordination, Monobloc with Le Fort II advancement enables effective, three-dimensional reconstruction of the complex Apert midface phenotype, reducing the need for staged procedures and improving long-term functional and aesthetic outcomes.

Outcome Highlights

Outcomes from the Monobloc + Le Fort II technique within our institutional cohort ($n = 41$ midface advancements) demonstrate notable improvements in facial projection, function, and proportion [49]. Among all osteotomy strategies studied, the Monobloc + Le Fort II subgroup demonstrated the greatest gain in facial convexity (median change of −34.9°), along with measurable improvements in nasofrontal angle, vertical facial height, and canthal orientation. These effects are illustrated in Fig. 20.7, which depicts preoperative and six-month postoperative soft tissue landmarks used for outcome analysis, including facial convexity angle, intercanthal distance, canthal tilt, and facial thirds.

Functionally, improvements in airway patency, occlusion, and ocular globe protection were observed. In some cases, postoperative orthognathic needs were eliminated due to early correction of the occlusal plane and sagittal relationship. Patients also demonstrated improved corneal protection, reduced globe prominence, and improved eyelid competence postoperatively.

Segmental osteotomies, including Monobloc + Le Fort II, were exclusively performed using external halo distraction, which facilitated refined vector control ($p = 0.047$). Although differences in operative time, blood loss, and pediatric intensive care unit (PICU) stay were not statistically significant, the LF II + ZR group demonstrated the lowest values across these metrics.

Figure 20.8 shows a representative case of segmental monobloc-based advancement. A nine-year-old female with Apert syndrome underwent monobloc with facial bipartition distraction. Her preoperative appearance (top row) and four-year postoperative follow-up (bottom row) highlight the stability, symmetry, and proportional improvement achievable with segmentation-based strategies.

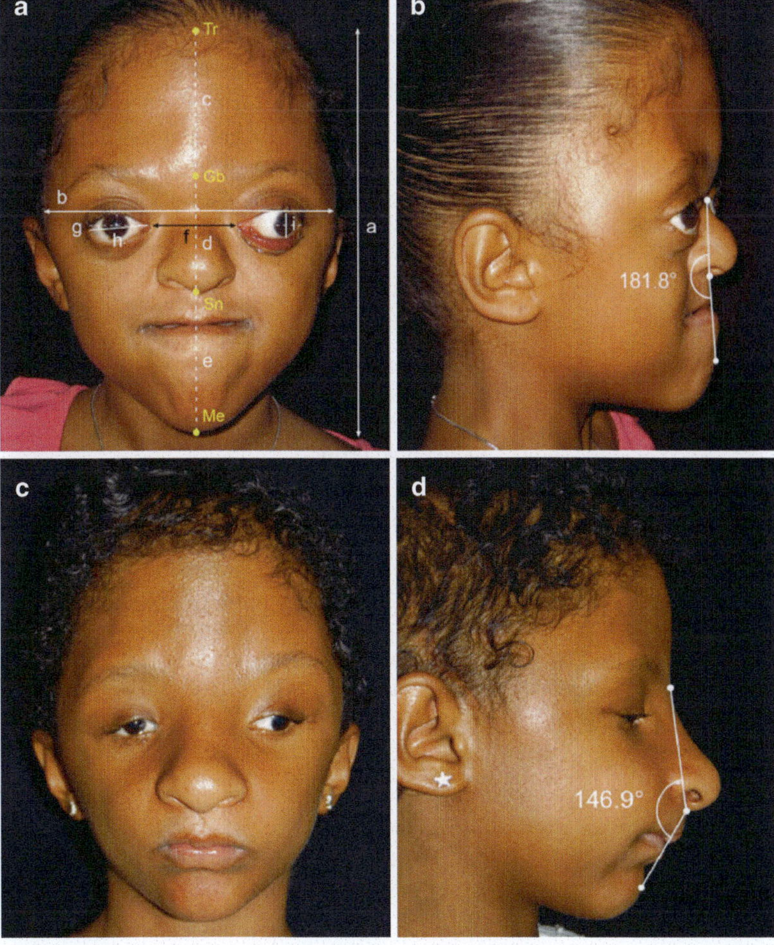

Fig. 20.7 Facial measurements used for the calculation of soft tissue ratios, demonstrated on the preoperative (top row) and six months postoperative (bottom row) photographs of an 11-year-old female patient who underwent monobloc with Le Fort II distraction: (**a**) facial height, (**b**) facial width, (**c**) upper third height, (**d**) middle third height, (**e**) lower third height, (**f**) intercanthal distance, (**g**) canthal tilt angle, (**h**) palpebral fissure width, (**i**) palpebral fissure height, (**j**) facial convexity angle. *Tr* trichion, *Gb* glabella, *Sn* subnasale, *Me* menton

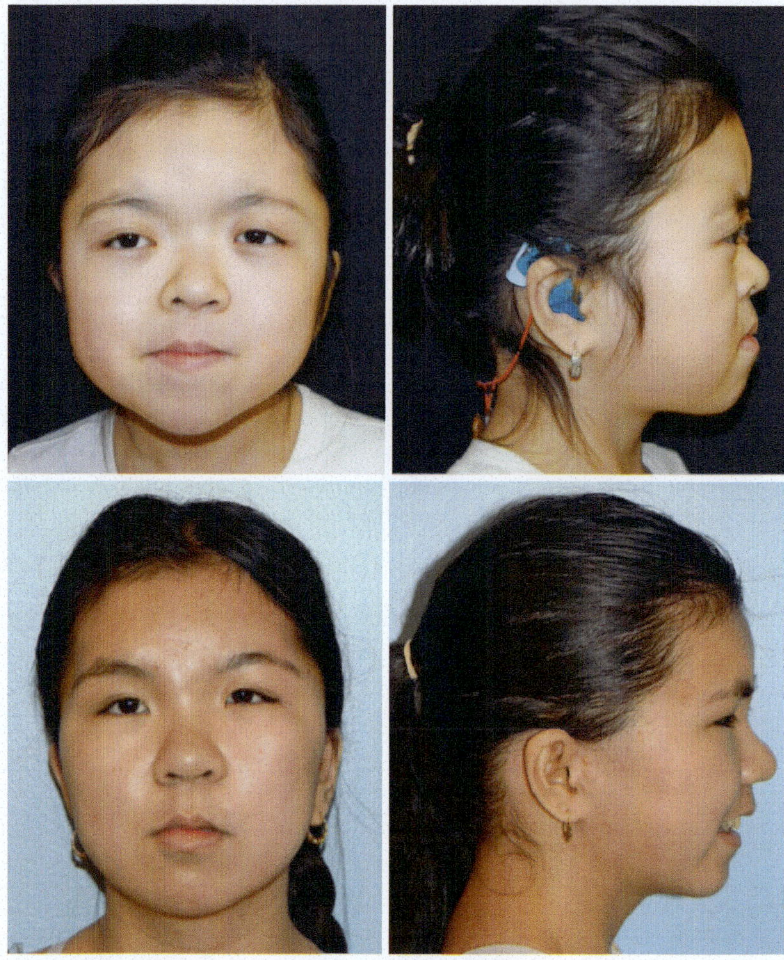

Fig. 20.8 A nine-year-old female with Apert syndrome who underwent monobloc with facial bipartition distraction is shown preoperatively (top row) and at four years postoperatively (bottom row)

Complications and Mitigation

Complication rates varied by osteotomy type, with Monobloc + Le Fort II showing a 67% complication rate, similar to LF II + ZR. However, complication severity differed. Only transcranial procedures (Monobloc-based) resulted in Clavien-Dindo grade IVa events, including one cerebrospinal fluid (CSF) leak requiring lumbar drainage and one ascending infection requiring operative re-exploration. Additional complications included infections and hardware migration, all of which were managed successfully.

Notably, segmental monobloc approaches did not show increased morbidity compared to monobloc alone, and Le Fort II + ZR demonstrated no higher complication rate than Le Fort III. This suggests that surgical segmentation can be achieved without a proportional increase in procedural risk, provided meticulous technique and close postoperative monitoring.

Long-term follow-up (mean > 24 months) has shown sustained skeletal and soft tissue stability in most patients, with no need for secondary midface advancement in those undergoing successful Monobloc + Le Fort II distraction. These results support the durability and efficacy of dual-vector midface correction when applied in appropriately selected patients with Apert syndrome.

Ultimately, this technique exemplifies how segmentation, external distraction, and individualized planning converge to optimize facial reconstruction in complex craniosynostosis. Through precise vector control and multidisciplinary management, Monobloc + Le Fort II advancement offers a comprehensive solution to a complex phenotype, improving function, aesthetics, and quality of life.

References

1. Hopper RA, Massenburg BB. Multisutural syndromic synostosis. In: Neligan PC, editor. Plastic Surgery 5th Edition: Volume 3: Craniofacial head and neck surgery, and pediatric plastic surgery. 5th ed. Elsevier; 2023.
2. Tahiri Y, Taylor J. An update on midface advancement using Le Fort II and III distraction osteogenesis. Semin Plast Surg. 2014;28(4):184–92. https://doi.org/10.1055/s-0034-1390171.
3. Massenburg BB, Susarla SM, Kapadia HP, Hopper RA. Subcranial midface advancement in patients with syndromic craniosynostosis. Oral Maxillofac Surg Clin North Am. 2022;34(3):467–75. https://doi.org/10.1016/j.coms.2022.01.002.
4. Kreiborg S, Cohen MM. Ocular manifestations of Apert and Crouzon syndromes: qualitative and quantitative findings. J Craniofac Surg. 2010;21(5):1354–7. https://doi.org/10.1097/SCS.0b013e3181ef2b53.
5. Hopper RA, Kapadia H, Morton T. Normalizing facial ratios in apert syndrome patients with Le fort II midface distraction and simultaneous zygomatic repositioning. Plast Reconstr Surg. 2013;132(1):129–40. https://doi.org/10.1097/PRS.0b013e318290fa8a.
6. Kakutani H, Sato Y, Tsukamoto-Takakusagi Y, Saito F, Oyama A, Iida J. Evaluation of the maxillofacial morphological characteristics of Apert syndrome infants. Congenit Anom (Kyoto). 2017;57(1):15–23. https://doi.org/10.1111/cga.12180.
7. McCarthy JG, Grayson B, Bookstein F, Vickery C, Zide B. Le fort III advancement osteotomy in the growing child. Plast Reconstr Surg. 1984;74(3):343–54. https://doi.org/10.1097/00006534-198409000-00003.
8. Taylor JA, Bartlett SP. What's new in syndromic craniosynostosis surgery? Plast Reconstr Surg. 2017;140(1):82e–93e. https://doi.org/10.1097/PRS.0000000000003524.
9. Carlson AR, Taylor JA. Discussion on distraction osteogenesis in craniofacial surgery: past, present, and future. J Craniofac Surg. 2021;32(Suppl 3):1228–30. https://doi.org/10.1097/SCS.0000000000007334.
10. Greig AVH, Britto JA, Abela C, et al. Correcting the typical Apert face: combining bipartition with monobloc distraction. Plast Reconstr Surg. 2013;131(2):219e–30e. https://doi.org/10.1097/PRS.0b013e3182778882.
11. Warren SM, Shetye PR, Obaid SI, Grayson BH, McCarthy JG. Long-term evaluation of midface position after Le Fort III advancement: a 20-plus-year follow-up. Plast Reconstr Surg. 2012;129(1):234–42. https://doi.org/10.1097/PRS.0b013e3182362a2f.
12. Yang R, Shakoori P, Lanni MA, et al. Influence of Monobloc/Le Fort III surgery on the developing posterior maxillary dentition and its resultant effect on orthognathic surgery. Plast Reconstr Surg. 2021;147(2):253e–9e. https://doi.org/10.1097/PRS.0000000000007539.
13. Ortiz-Monasterio F, del Campo AF, Carrillo A. Advancement of the orbits and the midface in one piece, combined with frontal repositioning, for the correction of Crouzon's deformities. Plast Reconstr Surg. 1978;61(4):507–16. https://doi.org/10.1097/00006534-197804000-00003.
14. Knackstedt R, Bassiri Gharb B, Papay F, Rampazzo A. Comparison of complication rate between LeFort III and Monobloc advancement with or without distraction osteogenesis. J Craniofac Surg. 2018;29(1):144–8. https://doi.org/10.1097/SCS.0000000000004132.
15. Schlieder D, Markiewicz MR. Craniofacial syndromes: the Le Fort III osteotomy for correction of severe midface hypoplasia. Atlas Oral Maxillofac Surg Clin North Am. 2022;30(1):85–99. https://doi.org/10.1016/j.cxom.2021.11.004.
16. van der Meulen JC. Medial faciotomy. Br J Plast Surg. 1979;32(4):339–42. https://doi.org/10.1016/0007-1226(79)90095-x.
17. Tessier P. Apert's syndrome: Acrocephalosyndactyly type I. In: Caronni EP, editor. Craniofacial surgery. Boston: Little, Brown and Company; 1985. p. 280–303.
18. Bradley JP, Gabbay JS, Taub PJ, et al. Monobloc advancement by distraction osteogenesis decreases morbidity and relapse. Plast Reconstr Surg. 2006;118(7):1585–97. https://doi.org/10.1097/01.prs.0000233010.15984.4d.
19. Dunaway DJ, Britto JA, Abela C, Evans RD, Jeelani NUO. Complications of frontofacial advancement. Childs Nerv Syst. 2012;28(9):1571–6. https://doi.org/10.1007/s00381-012-1804-y.
20. Smartt JM, Campbell C, Hallac R, Alford J, Derderian CA. A three-dimensional study of midfacial changes following Le Fort II distraction with zygomatic repositioning in syndromic patients. J Craniofac Surg. 2017;28(8):e728–31. https://doi.org/10.1097/SCS.0000000000003869.
21. Hammoudeh JA, Goel P, Wolfswinkel EM, et al. Simultaneous midface advancement and orthognathic surgery: a powerful technique for managing midface hypoplasia and malocclusion. Plast Reconstr Surg. 2020;145(6):1067e–72e. https://doi.org/10.1097/PRS.0000000000006816.
22. Boos Lima FBDJ, Hochuli Vieira E, Juergens P, Lima Junior SM. Is subcranial Le fort III plus Le Fort I osteotomy stable? J Craniomaxillofac Surg. 2017;45(12):1989–95. https://doi.org/10.1016/j.jcms.2017.09.004.
23. Yue OY, Kalra A, Eisemann BS, et al. Simultaneous Le Fort III and Le Fort I osteotomy: surgical outcomes and clinical parameters. J Craniofac Surg. 34(1):222–6. https://doi.org/10.1097/SCS.0000000000009066.
24. Paliga JT, Goldstein JA, Storm PB, Taylor JA. Monobloc minus Le Fort II for single-stage

treatment of the Apert phenotype. J Craniofac Surg. 2013;24(4):1380–2. http://www.ncbi.nlm.nih.gov/pubmed/24015416
25. Zimmerman CE, Sun J, Wes AM, et al. Long term speech outcomes following midface advancement in syndromic craniosynostosis. J Craniofac Surg. 2020;31(6):1775–9. https://doi.org/10.1097/SCS.0000000000006581.
26. Zhang RS, Lin LO, Hoppe IC, Swanson JW, Bartlett SP, Taylor JA. Retrospective review of the complication profile associated with 71 subcranial and transcranial midface distraction procedures at a single institution. Plast Reconstr Surg. 2019;143(2):521–30. https://doi.org/10.1097/PRS.0000000000005280.
27. Glass GE, Hon KAV, Schweibert K, et al. Ocular morbidity in the correction of orbital Hypertelorism and dystopia: a 15-year experience. Plast Reconstr Surg. 2017;139(4):967–75. https://doi.org/10.1097/PRS.0000000000003178.
28. Poole MD. Complications in craniofacial surgery. Br J Plast Surg. 1988;41(6):608–13. https://doi.org/10.1016/0007-1226(88)90168-3.
29. Britto JA, Greig A, Abela C, Hearst D, Dunaway DJ, Evans RD. Frontofacial surgery in children and adolescents: techniques, indications, outcomes. Semin Plast Surg. 2014;28(03):121–9. https://doi.org/10.1055/s-0034-1384807.
30. Glass GE, Ruff CF, Crombag GAJC, et al. The role of bipartition distraction in the treatment of Apert syndrome. Plast Reconstr Surg. 2018;141(3):747–50. https://doi.org/10.1097/PRS.0000000000004115.
31. Swanson JW, Samra F, Bauder A, Mitchell BT, Taylor JA, Bartlett SP. An algorithm for managing syndromic craniosynostosis using posterior vault distraction osteogenesis. Plast Reconstr Surg. 2016;137(5):829e–41e. https://doi.org/10.1097/PRS.0000000000002127.
32. Derderian CA, Wink JD, McGrath JL, Collinsworth A, Bartlett SP, Taylor JA. Volumetric changes in cranial vault expansion: comparison of fronto-orbital advancement and posterior cranial vault distraction osteogenesis. Plast Reconstr Surg. 2015;135(6):1665–72. https://doi.org/10.1097/PRS.0000000000001294.
33. Parthasarathy J. 3D modeling, custom implants and its future perspectives in craniofacial surgery. Ann Maxillofac Surg. 2014;4(1):9. https://doi.org/10.4103/2231-0746.133065.
34. Omara M, Ali S, Ahmed M. Accuracy of midface advancement using patient-specific surgical guides and pre-bent plates versus conventional interocclusal wafers and conventional plate fixation in quadrangular Le Forte II osteotomy. A randomised controlled trial. Br J Oral Maxillofac Surg. 2021;59(10):1253–8. https://doi.org/10.1016/j.bjoms.2021.05.002.
35. Gillies H, Harrison SH. Operative correction by osteotomy of recessed malar maxillary compound in a case of oxycephaly. Br J Plast Surg. 1950;3(2):123–7. https://doi.org/10.1016/s0007-1226(50)80019-x.
36. Tessier P. Total facial osteotomy. Crouzon's syndrome, Apert's syndrome: oxycephaly, scaphocephaly, turricephaly. Ann Chir Plast. 1967;12(4):273–86. http://www.ncbi.nlm.nih.gov/pubmed/5622570
37. Flores RL, Shetye PR, Zeitler D, et al. Airway changes following Le Fort III distraction osteogenesis for syndromic craniosynostosis: a clinical and cephalometric study. Plast Reconstr Surg. 2009;124(2):590–601. https://doi.org/10.1097/PRS.0b013e3181b0fba9.
38. Nout E, Bouw FP, Veenland JF, et al. Three-dimensional airway changes after Le Fort III advancement in syndromic craniosynostosis patients. Plast Reconstr Surg. 2010;126(2):564–71. https://doi.org/10.1097/PRS.0b013e3181de227f.
39. Arnaud E, Marchac D, Renier D. Reduction of morbidity of the frontofacial monobloc advancement in children by the use of internal distraction. Plast Reconstr Surg. 2007;120(4):1009–26. https://doi.org/10.1097/01.prs.0000278068.99643.8e.
40. Posnick JC, Al-Qattan MM, Armstrong D. Monobloc and facial bipartition osteotomies for reconstruction of craniofacial malformations: a study of extradural dead space and morbidity. Plast Reconstr Surg. 1996;97(6):1118–28. https://doi.org/10.1097/00006534-199605000-00005.
41. Cruz AAV, Akaishi PMS, Arnaud E, Marchac D, Renier D. Exorbitism correction of faciocraniosynostoses by monobloc frontofacial advancement with distraction osteogenesis. J Craniofac Surg. 2007;18(2):355–60. https://doi.org/10.1097/scs.0b013e3180333b3c.
42. Raposo-Amaral CE, Ghizoni E, Raposo-Amaral CA. Apert syndrome: selection rationale for midface advancement technique. Adv Tech Stand Neurosurg. 2023;46:245–66. https://doi.org/10.1007/978-3-031-28202-7_13.
43. Whitaker LA, Munro IR, Salyer KE, Jackson IT, Ortiz-Monasterio F, Marchac D. Combined report of problems and complications in 793 craniofacial operations. Plast Reconstr Surg. 1979;64(2):198–203. https://doi.org/10.1097/00006534-197908000-00011.
44. Forte AJ, Lu X, Hashim PW, et al. Airway analysis in Apert syndrome. Plast Reconstr Surg. 2019;144(3):704–9. https://doi.org/10.1097/PRS.0000000000005937.
45. Liu MT, Kurnik NM, Mercan E, Susarla SM, Purnell CA, Hopper RA. Magnitude of horizontal advancement is associated with apnea hypopnea index improvement and counter-clockwise maxillary rotation after subcranial distraction for syndromic synostosis. J Oral Maxillofac Surg. 2021;79(5):1133.e1–1133.e16. https://doi.org/10.1016/j.joms.2020.12.037.
46. Purnell CA, Evans M, Massenburg BB, et al. Lefort II distraction with zygomatic repositioning versus Lefort III distraction: a comparison of surgical outcomes and complications. J Craniomaxillofac Surg. 2021;49(10):905–13. https://doi.org/10.1016/j.jcms.2021.03.003.
47. Dunaway DJ, Budden C, Ong J, James G, Jeelani NUO. Monobloc distraction and facial biparti-

tion distraction with external devices. Clin Plast Surg. 2021;48(3):507–19. https://doi.org/10.1016/j.cps.2021.03.004.
48. Chen K, Duvvuri P, Gibstein A, et al. Hypertelorbitism corrected by facial bipartition improves exotropia. Plast Reconstr Surg. 2022;149(5):954e–61e. https://doi.org/10.1097/PRS.0000000000009041.
49. Wu M, Massenburg BB, Ng JJ, et al. The kaleidoscope of midface management in Apert syndrome: a 23-year single-institution experience. Plast Reconstr Surg. 2025;155(4):767e–79e. https://doi.org/10.1097/PRS.0000000000011415.

21 Hypertelorism Correction: Monobloc Facial Bipartition with Internal Distraction

Cassio Eduardo Raposo-Amaral,
Cesar Augusto Raposo-Amaral,
and Enrico Ghizoni

Introduction

Apert syndrome is characterized by a wide spectrum of clinical features including premature fusion of the cranial and facial sutures (craniofaciosynostosis) and complex syndactyly of the upper and lower limbs [1]. Patients with Apert syndrome always present abnormally retruded maxillary morphology, varying degrees of exophthalmos due to shallow orbits (exorbitism), and significant multilevel airway obstruction [2]. Additionally, patients with Apert syndrome frequently present elevated intracranial pressure due to craniosynostosis [3].

Based on a myriad of clinical features, comprehensive Apert syndrome management should begin at early infancy in a multidisciplinary setting [4]. The paramount surgical goals in Apert syndrome treatment are: (1) alleviation of elevated intracranial pressure, (2) protection of the ocular globe, (3) improvement in airway status, (4) reduction in facial morphologic disproportions without prejudicing maximum cognitive development, (5) achieving full use of upper and lower limbs, (6) providing 5-digit hand function and dexterity, and (7) improving facial and limb aesthetics [5, 6].

Prior to the start of the distraction osteogenesis (DO) era, monobloc facial bipartition was rarely performed to treat syndromic patients who presented midface retrusion accompanied by hypertelorism. Monobloc facial bipartition (hereafter referred to as MFB) represents the combined utilization of two landmark techniques: the frontofacial monobloc advancement as described by Ortiz-Monasterio [7] and facial bipartition described by Van der Muelen [8]. MFB adds facial bipartition to frontofacial monobloc advancement to address specific clinical features that cannot be resolved solely by monobloc advancement.

The treatment of midface retrusion accompanied by hypertelorism, as well as other less common syndromic conditions, experienced significant advancements in the late 1990s. This progress was achieved through the integration of distraction osteogenesis with monobloc facial bipartition, resulting in the development of a novel technique: monobloc and facial bipartition advancement with distraction osteogenesis (MFBDO) [9]. Distraction osteogenesis (DO) is increasingly recognized as a superior and comprehensive surgical technique resulting in increased bony stability and lower complication rates than immediate or acute movements. It can be performed mostly via internal and external halo distractor devices [10].

C. E. Raposo-Amaral (✉) · E. Ghizoni
Institute of Plastic and Craniofacial Surgery, SOBRAPAR Hospital, Campinas, São Paulo, Brazil

Department of Neurology, University of Campinas (UNICAMP), Campinas, São Paulo, Brazil

C. A. Raposo-Amaral
Institute of Plastic and Craniofacial Surgery, SOBRAPAR Hospital, Campinas, SP, Brazil

J. G. Meara et al. (eds.), *Apert Syndrome*, https://doi.org/10.1007/978-3-032-12551-4_21

MFBDO. was first described by the University of California, Los Angeles (UCLA) group in 2008 [11]. The Great Ormond Street Hospital (GOSH) group described a similar technique utilizing an external halo device and popularized the procedure worldwide with sequential studies [12–14].

MFBDO. is especially effective in treating syndromic patients concurrently presenting a combination of clinical features such as vertical orbital dystopia, palpebral fissure down slanting, divergent strabismus, and/or a collapsed maxillary arch with an inverted "V" shaped deformity. Medialization of the hemi-halves of the face, in combination with midface advancement in a single bloc, both of which are performed as part of the MFBDO technique, offers significant benefit to Apert, Crouzon, and Pfeiffer syndromic craniosynostosis (SC) patients with significant hypertelorism and/or vertical orbital dystopia [15].

It should be noted that patients with Apert syndrome will most frequently benefit from palatal expansion following hemifacial medialization as patients with this syndrome routinely present many of the clinical features that are characteristic of the syndromic face.

Although numerous studies in the applicable literature have already reported MFBDO as an effective technique for comprehensive treatment of the aforementioned clinical features in SC patients [12, 16, 17], it is not currently being performed in the majority of craniofacial centers worldwide.

MFBDO is indicated for SC patients with mild-to-severe exorbitism and/or midface retrusion, patients with recessive brow position accompanied by one or more of the following clinical features: hypertelorism, vertical orbital dystopia, marked down slanting of the palpebral fissure (even if unaccompanied by divergent strabismus), and a collapsed maxillary arch with an inverted "V" shaped deformity.

Surgical Technique

First Step: Craniofacial Skeleton Undermining

MFBDO is commenced by a combination of the gingivobuccal sulcus and coronal incisions to fully expose the midface, pyriform aperture, pterygomaxillary junction, and hard palate, immediately followed by a complete craniofacial skeletal undermining from the bottom to the top. Palatal incisions and harvesting are performed sequentially to prevent injury to the palatal mucosa during osteotomies.

Once the coronal incision has been made and the coronal flap has been sufficiently elevated, hemostatic sutures are placed to prevent excessive intraoperative bleeding.

To minimize blood loss, which is especially likely to occur in patients that have already undergone fronto-orbital and/or early midface advancement, subgaleal undermining is performed approximately 15 mm from the supraorbital nerve. To seal off communication between the oral/nasal cavities and the brain, and prevent cerebrospinal fluid (CSF) leakage, meningitis, and infection, the periosteal flap is elevated. Following flap elevation, the supraorbital nerve is released (using a 2 mm osteotome if needed), and the circumferential orbits, lateral orbital walls, and zygomatic arch are all exposed.

The temporalis muscle is released to enable insertion of the tip of the saw into the orbital fissure for subsequent performance of lateral orbital wall osteotomies. It is detached from the lateral orbital wall only. This technique also facilitates facial segment medialization following the bipartition maneuver. If any hollowing occurs, it is likely due to a bone gap resulting from medialization of the facial segments rather than temporalis muscle dissection. All steps described above must be completed, and the interorbital distance must be measured before performing any additional steps.

Second Step: Craniotomy

To enable dissection of the dura mater and exposure of the anterior cranial base, sphenoid, orbital roof, and cribriform plate, the senior plastic surgeon first marks the craniotomy site, and then the craniotomy is performed by the neurosurgeon. Dissection of the anterior cranial fossa should not extend beyond the crista galli. The craniotomy must be sufficiently large to ensure access for bone cuts and enable mitigation of forehead hollowing, which might result from monobloc advancement, but with due regard for the risk of residual bone loss and potential infection.

If sagittal sinus bleeding occurs, blood loss can be controlled via bipolar coagulation, sutures, and a dural patch superimposed onto the suture.

Third Step: Facial Osteotomies and Down-Fracture Maneuver

Once the orbital contents have been fully released, bilateral osteotomies are performed via reciprocating saw, starting from the anterior zygomatic arch, lateral orbital wall, and orbital roof, extending through the sphenoid bone, towards the anterior cranial base, and terminating anterior to the cribriform plate. A 5 mm osteotome is then used to perform orbital floor and posterior maxillary buttress osteotomies. A medial orbital wall osteotomy is performed behind the posterior lacrimal crest via a 3 mm osteotome to enable connection with the osteotomy performed across the orbital floor. The medial canthi are left attached. A pterygomaxillary osteotomy via Kawamoto osteotome is performed from the gingivobuccal sulcus incision toward the pterygomaxillary junction. An osteotome is then utilized to trim the septum and osteotomize the vomer transorally.

Confirmation of bilateral mobility and verification of the effectiveness of the posterior maxillary buttress osteotomy in the inferior lateral orbit are made via Tessier spreader insertion. A similar maneuver is performed at the pterygomaxillary junction via Kawamoto osteotome. A customized intraoral acrylic plate is placed inside the mouth to prevent inadvertent palatal fracture during craniofacial disjunction. To separate the cranium and the face, Rowe disimpaction forceps are placed, and the facial skeleton is downfractured. Stretching of the midface via side-to-side rocking is achieved via Rowe forceps.

Fourth Step: Facial Bipartition

Facial bipartition commences with a hard palate osteotomy at the midline, followed by an alveolar osteotomy between the frontal incisors via a small osteotome.

A caliper is used to measure the interdacryon distance, and a “V” shaped osteotomy is marked, and then performed via reciprocating saw from the upper medial orbital border towards the nasal bone. Between each medial orbital wall, a margin of approximately 7 mm of bone is maintained, leaving approximately 14 mm of bone between the medial canthi. The specific width of the midline “V” angle needed to medialize the hemifacial halves is determined by the individual patient’s degree of hypertelorism. Correction of associated vertical orbital dystopia can be achieved via an asymmetric “V” osteotomy. Our goal is to reduce the interorbital distance to a distance that varies from 11 to 19 mm.

After the above osteotomies have been performed, the pericranial flap is inserted into the midline to separate the oral and nasal cavities from the brain and then sutured into the dura mater. As an alternative, a periosteum patch can be sutured to the dura mater at the anterior cranial base to prevent cerebrospinal fluid (CSF) fistulae.

Fifth Step: Medialization of Facial Segments

To achieve facial convexity, the facial segments are moved medially and vertically as needed. To ensure maximum facial segment medialization, all bone in the midline, from the frontal bone of the supraorbital rim, across the ethmoid bone, towards and including the nasal bone, should be removed. Fixation at the midline with 2.0 mm titanium plates and screws, accompanied by maxillary fixation with wires, is necessary to maximize facial segment stability. Before insertion of distractor devices, interdacryon distance is re-measured. Kawamoto midface internal distraction devices (KLS Martin, Jacksonville, FL) are then placed anteriorly in the inferior region of the lateral orbital wall, posteriorly behind the zygomatic root, and above the auditory canal, as these areas of the craniofacial skeleton and cranial base are especially thick. Once the stability of the distractors is tested, two drains are placed in the subgaleal plane, and all incisions are sutured (Figs. 21.1, 21.2, 21.3 and 21.4).

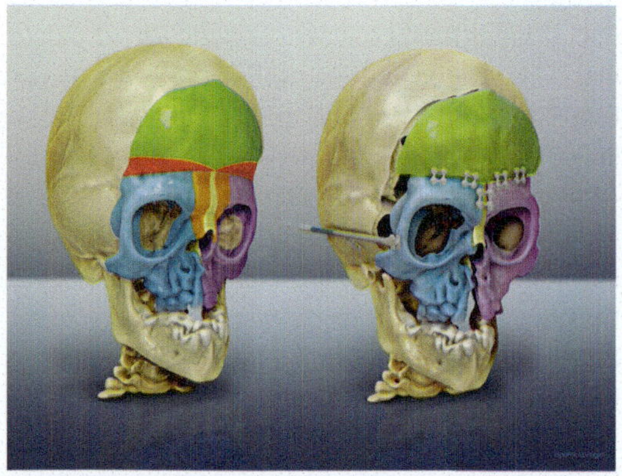

Fig. 21.1 Illustrative drawings of monobloc facial bipartition depicting the craniofacial skeleton of a 9-year-old patient with Apert syndrome (left). On the right, the craniofacial skeleton following hemi-facial medialization and subsequent fixation with plates and screws is shown. The resected midline bone can augment the nasal dorsum as a bone graft

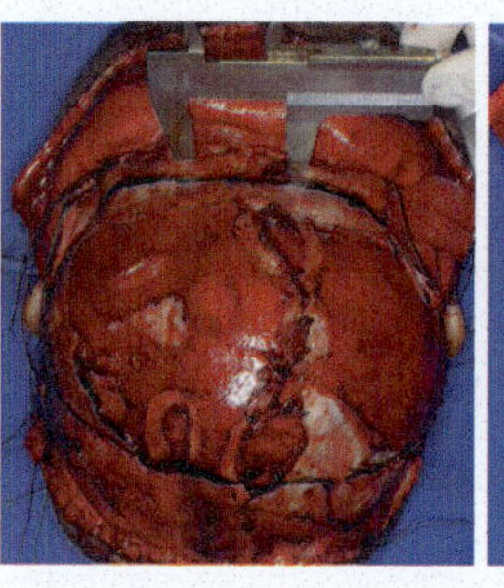

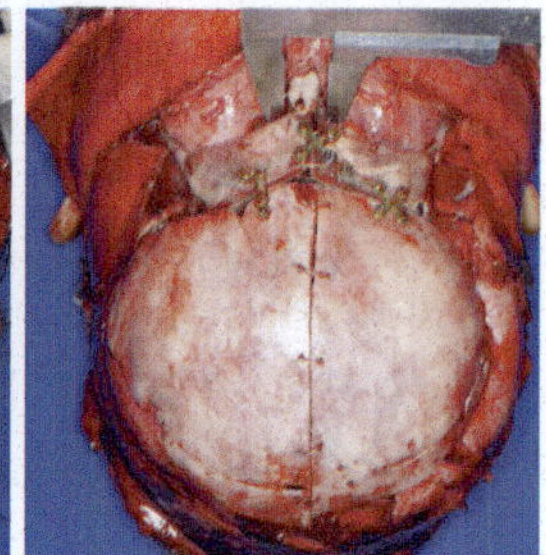

Fig. 21.2 Intraoperative photograph before craniotomy (left), showing an interorbital distance of 34 mm. The intraoperative photograph on the right depicts fixation at the midline with an interorbital distance of 14 mm (following a 20 mm midline resection)

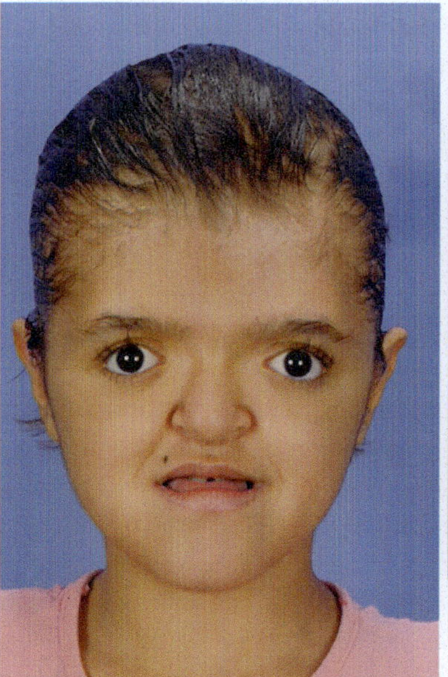

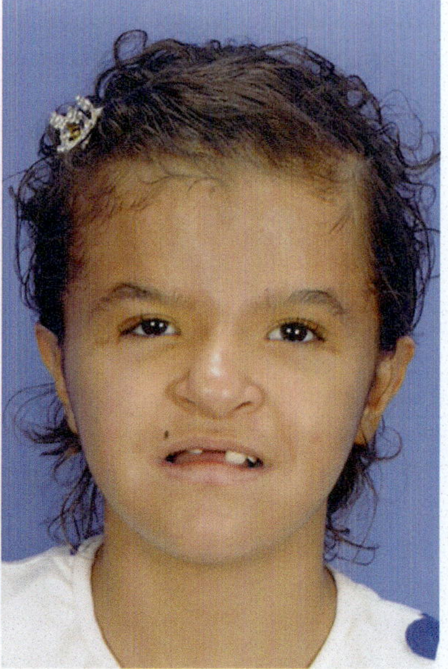

Fig. 21.3 Preoperative frontal photograph of a patient with Apert syndrome and the corresponding postoperative photograph

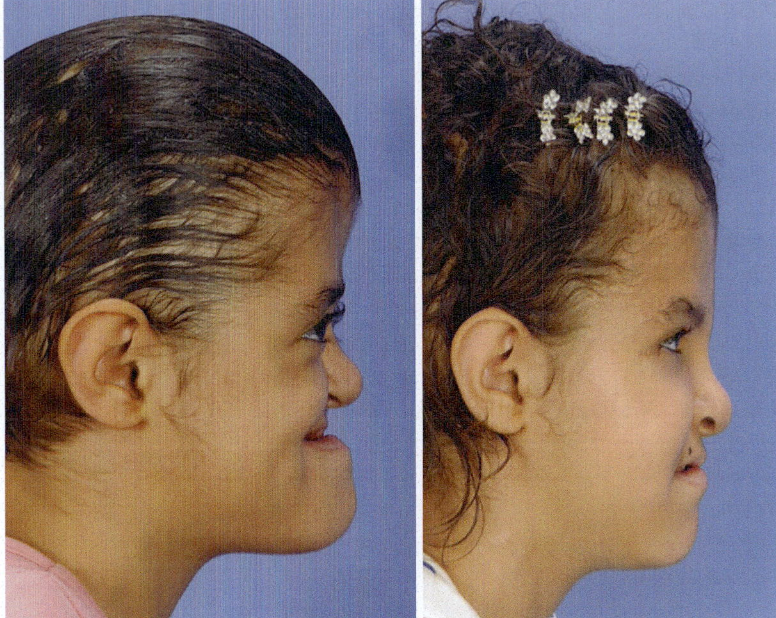

Fig. 21.4 Preoperative lateral photograph alongside the postoperative lateral photograph

Distraction End-Points

The end-point for distraction was the orbital level, which left those patients operated on at skeletal immaturity with mild enophthalmos. Conversely, patients who underwent surgery at skeletal maturity did not need subsequent overcorrection.

Distraction Protocol

Following distractor insertion and prior to any distractor activation, there is a latency period of 5–7 days to facilitate the sealing of the anterior cranial base. Once the latency period has been completed, there is a distractor activation period that may vary according to the patient's need, during which the midface is advanced at a rate of 1 mm per day. After completion of the activation period, there is an 8-week consolidation period.

There is no current consensus as to whether the distraction regimen's reconstructive and aesthetic benefits are best achieved by using internal distractors or external distractors.

Internal distractor device advantages include a longer utilization period if needed due to patient acceptance, improved device fixation and stability, and superior wound management before removal. In addition, the internal distractor device applies clockwise rotation, bringing greater sagittal movement on the lateral face in comparison to the central face [18, 19].

On the other hand, external distractor devices enable greater control of distraction vectors and easier removal. The external distractor devices apply counterclockwise rotation, bringing greater sagittal movement on the central face in comparison to the lateral face [16].

Complications and Patient Age

Serious complications associated with MFBDO include infection and frontal bone loss, CSF fistulae, meningitis, seizure, and major blood loss requiring massive transfusion of red blood cells during the distraction procedure as well as subdural hematoma. Fatality has also been reported in the literature.

Several studies have reported that midface growth appears to cease following the performance of midface advancement. Younger patients are more likely to require skeletal overcorrection via subsequent secondary procedures, as they are more prone to secondary procedures requiring additional midface advancement surgery at the end of craniofacial skeleton growth.

Monobloc Bipartition Distraction: Advantages and Disadvantages

The advantages and disadvantages to patients undergoing MFBDO appear to be syndrome-specific. Due to changes in lateral canthi position and orbital axis rotation, which is likely to fully address convergent strabismus, the ultimate surgical outcome for patients who undergo MFBDO will be true destigmatization of the syndromic face. Palatal expansion via bipartition within the MFBDO technique will correct classic Apert syndrome patient clinical features in the maxillary region, such as dental crowding and a high-arched palate. Frontal incisor diastema caused by MFBDO in patients with Apert syndrome is likely to improve over time, even without further orthodontia [18, 20]. On the other hand, patients with Crouzon syndrome usually do not require maxillary expansion via surgery, and a residual diastema caused by MFBDO facial bipartition would necessitate secondary orthodontic treatment.

Additionally, once a patient reaches adulthood, a patient who undergoes MFBDO (as with any other midface advancement technique) will still likely require orthognathic surgery, rhinoplasty, and soft-tissue refinements. Fat injection has gained momentum in mild and moderate facial deformities post-monobloc advancements [21].

Conflict of Interest The authors have no personal financial or institutional interests in any of the drugs, materials, or devices described in this article.

Funding None.

References

1. Taylor JA, Bartlett SP. What's new in syndromic Craniosynostosis surgery? Plast Reconstr Surg. 2017;140:82e–93e.
2. Allam KA, Wan DC, Khwanngern K, et al. Treatment of apert syndrome: a long-term follow-up study. Plast Reconstr Surg. 2011;127:1601–11.
3. Marucci DD, Dunaway DJ, Jones BM, Hayward RD. Raised intracranial pressure in Apert syndrome. Plast Reconstr Surg. 2008;122:1162–8; discussion 9–70.
4. Warren SM, Proctor MR, Bartlett SP, et al. Parameters of care for craniosynostosis: craniofacial and neurologic surgery perspectives. Plast Reconstr Surg. 2012;129:731–7.
5. Raposo-Amaral CE, Vincenzi-Lemes M, Medeiros ML, Raposo-Amaral CA, Ghizoni E. Apert syndrome: neurosurgical outcomes and complications following posterior vault distraction osteogenesis. Child's Nervous Syst: ChNS. 2024;40:2557–63.
6. Raposo-Amaral CE, Denadai R, Oliveira YM, Ghizoni E, Raposo-Amaral CA. Apert syndrome management: changing treatment algorithm. J Craniofac Surg. 2020;31:648–52.
7. Ortiz-Monasterio F, del Campo AF, Carrillo A. Advancement of the orbits and the midface in one piece, combined with frontal repositioning, for the correction of Crouzon's deformities. Plast Reconstr Surg. 1978;61:507–16.
8. van der Meulen JC. Medial faciotomy. Br J Plast Surg. 1979;32:339–42.
9. Cohen SR, Boydston W, Hudgins R, Burstein FD. Monobloc and facial bipartition distraction with internal devices. J Craniofac Surg. 1999;10:244–51.
10. Bradley JP, Gabbay JS, Taub PJ, et al. Monobloc advancement by distraction osteogenesis decreases morbidity and relapse. Plast Reconstr Surg. 2006;118:1585–97.
11. Bradley JP, Levitt A, Nguyen J, et al. Roman arch, keystone fixation for facial bipartition with monobloc distraction. Plast Reconstr Surg. 2008;122:1514–23.
12. Glass GE, Ruff CF, Crombag G, et al. The role of bipartition distraction in the treatment of Apert syndrome. Plast Reconstr Surg. 2018;141:747–50.
13. Greig AV, Britto JA, Abela C, et al. Correcting the typical Apert face: combining bipartition with monobloc distraction. Plast Reconstr Surg. 2013;131:219e–30e.
14. Khonsari RH, Way B, Nysjo J, et al. Fronto-facial advancement and bipartition in Crouzon-Pfeiffer and Apert syndromes: impact of fronto-facial surgery upon orbital and airway parameters in FGFR2 syndromes. J Craniomaxillofac Surg. 2016;44:1567–75.
15. Raposo-Amaral CE, Ghizoni E, Raposo-Amaral CA. Apert syndrome: selection rationale for midface advancement technique. Adv Tech Stand Neurosurg. 2023;46:245–66.
16. Dunaway DJ, Budden C, Ong J, James G, Jeelani NUO. Monobloc distraction and facial bipartition distraction with external devices. Clin Plast Surg. 2021;48:507–19.
17. Raposo-Amaral CE, Denadai R, Ghizoni E, Raposo-Amaral CA. Treating craniofacial Dysostoses with Hypertelorism by Monobloc facial bipartition

distraction: surgical and educational videos. Plast Reconstr Surg. 2019;144:433–8.
18. Raposo-Amaral CE, Vieira PH, Denadai R, Ghizoni E, Raposo-Amaral CA. Treating syndromic Craniosynostosis with Monobloc facial bipartition and internal distractor devices: destigmatizing the syndromic face. Clin Plast Surg. 2021;48:521–9.
19. Paternoster G, Haber SE, Khonsari RH, James S, Arnaud E. Craniosynostosis: Monobloc distraction with internal device and its variant for infants with severe syndromic Craniosynostosis. Clin Plast Surg. 2021;48:497–506.
20. Raposo-Amaral CE, Raposo-Amaral CA, Ghizoni E. Discussion of "Does the mutation type affect the response to cranial vault expansion in children with Apert syndrome?". J Craniofac Surg. 2023;34:913–5.
21. Denadai R, Raposo-Amaral CA, Raposo-Amaral CE. Fat grafting in managing craniofacial deformities. Plast Reconstr Surg. 2019;143:1447–55.

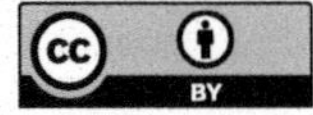

22 Hypertelorism Correction: Box Osteotomy

Mark Urata

Introduction and History

The term "ocular hypertelorism" was first introduced by David Greig in 1924 to describe a distinct craniofacial deformity characterized by excessive "breadth between the eyes." [1] Paul Tessier later refined this definition to clarify that orbital hypertelorism specifically refers to a skeletal anomaly characterized by an increased interorbital distance, typically associated with craniofacial malformations [2].

Early surgical approaches to orbital hypertelorism or hypertelorbitism involved soft tissue manipulation to simulate orbital medialization. In the 1950s, Webster and Deming described approaches such as the simple frontonasal skin resection or Z-plasty to reduce the intercanthal and interbrow distances, creating the illusion of closer-set eyes [3]. However, these techniques failed to correct the underlying skeletal deformity. In 1959, Converse and Smith attempted the first bony procedures using orbitonasal osteotomies to mobilize and approximate the medial orbital walls [4]. This technique yielded suboptimal results and was associated with injury to the lacrimal system, limiting its adoption. In 1966, Shmid was the first to fully mobilize the orbits in a single patient; however, this technique was not generalizable due to the unique anatomy of the patient's frontal sinus, which permitted uncomplicated access to the orbital roof [4, 5].

During the early 1960s, Tessier developed a series of extracranial techniques, known as the "B" techniques, which involved osteotomies of the medial orbital wall and floor. The "B" techniques did not fully mobilize the orbit, and in recognition of this limitation, Tessier introduced the "A" techniques in 1967. In collaboration with neurosurgeons Guiot and Derome, Tessier established a two-stage intracranial approach for severe orbital hypertelorism [6]. Using a frontal craniotomy for intracranial access, this technique involved the complete mobilization of the orbital box with osteotomies of the medial, lateral, superior, and inferior orbital walls, thus establishing the first box osteotomy [7]. Although more technically complex than previous surgical approaches for orbital hypertelorism, this technique offered greater control in the repositioning of the orbits, thereby improving safety and predictability [6]. Tessier's box osteotomy thus became the gold standard for surgical correction of orbital hypertelorism.

Subsequent refinements to Tessier's box osteotomy emerged in 1970, with Converse's modification permitting preservation of the cribriform plate and, accordingly, olfactory function, in a single-stage operation [8]. In the same year, Edgerton developed a single-stage intracranial box osteotomy that eliminated the need for a separate frontal bone flap [9, 10]. Marchac further

M. Urata (✉)
Children's Hospital of Los Angeles, University of Southern California, Los Angeles, CA, USA
e-mail: murata@chla.usc

J. G. Meara et al. (eds.), *Apert Syndrome*, https://doi.org/10.1007/978-3-032-12551-4_22

described the creation of lateral spurs of frontal bone to improve stabilization of the lateral orbits [11]. Others introduced a variety of minor modifications to surgical exposure and osteotomy design [9, 10, 12]. Nonetheless, the fundamental principles and surgical approach to the box osteotomy have remained largely unchanged since the late twentieth century.

The procedure has evolved more significantly through technical modernization than surgical technique. Surgical planning for early box osteotomies relied on cephalometric analysis from plain radiographs [13, 14]. In contrast, the introduction of three-dimensional (3D) computed tomography (CT) imaging significantly facilitated more thorough anatomical assessment and preoperative planning [13]. In particular, the advent of virtual surgical planning (VSP) has enabled the preoperative simulation of osteotomies and orbital movements, as well as the development of patient-specific cutting guides, thereby enhancing intraoperative precision and optimizing outcomes [13, 15]. Overall, the box osteotomy remains a cornerstone of craniofacial surgery for correcting orbital hypertelorism. Tessier's original approach has had a lasting impact on the field, while modern advancements in imaging and surgical planning have further refined its precision and efficiency.

All experienced craniofacial surgeons develop their algorithms for treating patients with Apert syndrome. Our center attempted to develop a simplified algorithm, only to discover that these patients exhibit significant variability in their presentation. This, combined with the complexity of their reconstruction, warrants a more complex decision-making tree. The value of describing our specific approach to hypertelorism in the patient with Apert syndrome is contingent on a baseline understanding of (1) our conceptual approach to these patients and (2) hypertelorism's place within the entire paradigm of our unique treatment for patients with Apert syndrome.

Surgical intervention for patients with Apert syndrome is best approached by considering the face in small units. While Hopper et al. have demonstrated their segmentation approach with Le Fort II distraction with simultaneous zygomatic repositioning (Le Fort II-ZF) [16, 17], we believe that addressing hypertelorism with box osteotomies and utilizing Le Fort III/Le Fort I/bilateral sagittal split osteotomy combinations on the lower and midface offers both functional and aesthetic advantages [18].

Algorithm and Indications

In our overall algorithm, patients undergo a fronto-orbital advancement at six to ten months of age. A posterior distraction may precede the fronto-orbital advancement in cases where the patient's initial presentation indicates clinical signs of severe brachycephaly or turricephaly, Chiari malformation, central sleep apnea, or elevated intracranial pressure (Fig. 22.1).

Around the age of four to five years, patients are evaluated for frontofacial hypoplasia. If the patient demonstrates isolated frontal hypoplasia, isolated midface hypoplasia, or an equivalent frontofacial hypoplasia, the patient will undergo readvancement or distraction of the fronto-orbital complex, midface distraction, or monobloc advancement or distraction, respectively.

The brain achieves most of its physical growth by the age of six to eight years. As such, this is the point at which we address hypertelorbitism in the algorithm. Hypertelorbitism is measured clinically by the intercanthal distance and on CT by the inter-dacryon distance. The average intercanthal distance in an adult is 25–28 mm [19]. The average inter-dacryon distance is 28 mm in the adult male and 25 mm in the female [20]. The ratio between the bony distance and the soft tissue intercanthal distance is nearly 1:1 in the normal patient. More variability is seen in patients with Apert syndrome, and the inter-dacryon distance is often increased in comparison to the intercanthal distance, which is often 40 mm or more. The inter-dacryon distance in a normal seven-year-old is 23 ± 4 mm, while the intercanthal distance is 30–31 mm [21].

Early on, the senior author was driven to perform the monobloc facial bipartition for hypertelorism. However, over time, we discovered at our institution that the operation lacked the efficacy, adaptability, and flexibility of box osteotomies. We have presented data to support that

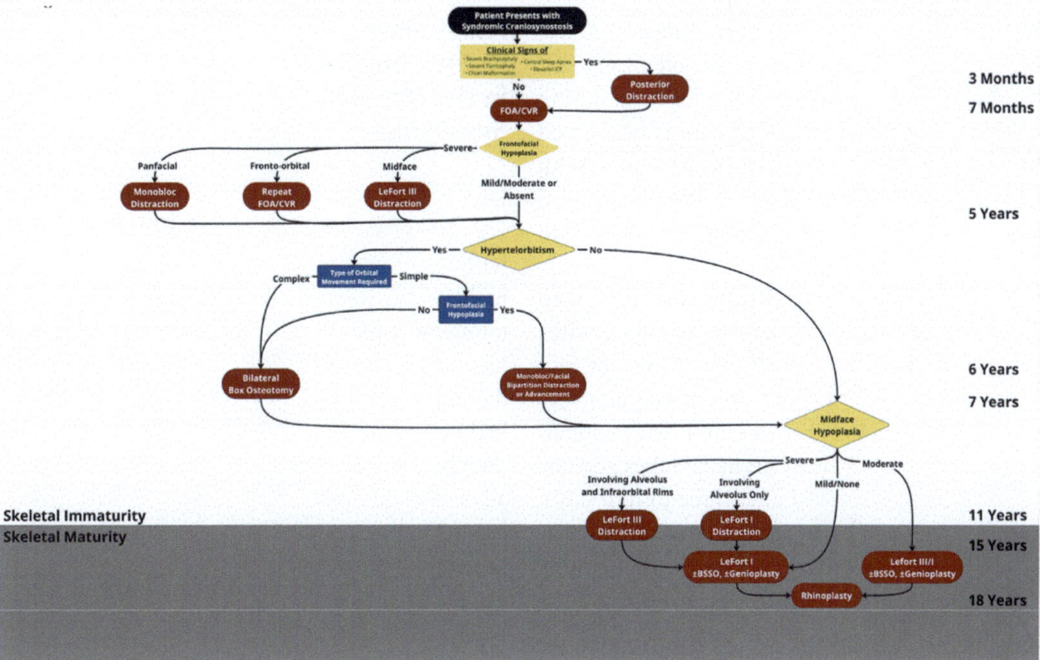

Fig. 22.1 Algorithm and indications for patients with Apert syndrome

Table 22.1 Intercanthal and inter-dacryon distances in patients with Apert syndrome compared with patients without Apert syndrome (i.e., Pfeiffer, Saethre-Chotzen, Crouzon, craniofrontonasal dysplasia)

	Apert ($n = 9$)	Non-Apert ($n = 19$)	p-value	Statistical power
Preop IDD, median	21.5 mm	33.1 mm	<0.001*	99%*
Preop ICD, median	42.6 mm	46.8 mm	0.037	66%
Preop IDD/ICD Ratio, median	0.52	0.69	<0.001*	99%*

Wilcoxon rank-sum test was used to compare the two groups

An asterisk (*) represents adequate statistical significance and/or power

Abbreviations: intercanthal distance (ICD); inter-dacryon distance (IDD)

the ratio of canthus movements to bone movement is superior in the box osteotomies when compared to the bipartition [22]. For every millimeter of bone resected, we decrease the telecanthus by 0.8 mm. By comparison, our studies demonstrate a 0.6 mm improvement in the telecanthus for every 1 mm of bony movement in the facial bipartition. This is particularly impactful in patients with Apert syndrome, as their inter-dacryon distance is often closer to normal even though their intercanthal distance is expanded.

In support of this finding, our institutional data confirms that Apert hypertelorism differs from other syndromes. The patient with Apert syndrome does demonstrate telecanthus, but the accompanying hypertelorbitism at the dacryon is significantly milder and often within a normal range. As such, we have less bone to remove while avoiding disruption to the medial canthus or to the integrity of the medial orbital bone; thus, our operation must be absolutely efficient in decreasing the soft tissue distance with the least amount of bony resection (Table 22.1).

Zide and colleagues published their work on the existence of three arms to the medial canthal tendon, in which they theorize that the superior medial limb may provide the strongest support for the elevation of the eyelids [23]. Other studies have reported that the posterior limb may be the weakest of the three [24]. In our own cadaver studies, we were able to locate the superior branch of the medial canthal tendon, which lies superior and is the most medial of the attachments. When a resection of over 1 cm is planned at the dacryon, the superior and medial location places the superior limb directly in the path of the wedge osteotomy of the facial bipartition (Fig. 22.2). By comparison, the box osteotomies require a straight resection in lieu of a wedge, and the superior tendon appears to be more often preserved with that same resection at the dacryon. We believe this may underlie the superior results achieved with box osteotomies, particularly in terms of the ratios of bone to soft tissue.

Even with these considerations, an indication for the monobloc facial bipartition remains in our current algorithm. Patients who (1) demonstrate hypertelorism along with an equivalent frontofacial hypoplasia (i.e., frontal and midface are equally hypoplastic) and (2) do not require complex orbital movements may be good candidates for monobloc facial bipartition. Complex movements of the orbit are classified as those that require:

1. A decrease at the dacryon of more than 1 cm
2. Elevation of the lateral canthi by more than 3–4 mm (via rotation of the box)
3. Vertical orbital repositioning
4. Anterior movement of the lateral orbital rims
5. Anterior repositioning of the supraorbital rims, or infraorbital rims

We have found that satisfying these parameters is increasingly rare, and box osteotomies now comprise 85% of our current hypertelorism approaches. The box is so versatile that it can obviate the need for a downstream Le Fort III in our algorithm. By performing the osteotomy caudad to include most of the malar prominence, we can then move the infraorbital rim, malar prominence, and the lateral orbital rim anteriorly, which are the principal visible achievements of a Le Fort III with respect to addressing midface hypoplasia (Fig. 22.3).

One of the most significant advantages of the box osteotomies is the ability to flare the lateral orbital rim anteriorly. This is a debilitating limitation of the facial bipartition. When a wedge is resected nasal frontally in the facial bipartition and the orbits are moved together, this necessarily constricts the facial width and creates an under projection of the lateral orbital rims. Yet, the lateral orbits cannot be flared anteriorly, as

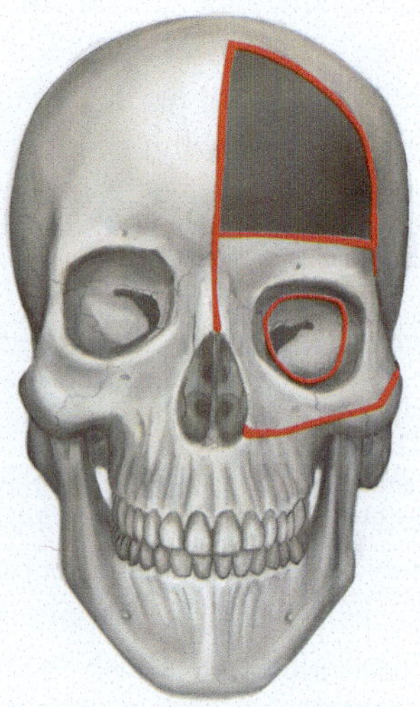

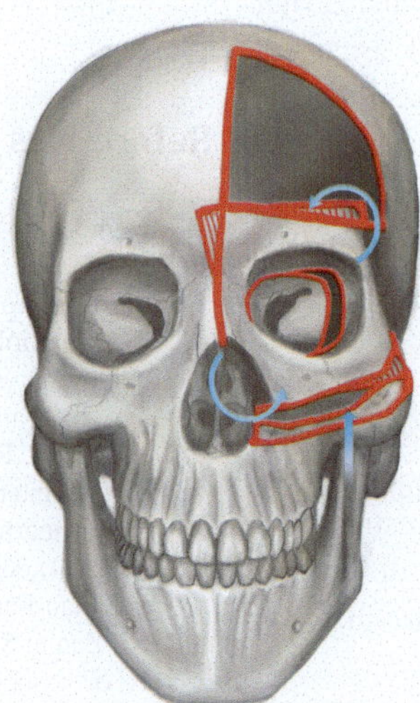

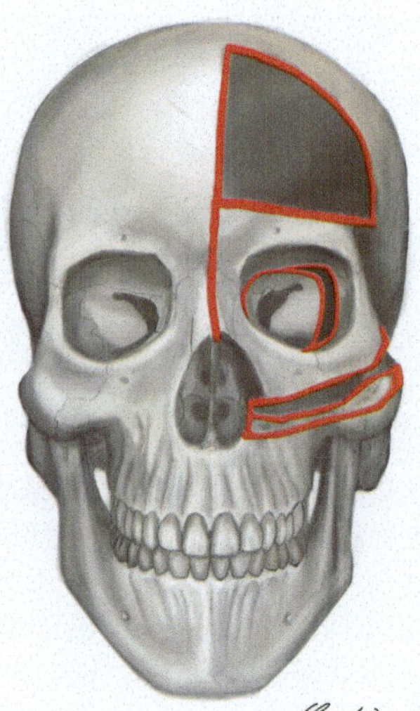

Fig. 22.2 In patients with asymmetric orbits, but symmetric malar prominences, the transverse maxillary cuts may be designed to be intra-malar, leaving the caudal malar prominence intact. This preserves malar symmetry while allowing the pinwheel rotation to adjust orbital positions and lateral canthal orientations without altering the malar prominences

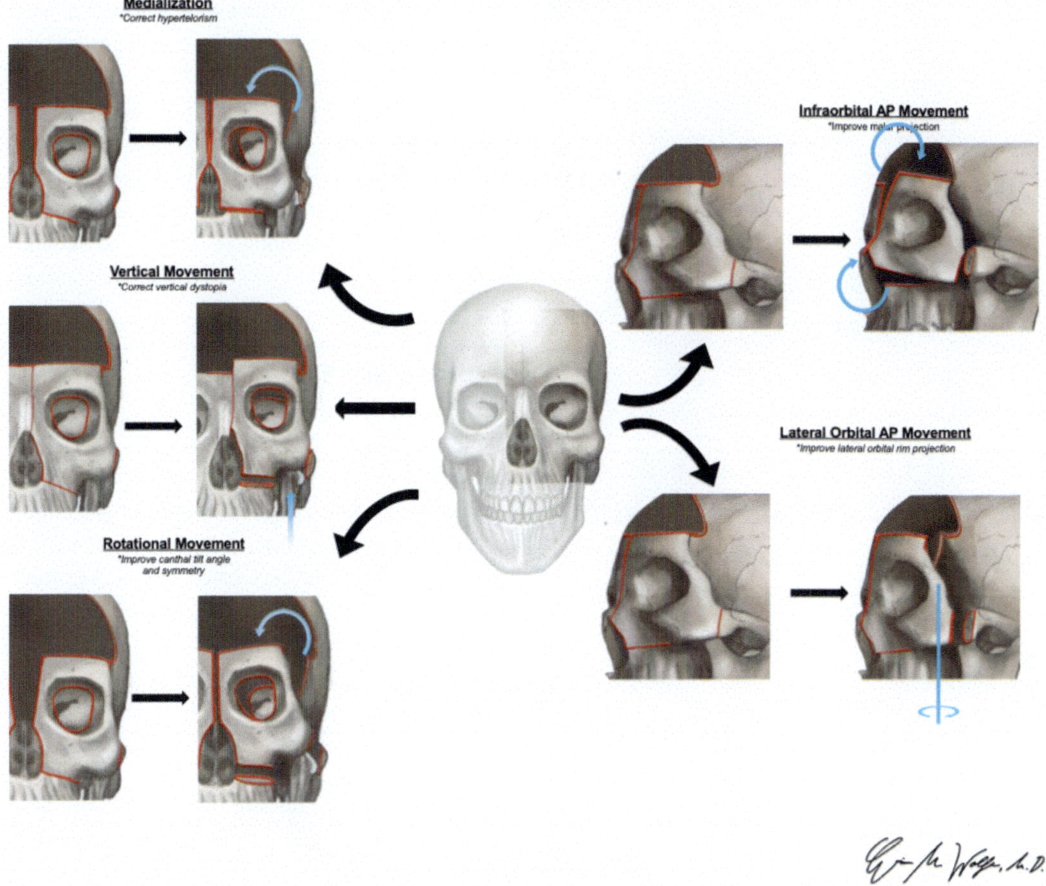

Fig. 22.3 Demonstrating the versatility of the box osteotomy movements

that requires a concomitant expansion of the posterior palate; this expansion is untenable due to limited mobility of the palatal mucosa and the bony construct. In fact, the lack of projection of the lateral orbital rims accentuates the hypertelorism appearance. The presence of visible soft tissue lateral to the orbits in the facial view gives the illusion that the eyes are closer together. Combined with the actual correction for the intercanthal appearance, this can significantly naturalize the face (Figs. 22.4 and 22.5).

Additionally, many patients with Apert syndrome demonstrate asymmetric vertical dystopia of the orbit, which often includes downslanting of the lateral canthi. As such, with the facial bipartition, this can require an asymmetric wedge resection, a procedure that is likely to compromise the medial canthal tendon on the side of larger wedge resection. Box osteotomies avoid this issue. In cases of asymmetric vertical dystopia, the more affected side can be differentially elevated and rotated without endangering the medial canthus. The rotation can most effectively address the lateral canthus, given that other surgical procedures addressing this area have substantial rates of relapse. In situations where the box will simultaneously address both a descended lateral canthus and a hypoplastic malar eminence, the fixation of the box must be such that the malar prominence is in a symmetric position to the contralateral side despite the rotation.

Some surgeons choose not to address the telecanthus or hypertelorism in patients with Apert syndrome, focusing solely on midface hypoplasia. As previously described, surgeons may base this decision on the fact that the telecanthus is not commensurate with significant bony hypertelorism in patients with Apert syndrome.

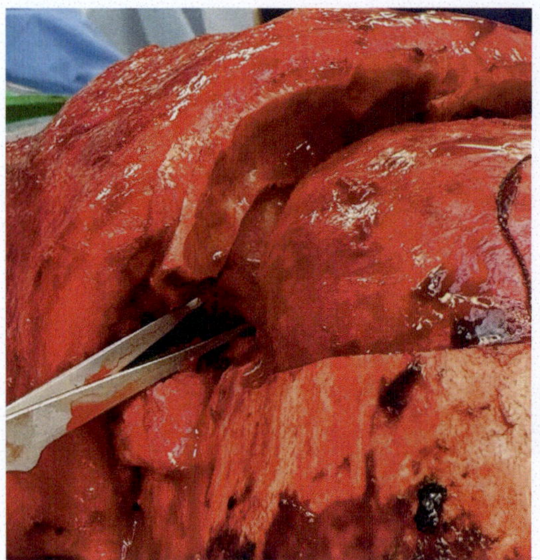

Fig. 22.4 From above, the Smith separators demonstrating the ability to flare anteriorly the lateral orbital rim

plasia in both the vertical and sagittal planes. However, we contend that the vertical nasomaxillary hypoplasia is primarily in the lower third of the face at the Le Fort I level. Thus, our approach allows us to address (1) the hypertelorism and midface hypoplasia with bilateral box osteotomies and (2) the para-pyriform advancement and elongation with orthognathic surgery at skeletal maturity.

Planning and Technique

The utilization of VSP can improve the efficiency of surgery, as has been clearly demonstrated for Le Fort I and bilateral sagittal split orthognathic surgery. However, we have not found that this advantage carries to box osteotomies. We have not yet developed the ability to accurately predict the movements of the soft tissues of the periorbital region in relation to the underlying bony movements. Thus, we are relegated to determining the position of the box in situ, where we can fixate the box based on the soft tissue changes.

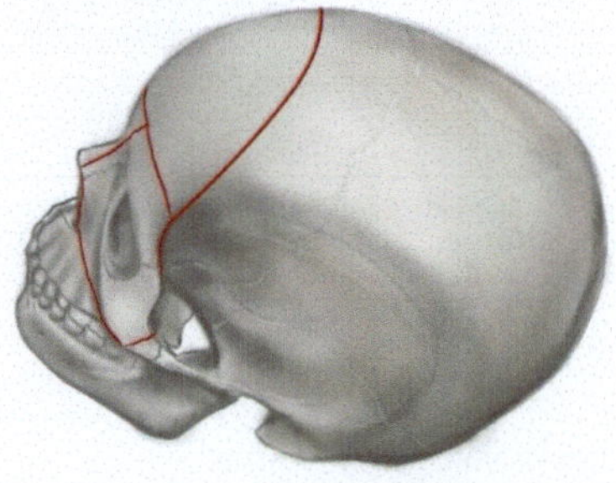

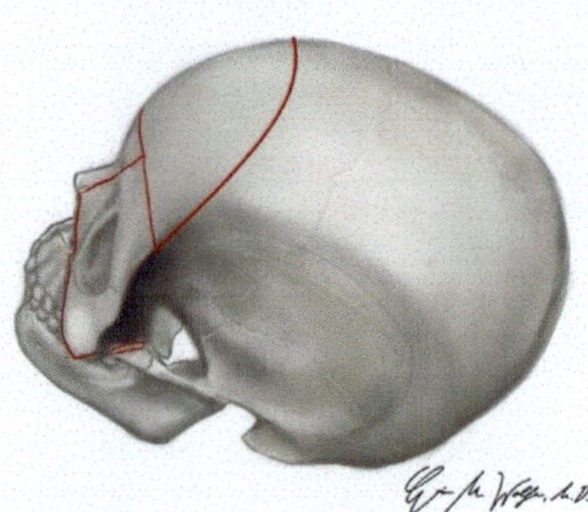

Fig. 22.5 Demonstrating the anterior flare of the lateral orbital rim

Addressing the telecanthus requires accepting that the bony reduction of a mildly expanded or normal inter-dacryon will further constrict the upper nasal vault. Typically, the Apert syndrome pyriform is already constricted, but at our institution, further constriction has not resulted in any measurable functional deficit. However, depending on the age and the disposition of the dentition, the pyriform can be widened at a later stage.

Hopper et al. described their Le Fort II-ZF approach to address nasomaxillary hypoplasia [16, 17]. However, a prior Le Fort II would make it almost challenging to develop intact bilateral box osteotomies, as the pathway of the prior Le Fort II osteotomies would have necessarily violated the framework. Patients with Apert syndrome inherently demonstrate hypoplasia in the bimalar region and exhibit nasomaxillary hypo-

Typically, our evaluation entails a CT scan axial and coronal of the brain and maxillofacial with fine cuts and 3D rendering. We also obtain an orthopantomogram or panorex. Between the ages of 6 and 11 years, the presence of unerupted premolars in the path of proposed osteotomies across the maxilla constitutes a rate-limiting step, and the panorex allows us to see the location of any unerupted teeth. Most premolars erupt into occlusion at 12–13 years of age, and the eruption sequence in the patient with Apert syndrome is often delayed by one to two years (Fig. 22.6).

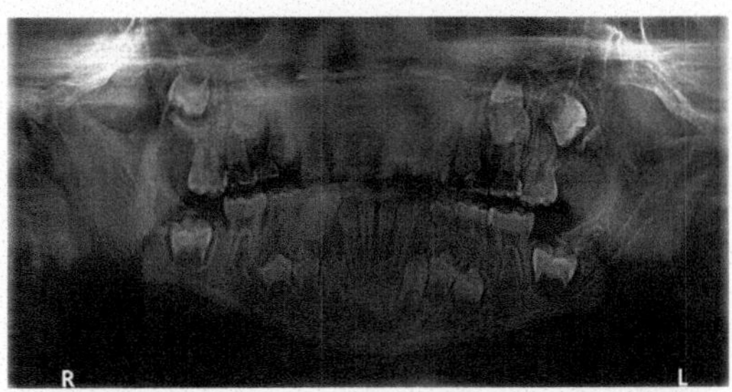

Fig. 22.6 Panorex of a 10-year-old male with Apert syndrome who has unerupted maxillary premolars that would make box osteotomies difficult without sacrificing those teeth

Thus, the presence of premolars high up in the maxilla may delay this surgery or prompt the decision to sacrifice premolars. In 34% of cases, current orthodontic treatment includes extraction of four premolars to provide space for alignment. As the patient with Apert syndrome has a narrower maxillary arch, the need to provide space with sequential extractions is commonplace. Therefore, a decision to sacrifice premolars enables box osteotomies to be performed earlier at 5–7 years old and may be executed with the treating orthodontist. In comparison, the facial bipartition requires eruption of the two maxillary permanent central incisors or visibility of an osteotomy pathway between the incisors. These teeth are fundamental to both oral health and facial aesthetics and should not be sacrificed.

The procedure begins with bilateral tarsorrhaphies to protect the eyes. Next, 0.1 cc of methylene blue is injected via a 1-cc syringe through the skin at the medial canthal tendons including the superior limb. This is accomplished by placing gentle lateral traction on the medial canthus, which allows it to be palpable. The dye alerts us that our dissection is nearing the location of the tendon, particularly at its most superior arm. We find that preserving these tendon attachments is critical for an optimal result.

A coronal approach is used to expose the calvarium. Centrally, we dissect in a subperiosteal plane. We clear the supraorbital neurovascular bundles from their respective notches or foramina and expose the orbital roof. We can dissect the periosteum away from the scalp flap should we need to incorporate a flap intracranially for cerebrospinal fluid (CSF) leaks.

Above the age of five years when we perform box osteotomies at our center, the temporalis muscle is only detached anteriorly for access to the lateral orbit; the muscle is not detached from the fossae at its origin. The superficial layer of the deep temporal fascia is dissected and elevated to allow entrance into the deep temporal fat pad and exposure of the zygomatic arch. Dissection is continued along the lateral orbital to the malar prominence. In sequence, exposure is performed on the lateral orbital wall extending caudad to demonstrate the lateral aspect of the inferior orbital fissure. Following that, the orbital floor is exposed from lateral to medial with gentle retraction of the globe. Then, while respecting the medial canthal attachments, we dissect the medial orbital wall with a Freer elevator posterior to the lacrimal groove and in continuity with the previously exposed orbital floor.

Next, we use a surgical marker to design the frontal craniotomy 1–1.25 cm superior to the supraorbital rim. We extend posterior to capture whatever aberrant deformity may be embedded in the anterior calvarial bone. We then create burr holes and dissect the dura in frontal and temporal lobes off the cranium with Penfield elevators and curved periosteal elevators. The frontal craniotomy is performed with a craniotomy, irrigation, and suction. After the craniotomy, and if deemed safe, we ask the anesthesiologists to lower the carbon dioxide to below 30 mm Hg to allow more laxity in the dural tent.

Freer and Penfield elevators are utilized to dissect the dura away from the fronto-orbital complex. If necessary, Kerrison elevators are used to remove the lip of the lesser wing of the sphenoids, which allows safer placement of retractors in the anterior middle cranial fossa. We then perform our initial osteotomy vertically through the zygomatic arch at the widest junction where it joins the zygoma. This encourages a bony bridge to form postoperatively, although many movements of the box may preclude formation of this bony bridge.

The next step—the lateral orbital osteotomy—is the same as that performed for monobloc or

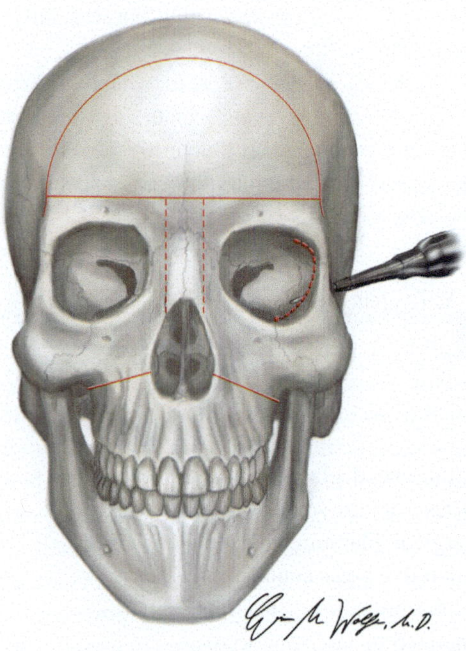

Fig. 22.7 From the temporal approach, the tip of the ultrasonic osteotome engages the lateral aspect of the inferior orbital fissure. The cut is then carried bodily in a superior direction, cutting the lateral orbital wall and roof, and simultaneously, the temporal bone to the junction with the frontal craniotomy

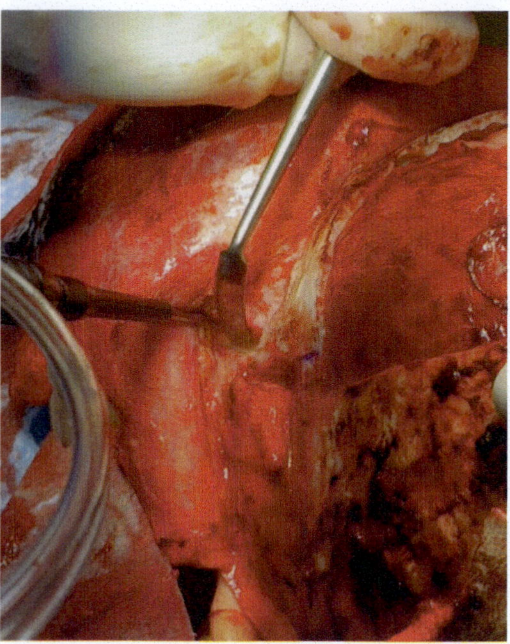

Fig. 22.8 Engaging the lateral aspect of the inferior orbital fissure and carrying the cut across the orbital floor with a posterior angle. A thin orbital retractor offers a better view to the operator than a larger one which will be restricted by the soft tissue envelope

subcranial Le Fort III procedures. We use an ultrasonic osteotome with a tapered 1.3 cm length cutting blade and embedded irrigation. The tip of the saw is engaged in the lateral aspect of the inferior orbital fissure (Fig. 22.7), while gentle traction is placed on the globe with a narrow orbital retraction. We find the narrowest, least intrusive retractor that provides visibility to be ideal; larger retractors place too much pressure on the globe and surrounding tissues, which paradoxically can decrease visibility and trigger the oculocardiac reflex.

Once the inferior orbital fissure is engaged, we advance the saw up the lateral orbit while retraction intracranially protects both the frontal and temporal lobes. The globe must also be protected, particularly as the cut approaches the orbital roof. Given that most of our patients have undergone a prior fronto-orbital advancement, we examine the zygomaticofrontal suture region for intact and robust bone. In cases where this region has a deficiency of bony continuity, a five- or six-hole plate is placed on the lateral orbital rim to bridge the region. The osteotomy of the lateral orbit will make this rim narrow, and therefore an added plate provides box integrity. The osteotomy continues cephalad near the junction of the frontal and temporal bones and is carried superiorly until it joins the frontal craniotomy. By nature of this three-dimensional cut, it traverses through the frontal bone laterally and simultaneously osteotomizes the lateral orbital roof.

Next, we elevate the globe with a small orbital retractor while engaging the lateral aspect of the inferior orbital fissure with the saw. The saw has a slight posterior angle (Fig. 22.8), as patients with Apert syndrome have a hypoplastic maxilla featuring an infraorbital rim the width of a knife edge. Making the osteotomy too anterior with no posterior angulation can result in mistakenly cutting off the infraorbital rim. This osteotomy is carried across the orbital floor to the junction of the floor with the medial wall.

Next, we perform the orbital roof osteotomy (Fig. 22.9). Again, this is completed after both sides have been addressed with the cuts described. The frontal and temporal lobes are retracted. The ultrasonic osteotome is used to engage the preexisting lateral orbital roof osteotomy, which was developed when the lateral orbital wall was cut. This roof osteotomy is continued across the orbital roof while a spoon retractor protects the globe. As the osteotome approaches the medial wall, it is lowered slightly causally into the orbit to engage the medial wall. The osteotomy is continued anterior to the cribriform plate and then across the other orbital roof to join with the cut on the lateral orbital roof.

Once the orbital roof osteotomy is complete, the remaining cuts through the coronal approach are (1) the medial wall of the orbits to join with the orbital-floor osteotomy and (2) the lateral nasal-wall osteotomy. Historically, these osteotomies have been poorly described and are difficult to conceptualize. Moreover, the development of the ultrasonic osteotome changed how these osteotomies are performed, and the procedure now looks quite different than when it was developed half a century ago. Prior to the ultrasonic osteotome—and as is the case for the orbital floor—the procedure typically utilized handheld osteotomes and a mallet and to create what amounted to controlled fractures, which diminished the potential for postoperative formation of bony bridges. Furthermore, the handheld osteotomes and reciprocating saw mandated a much broader dissection of soft tissue for exposure, avulsing some or all of the medial canthal tendon attachments and posing increased risk to the globe. Now, with more conservative retraction and the ultrasonic instrument, the procedure utilizes a fine cut that enables improved bone healing. At our institution, we address the medial wall of the orbit with an intracranial approach using the sharp portions at the side and end of the tapered ultrasonic osteotome while gently retracting the medial globe. The osteotome is inserted intranasally and carried laterally, cutting the medial orbital wall until it is in continuity with the orbital-floor cut.

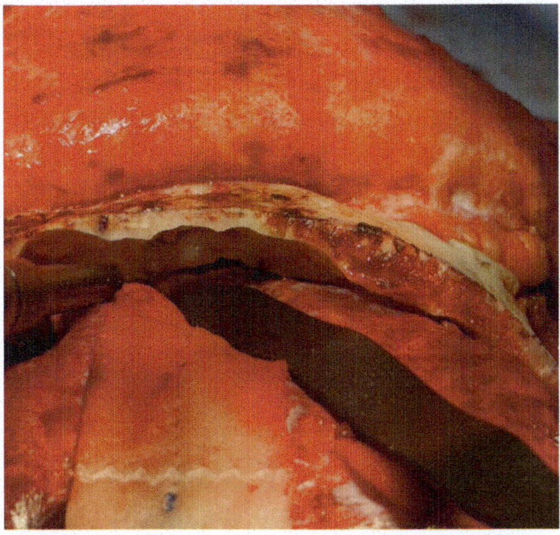

Fig. 22.9 Intracranial osteotomy across orbital roof, anterior to cribriform plate and joining with the lateral orbital wall osteotomy

Rather than continuing the cut down into the nose, we focus on the intraoral component of the procedure. After administering local anesthetic in the buccal sulcus, we make an incision from first molar to first molar. The dissection is performed subperiosteally, exposing the maxilla from caudad to cephalad. We identify and preserve the infraorbital nerves and dissect the lateral nasal mucosa. In cases where the planned movement of the boxes includes an anterior advancement, the precision of the horizontal osteotomy across the maxilla is not as critical, given that bony interference is not expected. However, in cases where the inferior aspect of the box is to remain in the same sagittal plane, the osteotomy across the maxilla must either be straight or divergent medially to enable the boxes to move medially without interference.

Again, we use the ultrasonic osteotome to perform the osteotomy from the lateral nasal wall across the mid-maxilla, including all or part of the zygoma, depending on the preoperative design. Historically, this portion of the procedure has not been well described. The horizontal maxillary osteotomy is carried onto the zygoma—to include part of it—or below the zygoma, to include all of it. In both cases, a separate osteotomy must be performed via the intra-oral approach to connect the horizontal maxillary osteotomy to the lateral aspect of the infraorbital fissure. This cut follows the path of the posterior aspect of the zygomaticomaxillary suture. This cut requires retraction of the globe from the coronal approach while the osteotomy is performed from the intraoral access.

The next osteotomy is performed from the coronal access using the end cutting portion of the ultrasonic osteotome. One surgeon visualizes the lateral nasal wall and the horizontal osteotomy of the maxilla. Concurrently, the other surgeon utilizes the ultrasonic osteotome to slowly proceed down the medial orbital wall and then the lateral nasal wall until it connects with the horizontal osteotomy of the maxilla.

Finally, through the coronal access, calipers and a surgical marker are used to mark the rectangle of the planned frontal nasal bone ostectomy. The ultrasonic osteotome is inserted via the intracranial access into the nasal vault and advanced outward toward the skin and the markings. The intracranial angulation allows the blade of the saw to parallel the nasal bones, safely making the cuts without violating the skin. Prior to the development of this technology and approach, use of a reciprocating saw necessitated a more aggressive soft tissue dissection superficial to the nasal bones to fit the blade; this process stretched or (more likely) avulsed a portion of the medial canthal tendon.

We use a Freer elevator to dissect the adherent soft tissues at the distal tip of the nasal bones, and a Coker elevator removes the segment, which is saved for potential bone grafting. A T-handled osteotome is used first to slowly complete the osteotomy intraorally at the pyriform aperture and then coronally at the lateral orbit, medial orbits, and lateral nasal walls. Completion of this step frees the box. After verifying the box remains in a single piece, we position it while appreciating the soft tissue improvements. If possible, we affix ladder plates to available points of fixation. The typical points of fixation are (1) intraorally at the pyriform and/or maxillary buttresses, (2) at the lateral orbits securing to the temporal bones, and (3) centrally, between the two boxes.

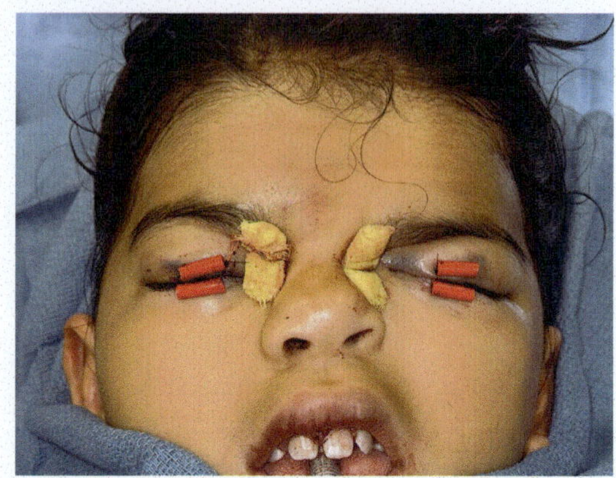

Fig. 22.10 Transcutaneous wires with Xeroform bolster dressings to protect the medial canthal attachments through peak edema stage. These are removed two weeks postoperatively

Our institution uses 28-gauge wire transnasally for a bolster dressing to protect the medial canthal tendons during peak edema (Fig. 22.10). The wire is passed through the skin above the medial canthal tendon, into the nasal vault, and exited through the skin above the medial canthal tendon on the opposite side. The wire is then turned back toward the skin, advanced through the skin below the tendon and into the nose and exited below the tendon on the opposite side. Xeroform cut into 2-cm strips is rolled and placed under the wire on both sides. The wire is then gently tightened until achieving light compression on the skin.

Finally, the frontal craniotomy bone is placed back in its original position and secured in place with plates and screws. In the case of nasal-base widening, an alar cinch suture is placed intraorally. Depending on the extent of box advancements and volume expansion, galeal scoring and scalp lengthening are performed. The scalp is then closed in a layered fashion.

Complications and Comparisons

Taylor et al. reviewed 11 prior studies on complications of box osteotomies and found a complication rate of 30% [25]. The most commonly reported complications were neurologic dysfunction (12.1%), ocular injury (5.8%), and infection

(5.2%). The neurologic complications included CSF leak, seizures, intracranial hematoma, hydrocephalus, and superior orbital fissure syndrome. Ocular complications included strabismus, ocular dyskinesia, and diplopia. Mortality was reported in three patients (0.9% of total patients) with intracranial hemorrhage and unilateral orbital edema leading to coma.

Reviewing their own experience performing "box-shift osteotomies," Jiang et al. followed 78 patients for a minimum of two years [26]. They reported early complications including strabismus (11.5%) and nasolacrimal duct obstruction (3.8%). Certainly, the horizontal osteotomy of the maxilla and accompanying lateral nasal-wall osteotomy require transection of the nasolacrimal apparatus, performed above its anterior exit beneath the inferior turbinate. Although the medial and orbital-floor osteotomies are posterior to the lacrimal groove, the 3D positioning of the box can place the lacrimal sac and accompanying canaliculi under so much tension as to render them less effective in their capacity to drain the tears. Thus, temporary obstruction to the nasolacrimal system is to be expected, and, surprisingly, our institution found this to be self-limiting. Additionally, the Jiang study identified infection (12.8%), CSF leak (29.5%), and epilepsy (2.6%) as labeled acute complications. Long-term complications included insufficient correction (55.1%), palpable hardware (92.3%), and drooping nasal tip (33.9%) [26].

In conducting our own comparison (unpublished data) of facial bipartitions and box osteotomies, we reviewed 45 cases between 2004 and 2023 that fit study criteria. We found no statistically significant difference in anesthesia time between the two procedures. Box osteotomies had an average blood loss of 400 cc, which was significantly less than the average blood loss for facial bipartitions (825 cc). As a result, box osteotomies had significantly lower blood transfusion requirements than facial bipartitions. Additionally, the box osteotomy cohort required an average of 5.5 postoperative inpatient days, compared to eight days for the facial bipartition group (Table 22.2).

Our review of our facial bipartitions and box osteotomies found postoperative complications in 33.3% of cases; however, 48.3% of the facial bipartition cohort had complications compared to only 6.2% of the box osteotomy group. This finding was statistically significant ($p = 0.004$). Box osteotomies had proportionally lower rates of major complications than facial bipartitions, at 6.2 and 24.1%, respectively ($p = 0.133$). Similarly, rates of minor complications were lower in box osteotomies (6.2%) than in facial bipartitions (27.6%) ($p = 0.087$). Two patients with facial bipartition and one patient with box osteotomy had a CSF leak, one of whom required an operation for persistent CSF leak after discharge. Additionally, two patients with facial bipartition (6.9%) experienced postoperative bleeding requiring craniotomy. One of these patients was found to have frontal intraparenchymal bleeding on postoperative CT, while the other patient experienced significant bleeding after a traumatic fall. One patient with facial bipartition required reoperation for orbital dystopia five months after the index procedure. Other complications included three cases (6.7%) of hardware exposure, three cases (6.7%) of wound infection, three cases (6.7%) of seromas, and one case (2.2%) of skin necrosis, all of which were experienced by the facial bipartition cohort. No significant differences between the two cohorts were observed in the occurrence of postoperative bleeding, CSF leak, seroma, wound infection, dehiscence, hardware exposure, or need for reoperation. Among the 15 patients who had complications, 11 experienced complications after hospital discharge (ten with facial bipartition, one with box osteotomy; however, 10 of 11 patients presented within three months postoperatively (Table 22.3).

Conclusion

Patients with Apert syndrome often demonstrate true telecanthus with normal or slightly increased inter-dacryon distance. This presentation is often seen in traumatic telecanthus with avulsed medial canthal tendons and would typically be treated by medial canthopexies using transosseous wire fix-

Table 22.2 Perioperative outcomes across the box osteotomy and facial bipartition cohorts

	Total median [IQR]	Facial bipartition median [IQR]	Box osteotomy median [IQR]	p-value
Number of cases	$n = 45$	$n = 29$	$n = 16$	
Weight at surgery (kg)	30.0 [24.6–43.1]	29.3 [25.6–37.1]	40.2 [21.8–59.2]	0.442
Anesthesia time (hours)	10.4 [9.3–10.8]	10.3 [9.4–10.8]	10.4 [8.5–11.0]	0.735
Operative time (hours)	7.8 [7.0–8.6]	7.9 [7.3–8.7]	7.6 [6.2–8.4]	0.154
Estimated blood loss (mL)	600 [400–1000]	825 [525–1250]	405 [355–575]	0.014*
Transfused packed RBCs (mL)	546 [282–895]	799 [509–1165]	296 [252–550.5]	0.003*
LOS following surgery (days)	8.0 [6.0–9.0]	8.0 [7.0–9.0]	6.0 [4.5–8.0]	0.017*
Length of ICU stay (days)	5.0 [2.0–6.0]	5.0 [4.0–7.0]	3.0 [1.5–5.5]	0.075

Abbreviations: intensive care unit (ICU); interquartile range (IQR); length of stay (LOS); milliliter (mL); red blood cell (RBC)

*Indicates statistical significance at p-value less than 0.05

Table 22.3 Comparison of postoperative complications between facial bipartition and box osteotomy cohorts

	Total	Facial bipartition	Box osteotomy	p-value
Number of cases	$n = 45$	$n = 29$	$n = 16$	
All complications				
Any complications	15 (33.3%)	14 (48.3%)	1 (6.2%)	0.004*
Any major complications[a]	8 (17.8%)	7 (24.1%)	1 (6.2%)	0.133
Any minor complications[b]	9 (20.0%)	8 (27.6%)	1 (6.2%)	0.087
Short-term complications[c]	7 (15.6%)	6 (20.7%)	1 (6.2%)	0.201
Major complications	2 (4.4%)	2 (6.9%)	0 (0.0%)	0.283
Minor complications	6 (13.3%)	5 (17.2%)	1 (6.2%)	0.299
Cerebrospinal fluid leak	3 (6.7%)	2 (6.9%)	1 (6.2%)	0.934
Postoperative bleeding	1 (2.2%)	1 (3.4%)	0 (0.0%)	0.453
Mortality	0 (0.0%)	0 (0.0%)	0 (0.0%)	–
Reoperation	0 (0.0%)	0 (0.0%)	0 (0.0%)	–
Seroma	0 (0.0%)	0 (0.0%)	0 (0.0%)	–
Skin necrosis/dehiscence	0 (0.0%)	0 (0.0%)	0 (0.0%)	–
Unplanned reintubation	0 (0.0%)	0 (0.0%)	0 (0.0%)	–
Vision loss	0 (0.0%)	0 (0.0%)	0 (0.0%)	–
Wound infection	0 (0.0%)	0 (0.0%)	0 (0.0%)	–
Long-term complications	11 (24.4%)	10 (34.5%)	1 (6.2%)	0.299
Major complications	6 (13.3%)	5 (17.2%)	1 (6.2%)	0.299
Minor complications	5 (11.1%)	5 (17.2%)	0 (0.0%)	0.078
Hardware exposure/displacement	3 (6.7%)	3 (10.3%)	0 (0.0%)	0.183
Wound infection	3 (6.7%)	3 (10.3%)	0 (0.0%)	0.183
Seroma	3 (6.7%)	3 (10.3%)	0 (0.0%)	0.183
Postoperative bleeding	1 (2.2%)	1 (3.4%)	0 (0.0%)	0.453
Skin necrosis/dehiscence	1 (2.2%)	1 (3.4%)	0 (0.0%)	0.453
Reoperation	1 (2.2%)	1 (2.2%)	0 (0.0%)	0.453
Cerebrospinal fluid leak	1 (2.2%)	0 (0.0%)	1 (6.2%)	0.173
Mortality	0 (0.0%)	0 (0.0%)	0 (0.0%)	–
Vision loss	0 (0.0%)	0 (0.0%)	0 (0.0%)	–

[a]Major complications required returning to the operating room
[b]Minor complications did not require returning to the operating room
[c]Short-term complications occurred before discharge
[d]Long-term complications occurred after discharge
e Indicates statistical significance at p-value less than 0.05

ation or an equivalent. However, this procedure has high rates of relapse and failure [27]. Therefore, many craniofacial surgeons do not include addressing telecanthus in their respective algorithms. This omission compromises the ultimate goal of achieving a natural-looking facial construct. Moreover, any prior osteotomies of the medial or infraorbital wall compromise the integrity and efficacy of the box osteotomy approach. We have found box osteotomies to be the most effective way to address the multi-planar deformities of the orbital region in patients with Apert syndrome. Most commonly, this approach involves addressing the telecanthus, hypoplastic midface, deficient lateral orbital rim projection, and downslanting of the lateral canthus. Given their versatility and ability to simultaneously address midface hypoplasia, box osteotomies potentially decrease the number of large-scale surgeries a patient will need. Thus, by avoiding another midface intervention, box osteotomies can fulfill the major surgical needs of the patient until skeletal maturity, when orthognathic surgery is indicated, as outlined in our algorithm.

The literature and our data verify that box osteotomies can be a safe and effective approach for the complex reconstruction of patients with hypertelorism and telecanthus. When viewed within the specific algorithm we designed for our patients with Apert syndrome, box osteotomies constitute a remarkably powerful tool in the armamentarium.

References

1. Greig DM. Hypertelorism: a hitherto undifferentiated congenital Cranio-facial deformity. Edinb Med J. 1924;31(10):560. https://www.ncbi.nlm.nih.gov/pmc/articles/PMC5294069/. Accessed 18 Nov 2022.
2. Tessier P, Orbital hypertelorism. I. Successive surgical attempts. Material and methods. Causes and mechanisms. Scand J Plast Reconstr Surg. 1972;6(2):135–55. https://doi.org/10.3109/02844317209036714.
3. Webster JP. The surgical treatment of the Bifid nose. 1950. https://books.google.com/books/about/The_Surgical_Treatment_of_the_Bifid_Nose.html?hl=&id=ZmbNzgEACAAJ
4. Converse JM, Smith B. An operation for congenital and traumatic hypertelorism. In: Troutman RC, Converse JM, Smith B, editors. Plastic and reconstructive surgery of the eye and adnexa. Butterworth Inc; 1962. p. 104–9.
5. Longacre JJ. Craniofacial anomalies: Pathogenesis and repair. 1968. https://books.google.com/books/about/Craniofacial_Anomalies.html?hl=&id=Q5tsAAAAMAAJ
6. Tessier P, Guiot G, Rougerie J, Delbet JP, Pastoriza J. Cranio-naso-orbito-facial osteotomies. Hypertelorism. Ann Chir Plast. 1967;12(2):103–18. https://europepmc.org/article/med/5595910.
7. Arnaud É. L'innovation en chirurgie craniofaciale: depuis Tessier jusqu'aux perspectives futures. D'après les témoignages de F. Ortiz-Monasterio, D. Marchac, F. Firmin et T. Wolfe. Ann Chir Plast Esthet. 2010;55(5):363–83. https://doi.org/10.1016/j.anplas.2010.07.016.
8. Converse JM, Wood-Smith D. A new technique for the correction of orbital hypertelorism. Laryngoscope. 1972;82(8):1455–62. https://doi.org/10.1288/00005537-197208000-00009.
9. Edgerton MT, Udvarhelyi GB, Knox DL. The surgical correction of ocular hypertelorism. Ann Surg. 1970;172(3):473–96. https://doi.org/10.1097/00000658-197009000-00012.
10. Marchac D, Renier D, Jones BM. Experience with the "floating forehead". Br J Plast Surg. 1988;41(1):1–15. https://doi.org/10.1016/0007-1226(88)90137-3.
11. Marchac D, Renier D. Congenital craniofacial malformations. In: Youmans JR, editor. Neurological Surgery. Saunders; 1996. p. 1012–34.
12. Whitaker LA, Munro IR, Salyer KE, Jackson IT, Ortiz-Monasterio F, Marchac D. Combined report of problems and complications in 793 craniofacial operations. Plast Reconstr Surg. 1979;64(2):198–203. https://doi.org/10.1097/00006534-197908000-00011.
13. Vannier MW, Marsh JL, Warren JO. Three dimensional CT reconstruction images for craniofacial surgical planning and evaluation. Radiology. 1984;150(1):179–84. https://doi.org/10.1148/radiology.150.1.6689758.
14. Firmin F, Coccaro PJ, Converse JM. Cephalometric analysis in diagnosis and treatment planning of craniofacial dysostoses. Plast Reconstr Surg. 1974;54(3):300–11. https://doi.org/10.1097/00006534-197409000-00007.
15. García-Mato D, Ochandiano S, García-Sevilla M, et al. Craniosynostosis surgery: workflow based on virtual surgical planning, intraoperative navigation and 3D printed patient-specific guides and templates. Sci Rep. 2019;9(1):17691. https://doi.org/10.1038/s41598-019-54148-4.
16. Hopper RA, Kapadia H, Morton T. Normalizing facial ratios in apert syndrome patients with Le Fort II midface distraction and simultaneous zygomatic repositioning. Plast Reconstr Surg. 2013;132(1):129–40. https://doi.org/10.1097/PRS.0b013e318290fa8a.
17. Hopper RA, Prucz RB, Iamphongsai S. Achieving differential facial changes with Le Fort III distraction osteogenesis: the use of nasal passenger grafts, cerclage hinges, and segmental movements. Plast

Reconstr Surg. 2012;130(6):1281–8. https://doi.org/10.1097/PRS.0b013e31826d160b.
18. Hammoudeh JA, Goel P, Wolfswinkel EM, et al. Simultaneous midface advancement and orthognathic surgery: a powerful technique for managing midface hypoplasia and malocclusion. Plast Reconstr Surg. 2020;145(6):1067e–72e. https://doi.org/10.1097/PRS.0000000000006816.
19. Farkas LG, Kolar JC. Anthropometrics and art in the aesthetics of women's faces. Clin Plast Surg. 1987;14(4):599–616. https://www.ncbi.nlm.nih.gov/pubmed/3652607.
20. AO Foundation. Classification of intraorbital hypertelorism. AO Surgery Reference; 2021. https://surgeryreference.aofoundation.org/cmf/congenital-deformities/hypertelorism/further-reading/classification-of-intraorbital-hypertelorism. Accessed 15 May 2025.
21. Farkas LG, Munro IR. Anthropometric facial Pproportions in medicine. Charles C. Thomas Publisher; 1987. https://books.google.com/books/about/Anthropometric_Facial_Proportions_in_Med.html?hl=&id=u5ppAAAAMAAJ
22. Roohani I, Moshal T, Lasky S, Jolibois M, Nagengast E, Hammoudeh J, Urata M. Bone to soft tissue changes following box osteotomy and facial bipartition for surgical correction of hypertelorism: a three-dimensional analysis. Plast Reconstr Surg Glob Open. 2024;12(Suppl 8):10–1. https://doi.org/10.1097/01.GOX.0001063864.68947.a4. PMCID: PMC11411976.
23. Zide BM, McCarthy JG. The medial canthus revisited--an anatomical basis for canthopexy. Ann Plast Surg. 1983;11(1):1–9. https://doi.org/10.1097/00000637-198307000-00001.
24. Anderson RL. Medial canthal tendon branches out. Arch Ophthalmol. 1977;95(11):2051–2. https://doi.org/10.1001/archopht.1977.04450110145019.
25. Go BC, Shakir S, Swanson JW, Bartlett SP, Taylor JA. A critical appraisal of surgical outcomes following orbital hypertelorism correction: what is the incidence of true bony relapse versus soft tissue telecanthus? Childs Nerv Syst. 2021;37(1):21–32. https://doi.org/10.1007/s00381-020-04890-2. Epub 2020 Sep 22. PMID: 32964257.
26. Jiang T, Yu Z, Chi TY, et al. Postoperative complications of box-shift osteotomy for orbital hypertelorism. J Craniofac Surg. 2020;31(2):385–8. https://doi.org/10.1097/SCS.0000000000006051.
27. Kelly CP, Cohen AJ, Yavuzer R, Moreira-Gonzalez A, Jackson IT. Medial canthopexy: a proven technique. Ophthalmic Plast Reconstr Surg. 2004;20(5):337–41. https://doi.org/10.1097/01.iop.0000139519.40976.28.

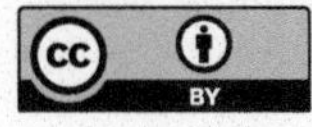

23 Segmental Subcranial Midface Osteotomies: Le Fort II with Zygomatic Repositioning

Richard A. Hopper

Introduction

Surgical pioneers developed the subcranial osteotomy into the standard of care for treating severe midface hypoplasia in syndromic craniosynostosis [1–5]. With early recognition of the need for differential movement of parts of the Le Fort III segment to achieve facial harmony in Apert syndrome, Obwegeser advocated combining segmental Le Fort osteotomies with differential mobilization in 1969 [6]. Polley revisited this differential concept through tiered midface osteotomies in a "piggyback" fashion for simultaneous correction of orbital, midface, and occlusal abnormalities [7]. Soft tissue resistance, the need for bone grafts, and the degree of subperiosteal degloving required limited the success of these traditional Le Fort III advancement techniques and contributed to relapse and soft tissue atrophy [8].

Midface advancement using distraction osteogenesis was developed in the early 1990s with reported benefits of greater advancement, less surgical dissection, improved stability, lower relapse, and superior airway outcomes [9–12]. With these advantages, single-piece Le Fort III distraction has largely replaced traditional subcranial advancements in treating Apert syndrome midface hypoplasia in adolescence [13]. As with what occurred with traditional surgery, there is now a resurgent awareness of the shortcomings of *en bloc* distraction movement in addressing multilevel asymmetries associated with the unique Apert facial dysmorphology compared to Crouzon syndrome. This has led to approaches that combine the benefits of distraction with the directional control of traditional techniques.

Combined distraction of Le Fort III and Le Fort I osteotomies has been described for the treatment of syndromic midface hypoplasia to differentially correct orbital and occlusal hypoplasia [14–17]. Appreciation of the distinct facial ratios of Apert syndrome has led to techniques such as Le Fort II distraction with zygomatic repositioning (LF2ZR) to correct greater central vertical and sagittal deficiency to normalize facial ratios in this unique condition [18–20]. Similarly, the bipartition monobloc distraction technique has combined a traditional midline osteotomy and wire fixation with the power of distraction to achieve favorable differential changes in Apert dysmorphology [21–25]. This chapter will focus on a segmental subcranial approach to treating the Apert midface and contrast it with the segmental transcranial option.

R. A. Hopper (✉)
Department of Surgery, Baylor College of Medicine, Houston, TX, USA

Texas Children's Hospital, Austin, TX, USA
e-mail: richard.hopper@bcm.edu

J. G. Meara et al. (eds.), *Apert Syndrome*, https://doi.org/10.1007/978-3-032-12551-4_23

Apert Syndrome Subcranial Dysmorphology

Segmental subcranial or transcranial procedures recognize that certain syndromes have differential hypoplasia of the facial skeleton that will not be fully treated by *en bloc* movements [26]. In patients with Apert syndrome, the degree of hypoplasia varies between the central nasomaxillary region and the lateral orbito-zygomatic region. The midface deformity is characterized by the presence of a central concavity in the setting of a retrusive midface. This is due to a severe deficiency in both the sagittal and vertical dimension of the central midface relative to the lateral midface compared to Crouzon dysmorphology and non-syndromic ratios [27] (Fig. 23.1). Unlike the midface hypoplasia associated with Crouzon syndrome, the Apert facial dysmorphology has been described as an abnormal face in an abnormal position [19].

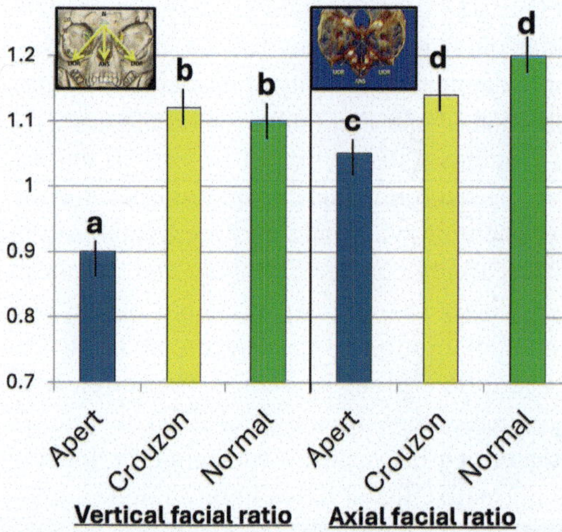

Fig. 23.1 Vertical (left) and axial (right) facial ratios of Apert, Crouzon, and normal controls (n = 7/group). Vertical facial ratio (VFR) was calculated as Nasion to anterior nasal spine distance divided by nasion to lateral orbital rim. Axial facial ratio (AFR) was calculated as distance from sella to anterior nasal spine divided by sella to lateral inferior orbital rim. Bars with the same letter were not significantly different (analysis of variance [ANOVA], $p < 0.05$). Apert AFR and VFR are significantly different from both Crouzon and normal control, which are not different from each other

The *en bloc* midface advancement achieved through Le Fort III distraction corrects exorbitism and malar hypoplasia through sagittal advancement of the inferior orbital rim and the body of the zygomas. The extent of sagittal advancement in the central nasomaxillary region with the Le Fort III operation is limited by the risk of causing enophthalmos. To avoid iatrogenic deformity, the advancement of the inferior orbital rim needs to stop when it reaches the level of the corneal surface. In Crouzon syndrome, this is not a concern since the central midface and lateral zygomas are equally retruded and, therefore equally treated with an *en bloc* movement. In Apert syndrome, however, the central deficiency is greater than the lateral retrusion, leaving the central midface under-treated when the inferior rim stops at the corneal surface. Similarly, vertical lengthening is limited by the risk of creating excessive orbital height. In Apert syndrome, the central midface is vertically deficient compared to the zygomas. If the midface was to be lengthened appropriately during distraction using an *en bloc* technique, the inferior movement of the zygomas and inferior orbital rim would disrupt lower lid support and malar aesthetics. Due to these limitations of *en bloc* Le Fort III distraction, the relative central midface vertical and axial deficiency have historically remained under-corrected in patients with Apert syndrome, resulting in favorable changes in lateral view but no change in the distinct Apert dysmorphology on frontal view (Fig. 23.2).

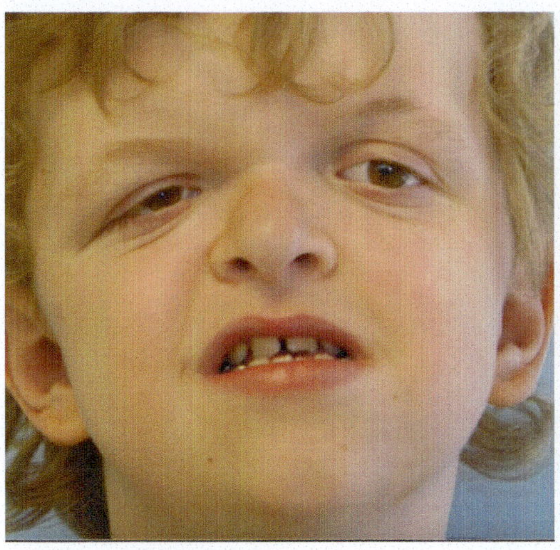

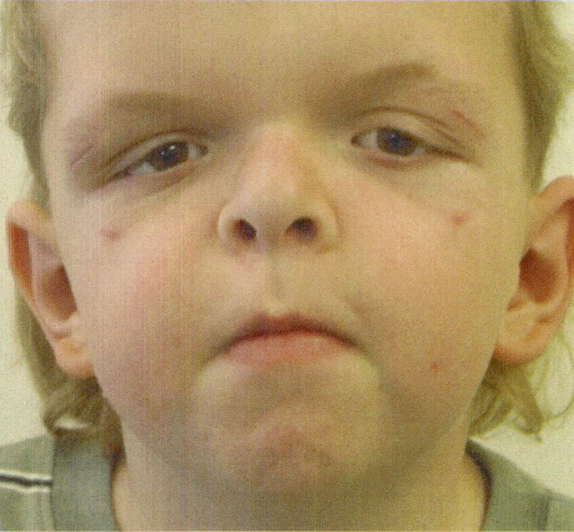

Fig. 23.2 Patient with Apert syndrome before (left) and after (right) *en bloc* Le Fort III midface distraction advancement. Although there was a difference in the patient's lateral profile with advancement (not shown), the frontal view has not appreciably changed

Segmental Osteotomies to Treat Apert Syndrome Subcranial Dysmorphology

The Le Fort II advancement with simultaneous zygomatic repositioning (LF2ZR) is a modification of the traditional LF3 distraction operation to treat patients with differential midface hypoplasia [19, 20, 28]. Through segmental distraction of the central nasomaxillary region and repositioning of the lateral orbito-zygomatic regions, the LF2ZR operation is intended to correct the facial bi-concavity present in Apert syndrome (Fig. 23.3). It is equally effective in other non-synostotic conditions with similar abnormal ratios such as Achondroplasia [20, 28]. The traditional zygomatic repositioning (ZR) and fixation portion of the operation improves the relationship between the orbit and the globe to correct exorbitism and malar hypoplasia. Since the central LF2 segment is then distracted independent of the zygomas, the vector and magnitude of advancement can be controlled without impacting the orbital morphology. This technique allows for not only correction of the severe central retrusion in the sagittal plane by greater magnitude of advancement but also closure of an anterior open bite, extension of the nasal length, and improvement in the palpebral fissure orientation through a downward vector of distraction.

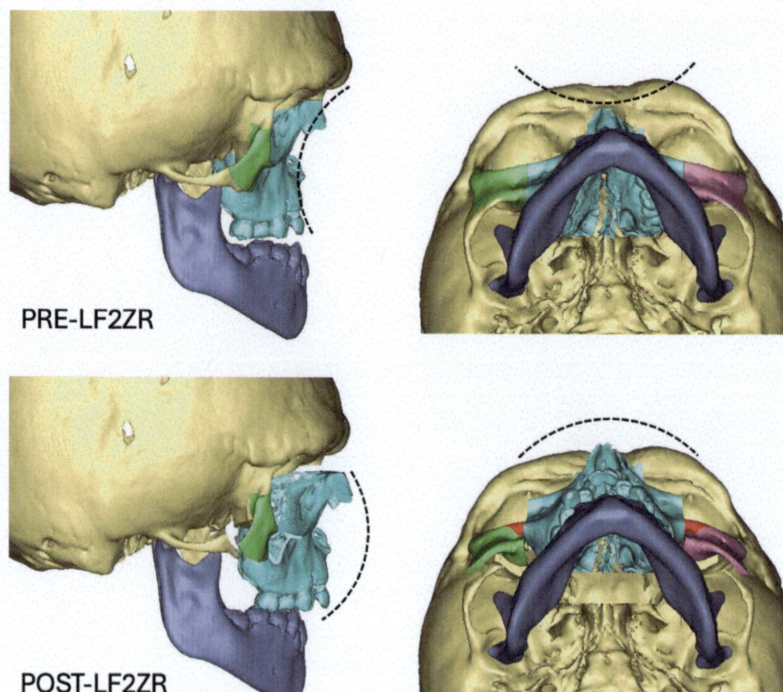

Fig. 23.3 Virtual surgical plan for Le Fort II distraction advancement (light blue segment) and simultaneous zygomatic repositioning (green segments) before (top) and after (bottom) the planned surgery. The differential movement of the zygomas and central midface segments corrects both the sagittal (left) and axial (right) convexities associated with Apert syndrome

Complications of Segmental Midface Surgery

A recent review we did of 53 subcranial distraction procedures describes a complication rate of 7/19 after LF2ZR and 12/39 after Le Fort III with no difference between the two techniques [29]. These rates are consistent with the other large series previously published on LF3 distraction with complication rates ranging from 29% to 33% [11, 30, 31].

Of the 19 LF2ZR cases in this series, two had eyelid retraction that resolved over time, three required external hardware adjustments in the operating room, one had a postoperative seroma over the forehead polyether ether ketone (PEEK) implant that resolved with compression, one had postoperative fevers that resolved with oral antibiotics, one had acute tracheitis requiring antibiotics, and one required removal of forehead implant 1 year after surgery due to infection.

Timing of Segmental Midface Surgery in Apert Syndrome

Non-syndromic facial growth curves demonstrate cessation of periorbital and malar growth by 7–8 years of age, with the remaining growth occurring in the maxilla–mandibular complex [32, 33] which also coincides with eruption of the permanent central incisors and first molars. As a result, most elective subcranial surgeries are performed between 6 and 8 years of age [11, 29, 34]. Le Fort III subcranial midface advancement can also take place at younger ages if needed for severe obstructive airway improvement. For segmental surgeries, however, to optimize the zygomatic repositioning part of the LF2ZR technique, we recommend the procedure is performed after 7 years of age. This will also ensure there is sufficient space to make the zygomaticomaxillary osteotomy without damage to permanent dentition.

Growth after midface or frontofacial advancement is diminished in the anterior direction, with only minimal vertical growth occurring in the subnasal spine region [8, 35, 36]. As a result, anticipated growth of the mandible and desired final anterior vertical facial height at maturity must be built into the advancement plan at mid-childhood as an overcorrection [11, 22]. If there is adequate projection of the orbito-zygomatic region in middle childhood, the patient may only require a Le Fort I procedure at skeletal maturity for malocclusion. However, there is an increased awareness of Apert syndrome having mandible hypoplasia that was not previously recognized when the greater midface deficiency was historically undertreated. Now that midface techniques can fully correct central midface retrusion in Apert syndrome, more patients are having a sagittal split advancement of the mandible built into their final orthognathic plan.

Technical Description of Subcranial Segmental LF2ZR Procedure

Le Fort III Osteotomy and Downfracture

The procedure starts with a standard Le Fort III osteotomy through a coronal incision (Fig. 23.4). The dissection is subperiosteal, with elevation of the anterior half of the temporalis muscles bilaterally as part of the composite scalp flap down to the inferior orbital rims and anterior aspect of the zygomatic arch. With reflection of the temporalis muscle, the zygomatic arch is cut with a piezoelectric saw just at the junction of the zygomatic body and anterior arch. Stepped bilateral osteotomies are then made through the lateral orbit from the frontozygomatic suture into the inferior orbital fissure. The step pattern will allow a stable anterior and superior movement of the zygomas once they are mobilized. The zygomatic retaining ligaments and periosteal vascular supply to the malar prominence must be maintained intact throughout the surgery.

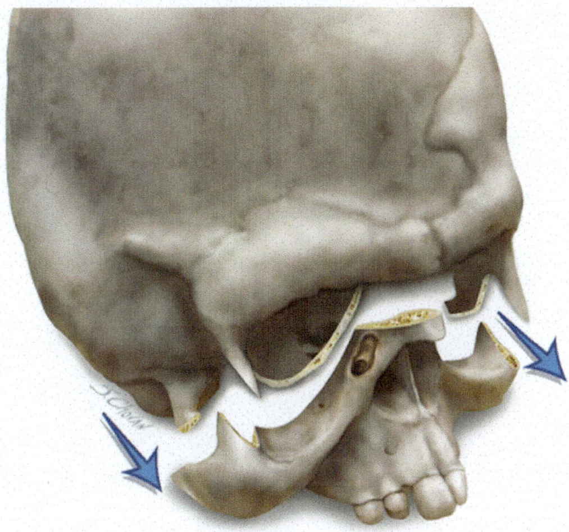

Fig. 23.4 Standard Le Fort III osteotomy down fracture with angled step osteotomies at the lateral orbital rims

Zygomatic Repositioning and Fixation

The disimpacted and mobilized Le Fort III segment can be manipulated by grasping the maxilla through the mouth. This allows the right lateral orbital step osteotomy to be transposed 7 mm anteriorly and 5 mm superiorly and fixated with 1.5-mm titanium plates (Fig. 23.5). Through an upper gingival labial sulcus incision, a limited subperiosteal exposure of the maxillary buttress lateral to the infraorbital nerve and foramen is performed but with care taken not to release the zygomatic retaining ligament (MacGregor patch) to avoid compromising vascularity to the zygoma. The repositioned and fixated right orbito-zygomatic complex can be released from the remainder of the Le Fort III segment using a piezoelectric saw intraorally, with the osteotomy located lateral to the infraorbital nerve, and continued into the orbital floor to join the transverse orbital floor cut. In this manner, the repositioned right zygoma is separated from the central Le Fort II midface (Fig. 23.6). The intact left zygoma is then repositioned, fixated, and released similarly. This staged repositioning is important to avoid strain and early fracture across the weak zygomaticomaxillary suture, which can occur if simultaneous zygomatic repositioning and fixation is attempted.

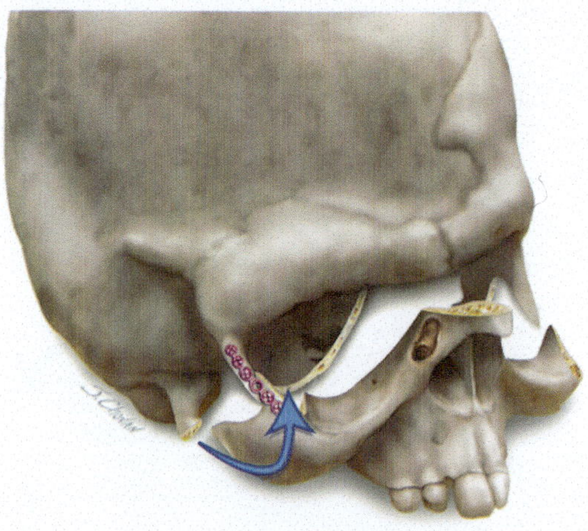

Fig. 23.5 With manual control of the maxilla through the mouth, the surgeon repositions the right zygoma anteriorly and superiorly by transposing the lateral orbital rim osteotomy and fixating with a single 1.5 mm titanium plate

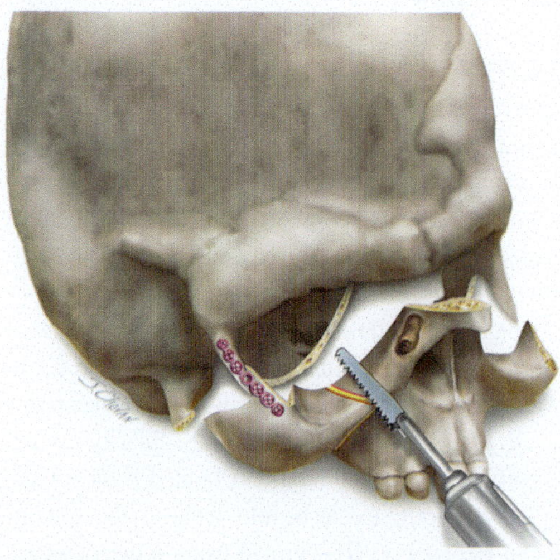

Fig. 23.6 Through an upper gingivobuccal intraoral approach, the surgeon releases the repositioned and fixated right zygoma just lateral to the infraorbital nerve using either a reciprocating or piezoelectric saw. This process is then repeated for the left zygoma repositioning (not shown)

Custom Forehead Implant and Halo Distraction Device Placement

After completing the zygomatic repositioning (ZR), the remaining mobile unit is a Le Fort II segment, which will be advanced in a forward and downward direction with distraction osteogenesis.

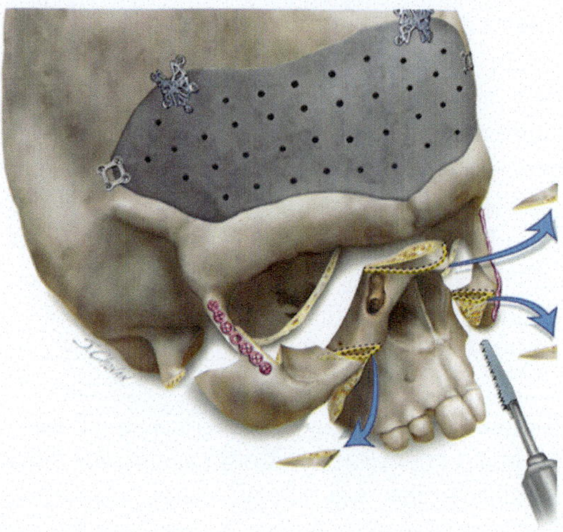

Fig. 23.7 To improve the esthetics of the central forehead concavity common in Apert syndrome, the surgeon has placed a custom made onlay implant (gray). The zygomas have been repositioned and are separate from the central Le Fort 2 segment. The surgeon anticipates any sharp bone edges that would be palpable after distraction advancement and removes them with a saw

Before placing the distraction device, a custom onlay forehead implant can be placed, if needed, for central contour irregularities that can commonly occur after anterior cranial expansion in Apert syndrome (Fig. 23.7). It is also important to anticipate bony step deformities that can occur along the Le Fort II osteotomies after a large-magnitude movement. Small triangles of bone are removed at the inferior orbital rim and the nasofrontal root to smooth the contour in anticipation of the future distraction movement (Fig. 23.7).

A lateral canthopexy is performed to re-secure the ligament to the posterolateral orbit and the medial canthus must remain attached to the upper portion of the mobile Le Fort II segment. In this way, the downward movement of the central Le Fort II midface during distraction will lower the medial palpebral fissure relative to the secured lateral canthopexy, improving the reverse canthal tilt frequently observed in patients with Apert syndrome. The exposed skull is irrigated thoroughly with antibiotic irrigation and the deep temporal fascia and muscle are reattached to drill holes in the lateral and superior orbital rims. The lateral splint is fixated to the lateral maxillary arch below the Le Fort II osteotomy with two pairs of 26-gauge suspension wires (Fig. 23.8).

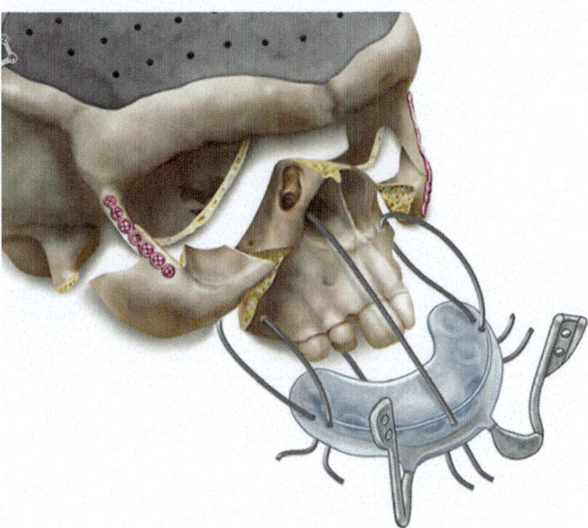

Fig. 23.8 Due to the higher soft tissue resistance to midface advancement in Apert syndrome, the oral traction splint must be firmly anchored to the Le Fort II segment with transosseous wires

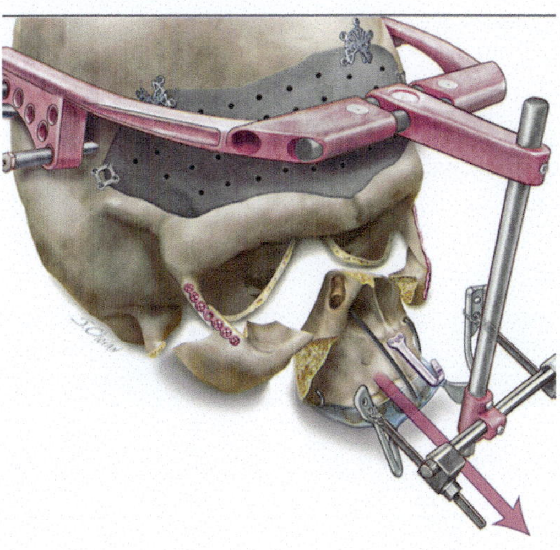

Fig. 23.9 A cranial based external distraction device creates a forward and downward traction on the oral traction splint to lengthen and advance the central midface. Note that the medial canthus attached to the lacrimal fossa will follow the same vector, while the lateral canthi will remain stable attached to the lateral orbital walls

The medial wires are passed through holes drilled in the lateral piriform rim. The intraoral wounds are irrigated thoroughly and closed with 4-0 chromic gut suture.

To control closure of the anterior open bite associated with Apert syndrome during the Le Fort II distraction, orthodontic bone anchors are placed in the midline maxillary splint and at the mandible midline for postoperative elastic control. A rigid external fixation traction device is applied with cranial pins, a vertical midface post, and a transverse activation arm with multi-vector control at the occlusal plane level. The distraction vector is 45° downward, and the activation arms are secured to the oral traction splint using 24-gauge hand-tied wires (Fig. 23.9). The activation posts are reversed turned at the end of the case to compress the midface subcranial separation during the acute swelling phase.

Postoperative Care and Distraction Protocol

Patients remain sedated and intubated for 2–3 days in the intensive care unit. Once an air leak is confirmed around the endotracheal tube, the patient is extubated. Distraction is started after a latency period of 3 days and proceeds at a rate of 2 mm per day. This faster rate is required to minimize the risk of premature consolidation due to the higher osteogenic potential in Apert syndrome. The distraction vector is chosen to achieve a balance of desired nasal dorsal length, anterior vertical maxillary length, and maxillary occlusal plane angle. The end-point of distraction is achieved when the desired overjet (usually an overcorrection of 3–5 mm) exists and the medial canthal position is neutral relative to the lateral canthal position. The critical point to watch to determine end of activation is the medial canthus. Over activation will pull the medial punctum away from the sclera. If this occurs, the device should be backed up until the punctum returns to its natural position. Once end activation is achieved, patients are kept in consolidation for 6 weeks before device removal.

Facial Ratio Changes with LF2ZR Procedure

Computed tomography scan analysis of patients with Apert syndrome who underwent LF2ZR has demonstrated significantly greater advancement

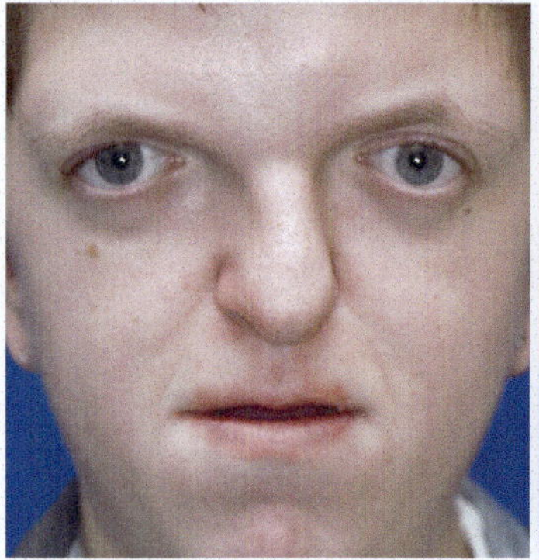
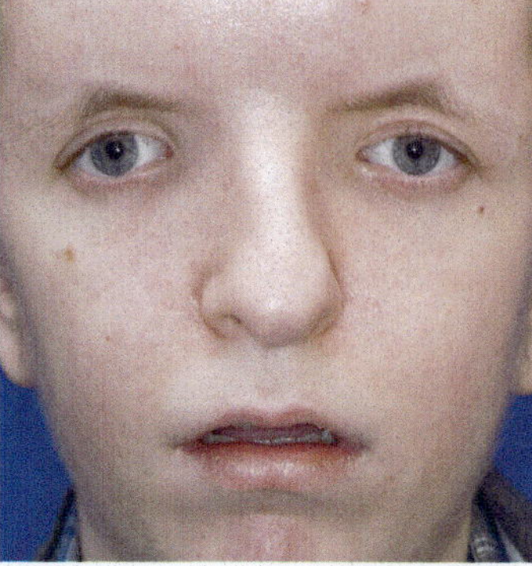
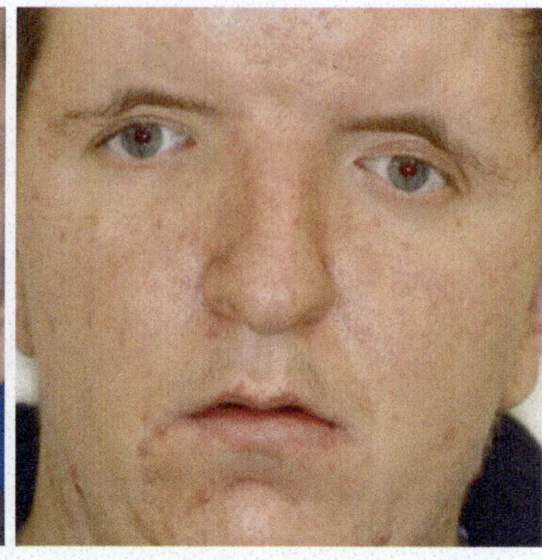

Fig. 23.10 A patient with Apert syndrome before (left), 1 year after (center), and 8 years after (right) LF2ZR surgery. Although the typical soft tissue changes associated with Apert syndrome have occurred with age, the facial ratio improvements achieved with the LF2ZR surgery are maintained

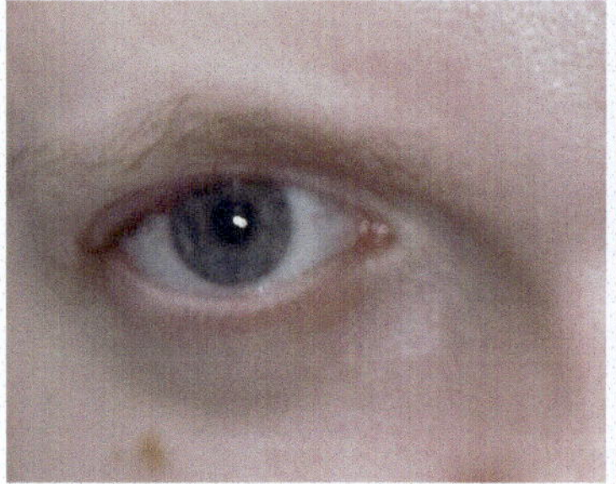
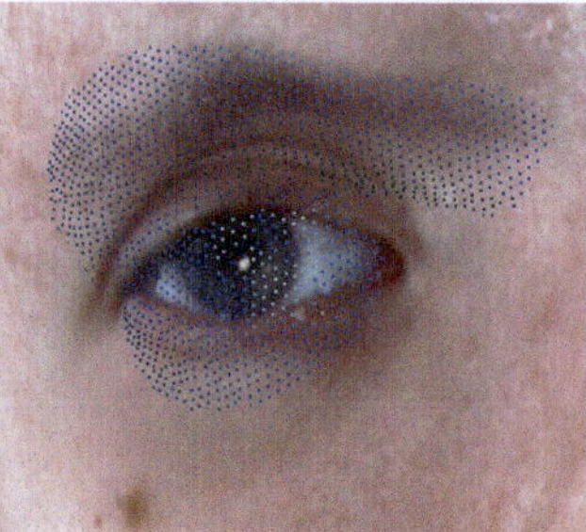
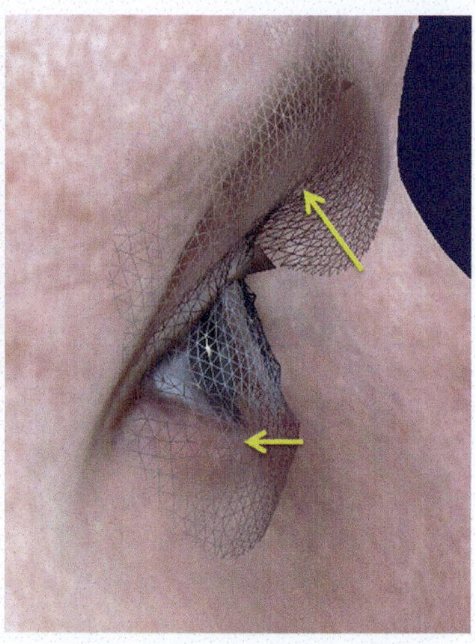

Fig. 23.11 Periorbital changes before (left) and after (center and right) LF2ZR surgery. The pre-operative soft tissue surface scan mesh (blue) is superimposed on the post-LF2ZR images. The periorbital changes include an increase in the supratarsal space, a leveling of the palpebral fissure, and decreased scleral show from increased lower lid support from the zygomatic repositioning

and lengthening of the central midface compared to the lateral orbits, resulting in normalization of the facial ratio [19]. These favorable facial ratios are maintained with age (Fig. 23.10). The aesthetic improvement following LF2ZR on frontal view includes nasal lengthening and improved biplanar facial convexity. The most dramatic change compared to *en bloc* Le Fort III, however, is in the palpebral shape. The inferior movement of the medial canthus on the Le Fort II segment levels the palpebral fissure, creating favorable changes in both the upper and lower lids (Fig. 23.11).

Segmental Subcranial Versus Transcranial Procedures

The craniofacial group at Great Ormond Street Hospital has proposed using bipartition monobloc advancement as an alternative technique for differential facial advancement [23]. This technique has the advantage of improving the hypertelorism that is present to different degrees in patients with Apert syndrome while also correcting the axial concave deformity. However, this technique requires a transcranial approach and the associated higher risk relative to subcranial

Table 23.1 Comparative effect of three midface advancement techniques on treating components of Apert facial dysmorphology

	Le Fort III advancement	Le Fort II advancement + zygomatic repositioning	Bipartition frontofacial advancement
Central midface retrusion	+[a]	++	++
Central midface vertical deficiency	–	++	–
Hypertelorism	–	–	+++
Palpebral fissure slant	–	+++[b]	+
Closure anterior open bite	–	+	–
Nasal lengthening	+	++	++[c]

(+) degree of positive effect
(–) no effect
[a]Limited by degree of one-piece zygoma advancement
[b]Secondary to lowering of medial canthi
[c]Secondary to nasal cantilever graft

surgery [30]. It corrects the width of the face but does not allow for differential vertical lengthening of the central midface or downward movement of the medial canthi. Bipartition can improve the facial height to width ratio by narrowing the face but does not normalize oculofacial morphology [24]. The bipartition monobloc approach would be indicated for patients with severe hypertelorism that would not be adequately corrected by the nasal dorsal lengthening and augmentation of LF2ZR, or for patients requiring simultaneous expansion of the anterior cranial fossa (Table 23.1).

Summary

It is now recognized that traditional *en bloc* Le Fort III movements have been undertreating critical parts of the Apert dysmorphology. Segmental procedures allowing differential movement of the facial bones will result in more favorable results. Although the Apert phenotype has a narrower spectrum compared to other conditions such as Pfeiffer and Crouzon syndromes, there is still variability that should be recognized, that will determine which of the current procedures is best suited to a particular patient. In patients where vertical midface compression is the primary deformity (small nose, palpebral slant, maxillary deficiency), a technique such as the LF2ZR procedure would address the primary deformity. In other cases of Apert syndrome where hypertelorism is more significant and contributes the most to the overall appearance, a technique such as bipartition frontofacial advancement would be appropriate.

Financial Disclosure Statement Dr. Hopper is an educational consultant for Integra Health Sciences. No funding was received for this chapter.

References

1. Gillies SH, Harrison SH. Operative correction by osteotomy of recessed malar maxillary compound in a case of oxycephaly. Br J Plast Surg. 1950:3. https://doi.org/10.1016/S0007-1226(50)80019-X.
2. Ortiz-Monasterio F, Del Campo AF, Carrillo A. Advancement of the orbits and the midface in one piece, combined with frontal repositioning, for the correction of Crouzon's deformities. Plast Reconstr Surg. 1978:61. https://doi.org/10.1097/00006534-197804000-00003.
3. Tessier P. Total facial osteotomy. Crouzon's syndrome, Apert's syndrome: oxycephaly, scaphocephaly, turricephaly. Ann Chir Plast. 1967;12:273.
4. Tessier P. The definitive plastic surgical treatment of the severe facial deformities of craniofacial dysostosis: Crouzon's and Apert's diseases. Ann Plast Surg. 1987:18. https://doi.org/10.1097/00000637-198704000-00012.
5. Tessier P. Total osteotomy of the middle third of the face for faciostenosis or for sequelae of Le fort III fractures. Plast Reconstr Surg. 1971;48 https://doi.org/10.1097/00006534-197112000-00003.
6. Obwegeser HL. Surgical correction of small or retrodisplaced maxillae: the "dish-face" defor-

mity. Plast Reconstr Surg. 1969;43 https://doi.org/10.1097/00006534-196904000-00003.
7. Polley JW, Figueroa AA. "Piggyback" osteotomies in craniomaxillofacial surgery. J Craniofac Surg. 1995;6 https://doi.org/10.1097/00001665-199505000-00005.
8. Warren SM, Shetye PR, Obaid SI, Grayson BH, McCarthy JG. Long-term evaluation of midface position after le Fort III advancement: a 20-plus-year follow-up. Plast Reconstr Surg. 2012;129 https://doi.org/10.1097/PRS.0b013e3182362a2f.
9. Ettinger RE, Hopper RA, Sandercoe G, Kifle Y, Saltzman B, Chen M, et al. Quantitative computed tomographic scan and polysomnographic analysis of patients with syndromic midface hypoplasia before and after le Fort III distraction advancement. Plast Reconstr Surg. 2011;127 https://doi.org/10.1097/PRS.0b013e318208d2de.
10. Fearon JA, Polley JW, Figueroa AA. The Le Fort III osteotomy: to distract or not to distract? Plast Reconstr Surg. 2001;107 https://doi.org/10.1097/00006534-200104150-00002.
11. Fearon JA. Halo distraction of the Le fort III in syndromic craniosynostosis: a long-term assessment. Plast Reconstr Surg. 2005;115 https://doi.org/10.1097/01.PRS.0000160271.08827.15.
12. Chin M, Toth BA. Le Fort III advancement with gradual distraction using internal devices. Plast Reconstr Surg. 1997;100 https://doi.org/10.1097/00006534-199709001-00001.
13. Saltaji H, Altalibi M, Major MP, Al-Nuaimi MH, Tabbaa S, Major PW, et al. Le Fort III distraction osteogenesis versus conventional le Fort III osteotomy in correction of syndromic midfacial hypoplasia: a systematic review. J Oral Maxillofac Surg. 2014;72 https://doi.org/10.1016/j.joms.2013.09.039.
14. Satoh K, Mitsukawa N, Hosaka Y. Dual midfacial distraction osteogenesis: Le Fort III minus I and Le fort I for syndromic craniosynostosis. Plast Reconstr Surg. 2003;111 https://doi.org/10.1097/01.PRS.0000047440.06788.72.
15. Takashima M, Kitai N, Murakami S, Takagi S, Hosokawa K, Kreiborg S, et al. Dual segmental distraction osteogenesis of the midface in a patient with apert syndrome. Cleft Palate Craniofac J. 2006:43. https://doi.org/10.1597/04-15R1.1.
16. Matsumoto K, Nakanishi H, Koizumi Y, Seike T, Okazaki M, Yokozeki M, et al. Segmental distraction of the midface in a patient with Crouzon syndrome. J Craniofac Surg. 2002;13 https://doi.org/10.1097/00001665-200203000-00015.
17. Lee DW, Ham KW, Kwon SM, Lew DH, Cho EJ. Dual midfacial distraction osteogenesis for Crouzon syndrome: long-term follow-up study for relapse and growth. J Oral Maxillofac Surg. 2012:70. https://doi.org/10.1016/j.joms.2011.11.010.
18. Hopper RA, Prucz RB, Iamphongsai S. Achieving differential facial changes with Le Fort III distraction Osteogenesis. Plast Reconstr Surg. 2012;130 https://doi.org/10.1097/prs.0b013e31826d160b.
19. Hopper RA, Kapadia H, Morton T. Normalizing facial ratios in apert syndrome patients with le fort ii midface distraction and simultaneous zygomatic repositioning. Plast Reconstr Surg. 2013;132 https://doi.org/10.1097/PRS.0b013e318290fa8a.
20. Hopper RA, Kapadia H, Susarla SM. Le Fort II distraction with zygomatic repositioning: a technique for differential correction of midface hypoplasia. J Oral Maxillofac Surg. 2018;76 https://doi.org/10.1016/j.joms.2018.04.023.
21. Visser R, Ruff CF, Angullia F, Ponniah AJT, Jeelani NUO, Britto JA, et al. Evaluating the efficacy of Monobloc distraction in the Crouzon-Pfeiffer craniofacial deformity using geometric Morphometrics. Plast Reconstr Surg. 2017;139 https://doi.org/10.1097/PRS.0000000000003016.
22. Gwanmesia I, Jeelani O, Hayward R, Dunaway D. Frontofacial advancement by distraction osteogenesis: a long-term review. Plast Reconstr Surg. 2015;135 https://doi.org/10.1097/PRS.0000000000001115.
23. Ponniah AJT, Witherow H, Richards R, Evans R, Hayward R, Dunaway D. Three-dimensional image analysis of facial skeletal changes after monobloc and bipartition distraction. Plast Reconstr Surg. 2008:122. https://doi.org/10.1097/PRS.0b013e3181774308.
24. Glass GE, Ruff CF, Crombag GAJC, Verdoorn MHAS, Koudstaal M, Anguilla F, et al. The role of bipartition distraction in the treatment of apert syndrome. Plast Reconstr Surg. 2018;141 https://doi.org/10.1097/PRS.0000000000004115.
25. Raposo-Amaral CE, Vieira PH, Denadai R, Ghizoni E, Raposo-Amaral CA. Treating syndromic Craniosynostosis with Monobloc facial bipartition and internal distractor devices: destigmatizing the syndromic face. Clin Plast Surg. 2021;48 https://doi.org/10.1016/j.cps.2021.03.002.
26. Hopper RA. New trends in cranio-orbital and midface distraction for craniofacial dysostosis. Curr Opin Otolaryngol Head Neck Surg. 2012;20 https://doi.org/10.1097/MOO.0b013e3283543a43.
27. Oberoi S, Hoffman WY, Vargervik K. Craniofacial team management in Apert syndrome. Am J Orthod Dentofacial Orthop. 2012;141 https://doi.org/10.1016/j.ajodo.2012.01.003.
28. Hopper RA, Kapadia H, Susarla SM. Surgical-orthodontic considerations in subcranial and Frontofacial distraction. Oral Maxillofac Surg Clin North Am. 2020;32 https://doi.org/10.1016/j.coms.2020.01.005.
29. Purnell CA, Evans M, Massenburg BB, Kim S, Preston K, Kapadia H, et al. Lefort II distraction with zygomatic repositioning versus Lefort III distraction: a comparison of surgical outcomes and complications. J Craniofac Surg. 2021;49 https://doi.org/10.1016/j.jcms.2021.03.003.
30. Zhang RS, Lin LO, Hoppe IC, Swanson JW, Bartlett SP, Taylor JA. Retrospective review of the complication profile associated with 71 subcranial and transcranial midface distraction procedures at a single

institution. Plast Reconstr Surg. 2019;143 https://doi.org/10.1097/PRS.0000000000005280.

31. Greig AVH, Davidson EH, Grayson BH, McCarthy JG. Complications of craniofacial midface distraction: 10-year review. Plast Reconstr Surg. 2012;130 https://doi.org/10.1097/PRS.0b013e31825900c4.
32. Buschang PH, Baume RM, Nass GG. A craniofacial growth maturity gradient for males and females between 4 and 16 years of age. Am J Phys Anthropol. 1983;61 https://doi.org/10.1002/ajpa.1330610312.
33. Ranly DM. Craniofacial growth. Dent Clin N Am. 2000;44:457–70.
34. Shetye PR, Davidson EH, Sorkin M, Grayson BH, McCarthy JG. Evaluation of three surgical techniques for advancement of the midface in growing children with syndromic craniosynostosis. Plast Reconstr Surg. 2010;126 https://doi.org/10.1097/PRS.0b013e3181e6051e.
35. Shetye PR, Kapadia H, Grayson BH, McCarthy JG. A 10-year study of skeletal stability and growth of the midface following le Fort III advancement in syndromic craniosynostosis. Plast Reconstr Surg. 2010;126 https://doi.org/10.1097/PRS.0b013e3181e60502.
36. Tonello C, Cevidanes LHS, Ruellas ACO, Alonso N. Midface morphology and growth in syndromic Craniosynostosis patients following Frontofacial Monobloc distraction. J Craniofac Surg. 2021;32 https://doi.org/10.1097/SCS.0000000000006997.

24 Le Fort III Distraction with or without Facial Bipartition

Roman H. Khonsari, Elle Vandervord, Giovanna Paternoster, Samer E. Haber, and Eric Arnaud

Introduction

Le Fort III osteotomy is the first major subcranial procedure proposed in the treatment plan of patients with Apert syndrome. The main functional benefit of this full maxillo-zygomatic osteotomy is respiratory as it is associated with significant improvement of obstructive sleep apnea syndrome (OSAS). The morphological changes secondary to Le Fort III osteotomy include a reduction of exorbitism, improvement in zygomatic projection, and correction of maxillary retrusion. When combined with facial bipartition, Le Fort III osteotomy can also contribute to simultaneously improving hypertelorism, palpebral fissure inclination, and a narrow maxillary arch.

The vast majority of patients with Apert syndrome require orthognathic, generally maxillo-mandibular, surgery after skeletal maturity. Le Fort III osteotomy is thus generally performed as late as possible to avoid relapse but earlier than 16 years of age to allow time for orthodontic preparation and orthognathic surgery [1].

In practical terms, after issues with intracranial pressure are managed (after the 6th year of life), the two main next functional questions for children with Apert syndrome are exorbitism with risks for corneal ulceration and obstructive sleep apnea before the orthognathic age. The indications for Le Fort III osteotomy are primarily based on these two factors, monitored with yearly polysomnography and ophthalmological screening examinations. For instance, a nine-year-old child with severe sleep apnea (apnea-hypopnea index = 35/h) will be proposed to undergo Le Fort III even if the risk of relapse is high at this age due to the remaining growth potential. When functional indications are absent, aesthetic demands are considered, with a constant preference for delaying the surgery as long as possible to optimize the stability of the results. Later Le Fort III provides better aesthetic results, but no compromise should be made on functional indications,

R. H. Khonsari (✉)
Craniofacial Surgery Unit, CRMR CRANIOST, Hôpital Necker–Enfants malades, Assistance publique–Hôpitaux de Paris, Paris, France

School of Medicine, Université Paris Cité, Paris, France

Craniofacial Growth and Form Laboratory, Imagine Institute, Paris, France
e-mail: roman.khonsari@aphp.fr

E. Vandervord
Children's Hospital Westmead, Sydney, NSW, Australia

G. Paternoster · S. E. Haber
Craniofacial Surgery Unit, CRMR CRANIOST, Hôpital Necker–Enfants malades, Assistance Publique–Hôpitaux de Paris, Paris, France

É. Arnaud
Craniofacial Surgery Unit, CRMR CRANIOST, Hôpital Necker–Enfants malades, Assistance Publique–Hôpitaux de Paris, Paris, France

Clinique Marcel Sembat (Ramsay Générale de Santé), CCMR CRANIOST, Boulogne-Billancourt, France

J. G. Meara et al. (eds.), *Apert Syndrome*, https://doi.org/10.1007/978-3-032-12551-4_24

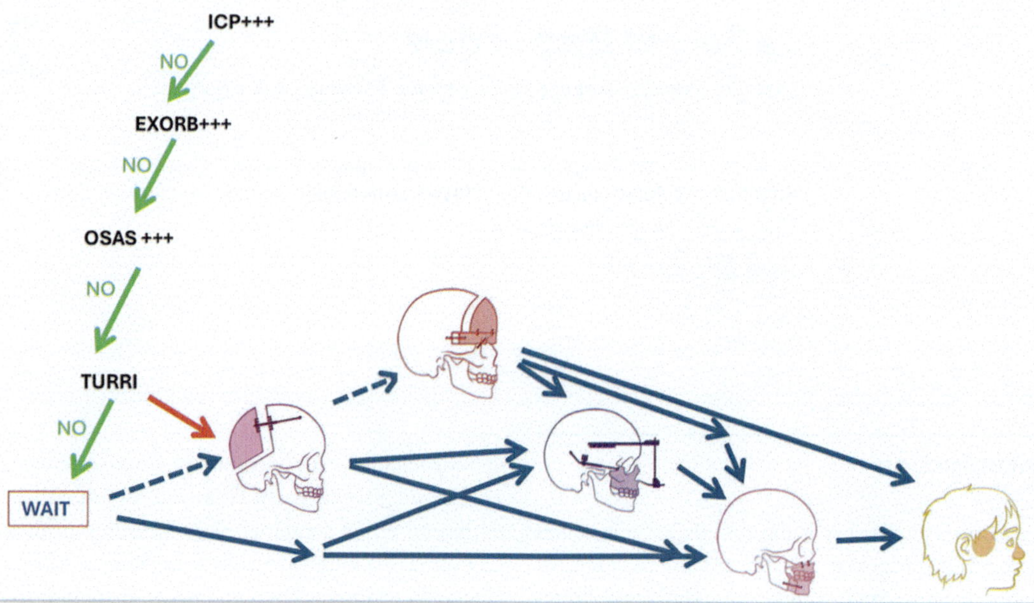

Fig. 24.1 The Arnaud algorithm for the management of mild cases of Apert syndrome with no indication for frontofacial monobloc advancement, after assessing intracranial pressure (*ICP*), exorbitism (*exorb*), and obstructive sleep apnea (*OSAS*). The main procedures are then: (1) posterior vault distraction in case of turricephaly (*turri*), (2) fronto-orbital advancement, (3) Le Fort III osteotomy, (4) maxilla-mandibular osteotomy, and (5) facial plastic surgery (temporal fat grafting and rhinoplasty). (Source: Dr. Éric Arnaud)

even if there is a risk of performing a second Le Fort III during pubertal growth (Fig. 24.1).

In this chapter, we provide an overview of the technique for Le Fort III osteotomy with and without facial bipartition and discuss the results of this technique in the management of Apert syndrome.

Le Fort III Osteotomy with and Without Facial Bipartition: Surgical Technique

Installation and Incision

The patient is positioned supine with oral intubation, securing the endotracheal tube to the lower jaw using non-absorbable braided sutures. A throat pack is placed with care to avoid excessive pressure on the tongue base and prevent postoperative macroglossia [2]. Bilateral tarsorrhaphies are placed using non-absorbable monofilament sutures to prevent postoperative chemosis. The patient is stabilized on a headrest with chest rolls under the thighs and shoulders, taped to the operating table to prevent sliding. An instrument table is positioned approximately 20–25 cm from the patient's chin. If present, scars from previous posterior vault expansion, fronto-orbital advancement, or frontofacial monobloc advancement (FFMBA) procedures are reused, employing a zigzag bi-coronal incision. A 3-cm-wide band of hair is shaved along the incision line. Subgaleal and subdermal infiltration with 1 mg/mL adrenaline solution is applied along the incision. The installation is similar to the protocol previously described for frontofacial monobloc advancement [3].

Exposure

Dissection proceeds in the subgaleal plane when feasible, extending to the superior orbital ridge and along the superficial layer of the deep temporal fascia, minimizing risk to the frontal branch of the facial nerve. Previous surgeries may complicate this dissection; care is taken to maintain adequate flap thickness to reduce the risk of alopecia and necrosis. The periosteum over the forehead is elevated, exposing the supraorbital ridge and orbital roofs. Small horizontal incisions in the superficial layer of the deep temporal fascia, perpendicular to the lateral orbital wall, facilitate the Tessier maneuver, exposing the zygoma and zygomatic arch [3]. The orbital roofs and lateral orbital walls are dissected with a periosteal elevator, while the temporal muscles are raised to expose the infratemporal fossa. A midline suspension is performed using thick (2.0) sutures and fixed to the instrument table.

Osteotomies and Craniofacial Disjunction

The lateral orbital wall is sectioned using a reciprocating saw, starting with an upward motion directed into the orbital cavity. The lateral orbital mobile segment should be about 3–5 mm thick to avoid the anterior translation of the globes during distraction, which is a specific risk in Apert syndrome due to the abnormal orientation of the orbital walls [4, 5]. Anterior down-slanting osteotomy of the upper aspect of the lateral wall achieves a smooth advancing segment border. The posterior attachment of the zygoma body is sectioned downward from an intra-orbital approach, and the zygomatic arch is cut near its attachment to the zygoma. The osteotomy of the orbital floor begins 1–2 mm anterior to the inferior orbital fissure using the saw, extending medially with a curved osteotome while avoiding the lower orbital rim. Due to shallow orbits in Apert syndrome [4], the osteotomy is set posteriorly enough to mitigate rim fracture risks. An illuminated retractor with suction facilitates visualization of the orbital floor during osteotomy. The contralateral side undergoes identical osteotomies. On the medial orbital wall, the lacrimal crest is identified, and the osteotomy is performed posterior to it, preserving the medial canthal ligament. The midline horizontal osteotomy at the frontonasal suture level involves sectioning the ethmoid and septum/vomer, using a reciprocating saw (and/or piezosurgery) and completing it with a curved osteotome down to the vomer.

Pterygomaxillary disjunction is achieved via an infra-temporal approach with an elevator or curved osteotome, verified using intra-oral palpation. In secondary cases with significant fibrosis, additional disjunction using an elevator in the pterygomaxillary junction may be required.

For craniofacial disjunction, Rowe forceps (with silicone sleeve protection for their intra-oral branch) are employed. A counterclockwise movement initiates disjunction, followed by controlled lateral and clockwise movements to complete posterior disjunctions in nasal and oral regions. The forceps are used in tandem to prevent midline disjunction and palatal lacerations. A custom-made palatal plate can be used to further protect the palatal mucosa.

Facial Bipartition

The nasal bones are dissected to the bone–cartilage junction, and the nasal mucosa is detached with blunt dissection using cotton strips. A triangular bone resection with a superior base with dimensions adapted to the correction of hypertelorism initiates the upper part of the bipartition procedure, maintaining a minimum 5 mm bone margin between the lateral osteotomy line and lacrimal fossa (Fig. 24.2).

To perform the lower part of the bipartition procedure, the maxillary vestibule is infiltrated with 1% lidocaine with adrenaline, followed by a Le Fort I incision. The maxillo-zygomatic surfaces and piriform aperture are exposed. If necessary, the choana can be expanded with a round burr, taking care to avoid central incisor root injury. A midline inter-maxillary osteotomy is performed, preferably with a piezoelectric saw, which minimizes incisor damage. Orthodontic alignment may be required preoperatively to accommodate the midline osteotomy by changing the orientation of incisor roots in a divergent manner. A pre-positioned maxillary plate with an activator can help to guide transverse maxillary expansion during the procedure and avoid over-expansion. After maxillary expansion, the two orbital fragments are approximated on the midline and fixed using three steel sutures (Fig. 24.2).

Two midface osteosynthesis plates are fixed to the maxillo-zygomatic surface on both sides of the piriform aperture. A single plate bridging the

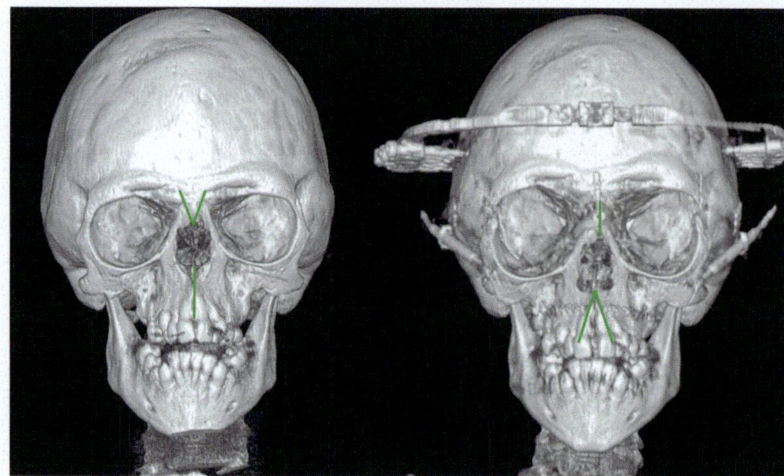

Fig. 24.2 Midline bone resection and intermaxillary osteotomy in facial bipartition associated with Le Fort III osteotomy leading simultaneously to a reduction in the internal intercanthal distance and to an increase of the transversal maxillary dimension. (Source: Craniofacial team, Necker—Enfants malades Hospital, AP-HP)

midline should be avoided in order to limit interferences with transversal maxillary growth. Screw should be positioned with care to avoid dental roots, notably the roots of the canines. One steel wire on each side is then positioned under the plate with a transcutaneous passage approximately 3 mm lateral to the lateral insertion of the *alae nasi* (Figs. 24.3 and 24.4).

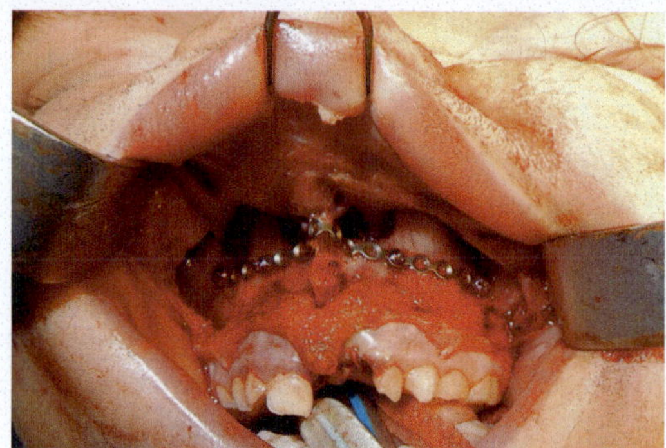

Fig. 24.3 Positioning of 2 maxillo-zygomatic plates to anchor the external distractor after facial bipartition. (Source: Craniofacial team, Necker—Enfants malades Hospital, AP-HP)

Facial Advancement and Internal Distractor Positioning

A midface plate (1.6 mm) is placed along the frontozygomatic suture, with an intra-operative advancement of approximately 1 cm. This plate is secured with a single 4–5 mm screw on the advancing segment (Fig. 24.5), which allows for rotation of the facial fragment during distraction.

Four external cortical bone grafts, approximately 1 × 4 cm, are harvested from the supraorbital rim (frequently hypertrophic in Apert syndrome, [6]). The extent and position of the frontal sinus are assessed prior to graft harvesting. Two triangular grafts cover the frontozygomatic plates, fixed with tissue glue and PDS sutures, while the remaining grafts form a butterfly shape on a T-plate to address midline and inner orbital wall defects, secured at the nasion with 1 or 2 4 mm screws (Fig. 24.6).

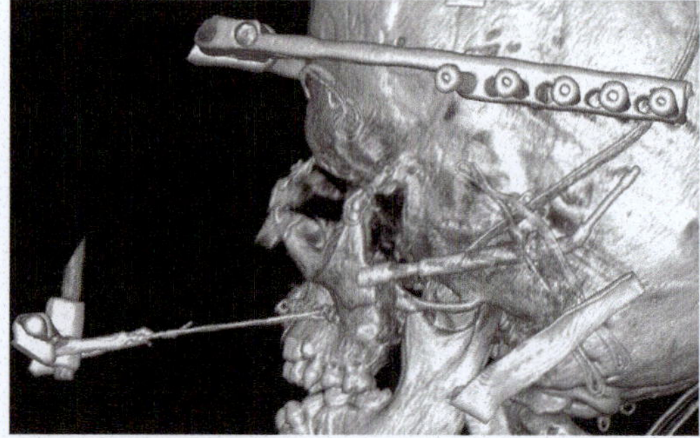

Fig. 24.4 The maxillo-zygomatic plates are used to anchor the facial fragment on the external distractor using steel wires. (Source: Craniofacial team, Necker—Enfants malades Hospital, AP-HP)

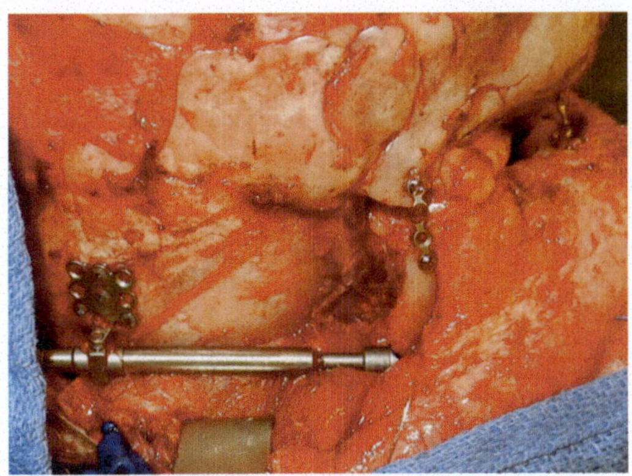

Fig. 24.5 Position of the frontozygomatic plate, with intraoperative advancement. Placement of a single screw on the mobile segment allows for both advancement and rotation during distraction. The internal distractor is positioned approximatively parallel to the zygomatic arch, with the anterior end as low as possible along the external orbital wall, immediately above the osteotomy line of the zygomatic arch. (Source: Craniofacial team, Necker—Enfants malades Hospital, AP-HP)

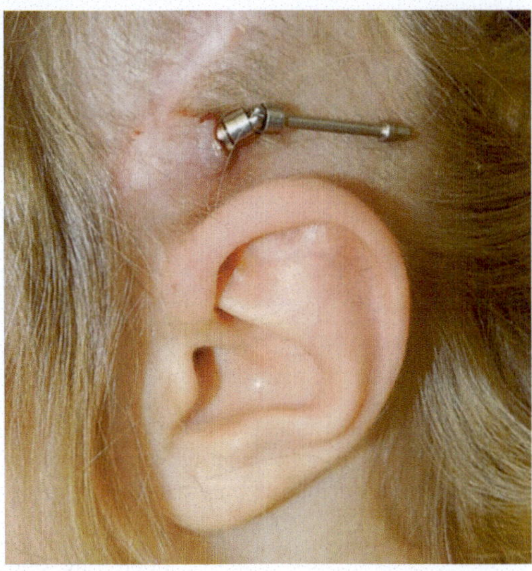

Fig. 24.7 Activation arm of the internal distractor exiting the skin above the external ear. (Source: Craniofacial team, Necker–Enfants malades Hospital, AP-HP)

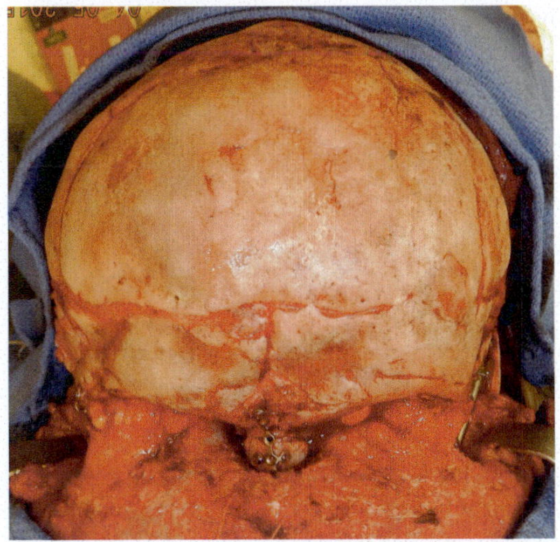

Fig. 24.6 Butterfly-shaped nasal graft extending to the inner orbital walls, obtained from bone fragments harvested at the level of the superior orbital rim. (Source: Craniofacial team, Necker—Enfants malades Hospital, AP-HP)

Internal temporo-zygomatic distractors are placed beneath the temporalis muscle, with only the superior fixation zone attached. The inferior fixation zone is removed from the distractor before positioning. The anterior distractor arm is positioned low on the zygoma, near the osteotomy line of the zygomatic arch, with a notch on the lateral orbital wall for stability. The main axis of the device is directed approximatively parallel to the zygomatic arch (by analogy with results on frontofacial monobloc advancement, [7]) (Fig. 24.5). Neuroscrews are used to minimize the risks of dural injuries. The activation arm extends through the skin postero-superiorly to the external ear and beyond the coronal incision (Fig. 24.7). A 2.1 mm Kirschner wire may be used for transfacial pinning through the zygoma to stabilize bipartitioned fragments, with high risks of morbidity on tooth germs depending on the age at surgery (by analogy with results on frontofacial monobloc advancement, [8]).

Closure and External Distraction

The temporalis muscle is repositioned and secured to prevent hollowing, occasionally requiring a posterior cut to facilitate rotation. External canthopexies are performed with moderate overcorrection using surgical stainless-steel sutures or non-absorbable monofilament sutures affixed to the frontozygomatic plates.

The periosteum is optimally positioned to cover bone fragments, using absorbable sutures for suspension where necessary. Bilateral drainage is implemented without suction in case of inadvertent cerebrospinal fluid leakage during distractor positioning. Skin closure is performed with 3-0 and 4-0 braided absorbable sutures, with minimal subcutaneous sutures. Nasopharyngeal tubes with transseptal fixation are placed to ensure airway patency.

An external distractor (RED frame) is applied post-closure, connecting the two maxillary wires (Fig. 24.8). Compressive dressings are not recommended. All patients are postoperatively admitted to the intensive care unit, with extubation on day 0 or 1. Nasopharyngeal tubes and tarsorrhaphies are removed after three to four days. Distraction typically commences on day 1 following a confirmatory computed tomography (CT) scan, generally performed before extubation during the transfer to intensive care.

The end-point of distraction is determined clinically, with specific attention being given to avoiding enophthalmos. This may limit the degree of occlusal over-correction. Plating at the frontozygomatic osteotomy with single-screw fixation on the mobile segment allows for rotation movement rather than linear advancement, allowing maximal occlusal correction with decreased risk of enophthalmos.

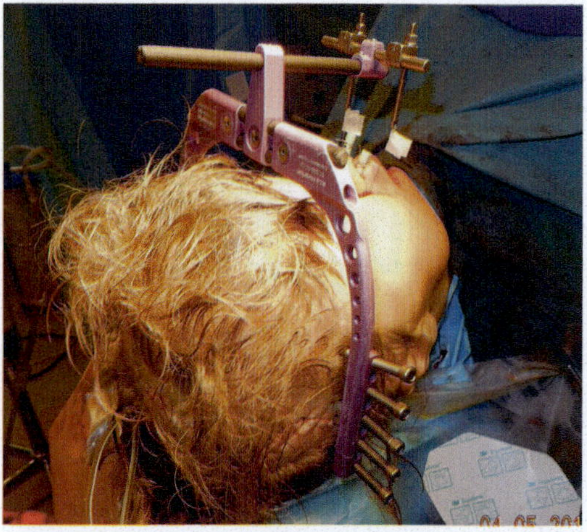

Fig. 24.8 Positioning of the external distractor with the anchoring of the two steel wires attached to the maxillo-zygomatic osteosynthesis plates. (Source: Craniofacial team, Necker—Enfants malades Hospital, AP-HP)

Assessment of the Le Fort III Osteotomy Results in the Management of Apert Syndrome

Due to the limits of retrospective real-life data collection, we assessed a cohort of 61 patients with Apert syndrome treated at Necker–Enfants malades Hospital since 1995 with available digital medical files. In this cohort, 19 patients who had undergone initial FFMBA underwent no further midface advancement procedure, whilst nine had Le Fort III osteotomy; 33 patients proceeded directly to Le Fort III osteotomy as the first facial advancement procedure, after initial fronto-orbital advancement. We assessed the reduction in AHI (Apnea–Hypopnea Index) among two groups of patients from this cohort undergoing Le Fort III advancement and for which we had complete pre- and postoperative polysomnography data: (1) patients who underwent two sequential procedures: a frontofacial monobloc advancement followed by a Le Fort III osteotomy (*FFMBA + LF3* group, 4 patients) (Figs. 24.9 and 24.10) and (2) patients who underwent a Le Fort III procedure after initial fronto-orbital advancement (*LF3* group, 19 patients) (Figs. 24.11 and 24.12). Pre- and postoperative AHI values were collected for each procedure in both groups, and the reduction in AHI was calculated. Age at surgery was included as a covariate to assess its influence on the magnitude of AHI reduction. Statistical analyses were performed using: (1) descriptive statistics for age and AHI values, (2) ordinary least squares (OLS) regression models to evaluate AHI reduction and its dependency on age for each procedure, and (3) analysis of covariance (ANCOVA) to compare AHI reductions between groups and assess the interaction between age and group membership.

In the *FFMBA + LF3* group, the age at surgery for frontofacial monobloc advancement was 3.39 ± 2.02 years (min. 1.1, max. 6.1), preoperative AHI was 37.83 ± 34.73 (min. 5.0; max. 105.0), and postoperative AHI was 10.00 ± 10.36 (min. 1.0; max. 30.0). The age at surgery for Le Fort III osteotomy was 11.88 ± 4.39 years (min. 5.8; max. 20.9), preoperative AHI was

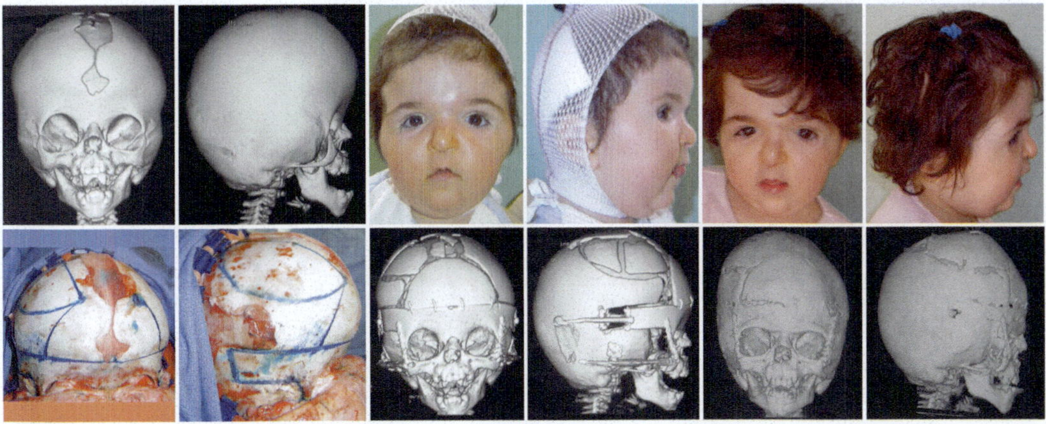

Fig. 24.9 Treatment sequence with frontofacial monobloc advancement followed by Le Fort III osteotomy: before/after frontofacial monobloc advancement. (Source: Craniofacial team, Necker—Enfants malades Hospital, AP-HP)

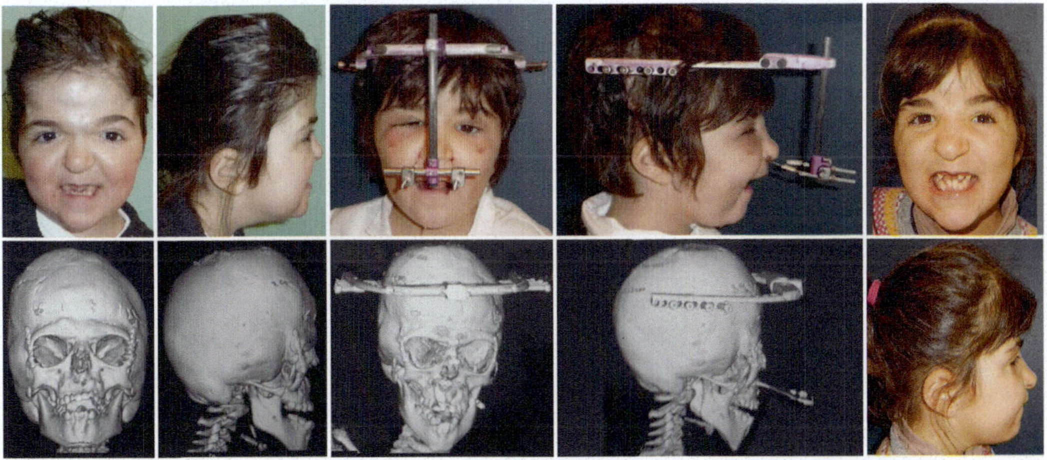

Fig. 24.10 Treatment sequence with frontofacial monobloc advancement followed by Le Fort III osteotomy: before/after Le Fort III osteotomy. (Source: Craniofacial team, Necker—Enfants malades Hospital, AP-HP)

13.25 ± 19.78 (min. 1.0; max. 52.0), and postoperative AHI was 3.25 ± 3.86 (min. 1.0; max. 9.0). In the *LF3* group, the age at surgery was 9.98 ± 4.15 years (min. 3.4; max. 18.0), preoperative AHI was 12.89 ± 14.20 (min. 0.0; max. 56.0), and postoperative AHI was 6.91 ± 8.92 (min. 0.0; max. 29.0). In the *FFMBA* + *LF3* group, AHI reductions were analyzed separately for frontofacial monobloc advancement and Le Fort III osteotomies. Frontofacial monobloc advancement significantly reduced AHI, particularly for older patients, highlighting its efficacy in addressing severe obstructive sleep apnea [9]. Le Fort III osteotomy performed after frontofacial monobloc advancement also reduced AHI, with younger patients showing slightly greater benefits, indicating a cumulative effect of the combined surgical approach. This confirmed previous results on a cohort including patients with both Apert and Crouzon syndromes [10]. In addition, there was no statistically significant impact of the time interval between frontofacial monobloc advancement and Le Fort III osteotomy on AHI reduction.

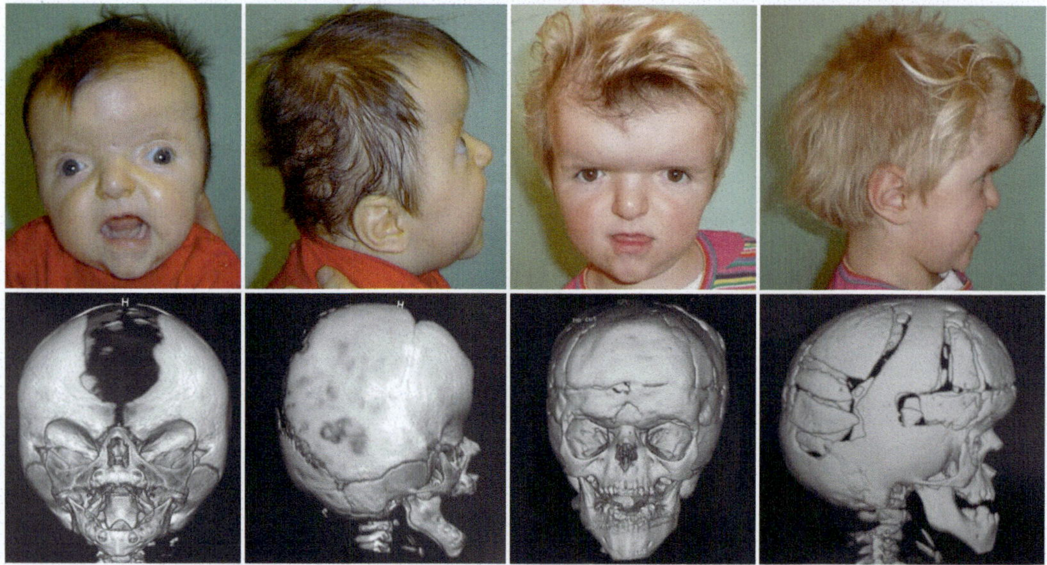

Fig. 24.11 Treatment sequence with fronto-orbital advancement followed by Le Fort III osteotomy: before/after fronto-orbital advancement. (Source: Craniofacial team, Necker—Enfants malades Hospital, AP-HP)

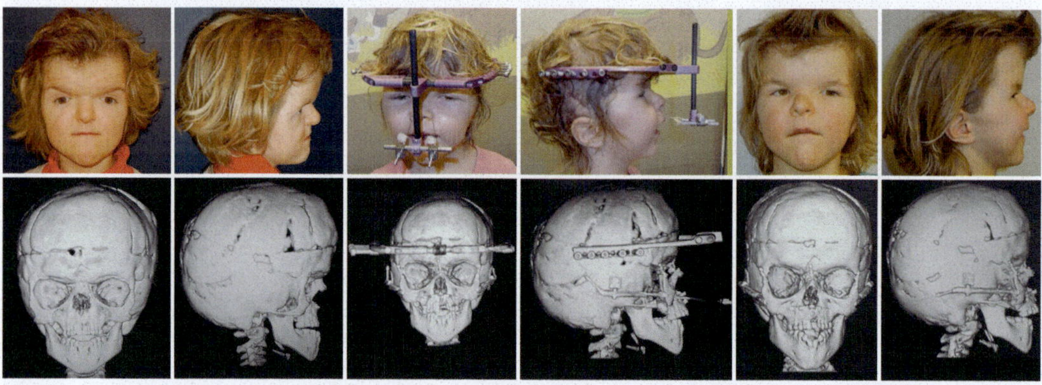

Fig. 24.12 Treatment sequence with fronto-orbital advancement followed by Le Fort III osteotomy: before/after Le Fort III osteotomy. (Source: Craniofacial team, Necker—Enfants malades Hospital, AP-HP)

For the *LF3* group, AHI was significantly reduced post-surgery, with the magnitude of reduction being independent of age. This indicates that Le Fort III osteotomy alone is effective for reducing AHI irrespective of the patient's age in this sub-group. When comparing the two groups, the *FFMBA + LF3* group demonstrated significantly greater reductions in AHI than the *LF3* group. Age was an influential factor in the *FFMBA + LF3* group, with younger patients benefiting more from the combined approach. This suggests that a staged surgical strategy involving frontofacial monobloc advancement followed by Le Fort III osteotomy is particularly effective for addressing severe cases, especially when performed at an earlier age. Of note, all Le Fort III cases in our unit are operated using the combination of two internal temporo-zygomatic distractors and one external distractor. This dual distraction approach allows to exert strong traction forces, necessary in cases with prior frontofacial monobloc advancement and pterygo-maxillary fibrosis, but also allows to remove the external distractor early after the end of the distraction process (approximately 2 weeks post-operatively), as the two internal distractors act as buttresses and prevent relapse [11].

Regarding the orbital parameters, the addition of a subcranial bipartition to the Le Fort III can be used as a tool to address hypertelorism and allow correction of palpebral fissure inclination simultaneously. We previously showed statistically significant improvement in palpebral fissure inclination, though we noted the difficulty in differentiating between the contribution of the bony movements and the canthopexy component of the procedure [12].

We do not have an assessment of the specific complications related to the associated bipartition compared to a standard subcranial Le Fort III osteotomy. Still, the main risk of this added step is an injury to the tooth buds of the permanent incisors, which occurred to our knowledge in one case of our cohort, requiring the placement of dental implants. Potential injuries to the palatal mucosa during the intermaxillary disjunction do not result to our knowledge in the development of a permanent fistula and heal spontaneously. In brief, based on our retrospective data, adding facial bipartition to a standard subcranial Le Fort III does not seem to increase the global morbidity of this procedure, but this point requires formal validation.

Based on retrospective real-life data, Le Fort III osteotomy efficiently tackles obstructive sleep apnea, especially when included in a two-step protocol involving an initial frontofacial monobloc advancement. Furthermore, associated subcranial bipartition efficiently corrects the specific orbital-palpebral anomalies of Apert syndrome.

Main Messages

- Le Fort III osteotomy has both functional and aesthetic indications.
- Le Fort III osteotomy should be delayed as long as possible and ideally performed around 14 years of age, without compromising on the functional indications.
- Le Fort III osteotomy is efficient for the management of OSAS.
- The addition of subcranial bipartition to Le Fort III can improve hypertelorism, palpebral fissure inclination, and a narrow maxillary arch.
- Facial bipartition does not add significant morbidity to the Le Fort III osteotomy.
- The combined use of internal distractors with rigid external distractor frame allows for early RED frame removal with minimal risks for relapse due to the buttress effect of the internal devices.
- Orthognathic surgery is required in the vast majority of cases following Le Fort III osteotomy, after orthodontic preparation, around the age of 18.

References

1. Kaban LB, Conover M, Mulliken JB. Midface position after Le Fort III advancement: a long-term follow-up study. Cleft Palate J. 1986;23(Suppl 1):75–7.
2. Bouaoud J, Joly A, Picard A, Thierry B, Arnaud É, James S, Hennessy I, McGarvey B, Cairet P, Vecchione A, Vergnaud E, Duracher C, Khonsari RH. Severe macroglossia after posterior fossa and craniofacial surgery in children. Int J Oral Maxillofac Surg. 2018;47(4):428–36.

3. Arnaud É, Paternoster G, Khonsari RH, Haber S. Frontofacial monobloc advancement with internal distraction. Tactics and strategy in faciocraniosynostosis. Berlin: Springer; 2023, 320 p.
4. Khonsari RH, Way B, Nysjö J, Odri GA, Olszewski R, Evans RD, Dunaway DJ, Nyström I, Britto JA. Fronto-facial advancement and bipartition in Crouzon-Pfeiffer and Apert syndromes: impact of fronto-facial surgery upon orbital and airway parameters in FGFR2 syndromes. J Craniomaxillofac Surg. 2016;44(10):1567–75.
5. Kogane N, Hennocq Q, Collet C, Touzé R, Arnaud É, Paternoster G, Khonsari RH. Optic nerve elongation during fronto-facial surgery for Crouzon syndrome: 3D quantification and clinical implications. J Neurosurg Pediatr. 2024;34(4):414–22.
6. Bouaoud J, Hennocq Q, Paternoster G, James S, Arnaud É, Khonsari RH. Excessive ossification of the bandeau in Crouzon and Apert syndromes. J Craniomaxillofac Surg. 2020;48(4):376–82.
7. Guérin J, Hennocq Q, Paternoster G, Arnaud É, Khonsari RH. Distractor position and distraction amplitude in fronto-facial monobloc advancement: a case series. J Stomatol Oral Maxillofac Surg. 2024;125(5S2):101942.
8. Sicard L, Hounkpevi M, Tomat C, James S, Paternoster G, Khonsari RH, Arnaud É. Dental consequences of pterygomaxillary dysjunction during fronto-facial monobloc advancement with internal distraction for Crouzon syndrome. J Craniomaxillofac Surg. 2018;46(9):1476–9.
9. Khonsari RH, Haber S, Paternoster G, Fauroux B, Morisseau-Durand MP, Cormier-Daire V, Legeai-Mallet L, James S, Hennocq Q, Arnaud É. The influence of fronto-facial monobloc advancement on obstructive sleep apnoea: an assessment of 109 syndromic craniosynostoses cases. J Craniomaxillofac Surg. 2020;48(6):536–47.
10. Haber SE, Leikola J, Nowinski D, Fauroux B, Morisseau-Durand MP, Paternoster G, Khonsari RH, Arnaud É. Secondary Le Fort III after early fronto-facial monobloc normalizes sleep apnoea in faciocraniosynostosis: a cohort study. J Plast Reconstr Aesthet Surg. 2022;75(8):2706–18.
11. Wall SA, Butler L, Byren J, et al. Combined internal and external Le Fort III distraction osteogenesis–the "elusive vector". J Craniofac Surg. 2009;20(Suppl 2):1806–8.
12. Chetty V, Haber SE, Khonsari RH, Arnaud É. Improvement of periorbital appearance in Apert syndrome after subcranial Le Fort III with bipartition and distraction. J Craniofac Surg. 2020;31(3):711–5.

Orthognathic Surgery I

25

Nicholas A. Han, Isabel A. Ryan, and Jesse A. Taylor

Key Points

- **Orthognathic surgery in Apert syndrome** addresses complex skeletal deformities resulting from *FGFR2* mutations, including midface hypoplasia, mandibular asymmetry, and severe malocclusion.
- **Midface hypoplasia**, due to early fusion of cranial base synchondroses, results in Class III skeletal relationships, airway obstruction, and dental crowding. Le Fort III, monobloc, and segmental osteotomies are often required for correction.
- **Mandibular anomalies** may include reduced length, asymmetry, and altered angulation. Though the mandible appears prognathic, it often requires repositioning or distraction osteogenesis to restore function and balance.
- **Extensive scarring** from previous surgeries complicates maxillary mobilization. Modified Le Fort I techniques and soft-tissue releases are essential to minimize relapse and enable advancement.
- **Computer-aided design and manufacturing technologies** enhance accuracy in osteotomy planning, guide fabrication, and patient-specific implant design; they are particularly valuable in double-jaw and multisegment procedures.
- **Multidisciplinary planning** with orthodontists, surgeons, and speech specialists ensures that timing and sequencing of interventions optimize both function and aesthetics.

Introduction

Apert syndrome is a complex craniofacial condition characterized by premature fusion of cranial sutures (i.e., craniosynostosis), midface hypoplasia, and various dental, palatal, and mandibular anomalies. These structural differences require comprehensive surgical intervention—including orthognathic surgery at skeletal maturity—to improve both function and aesthetics, which is explored herein. Advances in surgical techniques, particularly the use of computer-aided design and computer-aided manufacturing (CAD/CAM), have enhanced the precision and outcomes of orthognathic surgery and are a focus of this chapter.

Dental and Palatal Anomalies

Apert syndrome is marked by significant developmental anomalies affecting the maxilla and mandible, contributing to a range of craniofacial features and dental irregularities. These developmental anomalies are driven primarily by the *FGFR2* gene mutation, which leads to premature fusion of cranial sutures, significantly altering the

N. A. Han · I. A. Ryan · J. A. Taylor (✉)
Division of Plastic, Reconstructive, and Oral Surgery, Children's Hospital of Philadelphia, Philadelphia, PA, USA

J. G. Meara et al. (eds.), *Apert Syndrome*, https://doi.org/10.1007/978-3-032-12551-4_25

normal development of the skull and facial bones [1]. This mutation affects cranial development and the growth of the dental and alveolar structures [2]. Patients with Apert syndrome frequently present midface hypoplasia and Class III malocclusion that can be accompanied by significant dental crowding and an anterior open bite [3, 4]. Maxillary hypoplasia in the sagittal plane can lead to the appearance of mandibular prognathism, which may also be accompanied by mandibular asymmetry and maldevelopment [1, 5, 6].

The dentition in Apert syndrome is frequently characterized by crowding, delayed eruption, and hypodontia (i.e., congenital absence of teeth) [7]. Studies have shown that approximately 34.8% of patients with Apert syndrome are affected by hypodontia, a significantly higher prevalence compared to the general population [7, 8]. Hypodontia in Apert syndrome has been characterized by bilateral mandibular premolar agenesis [9] and maxillary lateral incisor agenesis [7]. The absence of these teeth may complicate orthodontic treatment, impeding the ability to establish a functional occlusion [7, 8]. In addition to missing teeth, delayed dental eruption can occur, with an average delay of 0.96 years previously reported. Orthodontic tooth movement in patients with Apert syndrome can be delayed or unpredictable due to hyperplastic gingiva and altered alveolar bone, and this can result in the potential for prolonged orthodontic treatment [1, 9–11]. These differences in eruption timing and altered orthodontic biomechanics can complicate orthodontic-treatment timelines and necessitate careful coordination between orthodontists and surgeons to optimize the sequence of interventions [9].

In many patients with Apert syndrome, the dental anomalies are compounded by palatal abnormalities, particularly the presence of a constricted, high-arched palate (Figs. 25.1 and 25.2) [4, 12]. This constriction is further exaggerated by lateral palatal swellings, giving rise to a characteristic pseudo-cleft appearance [4, 12]. Although this appearance may mimic a cleft palate, true clefts are less common in Apert syndrome than in other craniofacial conditions, such as Crouzon syndrome [4, 12]. These palatal anomalies affect the positioning of the teeth and contribute to functional difficulties, including feeding problems in infancy and subsequent speech articulation issues [11, 12]. The lateral palatal swellings are often filled with mucopolysaccharides, which contribute to their size and make the palate appear further constricted, reducing the available space for dental alignment [4, 12].

The presence of these palatal and dental anomalies necessitates a multidisciplinary approach to treatment that involves orthodontists, surgeons, and speech pathologists. Preoperative orthodontic intervention is critical in preparing patients for later surgical procedures (Fig. 25.3). The goal of orthodontic care is to alleviate crowding, align the teeth, and establish a stable occlusal relationship that will support subsequent surgical corrections, such as Le Fort I or higher level Le Fort (i.e., Le Fort II, Le Fort III, monobloc, monobloc+Le Fort II) osteotomies [3, 12]. Midface hypoplasia in the transverse plane and the associated narrow maxillary arch form may complicate orthodontic treatment. Expansion techniques—such as rapid maxillary expansion or surgically assisted rapid palatal expansion—are often employed to widen the maxillary arch and increase space for the teeth [13]. These appliances must be carefully adapted to the unique craniofacial structure of each patient, particularly given the slow and unpredictable nature of tooth movement in Apert syndrome [13].

One of the most significant challenges in orthodontic treatment for patients with Apert syndrome is the management of tooth movement, which is often delayed or unpredictable due to the thickened gingiva and abnormal bone structure around the alveolar ridges [11]. These factors can result in slow progress, requiring prolonged orthodontic treatment throughout the patient's development [11]. In many cases, early intervention is essential to reduce the severity of malocclusion and optimize surgical intervention timing. The collaboration between orthodontic and surgical teams is key to ensuring that the patient's occlusion is stable enough to support complex facial reconstructions while maintaining functional improvements in speech and feeding [3, 11].

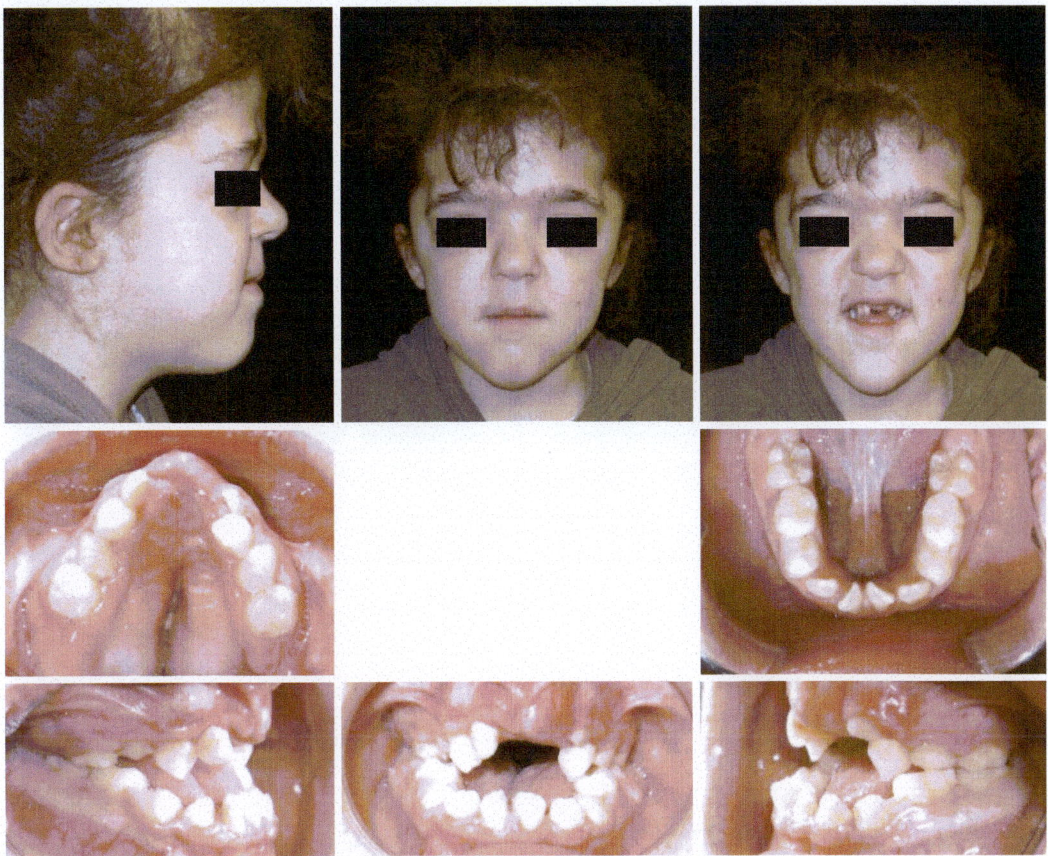

Fig. 25.1 An 8-year-old female (Patient 1) with Apert syndrome and orthodontic deformity including bilateral posterior crossbite, tapered maxilla, U-shaped mandible, dental crowding, and class 3 malocclusion

In addition to functional considerations, the dental and palatal anomalies in Apert syndrome have significant aesthetic implications, further emphasizing the importance of early and coordinated treatment [3, 11]. Patients with Apert syndrome often require multiple stages of orthodontic and surgical care, beginning in childhood and continuing into adulthood. Given the severe malocclusion and crowding, orthodontic treatment is essential not only for improving dental alignment but also for enhancing the overall success of orthognathic surgeries aimed at correcting midface hypoplasia and mandibular anomalies [3, 11].

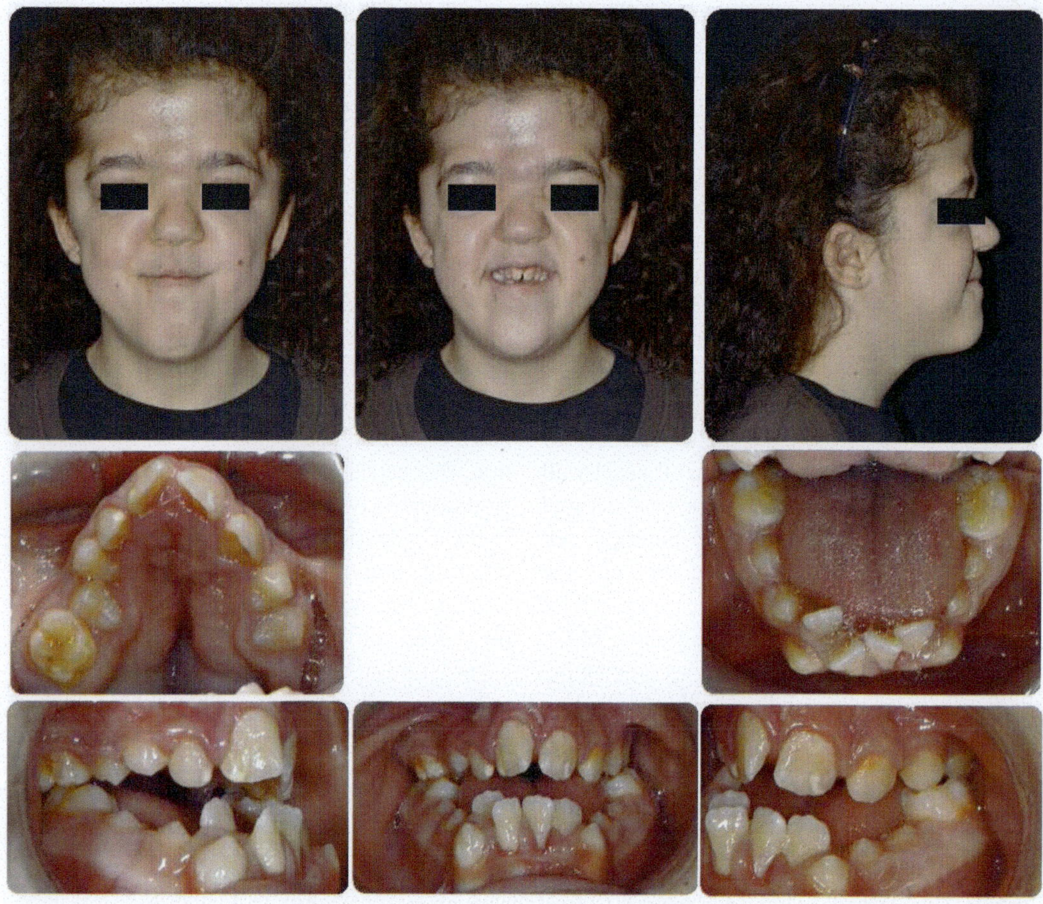

Fig. 25.2 Patient 1 at 11 years, in permanent dentition, with severe upper and lower crowding, hyperplastic gingiva, anterior crossbite, and class 3 malocclusion

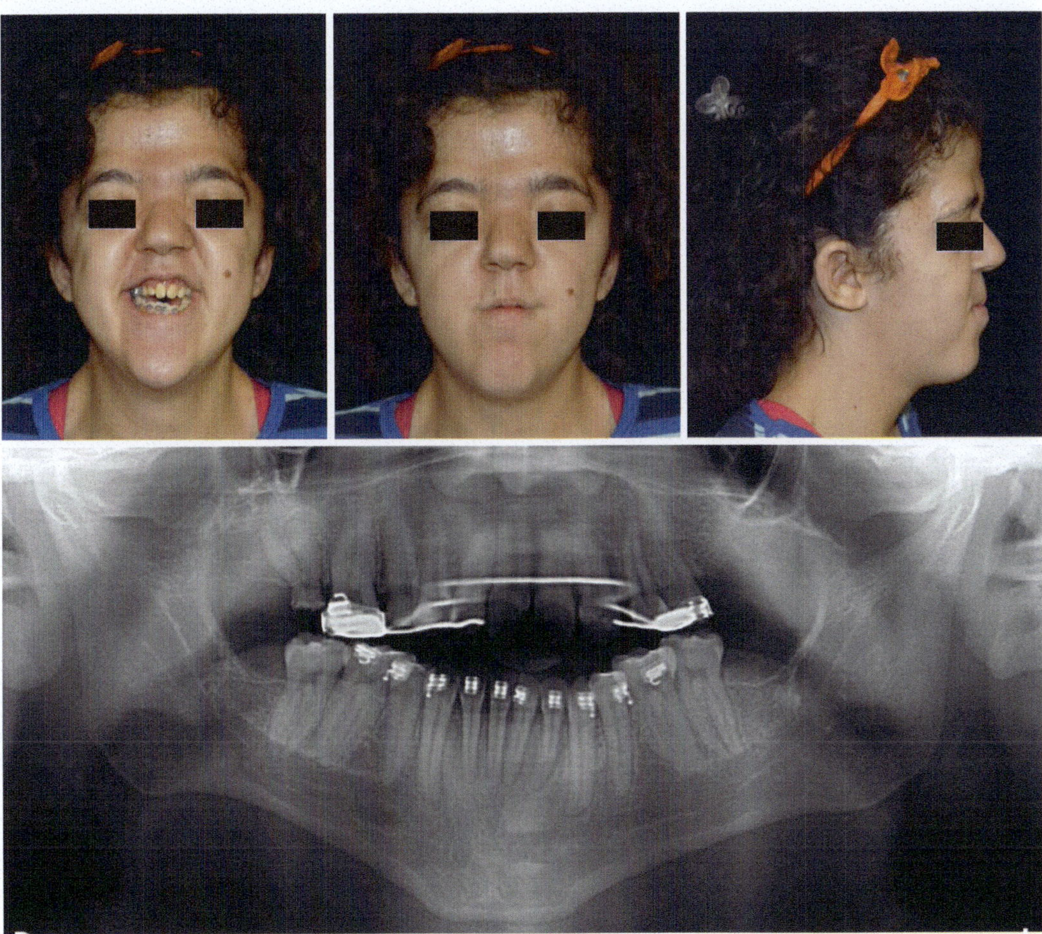

Fig. 25.3 Patient 1 at 14 years old, s/p extraction of teeth #1, 6, 11, 14, 15, 16, 17, 21, 28, 32 and initiation of palatal expansion and orthodontia

Maxillary Hypoplasia

Midface hypoplasia in patients with Apert syndrome presents significant structural and functional challenges due to the early fusion of cranial and cranial base sutures and synchondroses, notably the spheno-occipital synchondrosis, which affects maxillary growth across the anterior–posterior axis [14–16]. This synchondrosis, located at the junction of the sphenoid and occipital bones, typically supports midface growth into adolescence. However, in patients with Apert syndrome, this synchondrosis often fuses prematurely, sometimes as early as 2 years of age, as demonstrated in extensive radiographic reviews [15–17]. In both human studies and mouse models, early fusion is strongly linked to reduced midface projection, leading to a retruded maxilla that limits airway volume and exacerbates respiratory challenges, such as obstructive sleep apnea (OSA). This relationship between synchondrosis closure and hypoplasia reflects the central role of *FGFR2* mutations in altering cranial and facial growth dynamics.

Respiratory compromise in Apert syndrome often results directly from midface retrusion and the consequent reduction in nasopharyngeal airway volume. A study comparing *Ser252Trp* and *Pro253Arg* mutations found that patients with the *Ser252Trp* mutation exhibited nasopharyngeal airway volumes approximately 20–30% smaller than those with *Pro253Arg*, correlating with higher rates of severe OSA (62% in *Ser252Trp* versus 9% in *Pro253Arg*) [15]. This diminished airway capacity is compounded by additional nasal structural abnormalities—such as narrow nasal passages and septal deviations—and early midface advancement may be required in order to reduce respiratory complications and associated developmental delays [18, 19]. In younger patients, midface advancement through distraction osteogenesis is often preferred [20], as it allows for gradual skeletal movement while stretching the soft tissues to reduce relapse risk and improve airway function, as noted in long-term outcomes for distraction osteogenesis procedures [21].

In patients with Apert syndrome, the maxilla is often hypoplastic in vertical, sagittal, and transverse planes; this results in a Class III skeletal pattern, with a narrow high-arched palate and anterior open bite. As a result, the mandible can appear to be relatively prognathic compared to the hypoplastic maxilla. Beyond airway issues, the retruded maxilla also impacts dental and occlusal development, leading to pronounced malocclusion—typically a Class III pattern with anterior open bite—where the mandibular prominence exceeds the maxillary projection due to underdevelopment. This malocclusion creates functional challenges, such as difficulty with mastication, as well as differences in facial appearance, contributing to psychological and social challenges. Studies have shown that this Class III malocclusion, when accompanied by a high-arched, narrow palate, results in severe dental crowding, increased risk for anterior open bite, and difficulties with mastication [22]. The relationship between hypoplastic maxilla and palatal abnormalities, such as pseudo-clefts, indicates that these dental and skeletal issues are inextricably linked to the underlying genetic mutations driving premature synchondrosis fusion and altered cranial development [22].

Midface hypoplasia also significantly interferes with feeding, especially in infants and young children, as the structural limitations of the maxilla and high-arched palate impair tongue mobility and effective palatal closure. This challenge is particularly evident in infants with the narrow, high-arched palates common in Apert syndrome, who are frequently misdiagnosed as cleft palate or submucous cleft due to the lateral swellings of the palatal processes [22]. Up to 75% of patients with Apert syndrome display some form of palatal anomaly, with approximately 20–25% presenting a soft palate cleft [22]. Feeding difficulties are further compounded by mandibular prognathism and malocclusion, which affect lip seal and chewing mechanics and often require early feeding interventions, specialized orthodontic devices, or surgical corrections to enable adequate nutrition and avoid growth deficits [17, 18]..

Given these complexities, managing midface hypoplasia in Apert syndrome requires a multidisciplinary approach to address airway stability, dental occlusion, and feeding function concurrently, with careful consideration of the genetic profile and synchondrosis status for each patient. In recent years, segmental osteotomies—including Le Fort II with zygomatic repositioning, monobloc with Le Fort II, and monobloc with bipartition—have seen significant increase in use and have become preferred options. These multipiece procedures allow for targeted adjustments to specific facial features, such as intercanthal distance and bilateral canthal tilt, thus addressing unique midface imbalances in patients with Apert syndrome. Computer-aided design and manufacturing (CAD/CAM) technology and external halo distractors further support these complex procedures by enhancing precision during segmental mobilization. While transcranial techniques carry higher risks, such as infection and cerebrospinal fluid leak, options like monobloc with Le Fort II can achieve notable improvements in facial convexity and airway space, which are critical for both functional and aesthetic outcomes.

Mandibular Anomalies

The mandible in Apert syndrome presents a range of developmental anomalies that significantly impact both aesthetics and function. These anomalies stem largely from the *FGFR2* gene mutation, which disrupts the normal process of osteogenesis in craniofacial bones [23–26]. As a result, the mandible often develops in an altered manner, leading to reduced size, asymmetry, and abnormal growth patterns (Fig. 25.4). These deviations from typical mandibular development must be considered when planning surgical interventions, as they pose unique challenges for surgeons aiming to improve both the function and appearance of the lower face [27].

The literature reflects a debate regarding whether the mandible in patients with Apert syndrome is intrinsically abnormal or secondarily impacted due to maxillary hypoplasia. Recent advances in imaging and in the understanding of genetics and histology have offered insights about this question. One study published at the Children's Hospital of Philadelphia included two-dimensional (2D) and three-dimensional (3D) analysis of the mandible in 38 patients, finding significantly decreased mandibular length but no difference in mandibular volume, which suggests potential thickening of the bone [28]. Another study found narrower bicondylar width and increased ramus-to-intercondylar-plane angles compared to non-syndromic individuals, resulting in a micrognathic mandible with an inwardly torqued ramus [29]. This underdevelopment is particularly noticeable in the anterior–posterior dimension, where the reduced projection of the mandible may contribute to functional issues, such as difficulties with chewing and speech. While the mandible may appear prognathic due to the severe maxillary hypoplasia characteristic of Apert syndrome, this is often a relative prognathism, rather than true mandibular overgrowth [30].

In addition to differences in size, mandibular asymmetry may be seen in patients with Apert syndrome [31]. Asymmetry in the mandible is often the result of developmental instability,

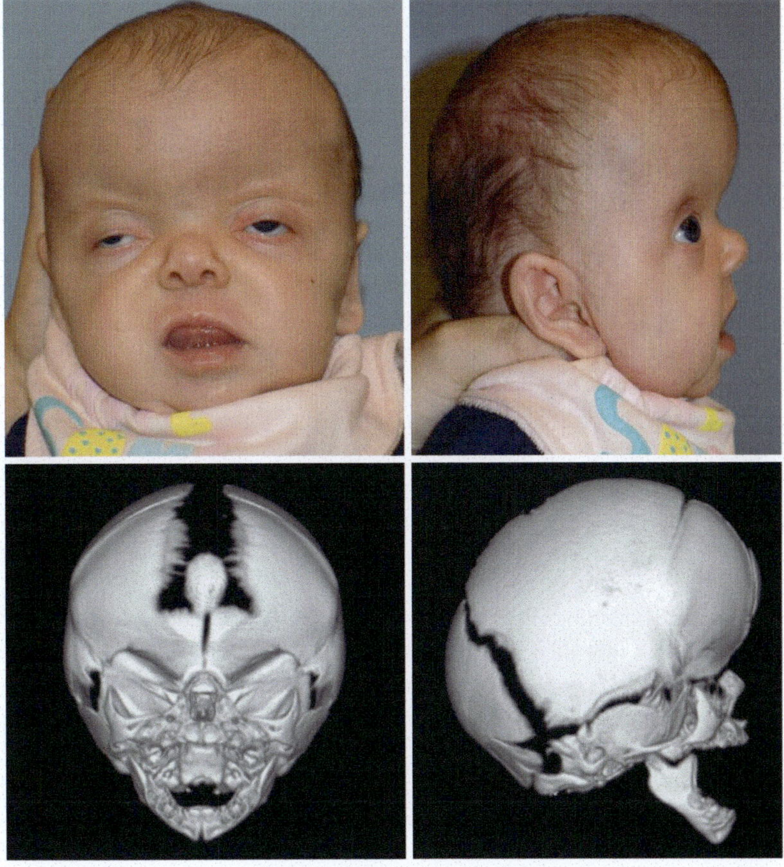

Fig. 25.4 A 2-month-old female (Patient 2) with Apert syndrome with characteristic maxillary hypoplasia and micrognathia. Severe tongue-base collapse on flexible laryngoscopy requiring CPAP

which arises from the disrupted osteogenesis that affects craniofacial growth. This instability in development, often reported as fluctuating asymmetry, has been associated with stress and disrupted developmental homeostasis [31]. This misalignment can cause functional problems, including malocclusion and jaw joint dysfunction, and often requires surgical correction.

The *FGFR2* mutation that drives the craniofacial abnormalities in Apert syndrome also contributes to altered bone mineralization and structural defects in the mandible. Histological studies have shown that the mandible in Apert syndrome exhibits increased osteoclastic activity and disrupted bone formation, leading to less dense bone tissue [25]. These defects affect the mandible's growth and increase susceptibility to fracture and malunion following surgical interventions. Surgeons must carefully consider these factors when planning osteotomies or other surgical procedures.

Surgical interventions typically involve procedures such as sagittal split osteotomy (SSO) or distraction osteogenesis (DO). SSO is commonly used to reposition the mandible and correct malocclusion, while DO may be employed to gradually lengthen the mandible in cases of severe underdevelopment. Careful preoperative planning is essential to account for the asymmetry and reduced bone density in the mandible [25].

Postoperatively, patients with Apert syndrome face additional challenges related to bone healing and soft-tissue adaptation. The disrupted osteogenesis in patients with Apert syndrome often leads to delayed bone healing, which can prolong the recovery period and increase the risk of complications such as nonunion or relapse. Additionally, the soft-tissue envelope, including the muscles and ligaments of the jaw, may also impact the stability of the new position of the midface and mandible. Long-term follow up is essential to monitor for issues such as relapse and to ensure that the surgical corrections are maintained over time.

The aesthetic implications of mandibular anomalies in Apert syndrome cannot be overlooked. The reduced size and asymmetry of the mandible contribute significantly to the overall facial appearance, and surgical correction must balance both functional and aesthetic goals. For many patients, improving mandibular structure through surgery not only enhances jaw function but also contributes to a more balanced and symmetrical facial profile.

Computer-Aided Design/Computer-Aided Manufacturing (CAD/CAM)

Offering precision and customization in surgical planning and execution, CAD/CAM technology has become an invaluable tool in orthognathic surgery [32, 33]. Its ability to model complex osteotomies, simulate surgical outcomes, and fabricate patient-specific guides and implants has transformed the approach to craniofacial surgery, particularly in cases like Apert syndrome, where the anatomy presents unique challenges (Figs. 25.5, 25.6 and 25.7). Widely used in craniofacial surgery, CAD/CAM is utilized in cases ranging from orthognathic surgery to hypertelorism correction to free-fibula mandible reconstruction [32].

Surgeons use 3D imaging to create digital reconstructions of the patient's craniofacial skeleton, which are then manipulated to simulate the desired surgical osteotomies and bone movements. This enables a precise analysis of both the skeletal deformities and the necessary corrections, ensuring that the surgery is meticulously planned before the operation (Figs. 25.8 and 25.9). Additionally, the process also allows for the design and fabrication of patient-specific cutting guides and implants (Figs. 25.10, 25.11 and 25.12). These guides are used intraoperatively to ensure that osteotomies are performed with the planned cuts from the CAD/CAM planning session, minimizing the risk of error and enhancing the accuracy of the procedure [34]. Facial disproportions related to Apert syndrome, such as midfacial hypoplasia and mandibular asymmetry, require complex and multi-plane corrections that are often difficult to visualize. The use of CAD/CAM technology for both midfacial advancement and orthognathic surgery allows for detailed visualization and preoperative planning that

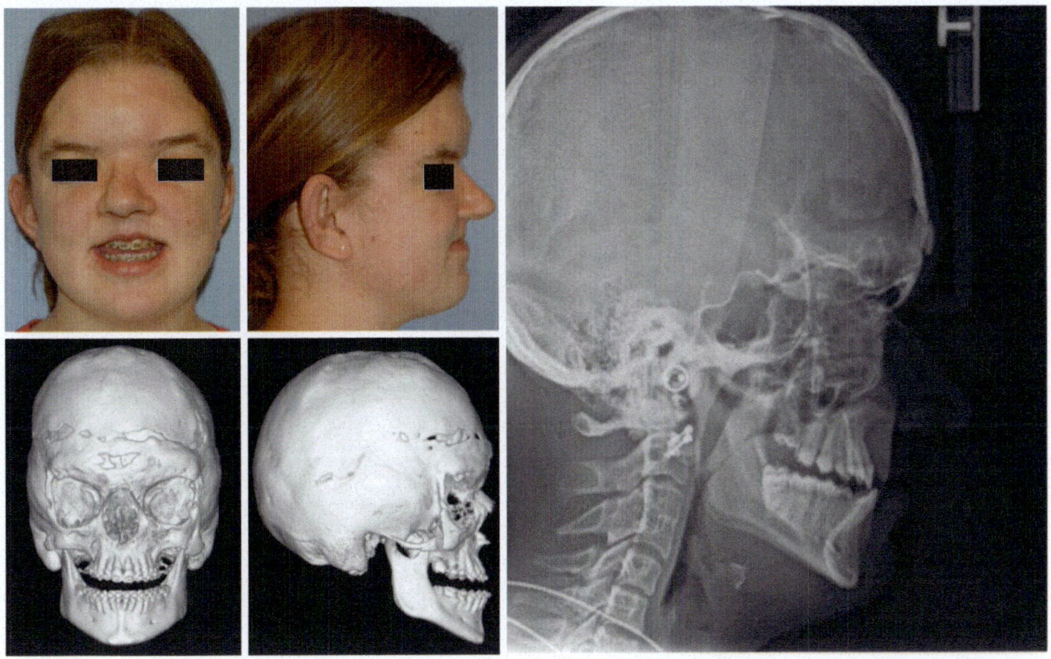

Fig. 25.5 A 14-year-old female (Patient 3) with apert syndrome with class III malocclusion presenting for orthognathic surgery

accounts for these differences. This process also reduces operative times, as plates are custom made and do not require manual bending.

In cases where the patient requires simultaneous corrections of the maxilla and mandible, CAD/CAM provides a platform for simulating the entire procedure and planning each osteotomy in relation to the others. This is particularly important for patients with Apert syndrome, who may require double jaw surgery subsequent to or concurrently with midfacial advancement. Moreover, CAD/CAM can assist in addressing the disproportionate size and asymmetry of the mandible in Apert syndrome, while patient-specific plates can aid in utilizing ideal bone stock for screw fixation. Achieving more precise bony movements intraoperatively reduces the risk of postoperative complications such as malocclusion or joint dysfunction, which are more common in patients with complex craniofacial deformities [28].

Maxillary procedures, such as Le Fort I osteotomies, are greatly enhanced by CAD/CAM technology. The underdeveloped midface in Apert syndrome often requires significant advancement, which can strain the surrounding soft tissues and lead to relapse if not carefully planned (Figs. 25.13 and 25.14). Orthognathic surgery is typically performed at growth completion, following other midface surgeries, and bone healing and scar formation can be unpredictable factors for the surgeon performing the orthognathic surgery. Furthermore, segmental osteotomies may be necessary to correct transverse discrepancies that persist despite orthodontics.

CAD/CAM technology has revolutionized orthognathic surgery, particularly in complex cases like Apert syndrome, where the craniofacial anatomy presents significant challenges. By providing precise preoperative simulations, customized implants, and detailed cutting guides, CAD/CAM optimizes both functional and aesthetic outcomes (Figs. 25.15, 25.16 and 25.17). Its ability to integrate with other advanced technologies, such as 3D printing, makes it an indispensable tool in the treatment of craniofacial syndromes. As CAD/CAM technology continues to evolve, it will likely play an even greater role

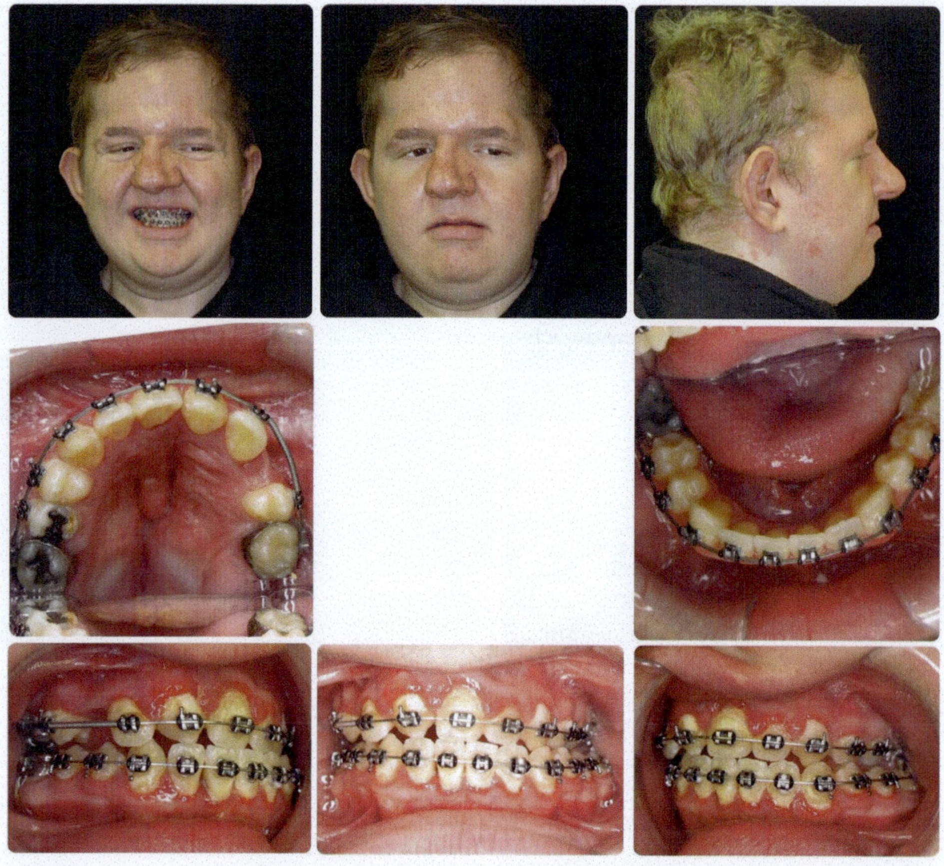

Fig. 25.6 A 16-year-old male (Patient 4) with a Apert syndrome undergoing pre-operative orthodontics prior to orthognathic surgery

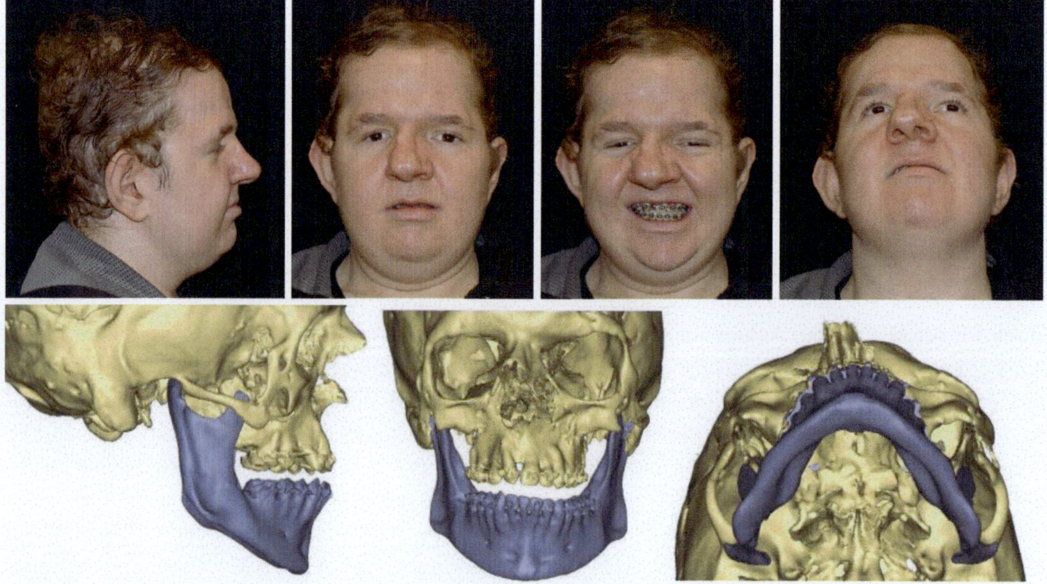

Fig. 25.7 Patient 4, pre-operative photos and 3D reconstructions before Lefort 1/BSSO

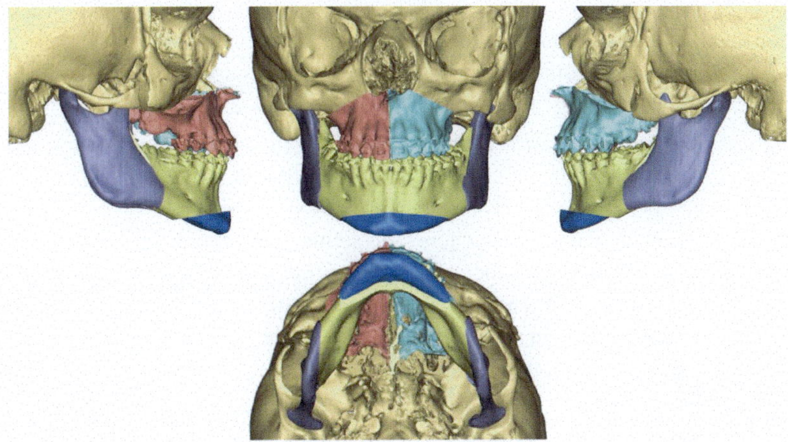

Fig. 25.8 Patient 3, planned final movements for Lefort I/BSSO/Genioplasty

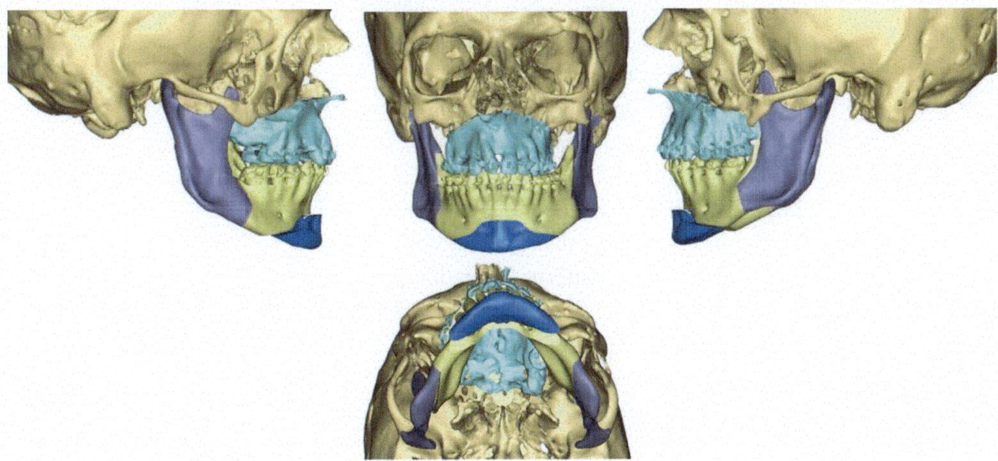

Fig. 25.9 Patient 4, planned final movements

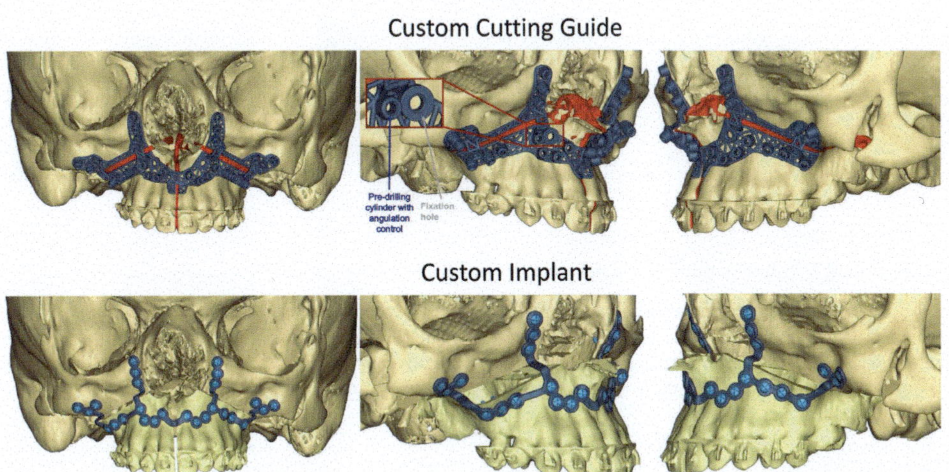

Fig. 25.10 Custom cutting guide and 3D-printed titanium implant for patient 3

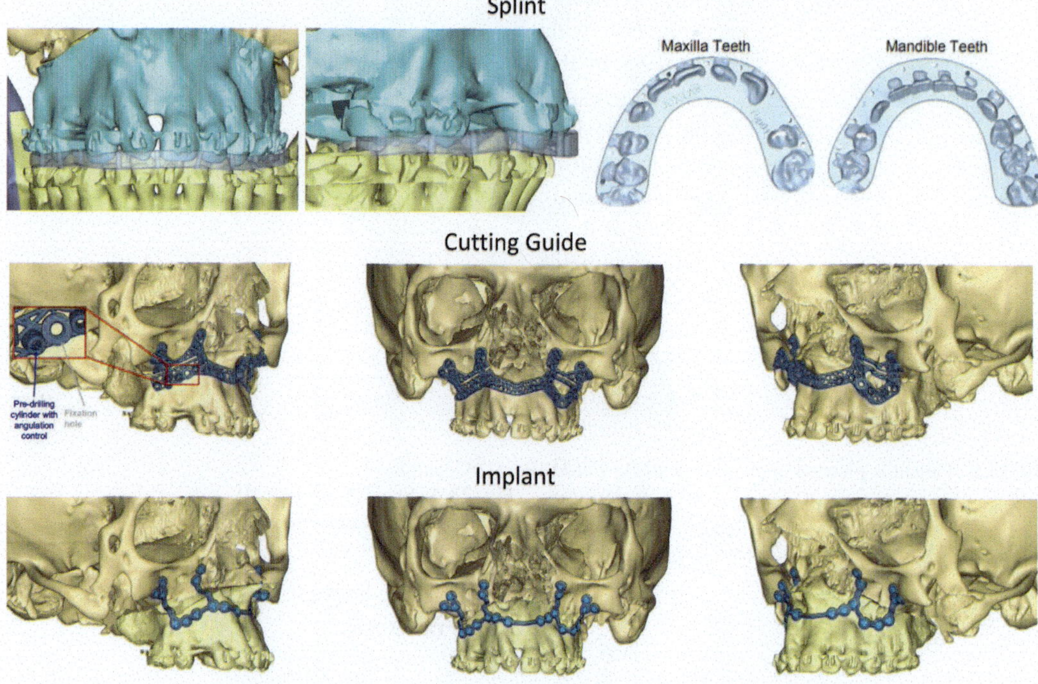

Fig. 25.11 Patient 4, custom splint, cutting guide, and implant for Lefort I

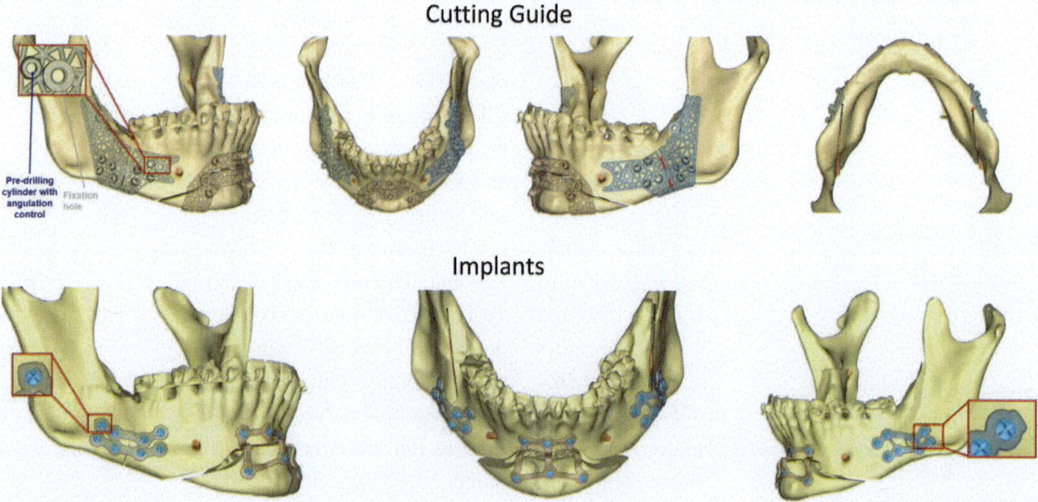

Fig. 25.12 Patient 4, custom cutting guide and implant for BSSO

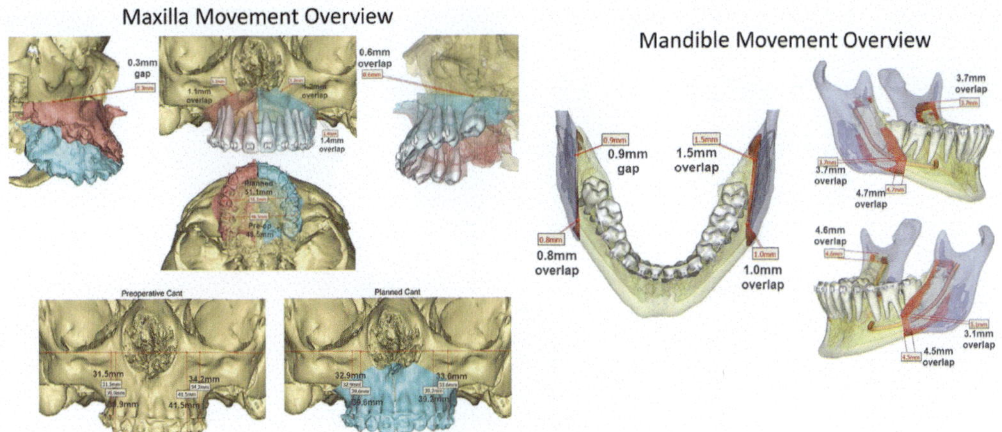

Fig. 25.13 Patient 3, planned movements of maxilla and mandible

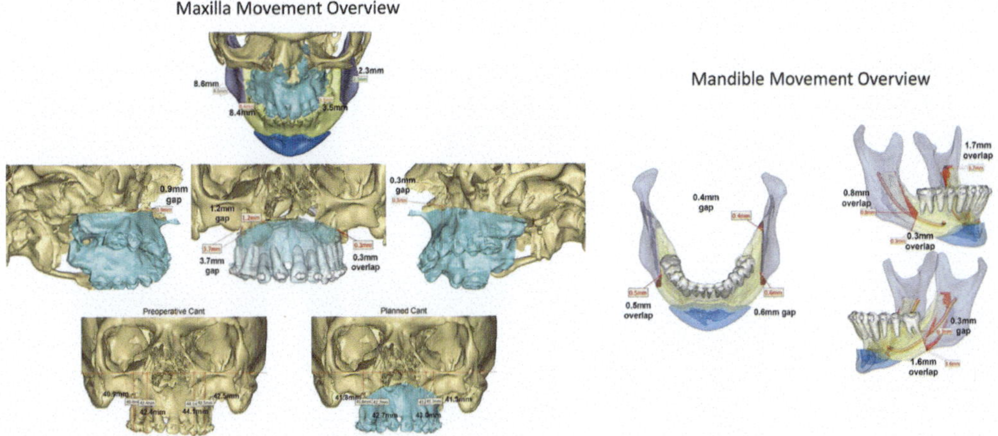

Fig. 25.14 Patient 4, planned movements of maxilla and mandible

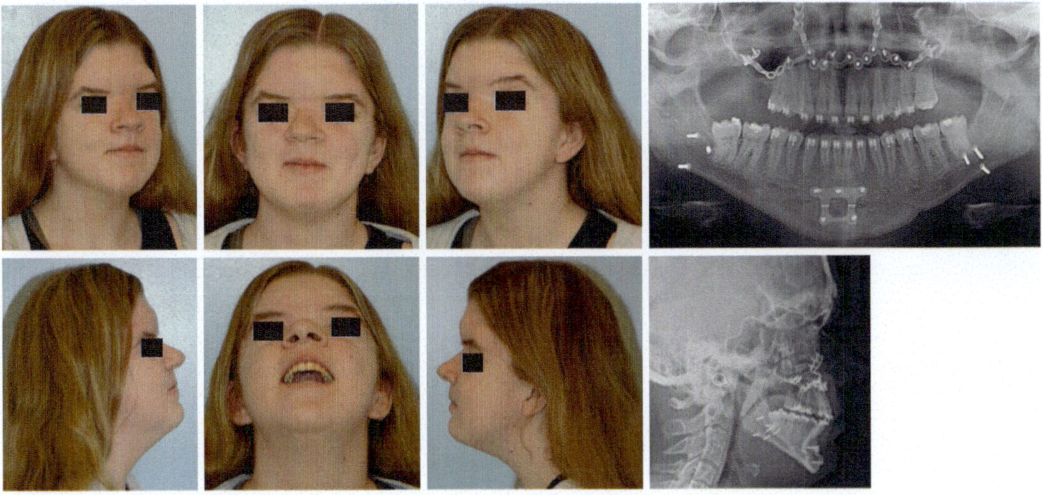

Fig. 25.15 (Left) 3-year post-op follow up photos and (Right) 1 year post-op follow up panoramic X-ray and lateral cephalogram for patient 3

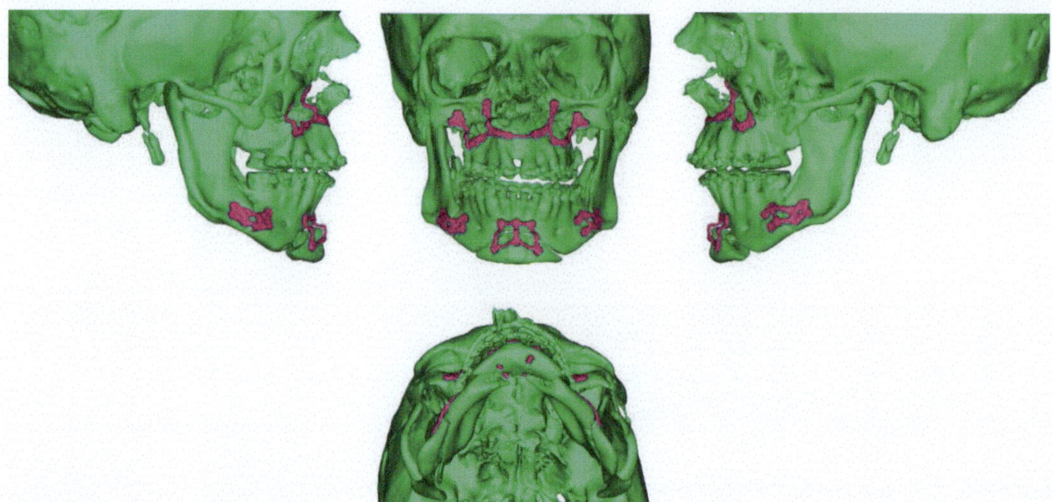

Fig. 25.16 Patient 4, post-operative positions

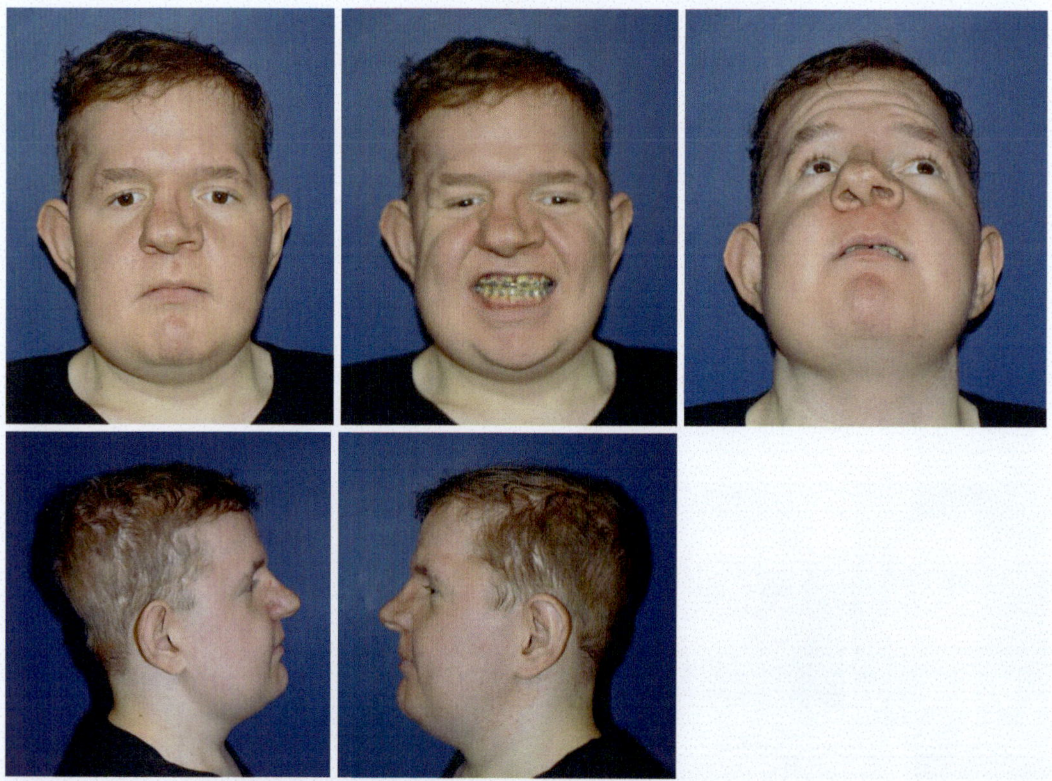

Fig. 25.17 Patient 4, post-operative photos

in improving the outcomes of orthognathic surgery for patients with Apert syndrome and other complex craniofacial conditions.

Scarring

Orthognathic surgery in patients with Apert syndrome presents a unique set of challenges due to the extensive scar tissue from prior surgeries, such as subcranial distractions and other craniofacial reconstructions [35]. Similar to patients with cleft palate, the increased scar burden, particularly around the posterior maxilla and soft tissues, significantly complicates mobilization during surgery [35–37]. Extensive scar release is often required to mobilize the maxilla for proper repositioning. Following tenets of cleft orthognathic surgery, fibrous tissue and periosteal scarring from prior surgeries that are tethering the maxilla require careful dissection and bone removal to free the soft-tissue attachments [35].

Cleft literature outlines technical modifications to orthognathic surgery specific to scar management [35], and these modifications remain relevant for patients with Apert syndrome undergoing orthognathic surgery [35]. Susarla et al. detailed several modifications to the Le Fort I osteotomy to account for and manage the increased scar tissue in the cleft population [37]. Specifically, the authors discussed the use of transmucosal pterygomaxillary separation and the release of the descending palatine vessels to mitigate the effects of scar tethering and allow for sufficient mobilization [37]. Further, they discuss the role of bony removal from the posterior maxillary wall to release soft-tissue tethers that would otherwise prevent the maxilla from moving freely during advancement, as well as gradual anterior and posterior traction to allow for advancement without surplus traction [37]. These modifications are equally crucial to achieving successful outcomes in patients with Apert syndrome.

Scar tissue also plays a critical role in the risk of relapse following orthognathic surgery, particularly in patients with craniofacial dysmorphologies—including Apert syndrome—secondary to a history of multiple craniofacial surgeries. Extensive scarring from previous procedures can create tension on the maxilla after advancement, hindering proper healing and increasing the likelihood of skeletal relapse [35, 38]. Studies have demonstrated that patients with a significant scar burden tend to experience higher rates of relapse, particularly when traditional maxillary advancement techniques are used without addressing the underlying soft-tissue restrictions [38]. Thus, techniques such as distraction osteogenesis, which allow for gradual skeletal advancement and soft-tissue accommodation, may be preferred to reduce the impact of scar-related tension and improve long-term stability [37, 38].

Despite the challenges, with careful preoperative planning and intraoperative techniques, significant maxillary advancements can be achieved in patients with Apert syndrome undergoing orthognathic surgery, even in the presence of extensive scarring. However, maintaining stability postoperatively remains a concern, as excessive tension on the soft-tissue envelope can lead to relapse.

Conclusion

Orthognathic surgery for patients with Apert syndrome presents a unique set of challenges due to the complex craniofacial anomalies associated with the condition. The combination of midface hypoplasia, mandibular asymmetry, and dental anomalies requires a multidisciplinary approach incorporating orthodontic and surgical interventions. Preoperative planning and the use of modern technologies, particularly patient-specific guides and implants, have dramatically improved the precision and outcomes of these procedures.

The management of dental and palatal anomalies is crucial in preparing patients for surgical interventions, as proper alignment of the teeth and expansion of the maxillary arch create a foundation for successful midface and mandibular corrections. Scarring, although minimized through intraoral incisions, remains a significant factor affecting both the aesthetic and functional results, particularly in complex cases involving midface advancement and distraction osteogenesis.

The integration of CAD/CAM technology has further revolutionized the field, providing surgeons with the tools to plan complex osteotomies, simulate outcomes, and produce patient-specific guides and implants that enhance both precision and predictability. This technology has proven particularly beneficial in addressing the unique challenges of Apert syndrome, allowing for more accurate corrections of skeletal deformities and minimizing the risk of postoperative complications such as relapse or asymmetry.

As surgical techniques and technologies continue to evolve, the outlook for patients with Apert syndrome undergoing orthognathic surgery is becoming increasingly optimistic. With the ongoing development of CAD/CAM and 3D printing, the ability to tailor surgical interventions to each patient's unique anatomy will only continue to improve, leading to better functional and aesthetic outcomes for these complex craniofacial cases.

References

1. Alam MK, Alfawzan AA, Srivastava KC, Shrivastava D, Ganji KK, Manay SM. Craniofacial morphology in Apert syndrome: a systematic review and meta-analysis. Sci Rep. 2022;12(1):5708. https://doi.org/10.1038/s41598-022-09764-y.
2. Blaser SI, Padfield N, Chitayat D, Forrest CR. Skull base development and craniosynostosis. Pediatr Radiol. 2015;45(Suppl 3):S485–96. https://doi.org/10.1007/s00247-015-3320-1.
3. Verdonck A, Bertrand J, Carels C, Swinnen S, Schoenaers J. Orthodontic and orthognathic management of a patient with Apert syndrome: a case report. J Orthod. 2010;37(2):121–7. https://doi.org/10.1179/14653121042984.
4. Ogura K, Kobayashi Y, Hikita R, Tsuji M, Moriyama K. Three-dimensional analysis of the palatal morphology in growing patients with Apert syndrome and Crouzon syndrome. Congenit Anom (Kyoto). 2022;62(4):153–60. https://doi.org/10.1111/cga.12470.
5. Varoli FP, Santos KCP, Costa C, Oliveira JX. Apert syndrome: clinical and radiographic features and case report. Revista Odonto Ciência. 2011;26:96–9.
6. Paula L, Cardoso IL. Apert syndrome and repercussions in dental medicine. J Med Biol. 2020;2(1):31–42.
7. Stavropoulos D, Bartzela T, Bronkhorst E, Mohlin B, Hagberg C. Dental agenesis patterns of permanent teeth in Apert syndrome. Eur J Oral Sci. 2011;119(3):198–203. https://doi.org/10.1111/j.1600-0722.2011.00821.x.
8. Reitsma JH, Ongkosuwito EM, van Wijk AJ, Prahl-Andersen B. Patterns of tooth agenesis in patients with Crouzon or Apert syndrome. Cleft Palate Craniofac J. 2014;51(2):178–83. https://doi.org/10.1597/12-180.
9. Reitsma JH, Balk-Leurs IH, Ongkosuwito EM, Wattel E, Prahl-Andersen B. Dental maturation in children with the syndrome of Crouzon and Apert. Cleft Palate Craniofac J. 2014;51(6):639–44. https://doi.org/10.1597/13-071.
10. Kaloust S, Ishii K, Vargervik K. Dental development in Apert syndrome. Cleft Palate Craniofac J. 1997;34(2):117–21. https://doi.org/10.1597/1545-1569_1997_034_0117_ddias_2.3.co_2.
11. Hohoff A, Joos U, Meyer U, Ehmer U, Stamm T. The spectrum of Apert syndrome: phenotype, particularities in orthodontic treatment, and characteristics of orthognathic surgery. Head Face Med. 2007;3:10. https://doi.org/10.1186/1746-160x-3-10.
12. Letra A, de Almeida AL, Kaizer R, Esper LA, Sgarbosa S, Granjeiro JM. Intraoral features of Apert's syndrome. Oral Surg Oral Med Oral Pathol Oral Radiol Endod. 2007;103(5):e38–41. https://doi.org/10.1016/j.tripleo.2006.04.006.
13. Meazzini MC, Corradi F, Mazzoleni F, et al. Circummaxillary sutures in patients with Apert, Crouzon, and Pfeiffer syndromes compared to nonsyndromic children: growth, orthodontic, and surgical implications. Cleft Palate Craniofac J. 2021;58(3):299–305. https://doi.org/10.1177/1055665620947616.
14. Goldstein JA, Paliga JT, Bartlett SP. Cranioplasty: indications and advances. Curr Opin Otolaryngol Head Neck Surg. 2013;21(4):400–9. https://doi.org/10.1097/MOO.0b013e328363003e.
15. Wagner CS, Wietlisbach LE, Kota A, et al. Genetic subtypes of Apert syndrome are associated with differences in airway morphology and early upper airway obstruction. J Craniofac Surg. 2023;34(7):1999–2003. https://doi.org/10.1097/SCS.0000000000009583.
16. Goldstein JA, Paliga JT, Wink JD, Bartlett SP, Nah HD, Taylor JA. Earlier evidence of spheno-occipital synchondrosis fusion correlates with severity of midface hypoplasia in patients with syndromic craniosynostosis. Plast Reconstr Surg. 2014;134(3):504–10. https://doi.org/10.1097/PRS.0000000000000419.
17. McGrath J, Gerety PA, Derderian CA, et al. Differential closure of the spheno-occipital synchondrosis in syndromic craniosynostosis. Plast Reconstr Surg. 2012;130(5):681e–9e. https://doi.org/10.1097/PRS.0b013e318267d4c0.
18. Kim BS, Shin HR, Kim HJ, et al. Septal chondrocyte hypertrophy contributes to midface deformity in a mouse model of Apert syndrome. Sci Rep. 2021;11(1):7979. https://doi.org/10.1038/s41598-021-87260-5.

19. Kim B, Shin H, Kim W, et al. PIN1 attenuation improves midface hypoplasia in a mouse model of Apert syndrome. J Dent Res. 2020;99(2):223–32. https://doi.org/10.1177/0022034519893656.
20. Wu M, Massenburg BB, Ng JJ, et al. The kaleidoscope of midface Management in Apert Syndrome: a 23-year single-institution experience. Plast Reconstr Surg. 2024; https://doi.org/10.1097/PRS.0000000000011415.
21. Zimmerman CE, Sun J, Wes AM, et al. Long term speech outcomes following midface advancement in syndromic Craniosynostosis. J Craniofac Surg. 2020;31(6):1775–9. https://doi.org/10.1097/SCS.0000000000006581.
22. Willie D, Holmes G, Jabs EW, Wu M. Cleft palate in Apert syndrome. J Dev Biol. 2022;10(3) https://doi.org/10.3390/jdb10030033.
23. Jiang Q, Mei L, Zou Y, et al. Genetic polymorphisms in FGFR2 underlie skeletal malocclusion. J Dent Res. 2019;98(12):1340–7. https://doi.org/10.1177/0022034519872951.
24. Morice A, Cornette R, Giudice A, et al. Early mandibular morphological differences in patients with FGFR2 and FGFR3-related syndromic craniosynostoses: a 3D comparative study. Bone. 2020;141:115600. https://doi.org/10.1016/j.bone.2020.115600.
25. Zhou X, Pu D, Liu R, et al. The Fgfr2(S252W/+) mutation in mice retards mandible formation and reduces bone mass as in human Apert syndrome. Am J Med Genet A. 2013;161A(5):983–92. https://doi.org/10.1002/ajmg.a.35824.
26. Motch Perrine SM, Wu M, Stephens NB, et al. Mandibular dysmorphology due to abnormal embryonic osteogenesis in FGFR2-related craniosynostosis mice. Dis Model Mech. 2019;12(5) https://doi.org/10.1242/dmm.038513.
27. Costaras-Volarich M, Pruzansky S. Is the mandible intrinsically different in Apert and Crouzon syndromes? Am J Orthod. 1984;85(6):475–87. https://doi.org/10.1016/0002-9416(84)90087-3.
28. Wink JD, Bastidas N, Bartlett SP. Analysis of the long-term growth of the mandible in Apert syndrome. J Craniofac Surg. 2013;24(4):1408–10. https://doi.org/10.1097/SCS.0b013e31828dcf09.
29. Boutros S, Shetye PR, Ghali S, Carter CR, McCarthy JG, Grayson BH. Morphology and growth of the mandible in Crouzon, Apert, and Pfeiffer syndromes. J Craniofac Surg. 2007;18(1):146–50. https://doi.org/10.1097/01.scs.0000248655.53405.a7.
30. Lu X, Forte AJ, Park KE, et al. Morphological basis for airway surgical intervention in Apert syndrome. Ann Plast Surg. 2021;87(1):59–64. https://doi.org/10.1097/SAP.0000000000002601.
31. Elmi P, Reitsma JH, Buschang PH, Wolvius EB, Ongkosuwito EM. Mandibular asymmetry in patients with the Crouzon or Apert syndrome. Cleft Palate Craniofac J. 2015;52(3):327–35. https://doi.org/10.1597/13-143.
32. Kalmar CL, Xu W, Zimmerman CE, et al. Trends in utilization of virtual surgical planning in pediatric craniofacial surgery. J Craniofac Surg. 2020;31(7):1900–5. https://doi.org/10.1097/SCS.0000000000006626.
33. Xun H, Yesantharao P, Kalmar C, Lopez J. Chapter 2: Computer-assisted design and computer-assisted manufacturing. In: Computer-assisted planning in craniofacial surgery. Elsevier; 2024. p. 11–7.
34. Kravchenko D, Lopez J, Steinbacher DM. Chapter 5: Computer-assisted surgical planning in orthognathic surgery: a practical workflow. In: Computer-assisted planning in craniofacial surgery. Elsevier; 2024. p. 43–52.
35. Han JT, Egbert MA, Ettinger RE, Kapadia HP, Susarla SM. Orthognathic surgery in patients with syndromic Craniosynostosis. Oral Maxillofac Surg Clin North Am. 2022;34(3):477–87. https://doi.org/10.1016/j.coms.2022.01.003.
36. Zaroni FM, Sales P, Maffia F, Scariot R. Complications of orthognathic surgery in patients with cleft lip and palate: a systematic review. J Stomatol Oral Maxillofac Surg. 2024;125(6):101795. https://doi.org/10.1016/j.jormas.2024.101795.
37. Susarla SM, Ettinger R, Preston K, Hitesh K, Egbert MA. Technical modifications specific to the cleft Le fort I osteotomy. J Craniofac Surg. 2020;31(5):1459–63. https://doi.org/10.1097/scs.0000000000006456.
38. Chaisiri S, Arayasantiparb R, Boonsiriseth K. Factors affecting the relapse of maxilla and soft tissues of nose, upper lip and velopharyngeal structures after maxillary advancement in cleft patients. PLoS One. 2023;18(11):e0294059. https://doi.org/10.1371/journal.pone.0294059.

Orthognathic Surgery II

26

Renato Yassutaka Faria Yaedú,
Isabela Toledo Teixeira da Silveira,
Caroline de Paula Oliveira Gringo,
and Mariela Peralta-Mamani

Orthognathic surgery is often one of the final interventions for patients with Apert syndrome. This procedure is indicated for correcting skeletal deformities across the three spatial planes, particularly when osteogenic distraction—such as Le Fort III or frontofacial advancement—does not provide sufficient correction. Moreover, this surgery is essential for addressing characteristic mandibular alterations in patients with Apert syndrome. The literature reflects significant debate on the relative merits of orthognathic surgery versus osteogenic distraction, especially in cases involving cleft lip and palate. However, this discussion is less pertinent to patients with Apert syndrome due to the typically marked clockwise rotation of the occlusal plane, making mandibular correction crucial for achieving satisfactory aesthetic and functional outcomes [6].

Osteogenic distraction during childhood and subsequent orthognathic surgery after skeletal growth completion are well-established steps in surgical protocols for rehabilitation of Apert syndrome [25].

R. Y. F. Yaedú (✉)
Department of Oral Surgery, Faculdade de Odontologia and Hospital de Reabilitação de Anomalias Craniofaciais HRAC, University of São Paulo, São Paulo, Brazil

I. T. T. da Silveira
Bauru School of Dentistry, Bauru, SP, Brazil

C. de Paula Oliveira Gringo · M. Peralta-Mamani
Hospital for Rehabilitation of Craniofacial Anomalies, University of São Paulo, Bauru, SP, Brazil

Objective of Orthognathic Surgery

Orthognathic surgery initially emerged with the exclusive purpose of achieving functional correction of occlusion, as described by Huliger in 1950 in Switzerland. At that time, the procedure was limited to single-segment surgeries focusing solely on occlusal alignment. Notably, Andrews's "Six Keys to Normal Occlusion" were documented only after the first orthognathic surgery had been performed [1, 20].

Over time, significant advancements in osteosynthesis materials, surgical instruments, general anesthesia, and surgical techniques have enabled orthognathic surgery to reach new heights. Today, modern orthognathic surgery is no longer limited to reestablishing occlusion—and is now guided by Andrews's occlusion keys—but also aims to restore functional occlusion. Additional key objectives include maintaining or expanding the patient's airway, achieving facial balance and harmony, and preserving or enhancing function while ensuring the absence of pain [5, 18].

Currently, the rising demand for aesthetics and the ongoing pursuit of facial balance and harmony have reshaped the indications for orthognathic surgery, which typically involves combined maxillary and mandibular procedures. The use of

J. G. Meara et al. (eds.), *Apert Syndrome*, https://doi.org/10.1007/978-3-032-12551-4_26

genioplasty for aesthetic purposes exemplifies this new approach of emphasizing both functional correction and improved facial aesthetics. Apert syndrome is characterized by a midface deficiency that significantly impacts the individual's growth and development and leads to functional issues in chewing, speech, and airway patency, as well as issues with facial balance and harmony [18]. Treatment during childhood includes frontofacial advancement or Le Fort III osteotomy via osteogenic distraction. In adulthood, orthognathic surgery is used to correct occlusion, increase facial volume, and expand the minimum cross-sectional area of the upper airway. This approach also aims to enhance facial balance and harmony [47, 21]. Addressing the complex aesthetic and functional demands of Apert syndrome cases and the broad scope of treatment objectives often necessitates bimaxillary surgeries [3].

Orthognathic Surgery Versus Osteogenic Distraction

The surgical approach for Apert syndrome should be planned in stages. The skeletal abnormalities in this patient group extend beyond the midface to affect the entire face. Thus,, osteogenic distraction is often more appropriate in the first stage of rehabilitation, as it addresses skeletal correction in both the midface and upper face (Fig. 26.1) [2, 19].

However, distraction through monobloc or Le Fort III advancement will only correct the skeletal positioning of the maxilla, potentially increasing the angle of the maxillary occlusal plane. Consequently, once skeletal maturation is reached, the patient will require a surgical procedure to correct occlusion [39, 40].

Orthognathic surgery is the preferred option in this context, given that it affords predictability and the capability for three-dimensional (3D) correction of the maxilla and mandible. The main challenges of this surgery involve extensive skeletal movement, particularly with rotation of the maxillary and mandibular occlusal planes. This type of movement is considered highly unstable and often presents intraoperative limitations for the passive mobilization of bone segments.

The literature recommends avoiding significant changes to the occlusal plane to ensure greater postoperative stability. Patients with Apert syndrome typically require adjustments to the maxillary and mandibular occlusal planes to close skeletal open bites, associating this surgery with high relapse rates [46].

A focus on bone segment mobilization is essential in preventing relapse, and required mobilization may exceed conventional movement. Moreover, this approach involves orthodontic preparation to ensure a stable final occlusion without premature contacts. Using high-quality—and preferably more rigid—fixation materials is crucial to prevent displacement or changes in positioning [41]. At this treatment stage, osteogenic distraction is challenging due to limited control over distractor movement in all

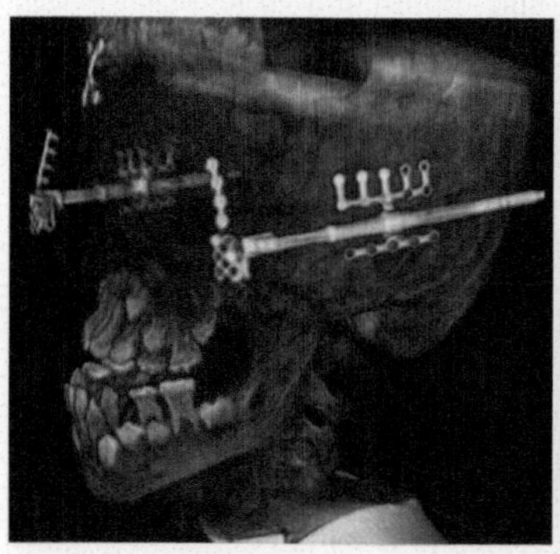
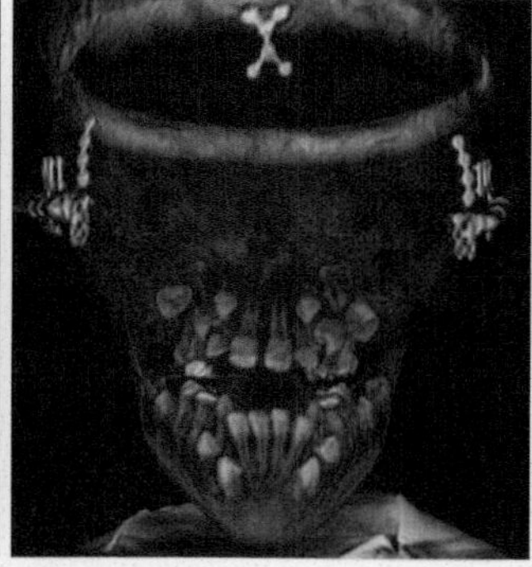
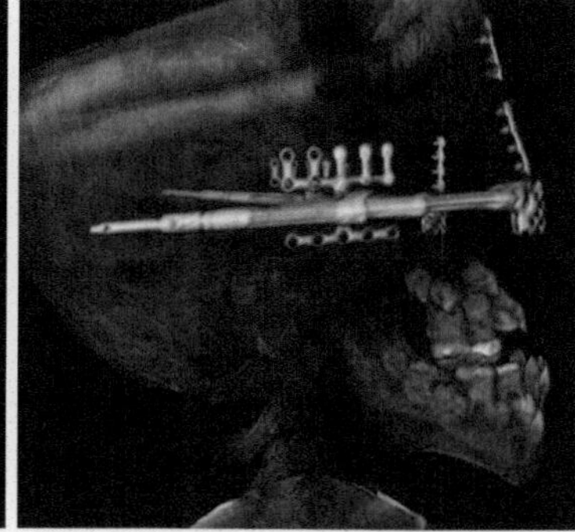

Fig. 26.1 Three-dimensional reconstruction from cone-beam computed tomography of a patient with osteogenic distraction. (Source: Image bank of the Oral Radiology and Craniofacial Surgery Department, HRAC/USP)

three spatial planes and the need to mobilize both the mandible and the maxilla.

Thus, osteogenic distraction and orthognathic surgery are complementary therapies in the rehabilitation process for Apert syndrome. A single procedure is insufficient for complete treatment in this patient group, requiring each technique to be strategically applied at specific stages to optimize surgical outcomes.

Orthodontic Preparation for Orthognathic Surgery

Phenotypes of Apert Syndrome

Apert syndrome is characterized by severe maxillary hypoplasia, leading to a concave facial profile, dental eruption anomalies, ectopic teeth, anterior open bite, dental crowding, cervical vertebrae fusion, clockwise mandibular rotation, and palatal development abnormalities [14, 16, 36].

The condition arises from a mutation in exon IIIa of the *FGFR2* gene, specifically *Ser252Trp* in 71% of cases and *Pro253*Arg in 26%. Although the literature has not identified statistically significant differences in the clinical phenotypes of these two mutations (*S252W* and *P253R*), notable differences in the maxilla are observed among these patients. These variations introduce distinct complexities in the orthodontic preparation for orthognathic surgery [34].

Mutations in the *FGFR2* gene have been linked to more severe palatal dysmorphisms, including more constricted and separated palatal plates and an increased tendency for palatal suture fusion. These mutations result in a distinctive adult phenotype. Wagner et al. report phenotypic differences in Apert syndrome between the *Ser252Trp* and *Pro253Arg* mutations. They conclude that compared to the *Pro253Arg* group, the *Ser252Trp* group exhibits more severe obstructive sleep apnea and shorter maxillary length (i.e., anterior nasal spine to posterior nasal spine), as well as a shorter distance from the basion to the anterior nasal spine [55].

Similarly, Lu et al. [33] proposed a classification of Apert syndrome subtypes based on the type of suture fusion. Later, the same research group described differences in cranial fossa depth in the anterior, middle, and posterior regions among three syndrome subtypes. These genetic and morphological variations may influence midface skeletal development and account for the range of maxillary transverse deficiencies, deep palate, and increased palatal mucosa volume seen in patients, resulting in variable degrees of skeletal anterior open bite. Notably, these traits appear even in patients who have not undergone frontofacial distraction, prompting questions about the origins of this phenotypic variability (Fig. 26.2).

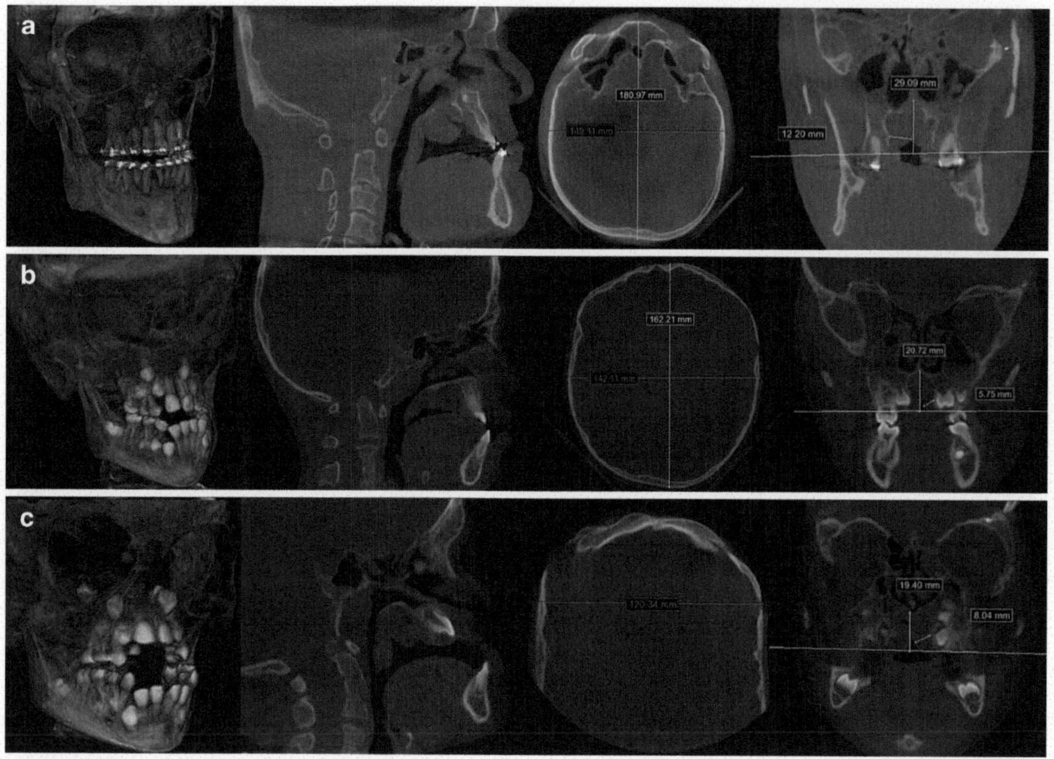

Fig. 26.2 Cone-beam computed tomography images of three patients with Apert syndrome reveal varying malocclusions and differences in palatal depth. (**a**) Patient presenting with a crossbite. (**b**) Patient presenting with an anterior open bite. (**c**) Patient presenting with a pronounced overjet combined with an anterior open bite. (Source: Image bank of the Oral Radiology and Craniofacial Surgery Department, HRAC/USP)

Dental Anomalies and Anterior Open Bite

Apert syndrome is often characterized by various dental anomalies, including tooth agenesis, which occurs in approximately 34.8–57.1% of patients, excluding third molars. The syndrome most commonly affects the lower second premolars and upper lateral incisors, displaying a symmetrical pattern that typically impacts two teeth, such as incisors 12 and 22 or premolars 35 and 45. Supernumerary teeth are less common, appearing in about 14.3% of cases [31, 48, 49].

In addition to agenesis, other common alterations include shovel-shaped incisors, severely delayed eruption, and ectopic eruption, particularly of the upper first molars. Enamel may also present with opacities (Fig. 26.3) [16, 32, 52].

These features pose challenges to orthodontic treatment, given that patients often present severe anterior crowding. In such cases, orthodontic preparation typically involves converting a premolar into a canine and performing dental extractions to reduce crowding and facilitate arch alignment and leveling [30, 22].

Treatment typically involves dental shortening, with instances of dental transposition, and aims for a stable occlusal finish. Due to the case complexity, caution with extractions is essential, as space loss may compromise treatment and result in significant arch shortening [30, 43].

Skeletal open bite is another prominent characteristic in Apert syndrome and can be quite pronounced. In such cases, the open bite may result from clockwise mandibular rotation due to growth patterns and/or the presence of a dual plane in the maxillary occlusal plane [28, 30].

Of note, and as supported by consensus in the literature, treating the maxilla in two planes is

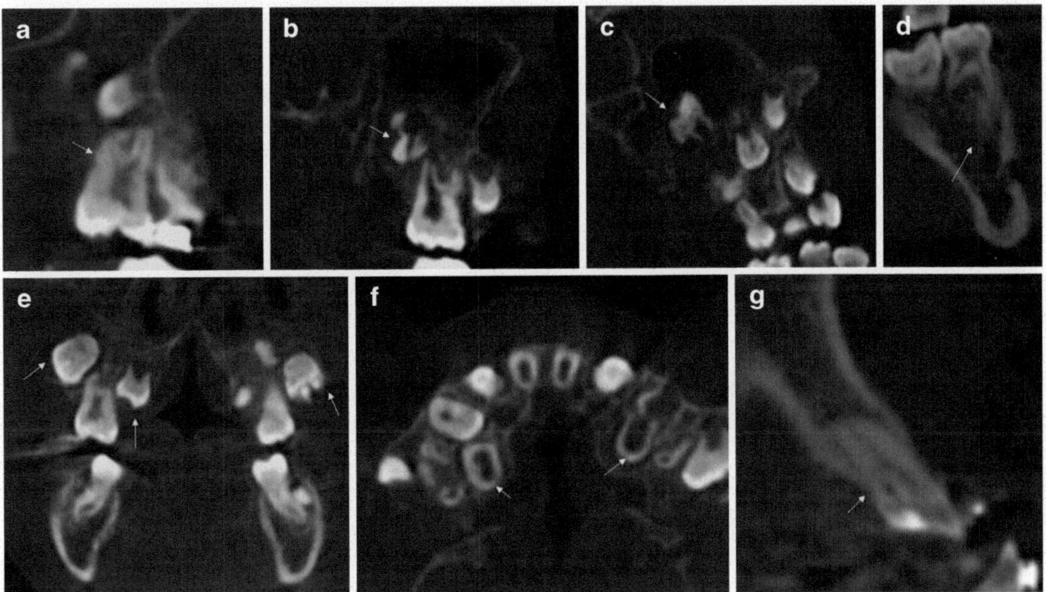

Fig. 26.3 Cone-beam computed tomography shows dental anomalies in Apert syndrome. (**a**) Taurodontism. (**b, c**) Ectopic eruption. (**d**) Agenesis of the right lower second premolar. (**e, f**) Bilateral ectopic eruption of premolars. (**g**) Dens in dente. (Source: Image bank of the Oral Radiology and Craniofacial Surgery Department, HRAC/USP)

necessary to prevent potential relapse. A one-plane maxilla does not allow for stable occlusion, as adjusting the occlusion in the posterior region leaves the anterior open bite unresolved; conversely, closing the anterior bite results in posterior opening. This condition should be carefully evaluated on study models before surgical planning [35, 24].

Orthodontic maxillary expansion during the mixed dentition phase can correct this feature before surgery by creating space to address dental crowding and reduce the need for excessive extractions. In cases where orthodontic maxillary expansion was not performed at the mixed dentition stage, techniques such as miniscrew-assisted rapid palatal expansion, surgically assisted rapid maxillary expansion, or multisegmented Le Fort I osteotomy may be used [17, 50, 35].

Ideally, the correction of maxillary transverse dimension should be performed during the mixed dentition phase, given that it creates space to resolve dental crowding and avoids serial extractions that shorten the dental arch. However, challenges in patient follow up and other issues can result in missing the optimal age window for this therapy. Such cases necessitate surgical alternatives and the potential for arch-length reduction [53].

Correction of skeletal anterior open bite should not solely rely on dental leveling when the maxilla presents in two planes. The stability of this approach is dependent on the appliance; after appliance removal or post-surgery, the maxillary anterior teeth tend to revert to their original position, reopening the anterior bite. In cases where anterior open-bite correction is achieved by dental leveling, cutting the wire between the lateral incisor and canine allows teeth to stabilize before surgery and is therefore advisable. If stability is achieved after 30–40 days, a single-segment Le Fort I osteotomy may be planned. In cases of persistent open bite, a multisegmented Le Fort I osteotomy should be considered to optimize postoperative stability.

The ideal treatment for skeletal anterior open bite should involve a segmented upper arch. However, this technique entails complex mechanical response and therefore demands greater expertise and control from the orthodontist. If the orthodontist is not confident in applying this approach, conventional orthodontic treatment can be chosen. The orthodontic wire should be cut at the end of the surgical preparation, allowing the open bite to relapse in the anterior teeth, which signals the need for maxillary segmentation to the surgeon [38].

Occlusal Plane

The occlusal plane is another critical factor directly related to orthognathic surgery planning. Clockwise mandibular rotation during growth is common in patients with Apert syndrome, worsening the anterior open bite and necessitating bimaxillary surgical planning. Similarly, individuals who have undergone frontofacial advancement may exhibit flattening of the maxillary occlusal plane, which exacerbates the anterior open bite and increases the need for significant clockwise rotation of the maxilla [13, 37, 56].

The literature consistently demonstrates that changes to the maxillary and mandibular occlusal planes are significant factors in reducing the stability of orthognathic surgery. In patients with Apert syndrome, maxillary occlusal plane flattening often intensifies anterior nasal spine retrusion, accentuating midface concavity. Meanwhile, the mandibular occlusal plane is notably steep, which contributes to a concave facial profile even in cases of normal mandibular growth. Therefore, precise alignment and leveling of the upper and lower arches are essential in enabling appropriate surgical movement and, ultimately, achieving stable occlusion and reducing the high recurrence rates in this patient group [57].

Challenges and Strategies for Intubation in Patients with Apert Syndrome During Orthognathic Surgeries

Apert syndrome causes reduced airway volume, a smaller cross-sectional area, a flattened occlusal plane, and altered relationships between the nostrils and the piriform fossa. Significant midface deformities make nasotracheal intubation challenging in patients with this syndrome [44].

Orotracheal intubation procedures generally do not present significant difficulties. Direct laryngoscopy typically achieves visibility of the epiglottis with relative ease, reassuring the anesthesiologist during orthognathic surgeries [42]. The greatest difficulty lies in passing the tube through the nose and reaching the oropharynx. In patients with Apert syndrome, alterations in the relationship of midface anatomical structures and narrow nostrils pose challenges to smooth tube passage [42, 51].

The use of equipment such as a videolaryngoscope, nasofibroscope, and guides like the Bougie are important auxiliary tools that should be available during intubation for orthognathic surgery. Apert syndrome causes anatomical variations in the midface that require adjustments to the tube path. This makes the intubation process more challenging and requires greater expertise from the anesthesiologist [8]. The anterior third of the nasal cavity often poses difficulties due to the bony relationship with the nostril. At this point, the tube must be directed upward to overcome the height difference between the nostril position and the piriform fossa until reaching the piriform fossa. After overcoming this anatomical variation, the tube should be angled posteriorly and downward until reaching the oropharynx (Fig. 26.4). After passing through the anterior third, the tube may encounter resistance at the curve from the nasopharynx to the oropharynx. At this point, a tube guide is extremely helpful for correctly directing the tube. Once the oropharynx is reached, further obstacles are unlikely, and intubation typically proceeds in a conventional manner.

The type of nasotracheal tube used in intubating patients with Apert syndrome for orthognathic surgery is important. Orthognathic surgery includes maxillary osteotomy reaching into the nasal cavity, and therefore pre-curved north-pole tubes, tubes with cuffs passing inside the tube, and silicone materials help prevent intraoperative issues like cuff rupture and the associated need for mid-surgery tube replacement [45].

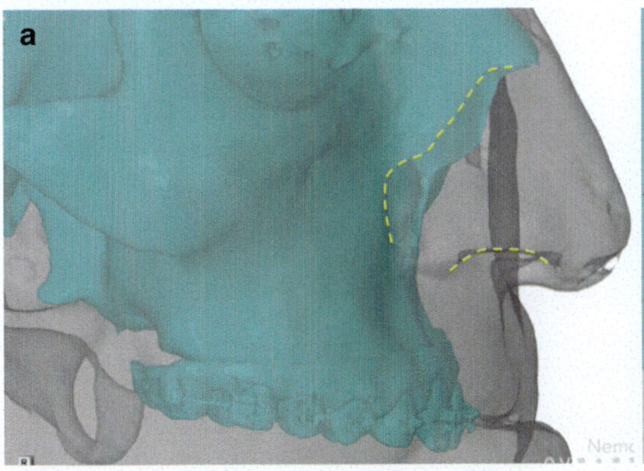

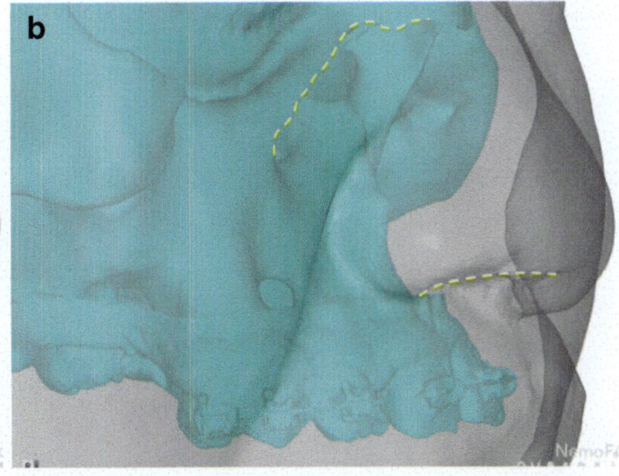

Fig. 26.4 Comparison of the vertical height between the nostril and the piriform fossa. (**a**) Height between the position of the nostril and the piriform fossa in a patient without Apert syndrome. (**b**) Height between the position of the nostril and the piriform fossa in a patient with Apert syndrome. (Source: Image bank of the Oral Maxillofacial Surgery Department, HRAC/USP)

Surgical Technique

The Le Fort I osteotomy is a surgical technique aimed at repositioning the maxilla and is widely indicated for correcting skeletal discrepancies such as open bite, prognathism, retrognathism, asymmetries, and vertical or transverse imbalances. This procedure is performed via an intraoral incision in the upper vestibular region, thereby avoiding external scars and allowing broad maxillary exposure. Following periosteal elevation and protection of the infraorbital nerve, a horizontal osteotomy is made 5–10 mm above the dental apices using specialized saws or piezoelectric devices; this enables 3D maxillary repositioning. For maxillae with two occlusal planes, segmentation is recommended to independently adjust bone segments, minimizing the "see-saw" effect associated with this structure. This adjustment corrects occlusal plane inclinations, facilitates anterior open-bite closure, and maintains posterior occlusion. The maxilla is then stabilized with titanium miniplates and screws, securing stability throughout healing. Complications can include bleeding, infection, and infraorbital nerve injury, making postoperative monitoring essential for safe recovery [9, 27].

Bilateral sagittal split osteotomy is recommended for the mandible. The "short split" technique, which involves a shorter bone splint, is used to optimize the procedure and reduce the likelihood of bony interference and torque on the proximal segment. This approach provides greater control and predictability in mandibular movement and decreases the risk of deviation in the proximal segment during repositioning [4].

Computed tomography evaluations during surgical planning can reveal anatomical variations that are characteristic of Apert syndrome, such as a maxillary characteristic in which the hard palate is significantly elevated and the alveolar ridge is high with a deep palate (Fig. 26.5). This requires a higher cut during Le Fort I osteotomy, shortening the midface and bringing the infraorbital foramen and orbital rims closer to the osteotomy area. Additionally, the absence of maxillary sinus pneumatization—with reduced sinus size and thicker or normal bony walls—often complicates the down-fracture phase of surgery in patients with Apert syndrome.

Due to the highlighted anatomical changes, osteotomies in patients with Apert syndrome are generally performed at a *steeper angle* and performed at a higher level than conventional osteotomies. The thicker maxillary sinus walls make the down-fracture phase more challenging, compounded by a longer and thicker pterygomaxillary suture. Manual maneuvers alone rarely achieve a complete down-fracture, thus chisels and a Smith spreader are often required to fully separate the maxilla.

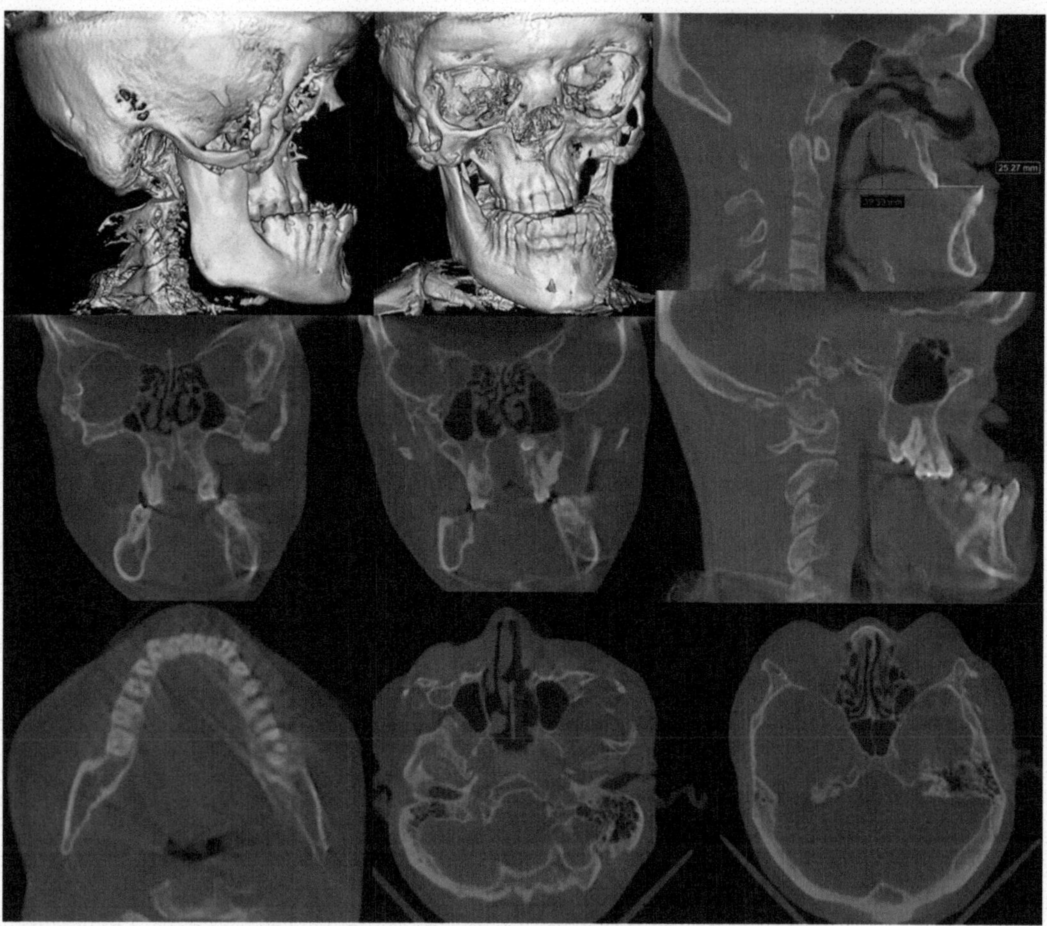

Fig. 26.5 Cone-beam computed tomography shows maxillomandibular discrepancy and a deep palate in a male patient with Apert syndrome. (Source: Image bank of the Oral Radiology and Craniofacial Surgery Department, HRAC/USP)

Of note, the nasal fossa space is often quite narrow. Moreover, the presence of the nasotracheal tube, inferior turbinate, and nasal–bone constriction complicate the positioning of the nasal guard for osteotomy and visualization of the lateral nasal wall osteotomy. Therefore, ensuring that the lateral nasal wall osteotomy is fully complete is essential, and this requires visual check or check with a chisel in cases where visualization is not possible.

Another important aspect of the surgical technique occurs during maxillary mobilization. Well-known and well-documented in the literature, passive bone repositioning is essential for skeletal stability. The maxilla must be fully released to allow passive movement, and mobilizing the maxilla presents additional challenges to those of the down-fracture. Notably, surgical planning for these patients generally requires significant clockwise rotation of the maxillary occlusal plane. Mobilization must enable this passive movement by removing bony interferences in the posterior maxilla.

Effective mobilization sometimes necessitates ligating the descending palatine artery on one or both sides to facilitate passive skeletal movement and positioning. Importantly, induced hypotension during general anesthesia is essential in safely and effectively performing these maneuvers, ensuring a surgical time that is compatible with maintaining safe hypotension for the patient.

The mandible in patients with Apert syndrome does not significantly differ from that of the general population. However, surgical planning typically involves substantial counterclockwise rotation of the mandibular occlusal plane. This rotation often necessitates first addressing the mandible, given occlusal interference from the surgical movement and the need for mouth opening and temporomandibular joint rotation. Such movement may result in a bimaxillary projection of the maxillary and mandibular segments. Upon mandibular repositioning after fixation, bimaxillary projection can cause immediate postoperative skeletal open bite.

Correct positioning of the condyle during osteosynthesis is of utmost importance. All records are made with the condyle in centric relation. Using an occlusal registration ensures that the mandible remains in the same position across records and allows for reproducibility under anesthesia while the patient is unconscious. To reposition the joint, we use the Peter Dawson maneuver to place one condyle in centric relation for fixation, then repeat on the opposite side for osteosynthesis. This technique enhances joint positioning security during surgery, and it allows verification of the condyle's correct placement post-osteosynthesis by observing its range of motion within the fossa.

This stage of surgery requires special attention. Normally, the joint fossa allows slight anterior–posterior condylar movement, which can lead to slight posterior displacement of the condyle by a few millimeters during proximal segment or maxilla repositioning. When this occurs after mandibular fixation, it can shift the entire plan slightly posteriorly and cause significant bony interference, especially in the posterior region. If this interference is not removed, application of excessive pressure during repositioning poses a high risk of relapse or unintended change in maxillary position during the immediate postoperative period (Figs. 26.6 and 26.7). Therefore, careful attention to condylar positioning during surgery is essential for [1] the fixation of the proximal and distal mandibular segments and [2] adjusting the maxilla, as slight condylar movements in the fossa can create interferences. The anatomical dimensions and relationships of the joint cavity and condyle vary from patient to patient and influence interferences.

Stability and Relapse of Surgical Movements

Orthognathic surgery is a predictable procedure with low complication rates. However, postoperative relapse is among the most common complications, especially in individuals with cleft lip and palate, Class II malocclusions, and craniofacial abnormalities. Causes of relapse include movements exceeding 7 mm, presence of cleft lip and palate, previous surgeries, scarring, limited maxillary mobilization, fibrosis, muscle forces, and non-compliance with postoperative guidelines. In patients with Apert syndrome, anatomical and biological peculiarities increase relapse risk, as they often require extensive surgical movements, such as occlusal plane rotation [29, 26].

The presence of scars from previous interventions, especially in the midface region, and increased bone thickness complicate mobilization and compromise bone stability. Additionally, craniofacial anomalies such as midface hypoplasia require substantial corrections, increasing postoperative instability. Abnormal bone characteristics such as high density and thickness hinder mobilization, and, when combined with reduced vascularization, limit bone remodeling. Respiratory disorders, like obstructive sleep apnea, lead to oral breathing patterns that heighten pressure on facial and mandibular muscles, further compromising stability. In the absence of rigorous, prolonged postoperative control, residual facial growth or late bone changes can also contribute to relapse. These factors underscore the need for detailed planning and strict postoperative adherence to ensure long-term stability [11, 30].

Before orthodontic treatment, adequate orthodontic preparation and a thorough assessment of the maxillary occlusal plane are essential in minimizing the possibility of relapse. Dental leveling performed with orthodontic appliances can result in open-bite relapse, as teeth often return to their

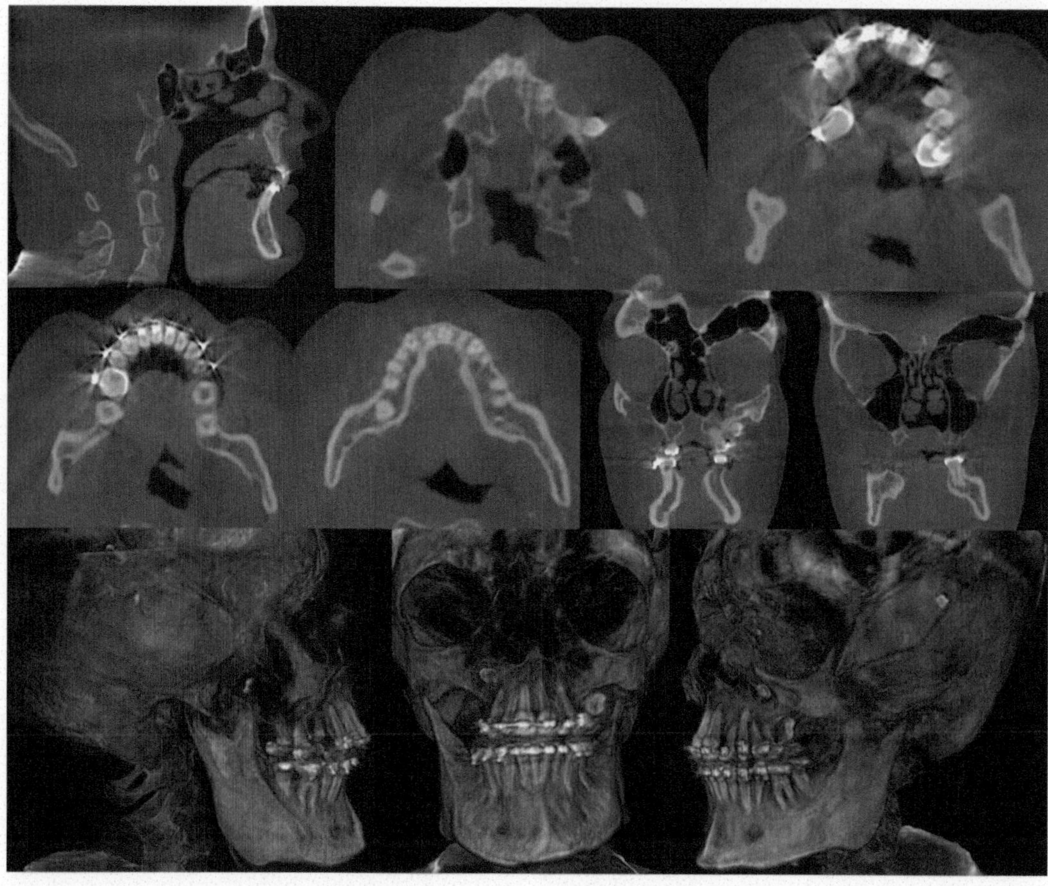

Fig. 26.6 Cone-beam computed tomography of the preoperative stage of orthognathic surgery in a patient with Apert syndrome. (Source: Image bank of the Oral Radiology and Oral and Maxillofacial Surgery Department, HRAC/USP)

initial position upon appliance removal. Coordination between orthodontics and surgery is crucial in planning the correction of skeletal open bite before Le Fort I osteotomy. If not done in time, maxillary segmentation should be considered for repositioning anterior teeth. However, segmentation should not be used indiscriminately, as it carries risks such as maxillary necrosis due to extensive mobilization. Moreover, segmentation complicates postoperative orthodontic finishing [23] (Kahnberg et al. 2010).

In orthodontic preparation, alignment and leveling should provide occlusal stability, either through a single or a segmented arch. Ideally, occlusion should be well-adjusted in a single position, with overjet, overbite, and incisor inclinations pre-determined during preoperative orthodontic planning. This careful preparation minimizes dental adjustments during surgery, enhancing occlusal stability and maintaining the orthodontist's planned position. This approach expedites surgery, prevents occlusal shifts during maxillomandibular fixation, and improves stability without premature contacts, thereby reducing relapse risk by distributing muscular forces evenly across a stable occlusion [7].

Rotation of the maxillary and mandibular occlusal planes is common in procedures for patients with Apert syndrome and is typically greater than that planned for non-syndromic patients. Studies find occlusal plane rotations to be unstable, thus passive mobilization and positioning of bone segments are essential, and effective osteosynthesis techniques are needed to maintain alignment [15]. In our practice, we secure the maxilla with 2.0 mm L-plates and

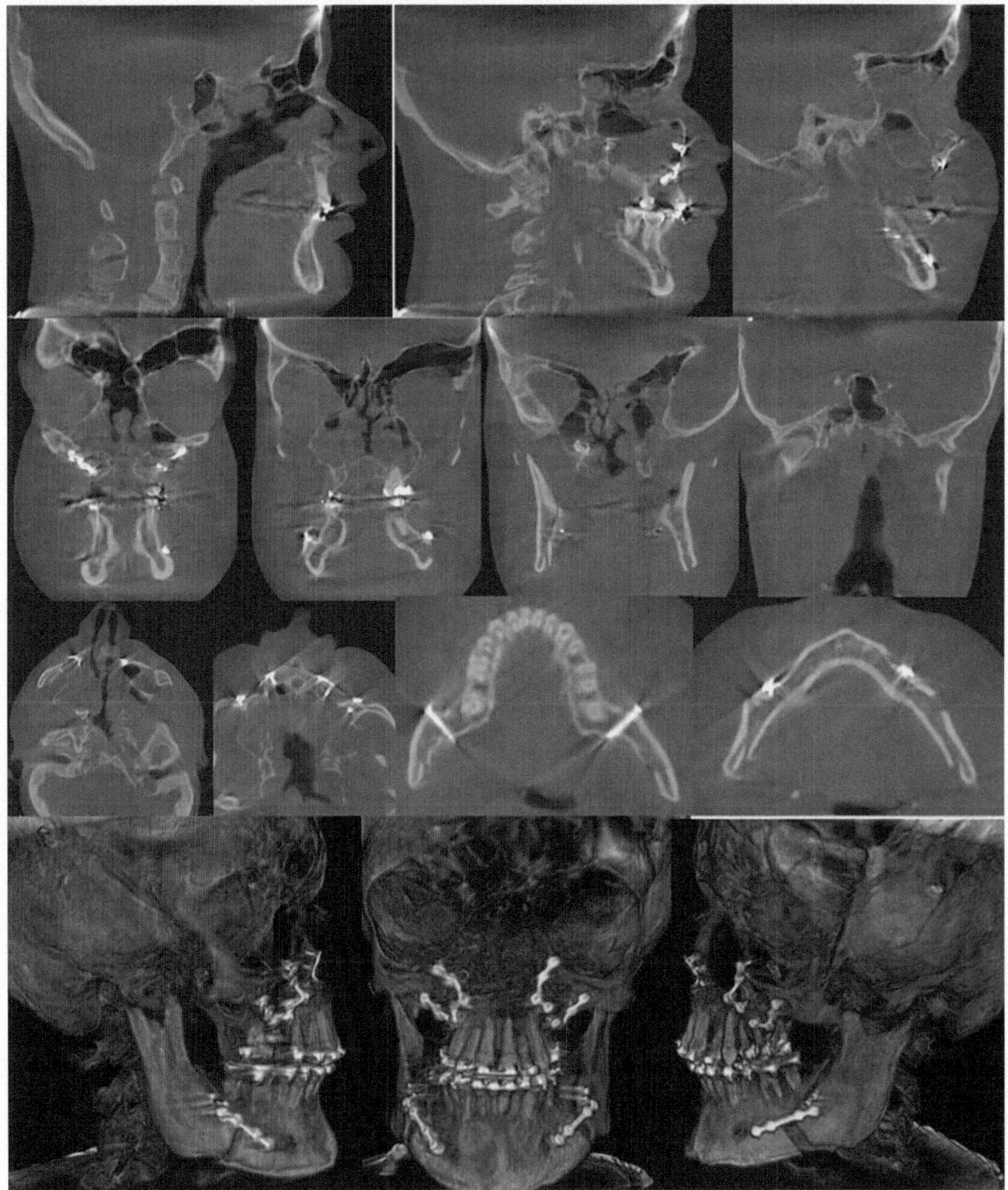

Fig. 26.7 Cone-beam computed tomography of the immediate postoperative stage of orthognathic surgery in a patient with Apert syndrome. (Source: Image bank of the Oral Radiology and Oral and Maxillofacial Surgery Department, HRAC/USP)

secure the mandible with a hybrid fixation comprising a 2.0 mm straight plate with a bridge and two positional bicortical screws to enhance stability.

In the context of mandibular occlusal plane rotation, careful attention to condylar positioning during surgery is critical. If the condyle is not properly seated in the fossa in centric relation, joint displacement within the articular fossa can occur, altering the mandible's final 3D position after fixation. Therefore, it is crucial that photographic and tomographic records be taken in centric relation, using an additional silicone occlusal registration to ensure consistent alignment [54].

Although patients present with a Class III malocclusion in molar and canine relationships, orthognathic surgery behaves like a Class II malocclusion due to mandibular occlusal plane rotation. This effect is caused by mandibular advancement at the vertical osteotomy site between the first and second molars, even without anterior mandibular displacement. This detail is crucial, particularly for repositioning the proximal segment, ensuring that the condyle is placed in centric relation within the articular fossa [10].

The mandibular condyle's position must remain consistent during both planning and surgery to ensure predictability in surgical planning. Small changes in its positioning can affect the final outcome of the mandible and, consequently, the maxilla.

Performing orthognathic surgery on a patient with Apert syndrome presents many challenges. Despite the complexities and specific requirements involved, this procedure yields undeniable patient benefits. Optimal surgical preparation entails orthodontics that precisely position and guide each tooth. The surgery itself poses challenges related to range of motion and anatomical variations. Individualized treatment is key and should employ the best surgical techniques and technological resources to enhance predictability and stability [12].

Case Report

This clinical case summarizes the surgical planning and immediate postoperative outcome of orthognathic surgery, focusing on the key anatomical considerations relevant to the procedure. The patient presents a reduced arch, slight open bite, flattened maxillary occlusal plane, and a steep mandibular occlusal plane. Notable anatomical variations include the midface structure and the relationship between the nasal fossa, orbit, infraorbital foramen, and the Le Fort I osteotomy area (Figs. 26.6, 26.7 and 26.8).

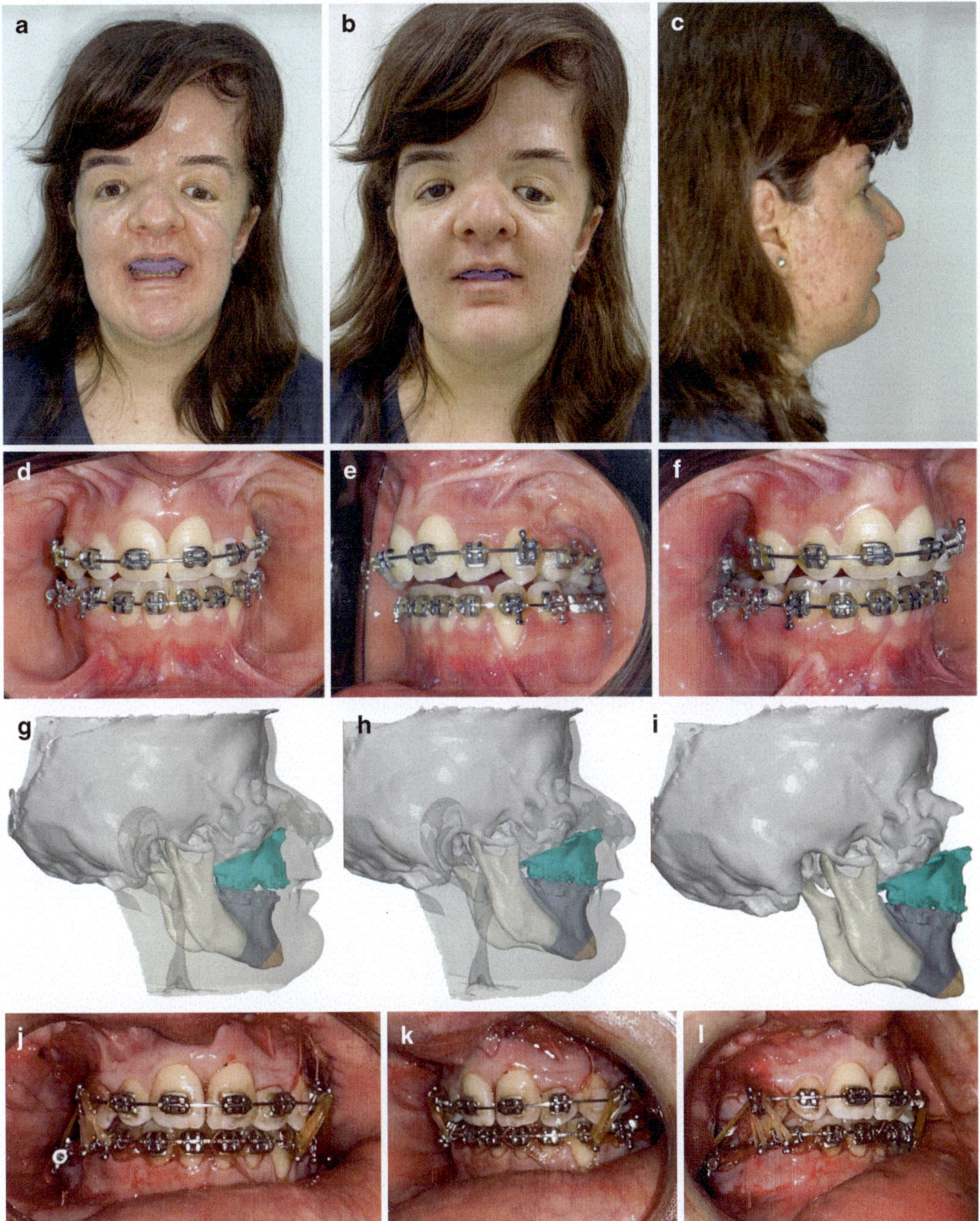

Fig. 26.8 Preoperative facial photographs and 1-year postoperative photographs. (Source: Image bank of the Maxillofacial Surgery Department, HRAC/USP)

m

Models Measurements

Maxilla		A-P		Vert		Side
ANS	→	8,7	↓	0,4	→	0,4
PNS	→	6,3	↑	7,2	→	1,1
Mx1R tip	→	3,8	↑	0,3	→	1,1
Mx1L tip	→	3,7	↓	0,1	→	1,1
R Canine	→	3,7	↑	0,7	→	1,1
L Canine	→	3,9	↑	1,9	→	1,2
Right Molar6 MB cusp tip	→	3,8	↑	2,9	→	1,2
Left Molar6 MB cusp tip	→	4,4	↑	4,9	→	1,2

Mandible		A-P		Vert		Side
Md1R tip	→	7,5	↑	4,2	→	0,1
Md1L tip	→	7,5	↑	4,0	→	0,1
B Point	→	7,2	↑	4,1	→	1,0
Pogonion	→	7,1	↑	4,1	→	1,3

Chin Osteotomy		A-P		Vert		Side
R Chin	→	7,0	↑	3,7	→	1,6
L Chin	→	7,1	↑	4,6	→	1,5
L Canine	→	7,5	↑	4,5	→	0,0
R Canine	→	7,5	↑	3,7	→	0,0
Left Molar6 MB cusp tip	→	7,4	↑	3,5	→	0,1
Right Molar6 MB cusp tip	→	7,5	↑	4,7	→	0,0

Pl. Oclu. Mx	Srg	Ini	Dif	Pl. Oclu. Md	Srg	Ini	Dif
MxOP R	83,3	91,1	-7,8	MdOP R	84,0	88,1	-4,2
MxOP L	77,9	87,0	-9,0	MdOP L	86,3	86,8	-0,5
MxOccPl	80,6	89,0	-8,4	MdOccPl	85,1	87,5	-2,4

Clipboard | Disk | Save as Image | OK

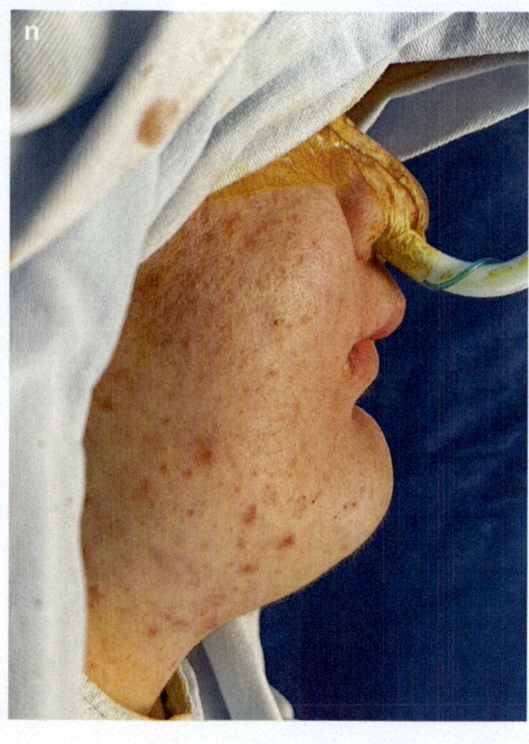

Fig. 26.8 (continued)

References

1. Andrews LF. The six keys to normal occlusion. Am J Orthod. 1972;62(3):296–309. https://doi.org/10.1016/s0002-9416(72)90268-0.
2. Al-Namnam NMN, Hariri F, Rahman ZAA. Distraction osteogenesis in the surgical management of syndromic craniosynostosis: a comprehensive review of published papers. Br J Oral Maxillofac Surg. 2018;56(5):353–66. https://doi.org/10.1016/j.bjoms.2018.03.002. Epub 2018 Apr 13
3. Allam KA, Wan DC, Khwanngern K, Kawamoto HK, Tanna N, Perry A, Bradley JP. Treatment of apert syndrome: a long-term follow-up study. Plast Reconstr Surg. 2011;127(4):1601–11. https://doi.org/10.1097/PRS.0b013e31820a64b6.
4. Arnett GW. Facial reconstruction and orthognathic surgery. Am J Orthod Dentofacial Orthop. 1999;115(6):680–90.
5. Arnett GW, Gunson MJ. Esthetic treatment planning for orthognathic surgery. J Clin Orthod. 2010;44(3):196–200.
6. Azoulay-Avinoam S, Bruun R, MacLaine J, Allareddy V, Resnick CM, Padwa BL. An overview of Craniosynostosis craniofacial syndromes for combined orthodontic and surgical management. Oral Maxillofac Surg Clin North Am. 2020;32(2):233–47. https://doi.org/10.1016/j.coms.2020.01.004.
7. Bailey LJ, Proffit WR, White RP Jr. Stability and predictability in orthognathic surgery: importance of orthodontic preparation for occlusal stability. Eur J Orthod. 2020;43(1):104–10. https://doi.org/10.1093/ejo/cjz062.
8. Barnett JS, Barnett JS, Barnett JS, Barnett JS, Barnett JS, Barnett JS. Soft tissue changes after mandibular setback and bimaxillary surgery in Class III patients. J Oral Maxillofac Surg. 2011;69(1):100–6.
9. Bell WH. Le Forte I osteotomy for correction of maxillary deformities. J Oral Surg. 1975;33(6):412–26.
10. Bergamo AZN, Andrucioli de Mattos JP, Pavan AJ. Changes in occlusal plane through orthognathic surgery: clockwise and counterclockwise rotations. Dent Press J Orthod. 2012;17(4):160–73. https://doi.org/10.1590/S2176-94512012000400022.

11. Breik O, Mahindu A, Moore MH, Molloy CJ, Santoreneos S, David DJ. Apert syndrome: surgical outcomes and perspectives. J Craniomaxillofac Surg. 2016;44(9):1238–45. https://doi.org/10.1016/j.jcms.2016.06.001.
12. Brock RA, Taylor SM, Lykins A. Role of muscle forces and bone remodeling in orthognathic surgery relapse: implications for craniofacial stability. Am J Orthod Dentofacial Orthop. 2021;160(4):516–23. https://doi.org/10.1016/j.ajodo.2021.02.026.
13. Choi JW, Jeong WS. Occlusal plane altering 2 jaw surgery based on the Clockwised rotational surgery-first Orthognathic approach. Plast Reconstr Surg Glob Open. 2017;5(10):e1492. https://doi.org/10.1097/GOX.0000000000001492. PMID: 29184726; PMCID: PMC5682162.
14. Cohen MM Jr, Kreiborg S. A clinical study of the craniofacial features in Apert syndrome. Int J Oral Maxillofac Surg. 1996;25(1):45–53. https://doi.org/10.1016/s0901-5027(96)80011-7.
15. da Silva WS, de Almeida ALPF, Pucciarelli MGR, Neppelenbroek KH, da Silva de Menezes JD, Yaedú RYF, Oliveira TM, Cintra FMRN, Soares S. Relapse after Le Fort I surgery in oral cleft patients: a 2-year follow-up using digitized and 3D models. Odontology. 2018;106(4):445–53. https://doi.org/10.1007/s10266-018-0351-8.
16. Dalben GS, Das NL, Gomide MR. Oral findings in patients with Apert syndrome. J Appl Oral Sci. 2006;14:465–9. https://doi.org/10.1590/S1678-77572006000600014.
17. Farronato G, Maspero C, Esposito L, Briguglio E, Farronato D, Giannini L. Rapid maxillary expansion in growing patients. Hyrax versus transverse sagittal maxillary expander: a cephalometric investigation. Eur J Orthod. 2011;33(2):185–9. https://doi.org/10.1093/ejo/cjq051.
18. Ferri J, Schlund M, Touzet-Roumazeille S. Orthognathic surgery in craniosynostosis. J Craniofac Surg. 2021;32(1):141–8. https://doi.org/10.1097/SCS.0000000000007154.
19. Fowler P, Hallang S, Snape L. Apert syndrome: an informative long-term dentofacial outcome. BMJ Case Rep. 2022;15(3):e245224. https://doi.org/10.1136/bcr-2021-245224. PMID: 35236672; PMCID: PMC8895904.
20. Gillies H, Harrison SH. Operative correction by osteotomy of recessed malar maxillary compound in a case of oxycephaly. Br J Plast Surg. 1950;3(2):123–7. https://doi.org/10.1016/s0007-1226(50)80019-x.
21. Guimarães Filho R, Oliveira Junior EC, Gomes TRM, de Souza TDA. Qualidade de vida em pacientes submetidos à cirurgia ortognática: saúde bucal e autoestima. Psicologia: Ciência E Profissão. 2014;34(1):242–51. https://doi.org/10.1590/S1414-98932014000100017.
22. Gugny M, Goudot P, Goudot P. Orthodontist's Role in Orthognathic Surgery. In: Goudot P, Goudot P, editors. Orthognathic Surgery: Principles and Practice. Springer. 2019;1–16.
23. Han JT, Egbert MA, Ettinger RE, Kapadia HP, Susarla SM. Orthognathic surgery in patients with syndromic Craniosynostosis. Oral Maxillofac Surg Clin North Am. 2022;34(3):477–87. https://doi.org/10.1016/j.coms.2022.01.003.
24. Hohoff A, Joos U, Meyer U, Meyer U. The spectrum of Apert syndrome: phenotype, particularities in orthodontic treatment, and characteristics of orthognathic surgery. Head Face Med. 2007;3(1):10.
25. Horiuchi S, Sato H, Iwasa A, Ichihara A, Tenshin H, Watanabe K, Hiasa M, Hashimoto I, Tanaka E. Long-term management of a patient with apert syndrome. J Contemp Dent Pract. 2021;22(10):1184–90.
26. Inchingolo F, Inchingolo F, Inchingolo F, Inchingolo F, Inchingolo F, Inchingolo F. Long-Term Follow-Up of Orthognathic Surgery in Patients with Cleft Lip and Palate. J Oral Maxillofac Res. 2023;14(4):e4.
27. Ismail IN, Leung YY. Anterior open bite correction by Le Fort I osteotomy with or without anterior segmentation: which is more stable? Int J Oral Maxillofac Surg. 2017;46(6):766–73. https://doi.org/10.1016/j.ijom.2017.02.1275.
28. Kahnberg KE, Hagberg C. Orthognathic surgery in patients with craniofacial syndrome. I. A 5-year overview of combined orthodontic and surgical correction. J Plast Surg Hand Surg. 2010;44(6):282–8. https://doi.org/10.3109/2000656X.2010.516594.
29. Kahnberg KE, Kahnberg KE, Kahnberg KE, Kahnberg KE, Kahnberg KE, Kahnberg KE. Stability of the anterior maxillary segment and teeth after segmental Le Fort I osteotomy. J Oral Maxillofac Surg. 2010;68(1):100–6.
30. Kaya D, Taner T, Aksu M, Keser EI, Tuncbilek G, Mavili ME. Orthodontic and surgical treatment of a patient with Apert syndrome. J Contemp Dent Pract. 2012;13(5):729–34. https://doi.org/10.5005/jp-journals-10024-1218.
31. Kobayashi Y, Ogura K, Hikita R, Tsuji M, Moriyama K. Craniofacial, oral, and cervical morphological characteristics in Japanese patients with Apert syndrome or Crouzon syndrome. Eur J Orthod. 2021;43(1):36–44. https://doi.org/10.1093/ejo/cjaa015.
32. Kreiborg S, Cohen MM Jr. The oral manifestations of Apert syndrome. J Craniofac Genet Dev Biol. 1992;12(1):41–8. PMID: 1572940
33. Lu X, Sawh-Martinez R, Jorge Forte A, Wu R, Cabrejo R, Wilson A, Steinbacher DM, Alperovich M, Alonso N, Persing JA. Classification of subtypes of Apert syndrome, based on the type of vault suture synostosis. Plast Reconstr Surg Glob Open. 2019;7(3):e2158. https://doi.org/10.1097/GOX.0000000000002158. PMID: 31044122; PMCID: PMC6467634.
34. Lunn JS, Fishwick KJ, Halley PA, Storey KG. A spatial and temporal map of FGF/Erk1/2 activity and response repertoires in the early chick embryo. Dev Biol. 2007;302:536–52. https://doi.org/10.1016/j.ydbio.2006.10.01.
35. Malara P, Malara P, Malara P, Malara P, Malara P, Malara P. Outcomes and Stability of Anterior Open

Bite Treatment with Skeletal Anchorage in Non-Growing Patients and Adults Compared to the Results of Orthognathic Surgery Procedures: A Systematic Review. J Clin Med. 2021;10(23):5682.
36. Marsh JL, Galic M, Vannier MW. The craniofacial anatomy of Apert syndrome. Clin Plast Surg. 1991;18(2):237–49.
37. Marchiori EC, Garcia RR, Moreira RW. Importance of occlusal plane reproduction on the semi-adjustable articulator in planning maxillary impactions for orthognathic surgery. Oral Maxillofac Surg. 2013;17(2):109–14. https://doi.org/10.1007/s10006-012-0353-6. Epub 2012 Aug 7. PMID: 23011674.
38. Matsumoto K, Matsumoto K, Matsumoto K, Matsumoto K, Matsumoto K, Matsumoto K. Changes in stomatognathic function induced by orthognathic surgery in patients with mandibular prognathism. J Oral Maxillofac Surg. 2012;70(1):125–31.
39. McCarthy JG, Stelnicki EJ, Mehrara BJ, Longaker MT. Distraction osteogenesis of the craniofacial skeleton. Plast Reconstr Surg. 2001;107(7):1812–27. https://doi.org/10.1097/00006534-200106000-00029. PMID: 11391207
40. Meling TR, Hans-Erik H, Per S, Due-Tonnessen BJ. Le Fort III distraction osteogenesis in syndromal craniosynostosis. J Craniofac Surg. 2006;17(1):28–39. https://doi.org/10.1097/01.scs.0000194177.21916.f1.
41. Moen K, Wisth PJ, Skaale S, Bøe OE, Tornes K. Dental or skeletal relapse after sagittal split osteotomy advancement surgery? Long-term follow-up. J Oral Maxillofac Surg. 2011;69(11):e461–8. https://doi.org/10.1016/j.joms.2011.02.086.
42. Nargozian C. Anesthesia for orthognathic surgery. Anesthesiol Clin North Am. 1991;9(3):575–91.
43. Ogura A, Wajima Z, Yoshikawa T, Ogura A, Shiga T, Shiga T. Is Preemptive Oral Tizanidine Effective on Postoperative Pain After Bimaxillary Orthognathic Surgery? A Randomized Clinical Trial. World J Plast Surg. 2022;11(3):3–10.
44. Pacheco A, Pacheco A, Pacheco A, Pacheco A, Pacheco A, Pacheco A. Iatrogenic Displacement of Lower Third Molar Roots Into the Sublingual Space. J Oral Maxillofac Surg. 2012;70(1):110–6.
45. Patel PK, Patel PK, Patel PK, Patel PK, Patel PK, Patel PK. Soft tissue cephalometric norms for orthognathic and esthetic surgery. J Oral Maxillofac Surg. 2013;71(1):100–6.
46. Proffit WR, Turvey TA, Phillips C. The hierarchy of stability and predictability in orthognathic surgery with rigid fixation: an update and extension. Head Face Med. 2007;3:21. https://doi.org/10.1186/1746-160X-3-21.
47. Ram A, Bharani A. Apert Syndrome. J Assoc Physicians India. 2020;68(9):70. PMID: 32798349
48. Reitsma JH, Ongkosuwito EM, van Wijk AJ, Prahl-Andersen B. Patterns of tooth agenesis in patients with crouzon or apert syndrome. Cleft Palate Craniofac J. 2014;51(2):178–83. https://doi.org/10.1597/12-180.
49. Stavropoulos D, Bartzela T, Bronkhorst E, Mohlin B, Hagberg C. Dental agenesis patterns of permanent teeth in Apert syndrome. Eur J Oral Sci. 2011;119(3):198–203. https://doi.org/10.1111/j.1600-0722.2011.00821.x.
50. Teixeira RAN, Ferrari Junior FM, Garib D. Influence of rapid maxillary expansion in the stability of anterior open bite treatment. Clin Oral Investig. 2022;26(10):6371–8. https://doi.org/10.1007/s00784-022-04592-w. Epub 2022 Aug 1. PMID: 35915261.
51. Tsukamoto Y, Yokoyama M. Long-term stability of mandibular setback surgery in patients with skeletal Class III malocclusion. J Oral Maxillofac Surg. 2015;73(1):135–42.
52. Vadiati Saberi B, Shakoorpour A. Apert syndrome: report of a case with emphasis on oral manifestations. J Dent (Tehran). 2011;8(2):90–5.
53. Verdonck A, Verdonck A, Verdonck A, Verdonck A, Verdonck A, Verdonck A. Surgical and prosthetic reconsiderations in patients with obturator prosthesis. Int J Oral Maxillofac Surg. 2010;39(1):1–7.
54. Vollmer A, Renner T, Müller-Richter U, Hartmann S, Brands R. Comparison of patient-specific condylar positioning devices and manual methods in orthognathic surgery: a prospective randomized trial. J Clin Med. 2024;13(3):737. https://doi.org/10.3390/jcm13030737.
55. Wagner JK, Cooper MK, Tolarova MM. Phenotypic variation in FGFR2-related craniosynostosis syndromes: analysis of the Ser252Trp and Pro253Arg mutations in Apert syndrome. Clin Genet. 2013;84(4):346–52. https://doi.org/10.1111/cge.12185.
56. Wolford LM, Chemello PD, Hilliard FW. Occlusal plane alteration in orthognathic surgery. J Oral Maxillofac Surg. 1993;51(7):730–40; discussion 740-1. https://doi.org/10.1016/s0278-2391(10)80410-0. PMID: 8509911.
57. Wolford LM. Comprehensive Post Orthognathic Surgery Orthodontics: Complications, Misconceptions, and Management. Oral Maxillofac Surg Clin North Am. 2020;32(1):135–51.

27 Virtual Surgical Planning for Orthognathic Surgery

Renato Yassutaka Faria Yaedú,
Isabela Toledo Teixeira da Silveira, Caroline de Paula Oliveira Gringo, Mariela Peralta-Mamani, and Roman H. Khonsari

Introduction

Virtual surgical planning (VSP) involves the intraoperative implementation of surgical decisions based on preoperative data primarily derived from three-dimensional (3D) imaging. In most cases, the decision-making process requires predicting an ideal surgical outcome. In Apert syndrome, the most common craniofacial procedures performed before orthognathic surgery include posterior vault expansion (PVE), fronto-orbital advancement (FOA), frontofacial monobloc advancement (FFMBA), and Le Fort III (LFIII) osteotomy with or without facial bipartition [5]. Conducted for both functional and morphological purposes in young children with growth potential, these procedures necessitate consideration of the altered growth dynamics caused by activating *FGFR* mutations [43]. Additionally, these procedures affect both craniofacial bones and soft tissues, making outcome prediction particularly challenging. This chapter will examine the specific challenges associated with using VSP in younger patients with Apert syndrome, current applications, and recent innovations and future perspectives in this field.

Specific Challenges in Outcome Prediction for Virtual Surgical Planning (VSP) in Apert Syndrome

A clear definition of surgical outcomes guides both VSP design of osteotomies and production of cutting and positioning guides. In orthognathic surgery performed after growth completion, occlusion is a reliable end-point for determining bone displacements. However, PVE, FFMBA, FOA, and LFIII present unique challenges in defining surgical outcomes.

Determining the final positions of the skull vault or facial bones at a specific age in a patient with Apert syndrome requires first establishing the normal anatomical position of these structures. This task is particularly complex in syndromic patients with significantly altered craniofacial anatomy and disrupted growth

R. Y. F. Yaedú (✉)
Department of Oral Surgery Faculdade de Odontologia and Hospital de Reabilitação de Anomalias Craniofaciais HRAC, University of São Paulo, São Paulo, São Paulo, Brazil

I. T. T. da Silveira
Bauru School of Dentistry, Bauru, SP, Brazil

C. de Paula Oliveira Gringo · M. Peralta-Mamani
Hospital for Rehabilitation of Craniofacial Anomalies, Bauru, SP, Brazil

R. H. Khonsari
Service de chirurgie maxillofaciale et chirurgie plastique, Hôpital Necker–Enfants malades, Assistance publique–Hôpitaux de Paris, Paris, France

J. G. Meara et al. (eds.), *Apert Syndrome*, https://doi.org/10.1007/978-3-032-12551-4_27

potential. Recent studies have developed growth models for the normal skull, such as Liang et al. [55], but detailed analyses of pre- and post-surgery craniofacial growth dynamics in Apert syndrome remain limited and exhibit high variability [38, 43].

In addition to bony repositioning, to determine the surgical outcome, you need to understand how much the soft tissue will move in relation to the bone movement. Soft-tissue considerations are especially important for morphological aspects—such as nasal and upper lip aesthetics in LFIII procedures—and for functional outcomes, including brain development in PVE and upper airway function in FFMBA and LFIII procedures. Unfortunately, predicting post-surgery soft-tissue changes remains rudimentary, particularly in syndromic cases [66].

Finally, many craniofacial advancement procedures involve distraction osteogenesis, introducing additional complexities to outcome prediction. The postoperative period in these cases is dynamic, given that the end-point of procedures like FFMBA and LFIII is typically determined by the correction of exorbitism and malocclusion during the distraction process [5].

Applications of VSP for Apert Syndrome Before Orthognathic Surgery

Given these limitations, early adopters of VSP in craniofacial surgery primarily used it to aid in designing standard osteotomies based on 3D visualization and/or 3D-printed skull models and simple cutting and positioning guides [1, 68, 70]. Similarly, over the past decade, several authors have reported case series involving virtual osteotomies planned on 3D imaging and 3D-printed surgical guides (e.g., [14, 53, 62]). As described in the literature, these guides can be classified into three main types: [1] cutting guides, which are typically secured to the skull with screws and are especially useful when piezosurgery is employed for osteotomies (Fig. 27.1) [2, 75] remodeling guides, which are particularly advantageous for shaping the forehead and bandeau in fronto-orbital reconstruction procedures [69]; and [3] guides designed to transfer the positions of surgical instruments or the vectors of distractors (Figs. 27.2 and 27.3) [75].

VSP facilitates knowledge dissemination and supports high-quality data collection. Given the limited ability to predict soft-tissue behavior and the incomplete understanding of postoperative growth dynamics, these approaches can be considered educational tools and are particularly useful in academic settings. Moreover, precise bone and implant positioning is generally less critical in craniofacial surgery than orthognathic surgery, especially in younger patients with substantial growth potential and significant remodeling capacity. For example, the parallel alignment of internal distractors—and thus precise vector directions—does not affect morphological outcomes in FFMBA procedures significantly [34].

Numerous studies have highlighted that VSP reduces surgical time, hospital stays, and blood loss while improving reconstruction accuracy [2,

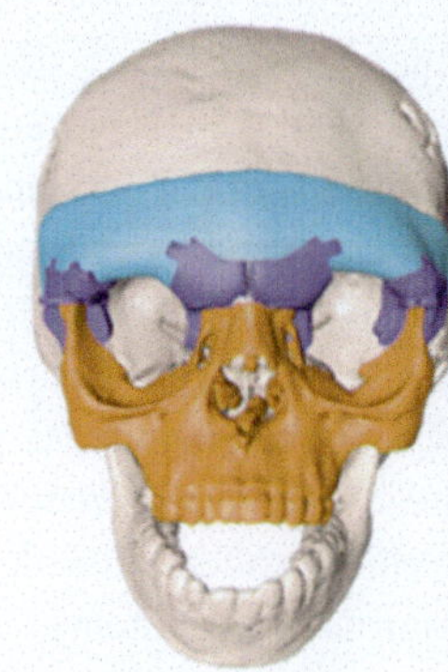
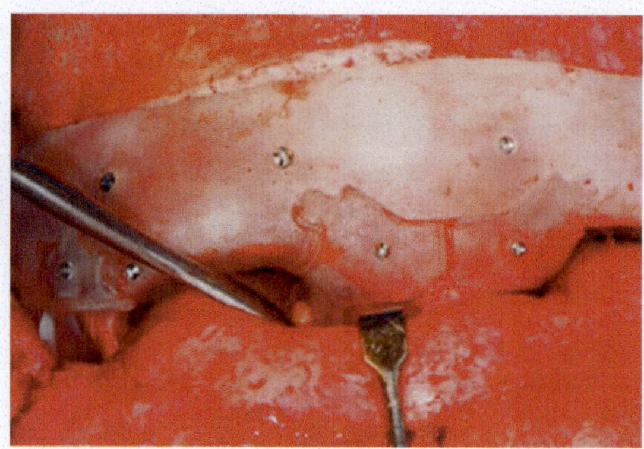

Fig. 27.1 (**a**) All cutting guides connect to a supraorbital reference bar with puzzle connections and indicate the planned orbital, nasal, septal, and pterygomaxillary osteotomy cuts. (**b**) Intraoperative view of the positioning of the guides. (Adapted from [74])

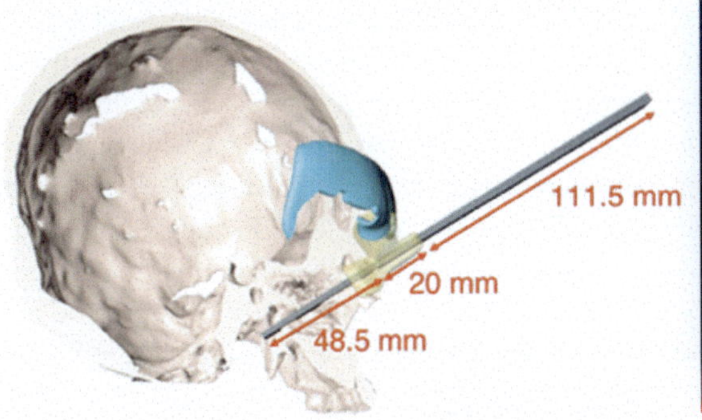

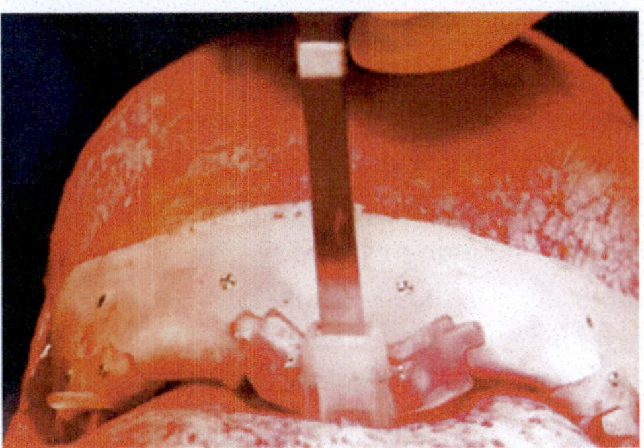

Fig. 27.2 Guide for the septal osteotomy designed to avoid the palate or the cranial base. (Adapted from [74])

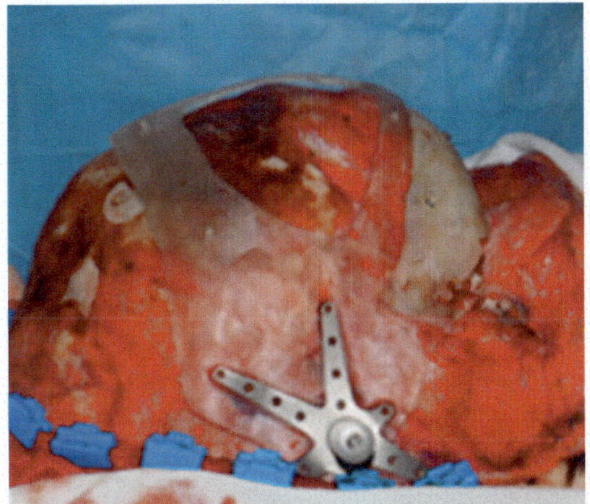
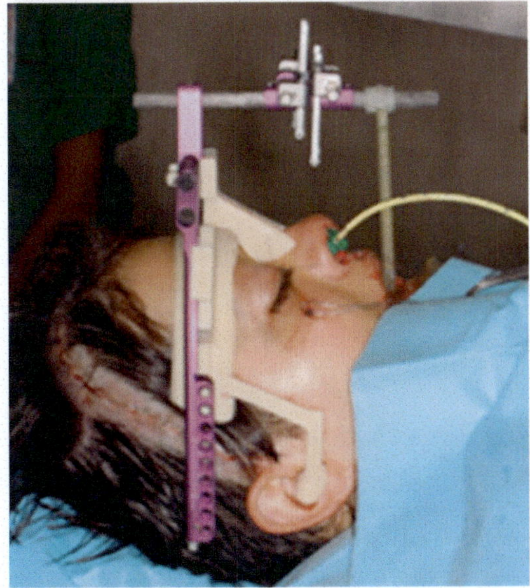

Fig. 27.3 Transfer systems: (*upper*) patient-specific footplates for external distractor fixation and (*lower*) face-bow method with occlusal guide. (Adapted from Vercryusse et al. 2021)

4, 76], making a compelling case for VSP integration into standard care. However, controlled studies are still needed to definitively validate its clinical benefits [18]. Improving outcome prediction—particularly for soft tissues—could greatly enhance the clinical applicability of virtual surgical planning (VSP) in young patients with Apert syndrome, by adding meaningful value to the concept of surgical accuracy.

Currently, the main method for transferring virtual planning into the operating room is using physical 3D-printed surgical guides [62]. However, high cost and complex regulatory requirements, particularly those in the European Union, limit adoption [44]. Additionally, the widespread use of 3D printing raises environmental concerns, given that reusable raw materials have not yet been developed for 3D printing [45].

Future advances in virtual surgical planning (VSP) for growing patients are expected to focus on two key challenges: [1] improving outcome prediction—particularly regarding soft tissue response and long-term skeletal stability—to support a clinically meaningful understanding of surgical accuracy, and [2] enhancing the transfer of digital plans into the operating room.

Opportunities for VSP for Apert Syndrome

Osteotomy VSP design relies on outcome prediction and integrates specific anatomical features of individual patients, such as bone defects, the position of the sagittal sinus, brain expansion capacity, and bone thickness. Geometric growth models of the skull are becoming increasingly complex [55], and the future development of inclusive craniofacial digital twins will further advance planning capability. These models will replicate both the morphological and biomechanical characteristics of the infant head—incorporating bone and soft tissues—and enable the simulation of various osteotomy patterns. Such multimodal models will optimize the reliability of osteotomy design by virtually testing the immediate and long-term outcomes of different cuts [20].

The development of automated tools that propose optimal cut designs is another promising direction for improving osteotomy design. These approaches utilize [1] geometry-based methods that achieve the desired outcome by accounting for necessary shape transformations and incorporating predefined parameters, such as sagittal sinus position or bone defects, and [2] artificial-intelligence-based methods trained on large datasets of expert-designed osteotomy patterns (Fig. 27.4) [26, 29].

Augmented reality (AR) holds significant potential for transferring information to the operating room and minimizing reliance on physical surgical guides. The craniofacial region is particularly well-suited for AR—especially in open skull vault procedures—due to its large, uniform surfaces and readily available anatomical landmarks for registration [13]. Ranging in complexity, AR solutions include sophistical systems [13] and simple mobile phone applications that enable cost-effective workflows but pose complex regulatory challenges, particularly within the European Union [3]. The combination of AR with intraoperative navigation can enhance precision by optimizing the final positioning of bone fragments (Fig. 27.5). Future advances could include automated osteotomies performed by robots equipped with bone-cutting lasers, a development that would enable intricate and counterintuitive designs (Fig. 27.6) [59].

Soon, the VSP workflow for patients with Apert syndrome could incorporate advanced prediction tools based on comprehensive craniofacial digital twins, algorithms for automated osteotomy design, and AR-enhanced navigation for the intraoperative transfer of planning information. These innovations could be followed by robot-assisted osteotomies, offering a seamless integration of prediction, planning, information transfer, and surgical execution.

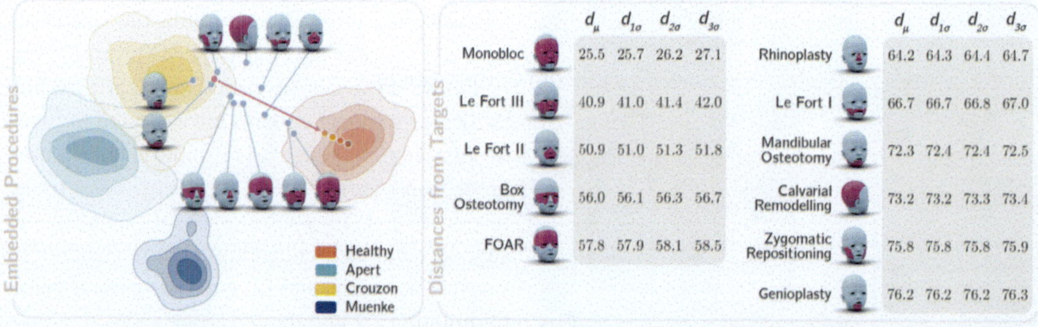

Fig. 27.4 Artificial intelligence-based simulation of various surgical procedures on a patient with *FGFR*-related craniosynostosis (here, Crouzon syndrome). The pink arrow represents the ideal interpolation trajectory from the original Crouzon anatomy toward the distribution of healthy subjects. Procedures are ranked from most to least effective in terms of distance to the target (i.e., healthy anatomy). (Adapted from [26])

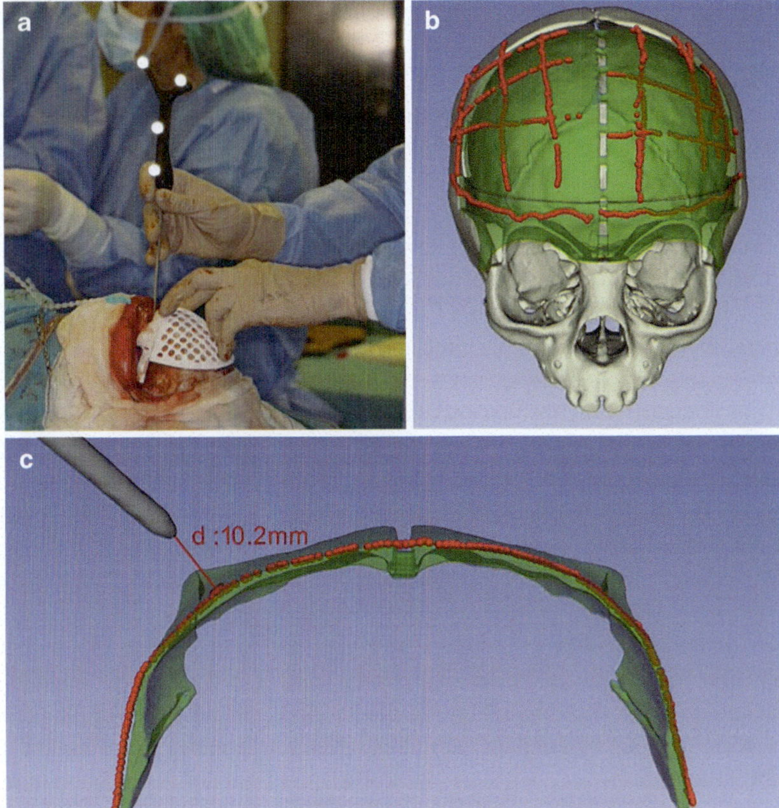

Fig. 27.5 (**a**) Recording of registration points on three-dimensional printed osteotomy guides using the tracked pointer. (**b**) Navigation points on remodeled bone surface (red) and virtual surgical planning (green). (**c**) Navigation on the supraorbital bar region

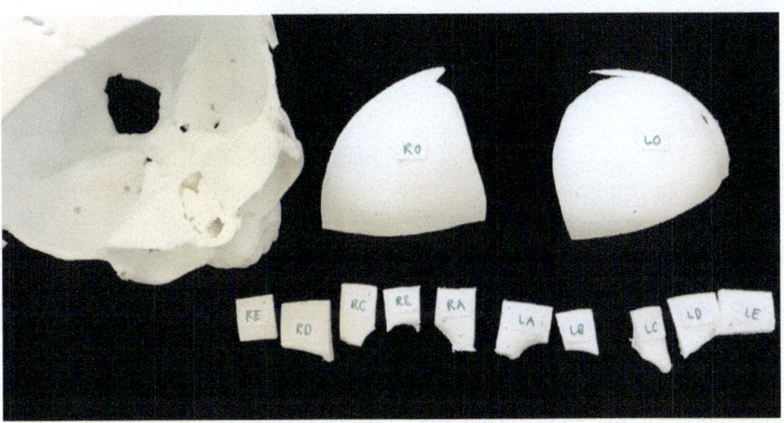

Fig. 27.6 Bony segments on three-dimensional-printed skulls after laser osteotomy. The use of this specific type of osteotomy device, navigation, and patient-specific osteosynthesis allows complex, counterintuitive, designs. (RO: right Os frontale, LO: left Os frontale, RA-RE: segments of the right supraorbital bandeau, LA-LE: segments of the left supraorbital bandeau). (Adapted from [59])

VSP for Orthognathic Surgery in Apert Syndrome

As crucial step in VSP, intraoral scanning allows for the precise digital capture of the patient's teeth and facilitates the creation of digital dental models. These digital models are combined with tomography to create a detailed 3D visualization of the bone and dental structures. Custom 3D surgical guides can be printed from these models to assist the surgeon during the procedure, ensure greater accuracy, and minimize errors.

In comparison with conventional planning, which relies on physical dental models and manual techniques, VSP offers several advantages. The traditional method requires creating models from impressions, manually simulating osteotomies, and fabricating surgical guides. In contrast, VSP uses 3D digital models overlaid on tomography, allows for quick and precise adjustments, reduces planning time, and increases surgical accuracy. Additionally, 3D printing efficiently creates surgical guides. Specialized software, such as NemoFAB, is widely used to create detailed 3D models, simulate osteotomies, adjust occlusion, and predict aesthetic outcomes.

Acquisition of Images

Strict standardizations in acquiring preoperative documentation ensures that the process is reproducible and predictable regarding expected surgical outcomes. While performing all steps for obtaining records and documentation, the ideal position of the condyle is centric relation. The patient is under general anesthesia during surgery, which typically results in the loss of habitual maximum intercuspation. Thus, the only reproducible position during the surgical procedure is the centric relation [50, 73].

To ensure that the centric relation is recorded in the same position throughout all surgical phases, it is essential to use an occlusal registration made with additional silicone specifically designed for this purpose, given that the setting time and flow of the silicone for molding differ from those of silicone used for occlusal registration [22]. The setting time for the additional silicone used for occlusal records is approximately 1 min, which is sufficient to apply the material to the occlusal surfaces and manipulate the patient's mandible into centric relation.

An occlusal record is obtained at the end of this process that will be used in all subsequent stages. Of note, this method allows the position and centric relation to be verified as often as necessary. Should the record be incorrect, the procedure can be repeated or the existing record adjusted, as appropriate. In the case of occlusal record-breaking during removal—a common issue—the maneuver can be repeated, and silicone can be added only to the fractured area, minimizing wasted material and time.

The use of wax for occlusal registration is not recommended, especially in hot regions, given that heat can soften the wax and allow the patient to move their mandible during the procedure, thereby altering the desired position. Additionally, because adapting the molding material to the model typically requires slight pressure for fitting, the use of wax could result in a distorted record [11].

Photographs

Photographs that adhere to a standardized protocol enable consistent comparisons during patient evaluations. Surgical planning can utilize both intraoral and extraoral images. All photographs must be taken with the occlusal record in position to prevent changes in mandibular positioning and ensure that the lips are relaxed. Of note, lip relaxation is fundamental for the predictability of soft tissues in surgical planning [17].

The patient's head should be in the natural head position (NHP), as it is more reproducible and reduces the risk of error. To achieve NHP, the patient looks straight ahead at the horizon or, for more accurate recording, at the reflection of their eye within a flat mirror placed in front of them. The latter method helps to prevent the head from tilting up or down, resulting in a more precise record of NHP [39].

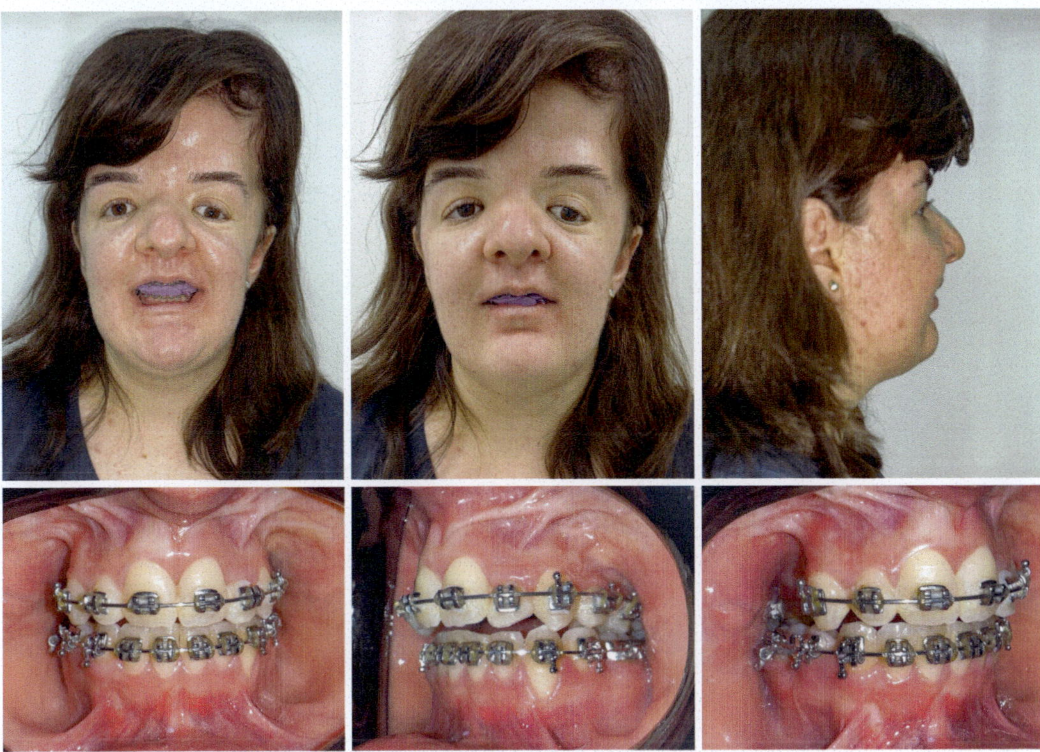

Fig. 27.7 Photography workflow used for postoperative planning and monitoring. Source: Image bank of the Oral and Maxillofacial Surgery Department, HRAC/USP

In contrast to using the Frankfurt plane, a position that the literature associates with an error of 6–8°, the NHP has a much lower error of only 2° [52, 58]. Therefore, NHP is preferred for imaging records in surgical patients, as it provides greater accuracy than cranial cephalometric points. This practice enhances the reliability of surgical planning and assessments [16].

Photogrammetry combined with computed tomography (CT) is another valuable resource that significantly aids in the planning and predictability of orthognathic surgery. This technique allows for 3D imaging of the patient in both resting and smiling positions, providing a more precise 3D visualization of the patient's face. This enhanced representation is beneficial for tailoring surgical approaches and improving outcomes [63].

Below, we present the workflow of photographs we utilize for surgical planning and postoperative monitoring (Fig. 27.7).

Dental Cast Study

Study models are crucial in orthodontic and surgical planning, physically representing dental and skeletal relationships. Digital scanning of the maxillary and mandibular teeth is now preferred over traditional impressions. Scanning only the crowns of the teeth is sufficient for VSP, as this allows for accurate overlay with CT data, facilitating effective treatment planning and outcome evaluation (Fig. 27.8).

Once scanning is complete, digital meshes (i.e., 3D representations of patient anatomy) are used to create 3D prints. Although VSP software provides tools for fully virtual occlusion, physical dental casts are important for finding the most stable position during manipulation, especially in cases where orthodontic preparation is not ideal. The need for physical dental casts is even more pronounced in patients with Apert syndrome due to reduced arch, dental transposition, and distinct occlusal relationships. Thus,

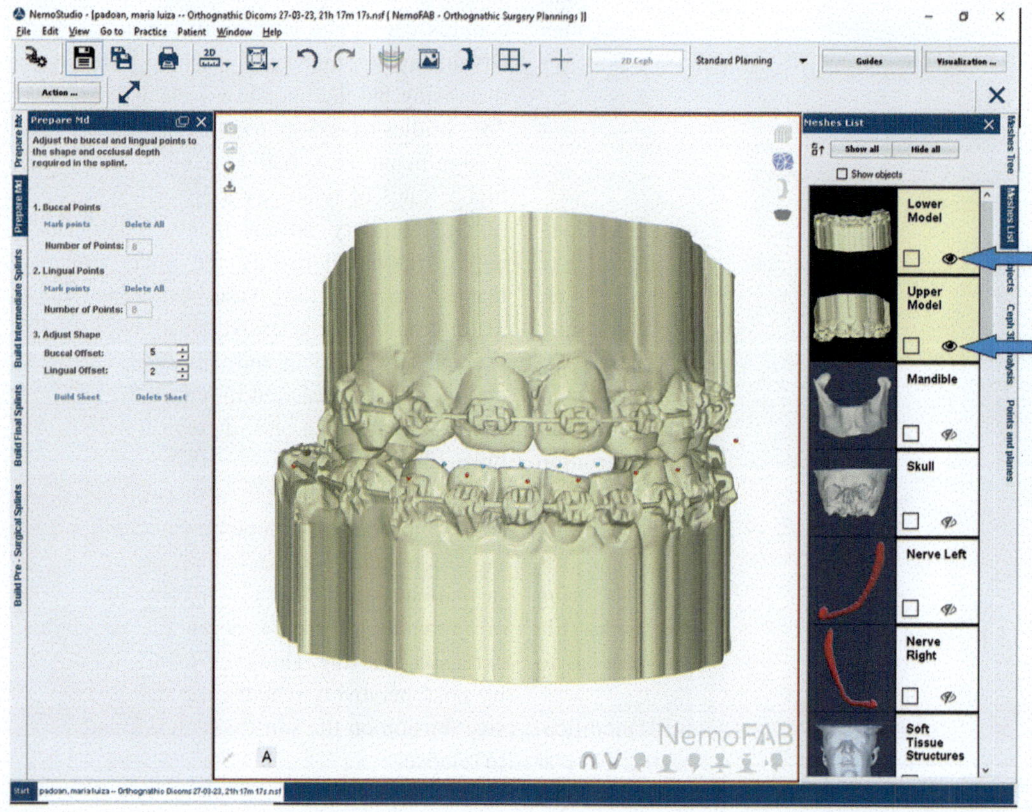

Fig. 27.8 Digital scanning of maxillary and mandibular teeth. Source: Image bank of the Oral and Maxillofacial Surgery Department, HRAC/USP

3D-printed dental casts are essential for effective planning and should be used to complement virtual methods.

Our facility's high volume of surgical patients requires optimized preparation and planning time. To this end, we have established printing configurations allowing dental cast production in 20–30 min. Although this process speeds up the evaluation of the dental cast and subsequent planning, it sacrifices the quality of the dental cast.

Computed Tomography (CT)

With the advancement of cone-beam CT (CBCT) in dentistry, VSP for orthognathic surgery has evolved from concentrating solely on occlusion to emphasizing the simulation of osteotomies and mandibular positioning. This technology allows for the integration of dental casts created through 3D scanning and photographs, yielding valuable insights for analyzing dental casts, assessing the temporomandibular joint (TMJ), and enhancing facial aesthetics [21, 67].

At this stage, the patient must stand while maintaining a relaxed lip position, with the occlusal record adjusted to ensure the mandible remains in centric relation. Also important, chin supports and head fixation at the glabella region should be avoided during the imaging process—especially with CBCT—as these devices can cause distortions during the exam, potentially compromising surgical planning [21].

The advantages and disadvantages of CBCT and multislice CT (MSCT) should be considered when selecting these technologies. The primary differences relate to patient posi-

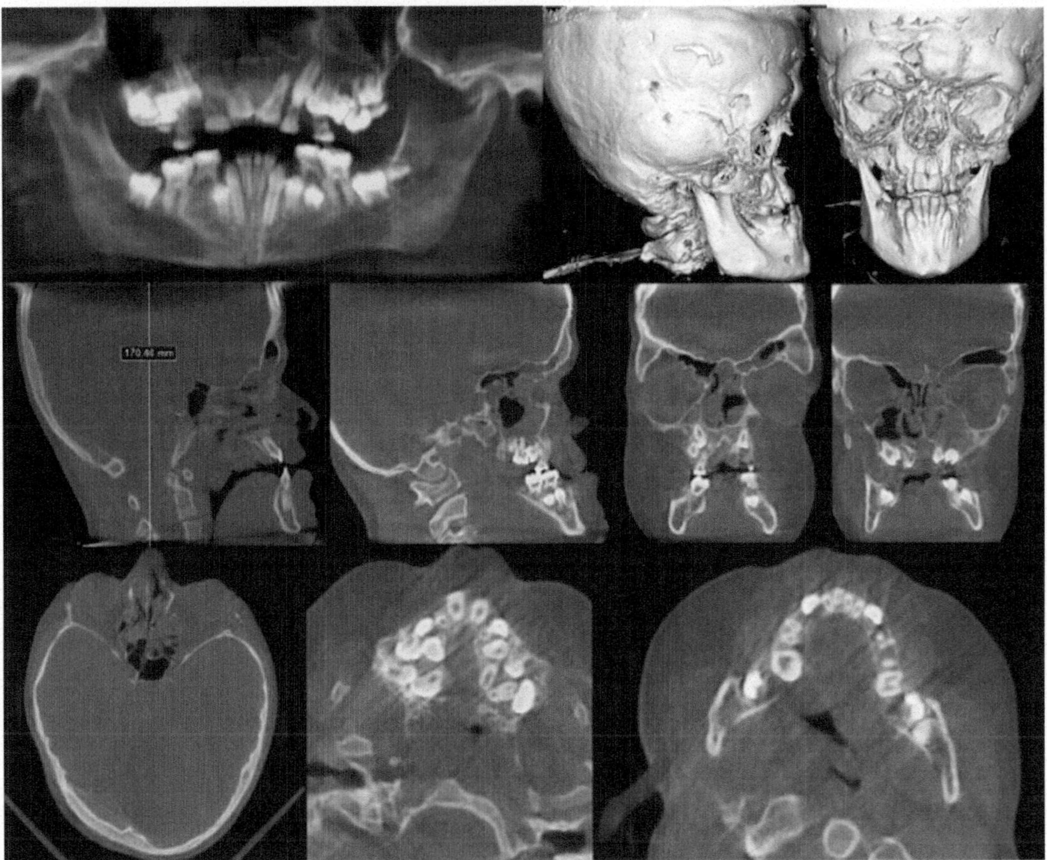

Fig. 27.9 Cone-beam computed tomography shows a female patient with Apert syndrome presenting with maxillary atresia and multiple dental anomalies. Field of view of 17 cm. Source: Image bank of the Oral Radiology and Craniofacial Surgery Department, HRAC/USP

tioning, with the patient seated or standing for CBCT and lying down for MSCT. Notable for its quicker image acquisition and lower ionizing radiation exposure, CBCT is advantageous in certain cases. Conversely, MSCT provides superior image resolution for soft tissues, making it better suited for situations requiring detailed anatomical information [49, 28].

Another factor to consider is the field of view (FOV) size in CBCT devices. Dental imaging clinics often use equipment with a smaller FOV that may be insufficient for scanning the entire face. Orthognathic surgery planning typically requires a minimum FOV of 17–23 cm for CBCT (Fig. 27.9) [37].

Superimposition Model on CT

The analysis of dental casts is crucial for generating surgical occlusion and defining the final position of the maxillae, a fundamental step in orthognathic surgery planning. Enabling virtual occlusion, intraoral digital scanning is indispensable. The 3D planning software integrates the bone anatomy from CBCT images with scanned models that contain information about the patient's occlusion, thereby ensuring accuracy in dento-skeletal relationships. This integration allows for virtual adjustments to occlusion and verification of premature contacts, cusp positions, and occlusal force distribution. Enabling more precise and effective planning, this integration is essential for detailed osteotomy planning [21].

Model movements can be performed manually, with consideration given to dental relationships and occlusal interferences. This can be achieved by [1] scanning the models in their final occlusion or [2] using printed configurations manipulated during planning to position the final models [56, 60]. These methods may result in slight variations in the actual position of surgical movements. Importantly, the surgical procedure must be considered when evaluating the positioning of models, as each step presents small differences that can impact results [71]. The preferred method for high surgery volume is positioning the models in final occlusion based on printed models. This approach ensures accuracy in occlusal positioning, along with reproducibility and predictability in outcomes [77, 80].

Analysis of the Temporomandibular Joint

TMJ analysis is essential for predicting the impact of maxillomandibular repositioning. The integrity of the mandibular head and the joint complex must be assessed to ensure predictability and safety in preserving or improving joint function, thereby reducing the risk of complications and optimizing functional and aesthetic outcomes. Additionally, monitoring the dentoarticular relationship is vital in ensuring that the new positioning of the maxillomandibular complex promotes healthy TMJ function (Fig. 27.10) [30].

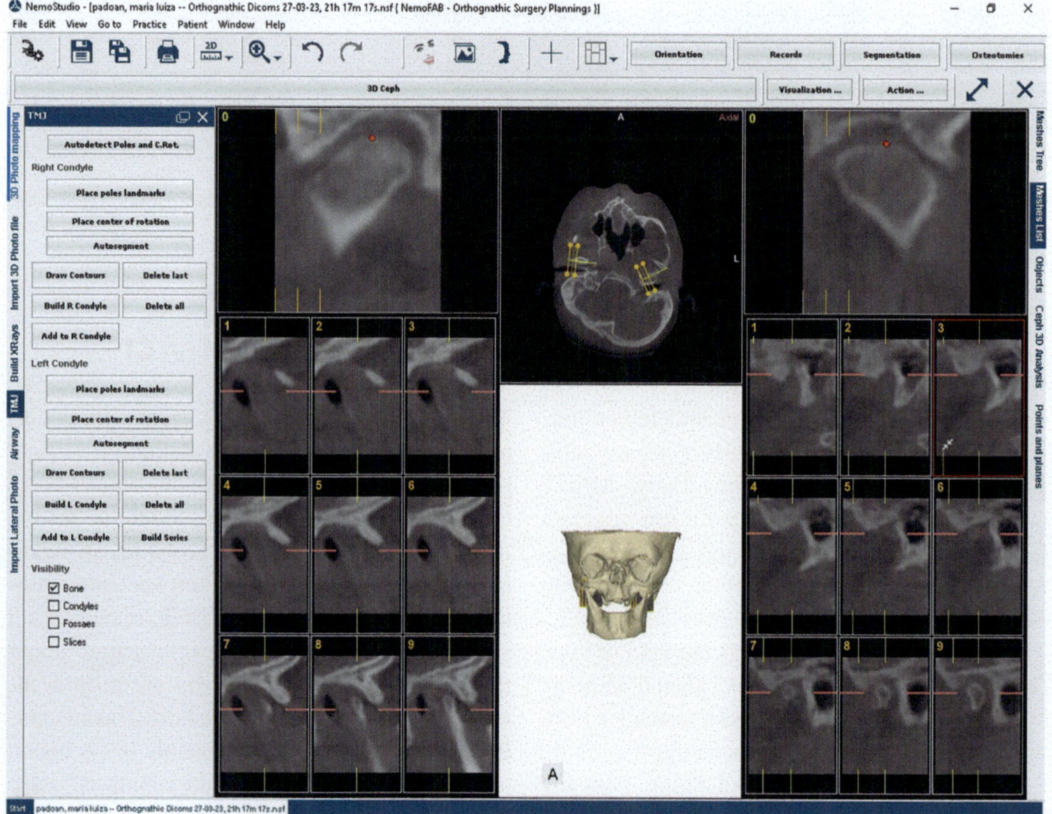

Fig. 27.10 Analysis of the temporomandibular joint. Source: Image bank of the Oral Maxillofacial Surgery Department, HRAC/USP

Profile	Occlusion Classification	Face front	Lower third	Exhibition IS	Cant	Middle line
Me-neck line	Overjet	Nasal wing	Right molar exposure	1 Relaxed	Mark the lowest	Nose
	Overbite	Vermilion of the upper lip	Left molar exposure	1 Smile		IS II Chin
		Vermilion of the lower lip	Upper lip length	2 Relaxed		
			Lower lip length	2 Smile		
			GAP	3 Relaxed		
				3 Smile		
				Length		

Fig. 27.11 Table outlining the measurements we utilize for facial analysis, as described by Arnett

Facial Analysis

Measuring changes in the patient's profile is essential in facial analysis; it involves evaluating both frontal and lateral views in resting and smiling positions. This comprehensive approach helps identify key issues that orthognathic surgery must address. Measurement selection is not governed by fixed rules, and each surgeon tailors the facial analysis to their specific needs and planning models. Although professionals may vary in the measurements and information they collect, their focus should be on recording useful data to guide surgical planning and to address all identified problems in the facial analysis [7]. The analysis should be comprehensive and as dynamic as possible, allowing for quick and systematic execution. Each recorded value must have a clear purpose for decision making during surgical planning and execution. Measurements that lack clinical rationale or do not contribute to planning or surgery are unnecessary and should be removed to optimize the analysis and enhance facial accuracy. Below is a table outlining the measurements we utilize for facial analysis, as described by Arnett (Fig. 27.11).

VSP Versus Conventional Planning

Conventional planning for orthognathic surgery involves manually handling physical dental casts and using analog techniques to determine bone movements. In contrast, VSP employs intraoral scanning to create models and then integrates these models and CBCT imaging into 3D planning software. By allowing for greater precision in simulating osteotomies and maxillomandibular repositioning, this digital approach provides a more detailed and predictable surgical plan.

The conventional planning process begins with taking an impression of the patient's dental arches. These impressions are used to create the dental casts that are the foundation for surgical planning. The dental casts are mounted in a mechanical articulator in the preoperative position, which simulates occlusion and mandibular movements and allows for the determination of the preoperative relationship between the upper and lower arches. Osteotomies are then simulated by making manual cuts directly on the dental casts to reproduce the planned bone movements for surgery. The cut sections are repositioned to visualize adjustments to the maxilla and mandible. These adjustments to the dental casts are then used to manually craft intermediate and final dental splint guides to assist the surgeon during the procedure.

In VSP, models are obtained through intraoral scanning and integrated with CBCT examinations using 3D planning software. This method eliminates the need for dental casts and surgeries on physical models, thereby significantly reducing the time required for surgical planning. Additionally, 3D-printed surgical guides and patient-specific implants can be created, ensuring greater precision and efficiency in the surgical process.

The manual manipulation of models used in the conventional method is less precise than the VSP 3D simulation, which provides high accuracy. Precision is directly linked to the operator's training and experience. Although both methods involve a learning curve, conventional planning demands significantly more training and experience. Moreover, the virtual model allows for quick adjustments—such as starting surgery with either the maxilla or mandible—whereas the conventional method requires additional time-consuming movements [31.

In terms of planning time, the conventional method entails time-consuming steps in molding, creating dental casts, and manual simulation of the surgery. Conversely, the VSP is faster in utilizing digital scanning and surgical simulation directly within the software. Potential distortions in physical models limit the visualization of results in the conventional method, while VSP offers more precise visualization. However, the final outcome of VSP is only confirmed during surgery. Whereas orthodontic planning is manual in the conventional method, in VSP, it is streamlined through digitalization, allowing for a more efficient workflow [54, 65].

Surgical Planning Software

Various VSP software options are available for orthognathic surgeries, each offering specific functionalities to enhance diagnosis, simulation, and execution. Some of the most widely used software include NemoFAB, Dolphin 3D Surgery™, ProPlan CMF™, VSP® by 3D Systems, IPS® CaseDesigner, Planmeca Romexis®, and InVivoDental™ by Anatomage. These programs provide advanced features for creating detailed 3D models, integrate imaging exams, and accurately simulate surgical outcomes, thereby facilitating communication between surgical and orthodontic teams.

NemoFAB by Nemotec is specifically designed for orthognathic surgery planning, encompassing 3D cephalometric analysis, bone segmentation, osteotomy planning, and the creation of cutting guides and surgical templates.

Dolphin 3D Surgery™ provides advanced tools for simulating orthognathic surgeries focused on aesthetic outcomes. Key features include precise 3D modeling of craniofacial structures, osteotomy planning tools, visualization of post-surgery soft-tissue change, comprehensive cephalometric analysis, and compatibility with various imaging capture systems. These characteristics make Dolphin a versatile and effective option for integrated surgical and orthodontic treatment planning.

ProPlan CMF™ focuses on craniomaxillofacial operations and is widely used for VSP and the fabrication of custom surgical guides. Key features include planning for orthognathic osteotomies and bone movements, simulating soft-tissue movements, and creating surgical guides. Additionally, ProPlan CMF™ integrates with 3D printing technologies for producing guides and physical models, making it a robust solution for optimizing precision and effectiveness in craniomaxillofacial surgeries.

In addition to software specialized for orthognathic surgery planning, 3D modeling and engineering software can be used to customize planning. For example, Blender software, which is free and open source, can be enhanced with the OrtogOnBlender add-on to facilitate orthognathic surgery planning. This flexibility provides customizable, accessible options for professionals looking to optimize their surgical preparation.

The role of software in surgical planning is to produce intermediate and/or final surgical guides. Software that allows for the segmentation of models to create a composite skull model—enabling the repositioning of segmented parts—aids in effective orthognathic surgery. However, planning and identifying the 3D locations for maxillary and mandibular movement are insufficient. Orthognathic surgery planning requires predictability, reproducibility, and minimal operator dependence. Many software programs facilitate planning but do not provide reproducible and predictable references and criteria, making them unsuitable for surgical application.

A user-friendly and intuitive software interface is crucial in lengthy processes such as preparing the composite skull for surgical manipulation. Specifically designed for orthognathic surgery planning, NemoFAB is our software of choice. NemoFAB features a sequential layout for preparing the composite skull and has proven to be accessible for surgical planning once users develop familiarity with the software.

From this point forward, we will outline VSP steps using the NemoFAB software. All surgical planning software options present similar functionalities, but each has specific features and sequence.

Virtual Planning Workflow for Orthognathic Surgery

Importing Tomography, Models, and Photos

The first step in VSP involves importing tomography—whether from MSCT, CBCT, or stereo lithography/polygon file format models—and conventional or 3D photos. NemoFAB streamlines this process by entering the locations of the tomography, upper, and lower models, which are then automatically stored in the patient's folder. Since the software utilizes cloud storage, this step is entirely dependent on Internet speed and can be time-consuming (Fig. 27.12).

Superpositioning Scan Models in Tomography

After importing the files, the patient's intraoral scan is overlaid onto the tomography. This step is crucial because tomography images often lack adequate resolution for surgical guide fabrication. While technology exists to enhance resolution, it increases radiation doses, especially in large FOV examinations. Instead, the patient's dental scan is overlaid onto the CT to achieve the detail required for effective planning. This manual step is operator-dependent, and aligning all planes when overlaying 3D structures can be challenging. Thus, this step entails a significant margin of error directly related to the professional's experience and knowledge of the patient's anatomy and dental relationships.

This issue becomes more pronounced in patients with Apert syndrome due to a significant open bite and numerous skeletal and dental anatomical alterations. These features complicate the overlaying of structures, posing challenges to accurate planning and increasing reliance on operator expertise.

To address this issue, companies including Nemotec have developed automatic overlay capabilities. The software automatically positions models over the tomography, greatly enhancing overlay accuracy and standardizing error. This automated process ensures consistent results with each overlay. However, the operator is responsible for verifying that the overlay has been correctly performed and that the maxillary and mandibular models align with the facial analysis in all three spatial planes.

NemoFAB added this functionality 2 years ago, and in that time, we have performed more than 200 automatic overlays of distinct patients. Errors occurred in only two instances and necessitated manual positioning. In both cases, the patient was missing multiple teeth, which complicated the automatic positioning of the models. All other models were completed to our satisfaction.

In cases requiring manual overlay, the quickest and most efficient method involves marking reference points on both the tomography and the model and then allowing the software to overlay

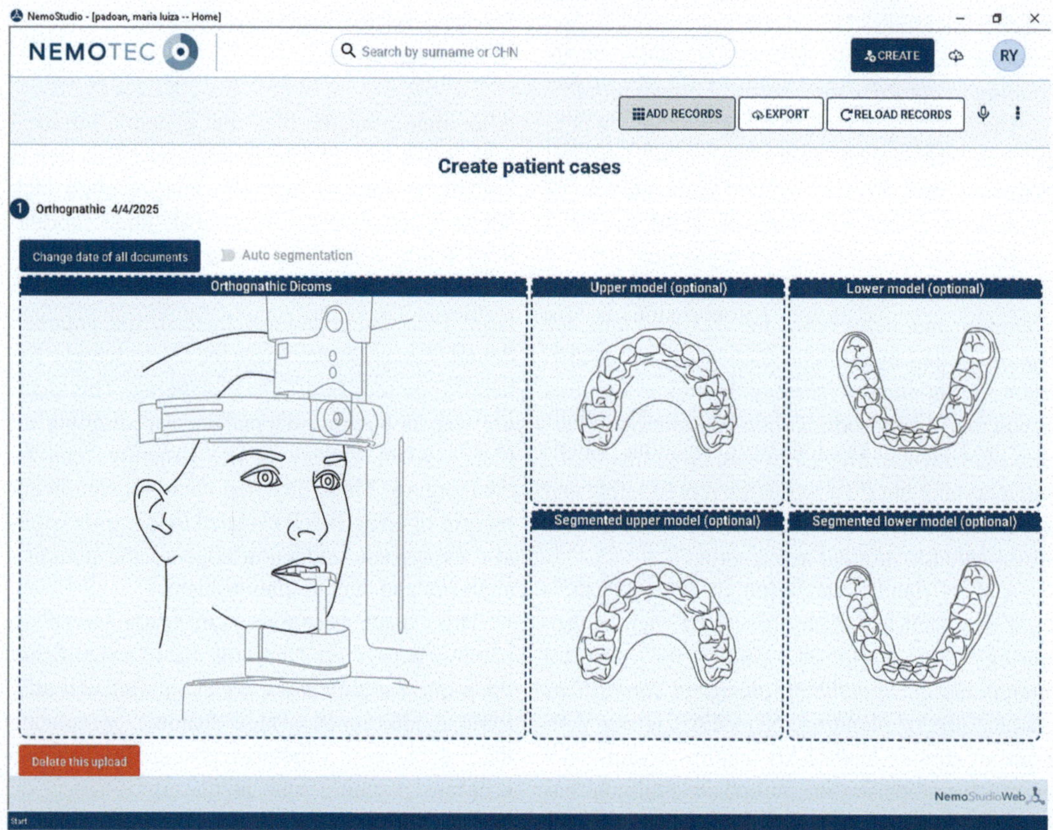

Fig. 27.12 Importing tomography from multislice cone beam or stereo lithography/polygon file format model and conventional or three-dimensional photos

the two structures automatically. Marking easily identifiable distant reference points on the tomography and models is essential in optimizing overlay. Typically, references for the maxilla and mandible include the mesiobuccal cusp of the second or first molar on both sides and the mesial angle of the right incisor. If clear identification is not possible due to unreliable points or artifacts in the tomography, another posterior cusp tip can be chosen as a reference. After the overlay, minor manual corrections are always required, and this stage of fine manual adjustments often entails errors (Fig. 27.13). The ability to visualize the 3D overlay plays an important role in facilitating the manual overlay of models. Adjusting the threshold enables highlighting the teeth in the tomography, providing a clear view of the model overlay and reducing the chances of error during the process.

Head Orientation

The skull must be oriented in the same position in the photographic records, facial analysis, and tomography to ensure proper VSP reproduction. Verifying and positioning the skull in NHP across all three spatial planes are essential, regardless of whether a cephalostat is used to achieve adequate orientation during tomography. Placing metal markers on the patient's reference points before the tomography enhances accuracy and allows for easier alignment during the orientation stage, facilitating the positioning process (Fig. 27.14). Nonetheless, the patient's head position can also be satisfactorily achieved without markers, relying solely on anatomical references, photographic records, and acquired facial analysis.

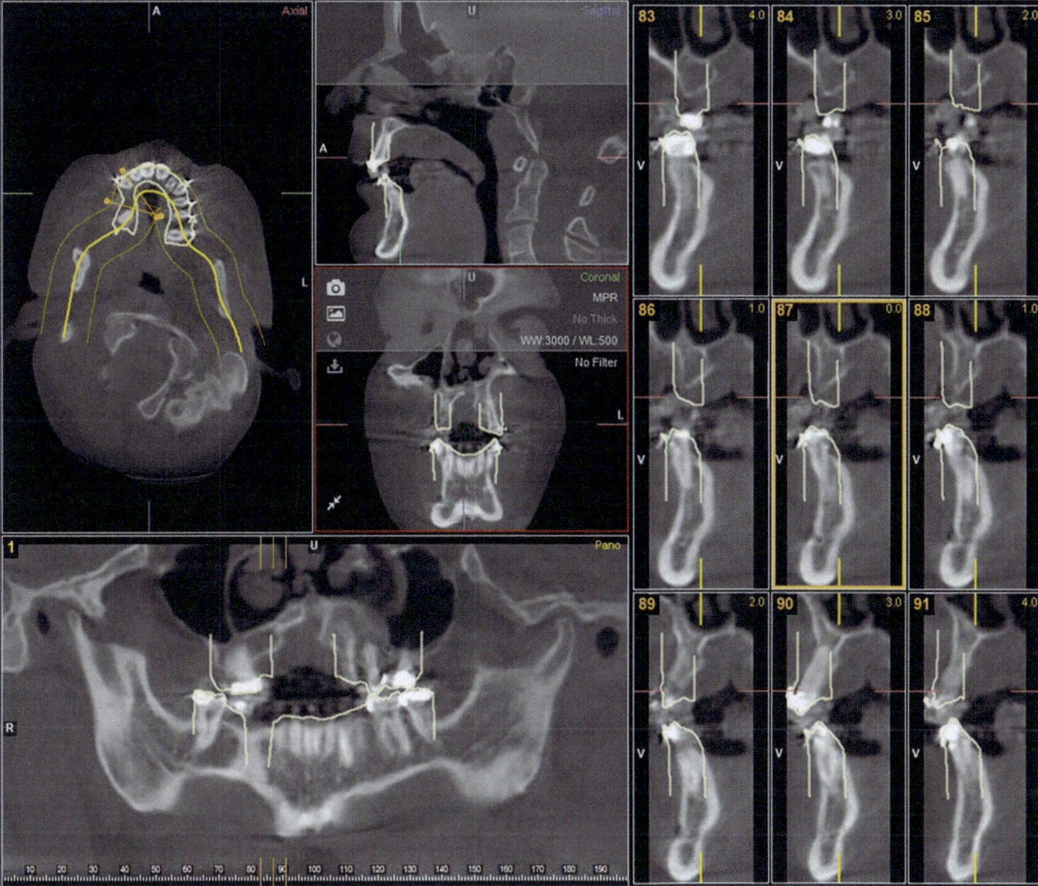

Fig. 27.13 Identifiable landmarks on both the computed tomography scan and the models. Source: Image bank of the Oral Radiology and Craniofacial Surgery Department, HRAC/USP

The frontozygomatic process can be used to orient yaw, and the inferior orbital rims can be used to orient the roll of the patient. The Frankfort horizontal plane is commonly used to ensure the patient is in NHP. After this, the distance from the glabella to a vertical reference line is adjusted to match the photographic positioning. Midlines and their deviations are established at this stage (Fig. 27.14). The orientation can be performed manually or by inputting facial analysis measurements into the software, which then aligns the skull. The preferred method is to conduct manual orientation first, and then enter the measurements obtained from the facial analysis into the automatic method to fine tune the orientation. This approach ensures the most accurate positioning (Fig. 27.15).

Mandible Segmentation

During the preparation of the composite skull, the segmentation of the mandible from the rest of the skull can lead to errors. The TMJ is a complex structure, and the mandible can be difficult to separate given the small distance between the glenoid fossa and the condyle. Moreover, the occlusal contact of the teeth and the density of the occlusal record can further hinder this separation.

Most software programs adjust the threshold of the bony mesh to create space between the articular cavity and the condyle while also eliminating the occlusal record. However, this process may reveal flaws in the mesh related to the density of the maxillary bone, especially in the ante-

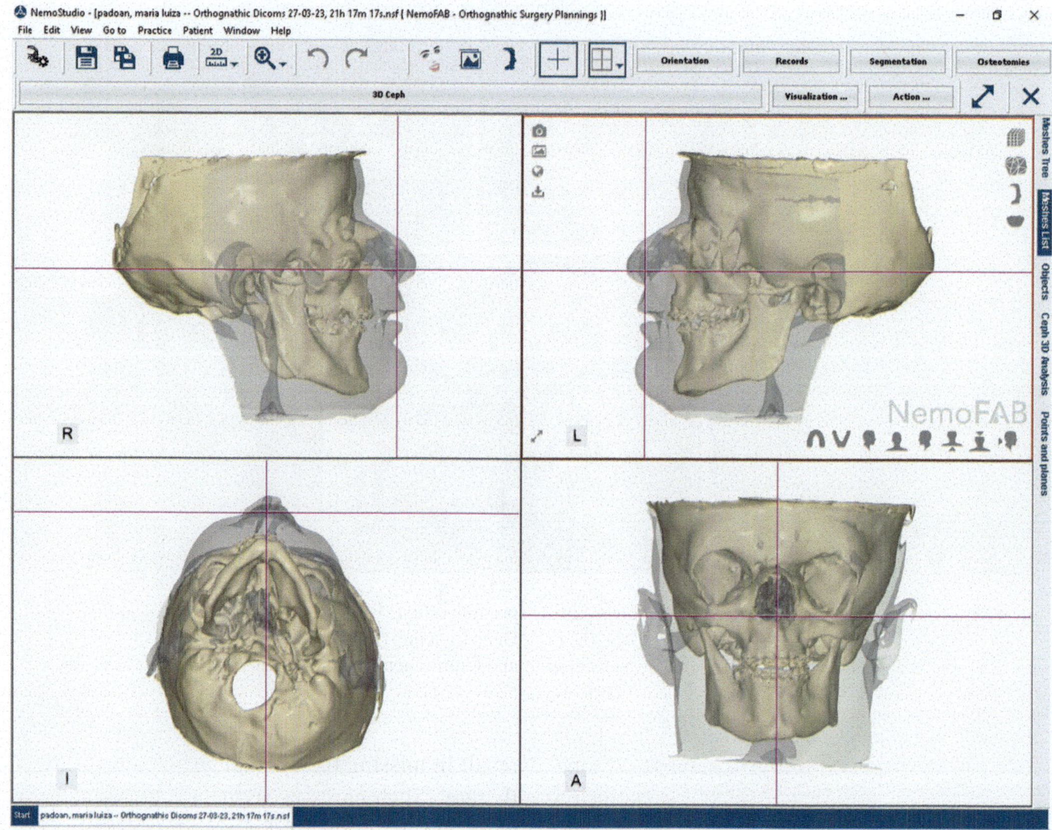

Fig. 27.14 Alignment of the frontozygomatic processes, inferior orbital margins and Frankfurt plane. Adjustment of the distance from the glabella to a vertical reference line. The midlines and their deviations are positioned at this stage. (Source: Image bank of the Oral Maxillofacial Surgery Department, HRAC/USP)

rior maxillary sinus region and the lateral nasal wall. In such situations, the mesh must be corrected to prevent complications during the osteotomy.

Technological advancements have made it possible to perform this step automatically, simplifying and optimizing the preparation of the composite skull. Similar to the process for models, a tool in NemoFAB automatically segments the mandible. This step takes approximately 5–10 min and creates a new file containing the segmentation of the skull, skin, mandible, maxilla, inferior alveolar nerves, teeth, maxillary sinus, airway, and teeth (Fig. 27.16).

Principles of Osteotomy Creation

The mandible must be segmented before the osteotomies can be performed to obtain the composite skull. The osteotomy design is typically more inclined for the maxilla in patients with Apert syndrome than in those without the syndrome [40]. Consideration of the anatomical variations characteristic of the syndrome is essential, especially given the likelihood that patients with Apert syndrome have previously undergone frontofacial advancement or LFIII surgery [41]. Anatomical changes associated with Apert syndrome—such as decreased mid-

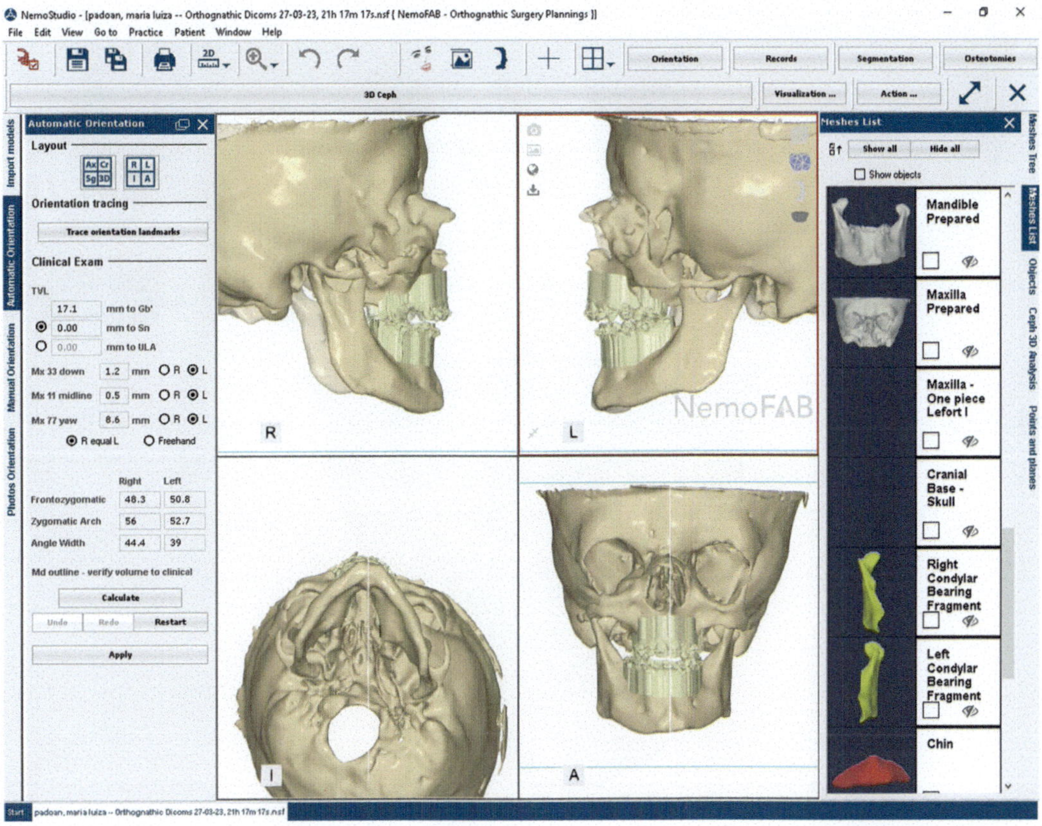

Fig. 27.15 Orientation performed automatically in the software. (Source: Image bank of the Oral Maxillofacial Surgery Department, HRAC/USP)

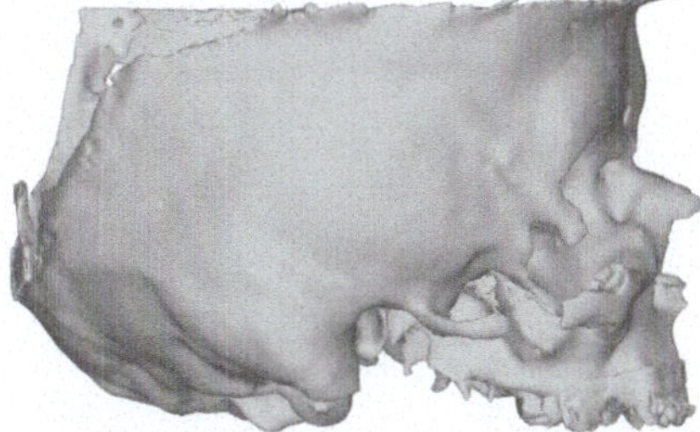
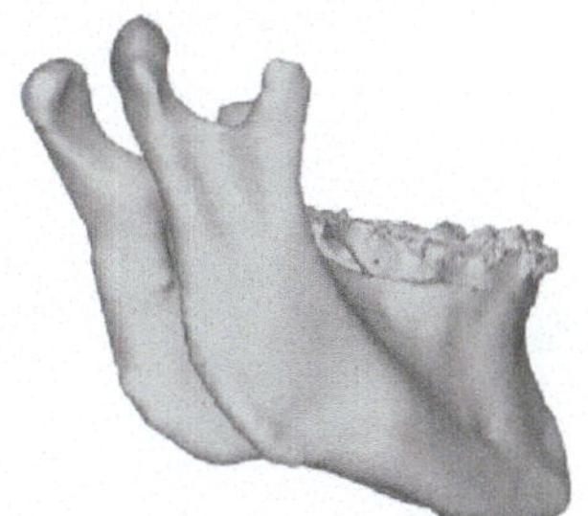

Fig. 27.16 Automatic segmentation of the mandible. (Source: Image bank of the Oral Maxillofacial Surgery Department, HRAC/USP)

face height, significantly increased palatal depth, reduced and elevated maxillary sinuses, and enlarged pterygomaxillary sutures—must be considered in both the design and execution of the osteotomy (Fig. 27.17). These variations are crucial for effective surgical planning and performance [57].

A distance of 3–5 mm from the apices of the molars to the piriform fossa serves as a reliable reference for designing the Le Fort I osteotomy. The design of the sagittal split osteotomy for the mandible follows the short-split technique described by Arnett in 1993 [6]. Although this type of osteotomy reduces the risk of unfavorable splits and facilitates mobilization, it also decreases the bony contact surface, making it challenging to use three bicortical screws for fixation. This type of osteotomy is particularly advantageous for patients with Apert syndrome, as it allows rotation of the occlusal plane to close

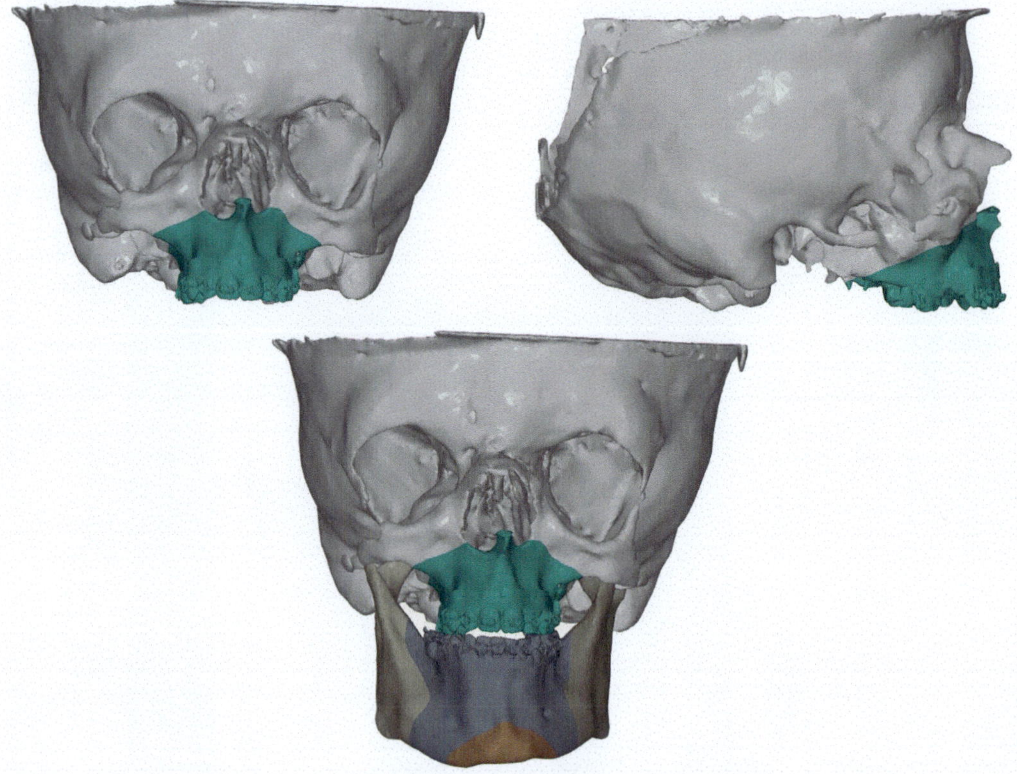

Fig. 27.17 Segmentation of the maxilla, mandible and chin. (Source: Image bank of the Oral Maxillofacial Surgery Department, HRAC/USP)

the anterior open bite while correcting the cant with minimal bony interference.

Three-Dimensional Cephalometric Analysis

Cephalometric analysis focuses on soft tissues and uses an extracranial reference line. The skull base has proven inefficient as a reference in orthognathic patients, as variations in the angulation of the skull base can lead to different therapeutic approaches. In the soft-tissue cephalometric analysis, the true vertical line is utilized as a reference, allowing for the repositioning of the maxillomandibular complex using an extracranial point [79]. Given that craniosynostosis causes alterations in the cranial vault and often in the skull base, relying solely on intracranial references can be problematic. In such cases, using stable extracranial reference points becomes even more critical for accurately repositioning the maxillomandibular complex and optimizing surgical outcomes [35].

By considering each side separately, 3D analysis facilitates the skeletal positioning of the maxillomandibular complex. This analysis provides measurements for cant correction and yaw adjustments, which are more difficult and less precise to observe in two-dimensional measurements. This approach enhances the accuracy of surgical planning and improves the overall outcome in patients with complex anatomical variations [48].

Cephalometric analysis can be customized to suit the surgeon's preferences. A few criteria must be observed to ensure surgical predictability and reproducibility of planning. These criteria include using extracranial references for repositioning the maxillomandibular complex, identifying reference points for accurate maxillary positioning in all three spatial planes, and ensuring that the cephalometric analysis aligns with facial analysis. This alignment is crucial for balancing clinical assessment with cephalometric measurements during surgical planning [42].

For maxillary positioning, the sagittal view assesses the anteroposterior distance of the incisors relative to the true vertical line. Vertical evaluation in the frontal view considers the relaxed and smiling exposure of the upper incisor, upper lip length, and anterior and posterior gingival exposure at the first molar while smiling. The frontal view also aligns the incisor midline with the facial midline and corrects canine cant. In the axial view, yaw is corrected using the mandible as a reference to minimize large lateral movements of the mandibular proximal segment and condylar torque.

Surgical Planning

Establishing the ideal positioning of the maxilla in patients with Apert syndrome is essential, as this allows for the subsequent positioning of the mandible and chin. Orthognathic surgery typically complements frontofacial advancement or LFIII procedures in this patient group, and therefore significant anteroposterior discrepancies are usually absent. The primary correction addresses the rotations of the maxilla and the mandible's occlusal planes [81].

Posterior maxillary impaction is often required to correct an anterior open bite. Thus, even in the absence of indications for profile alteration, a slight advancement of the maxilla should always be considered to mitigate interferences from the pterygoid plates. Advancements of up to 5 mm do not cause significant changes in patients with cleft lip and palate or syndromes, as the soft tissues provide a poorer response to skeletal movement [36]. This understanding can be leveraged to facilitate the surgical movement of maxillary impaction [8].

Another important consideration, the desired orthodontic decompensation is not always achieved due to limitations in dental movement, as previously discussed in the orthognathic surgery literature [12]. The less dental decompensation, the greater the rotation of the maxillary occlusal plane for projecting the base of the nose and the subnasal area. In the vertical dimension, the normal length of the upper lip allows for a downward movement of the maxilla by 1–2 mm, which aids in the rotation of the occlusal plane. While larger movements are possible, they require bone or materials to support the maxilla and maintain contact with its supporting pillars. We typically do not perform movements greater than 1–2 mm in our practice, as this range is sufficient to enhance incisor exposure and minimizes complications related to biomaterials [27].

With the anteroposterior and vertical relationships established, the canine cant and maxillary midline are corrected in the frontal view. Next, the mandibular midline is aligned with the facial midline, and the mandibular cant is adjusted. The mandible is positioned to correct the overjet, overbite, and expected final occlusion, ensuring proper dental contacts. This process results in the correct positioning of both the maxilla and mandible across all three spatial planes. To finalize the planning, the occlusal plane of the maxilla should be adjusted by moving the maxillomandibular complex. Lastly, a genioplasty can be performed if necessary (Figs. 27.18 and 27.19).

In our routine, surgical movements are guided by aesthetic and functional needs, without the need for compensatory skeletal adjustments due to constraints in maxillary advancement caused by velopharyngeal dysfunction or surgical limitations. A trained team is essential for managing anesthesia and inducing hypotension, allowing an additional 15–20% movement beyond the originally planned range to achieve passive movement and facilitate muscle lengthening [15]. Consequently, compensatory planning is unnecessary, particularly in patients with Apert syndrome [40, 47, 61].

Surgical Guide

Orthognathic surgery for patients with Apert syndrome invariably involves bimaxillary procedures, even though the anteroposterior correction

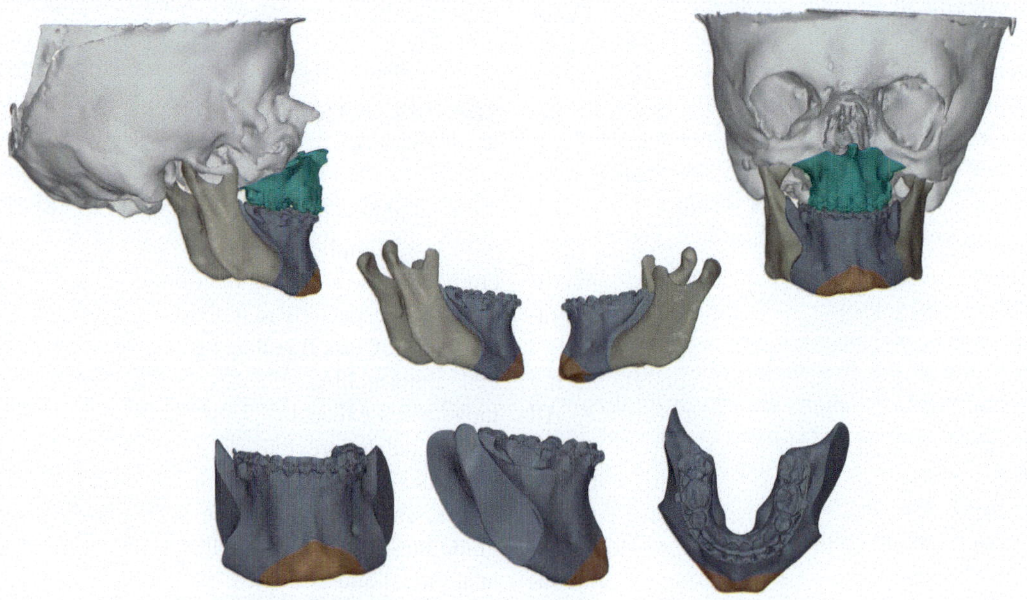

Fig. 27.18 Surgical Planning. (Source: Image bank of the Oral Maxillofacial Surgery Department, HRAC/USP)

Models Measurements

Maxilla		A-P		Vert		Side
ANS	→	8,7	↓	0,4	→	0,4
PNS	→	6,3	↑	7,2	→	1,1
Mx1R tip	→	3,8	↑	0,3	→	1,1
Mx1L tip	→	3,7	↓	0,1	→	1,1
R Canine	→	3,7	↑	0,7	→	1,1
L Canine	→	3,9	↑	1,9	→	1,2
Right Molar6 MB cusp tip	→	3,8	↑	2,9	→	1,2
Left Molar6 MB cusp tip	→	4,4	↑	4,9	→	1,2

Mandible		A-P		Vert		Side
Md1R tip	→	7,5	↑	4,2	→	0,1
Md1L tip	→	7,5	↑	4,0	→	0,1
B Point	→	7,2	↑	4,1	→	1,0
Pogonion	→	7,1	↑	4,1	→	1,3

Chin Osteotomy		A-P		Vert		Side
R Chin	→	7,0	↑	3,7	→	1,6
L Chin	→	7,1	↑	4,6	→	1,5
L Canine	→	7,5	↑	4,5	→	0,0
R Canine	→	7,5	↑	3,7	→	0,0
Left Molar6 MB cusp tip	→	7,4	↑	3,5	→	0,1
Right Molar6 MB cusp tip	→	7,5	↑	4,7	→	0,0

Pl. Oclu. Mx	Srg	Ini	Dif	Pl. Oclu. Md	Srg	Ini	Dif
MxOP R	83,3	91,1	-7,8	MdOP R	84,0	88,1	-4,2
MxOP L	77,9	87,0	-9,0	MdOP L	86,3	86,8	-0,5
MxOccPl	80,6	89,0	-8,4	MdOccPl	85,1	87,5	-2,4

Clipboard | Disk | Save as Image | OK

Fig. 27.19 Measurements. (Source: Image bank of the Maxillofacial Surgery Department, HRAC/USP)

of the maxilla is often performed beforehand. Therefore, the choice between performing maxillary or mandibular surgery first is crucial. The literature discusses various arguments for commencing with each option. In this section, we will highlight the reasons for beginning with the mandible, as the authors find this approach easier and more predictable in patients with Apert syndrome.

First, we consider the planned skeletal movement. This patient group typically requires rotations of the occlusal plane in both the maxilla and mandible. Interferences in the surgical guide and planned surgical movement that require mouth opening are common. While smaller rotations may not pose significant issues due to the compensatory anterior open bite, larger rotations lead to considerable dental interference, making it impractical to start surgery with the maxilla [24, 78].

Additionally, the greater movement typically occurs in the mandible, which has not been previously corrected. Previous advancement of the maxilla can result in more significant skeletal movement of the mandible [51]. Moreover, since the mandible is a movable bone, positioning it first in relation to the fixed maxilla bone is safer and facilitates evaluation of whether the procedure was performed correctly during the surgery [9, 72].

On the other hand, this choice must be made cautiously, particularly regarding the positioning of the proximal segment (i.e., condyle). During lengthy surgeries with challenging osteotomies, swelling in the TMJ can result in an anterior positioning of the mandible, affecting desired post-surgical occlusal movement. Similarly, unsatisfactory performance of the maneuver to place the condyle in centric relation can lead to posterior positioning of the mandible, which complicates maxillary movement and necessitates additional adjustments, such as removing part of the pterygoid process for passive maxillary repositioning [33].

Finally, the maxilla should be positioned passively, without applying force to maintain its position. Bony interferences can lead to postoperative instability and may result in the recurrence of anterior open bite, which often necessitates further surgical intervention (Fig. 27.20).

In the example below, starting the surgery with the maxilla is more appropriate, given the need for greater horizontal advancement of the maxilla and the absence of significant occlusal plane rotations.

Predictability of VSP

VSP offers a high degree of predictability, as demonstrated by numerous reports in the literature [64]. For patients with Apert syndrome, this technology is particularly valuable in managing bony interferences resulting from surgical movements. Additionally, VSP facilitates a shorter learning curve and aids in creating cutting guides; this benefits less experienced surgeons, especially in the context of Apert syndrome [35]. Conventional orthognathic surgery planning for patients with Apert syndrome involves anticipating all potential interferences and skeletal movements, thereby requiring extensive knowledge and experience and posing challenges to even experienced surgeons (Fig. 27.21).

Utilizing all available knowledge and technology is crucial in treating patients with Apert syndrome, given the high rate of orthognathic surgery in this patient group, the associated complexity of these procedures, and the elevated rates

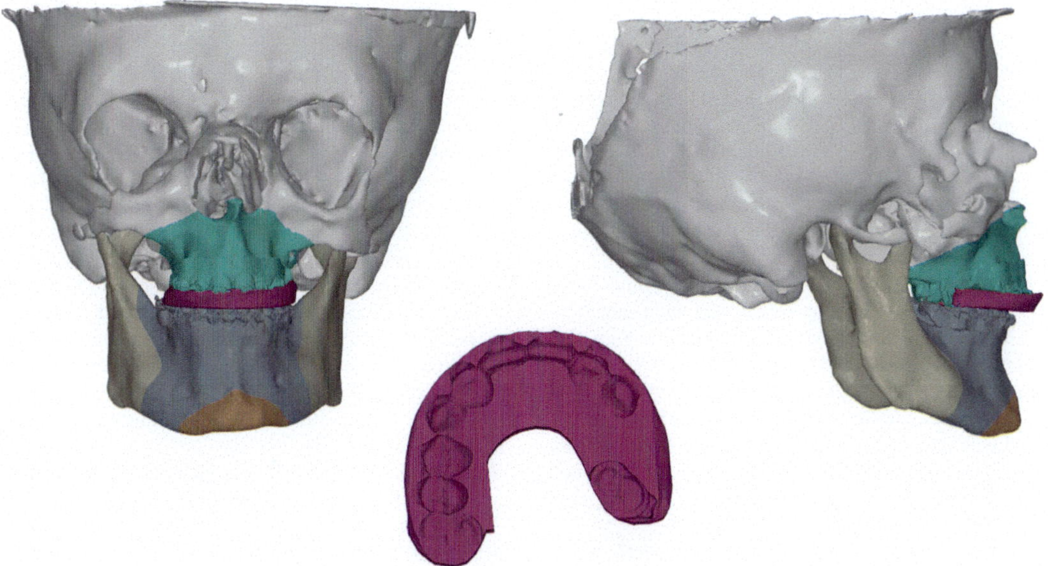

Fig. 27.20 Surgical guide. (Source: Image bank of the Oral Maxillofacial Surgery Department, HRAC/USP)

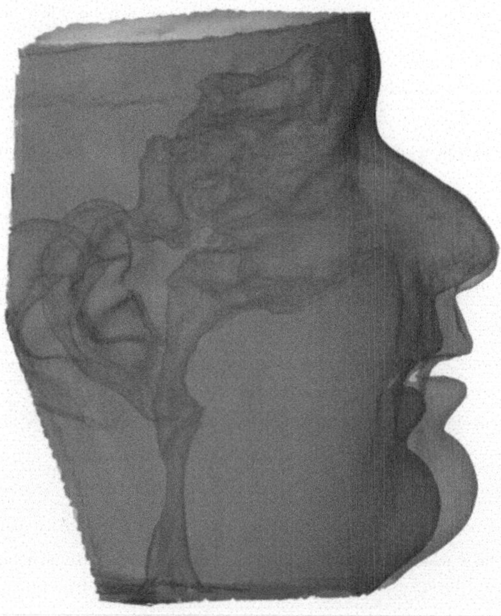

Fig. 27.21 Predictability of virtual planning. (Source: Image bank of the Oral Maxillofacial Surgery Department, HRAC/USP)

of relapse. Thus, VSP is an indispensable tool for enhancing predictability and stability in surgeries for patients with Apert syndrome [35].

References

1. Adolphs N, Haberl EJ, Liu W, Keeve E, Menneking H, Hoffmeister B. Virtual planning for craniomaxillofacial surgery–7 years of experience. J Craniomaxillofac Surg. 2014;42:e289–95.
2. Almeida MN, Alper DP, Williams MCG, Ihnat JMH, Parikh N, Diluna M, Alperovich M. Virtual surgical planning in craniosynostosis reduces operative time and length of stay for cranial vault remodeling. J Craniofac Surg. 2023;34:1931–3.
3. Alshomer F, Alazzam A, Alturki A, Almeshal O, Alhusainan H. Smartphone-assisted augmented reality in craniofacial surgery. Plast Reconstr Surg Glob Open. 2021;9(8):e3743.
4. Andrew TW, Baylan J, Mittermiller PA, Cheng H, Johns DN, Edwards MSB, Cheshier SH, Grant GA, Lorenz HP. Virtual surgical planning decreases operative time for isolated single suture and multi-suture craniosynostosis repair. Plast Reconstr Surg Glob Open. 2018;6:e2038.
5. Arnaud E, Paternoster G, Khonsari RH, Haber S. Frontofacial monobloc advancement with internal distraction. In: Tactics and strategy in faciocraniosynostosis. Springer; 2023. p. 59–81.
6. Arnett GW. A redefinition of bilateral sagittal osteotomy (BSO) advancement relapse. Am J Orthod Dentofacial Orthop. 1993;104(5):506–15. https://doi.org/10.1016/0889-5406(93)70076-Z.
7. Arnett GW, Gunson MJ. Facial planning for orthodontists and oral surgeons. Am J Orthod Dentofacial Orthop. 2004;126(3):290–5. https://doi.org/10.1016/j.ajodo.2004.06.006.
8. Azoulay-Avinoam S, Bruun R, MacLaine J, Allareddy V, Resnick CM, Padwa BL. An overview of Craniosynostosis craniofacial syndromes for combined orthodontic and surgical management. Oral Maxillofac Surg Clin North Am. 2020;32(2):233–47. https://doi.org/10.1016/j.coms.2020.01.004.
9. Badiali G, Bevini M, Lunari O, Lovero E, Ruggiero F, Bolognesi F, Feraboli L, Bianchi A, Marchetti C. PSI-guided mandible-first orthognathic surgery: maxillo-mandibular position accuracy and vertical dimension adjustability. J Pers Med. 2021;11(11):1237. https://doi.org/10.3390/jpm11111237. PMID: 34834588; PMCID: PMC8622626.
10. Bell WH. Le Forte I osteotomy for correction of maxillary deformities. J Oral Surg. 1975;33(6):412–26.
11. Bergamo AZN, de Andrucioli Mattos JP, Pavan AJ. Changes in occlusal plane through orthognathic surgery: clockwise and counterclockwise rotations. Dent Press J Orthod. 2012;17(4):160–73. https://doi.org/10.1590/S2176-94512012000400022.
12. Breuning KH, van Strijen PJ, Prahl-Andersen B, Tuinzing DB. Duration of orthodontic treatment and mandibular lengthening by means of distraction or bilateral sagittal split osteotomy in patients with Angle Class II malocclusions. Am J Orthod Dentofacial Orthop. 2005;127(1):25–9. https://doi.org/10.1016/j.ajodo.2003.11.024.
13. Cai EZ, Yee TH, Gao Y, Lu WW, Lim TC. Mixed reality guided advancement osteotomies in congenital craniofacial malformations. J Plast Reconstr Aesthet Surg. 2024;98:100–2.
14. Calluaud G, Pare A, Kulker D, Listrat A, Laure B. Computer-assisted frontofacial monobloc advancement and facial bipartition for Pfeiffer syndrome: surgical technique. World Neurosurg. 2022;161:97–102.
15. Carlos E, Monnazzi MS, Castiglia YM, Gabrielli MF, Passeri LA, Guimarães NC. Orthognathic surgery with or without induced hypotension. Int J Oral Maxillofac Surg. 2014;43(5):577–80. https://doi.org/10.1016/j.ijom.2013.10.020. Epub 2013 Dec 9
16. Cassi D, De Biase C, Tonni I, Gandolfini M, Di Blasio A, Piancino MG. Natural position of the head: review of two-dimensional and three-dimensional methods of recording. Br J Oral Maxillofac Surg. 2016;54(3):233–40. https://doi.org/10.1016/j.bjoms.2015.12.020.
17. Cintra O, Coachman C. Standardized digital photography for virtual orthognathic surgical planning. Sel Read Oral Maxillofac Surg. 2020;20(3):7–8.
18. Clegg DJ, Deek AJ, Blackburn C, Scott CA, Daggett JR. The use and outcomes of 3D printing in pediatric craniofacial surgery: a systematic review. J Craniofac Surg. 2024;35:749.

19. Day KM, Gabrick KS, Sargent LA. Applications of computer technology in complex craniofacial reconstruction. Plast Reconstr Surg Glob Open. 2018;6:e1655.
20. Deliege L, Carriero A, Ong J, James G, Jeelani O, Dunaway D, Stoltz P, Hersh D, Martin J, Carroll K, Chamis M, Schievano S, Bookland M, Borghi A. A computational modelling tool for prediction of head reshaping following endoscopic strip craniectomy and helmet therapy for the treatment of scaphocephaly. Comput Biol Med. 2024;177:108633.
21. De Vos W, Casselman J, Swennen GRJ. Cone-beam computerized tomography (CBCT) imaging of the oral and maxillofacial region: A systematic review of the literature. Int J Oral Maxillofac Surg. 2009;38(6):609–25
22. Díaz-Cárdenas S, Pérez-Sayáns M, Gándara-Vila P. Accuracy of silicone versus wax in occlusal registrations for orthognathic surgery. J Prosthet Dent. 2021;126(3):377–84. https://doi.org/10.1016/j.prosdent.2021.03.002.
23. Farrell BB, Franco PB, Tucker MR. Virtual surgical planning in orthognathic surgery. Oral Maxillofac Surg Clin North Am. 2014;26(4):459–73. https://doi.org/10.1016/j.coms.2014.08.011. Epub 2014 Sep 22
24. Farrell G, Tseloni, A, Tilley N. Why the crime drop? Crime and Justice. 2014;43(1):421–494.
25. Ferri J, Schlund M, Touzet-Roumazeille S. Orthognathic surgery in Craniosynostosis. J Craniofac Surg. 2021;32(1):141–8. https://doi.org/10.1097/SCS.0000000000007154.
26. Foti S, Rickart AJ, Koo B, O' Sullivan E, van de Lande LS, Papaioannou A, Khonsari R, Stoyanov D, Jeelani NUO, Schievano S, Dunaway DJ, Clarkson MJ. Latent disentanglement in mesh variational autoencoders improves the diagnosis of craniofacial syndromes and aids surgical planning. Comput Methods Programs Biomed. 2024;256:108395.
27. Freitas JA, Garib DG, Trindade-Suedam IK, Carvalho RM, Oliveira TM, de Lauris RC, Almeida AL, Neves LT, Yaedú RY, Soares S, Mazzottini R, Pinto JH. Rehabilitative treatment of cleft lip and palate: experience of the Hospital for Rehabilitation of Craniofacial Anomalies-USP (HRAC-USP)–part 3: oral and maxillofacial surgery. J Appl Oral Sci. 2012;20(6):673–9. https://doi.org/10.1590/s1678-77572012000600014. PMID: 23329251; PMCID: PMC3881850.
28. Froehler MT, Saver JL, Zaidat OO, Jahan R, Jovin TG, Levy EI. Interhospital Transfer Before Thrombectomy Is Associated With Delayed Treatment and Poorer Outcomes: Results From the STRATIS Registry. Circulation. 2017;136(13):1198–1208.
29. García-Mato D, Porras AR, Ochandiano S, Rogers GF, García-Leal R, Salmerón JI, Pascau J, Linguraru MG. Effectiveness of automatic planning of fronto-orbital advancement for the surgical correction of metopic craniosynostosis. Plast Reconstr Surg Glob Open. 2021;9:e3937.
30. Gateno J, Teichgraeber JF, Xia JJ. Three-dimensional surgical planning for maxillofacial surgery. J Oral Maxillofac Surg. 2011;69(3):662–71. https://doi.org/10.1016/j.joms.2010.10.006.
31. Ghanem AA, Hamad OA, Almukhtar AM, Sleem HA. Physical versus digital Orthognathic surgical planning. J Craniofac Surg. 2022;33(6):1816–9. https://doi.org/10.1097/SCS.0000000000008462. Epub 2022 Jan 7
32. Gillies H, Harrison SH. Operative correction by osteotomy of recessed malar maxillary compound in a case of oxycephaly. Br J Plast Surg. 1950;3(2):123–7. https://doi.org/10.1016/s0007-1226(50)80019-x.
33. Glovsky TE, Iwasaki LR, Wu Y, Liu H, Liu Y, Sousa Melo SL, Nickel JC. Orthognathic surgery effects on temporomandibular joint compressive stresses. Orthod Craniofac Res. 2023;26(Suppl 1):142–50. https://doi.org/10.1111/ocr.12659. Epub 2023 Apr 7
34. Guérin J, Hennocq Q, Paternoster G, Arnaud É, Khonsari RH. Distractor position and distraction amplitude in fronto-facial monobloc advancement: a case series. J Stomatol Oral Maxillofac Surg. 2024;125:101942.
35. Han JT, Egbert MA, Ettinger RE, Kapadia HP, Susarla SM. Orthognathic surgery in patients with syndromic Craniosynostosis. Oral Maxillofac Surg Clin North Am. 2022;34(3):477–87. https://doi.org/10.1016/j.coms.2022.01.003.
36. Harjunpää R, Alaluusua S, Leikola J, Heliövaara A. Le Fort I osteotomy in cleft patients: maxillary advancement and velopharyngeal function. J Craniomaxillofac Surg. 2019;47(12):1868–74. https://doi.org/10.1016/j.jcms.2019.11.017. Epub 2019 Nov 29
37. Hassan B, van der Stelt P, Sanderink G. Accuracy of three-dimensional measurements obtained from cone-beam computed tomography surface-rendered images for cephalometric analysis: influence of patient scanning position. Oral Surg Oral Med Oral Pathol Oral Radiol Endod. 2009;107(6):801–13. https://doi.org/10.1016/j.tripleo.2008.11.021.
38. Hennocq Q, Paternoster G, Collet C, Amiel J, Bongibault T, Bouygues T, Cormier-Daire V, Douillet M, Dunaway DJ, Jeelani NO, van de Lande LS, Lyonnet S, Ong J, Picard A, Rickart AJ, Rio M, Schievano S, Arnaud E, Garcelon N, Khonsari RH. AI-based diagnosis and phenotype – genotype correlations in syndromic craniosynostoses. J Craniomaxillofac Surg. 2024;52:1172–87.
39. Hernández-Alfaro F, Guijarro-Martínez R, Peiró-Guijarro MA. An overview of surgery-first orthognathic approach: History, indications and limitations, protocols, and dentoskeletal stability. J Oral Maxillofac Surg. 2021;79(6):1275–1284.
40. Hohoff A, Joos U, Meyer U, Ehmer U, Stamm T. The spectrum of Apert syndrome: phenotype, particularities in orthodontic treatment, and characteristics of orthognathic surgery. Head Face Med. 2007;3:10.

https://doi.org/10.1186/1746-160X-3-10. PMID: 17286873; PMCID: PMC1821014.
41. Hu CH, Wu CT, Ko EW, Chen PK. Monobloc frontofacial or Le fort III distraction Osteogenesis in syndromic craniosynostosis: three-dimensional evaluation of treatment outcome and the need for central distraction. J Craniofac Surg. 2017;28(5):1344–9. https://doi.org/10.1097/SCS.0000000000003570.
42. Kahnberg KE, Hagberg C. Orthognathic surgery in patients with craniofacial syndrome. I. A 5-year overview of combined orthodontic and surgical correction. J Plast Surg Hand Surg. 2010;44(6):282–8. https://doi.org/10.3109/2000656X.2010.516594.
43. Khonsari RH, Way B, Nysjö J, Odri GA, Olszewski R, Evans RD, Dunaway DJ, Nyström I, Britto JA. Fronto-facial advancement and bipartition in Crouzon-Pfeiffer and Apert syndromes: impact of fronto-facial surgery upon orbital and airway parameters in FGFR2 syndromes. J Craniomaxillofac Surg. 2016;44:1567–75.
44. Khonsari RH, Adam J, Benassarou M, Bertin H, Billotet B, Bouaoud J, Bouletreau P, Garmi R, Gellée T, Haen P, Ketoff S, Lescaille G, Louvrier A, Lutz JC, Makaremi M, Nicot R, Pham-Dang N, Praud M, Saint-Pierre F, Schouman T, Sicard L, Simon F, Wojcik T, Meyer C, French Society of Stomatology, Maxillo-Facial Surgery and Oral Surgery (SFSCMFCO). In-house 3D printing: why, when, and how? Overview of the national French good practice guidelines for in-house 3D-printing in maxillo-facial surgery, stomatology, and oral surgery. J Stomatol Oral Maxillofac Surg. 2021;122:458–61.
45. Khonsari RH. Emergency medical 3D printing – a case study during the COVID19 pandemic. L'Harmattan; 2023. p. 298.
46. Khonsari RH. Digital fabrication in craniofacial surgery. In: Mallakpour S, Hussain CM, editors. Medical additive manufacturing. Concepts and fundamentals. Elsevier; 2024. p. 251–66.
47. Ko EW, Huang CS, Chen YR. Characteristics and corrective outcome of face asymmetry by orthognathic surgery. J Oral Maxillofac Surg. 2009;67(10):2201–9. https://doi.org/10.1016/j.joms.2009.04.039.
48. Kogou T, Takaki T, Shibahara T. Three-dimensional analysis and evaluation in Orthognathic surgical cases with facial asymmetry. Bull Tokyo Dent Coll. 2018;59(3):147–61. https://doi.org/10.2209/tdcpublication.2017-0008.
49. Kortesniemi M, De Foer B. Cone beam computed tomography versus multislice CT in diagnostic imaging: comparative advantages and limitations. J Int Adv Otol. 2023;16(2):222–6.
50. Kusnoto P, Kaur A, Salem, et al. Implementation of ultra-low-dose CBCT for routine 2D orthodontic diagnostic radiographs: cephalometric landmark identification and image quality assessment. Semin Orthod. 2015;21(4):233–47.
51. Lande R, Engen S, Sæther BE. Corrigendum: Phenotypic selection in natural populations: what have we learned? Ecology Letters. 2021;24(10):2259–60
52. Larrabee WF Jr, Maupin G, Sutton D. Profile analysis in facial plastic surgery. Arch Otolaryngol. 1985;111(10):682–7. https://doi.org/10.1001/archotol.1985.00800120076010.
53. Laure B, Louisy A, Joly A, Travers N, Listrat A, Pare A. Virtual 3D planning of osteotomies for craniosynostoses and complex craniofacial malformations. Neurochirurgie. 2019;65:269–78.
54. Lee YC, Kim SG. Redefining precision and efficiency in orthognathic surgery through virtual surgical planning and 3D printing: a narrative review. Maxillofac Plast Reconstr Surg. 2023;45(1):42. https://doi.org/10.1186/s40902-023-00409-2. PMID: 38108939; PMCID: PMC10728393.
55. Liang C, Profico A, Buzi C, Khonsari RH, Johnson D, O'Higgins P, Moazen M. Normal human craniofacial growth and development from 0 to 4 years. Sci Rep. 2023;13:9641.
56. Liu C, Lin Y, Lin S, Yao C. Accuracy and clinical efficacy of computer-assisted orthognathic surgery: A systematic review and meta-analysis. Int J Oral Maxillofac Surg. 2021;50(7):911–23. https://doi.org/10.1016/j.ijom.2020.11.002.
57. Lu X, Forte AJ, Sawh-Martinez R, Wu R, Cabrejo R, Wilson A, Steinbacher DM, Alperovich M, Alonso N, Persing JA. Spatial and temporal changes of midface in Apert's syndrome. J Plast Surg Hand Surg. 2019;53(3):130–7. https://doi.org/10.1080/2000656X.2018.1541324. Epub 2019 Feb 19
58. Lundström F, Lundström A. Natural head position as a basis for cephalometric analysis. Am J Orthod Dentofacial Orthop. 1992;101(3):244–7. https://doi.org/10.1016/0889-5406(92)70093-P.
59. Maintz M, Desan N, Sharma N, Beinemann J, Beyer M, Seiler D, Honigmann P, Soleman J, Guzman R, Cattin PC, Thieringer FM. Fronto-orbital advancement with patient-specific 3D-printed implants and robot-guided laser osteotomy: an in vitro accuracy assessment. Int J Comput Assist Radiol Surg. 2024. (in the press);20:513.
60. Metzger MC, Hohlweg-Majert B, Schwarz U, et al. Manufacturing splints for orthognathic surgery using three-dimensional printer technology. J Oral Maxillofac Surg. 2008;66(6):1446–52. https://doi.org/10.1016/j.joms.2007.12.022.
61. Nout E, Koudstaal MJ, Wolvius EB, Van der Wal KG. Additional orthognathic surgery following Le Fort III and monobloc advancement. Int J Oral Maxillofac Surg. 2011;40(7):679–84. https://doi.org/10.1016/j.ijom.2011.02.014. Epub 2011 Mar 12

62. Parikh N, Aral A, Lewis K, Alperovich M. Application of computerized surgical planning in craniosynostosis surgery. Semin Plast Surg. 2024;38:214–23.
63. Park JU, Lee JS, Kim YI, Son WS. Photogrammetric analysis in orthognathic surgery: benefits and reliability. Pocket Dentistry; 2022.
64. Quast A, Santander P, Kahlmeier T, Moser N, Schliephake H, Meyer-Marcotty P. Predictability of maxillary positioning: a 3D comparison of virtual and conventional orthognathic surgery planning. Head Face Med. 2021;17(1):27. https://doi.org/10.1186/s13005-021-00279-x. PMID: 34256775; PMCID: PMC8276391.
65. Resnick SM, Cheng R, Simpson M, Lourenco F. Marketing in SMEs: a "4Ps" Self-Branding Model. Int J Entrep Behav Res. 2016;22(2):229–48.
66. Rostamzad P, Abdel-Alim T, Wolvius EB, Roshchupkin G, van Veelen ML, Pleumeekers MM. Three-dimensional quantification of soft tissue changes and its relationship to skeletal changes after Le Fort III, monobloc, and facial bipartition in syndromic craniosynostosis. Int J Oral Maxillofac Surg. 2024;53:989–96.
67. Sánchez Carretero D, Carretero M. Low-Carbon Planning for A Solar Energy Future. SSRN Electronic Journal. 2022.
68. Seruya M, Borsuk DE, Khalifian S, Carson BS, Dalesio NM, Dorafshar AH. Computer-aided design and manufacturing in craniosynostosis surgery. J Craniofac Surg. 2013;24:1100–5.
69. Soleman J, Thieringer F, Beinemann J, Kunz C, Guzman R. Computer-assisted virtual planning and surgical template fabrication for fronto-orbital advancement. Neurosurg Focus. 2015;38(5):E5.
70. Steinbacher DM. Three-dimensional analysis and surgical planning in craniomaxillofacial surgery. J Oral Maxillofac Surg. 2015;73:S40–56.
71. Stokbro K, Tostevin A, Thygesen T, Bell RB. Virtual planning in orthognathic surgery. Int J Oral Maxillofac Surg. 2014;43(8):933–940.
72. Stokbro K, Liebregts J, Baan F, de Koning M. Does Mandible-First Sequencing Increase Maxillary Surgical Accuracy in Bimaxillary Procedures? J Oral Maxillofac Surg. 2019;77(10):2137–44.
73. Vollmer H, Ahblom P, Cederberg E. Where the value is: Accounting and the shifting spheres: The economic, the public, the planet. Accounting, Organizations and Society. 2024;113:101675.
74. Vercruysse F, Naud R, Sprekeler H. Self-organization of a doubly asynchronous irregular network state for spikes and bursts. PLoS Comput Biol. 2021;17(11):e1009478.
75. Vercruysse H Jr, Rubio-Palau J, Van de Casteele E, Nadjmi N, De Praeter M, Dunaway D. Virtual planning in Le Fort III distraction osteogenesis: a case series. J Craniomaxillofac Surg. 2021;49:341–6.
76. Wu KL, Lu TC, Lin TC, Chan CS, Wu CT. Application of virtual planning and 3-dimensional printing guide in surgical management of craniosynostosis. World Neurosurg. 2024;194:123475.
77. Xia JJ, Phillips CV, Gateno J. A new paradigm for planning orthognathic surgery: the use of digital technology and 3D printing. J Oral Maxillofac Surg. 2015;73(7):1405–19. https://doi.org/10.1016/j.joms.2015.01.034.
78. Xue A, Wu Y, Zhu Z, Zhang F, Kemper KE, Zheng Z, Visscher PM. Genome-wide association analyses identify 143 risk variants and putative regulatory mechanisms for type 2 diabetes. Nat Commun. 2018;9(1):2941
79. Yoshikawa H, Tanikawa C, Ito S, Tsukiboshi Y, Ishii H, Kanomi R, Yamashiro T. A three-dimensional cephalometric analysis of Japanese adults and its usefulness in orthognathic surgery: A retrospective study. J Craniomaxillofac Surg. 2022;50(4):353–63. https://doi.org/10.1016/j.jcms.2022.02.002. Epub 2022 Feb 18
80. Zhang N, Liu S, Yu H, Shen SGF. Three-dimensional printing technology in orthognathic surgery: A systematic review. Int J Oral Maxillofac Surg. 2019;48(7):973–82. https://doi.org/10.1016/j.ijom.2019.01.029.
81. Zhao C, Teng L. Application and development of orthognathic surgery in treatment of syndromic craniosynostosis. Zhongguo Xiu Fu Chong Jian Wai Ke Za Zhi. 2023;37(7):879–84. https://doi.org/10.7507/1002-1892.202302102. Chinese. PMID: 37460186; PMCID: PMC10352517.

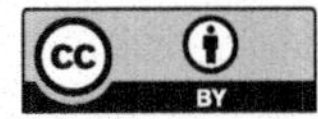

28 Aesthetic Refinements

Eric Arnaud

Introduction

Unless significant cognitive deficits are at play, almost all children with Apert syndrome express the need for cosmetic improvement before reaching adulthood. Early aggressive surgical treatment and strong family support play important roles in achieving better psychosocial outcomes. Aesthetic refinements in faciocraniosynostoses are usually requested around adolescence or later [1]. No usual protocol or predefined sequence of interventions has been established; instead, a variable set of ancillary procedures is available.

An orthognathic procedure is often necessary for patients with Apert syndrome. After 14 years of age, the orthognathic procedure should be performed before other aesthetic procedures, particularly rhinoplasty and other soft tissue improvements.

The non-exhaustive list of possible improvements for faciocraniosynostoses includes:

A. Bicoronal scar revision
B. Frontal sinus reduction (particularly in Apert syndrome)
C. Correction of frontal/calvarial irregularities
D. Lateral/medial canthopexies
E. Genioplasty (advancement)
F. Rhinoseptoplasty (especially after Le Fort III (LFIII), which disrupts the nasal dorsum)
G. Fat grafting in the temporal and zygomatic regions

Figures 28.1, 28.2, 28.3, 28.4, 28.5, 28.6, and 28.7, which show various patterns of surgical strategy, will describe and illustrate these techniques.

E. Arnaud (✉)
Craniofacial Unit, Hôpital Necker–Enfants malades, Paris, France

Craniofacial Rare Diseases Competence Center, Clinique Marcel Sembat, Ramsay, Boulogne Billancourt, France

J. G. Meara et al. (eds.), *Apert Syndrome*, https://doi.org/10.1007/978-3-032-12551-4_28

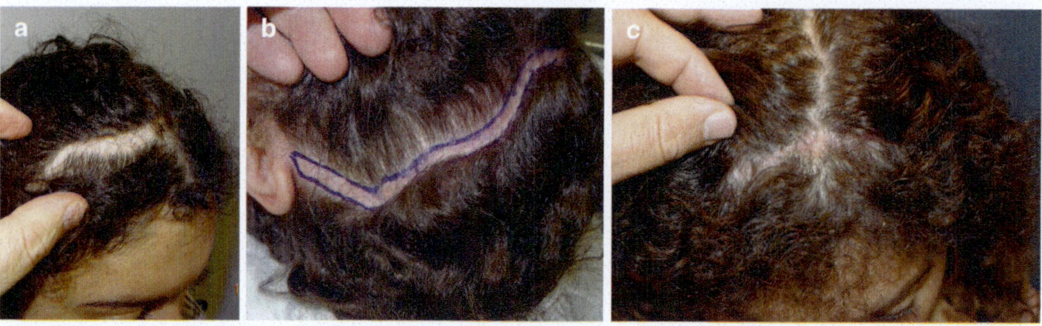

Fig. 28.1 (**a–c**) Patient reaching adulthood with a 1-cm wide coronal scar. (**a**) Before surgery. (**b**) Design of scar resection before infiltration. Avoid cautery and use 3/0 Rapide Vicryl to close the wound. (**c**) Result at six months

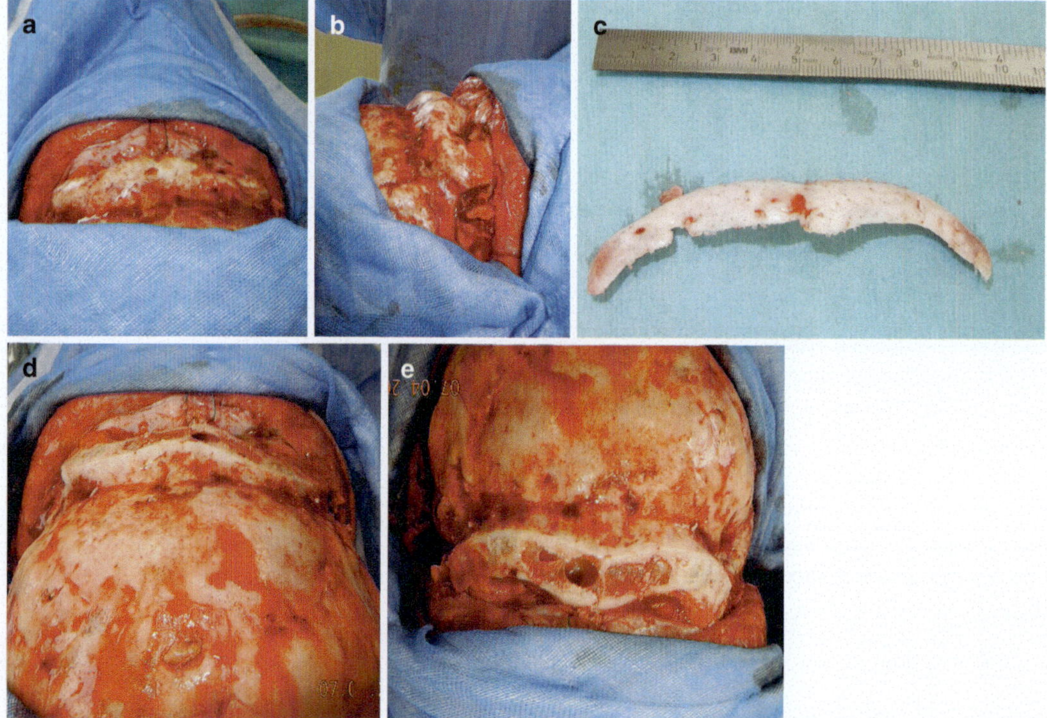

Fig. 28.2 (**a**, **b**) Preoperative view showing the bulging of the supraorbital bar. (**c**) Longitudinal osteotomy of the supraorbital bar. (**d**, **e**) The supraorbital bar after the osteotomy indicated that the bulging was primarily the result of frontal sinus hyperpneumatization. (**f**, **g**, **h**, **i**) Fixation of the supraorbital bar using miniplates after volume reduction

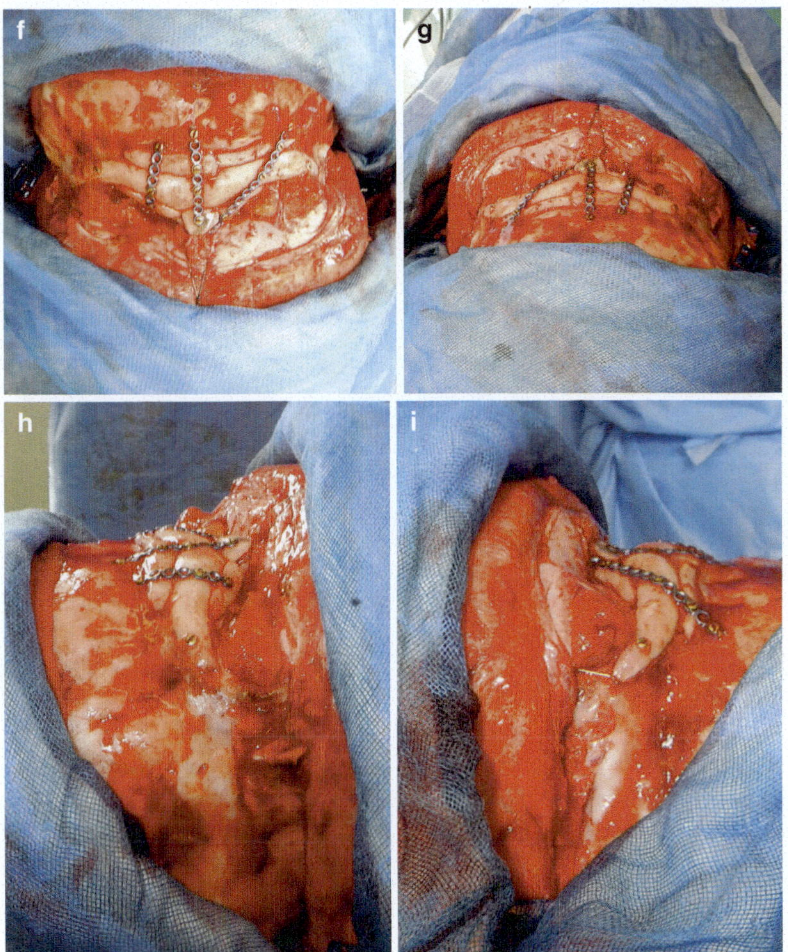

Fig. 28.2 (continued)

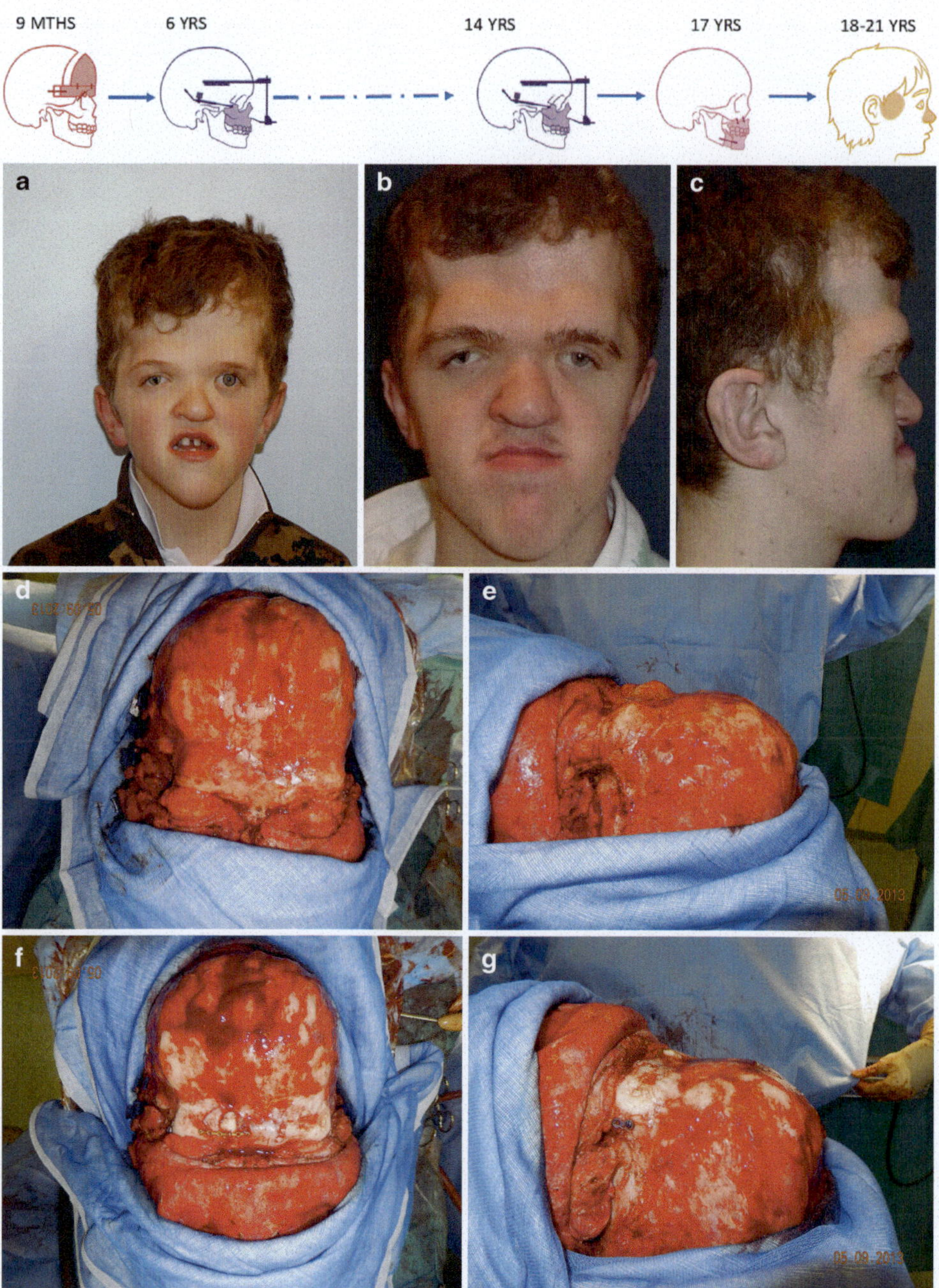

Fig. 28.3 Child with Apert syndrome treated with a two-stage strategy starting with a fronto-orbital advancement in infancy followed by Le Fort III at adolescence. (**a**) Child with Apert syndrome at the age of six years before first Le Fort III. (**b**, **c**) At the age of 15 years, before a second Le Fort III, frontal sinus reduction, and correction of frontal irregularities by burring. (**d**, **e**) Front and profile view of frontal irregularities. (**f**, **g**) Front and profile view after frontal sinus reduction. (**h**, **i**) Postoperative clinical results after Le Fort III and frontal sinus reduction. (**j**, **k**) At the age of 17 before augmentation rhinoplasty. (**l**) Harvesting of sixth left chondrocostal rib graft before sculpting. (**m**) Dorsal graft and columellar strut in a tongue and groove connection. (**n**) Insertion of both grafts through a closed approach. (**o**, **p**) Immediate result of augmentation rhinoplasty. (**q**, **r**) Result at the age of 18 years. (**s**, **t**) Stable result at the age of 21 years

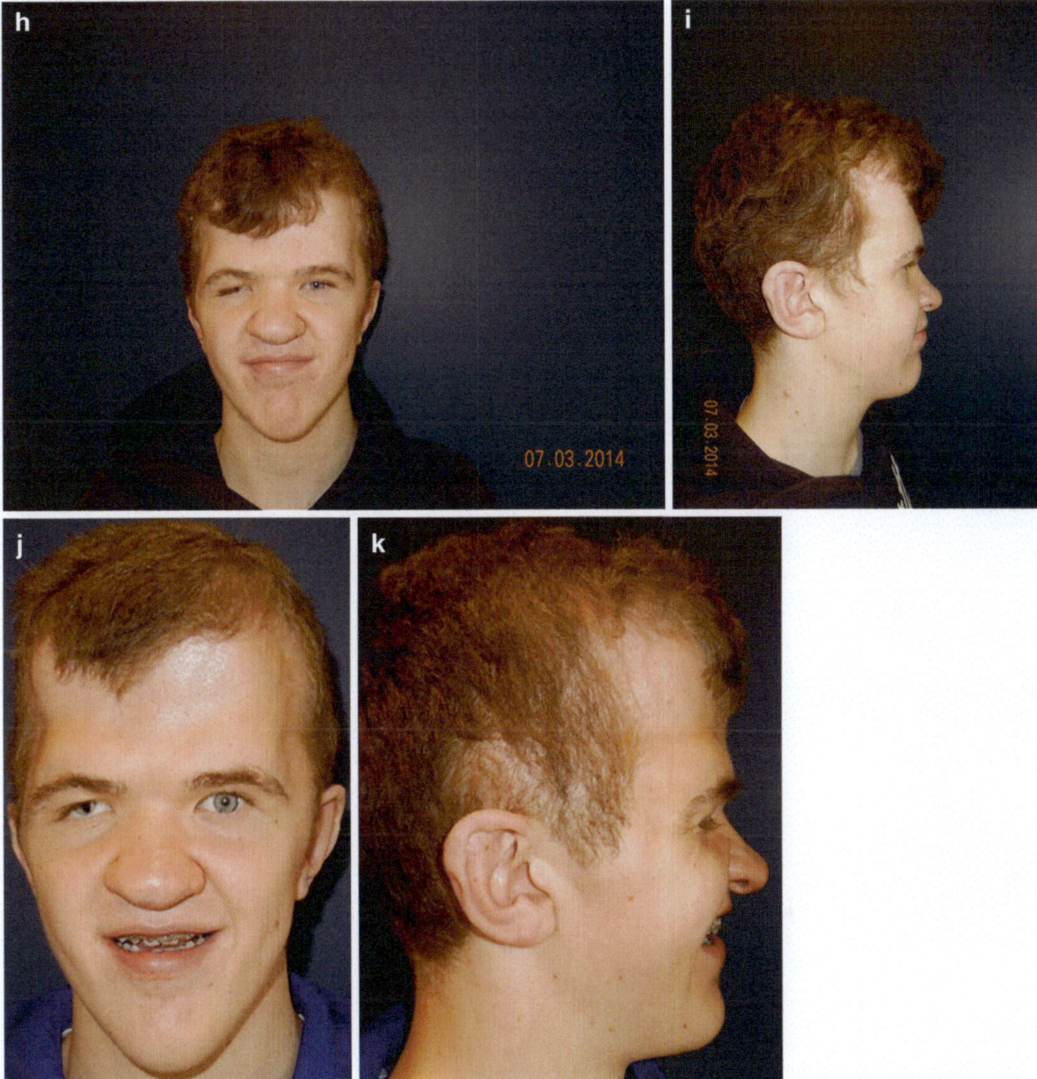

Fig. 28.3 (continued)

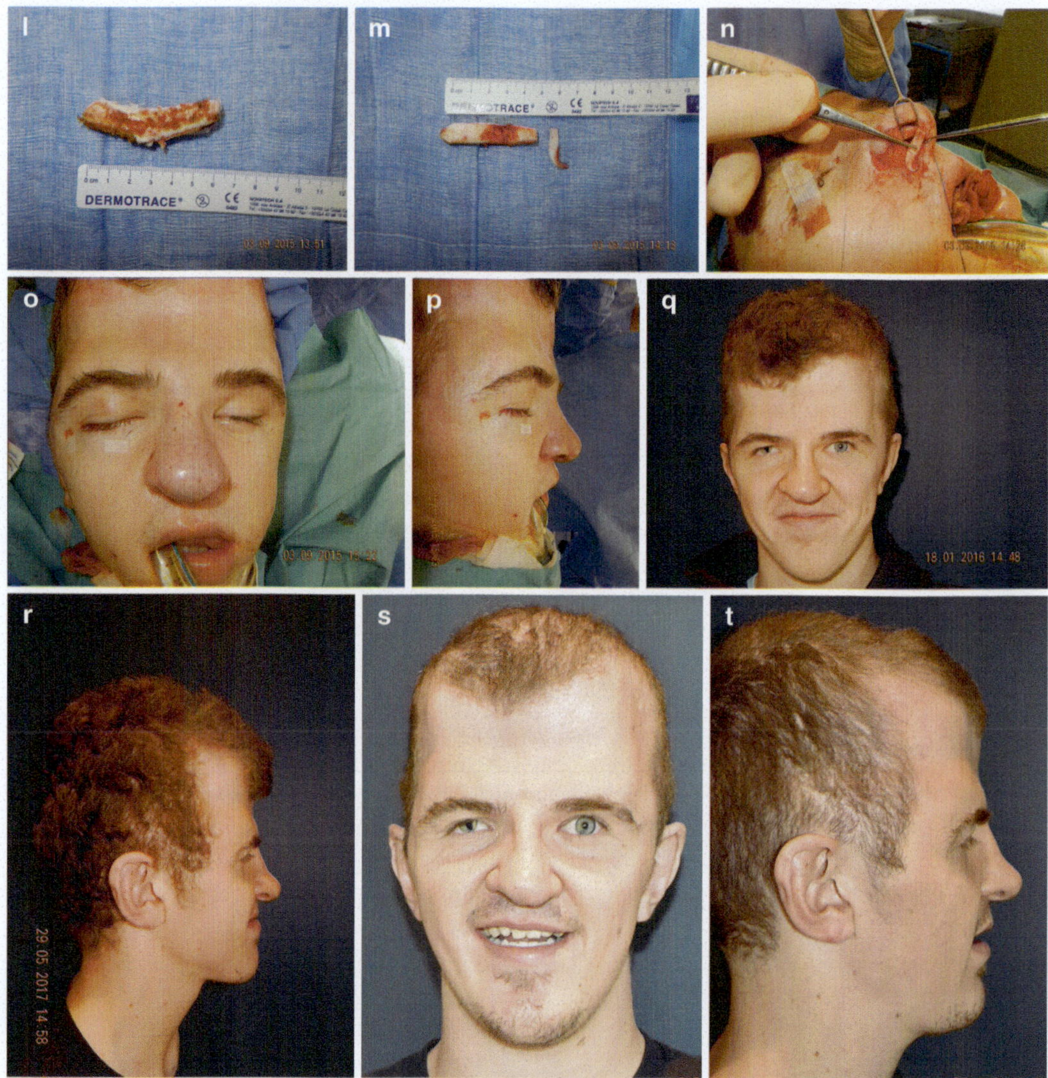

Fig. 28.3 (continued)

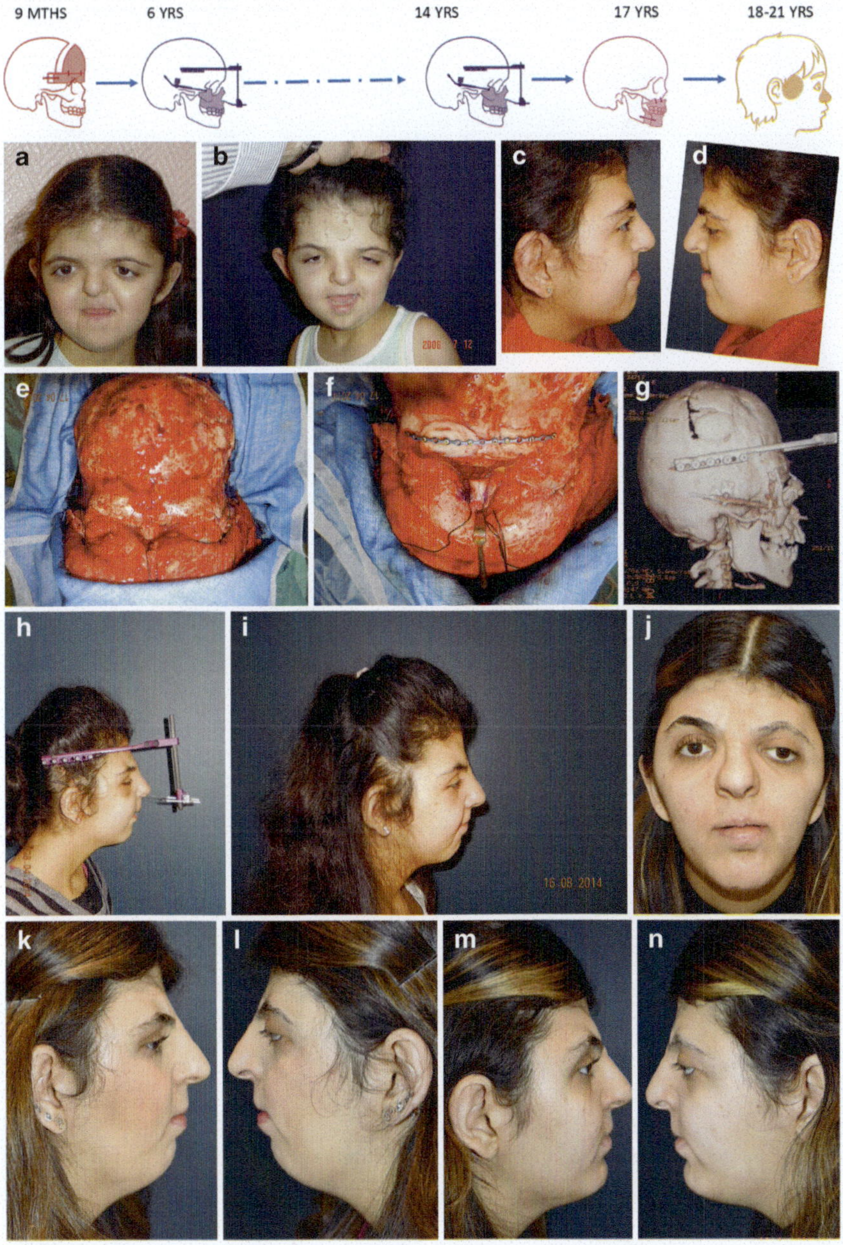

9 MTHS 6 YRS 14 YRS 17 YRS 18-21 YRS

Fig. 28.4 Surgical sequence without monobloc. (**a**) Young child with Apert syndrome at the age of two years after fronto-orbital advancement. (**b**) At the age of six years. (**c, d**) At the age 12 years before Le Fort III and correction of frontal irregularities. (**e**) Frontal aspect with hypertrophic supraorbital bar. (**F**) Frontal aspect after frontal reduction and osteosynthesis at the time of Le Fort III. (**g**) Profile view of computed tomography scan after osteotomy with internal and external distractors. (**h**) Profile view of patient with both distractors. (**i**) Profile view six months after removing the distractors.. (**j**) Front view before genioplasty and fat grafting. (**k, l**) Lateral view before genioplasty and fat grafting. (**m, n**) Lateral view after advancement genioplasty. (**o**) Rhinoplasty and fat grafting. (**p–r**) Front and profile view after rhinoplasty, temporal fat grafting, and left lateral canthopexy. (**s, t**) Final results of computed tomography scan at the age of 21 years. (**u, v**) Final clinical result front and profile at the age of 21 years

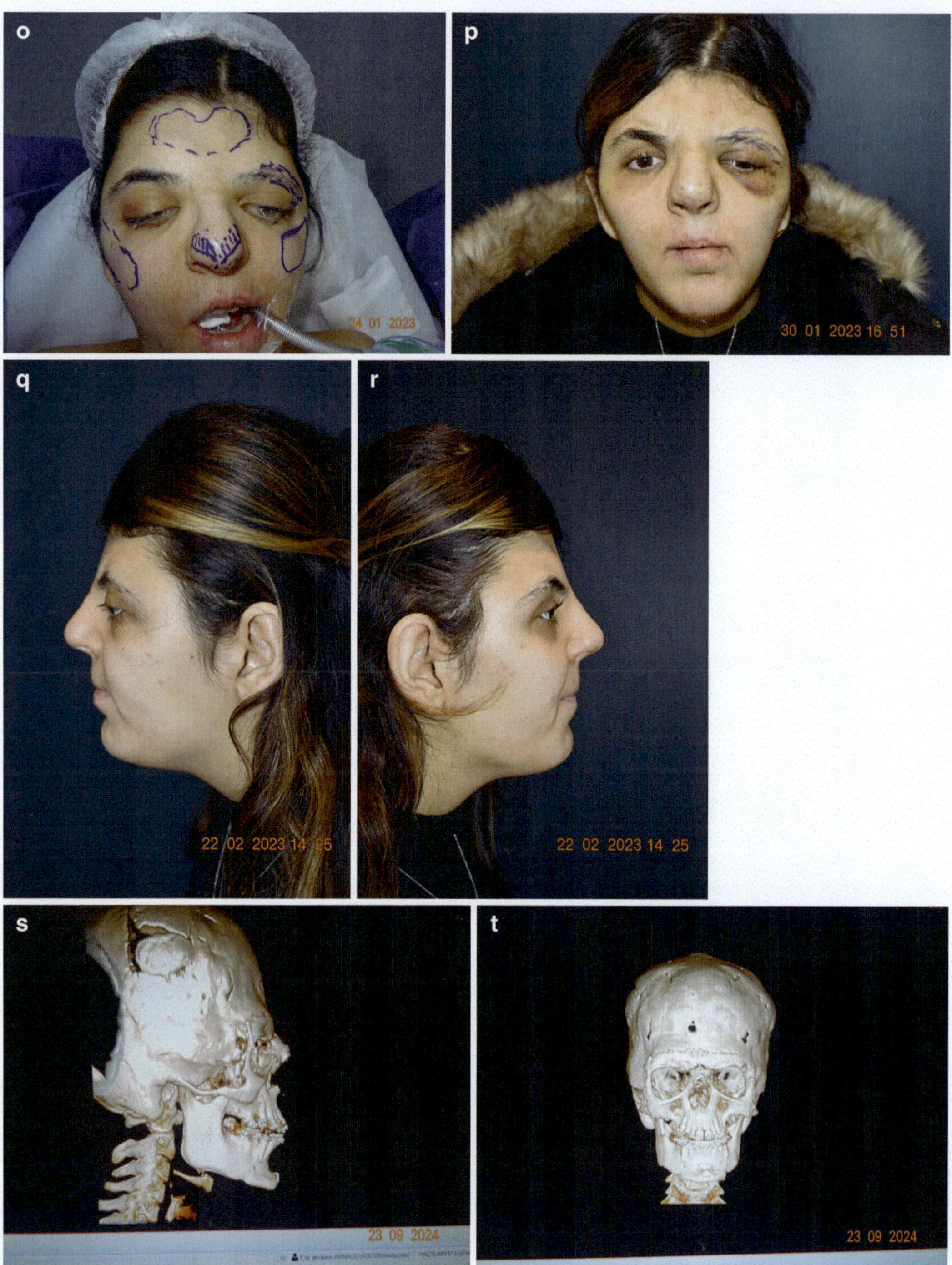

Fig. 28.4 (continued)

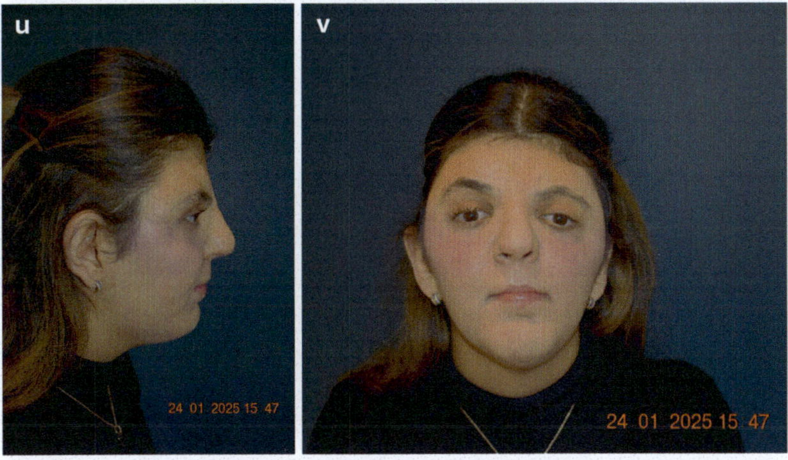

Fig. 28.4 (continued)

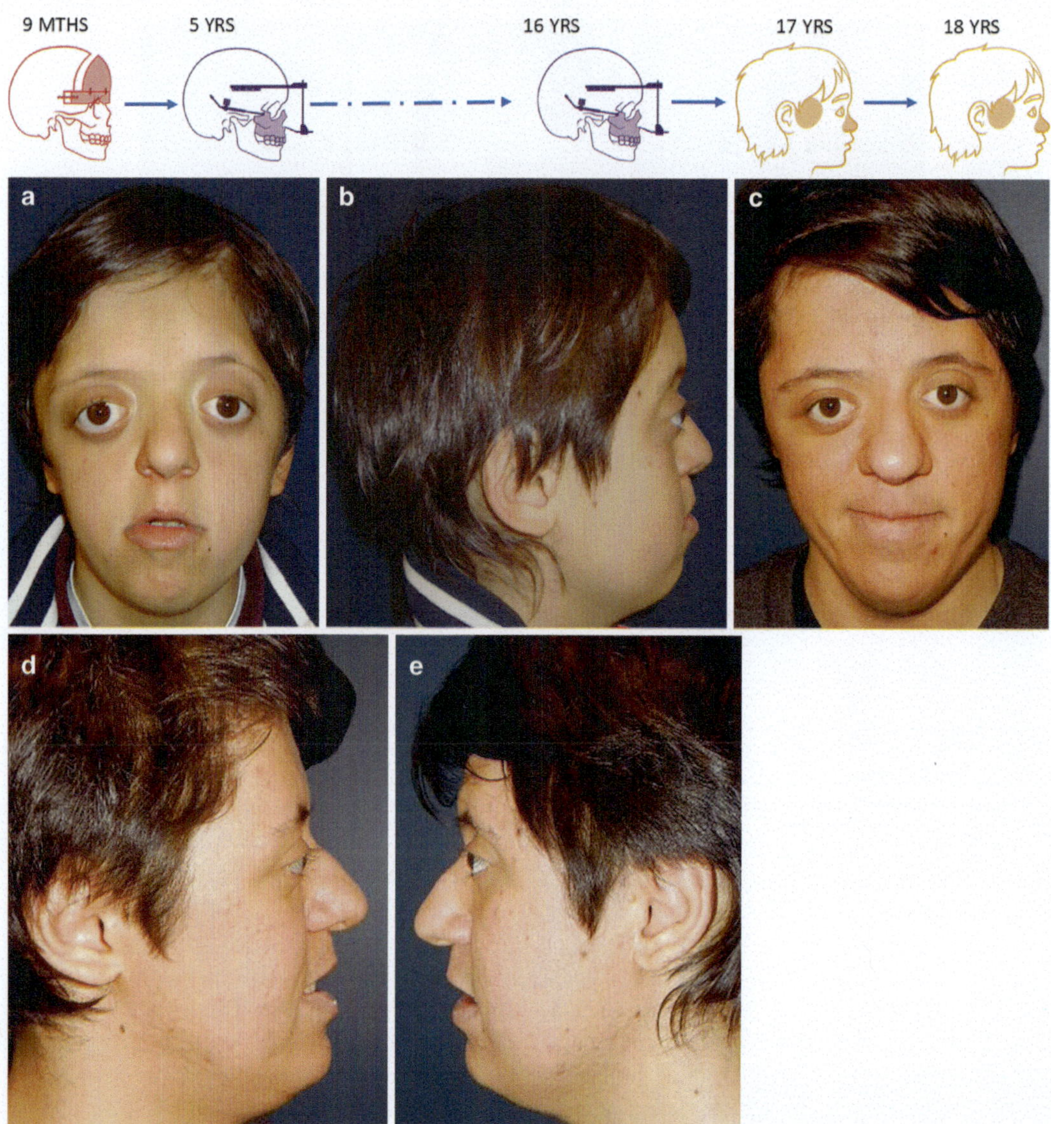

Fig. 28.5 Apert syndrome treated by a sequence without monobloc. (**a**, **b**) At the age of seven years. Front and profile view after fronto-orbital advancement in infancy and early Le Fort III with internal distractor at five years. (**c–e**) Clinical view at the age of 16 years before Le Fort III. Observe asymmetry. (**f**, **g**) Per operative view before and after burring as well as saw reduction in glabellar prominence at the time of Le Fort III. (**h**, **i**) Final result on computed tomography scan, without need of orthognathic surgery. (**j**, **k**) Final clinical result at the age of 21 years after fat grafting and rhinoplasty

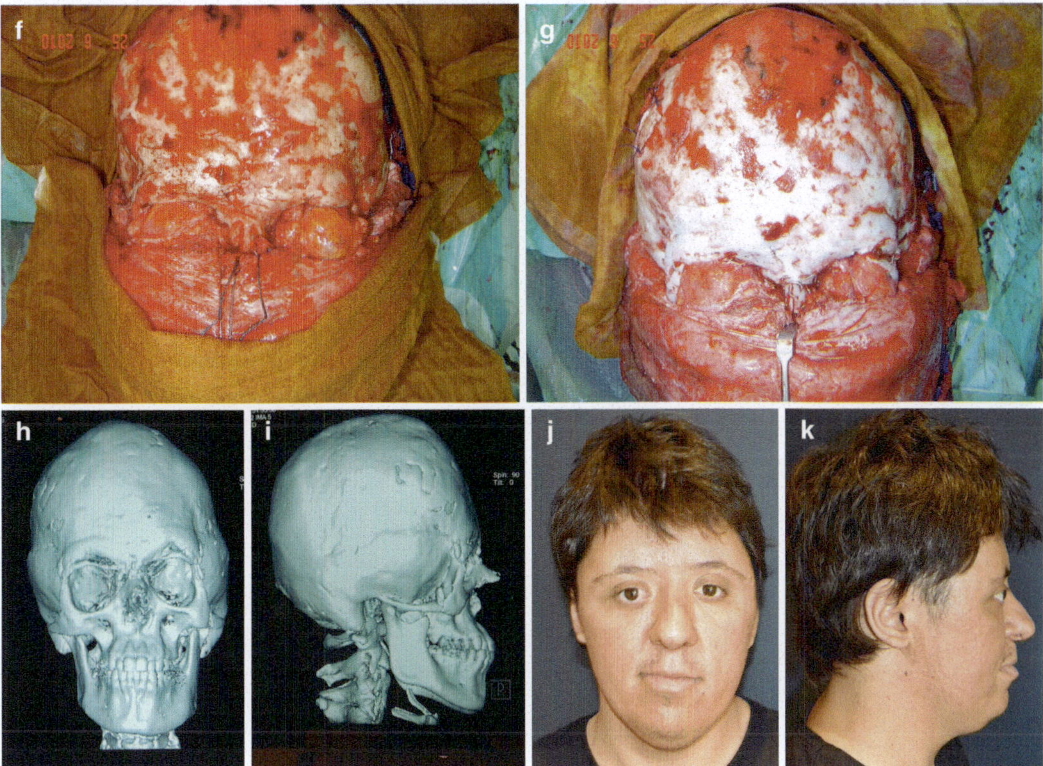

Fig. 28.5 (continued)

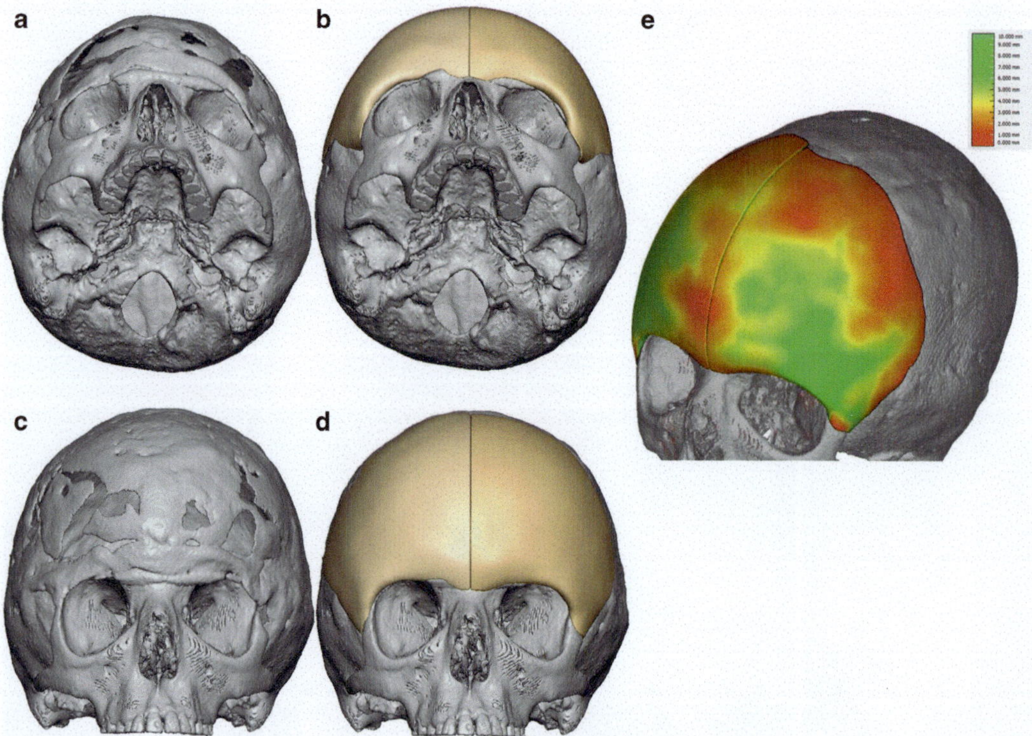

Fig. 28.6 (**a**–**d**) Polyetheretherketone implants covering frontal irregularities. (**e**) Heat map showing the depth of the implants for safe and proper screw fixation

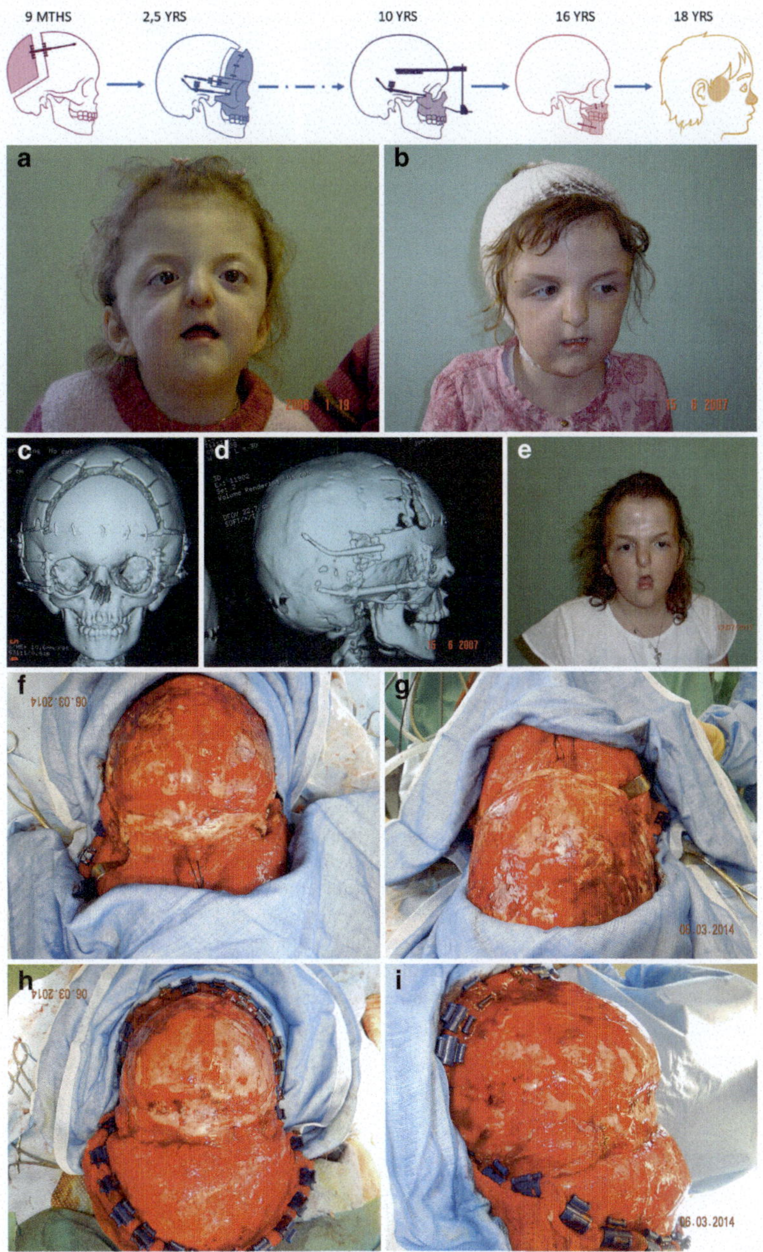

Fig. 28.7 Apert syndrome treated initially by monobloc. (**a**) At the age of 18 months after posterior distraction. (**b**) At the age of three years, six months after monobloc at the time of distractor removal. (**c, d**) Computed tomography scan at the time of distractor removal. (**e**) Clinical view at the age of eight years showing frontal irregularities. (**f, g**) Per operative view at the age of ten years before removing frontal irregularities. (**h, i**) Preoperative view after removal of frontal irregularities harvested for bone grafting. (**j**) Clinical view with external distractors, with internal distractors in place. (**k**) Clinical view two years after Le Fort III, before orthognathic surgery. (**l**) Computed tomography scan after orthognathic surgery and before rhinoplasty. (**m**) Clinical view at 17 years of age before rhinoplasty and fat grafting. (**n, o**) Final clinical result at 19 years of age

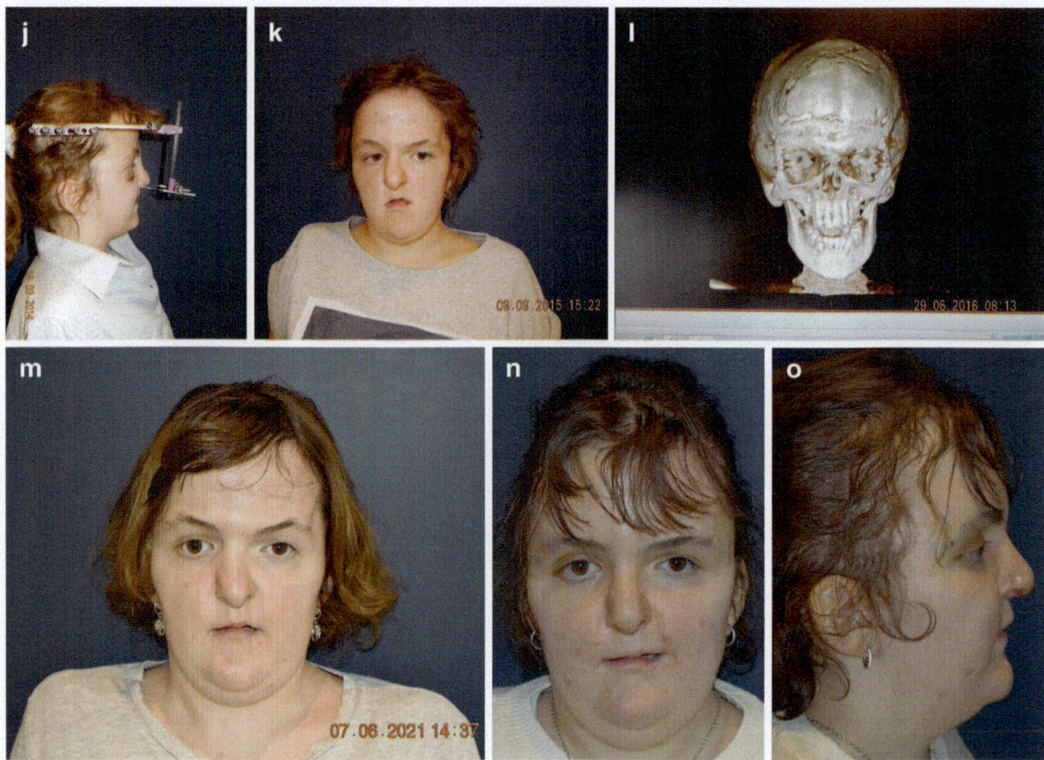

Fig. 28.7 (continued)

A. Bicoronal Scar Revision

Bicoronal scar widening is typically bitemporal but can occur at the vertex. Patients with Apert syndrome often present hyperlaxity, and hypertrophic scarring is less common. Both conditions may demand aesthetic scar improvement in adolescence or adulthood. Given the thick dermis of the scalp, scar revision may or may not achieve improvement, making patient information crucial in managing expectations. Generally, a 50% width reduction is possible after completion of skull growth (Fig. 28.1). Skull growth is an intrinsic factor of coronal scar enlargement—explaining why scalp surgery in infancy evolves toward constant enlargement—and therefore scar reduction is not advised in patients younger than six years old.

B. Frontal Sinus Reduction

Frontofacial monobloc advancement (FFMBA) can lead the supraorbital ridge to overproject and/or become hypertrophic, particularly in patients with Apert syndrome. This hypertrophy can be purely bony or associated with an over-pneumatized frontal sinus. Frequently encountered in Apert syndrome, an enlarged frontal sinus may be related to the FFMBA (Fig. 28.2a–e). The procedure preserves the vascularization of the supraorbital ridge and is associated with a consistent decrease in raised intracranial pressure. However, an enlarged frontal sinus is also encountered after single fronto-orbital advancement with bone devascularization.

The consequences of enlarged frontal sinus are strictly aesthetic; the over-projecting glabellar region and supraorbital ridge cause masculinization of the face in women and a dysmorphic appearance in men. Surgical treatment is performed through the pre-existing bicoronal scar. Once the forehead bone is exposed, the reciprocating saw is used to carefully harvest an oval-shaped bony cap spanning the glabella and both supraorbital regions. The underlying bone projection is then uniformly reduced with a surgical bur. Typically, the frontal sinus is widely exposed in this process. The entire sinus mucosa is removed with a microdiamond bur. Abundant irrigation with normal saline is applied to avoid debris blocking sinus drainage at the level of the frontal ostium.

Care is taken to avoid excessive widening of the sinus opening, as this can cause the bony cap to fall into the sinus cavity. The surgical bur is used to thin the bony cap, which is ultimately repositioned using titanium microplates and screws. In cases where thickening is strictly bony, the prominent area is burred to an acceptable level. It is critical to provide a stable metallic osteosynthesis with a titanium microplate to immobilize the segmental tap (Figs. 28.3b–i and 28.4e, f). Given the risk of contamination, we do not advise using resorbable plates.

C. Burring of Frontal/Calvarial Irregularities

Bony forehead or irregularities in the hair-bearing region are frequently palpable in patients with Apert syndrome who have undergone surgery. For unclear reasons, such irregularities are more frequent in this patient group than in non-Apert post-surgical faciocraniosynostoses. Surgery is only justified if the irregularities cause visible deformity or asymmetry with meets aesthetic demands. In such cases, surgery is indicated using the pre-existing bicoronal approach to flatten the bony lumps with a surgical bur (Figs. 28.5f, g and 28.7f–i). This procedure can be complemented with frontal sinus reduction, detailed in the previous paragraph, which is more anatomical and avoids alloplastic material. Saw reduction in irregularities and frontal sinus reduction can be performed in conjunction with LFIII advancement, as these steps can provide the bone grafts used at the orbital level.

Although alloplastic onlay implants have been used in cases of significant frontal irregularities, we have ceased this practice due to possible risks of infections. Made on location in real time with modeled polymethylmethacrylate, these implants join with the native forehead in a junction that is often visible. More recently, polyetheretherketone was introduced in craniofacial surgery and is used in patient-specific implants. These alternative implants provide excellent contour and fit with a low complication rate (Fig. 28.6a–e) [2, 3].

D1. Lateral Canthopexy

Patients with Apert syndrome frequently present with downward slanting of the palpebral fissures. The lateral canthal descent is related to the syndrome or the subperiosteal undermining, causing soft tissues to sag. This inferior displacement could be caused by gravity and/or the inelastic maxillary periosteal downward traction during maxillary distraction.

The indication for lateral canthopexy can be curative in patients who display slanting of the palpebral fissures or prophylactic during FFMBA or LFIII to prevent this type of deformity [4].

Technically, the lateral canthopexies have been detailed in chapter Peri ophtalmologic improvement on ophthalmic and periorbital procedures. When a coronal approach is used for the aesthetic revision, the lateral and medial canthopexies can be performed from a superior approach. Otherwise, the canthopexies have to be performed through minimal palpebral approaches. Complications of lateral canthopexy include relapse and extrusion of the suture material.

D2. Medial Canthopexy

The main objective of medial canthopexy in patients with Apert syndrome is reducing intercanthal distance. Indicated in patients with hypertelorism and telecanthus, the procedure is usually performed in patients with Apert syndrome during bipartition and medial rotation of the LFIII segments.

Stainless steel wires are used transnasally to medialize the medial canthi. When performed bilaterally, the canthopexy wires can be tied together transnasally or at the base of the nasal root. Otherwise, the wire is anchored contralaterally around a bone graft or a twisted locking wire. This procedure is standard during the LFIII (Fig. 28.4t) or may complement an augmentation rhinoplasty.

E. Genioplasty (Advancement Type)

Overcorrection during LFIII can lead to the development of mandibular retrusion with retrogenia in children with Apert syndrome. Although orthognathic surgery usually addresses the mandibular malposition, in many cases genioplasty remains necessary for optimal projection after LFIII. The inferior vestibular surgical approach is classically used with horizontal suprabasilar osteotomy, advancement, and osteosynthesis with locking plates and/or lag screws [5]. Genioplasty is typically performed during orthognathic surgery but may be performed separately at the time of rhinoplasty (Fig. 28.4l, m).

F. Rhinoseptoplasty

Rhinoseptoplasty is usually the last procedure to be performed on the face for patients with Apert syndrome. Commonly described as a finishing touch, the procedure yields significant aesthetic improvement and entails relatively minimal downtime compared to preceding facial advancements that are far more invasive. After FFMBA and LFIII, the nasal septum is characteristically deviated. The septum often presents a longitudinal fibrous fracture corresponding to the transnasal osteotomy line. When possible, dissecting the septal cartilage through this fibrous barrier should be avoided to preserve mucosal integrity (Fig. 28.4o–r). The dorsal hump is separated and removed as usual, regardless of the glabellar titanium plate previously inserted during LFIII facial advancement [1]. Despite the LFIII, an augmentation rhinoplasty with a chondral or osteochondral rib graft remains an excellent treatment for Apert nasal deformity, as it significantly enhances the medialization of the medial canthi (Fig. 28.3l–n).

G. Fat Grafting in the Temporal and Zygomatic Regions

Fat grafting to enhance the aesthetics of patients with Apert syndrome reaching adult age has become almost systematic. Mandatory limiting factors are the existence of a donor site and the absence of severe acne in the face.

Typical locations requiring fat grafting are the zygomatic regions and temporal regions, as previous distractions can cause retraction and hypotrophy of the temporal muscles (Fig. 28.4o). Given the resorption of fat in these locations, treatment often entails more than one session.

Typically, fat is aspirated manually in the periumbilical region or from the inner thigh using a super-wet technique and a 3-mm cannula. The harvested fat is typically processed on a back table, while other ancillary procedures, such as genioplasty and rhinoplasty, are performed on the face. The fat can be separated in a syringe via gravity or with centrifugation, which is limited to two minutes at 2000 revolutions per minute. Care is taken during this process to avoid direct exposure to air. The prepared fat is placed in 1-mm syringes. Stab puncture wounds are then used to introduce a 16-gauge cannula in the subcutaneous plane and/or in the plane of the superficial muscular aponeurotic system. Fat is injected as the cannula is withdrawn to avoid intravascular fat migration. Postoperative fat resorption is approximately 50%, and aesthetic improvement is stable in the long term [6, 7]. Acne must be treated before the procedure, as its presence increases the risk of fat infection. Given that the only limitation is the absence of a fat donor site, almost all patients can benefit from fat grafting in the temporal and zygomatic region.

References

1. Arnaud E, Haber SE, Paternoster G, et al. Secondary surgeries in craniosynostosis and faciocraniosynostosis. Ann Chir Plast Esthet. 2019;64(5–6):494–505.
2. Scolozzi P, Martinez A, Jaques BJ. Complex orbito-fronto-temporal reconstruction using computer-designed PEEK implant. Craniofac Surg. 2007;18(1):224–8. https://doi.org/10.1097/01.scs.0000249359.56417.7e. PMID: 17251868.
3. Gugliotta Y, Zavattero E, Ramieri G, Borbon C, Gerbino G. Cranio-maxillo-facial reconstruction with polyetheretherketone patient-specific implants: aesthetic and functional outcomes. J Pers Med. 2024;14(8):849. https://doi.org/10.3390/jpm14080849.
4. Chetty V, Haber SE, Khonsari RH, et al. Improvement of periorbital appearance in apert syndrome after subcranial Le Fort III with bipartition and distraction. J Craniofac Surg. 2020;31(3):711–5.
5. Ousterhout DK, Vargervik K. Aesthetic improvement resulting from craniofacial surgery in craniosynostosis syndromes. J Craniomaxillofac Surg. 1987;15(4):189–97.
6. Cervelli D, Tambasco D, Grussu F, et al. Fat grafting as adjunct refinement procedure in craniosynostosis management. J Craniofac Surg. 2013;24(2):691–2.
7. Fahradyan A, Goel P, Williams M, et al. Temporal fat grafting in children with craniofacial anomalies. Ann Plast Surg. 2020;85(5):505–10.

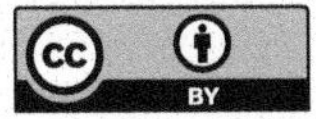

29 Aesthetic Refinements During Adolescence

Fernando Molina

Introduction

Apert syndrome in adolescence is aesthetically characterized by varying degrees of midface hypoplasia, exorbitism, and Class III malocclusion. In the first months of life, surgical treatment should focus on addressing neurological, optical, and respiratory deficits. Ideally, early operations should aim to avoid functional losses, developmental delays, and detriment to vision and hearing. Normalization of appearance should be performed in as few operations as possible. This chapter describes aesthetic refinements available to the adolescent patient with Apert syndrome. In large part, aesthetic refinements can be achieved with orthognathic surgery, an effective means to correct central midface hypoplasia, a concave profile, short-face deformity, open bite, and other malocclusions. Additionally, this chapter addresses adjunct procedures including autologous fat grafting, lateral canthopexy, and rhinoplasty.

F. Molina (✉)
Plastic Surgery and Craniofacial Surgery, Universidad Nacional Autónoma de Mexico, Mexico City, Mexico

Medicine Faculty, Postgraduate Division, Fundación Fernando Ortiz Monasterio for Craniofacial Anomalies, at Hospital Angeles del Pedregal, CDMX, Mexico City, Mexico

Orthognathic Surgery

Apert syndrome, associated with one of two autosomal dominant mutations in the *FGFR2* gene, accounts for roughly 5% of all craniosynostosis syndromes [1]. The bone facial structure of patients with Apert syndrome is especially distinguished by midface hypoplasia, which is more pronounced in the central face and occurs in the sagittal, transverse, and vertical planes [2]. This results in a biconcave appearance with significantly more nasomaxillary than orbito-zygomatic hypoplasia, which manifests as a depressed nasal bridge and "parrot-beak" nose, retruded maxilla with counterclockwise rotation of the occlusal plane, and decreased midface-to-orbital height ratio [3, 4]. The sagittal disharmony between maxillary and mandibular growth may lead to an anterior open bite and inverted V maxilla [5, 6]. Characteristic periorbital features include down-slanting palpebral fissures and shallow orbits with ocular proptosis. Moreover, patients with Apert syndrome can present with hypertelorism, characterized by a negative canthal axis and counterrotated orbits [7].

As they grow, patients with Apert syndrome may develop differential bone growth in the orbits and middle third of the face. In addition to developing thicker skin that often features severe facial acne, these patients experience facial bone changes to their bone structure, as indicated on X-rays, upon reaching puberty. In young adults with Apert syndrome, the discrepancy between

J. G. Meara et al. (eds.), *Apert Syndrome*, https://doi.org/10.1007/978-3-032-12551-4_29

the maxilla and the mandible becomes accentuated in the anteroposterior, transverse, and vertical dimensions.

Dental occlusion analysis reveals several problems including an incomplete number of teeth, anterior open bite, severe high-arched palates, and poor position of the molar and incisor roots. Although continuous functional orthodontics helps to prevent severe deformities of the maxilla and, secondarily, of the mandible, this intervention is insufficient to address all issues. Occlusion, maxillary structure, numerous functional problems, and facial aesthetics pose challenges to both patients and surgeons.

No single osteotomy pattern can adequately address this range of problems. Effects from Apert syndrome and from the patient's particular surgical history combine to result in varying types of midface hypoplasia. Analysis of facial morphology during the periods of mixed dentition and adolescence can produce a final analysis of differential midface hypoplasia type. An experienced surgical team can then employ an array of techniques to optimize final outcomes.

Over the past two decades, techniques utilizing segmental osteotomies have seen increasing observations of benefit in Apert midface treatment. The osteotomies and their segmentation allow for greater normalization of midfacial dysmorphology. Moreover, virtual surgery three-dimensional (3D) planning aids in determining the best surgical options for complex deformities [8].

The abilities to perform multipiece osteotomies and to combine osteotomies and bone distraction enable simultaneous soft-tissue expansion and increases the quality of the result. Moreover, this process avoids complications secondary to poor vascularity of small bone segments with recurrences in the medium term. Using osteotomies plus distraction in well-selected cases offers more straightforward and logical surgical procedures that can increase the osteotomy's stability and improve the quality of the functional result, the occlusal relationship, and face aesthetics.

Careful patient selection is essential in determining whether a young adult with Apert syndrome will undergo orthognathic surgery and other associated aesthetic procedures. Historically, parent metrics indicate low patient scores on metrics of emotional functioning, behaviors, self-esteem, and time required from parents. Despite potential complications, surgical intervention in well-selected patients can lead to improved psychological, social, and daily functioning [9, 10]. Additionally, most studies report lower overall intelligence quotient (IQ) scores and higher rates of depression and bullying in this patient group than in the general population. These factors contribute to patients with Apert syndrome obtaining lower overall levels of education and employment, as well as increased need for assistance in daily tasks [11, 12].

Planning surgical intervention in a young adult with Apert syndrome should include several points of consideration:

- Surgical decision-making must be individualized. The surgeon must differentiate two problems: visual perception versus the quantitative reality of facial bone structure. This implies that the visual perception of certain facial relationships may be quite disparate from its quantitative measurement [13].
- In the author's experience, visual perception must always take precedence. Very frequently, patients with Apert syndrome are observed to have excessive projection and height of the lower face. These differences produce an excessive concavity of the profile and an abnormal relationship of the lips in which the lower lip protrudes in relation to the upper lip.
- In cases of severe hypoplasia of the upper jaw, associated anterior open bite of highly variable degrees is commonly observed. These fundamental anatomical abnormalities are cause for planning segmental osteotomies.
- Combining osteotomies and bone distraction minimizes surgery, preserves bone vascularity, and adds the advantages of simultaneous tissue expansion and—with the new bone formation—more bone volume, allowing the orthodontist to obtain greater occlusal stability.

Fat Grafting

Autologous fat grafting is an efficacious volumizing and contouring procedure. Often regarded as the ideal biological filler, its permanence has made fat grafting an attractive soft-tissue reconstructive option. Additionally, autologous fat grafting utilizing adipose-derived stem cells exhibits remarkable regenerative potential, effectively improving skin quality, decreasing skin pigmentation, and softening scars. Today, autologous fat grafting is used in young adults with Apert syndrome to correct facial asymmetry, forehead contour irregularities, and the lack of facial angularity.

Predictive factors for fat graft retention include surgical technique, age, body mass index, donor site, and recipient site. Our preferred methodologies for optimizing the number of viable cells are gravity separation and strainer filtration. We aim to maintain greater concentrations of stromal vascular fraction cells and adipose stem cells in the supernatant to enhance the fat graft. Other options include elements like platelet-rich plasma and cell protectants.

In the author's experience, fat-grafted volumes range from 8 to 60 mL. The lower abdomen is the most common donor site. Patients most commonly undergo two to five rounds of fat grafting, which are spaced apart by a minimum of four months. The author's maximum long-term follow up is 12 years.

In Apert syndrome, the upper third of the face is the main anatomical treatment area, primarily to camouflage underlying abnormalities in bony contour. Select patients have also had enhancement in the malar-zygoma region to augment soft-tissue volume in the retrusive midface.

Using blunt cannulas, fat is injected into multiple tissue planes via a series of passes. This method maximizes grafted fat contact with native vascularized tissues. Additionally, various implications and benefits are gained in each tissue plane. Fat placement into the supraperiosteal plane is fundamental in treating patients with Apert syndrome, and 50% of the total fat volume is injected here. Next, we insert 30% of the fat volume into the muscle plane. Subdermal plane fat placement is necessary for patients with scar or fibrous tissue. First, adhesions are released, and pre-tunneling is performed. A liquefied fat graft should then be injected as the cannula is withdrawn. If over-injection occurs and a clump forms, digital manipulation is sometimes able to smooth minor flaws. Additionally, cross-hatching the fat-grafted area may help blunt contour irregularities (Fig. 29.1a–d).

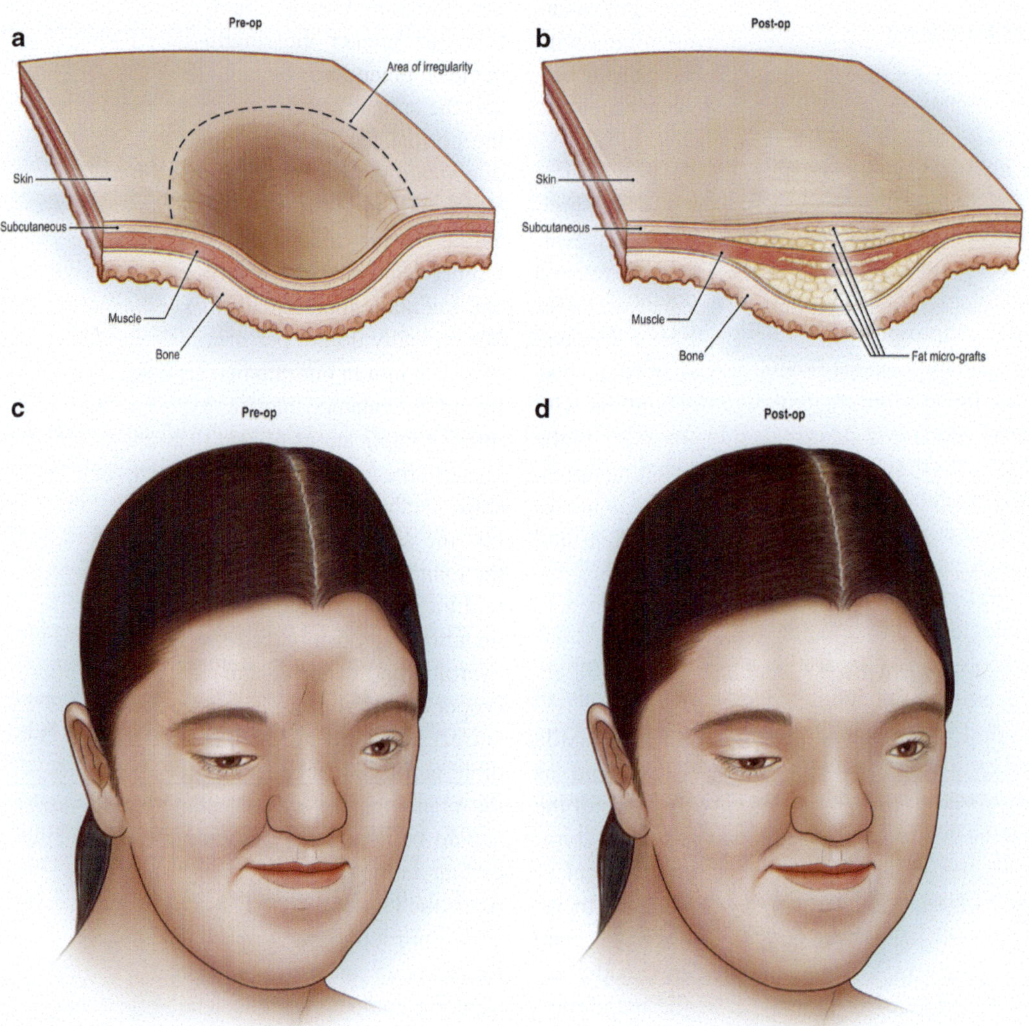

Fig. 29.1 (**a**) Note the area of depression and irregularity due to underlying bony depression. (**b**) Injection of fat cells into multiple layers directly superficial to the bone, in the muscle and in the subcutaneous tissue camouflages the bony depression and gives the overlying skin a more natural contour. (**c**, **d**) Pre- and post-operative drawings of contour correction with fat injection in the glabellar region

Lateral Canthopexy

An effective lateral canthopexy is a versatile tool that can address negative canthal tilt, correct inferior eyelid malposition/laxity, and restore the integrity of the lower lid to produce a more aesthetic appearance. A correct lower-lid position can enhance the globe's and periorbita's integrity, position, and function. The structures of the lateral retinaculum coalesce at the lateral orbit and support the globe and eyelids like a hammock. The lateral retinaculum comprises the lateral canthal tendon, the lateral horn of the levator aponeurosis, Lockwood's ligament, and the check ligaments. They converge and insert securely into the thickened orbital periosteum overlying Whitnall's tubercle. (Fig. 29.2a)

The lateral canthal tendon has superficial, deep (or anterior and posterior), and superior and inferior attachments to the orbital rim. A highly effective lateral canthopexy necessitates full release of the labyrinth of connective tissue around the orbit, including the orbital septum, lateral horn of the levator aponeurosis, and orbital rim periosteum.

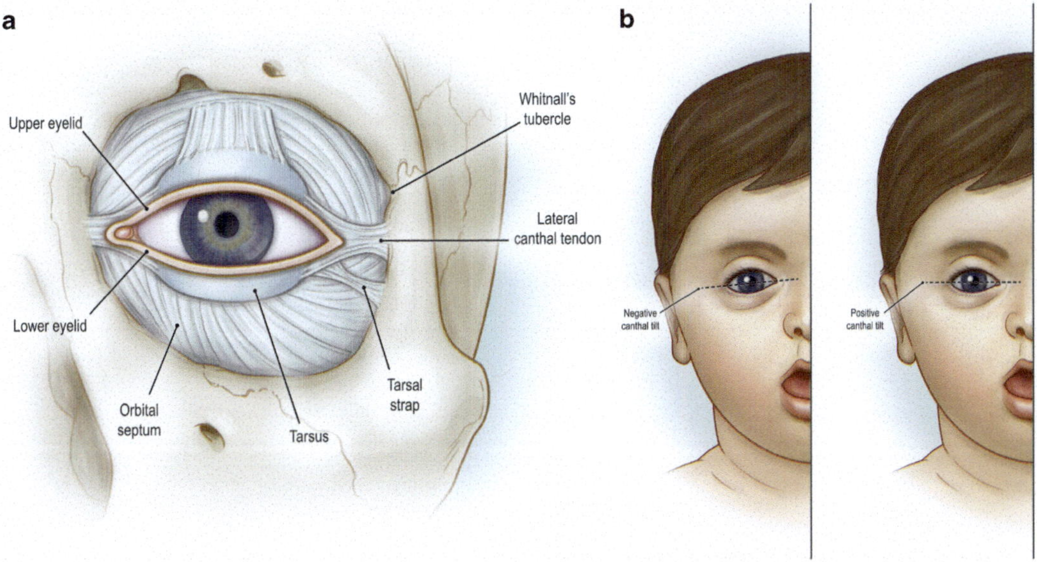

Fig. 29.2 (**a**) Note the lateral canthal tendon attaching on Whitnalls' tubercle. (**b**) Note the negative canthal tilt on the left and the improvement of the lateral canthal position on the right after canthopexy

Applying upward traction on the lower lid with a hook, the surgeon can observe how dramatically the untethered lateral canthus elevates. In patients with Apert syndrome featuring a severe negative canthal tilt, this position must be overcorrected. For this, the author uses a 3–0 nylon suture. The structures are sutured superiorly using a vertical vector into the deep temporal fascia. Then, a second suture—4 mm below and to the canthus side—is added on the orbicularis oculi muscle and orbital septum to ensure that full reticulum elements are easily elevated, producing a successful and long-lasting canthopexy (Fig. 29.2b).

Apert Rhinoplasty

In young adults with Apert syndrome, the nose is often small in relation to the face, and nasal skin is frequently thick and sebaceous. Furthermore, the nose is supported on a three-dimensionally hypoplastic maxilla. The goals of Apert rhinoplasty include increasing the nasal size (i.e., augmentation rhinoplasty) and improving nasal tip definition, projection, and rotation.

The author's practice utilizes a closed manner with bilateral rim incisions for rhinoplasty procedures. Extensive dissection is performed to completely liberate the native cartilaginous structures. Costal cartilage is harvested, and two grafts are designed. The graft for the nasal tip recreates the deep structural subunit corresponding to the columella skin subunits, soft triangles, and the tip itself. This graft is a short pyramid with an isosceles triangle as its base. The equal sides of the base triangle correspond to the distance from the anterior nasal spine to the light reflex on each side of the tip (16–22 mm). The third side is the width of the tip (8–10 mm) (Fig. 29.3a–c). The superior face of this pyramidal graft recreates the dome tip properly. For the nasal dorsum, a second graft re-establishes nasal length by coursing from the radix to the posterior surface of the tip graft. In patients with Apert syndrome, the step-off between the dorsum and the tip graft should be 8–10 mm due to the thick skin. In cases where the internal nasal valve is compromised, a third set of grafts (i.e., spreader grafts) are added.

This technique results in aesthetic improvements in nasal size and enhances nasal dorsum projection such that any apparent hypertelorism is obscured. The step-off between the two grafts prevents the production of a scarred supra-tip. The nasal tip is strong and well-structured, with good morphology, excellent definition, and projection.

By restoring two deep structural subunits and blending soft-tissue contours, this technique improves the aesthetics of the nose in this

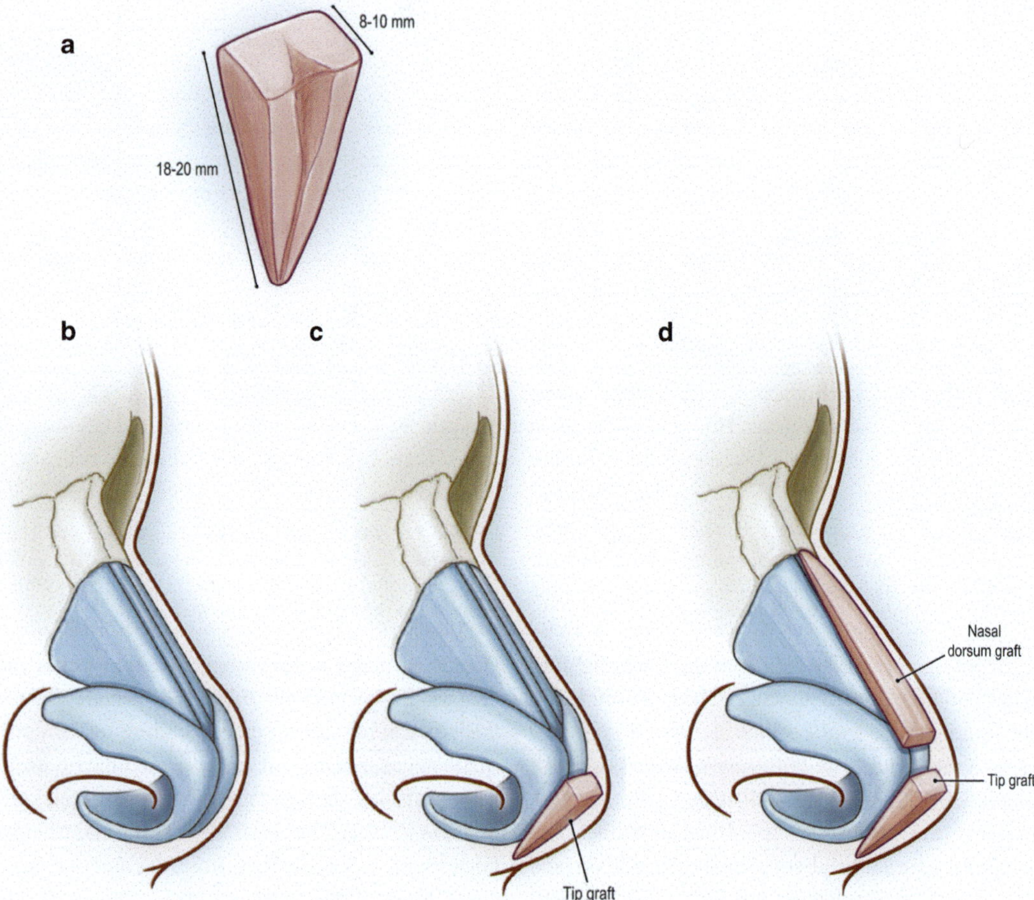

Fig. 29.3 (**a**-**c**) Note the tip graft geometry and placement. (**d**) The dorsal nasal graft is thinner and narrower at the cephalic end

extremely challenging patient subpopulation. Advantageous in more complex frameworks, the two-subunit system for the deep nasal structures can recreate all cutaneous subunits. Secondarily, these grafts are thick, structurally robust, and able to resist the unique demands of the scarred inelastic soft-tissue envelope seen in this patient group.

A typical graft for a nasal dorsum: the thinnest part is positioned toward the cephalic, and it is sometimes thicker in the patient with Apert syndrome (Fig. 29.3d).

Clinical Case Examples

Clinical Case No. 1

An 18-year-old female patient with Apert syndrome and a severe facial bone deformity. At 14 months of age, a monobloc advancement was performed with a highly satisfactory functional and aesthetic result. Orthodontic therapy was performed throughout childhood without success in normalizing maxillary growth. Severe acne began at 14 years of age, for which she received dermatological treatment.

Upon reaching 18 years of age, her upper facial third was flat and with non-prominent supraorbital ridges. The frontal and procerus muscles were highly contractile. The skin was thick, with acne and abundant sebaceous glands. There were indentations in the temporal area, likely attributable to muscle atrophy or problems with post-monobloc bone healing. The eyes showed slight exorbitism and strabismus, which were more severe in the left eye. The middle third of the face was severely hypoplastic. The malar bones and the lower orbital rim were deficient in volume and projection. Midface bone deficiency was camouflaged by thick and heavy soft tissues that highlighted the acne-prone skin and produced discreet jowls on the cheeks, deep nasolabial folds, and a nose of good size and projection. The lower third of the face was long and over-projected. The mandibular angles and the border of the mandibular body were not defined. The chin was long and had ill-defined contours. She had an exaggerated prominence of the lower lip resulting from the push produced by the inferior dental arch (Fig. 29.4a, b).

The surgical plan focused on solving the functional problems of sleep apnea and digestive disorders caused by dental malocclusion. Employing the philosophy of avoiding extensive and more traumatic maxillo-mandibular osteotomies, the surgical plan included an 8 mm Le Fort I advancement and 5 mm of anterior maxillary vertical elongation. The Le Fort I was midline segmented to allow horizontalization of the two hemi-maxillary segments—which corrects the anterior open bite and horizontalizes the occlusal plane—simultaneously with the A-P advancement-elongation of the entire maxilla. Properly rigid fixation was used to keep the segments in the correct position.

Then, a central mandibular body linear osteotomy was performed between the second premolar and the first molar. Four days later, elastic bands produced a distraction vector to elevate the full anterior mandibular segment. The mandible was slowly adapted to the already-corrected new maxillary position, and the severe anterior open bite was closed, allowing final orthodontics refinements. Important to note, this mandible osteotomy modality preserves the patient's stable posterior molar occlusal contact and avoids prolonged orthodontic therapy. The incorporated newly generated bone in the central mandibular body serves to increase bone volume and better accommodate teeth in the lower dental arch. Simultaneous expansion of the floor of the mouth muscles assists in alleviating sleep apnea.

The time for adaptation of the mandible to the maxilla and final occlusal orthodontic refinements was two weeks. Then, a four-week intermaxillary fixation completes final result stability. Visually, the patient's facial proportions are much improved. Midface fullness has been added, the columella and the nasal tip of the nose are more projected, and the lips are in a better relationship and are able to close passively. Soft-tissue components and skin quality are important in the final result. Unfortunately, severe acne is still present.

Her profile is now convex, and the lower third of the face is visually shorter. Anteriorly, a minor anterior mandibular rotation is produced, which automatically reduces the vertical dimension of

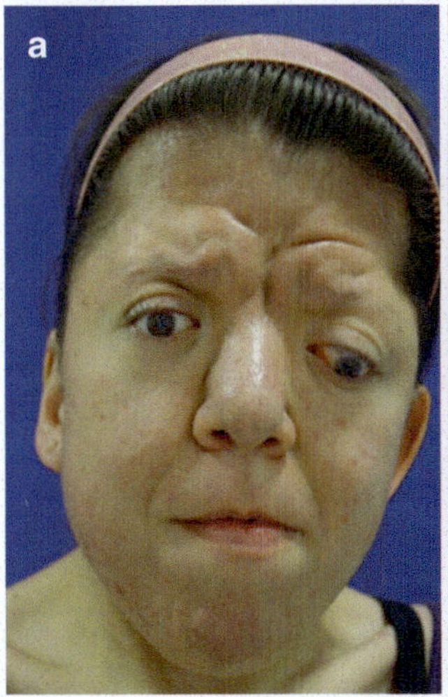

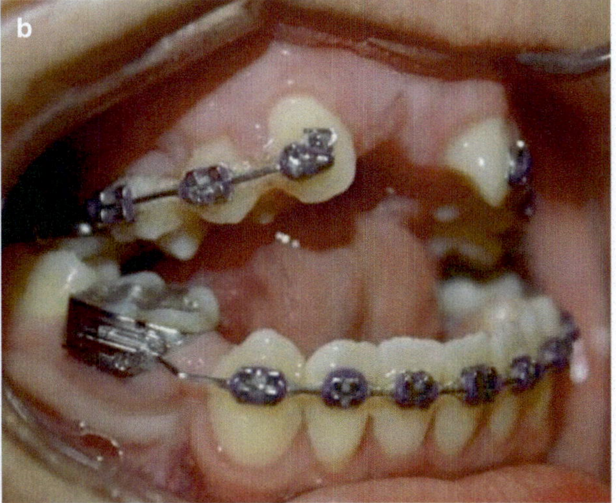

Fig. 29.4 (**a**, **b**) 18 y/old female with Apert syndrome. Her facial appearance shows the natural evolution of the syndrome and the long-term sequels of a monobloc advancement done early in life. Dental occlusion is class III associated with a severe open bite "V" shaped due to maxillary hypoplasia and anatomical malposition

the lower third face. The new bone volume added to the midface produces a more efficient expansion of the muscles and facial skin—which is heavy and thick—and overall enhances the patient's result. Visual perception can vary from the bone structure quantitative reality. This sometimes results in observers attributing typical, preoperative Apert syndrome face deformities to negative emotional states such as sadness, sullenness, anger, or discontent (Fig. 29.5a–h).

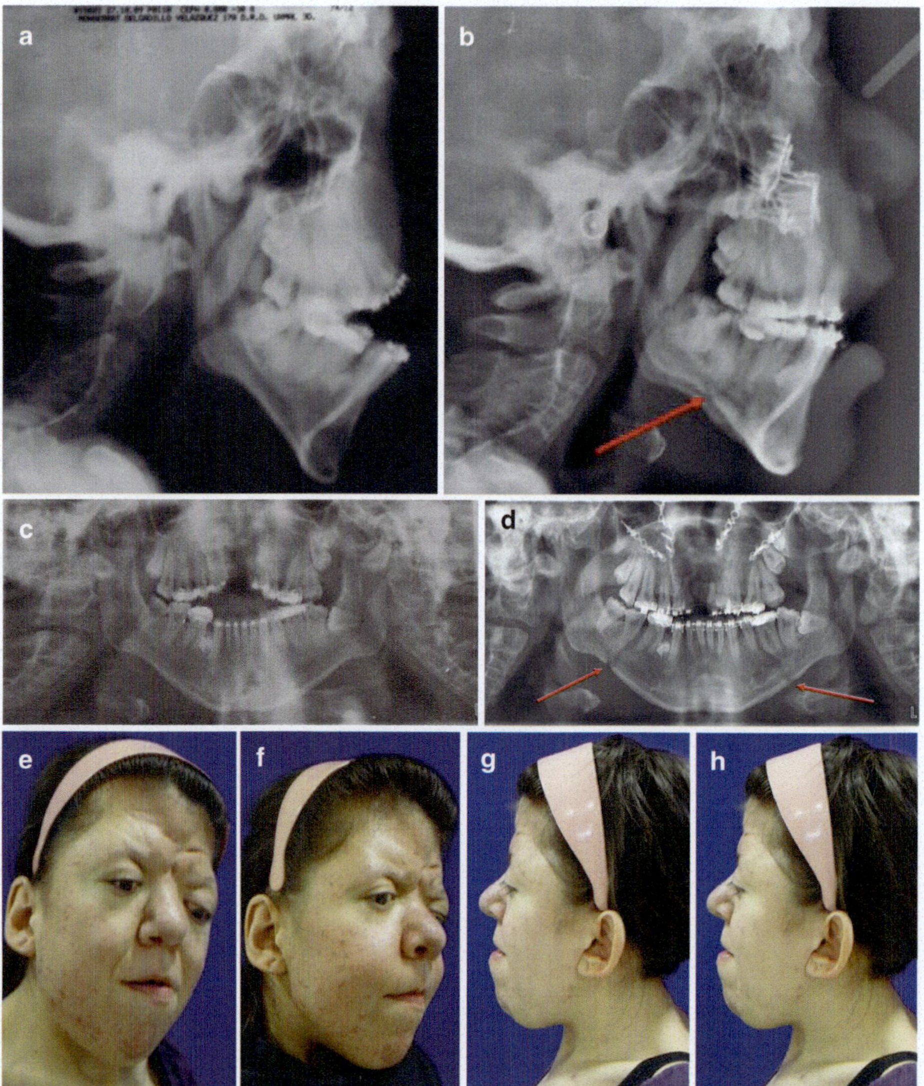

Fig. 29.5 (**a**, **b**) Pre- and post-operative lateral cephalograms. The segmented Le Fort I horizontalized the maxillary occlusal plane. Red arrow shows the osteotomy site and mandibular bone neoformation. The anterior open bite was corrected by cephalad movement of the anterior mandibular segment. Note the dramatic changes in the post-maxillary airway dimension and note the position and new dimension of the post-tongue airway. Post-op studies demonstrate normal blood oxygenation during sleep. (**c**, **d**) Pre- and post-operative panorex radiographs showing the two maxillary segments in horizontal position. Note the mandible has been adapted to the maxilla, closing the anterior open bite and achieving satisfactory occlusal stability. The red arrows show the bone neoformation. The preservation of the posterior molar occlusion also means that the ascending ramus and the condyle-glenoid fossa relationship are not modified. This anatomical preservation prevents future problems in the TM joint function and mouth opening. (**e**, **f**) Patient's face is much better proportioned. Midface fullness after the new maxillary position has been added, and the lips are close in a passive way. Soft tissue components and skin quality are important in the result. Severe acne persists. (**g**, **h**) Her profile is now convex, a new volume has been added to the

Clinical Case No. 2

A 19-year-old female patient with Apert syndrome and a severe facial bone deformity. At 16 months of age, a monobloc advancement with 24 mm at the orbital–frontal level was performed without bipartition. The patient did well functionally from a respiratory, ophthalmological, neurological, and digestive standpoint.

Due to the severity of the case, sleep apnea recurred at the eight years of age. To address this, a subcranial Le Fort III was performed using a transmalar pin, and A-P advancement achieved an overcorrected dental arch maxillomandibular relationship. Notably, from the age of four years old the patient had functional orthodontic treatment that was suspended at various periods during her growth years; thus, orthodontics lacked optimal continuity.

The patient had a short face with a severe Class III malocclusion and a discrete hypertelorism, optically more accentuated by a low nasal dorsum (Fig. 29.6a–c). Cephalometric measurements show a midface height of 54 mm compared with a lower face height of 66 mm). A surgical distraction procedure for skeletal correction was projected; it included 15-mm maxillary advancement and 4-mm maxillary elongation using distraction forces and a facial mask. Additional aesthetic procedures were performed at the same time, including augmentation rhinoplasty and frontotemporal fat grafting to correct indentations and irregularities.

A Le Fort I high osteotomy was performed to create a new vertical face proportion by (a) moving the midface forward and lengthening it, and (b) producing a shorter inferior face achieved via a different mandibular clockwise rotation that visually changes the vertical dimension of the lower third.

Bone distraction was initiated six days after surgery. Initially, a strictly horizontal vector was used. Once 10 mm of A-P advancement was achieved, the direction of the distraction vector was changed into a caudal and oblique position to both avoid producing an anterior open bite and to sufficiently elongate the vertical dimension of the maxilla. The final procedure produced a 12% midface structural overcorrection. The orthodontist used elastic bands in Class II to

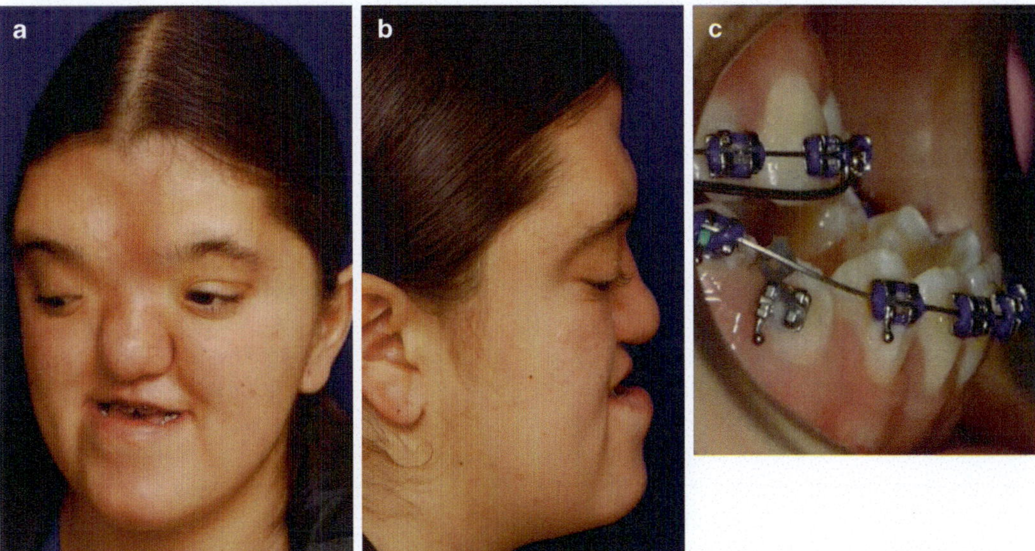

Fig. 29.6 (a–c) 19 y/old female patient with Apert syndrome after two surgical procedures performed during her years of growth. A monobloc at 16 months of age and a subcranial Le Fort III at 8 years. Functional orthodontic treatment without continuity corrected the anterior openbite; however, it did not prevent A-P maxillary growth failure, which was associated with obstructive sleep apnea with a 14 mm A-P jaw discrepancy

Fig. 29.5 (continued) midface, and her labial relationships are normal. Visual perception can be very different from the quantitative reality of the bone structure. This is relevant because ordinary people, as observers of a typical Apert face deformity patient, preoperatively will not infrequently attribute them with negative emotional characteristics such as sadness or sullenness, anger, or discontent

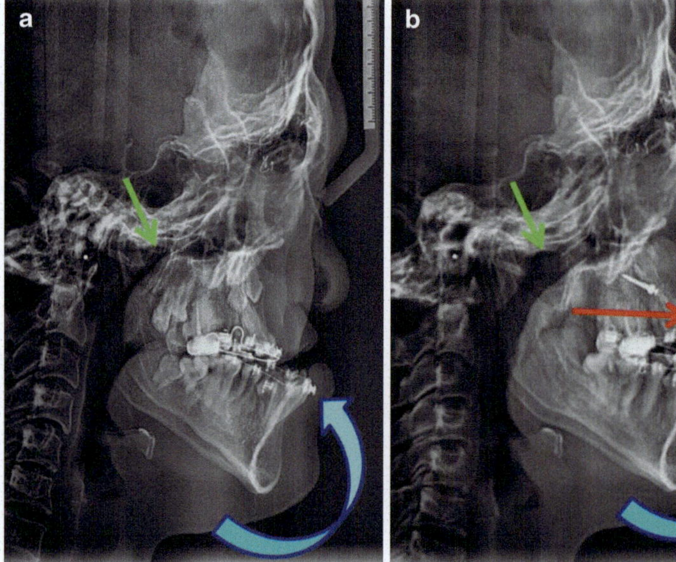

Fig. 29.7 (**a**, **b**) Pre- and post-lateral cephalograms show a 15 mm advancement and 3 mm anterior elongation of the maxilla. A solid and healthy mass of new bone can be observed at the pterygomaxillary regions. Two screws were inserted into the piriform regions from which the maxilla was properly pulled. The red arrow indicates the horizontal distraction vector parallel to the occlusal plane that was initially used. X-rays show a prominent anterior maxillary vertical elongation. Also, the new dimension and position of the maxilla naturally changes the anterior mandibular clockwise rotation, which automatically shortens the lower third of the face. The airway dimension at the posterior maxillary portion and at the velopharyngeal area and posterior tongue has changed dramatically. The obstructive sleep apnea has been completely corrected, and the apnea-hypopnea index is now normal

establish a Class I occlusal relationship and good stability.

The pre- and post-lateral cephalograms show midfacial bone structure that is more prominent, vertically longer, and forward positioned. A solid and healthy new bone structure is observed at the pterygomaxillary regions, maintaining the new position of the maxillae for the long term (Fig. 29.7a, b). Initially, a horizontal distraction vector was strictly parallel to the maxillary occlusal plane. Then, after elongating the maxilla anteriorly, the initial vector was changed to an oblique and inferior direction, a maneuver that also prevents the production of an anterior open bite. The changes to facial structure also shifted the airway dimension. Demonstrating the advantages of associating bone distraction changes, the soft-tissue expansion produced significant 3D modification in neighboring areas. Drastic changes were seen in the patient's airway dimension at the posterior maxillary portion, the velopharyngeal area, and the posterior tongue. The air column from the nose changed from a curved, caudal shape to completely horizontal. Physiologically, this significantly improves blood oxygenation during sleep. Functionally, the obstructive sleep apnea was completely corrected, and the apnea–hypopnea index is now normal.

Postoperative clinical analysis of the patient confirms the absence of visual disproportions that suggest the face is short, despite the quantitative vertical facial dimension. A normal labial relationship is established with no lip strain. The mouth shows 1.0 mm of incisal exposure with the lips relaxed, and smiling results in full anterior dentition and normal gingiva exposure. The midface's new volume, position, and vertical increase have produced a better facial aesthetic, with a more oval face and improved proportion between the facial thirds. The augmentation rhinoplasty has produced a thinner, longer, and larger nose, with a reasonable definition of the dorsum and the tip. The mouth shows an upper dental arch in a correct position. Laterally, the buccal commissures have shifted superiorly, the marked nasolabial fold now looks normal, and the lower lip has

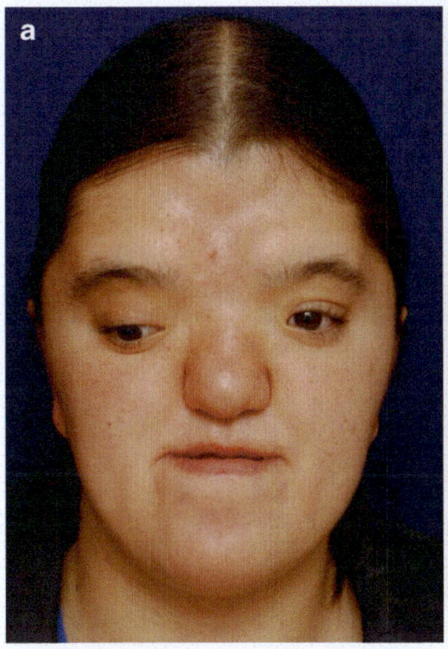

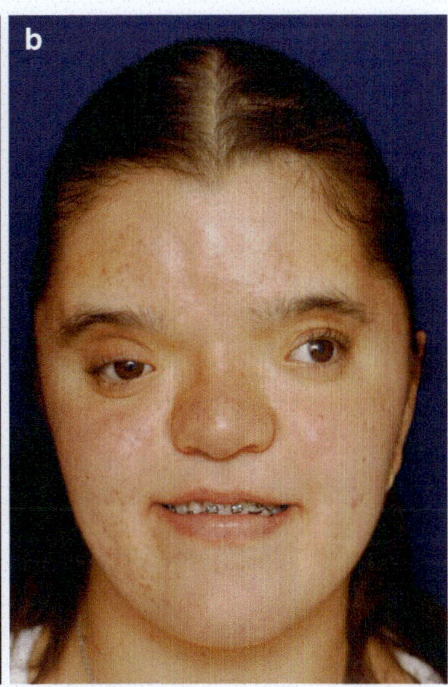

Fig. 29.8 (**a**, **b**) Pre- and post-frontal views demonstrating the fundamental changes obtained with the correction of a short and retruded middle third of the face. The midface's new volume, anterior maxillary position, and elongated vertical dimension produce a better facial aesthetic, with a more oval face and good proportion between the facial thirds. The nose is thinner, longer, and larger with a reasonable definition of the dorsum and the tip. The upper lip shows 1 mm of gingiva over an upper dental arch in the correct position. The corners of the mouth have shift superiorly, the marked nasolabial fold now looks normal, and the lower lip has become less prominent

become less prominent. No change is observed at the labio-mental fold; it preserves an adequate depth and definition. Therefore, strict adherence to these aesthetic conditions widely justifies treatment plans that result in a well-proportioned vertical face (Fig. 29.8a, b).

The frontal and temporal regions now appear regular, with better definition and shape. With the micro-fat grafts, the frontal region is rounder and more feminine. Hypoplasia and temporal muscle wasting were also satisfactorily corrected.

The nose is a fundamental facial aesthetic element, and its aesthetic correction contributes significantly to normalization of the face. In young adults, Apert costal cartilage grafts are properly carved and inserted into the nose dorsum. The tip can produce a more prominent nose that is harmoniously proportioned to the rest of the face.

Augmentation rhinoplasty to provide structural support to the tip and columella entails designing a long single-piece graft. Supported inferiorly on the anterior nasal spine, the graft extends to the columella and to the nasal tip. In the author's experience, the proper carving of a cartilage graft can produce an anatomically complete, well-projected, and defined nasal tip, despite thick skin dense with oil glands. Equally aesthetically important, a second one-piece graft establishes a nasal dorsum. The patient achieved adequate new projection of the nasal dorsum, and the inserted cartilage graft produced a structurally important nose to counterbalance the new dimension and projection of the lower face (Fig. 29.9a, b).

Using the conventional orthognathic concept, analyzing this result suggests that these perioral changes are caused by a static re-draping of the soft tissues over an expanded skeletal mass after standard osteotomies. Also, these changes are attributable, at least in part, to obligatory alterations in the resting tone of the perioral musculature, which occur to accommodate changes in skeletal volume. In this specific case, distraction osteogenesis was used, and the skeletal volume was notably increased by newly formed bone and by adding projection and height to the midface. Additionally, distraction has produced midface soft-tissue expansion. Subsequently, the resting

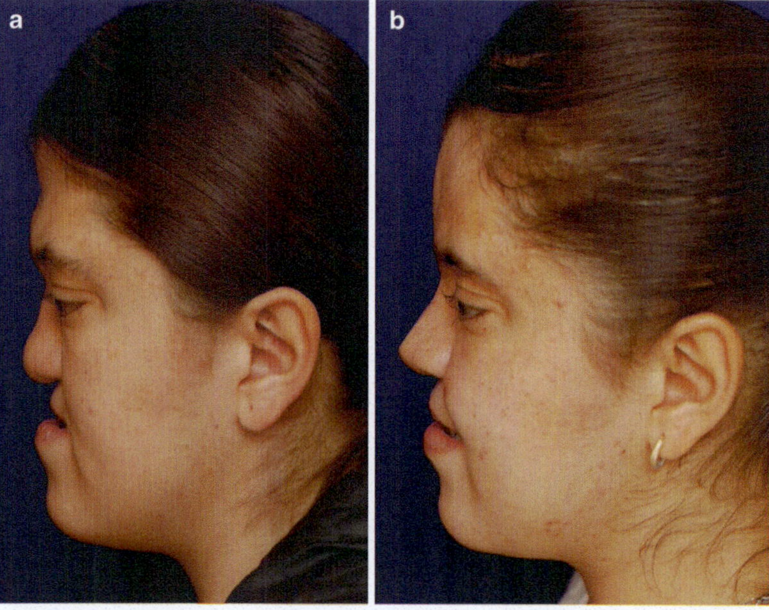

Fig. 29.9 (**a**, **b**) Pre- and post-lateral views showing a nice, rounded forehead with a regular surface. The bony changes in volume and dimension of the maxilla allow the soft tissues to be redistributed satisfactorily. The costal cartilaginous grafts inserted into the nose produce a dorsum, reconstructing an aesthetically pleasing frontal-nasal angle. Projection, definition and angularity were achieved at the nasal tip despite very thick skin

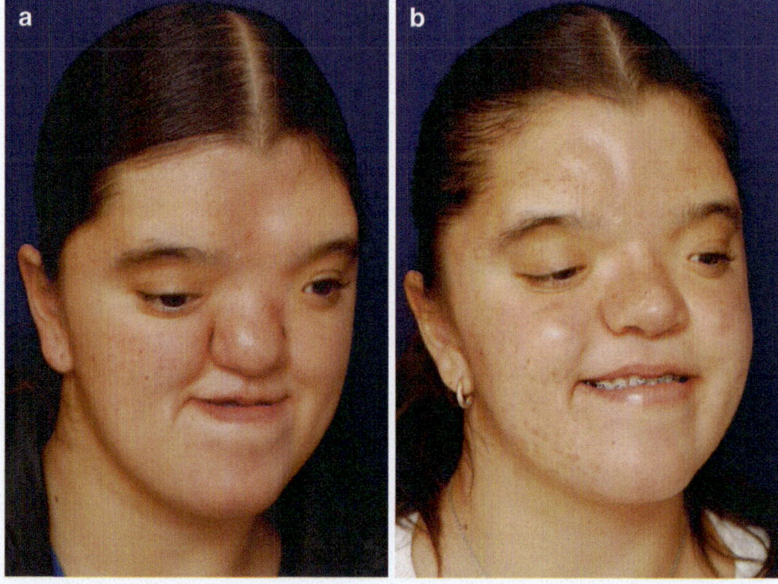

Fig. 29.10 (**a**, **b**) The three-quarters pre- and post-views show a smiling patient and all the changes obtained after 15 mm forward distraction midface at the central incisors with simultaneous augmentation rhinoplasty and fat grafts in the frontal region

musculature tone increases, and oral competency is maintained. The ability to increase resting perioral muscular tone may produce additional facial changes, including decreased width of the mouth, fuller lips, inclination of the oral commissures to shift superiorly, a less procumbent lower lip, and relaxation and redistribution of labio-mental muscles resulting in a shortened chin (Fig. 29.10a, b). The greater the increase in skeletal volume through new bone formation, the greater the change in perinasal and perioral soft tissues. These beneficial effects on the facial aesthetics of patients with Apert syndrome will produce a sense of lightness and elegance in the final result.

In this patient, the facial bone condition, malocclusion, and associated functional problems could likely be corrected with a bimaxillary and chin osteotomy. The rising popularity of virtual surgical planning has enabled greater accuracy and intraoperative time savings, increasing the feasibility of such procedures. Although custom-fabricated plates remain cost-prohibitive in many cases, they are likely justified in highly complex cases.

Recent studies show that extensive orthognathic surgery and segmental osteotomies reduce vascularity. Thus, these procedures carry risk of multiple complications, including bleeding, infection, scarring, malunion, nonunion, and bony or dental relapse [14, 15].

Mandibular osteotomies should be avoided in many patients with Apert syndrome with severe midface retrusion due to issues related to bone structure and to soft tissue changes of the lower third of the face. Regarding bone structure, the rate of a "bad split" during bilateral sagittal split osteotomy is reported to be approximately 2.3% [16]. In the complex cases of patients with Apert syndrome presenting abnormal intra-bone histology, the incidence of "bad split" could be higher. Causes and risk factors include inadequate vertical osteotomy at the inferior border, horizontal osteotomy performed too high above the lingula, exertion of excess force when separating the proximal and distal segments, and impacted third molars [17–20]. Avoiding early relapses after bimaxillary osteotomies is another important consideration. Multiple factors contribute to early relapses, including muscle-related physiologic effects, changes in the position of dentition after surgery, condylar position changes at the time of intraoperative fixation, articular disc problems, type of fixation, the creation of gaps between bony mandibular segments, and secondary condylar resorption [21–23]. Many of these factors also pertain to late pathology.

Soft-tissue considerations also play a role in selecting surgical candidates for mandibular osteotomies. A mandibular setback osteotomy can lead to changes in the physiologic equilibrium of the pterygomasseteric sling, which may subsequently affect the functioning of the mastication muscles. These muscle changes tend to rotate the proximal segment counterclockwise to restore its original position. The efficacy of bilateral sagittal split osteotomy decreases with increased counterclockwise rotation of the proximal segment [24–27]. Additionally, when considering facial balance and aesthetics, soft tissue changes that frequently accompany lower face reductions in skeletal size may result in an older appearance. Negative perioral and superior neck soft-tissue changes are always present. Skeletal support to the soft tissues decreases when reducing projection and/or height, and this issue is more pronounced with soft tissues that are heavy, fleshy, and have thick skin. In patients with Apert syndrome, bone reduction risks creating an imbalance between skeletal and soft-tissue masses or worsening a preexisting imbalance.

For this reason, it is logical that distraction increases bone volume, corrects the position of the maxilla, increases vertical growth, and expands all soft tissues, adding functional and aesthetic benefits.

For young adults with Apert syndrome, associated aesthetic procedures—performed in conjunction with correction of severe short midface and related secondary functional problems—are important improvements. Currently, these young adults belong to the millennial and generation Z cohorts, whose lives are characterized by computer, cell phone, and social media use and the emphasis these platforms place on image. Therefore, self-image is essential to self-esteem, and the craniofacial surgeon should consider pursuing more comprehensive facial aesthetics. Patients with normal IQ scores who are integrated into social groups, participate in school activities, and have developed psychomotor skills should be given particular consideration as surgical candidates.

Important Messages

1. A wide expansion soft-tissue procedure should always be considered if an aesthetic option exists. For instance, in patients with moderate-to-severe degrees of mandibular excess, a more ambitious maxillary advancement may be more appropriate both aesthetically and functionally. From this perspective, the advantages of distraction osteogenesis

include the generation of new bone, the progressive expansion of all soft tissues, the correct management of vectors, and the possibility of modifying all these factors to mobilize the maxilla correctly.
2. Planning the occlusal result should consider both the final aesthetic and functional outcomes. A low threshold for using a double-jaw procedure is practical in cases where a better soft-tissue outcome can be achieved. With this philosophy in mind, this approach can eliminate the aesthetic limitations of establishing a normal occlusion using single-jaw surgery.
3. Use proper vectors to produce different skeletal movements, when indicated, to better control lower face projection and height. Once the maxillary structure is correctly positioned, mandibular clockwise rotation can produce a different inferior height, which conveniently reduces height and re-drapes soft tissues in a patient with Apert syndrome and short face.

References

1. Cohen MM, Kreiborg S. New indirect method for estimating the birth prevalence of the Apert syndrome. Int J Oral Maxillofac Surg. 1992;21(2):107–9.
2. Massenburg BB, Susarla SM, Kapadia HP, Hopper RA. Subcranial midface advancement in patients with syndromic craniosynostosis. Oral Maxillofac Surg Clin North Am. 2022;34(3):467–75.
3. Kreiborg S, Cohen MM. Ocular manifestations of Apert and Crouzon syndromes: qualitative and quantitative findings. J Craniofac Surg. 2010;21(5):1354–7.
4. Hopper RA, Kapadia H, Morton T. Normalizing facial ratios in apert syndrome patients with Le Fort II midface distraction and simultaneous zygomatic repositioning. Plast Reconstr Surg. 2013;132(1):129–40.
5. Kakutani H, Sato Y, Tsukamoto-Takakusagi Y, Saito F, Oyama A, Iida J. Evaluation of the maxillofacial morphological characteristics of Apert syndrome infants. Congenit Anom (Kyoto). 2017;57(1):15–23.
6. McCarthy JG, Grayson B, Bookstein F, Vickery C, Zide B. Le Fort III advancement osteotomy in the growing child. Plast Reconstr Surg. 1984;74(3):343–54.
7. Crombag GA, Verdoorn MH, Nikkhah D, Ponniah AJ, Ruff C, Dunaway D. Assessing the corrective effects of facial bipartition distraction in Apert syndrome using geometric morphometrics. J Plast Reconstr Aesthet Surg. 2014;67:e151–61.
8. Wu M, Massenburg BB, Ng JJ, Romeo DJ, Swanson JW, Bartlett SP, Taylor JA, Division of Plastic, Reconstructive, and Oral Surgery, Children's Hospital of Philadelphia, Philadelphia PA, USA. The Kaleidoscope of Midface Management in Apert Syndrome: a 23-year single institution experience. Plast Reconstr Surg. 2025; Advance Online Article.
9. Allam KA, Wan DC, Khwanngern K, Kawamoto HK, Tanna N, Perry A, Bradley JP. Treatment of apert syndrome: a long-term follow-up study. Plast Reconstr Surg. 2011;127(4):1601–11.
10. Raposo-Amaral CE, Neto JG, Denadai R, Raposo-Amaral CM, Raposo-Amaral CA. Patient-reported quality of life in highest-functioning Apert and Crouzon syndromes: a comparative study. Plast Reconstr Surg. 2014;133(2):182e–91e.
11. Tovetjarn R, Tarnow P, Maltese G, Fischer S, Sahlin PE, Kölby L. Children with Apert syndrome as adults: a follow-up study of 28 Scandinavian patients. Plast Reconstr Surg. 2012;130(4):572e–6e.
12. Visram SM, Gill D, Shute JT, Cunningham SJ. Qualitative study to identify issues affecting quality of life in adults with craniofacial anomalies. Br J Oral Maxillofac Surg. 2019;57(1):47–52.
13. Rosen HM. Evolution of a surgical philosophy in orthognathic surgery. Plast Reconstr Surg. 2017;139:978–90.
14. Thastum M, Andersen K, Rude K, Nørholt SE, Blomlöf J. Factors influencing intraoperative blood loss in orthognathic surgery. Int J Oral Maxillofac Surg. 2016;45:1070–3.
15. Steel BJ, Cope MR. Unusual and rare complications of orthognathic surgery: a literature review. J Oral Maxillofac Surg. 2012;70:1678–91.
16. Steenen SA, Becking AG. Bad splits in bilateral sagittal Split osteotomy: systematic review of fracture patterns. Int J Oral Maxillofac Surg. 2016;45:887–97.
17. Taylor JA, Naran S, Steinbacher DM. Current concepts in orthognathic surgery. Plast Reconstr Surg. 2018;141(6):925e–36e.
18. Posnick JC, Choi E, Liu S. Occurrence of a 'bad' split and success of initial mandibular healing: a review of 524 sagittal ramus osteotomies in 262 patients. Int J Oral Maxillofac Surg. 2016;45:1187–94.
19. Steenen SA, van Wijk AJ, Becking AG. Bad splits in bilateral sagittal split osteotomy: systematic review and meta-analysis of reported risk factors. Int J Oral Maxillofac Surg. 2016;45:971–9.
20. Schwartz HC. Simultaneous removal of third molars during sagittal split osteotomies: the case against. J Oral Maxillofac Surg. 2004;62:1147–9.
21. Moroi A, Yoshizawa K, Iguchi R, et al. Comparison of the computed tomography values of the bone fragment gap after sagittal split ramus osteotomy in mandibular prognathism with and without asymmetry. Int J Oral Maxillofac Surg. 2016;45:1520–5.
22. Kang MG, Yun KI, Kim CH, Park JU. Postoperative condylar position by sagittal split ramus osteotomy with and without bone graft. J Oral Maxillofac Surg. 2010;68:2058–64.

23. Yang HJ, Hwang SJ. Evaluation of postoperative stability after BSSRO to correct facial asymmetry depending on the amount of bone contact between the proximal and distal segment. J Craniomaxillofac Surg. 2014;42:e165–70.
24. Yang HJ, Hwang SJ. Contributing factors to intraoperative clockwise rotation of the proximal segment as a relapse factor after mandibular setback with sagittal split ramus osteotomy. J Craniomaxillofac Surg. 2014;42:e57–63.
25. Han JJ, Park MW, Park JB, Park HS, Paek SJ, Sul H. Evaluation of dominant influencing factor for postoperative relapse after BSSRO for mandibular prognathism. Recent Adv Orthod Orthognath Surg. 2014;1:27–36.
26. Jakobsone G, Stenvik A, Sandvik L, Espeland L. Three-year follow-up of bimaxillary surgery to correct skeletal class III malocclusion: stability and risk factors for relapse. Am J Orthod Dentofacial Orthop. 2011;139:80–9.
27. Han JJ, Lee SY, Hwang SJ. Postoperative stability after SSRO in mandibular prognathism in relation to rotation of proximal segment. Recent Adv Orthod Orthognath Surg. 2013;2:1–8.

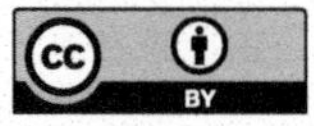

Innovations and Emerging Technologies in Craniofacial Surgery

30

William Cobb, Rose Meltzer, Andrew Willmer, and Rajendra Sawh-Martinez

Introduction

Craniofacial surgery has radically transformed since its formal inception in the 1960s. In the years since Dr. Paul Tessier paved the way for our contemporary practices, pioneering efforts have allowed us to integrate advanced technologies to address complex craniofacial anomalies [1]. The evolution from traditional surgical methods to the incorporation of virtual surgical planning (VSP), augmented reality (AR), robotics, and artificial intelligence (AI) holds promise for enhancing our surgical precision, improving patient outcomes, and expanding into all areas of surgical care.

The authors have no financial disclosures. We do present unpublished data and representative images of novel technologies and their applications.

W. Cobb
Department of General Surgery, AdventHealth Orlando, Orlando, FL, USA

R. Meltzer · A. Willmer
University of Central Florida School of Medicine, Orlando, FL, USA

R. Sawh-Martinez (✉)
Department of General Surgery, AdventHealth, Orlando, FL, USA

University of Central Florida School of Medicine, Orlando, FL, USA

Plastic and Reconstructive Surgery, AdventHealth for Children, Orlando, FL, USA

This chapter delves into key historical milestones and current innovations in craniofacial surgery, emphasizing the comprehensive management of syndromic craniosynostosis, such as Apert syndrome, with the application of these novel surgical methods and complex surgical decisions. Additionally, this chapter discusses the possible future integration of robotic systems and the prospective role of AI in the continued advancement of our field.

The field has evolved from its early days of reconstructive techniques to a sophisticated, technology-driven discipline that leverages advanced imaging, computer-assisted planning, and precision surgical tools, thereby revolutionizing the management of congenital and acquired craniofacial anomalies. The pioneering contributions of Tessier—regarded as the father of modern craniofacial surgery—laid the foundation for innovative approaches that continue to shape contemporary surgical practice.

Tessier's groundbreaking work in orbitofacial advancements and midface reconstruction provided the conceptual framework for correcting complex craniofacial deformities. Underpinning every technological advance aimed at "restoring normal," his meticulous approach to addressing craniosynostosis, cleft anomalies, and traumatic injuries emphasized function and aesthetics. In the decades since, advancements in three-dimensional (3D) imaging, biomaterials, and surgical techniques have transformed how craniofacial surgery is conceptualized and performed.

J. G. Meara et al. (eds.), *Apert Syndrome*, https://doi.org/10.1007/978-3-032-12551-4_30

Historical Context and Evolution of Craniofacial Surgery

In the early twentieth century, craniofacial surgery was largely limited to basic reconstructive efforts following trauma or congenital malformations. Techniques such as simple bone grafting and soft tissue rearrangement were primary tools available to surgeons. The mid-twentieth century witnessed the introduction of more sophisticated surgical approaches, thanks to advancements in anesthesia, microsurgical techniques, and imaging modalities such as X-rays and computerized tomography (CT) scans.

By the 1970s and 1980s, advances in CT scanning enabled better preoperative planning, providing 3D views of complex craniofacial anatomy. These developments set the stage for the introduction of computer-assisted surgical planning (CASP), which emerged in the 1990s and significantly enhanced the precision of craniofacial reconstructions [2]. Innovations such as distraction osteogenesis—first introduced by McCarthy et al. in 1992 for mandibular lengthening—further expanded the possibilities in the field by allowing gradual bone lengthening without the need for extensive grafting [3, 4].

More recently, the integration of VSP, AR, robotics, and AI has paved the way for highly individualized and precise surgical interventions. These technologies promise improved surgical accuracy, reduced operative times, minimized complications, and enhanced patient satisfaction [5–9]. As these technologies continue to evolve, their full potential and impact remain controversial, with safety, adaptability, cost, workflows, and learning curves at the forefront of critical issues that warrant paramount attention [10, 11].

Virtual Surgical Planning

Historical Background and Evolution

Virtual surgical planning (VSP) is a preoperative planning method that uses 3D imaging computer software to visualize a surgical procedure and enables surgeons to predefine their surgical maneuvers [12, 13]. VSP allows for precise preoperative planning, efficient intraoperative correction of cranial deformity, and objective surgical outcome assessment. Integration of VSP in craniosynostosis operations enables individualized correction for each patient, with reduced operation times and hospital admissions [14]. The origins of modern VSP in the craniofacial literature are found in various operations of the jaw—including distraction osteogenesis, orthognathic surgery, and microvascular mandibular reconstruction [15]—and can be traced back to the 1980s, when models of the patient's skull, based on CT data, were used for preoperative model planning and simulation surgery in maxillofacial surgery [16]. Early depictions of VSP can be seen in Figs. 30.1 and 30.2 by Marmulla et al. and Carpentier et al. [17, 18]. The phases of VSP evolution include (1) early foundations between 1999 and 2004, (2) expansion of applications and improved accuracy between 2005 and 2014, and (3) advanced integration between 2015 and 2024 [19]. Widely implemented in craniomaxillofacial surgery, VSP is commonly used in mandibular reconstruction, orthognathic surgery, maxillofacial trauma, and temporomandibular joint reconstruction, with a growing use in cranial vault remodeling and midface advancement [12]. Computer-assisted or virtual planning in surgery is intended to reduce intraoperative subjectivity, increase surgical accuracy, decrease surgical time, produce consistent results, and predict or obviate anatomical complications and difficulties, thereby accurately designing a precise

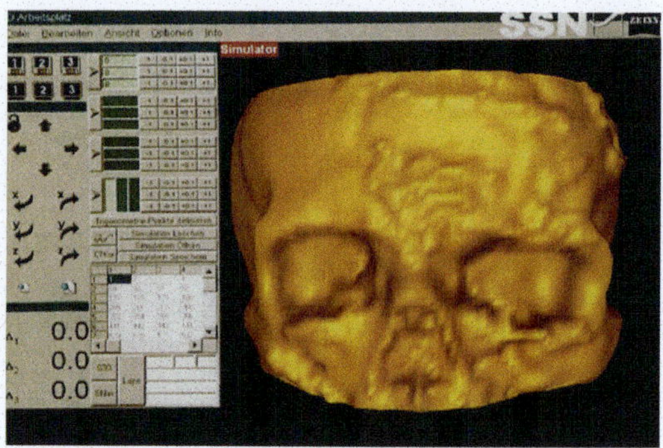

Fig. 30.1 Early reports of three-dimensional reconstruction of computerized tomography scan [17]

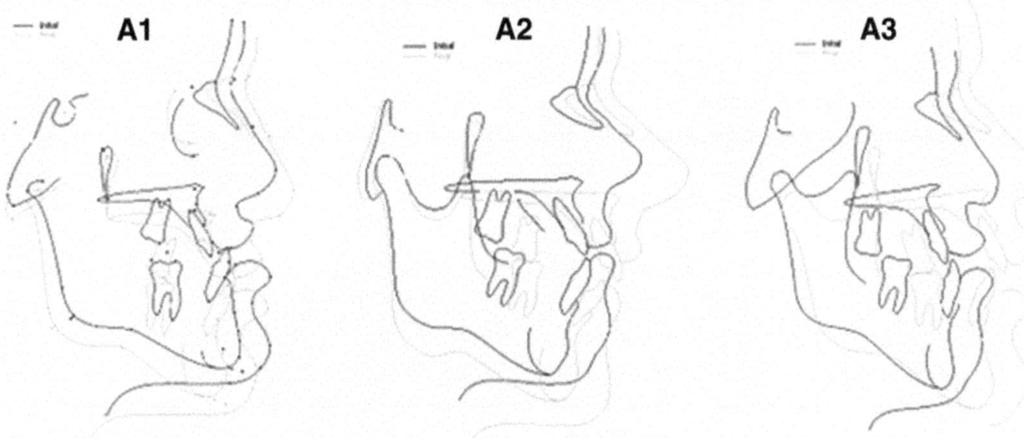

Fig. 30.2 Early utilization of virtual surgical planning for superimposition (black is pre-treatment and gray is post-treatment) of three patients with Apert syndrome who underwent either Le Fort (LF) I or Le Fort III. Patient 1 (A1), patient 2 (A2) and patient 3 (A3) [18]

and adequate surgical plan preoperatively [12, 13, 20].

Virtual Surgical Planning Process in Apert Syndrome and Craniosynostosis

VSP serves as a stimulator wherein the surgeon can outline the existing and potential problems, visualize the skull anatomy and deviations, plan the degree of bony resection/remodeling, and determine the precise desired degree of reconstruction. This enables the surgeon to visualize complex defects and variable anatomy to more accurately predict the unique reconstruction and treatment requirements of each patient. This enables high-fidelity transfer of preoperative surgical plans carefully derived from clinical and radiographic assessment to intraoperative maneuvers [12, 21].

The planning process is commonly divided into seven phases: (1) image acquisition, (2) planning session, (3) patient consultation, (4) computer-aided manufacturing, (5) delivery, (6), surgery, and (7) postoperative verification of results [15]. Preoperative planning of osseous maneuvers may be guided by using "standardized" age-matched infant skulls as a reference of "normal," or by using mirror image overlays to create symmetry and volume expansion. Superimposing 3D CT scan reconstructions of a representative age-matched patient's skull facilitates identification of the precise areas of modification of the underlying craniofacial skeleton [21]. Examples of VSP for patients undergoing Le Fort (LF) I, LF III, fronto-orbital advancement (FOA), LF II distraction with zygomatic repositioning, and cranial vault remodeling can be seen in Figs. 30.2, 30.3, 30.4, and 30.5 [18, 22, 23].

Prior to the advent of VSP, surgeons engaged in a preoperative planning process whereby judgments and measurements relied on cephalometric landmarks and measurements from normalized skulls. When applied to the malformed skull, slight measurement discrepancies or inaccurate assessments can lead to error transmission in surgical maneuvers and potential under-corrections or incomplete corrections [24–30].

The added ability to directly superimpose a virtual surgical plan on the individual child's skull—via 3D printed surgical cutting and remodeling guides—further reduces potential subjectivity during surgery. Critically, any errors of judgment in the virtual preplanning process carry forward to the manufacturing and surgical phases [15]. Although the virtual space allows for infinite options, it

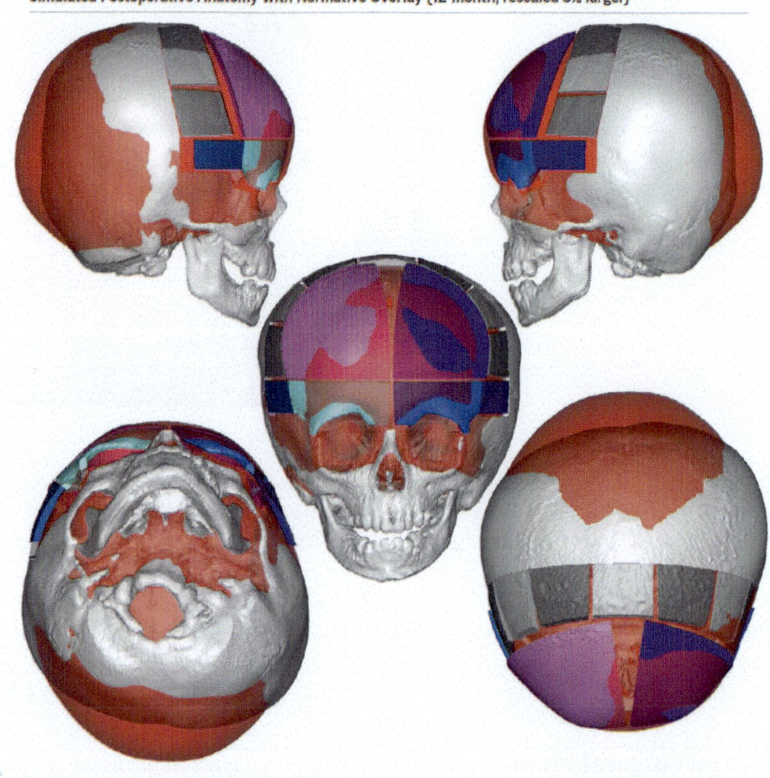

Fig. 30.3 Sample skull overlay for fronto-orbital advancement (FOA). This allows for adjusting and matching the "normal" anatomy with planned expansion or over-correction as desired for FOA. Visualized is a representative demonstration of a planned correction of a patient with syndromic presentation of metopic craniosynostosis via FOA

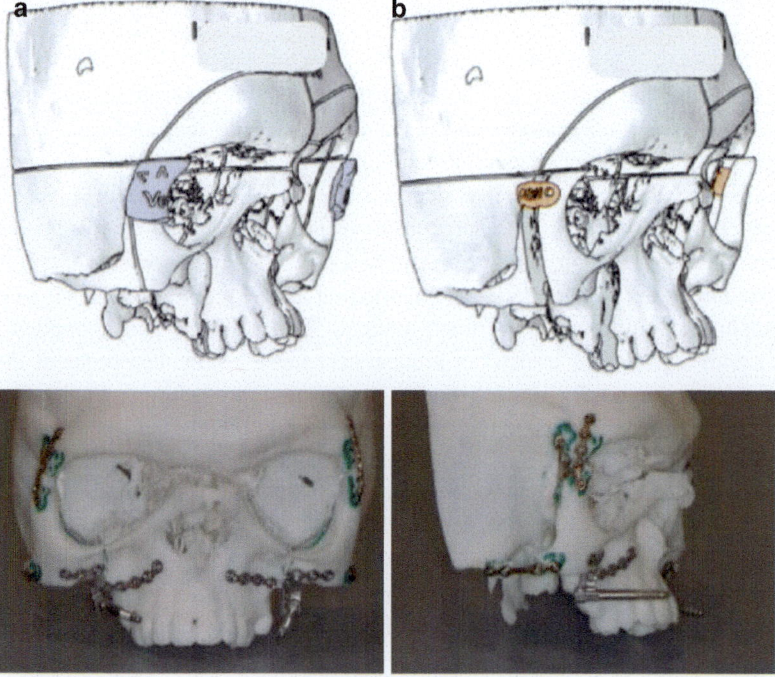

Fig. 30.4 The use of virtual surgical planning (VSP) tools by Nørholt et al. for Le Fort II distraction with zygomatic repositioning in a patient with Apert syndrome. (**a**) VSP design cutting guides (purple). (**b**) VSP design spaces (orange). (**c**) Preoperative planning with simulation of distraction [22]

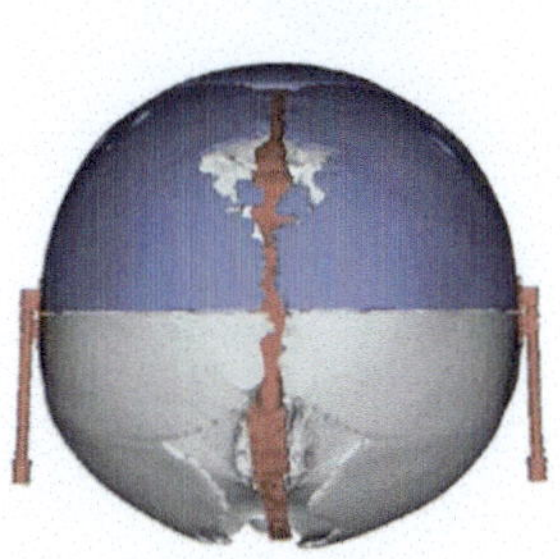

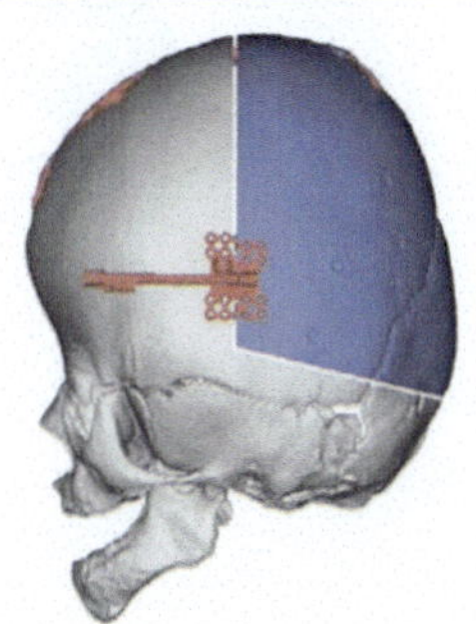

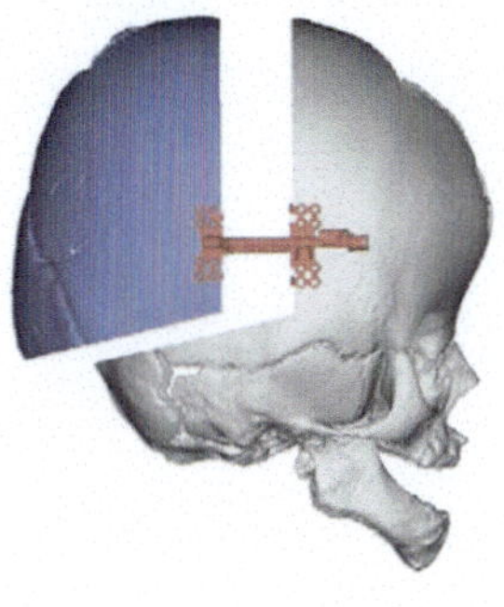

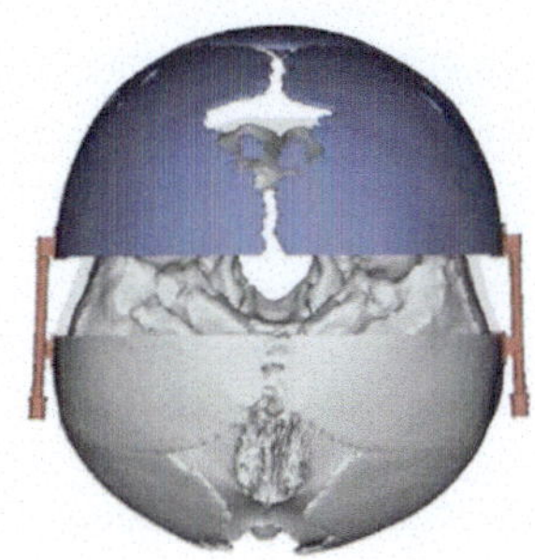

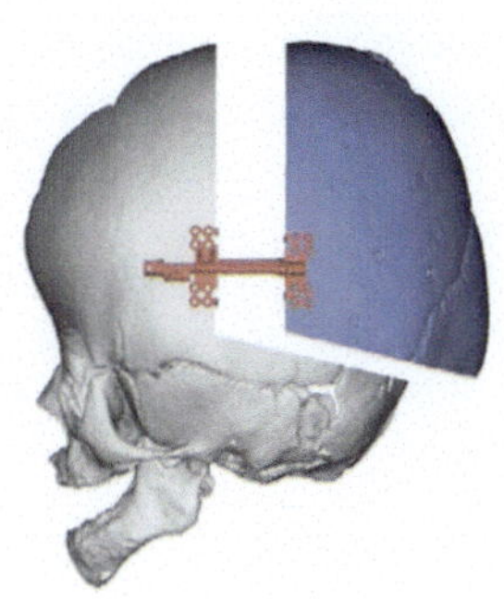

Fig. 30.5 Imahiyerobo et al. utilizing virtual surgical planning to demonstrate placement of cranial distractors and subsequent movement with (**a**) initial position and (**b**) final position in a patient with Apert syndrome undergoing cranial vault remodeling [23]

remains the domain of expert surgeons to use their judgement and expertise to ensure the surgical plan is safe and achievable. Thus, surgical trainees and junior surgeons are tasked with mastering complex anatomical cephalometric principles, understanding of the panoply of surgical options, and developing a clear, robust understanding of what constitutes a realistic, achievable surgical plan (Fig. 30.6).

Free-access software and low-cost in-house printing equipment currently on the market make VSP more accessible globally. However, third-party industry solutions remain a cornerstone of the surgical process for complex cases and for the operating-room-safe fabrication of patient-specific guides and implants. Novel surgical planning applications, surgical simulation software, and 3D printers continue to arrive in the marketplace, each with varying costs and nuances in workflows aimed at improving surgeon interaction with patient-specific virtual models [12].

Advantages of Virtual Surgical Planning

Several advantages of VSP have been touted in the literature, such as decreased surgical time, decreased preoperative planning time, and improved surgical accuracy (see Table 30.1). Guruprasad et al. found that VSP decreased operative time as compared to conventional planning in maxillofacial reconstruction surgery [13]. Lin et al. performed a systematic review of 78 articles regarding applications of 3D printed technology in orthognathic surgery with the use of occlusal splints, osteotomy guides, positioning guides, spacers, fixations (e.g., plates and implants), and 3D printed models. They found this technology to be beneficial to both the clinician and the patient, reducing both preoperative planning time and overall surgical time [32]. In their systematic review,

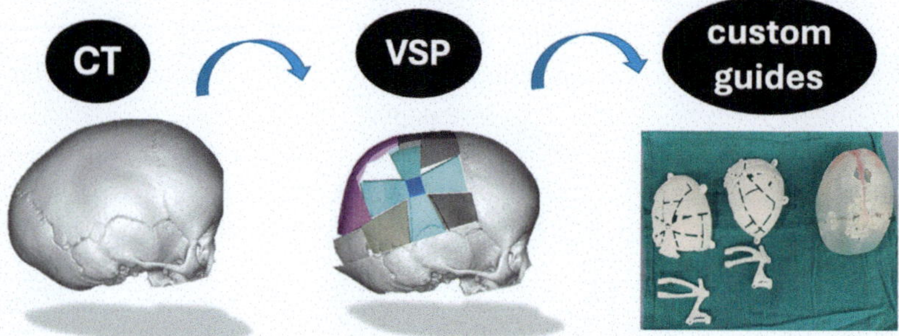

Fig. 30.6 Virtual surgical planning workflows are critically reliant on surgeon expertise to define the parameters of a safe and achievable surgery. Surgical plans are aided by custom three-dimensional printed guides, which can be sterilized and used intraoperatively to guide surgical decision making and visualize challenging anatomy

Table 30.1 Summary of recent advantages to VSP

Author	Year	Major findings
Lin	2018	Reduced preoperative planning time and overall surgical time
Alkhaver	2020	Virtual planning leads to increased surgical accuracy
Kalmar	2020	Increased utilization of VSP for pediatric craniofacial procedures
Pampin-Martinez	2022	Overall acceptable predictability of virtual surgical planning accuracy
Guruprasad	2024	VSP decreased time of surgery compared to conventional

Alkhayer et al. analyzed 12 manuscripts regarding the accuracy analysis of VSP. They observed that the calculation of the linear and angular differences between the virtual plans and postoperative outcomes was the method most frequently used for accuracy assessment, and a difference of less than 2 mm/° was considered acceptable. They concluded that VSP led to increased accuracy [33]. In evaluating the accuracy of VSP, Pampin Martinez et al. found the differences between the surgical simulation and the actual postoperative results were less than 1 mm for most cephalometric landmarks, indicating overall acceptable predictability of the virtual surgery [20]. Kalmar et al. found that utilization of VSP for pediatric craniofacial procedures is increasing, especially for complex orthognathic procedures and osteocutaneous free tissue transfers [31] (Figs. 30.7, 30.8, and 30.9).

To date, VSP has been used in planning operations on the calvarium, cranial vault, orbit, nasoethmoid bone, zygomatic bone, zygomatic-orbital-maxillary complex, zygomaticomaxillary complex, midface, temporo-mandibular joint, masseter muscle, maxilla, mandible, dental arches, skull base, upper airway, and fibula [34].

Challenges in Virtual Surgical Planning

Noted drawbacks and critiques of VSP merit strong consideration: surgeon learning curve, cost, planning time, preparation time, and additional training must be accounted for in considering its use. Critically, VSP cannot guarantee successful surgical outcomes and is wholly reliant on surgeon expertise to fully analyze the existing anatomy and variability, then to review all variables that could lead to errors at any point in the process. These include 3D integration with patient's anatomical data, segment identification and mobilization, computer-aided surgical simulation, fabrication of splints and surgical guides,

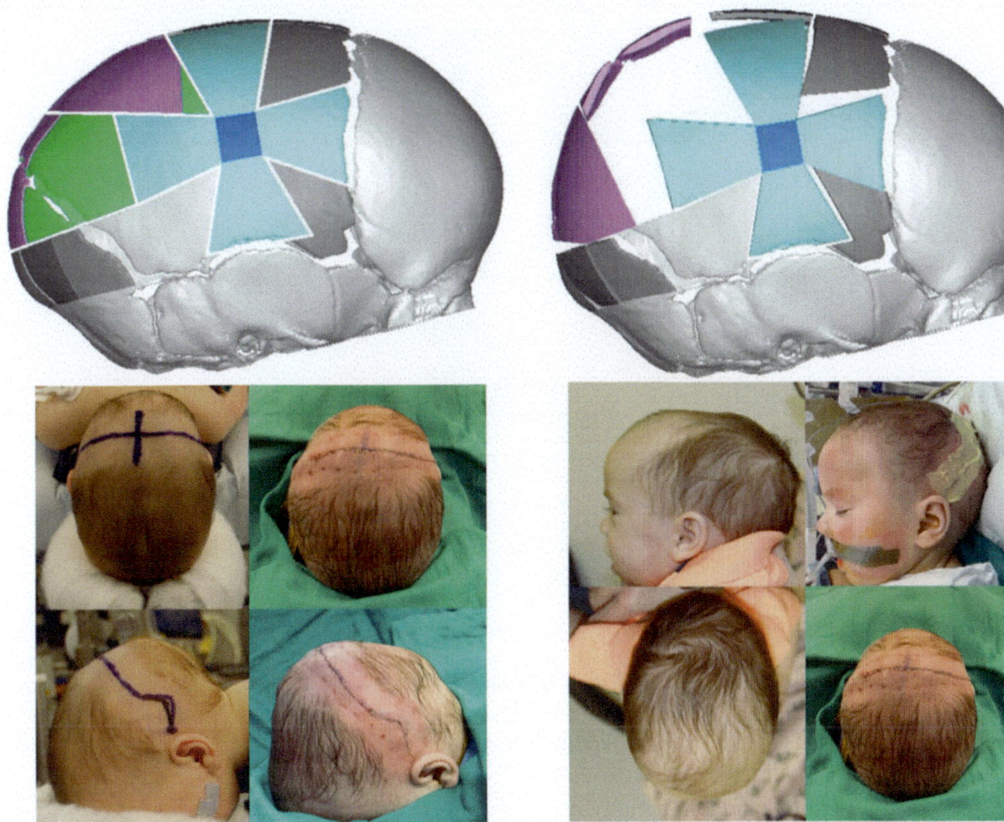

Fig. 30.7 Clinical examples of surgical outcomes aided by virtual surgical planning (VSP). Complex anatomy and patient-specific landmarks are visualized and accounted for, allowing for customized and optimized surgical corrections. Clinical example of VSP in single suture craniosynostosis with customized plan accounting for individual variation

3D image superimposition, and determination in virtual space [12]. Expert surgeons must also have robust "back-up" plans, be able to anticipate failures and inaccuracies, and account for growth as they perform surgeries in the growing skeleton.

Conclusion

Overall, VSP has facilitated accurate diagnoses and detailed treatment planning through improved visualization in 3D space of phenotypic changes, allowing for a precise preoperative surgical plan using a computerized 3D environment. Over the past 10 years, the development of 3D printed models and patient-specific guides has significantly improved surgical planning and transfer of the surgical plan into the operating room [20]. Much of the current published literature on this topic focuses on workflow, technology, and protocols necessary for its integration into clinical practice [34]. As an increasing number of centers around the world adopt and optimize workflows, technological costs may continue to decrease and allow for widespread adoption of this surgical tool.

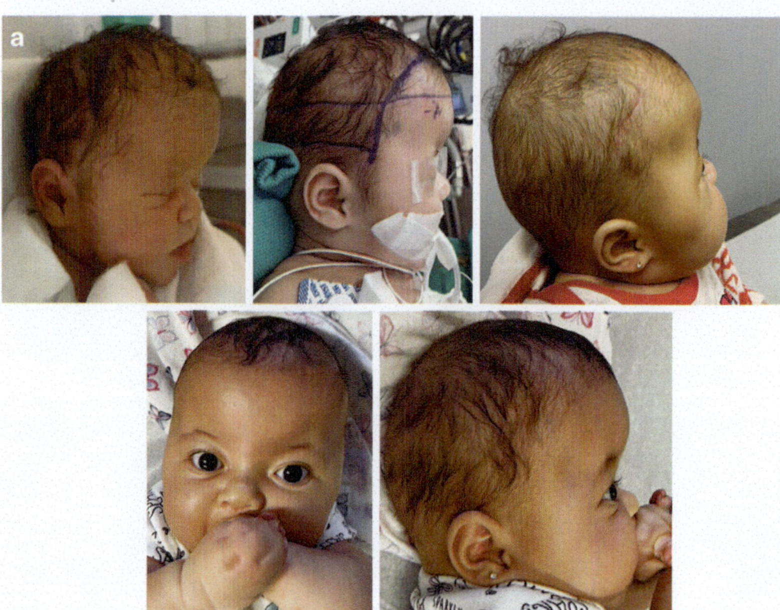

Fig. 30.8 Apert virtual surgical planning case (**a**) Infant with Apert syndrome and bicoronal craniosynostosis undergoing planned staged approach (strip craniectomy and posterior vault distraction osteogenesis). *Top left,* initial presentation. *Top middle,* surgical plan at strip craniectomy. *Top right,* clinical improvement in cranial shape after strip craniectomy. *Bottom left and right,* three-month post-strip craniectomy. (**b**) *Left,* virtual surgical planning images with highlights of avoidance of cranial defects from prior strip craniectomy and demonstration of the osteotomy and three-dimensional printed guides. *Right,* detailed anatomical planning and heat maps of bone thickness allow for optimal distractor placement. (**c**) *Top left,* demonstration of incision placement. *Top center,* osteotomy guides. *Top and bottom right,* pre- and postoperative surgical models. *Bottom middle,* pericranial flaps and intraoperative placement of distractor devices. *Bottom left,* immediate postoperative result with exposed distractor arms. (**d**) Clinical progression over time and long-term outcomes of cranial morphology. *Top left,* initial presentation and morphology at time of strip craniectomy. *Top right,* cranial morphology after strip craniectomy (eight months of age). *Bottom left,* result at six months post-operation. *Bottom right,* result of long-term correction (four years of age) without additional intervention

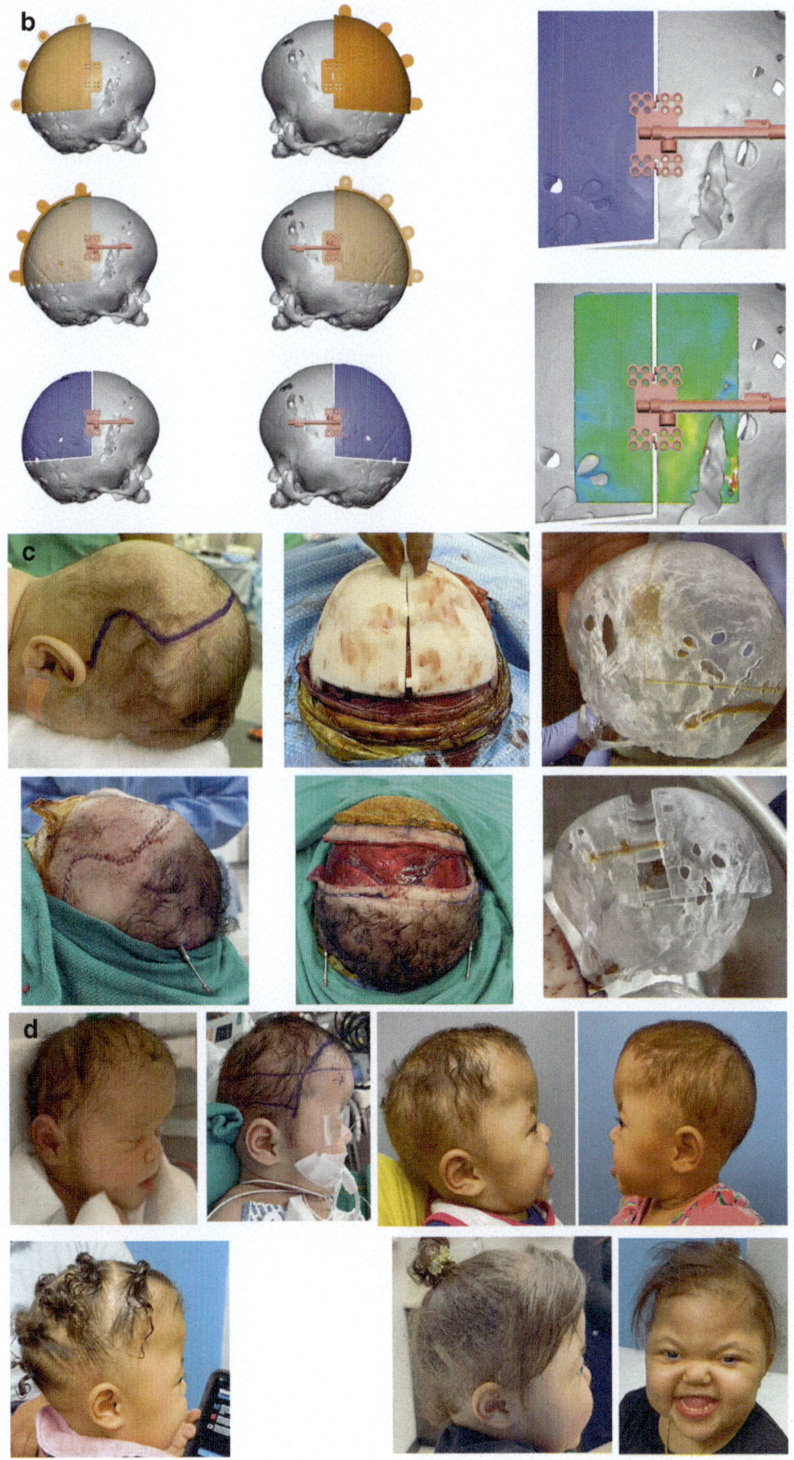

Fig. 30.8 (continued)

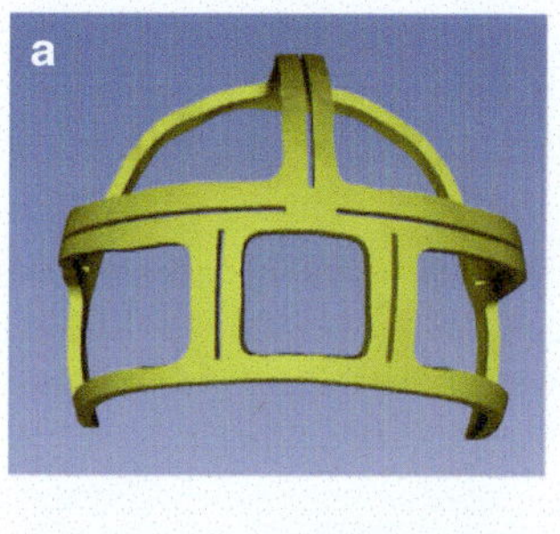

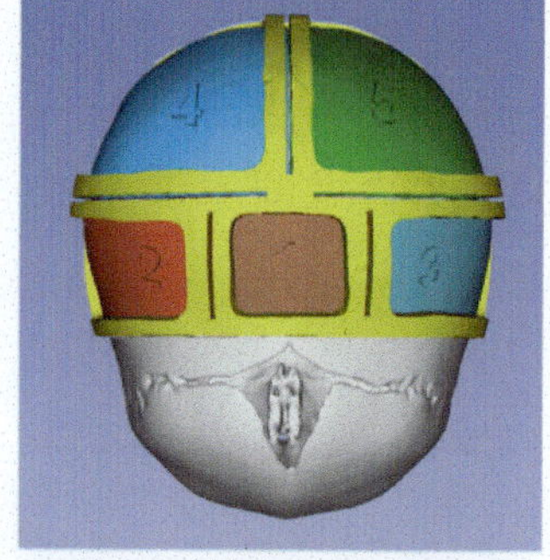

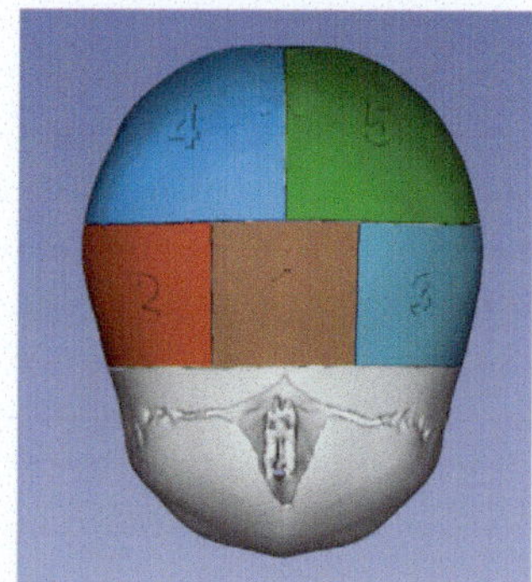

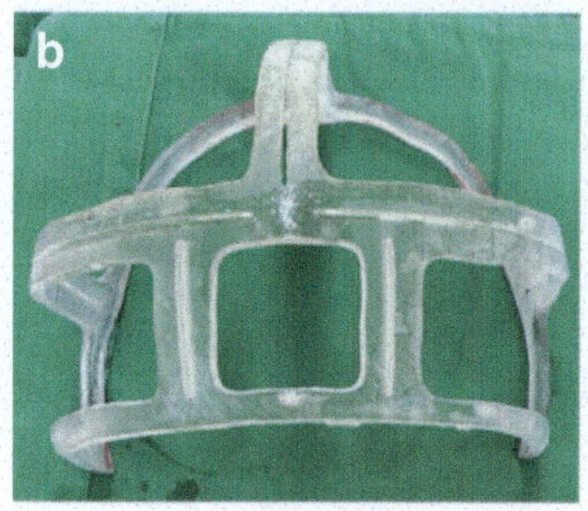

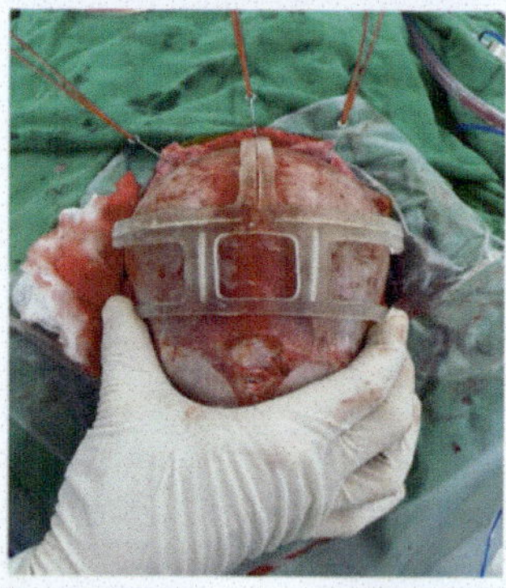

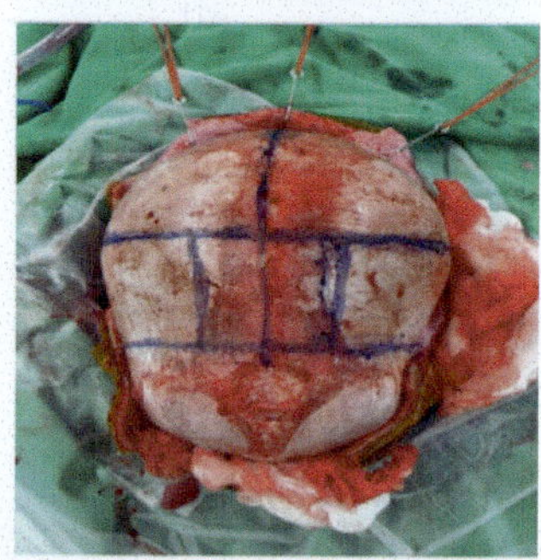

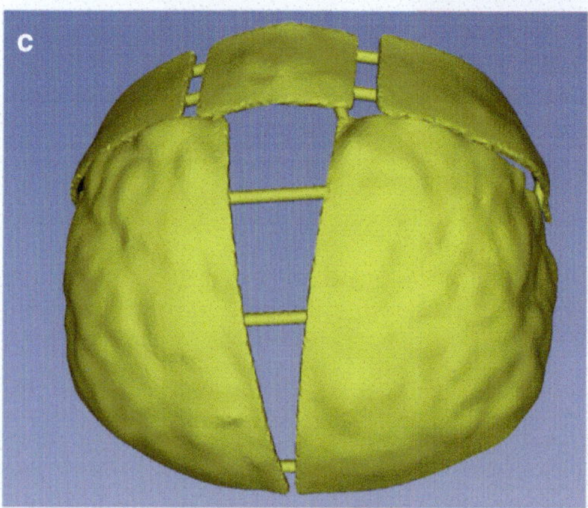

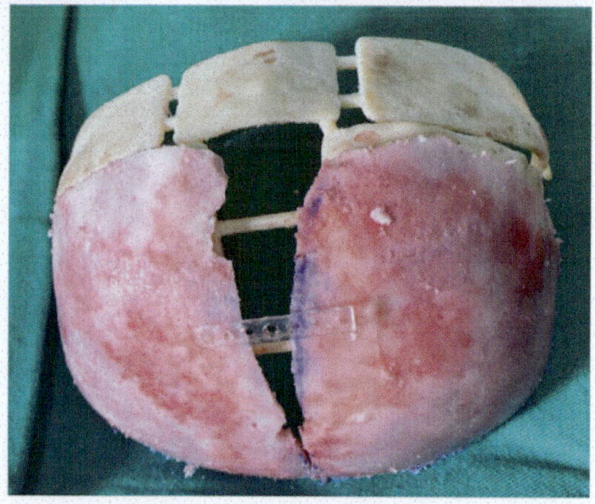

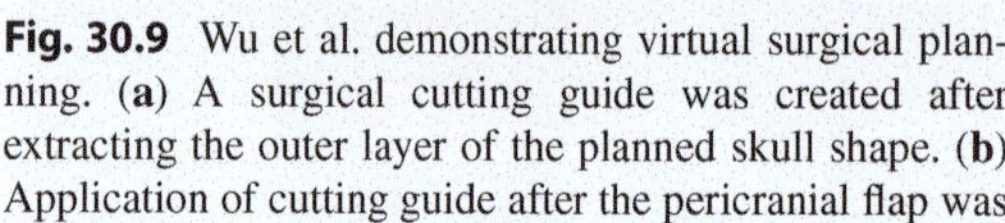

Fig. 30.9 Wu et al. demonstrating virtual surgical planning. (**a**) A surgical cutting guide was created after extracting the outer layer of the planned skull shape. (**b**) Application of cutting guide after the pericranial flap was lifted. (**c**) A surgical reconstruction guide was created after extracting the inner layer of the planned skull shape. Bone flaps were assembled according to the reconstruction guide [14]

Augmented Reality (AR)

"The eye sees only what the mind is prepared to comprehend"—Robertson Davies

Current State of AR in Surgery

Augmented reality (AR) has potential to enhance intraoperative visualization by overlaying 3D holographic virtual information onto the surgical field, providing surgeons with real-time guidance and improved spatial awareness [35]. AR is distinct from virtual reality (VR), which creates a wholly contained virtual interaction and does not engage with "real" space. Most surgical VR applications find their niche in the surgical planning, education, and training paradigms. Herein, we are focused on AR, which aims to engage directly with our surroundings and holds the promise to improve our real-time visualization of "hidden" anatomy in surgery.

As technology continues to evolve, both software and hardware used for displaying and analyzing patient data remain dynamic. The development of AR solutions in surgery requires close collaboration between technology companies, academic institutions, and health systems to ensure the safety and efficacy of their products [36]. Given the nature of its application, continued study is required before AR can be routinely utilized in the operating room [37]. Various companies (e.g., Novarad, Medivis, Sira Medical) have dedicated resources and partnered with surgeons to specifically develop AR applications for surgery using commercially available headsets (e.g., Microsoft HoloLens, Apple Vision Pro) [38]. Other strategies aim to streamline AR technology specifically for surgical applications by developing solutions that integrate both hardware and software on proprietary headsets [37, 39–41].

Applications of AR in the Operating Room

A critical application of AR in surgery is the integration of patient scans, such as magnetic resonance imagings (MRIs) or CTs, directly onto the patient during the procedure [40]. This allows surgeons to visualize deeper anatomical structures without repeated imaging, thereby reducing radiation exposure and operative time [42, 43]. Additionally, MRI scans and computer-aided design (CAD) models can be directly visualized throughout the surgery, making established imaging tools more accessible for preoperative planning [44]. This enhances the surgeon's ability to perform the procedure with minimal need for cross-referencing external planning materials. However, accurate image registration is essential to prevent surgical errors. Solutions to this challenge include mapping images to anatomical landmarks, using fiducial markers placed on the patient and within virtual planning software, using manual registration, and evolving use of digital (QR) registration codes [41]. Static scans may not always reflect the patient's growth and real-time positioning, requiring the surgeon to remain vigilant to anatomical differences that may arise during patient preparation or when adjusting patient orientation after registration (Fig. 30.10).

AR for Craniofacial Surgery

Given the broad applications of AR, research continues to highlight innovative uses across nearly all surgical subspecialties [37]. Recent studies emphasize the potential of AR to improve outcomes in craniosynostosis repair, orthognathic surgery, and trauma reconstruction. The skull provides an excellent model for overlaying holograms of patient data in the operating room, as cranial cephalometric landmarks remain mostly stable regardless of patient positioning. For example, in posterior vault distraction osteogenesis, VSP can define the precise locations of cuts along the posterior vault. The portions of the skull intended for removal can then be highlighted or made to disappear from the hologram, depending on the surgical stage. In orthognathic or midface advancement surgeries, pre-planned realignment of the facial profile can be visualized before surgery, while real-time holographic overlays of pre- and postoperative images aid in assessing the accuracy of corrections intraopera-

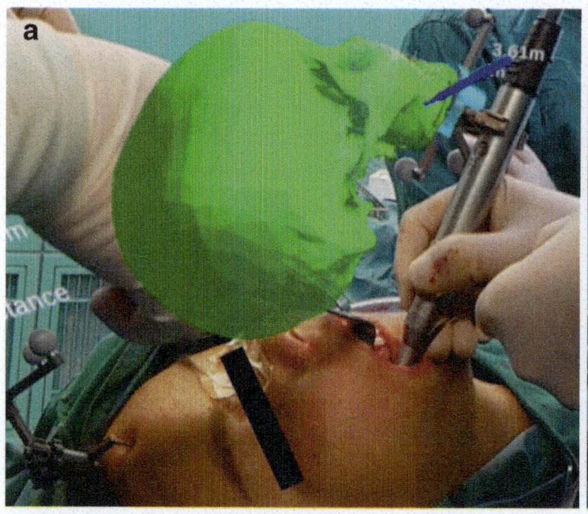

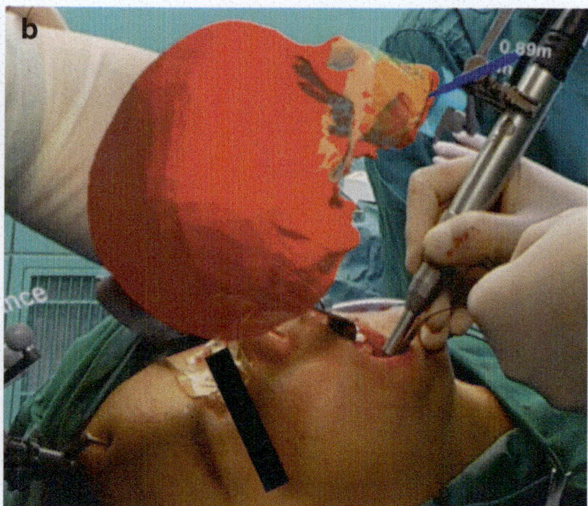

Fig. 30.10 Lui et al. demonstrating different stages of intraoperative guidance with augmented reality: (**a**) When the drill remains at a large distance from the designed surface (>1 mm), the model is rendered in green, displaying real-time data. (**b**) When the drill is about to reach the designed surface (≤1 mm), the model is rendered in red, displaying real-time data [45]

tively. In trauma reconstruction, patient-specific prosthetics can be incorporated into the hologram, guiding the surgeon in positioning and installing the device correctly (Fig. 30.11).

Currently, AR applications in the operating room are being tested and explored, with constant advancement of application tools, processing speed of digitized registration, and novel approaches to image registration. Best practices in craniofacial surgery revolve around dedicated surgeons collaborating with software engineers to continue the iterative process of improvement to allow for a functional clinical solution. Major challenges in adopting AR include reliance on headsets, requirements for lighting and transparency, a steep learning curve for surgeons, improving registration accuracy, maintaining image stability under changing conditions, minimizing image lag, high costs, and limited clinical data on safety and outcomes (Fig. 30.12).

Despite these challenges, the longstanding promise of AR technology continues to near realization. As our technological capabilities evolve—coupled with burgeoning integration with AI, improved image registration techniques, and expansion into new surgical domains—AR has the potential to revolutionize modern surgery by enhancing precision, increasing efficiency, and improving patient outcomes.

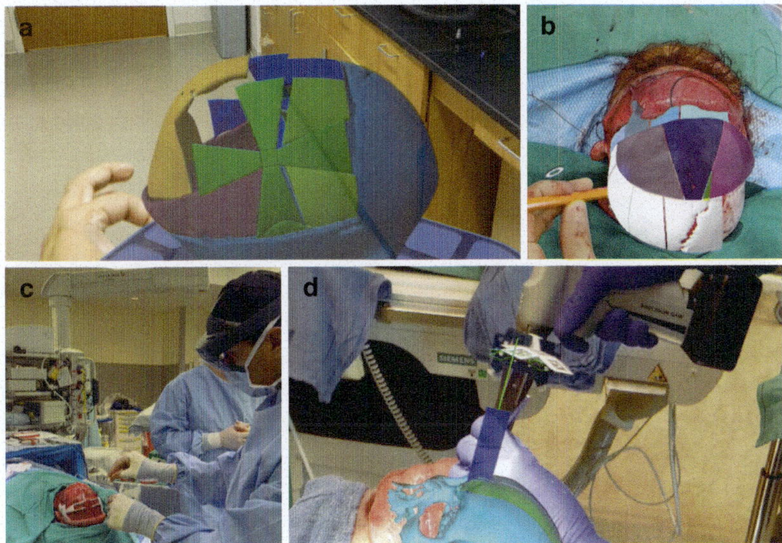

Fig. 30.11 Augmented reality (AR) applications in craniofacial surgery are in development. (**a**) The ability to overlay digital representations of virtual plans and manipulate them with 360-degree visualization allows for nuanced pre-surgical understanding. (**b**) Intraoperative view through the HoloLens of a "cutting guide" allows for the evaluation and testing of this technology as compared to traditional methods. (**c**) External view of the surgeon using AR to ensure correct positioning of bony reconstruction. (**d**) Development of next-generation AR tools, including drill guidance and fiducials using QR codes

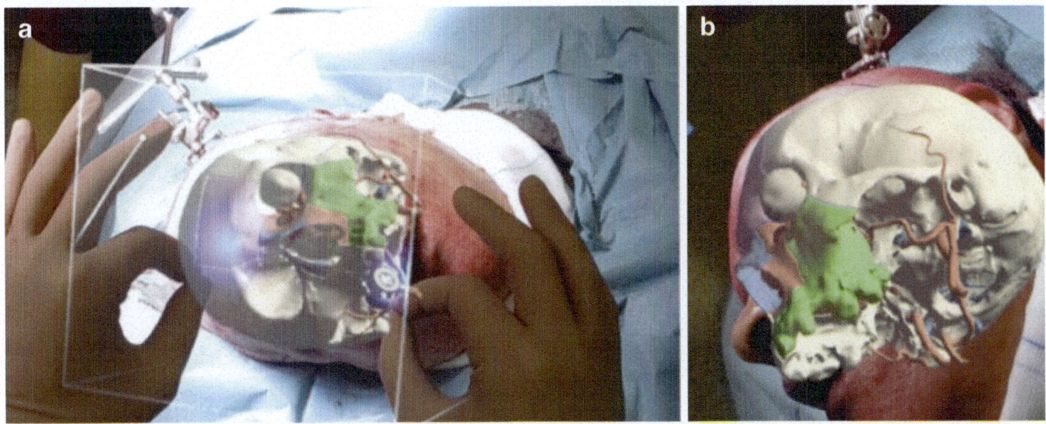

Fig. 30.12 Tel et al. demonstrate the use of augmented reality (AR) intraoperatively. (**a**) Interactive overlap of the AR image within the surgical field. (**b**) Observing the alignment from multiple perspectives while the AR projection remains stable [46]

Robotic-Assisted Surgery

Historical Background and Evolution

The incorporation of robotic systems in surgery dates to the 1980s, with the development of the PUMA 560, one of the first robotic-assisted surgical devices used for neurosurgical biopsies. Robotic surgery has advanced drastically in the years since, particularly with the advent of the da Vinci Surgical System that revolutionized minimally invasive surgery.

In 2000, Steiner advocated for transoral laser microsurgery but encountered issues with obstruction in the line of sight, as well as resection complications in the cranial and axial axes. To overcome these limitations, transoral robotic surgery (TORS) was proposed and first applied clinically in maxillofacial surgery by McLeod and Melder to excise a vallecular cyst. This procedure was approved by the US Food and Drug Administration in 2009 for use in stage T1 and T2 oropharyngeal cancer. Since that time, robot-assisted maxillofacial surgery has grown steadily and holds promise in the treatment of craniofacial conditions, head and neck neoplasms, cleft lip and palate, and craniofacial dysmorphologies [47–49].

In craniofacial surgery, robotics have primarily been utilized for microsurgical reconstruction, with an increasing interest in applying robotic precision to osteotomies, implant positioning, and distraction osteogenesis. The emergence of supermicrosurgery robots (e.g., Symani Surgical System, MUSA) has further expanded the possibilities for delicate procedures.

Pioneering work for robotic craniofacial surgery started on animal models [50–52] (Figs. 30.13, 30.14, and 30.15).

Current Applications in Craniofacial Surgery

Robotic technology is currently being used in the following areas of craniofacial surgery: microsurgical free flap reconstruction, orthognathic surgery, and pediatric craniofacial surgery. The delicate nature of pediatric craniofacial anatomy makes robotics an attractive option for improving

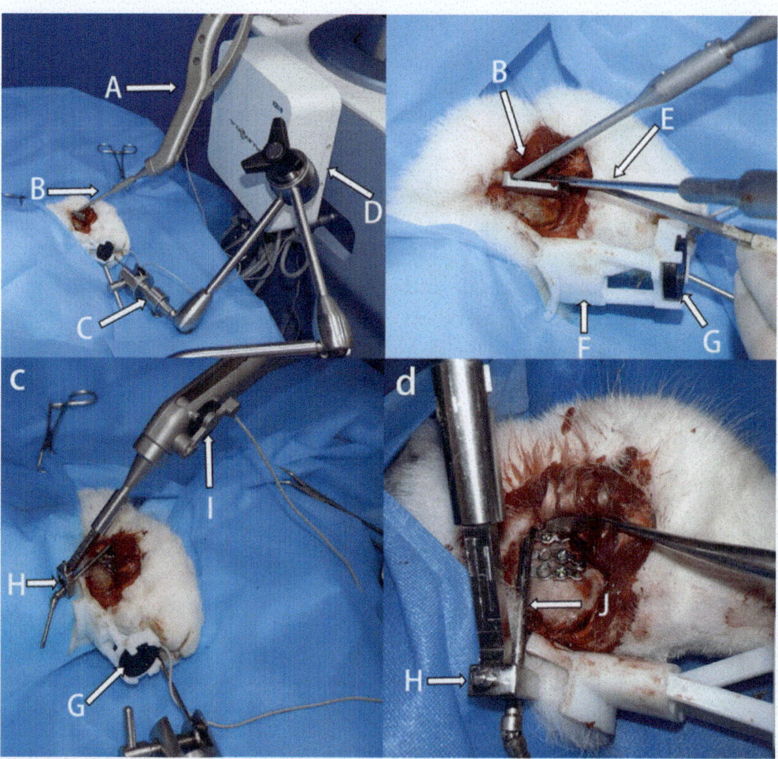

Fig. 30.13 Robotic-assisted osteotomy and distractor positioning. (A) The template is at the initial target position. (B) Robotic-assisted osteotomy under electromagnetic navigation. The saw blade is against the template. The robot moves continuously from the initial position to the second position along the osteotomy line, with the saw blade following it forward. (C) The template has been replaced with the clamp, which holds the distractor in motion to the expected position. (d) Distractor implantation is completed after drilling and tightening the screws. (A) robotic arm sub-end, (B) template, (C) fixator, (D) electromagnetic generator, (E) bone saw, (F) registration complex, (G) electromagnetic sensor connected to the mandible, (H) clamp, (I) electromagnetic sensor connected to the robotic arm, (J) distractor [50]

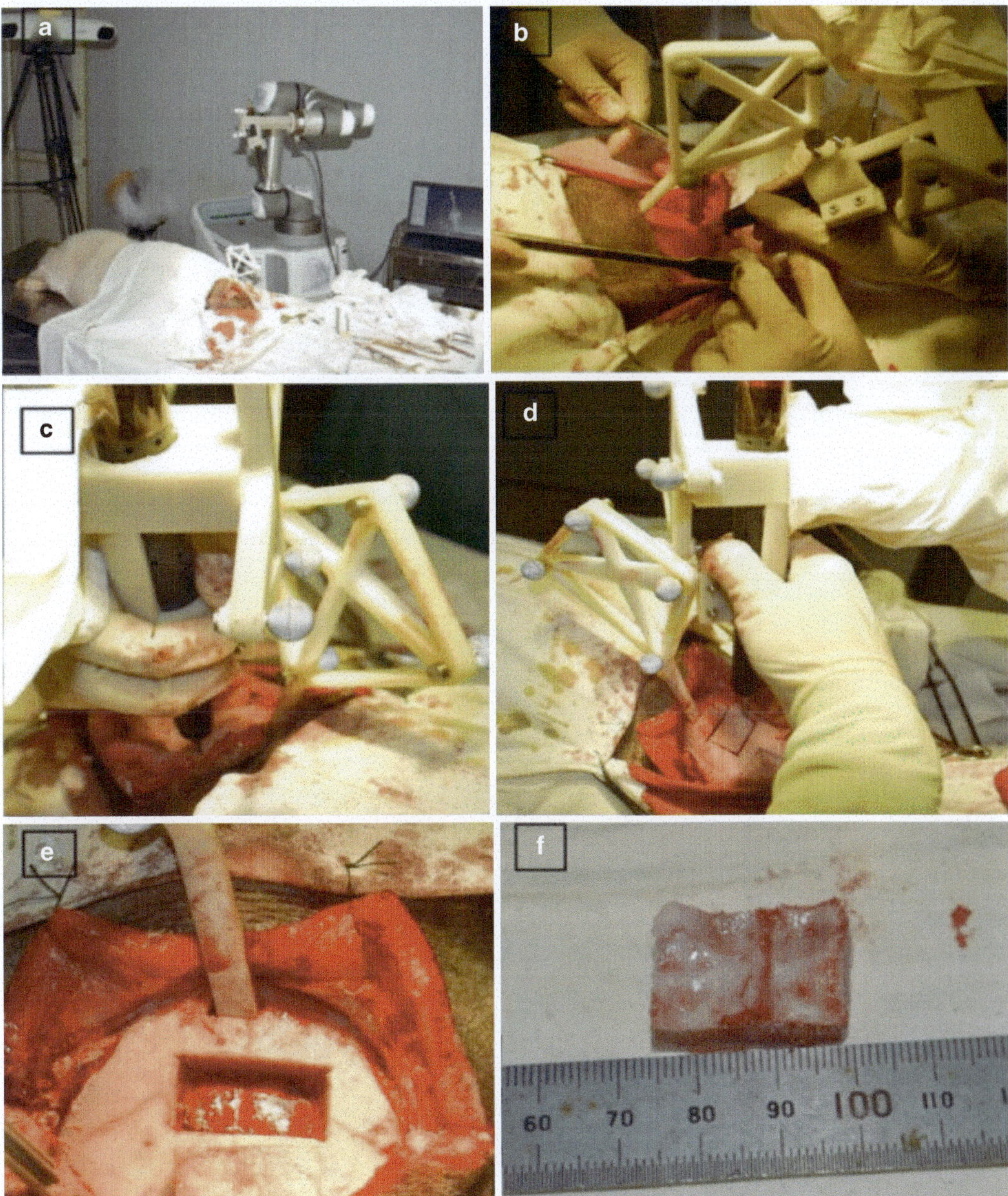

Fig. 30.14 (**a**) Preparation for surgery on an animal with a craniomaxillofacial plastic surgery robot. (**b–d**) Osteotomy with craniomaxillofacial plastic surgery robot on the animal. (**e**) Frontal bone flap and dura mater without injury. (**f**) The frontal bone flap from the osteotomy with craniomaxillofacial plastic surgery robot [51]

surgical precision. Robotic-assisted distraction osteogenesis has been explored to correct conditions such as Pierre Robin sequence and severe mandibular hypoplasia. Khan et al. first reported the theoretical feasibility of robotic intraoral cleft surgery and Hynes pharyngoplasty in a pediatric airway manikin and human cadaver in 2015 [53]. Nadjmi demonstrated the technical feasibility and safety of robot-assisted soft palate muscle reconstruction in ten consecutive patients with palatal clefts after cadaveric TOR [54] (Fig. 30.16).

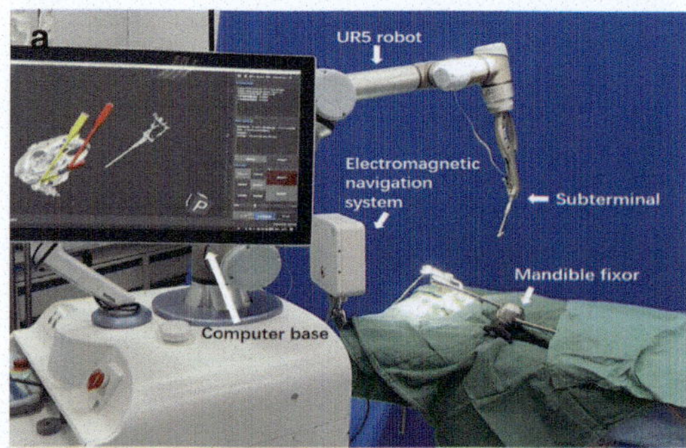

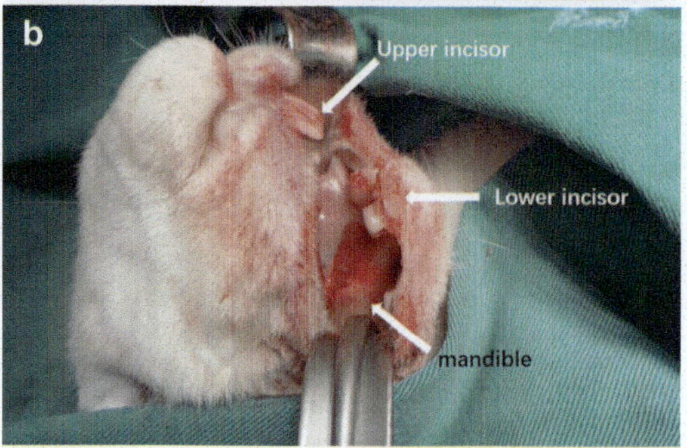

Fig. 30.15 (**a**) The maxillofacial surgical robotic system used by Han et al. (**b**) Intraoral exposure of the mandible [52]

Other clinical applications of these robotic technologies include surgical treatment for head and neck cancers, thyroid and parathyroid dissection, lingual thyroglossal duct cyst, salivary gland removal, neck dissection, post-ablative reconstruction, cleft lip and palate, maxillofacial fractures, craniofacial asymmetry, laryngeal clefts and laryngocele [47].

Advantages of Robotic Surgery

The key advantages of robotic systems in craniofacial surgery include increased precision, enhanced visualization, and a minimally invasive approach. Fine motor control and tremor elimination allow for more delicate and intricate procedures. Robotic systems offer high-definition, 3D visualization while improving the surgeon's ability to navigate complex anatomy. Additionally, robotic systems improve ergonomics for the surgeon. The smaller incisions and reduced soft-tissue disruption achieved with robotic systems

Fig. 30.16 (**a**) Raising left Hynes pharyngoplasty flap (dental rubber template) in the posterior pharynx. (**b**) Unconventional view with patient anatomy "correct side up" demonstrating potential access to palate [50]

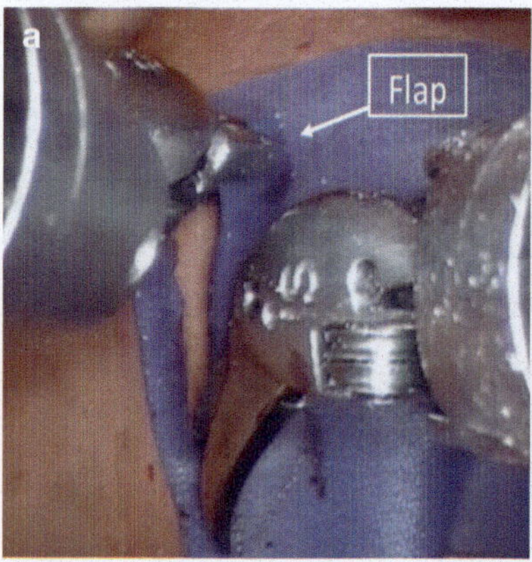

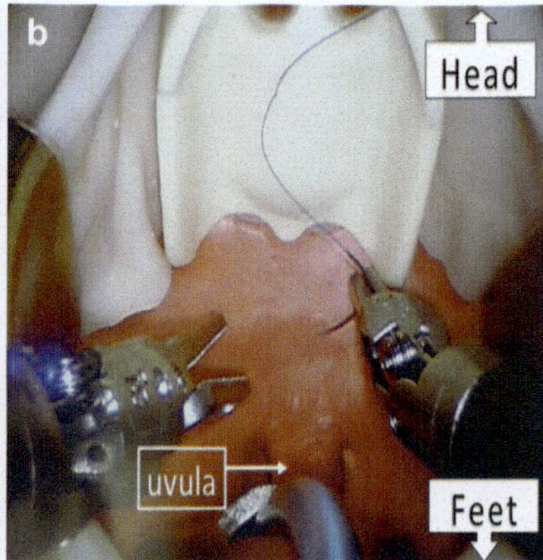

enable faster recovery times [55, 56]. The high precision and accuracy of robotic surgery could improve patient care overall, as reflected in the lower rate of reported complications, reduced blood loss, and reduced postoperative pain [55]. Although patient benefits include lower rate of complications and quicker recovery, some categories entail longer operative duration [55]. Robots enhance precision during microvascular anastomosis by reducing human tremor, improving suture placement accuracy, and reducing the variability in manual osteotomies, leading to fewer postoperative complications. Studies by Davison et al. demonstrated that robotic-assisted free flap reconstruction resulted in a 20% improvement in patency rates compared to manual techniques. Robot-assisted osteotomies potentially allow for highly precise and reproducible bone cuts, although these have yet to be reported. Robotic assistance in craniofacial surgery holds promise in preventing iatrogenic injury from more traditional methods and could allow for operations to proceed earlier in life in the management of midface distraction [56] (Fig. 30.17).

In 2025, Li et al. reported that robotic-assisted procedures in mandibular osteotomy surgery can reduce osteotomy length error by an average of 2.2 mm and mandibular angle error by 9.09°, while decreasing the average surgery time by 10.43 minutes. In hemifacial microsomia distraction osteogenesis surgery, robotic-assisted surgery can reduce osteotomy length error by an average of 4.6 mm and shorten the average surgery time by 60 minutes, with better perioperative outcomes for patients. Overall, robot-assisted procedures improved surgical precision and significantly reduced postoperative complications [57].

Challenges in Robotic-Assisted Craniofacial Surgery

Despite its promise, robotic craniofacial surgery faces several challenges including high costs, a steep learning curve, and lack of haptic feedback during the operation. Most current systems do not provide tactile feedback, which is critical for certain surgical tasks. Robotic systems are also expensive to acquire and maintain, limiting their widespread adoption. Moreover, surgeons require extensive training to master robotic-assisted techniques effectively [47, 55].

Future Prospects of Robotics in Craniofacial Surgery

As robotic technology continues to evolve, future applications may include autonomous robotic systems capable of executing pre-

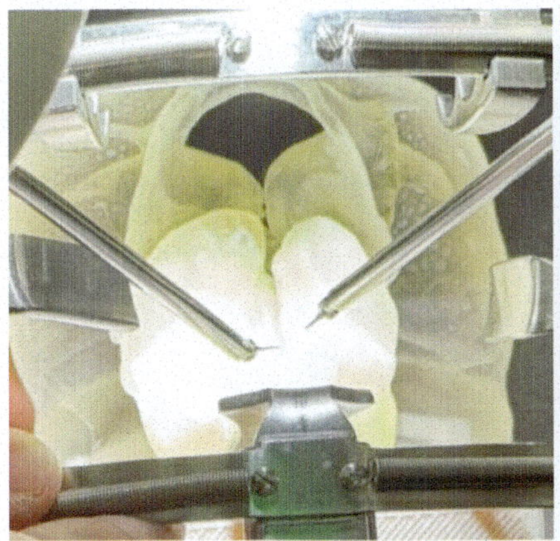

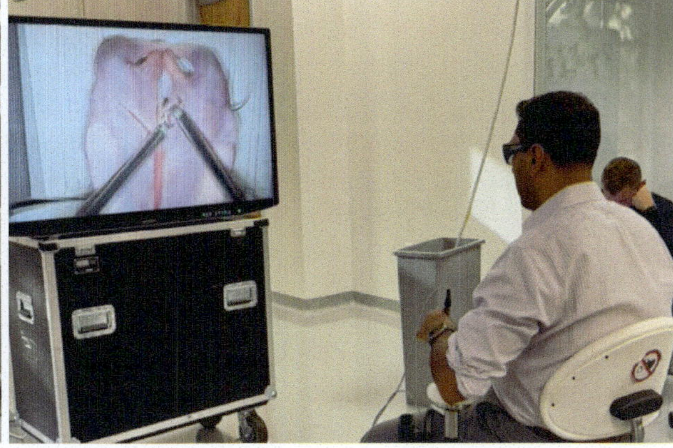

Fig. 30.17 Robotic applications in craniofacial surgery are in development. Model and cadaveric studies with novel surgical robots allowing for smaller entry profiles and pediatric craniofacial applications hold tremendous promise. Clinical applications remain to be proven, but carry the promise of increased precision, improved ergonomics, reduction of tremor, and improved visualization

planned osteotomies. Integration with AR could enhance intraoperative guidance and decision-making, while AI integration for outcome analysis, systematic learning, and improvements may yield systems that critically reduce complications.

Artificial Intelligence (AI)

Beginnings of AI

The advent of the twenty-first century witnessed a paradigm shift driven by advancements in computational capabilities, data availability, and integration of algorithmic development into medicine. These advancements have demonstrated transformative potential, fostering further advancements in diagnostic accuracy, therapeutic precision, and healthcare delivery [54]. As AI advances its integration, the potential medical and surgical applications are vast.

Most successful clinical applications of AI are seen in medical specialties that inherently collect standardized data, such as radiology, pathology, ophthalmology, and dermatology [60]. Most of the identified literature focuses on applications of AI in plastic surgery—primarily aesthetic and breast surgery—followed by craniofacial surgery. Successful integration of AI into plastic surgery is seen in fields within plastic surgery that collect large amounts of standardized data and utilize AI to perform either inherently subjective or time-consuming tasks [61]. AI models can alleviate cognitive tasks in plastic surgery with high accuracy in predicting diagnosis and outcomes, streamlining preoperative surgical planning, and evaluating postoperative outcomes [61]. Additionally, AI allows for medical applications based on deep learning that include image recognition, classification, detection, and segmentation; face recognition; visual tracking; video classification; speech recognition; and natural language processing [61].

Theoretical Applications and Current Developments

Integration of AI in craniofacial surgery is still in its early stages, but its potential impact is substantial. Machine learning algorithms have the capacity to analyze vast amounts of patient data, identify patterns, and assist in decision-making. AI's robust automated computing power can reduce diagnostic errors, conserve resources, and increase efficiency [60]. Some promising applications of AI in craniofacial surgery include predictive analytics, automated image analysis, and personalized treatment plans. AI's ability to predict surgical outcomes based on patient-specific data could tailor treatment plans more effectively. Algorithms can analyze past surgical outcomes to refine current techniques and reduce complications. The use of deep learning models to analyze radiographic images and detect abnormalities can assist in preoperative planning. AI-assisted image segmentation can streamline VSP workflows. AI models can consider patient-specific factors such as age, bone density, and growth potential to optimize surgical interventions. Additionally, AI-driven data analytics and machine learning algorithms are being utilized to optimize surgical planning, predict outcomes, and enhance postoperative care. AI applications in craniofacial surgery include automated diagnostic tools for syndromic conditions, outcome predictions based on large datasets, and personalized treatment planning. As VSP and 3D printing become essential components in craniofacial and orthognathic surgery, additional opportunities for data entry points for AI systems may usher in a new era of data processing and clinical understanding [62] (Fig. 30.18).

Applications of AI

AI has been shown to aid in diagnosis, imaging, preoperative planning, prognosis, and postoperative management. In future, it could potentially be used to detect and classify craniofacial

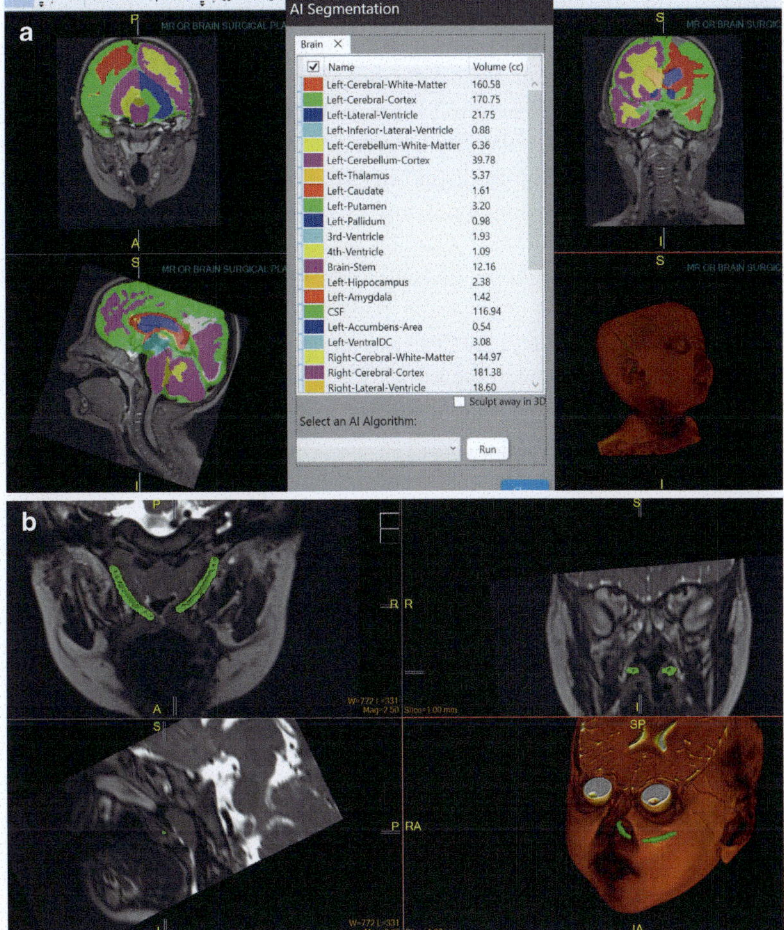

Fig. 30.18 (**a**) Artificial intelligence (AI) driven auto-segmentation of an MRI brain in an infant. (Novarad). (**b**) Novel segmentation of critical anatomy (Levator Veli palatini in this example) can be used to train AI models to auto-segment

anomalies, identify facial phenotypes of genetic disorders, predict genetic risk of non-syndromic oral clefts, and assist with surgical treatment/rehabilitation. These algorithms have demonstrated an accuracy of over 85% in identifying facial phenotypes associated with genetic syndromes [58]. For example, DeepGestalt is a deep convolutional neural network (CNN) trained on tens of thousands of images to identify facial phenotypes for genetic disorders [59]. In 2024, Hennocq et al. reported on an innovative model that uses AI-based methods on two-dimensional (2-D) facial frontal, lateral, and external ear photographs to assist diagnosis for syndromic craniosynostoses such as Apert syndrome. The model correctly diagnosed 70% of patients in the validation set [63]. Rickart et al. utilized AI to assess the regional movements achieved during surgery [64]. A process using linear discriminant analysis to project the high-dimensional vectors onto a 2D space demonstrates how surgery elicits global shape changes in each patient and how the shape properties of Apert and Crouzon syndromes can be visualized in relation to the healthy population.

Facial recognition neural networks have also shown improved gender-typing of transgender women from preoperative facial feminization surgery to postoperative facial feminization surgery [56]. Within pediatric otolaryngology, a growing body of evidence illustrates the role of AI in diagnosis and triaging of acute otitis media and middle ear effusion, pediatric sleep disorders, and syndromic craniofacial anomalies [60]. Moreover, there is potential to develop an algorithm using a recurrent neural network to extract characteristic voice features from a picture or sentence pronunciation test using spectral analysis. Because cleft palate and velopharyngeal insufficiency are both closely related to speech, these technologies could play an integral role in surgical intervention [61]. In diagnosing craniofacial trauma, the most important tool is a CT scan. Using convolutional neural network (CNN)-based classification or detection mechanisms, AI can diagnose craniofacial bone fractures automatically. Several studies have already found CNN-based imaging diagnostics for bone fractures in the extremity, spine, and hip to be effective [61] (Fig. 30.19).

Machine learning is a branch of AI designed to rapidly analyze massive amounts of data and make predictions based on pattern recognition. This technology has the potential to create a powerful, automated method of screening and classification of craniofacial anomalies based on standard digital photographs [65]. In 2024, Luo et al. performed a systematic review of machine learning on the identification and treatment of craniosynostosis and found promising accuracy of machine learning models in diagnosing craniosynostosis types [66]. These findings underscore the opportunity for machine learning to revolutionize the management of craniosynostosis. Potential advantages of this technology include individualized treatment strategies and diagnostic approaches that are efficient, radiation-free, and automated with technologies such as 3D imaging [66].

Other potential applications of AI in craniofacial surgery include eliminating inter-observer variability between surgeons, creating screening and point-of-care diagnosis tools to aid primary care providers in identifying patients who require specialist assessment, and developing surgical education algorithms to train junior surgeons in craniofacial surgery [67] (Table 30.2).

Limitations of AI

An evolving tool into the surgeon's armamentarium, AI carries ethical implications that are wide, varied, and paramount for consideration. Broader social implications, regulations, safety, and widespread adoption by industry will undoubtedly influence AI adoption. Ultimately, machine learning and AI rely on robust data inputs, but in craniofacial surgery, the scarcity of pooled datasets poses a significant limitation. As our integration carries forward, we must continue to stay vigilant as early AI applications and models are likely to have significant errors.

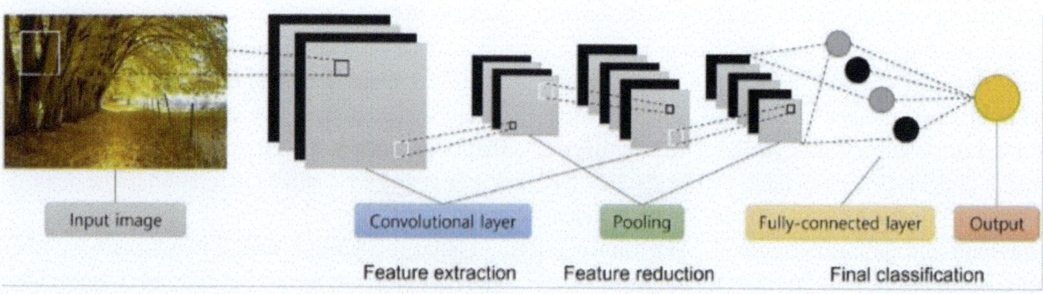

Fig. 30.19 Basic structure of a convolutional neural network consisting of feature extraction, feature reduction, and final classification [61]

Table 30.2 Adapted from Harrison et al. AI applications in Pediatric Craniofacial Surgery. 2025

Domain	AI applications	Key findings
Cleft lip and palate	AI-assisted genetic analysis (CNNs for SNPs)	Improved SNP-based prediction of cleft risk (Pearson correlation 0.50–0.83)
	AI for prenatal and postnatal diagnosis (ultrasound, clinical photos)	Enhanced ultrasound-based detection accuracy (92.5%)
	Automated nasoalveolar molding device design	CAD-generated NAM devices optimized treatment (91% success rate)
	AR for surgical training and telemedicine	AR-supported global outreach programs enhanced training outcomes
Velopharyngeal insufficiency (VPI)	AI-driven speech analysis for hypernasality	Deep learning models achieved clinician-level accuracy in speech assessment ($r = 0.81–0.89$)
	AI-assisted nasopharyngeal imaging	AI-enhanced imaging segmentation for VPI evaluation (Dice score 0.92–0.97, detected 90% of closures)
	AI-based OSA risk screening	AI models improved OSA screening before VPI surgery (accuracy, sensitivity, and specificity >85%)
Orthognathic surgery	AI-driven skeletal maturity assessment	AI-improved surgical timing and decision-making (sensitivity 95.5%, specificity 95.2%, simulation error 1.1 mm)
	AI-assisted cephalometric analysis	CNN models classified skeletal discrepancies with high accuracy
	AI for predicting orthognathic surgery need and outcome	AI-predicted post-surgical facial changes improved patient counseling
Craniosynostosis	AI-based skull morphology classification	AI algorithms classified craniosynostosis with 90.6% accuracy
	AI-assisted severity scoring and surgical indication	AI-based severity scores correlated with surgical decision-making (96% concordance)
	AI-powered AR for intraoperative guidance	AR-assisted suture mapping (error 2.4 mm)
Craniofacial microsomia and microtia	AI-driven classification models (clinical photos, cephalometrics)	CNN-based classification models achieved 94–99% accuracy
	AI-assisted mandibular osteotomies and distractor placement	AR-guided osteotomies enhanced surgical precision ($p < 0.05$)
	AR for microtia reconstruction planning	AR improved ear positioning accuracy within 2 mm

Summary and Vision for the Future

While these technologies offer immense potential, their widespread adoption faces several challenges related to cost and accessibility, learning curve, and regulatory and ethical considerations. The high cost of implementing these technologies may limit their use in resource-limited settings, making equitable access a concern. Advanced technologies require significant training and adaptation by surgical teams, necessitating dedicated educational programs. The integration of AI in surgical decision-making raises ethical and legal concerns, including data privacy, liability, and informed consent.

However, as these technologies evolve, their intersections are likely to catalyze innovation. Emerging applications of AR and its integration with AI will likely further enhance its utility in the operating room [36]. When used to identify and display structures during preoperative planning, AI is particularly valuable in scenarios requiring rapid preparation, such as trauma surgery. Taking this a step further, AI has the potential to assist in the real-time identification of anatomical structures during surgery, highlighting relevant tissues and helping the surgeon distinguish critical areas relevant to the procedure [44].

Looking ahead, seamless integration of these technologies will likely shape the future of craniofacial surgery. The convergence of robotics, AR, and AI, admixed with VSP, may enable a fully personalized, minimally invasive surgical experience that prioritizes both functional outcomes and aesthetic harmony. We envision a future where patient-specific implants are 3D-printed based on AI-driven analysis, surgical procedures are guided by AR overlays, and robotic systems perform complex osteotomies with unparalleled precision.

Conclusion

The journey of craniofacial surgery from its humble beginnings to its current technological sophistication is a testament to the relentless pursuit of innovation in the field. By harnessing the power of VSP, AR, robotics, and AI, craniofacial surgeons can achieve unprecedented levels of precision and patient-specific care. As these technologies continue to evolve, they will undoubtedly redefine the standards of excellence in craniofacial surgery, making complex procedures safer, more predictable, and more accessible to a broader patient population.

References

1. Tessier P. Total facial osteotomy. Crouzon's syndrome, Apert's syndrome: oxycephaly, scaphocephaly, turricephaly. Ann Chir Plast. 1967;12:273.
2. Woodcock M. Development of a virtual surgery environment. Proceedings of Third Australian and New Zealand Conference on Intelligent Information Systems ANZIIS-95. 1995. https://doi.org/10.1109/ANZIIS.
3. McCarthy JG, Schreiber J, Karp N, Thorne CH, Grayson BH. Lengthening the human mandible by gradual distraction. Plast Reconstr Surg. 1992:89. https://doi.org/10.1097/00006534-199289010-00001.
4. McCarthy JG, Katzen JT, Hopper R, Grayson BH. The first decade of mandibular distraction: lessons we have learned. Plast Reconstr Surg. 2002;110:1704–13. https://doi.org/10.1097/01.PRS.0000036260.60746.1B.
5. Suchyta MA, et al. Utilizing "Black Bone" MRI in craniofacial virtual surgical planning: a comparative cadaver study. Plast Reconstr Surg. 2018; https://doi.org/10.1097/PRS.0000000000004396.
6. Andrew TW, et al. Virtual surgical planning decreases operative time for isolated single suture and multi-suture craniosynostosis repair. Plast Reconstr Surg Glob Open. 2018:6. https://doi.org/10.1097/GOX.0000000000002038.
7. Sawh-Martinez R, et al. Improved temporomandibular joint position after 3-dimensional planned mandibular reconstruction. J Oral Maxillofac Surg. 2017;75:197–206. https://doi.org/10.1016/j.joms.2016.07.032.
8. Gray R, Gougoutas A, Nguyen V, Taylor J, Bastidas N. Use of three-dimensional, CAD/CAM-assisted, virtual surgical simulation and planning in the pediatric craniofacial population. Int J Pediatr Otorhinolaryngol. 2017:97. https://doi.org/10.1016/j.ijporl.2017.04.004.
9. Franco PB, Farrell BB. Inverted L osteotomy: a new approach via intraoral access through the advances of virtual surgical planning and custom fixation. J Oral Maxillofac Surg. 2016;2:1.
10. Kwon. Considerations for virtual surgical planning and simulation in orthognathic surgery—a narrative review.
11. Alotaibi NM, Ayoub AF. In: Khojasteh A, Ayoub AF, Nadjmi N, editors. Emerging technologies in oral and maxillofacial surgery. Springer Nature Singapore; 2023. p. 169–98.
12. Velarde K, Cafino R, Isla A Jr, et al. Virtual surgical planning in craniomaxillofacial surgery: a structured review. Comput Assist Surg (Abingdon). 2023;28(1):2271160.
13. Guruprasad Y, Laskar S, Patadiya MMM, et al. Exploring the use of virtual surgical planning (VSP) in maxillofacial reconstructions. J Pharm Bioallied Sci. 2024;16(Suppl 3):S2312–4.
14. Wu KL, Lu TC, Lin TC, Chan CS, Wu CT. Application of virtual planning and 3-dimensional printing guide in surgical management of craniosynostosis. World Neurosurg. 2024;194:123475.
15. Day KM, Kelley PK, Harshbarger RJ, et al. Advanced three-dimensional technologies in craniofacial reconstruction. Plast Reconstr Surg. 2021;148(1):94e–108e.
16. Robiony M, Salvo I, Costa F, et al. Virtual reality surgical planning for maxillofacial distraction osteogenesis: the role of reverse engineering rapid proto-

typing and cooperative work. J Oral Maxillofac Surg. 2007;65:1198–208.
17. Marmulla, et al. Surgical Planning of Computer-assisted repositioning osteotomies. Plast Reconstr Surg. 1999;104(4):938–44.
18. Carpentier S, Schoenaers J, Carels C, Verdonck A. Cranio-maxillofacial, orthodontic and dental treatment in three patients with Apert syndrome. Eur Arch Paediatr Dent. 2014;15(4):281–9.
19. Joachim MV, Miloro M. The evolution of virtual surgical planning in craniomaxillofacial surgery: a comprehensive review. J Oral Maxillofac Surg. 2024:S0278-2391(24)00926-1.
20. Pampín Martínez MM, Gutiérrez Venturini A, Díaz G, de Cevallos J, et al. Evaluation of the predictability and accuracy of orthognathic surgery in the era of virtual surgical planning. Appl Sci. 2022;12(9):4305.
21. Cronin BJ, Lee JC. Preoperative radiology and virtual surgical planning. Oral Maxillofac Surg Clin North Am. 2024;36(2):171–82.
22. Nørholt SE, Sköldstam J, Blomlöf J, Karunahara S, Pedersen TK. Zygomatic repositioning and Le Fort II distraction with intraoral devices in Apert syndrome: a case report. J Craniomaxillofac Surg. 2022;50(4):364–70.
23. Imahiyerobo TA, Valenti AB, Guadix S, LaValley M, Asadourian PA, Buontempo M, Souweidane M, Hoffman C. The role of virtual surgical planning in surgery for complex craniosynostosis. Plast Reconstr Surg Glob Open. 2024;12(1):e5524.
24. Sawh-Martinez R, Steinbacher DM. Syndromic craniosynostosis. Clin Plast Surg. 2019;46(2):141–55. https://doi.org/10.1016/j.cps.2018.11.009.
25. Kutkowska-Kaźmierczak A, Gos M, Obersztyn E. Craniosynostosis as a clinical and diagnostic problem: molecular pathology and genetic counseling. J Appl Genet. 2018;59(2):133–47. https://doi.org/10.1007/s13353-017-0423-4.
26. Udayakumaran S, Krishnadas A, Subash P. Multisuture and syndromic craniosynostoses: simplifying the complex. J Pediatr Neurosci. 2022;17(Suppl 1):S29–s43. https://doi.org/10.4103/jpn.JPN_26_22.
27. Kalmar CL, Zapatero ZD, Kosyk MS, et al. Elevated intracranial pressure with craniosynostosis: a multivariate model of age, syndromic status, and number of involved cranial sutures. J Neurosurg Pediatr. 2021;28(6):716–23. https://doi.org/10.3171/2021.6.PEDS21162.
28. Hayward R, Britto J, Dunaway D, Jeelani O. Connecting raised intracranial pressure and cognitive delay in craniosynostosis: many assumptions, little evidence. J Neurosurg Pediatr. 2016;18(2):242–50. https://doi.org/10.3171/2015.6.PEDS15144.
29. Hersh DS, Hughes CD. Syndromic craniosynostosis: unique management considerations. Neurosurg Clin N Am. 2022;33(1):105–12. https://doi.org/10.1016/j.nec.2021.09.008.
30. Chiang SN, Skolnick GB, Naidoo SD, Smyth MD, Patel KB. Outcomes after endoscope-assisted strip craniectomy and orthotic therapy for syndromic craniosynostosis. Plast Reconstr Surg. 2023;151(4):832–42. https://doi.org/10.1097/prs.0000000000010006.
31. Kalmar CL, Xu W, Zimmerman CE, et al. Trends in utilization of virtual surgical planning in pediatric craniofacial surgery. J Craniofac Surg. 2020;31(7):1900–5.
32. Lin HH, Lonic D, Lo LJ. 3-D printing in orthognathic surgery—a literature review. J Formos Med Assoc. 2018;117:547–58.
33. Alkhayer A, Piffkó J, Lippold C, Segatto E. Accuracy of virtual planning in orthognathic surgery: a systematic review. Head Face Med. 2020;16:1–9.
34. Wang L, Kreutz-Rodrigues L, Gibreel W. Virtual surgical planning in craniofacial surgery: the top 50 most frequently cited papers. Plast Surg (Oakv). 2024:22925503241305638.
35. U.S. Food and Drug Administration. Augmented reality and virtual reality in medical devices. n.d.. Retrieved from fda.gov.
36. Zco Corporation. Revolutionary Applications of Microsoft HoloLens and Apple Vision Pro. 2024, March 20. Retrieved from zco.com.
37. Augmedics. Augmedics marks record-setting 5,000 spine patients treated in another first for augmented reality surgery. 2023, December 22. Retrieved from augmedics.com.
38. FDA Reporter. Medivis Wins FDA Clearance for Breakthrough Augmented Reality Surgical System. 2018, May 30. Retrieved from fdareporter.com.
39. Radiology Business. FDA updates list of cleared VR, augmented reality devices, with radiology leading way. 2023, August 15. Retrieved from radiologybusiness.com.
40. Augmedics. Augmedics announces FDA clearance, completion of first surgery for new CT-Fluoro registration. 2024, November 19. Retrieved from businesswire.com.
41. Novarad. VisAR: Augmented Reality Surgical Navigation. n.d. Retrieved February 15, 2025, from https://www.novarad.net/visar.
42. Hamilton A. The future of artificial intelligence in surgery. Cureus. 2024;16(7):e63699. https://doi.org/10.7759/cureus.63699. PMID: 39092371; PMCID: PMC11293880.
43. Żelechowski M, Zubizarreta-Oteiza J, Karnam M, Faludi B, Zentai N, Gerig N, Rauter G, Thieringer FM, Cattin PC. Augmented reality navigation in orthognathic surgery: comparative analysis and a paradigm shift. Healthc Technol Lett. 2024;12(1):e12109. https://doi.org/10.1049/htl2.12109. PMID: 39816699; PMCID: PMC11730987.
44. Krilavičius T, De Paolis LT, De Luca V, et al. eXtended reality and artificial intelligence in medicine and rehabilitation. Inf Syst Front. 2025; https://doi.org/10.1007/s10796-025-10580-8.
45. Liu K, Gao Y, Abdelrehem A, et al. Augmented reality navigation method for recontouring surgery of craniofacial fibrous dysplasia. Sci Rep. 2021;11:10043.
46. Tel A, Raccampo L, Vinayahalingam S, Troise S, Abbate V, Orabona GD, Sembronio S, Robiony M. Complex craniofacial cases through augmented

reality guidance in surgical oncology: a technical report. Diagnostics (Basel). 2024;14(11):1108.
47. Liu HH, Li LJ, Shi B, Xu CW, Luo E. Robotic surgical systems in maxillofacial surgery: a review. Int J Oral Sci. 2017;9(2):63–73. https://doi.org/10.1038/ijos.2017.24.
48. Steiner W. Endoscopic laser surgery of the upper aerodigestive tract. New York: Georg Thieme; 2000.
49. Mcleod IK, Melder PC. Da Vinci robot-assisted excision of a vallecular cyst: a case report. Ear Nose Throat J. 2005;84(3):170–2.
50. Zhang Z, Kim BS, Han W, et al. Preliminary study of the accuracy and safety of robot-assisted mandibular distraction osteogenesis with electromagnetic navigation in hemifacial microsomia using rabbit models. Sci Rep. 2022;12:19572.
51. Lei B, Sun T, Ma H, Li B, Yang B. Application and accuracy of craniomaxillofacial plastic surgery robot in congenital craniosynostosis surgery. J Craniofac Surg. 2023;34(5):1371–5.
52. Han W, Yan Y, Sun M, Zhang Z, Lin L, Zhang Y, Chai G. Evaluating robotic assistance on the learning curve and efficiency of mandibular angle ostectomy: an animal model study. Front Surg. 2024;11:1453135.
53. Khan K, Dobbs T, Swan MC et al. Trans-oral robotic cleft surgery (TORCS) for palate and posterior pharyngeal wall reconstruction: a feasibility study. J Plast Reconstr Aesthet Surg. 2015.
54. Nadjmi N. Transoral robotic cleft palate surgery. Cleft Palate Craniofac J. 2015;44:e114–5.
55. Awad L, Reed B, Bollen E, Langridge BJ, Jasionowska S, Butler PEM, Ponniah A. The emerging role of robotics in plastic and reconstructive surgery: a systematic review and meta-analysis. J Robot Surg. 2024;18(1):254. https://doi.org/10.1007/s11701-024-01987-7.
56. Whiteman E, Rehman U, Hussien M, Sarwar MS, Harsten R, Brennan PA. The implementation of robotic systems in paediatric craniofacial and head and neck surgery: a narrative review of the literature. Br J Oral Maxillofac Surg. 2024; https://doi.org/10.1016/j.bjoms.2024.11.011.
57. Li L, Lin L, Xu H, Zhang Y, Chai G. New productive force: the preliminary report of first craniofacial surgical robot IST multicenter clinical trial in China. J Craniofac Surg. 2025;36(1):21–5.
58. Dang RR, Kadaikal B, Abbadi SE, Brar BR, Sethi A, Chigurupati R. The current landscape of artificial intelligence in oral and maxillofacial surgery- a narrative review. Oral Maxillofac Surg. 2025;29(1):37. https://doi.org/10.1007/s10006-025-01334-6.
59. Gurovich Y, et al. Identifying facial phenotypes of genetic disorders using deep learning. Nat Med. 2019;25:60–4.
60. Spoer DL, Kiene JM, Dekker PK, Huffman SS, Kim KG, Abadeer AI, Fan KL. A systematic review of artificial intelligence applications in plastic surgery: looking to the future. Plast Reconstr Surg Glob Open. 2022;10(12):e4608. https://doi.org/10.1097/GOX.0000000000004608.
61. Ryu JY, Chung HY, Choi KY. Potential role of artificial intelligence in craniofacial surgery. Arch Craniofac Surg. 2021;22(5):223–31. https://doi.org/10.7181/acfs.2021.00507.
62. Huang AE, Valdez TA. Artificial intelligence and pediatric otolaryngology. Otolaryngol Clin N Am. 2024;57(5):853–62. https://doi.org/10.1016/j.otc.2024.04.011.
63. Hennocq Q, Paternoster G, Collet C, Amiel J, Bongibault T, Bouygues T, Cormier-Daire V, Douillet M, Dunaway DJ, Jeelani NO, van de Lande LS, Lyonnet S, Ong J, Picard A, Rickart AJ, Rio M, Schievano S, Arnaud E, Garcelon N, Khonsari RH. AI-based diagnosis and phenotype - genotype correlations in syndromic craniosynostoses. J Craniomaxillofac Surg. 2024;52(10):1172–87.
64. Rickart AJ, Foti S, van de Lande LS, Wagner C, Schievano S, Jeelani NUO, Clarkson MJ, Ong J, Swanson JW, Bartlett SP, Taylor JA, Dunaway DJ. Using a disentangled neural network to objectively assess the outcomes of midfacial surgery in syndromic craniosynostosis. Plast Reconstr Surg. 2024.
65. Geisler EL, Agarwal S, Hallac RR, Daescu O, Kane AA. A role for artificial intelligence in the classification of craniofacial anomalies. J Craniofac Surg. 2021;32(3):967–9.
66. Luo A, Gurses ME, Gecici NN, Kozel G, Lu VM, Komotar RJ, Ivan ME. Machine learning applications in craniosynostosis diagnosis and treatment prediction: a systematic review. Childs Nerv Syst. 2024;40(8):2535–44.
67. Qamar A, Bangi SF, Barve R. Artificial intelligence applications in diagnosing and managing nonsyndromic craniosynostosis: a comprehensive review. Cureus. 2023;15(9):e45318.

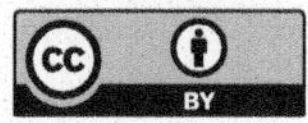

Surgical Treatment of the Apert Hand

31

Brian I. Labow, Amir Taghinia, Stéphane Guero, Hugo Nakamoto, Edgard Novaes França Bisneto, and Marcelo Rosa Rezende

Introduction

Unlike other forms of syndromic craniosynostosis, Apert syndrome invariably involves the limbs. All patients present with various forms of complex syndactyly of all four limbs, including soft-tissue, bone, and joint differences that manifest throughout the upper and lower extremities. Given the hand's role as a major sensory organ in early childhood development and its central role in our daily lives, optimizing hand function in patients with Apert syndrome should be viewed as a primary goal of treatment rather than a secondary concern.

B. I. Labow (✉) · A. Taghinia
Department of Plastic and Oral Surgery, Boston Children's Hospital, Boston, MA, USA
e-mail: Brian.Labow@childrens.harvard.edu

S. Guero
Institut de la Main, Paris, France

Hôpital Necker–Enfants malades, Université Paris Centre, Paris, France

H. Nakamoto
Department of Orthopedics, Hand and Microsurgery Group, Hospital das Clinicas, University of São Paulo, São Paulo, Brazil

E. N. F. Bisneto
Department of Orthopedics and Traumatology, Universidade de São Paulo, São Paulo, Brazil

M. R. Rezende
Department of Orthopedics, Hand and Microsurgery Group, Hospital das Clinicas, Universidade de São Paulo, São Paulo, Brazil

Considering the rarity of this condition, most of the literature reports short-term outcomes in small- to medium-sized cohorts. As such, this chapter should be viewed as the authors' experience and general rationale for treating the Apert hand. In general, this group of authors' philosophy has been to individualize treatment with a problem-based longitudinal approach throughout development, up to and beyond skeletal maturity. Although most clinicians and parents focus on the syndactyly release, it should be noted that a number of adjunct procedures exist to refine patients' hands as they age. Not all patients require or want all available procedures, and it is the role of the hand surgeon to guide parents and older patients through the reconstructive process.

It should also be noted that the authors of this chapter live and work primarily in large urban centers in developed countries. Not all patients with Apert syndrome can access these resources and, particularly for hand surgery, may need to be treated in more remote settings. At least one member of our authorship group (SG) has treated the hands of many patients with Apert syndrome in the developing world. In these instances, as is often the case with global surgery, standard treatment algorithms and techniques may need to be adapted to the realities of the environment.

This chapter aims to provide an in-depth review of the surgical treatment options available for managing hand abnormalities in Apert syndrome, emphasizing both surgical techniques and

J. G. Meara et al. (eds.), *Apert Syndrome*, https://doi.org/10.1007/978-3-032-12551-4_31

Table 31.1 Published studies on the treatment of the Apert hand

Year	Author(s)	Number of patients	Summary
1970	Hoover	20 (65 papers reviewed)	Anatomy, early surgical recommendations, outcomes
1986	Barot & Caplan	10	Early surgical release
1991	Upton	68	Classification, anatomy
1997	Holten	45	Detailed anatomy, pathology
2003	Fearon	57	Two procedures, early release/late osteotomy
2004	Guero	52	Treatment schedule based on type, early straightening of thumb
2018	Raposo-Amaral et al.	41	Treatment schedule based on type, revision rates by type

outcomes to facilitate decision-making in the care of children with Apert syndrome.

Background

Historical Perspective

Apert syndrome was first described by the French physician Eugène Apert in 1906 [1, 2]. However, over the past 120 years, relatively few studies have been dedicated to the treatment of the hand differences associated with this syndrome (Table 31.1) [3–9]. Upton's publication in 1991 provides an extensive description of the various limb differences that may be present [5]. Despite the relatively restricted genotypic presentation, it remains unclear how the phenotypic variations arise.

Anatomy of the Upper Limb

Tissues

Skin

The skin of patients with Apert syndrome differs from unaffected children. In the hand, the palmar skin is thinner with increased apocrine activity. Hyperhidrosis is common and hand hygiene can be challenging in babies with very concave hands. Moreover, when these patients undergo surgical release of their syndactylies, hyperhidrosis can lead to maceration beneath the dressings that can compromise skin grafts' take and complicate wound healing. Beyond the hand, acne can be severe in these patients during adolescence, presumably due partly to increased apocrine function in affected areas.

Nails

The distal elements of the fingers are invariably conjoined to a variable degree. In more severe forms, fusion of the nail plates (synonychia) will be encountered. In the most severe cases, a single nail plate can extend from the thumb to the fifth finger. With increasing degrees of palmar concavity, ingrown nails or irritation between difficult-to-trim nail plates and adjacent skin can lead to paronychia, inflammation, or infection (Fig. 31.1). Although the nail plates may be conjoined, longitudinal ridges provide useful topographical markings to the ideal cleavage plains between conjoined distal phalangeal elements below. Once digital separation has occurred, problems with nail trimming and infection decrease dramatically. Long-term issues with retained germinal matrix or chronic hang nails can certainly occur, although these can usually be dealt with selectively. Prior to syndactyly release, antibiotics and meticulous nail care can typically obviate the need for an extra trip to the operating room, but in some cases, this cannot be avoided.

Bone

Plain radiographs of the hand of a patient with Apert syndrome may demonstrate an array of anomalies. In addition, patients may manifest these differences to varying degrees. In some patients, these changes can produce function-limiting changes, whereas in others they can be noted but not require surgical intervention.

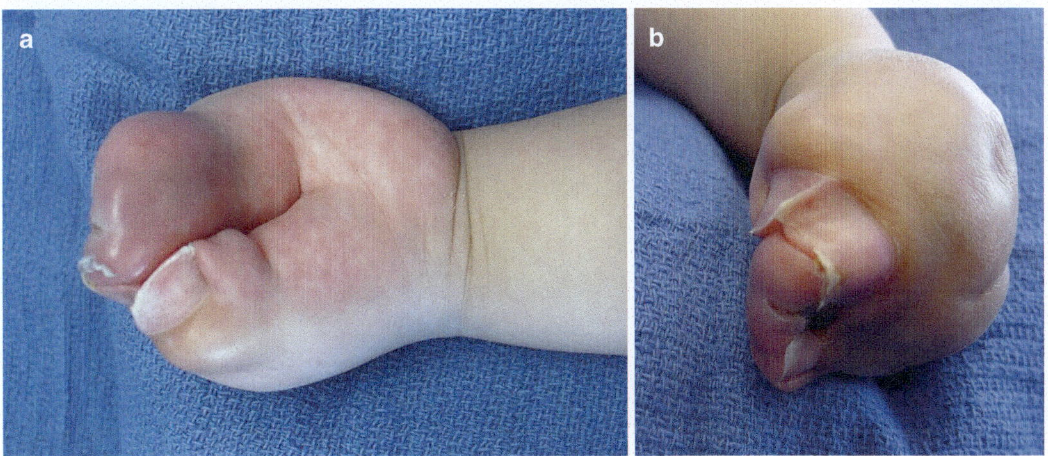

Fig. 31.1 (**a**, **b**) Type III hand with inflammation of the fingertips due to maceration and ingrown nails

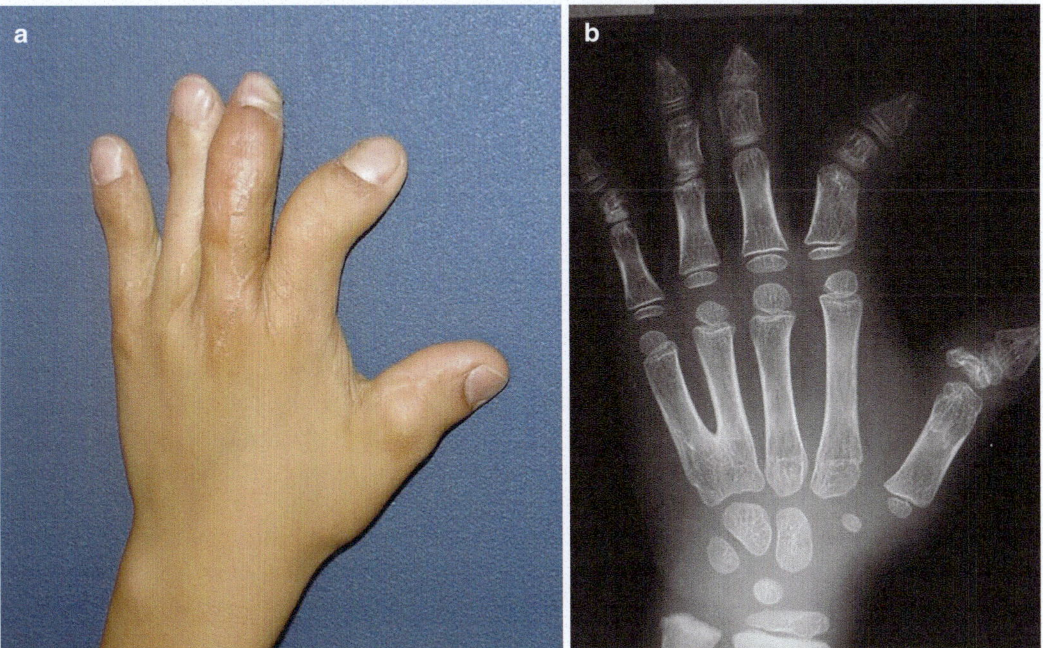

Fig. 31.2 (**a**, **b**) Clinodactyly of the index finger. Note the partial closure of the physeal plate of the proximal phalanx, and the synostosis on the base of the fourth and fifth digit

Synostosis

One of the most striking features of an Apert hand radiograph is the synostoses between digital rays. All patients with Apert syndrome present with some degree of distal phalangeal coalition, which may extend to more proximal phalangeal segments. Metacarpal synostosis is usually limited to the base of the fourth and fifth digits. It may develop over the first decade of life: 77% for Dao et al. and over 80% for Upton and Khoury (Fig. 31.2) [10, 11]. "Tight" synostosis with overlapping fourth and fifth metacarpals can narrow the hand and produce or exacerbate abduction deformities in the small finger. If this becomes problematic (e.g., unable to wear gloves, put hands in pockets, adequately position small finger), aggressive osteotomy/ostectomy of the synostosis with placement of a spacer can dramatically address this problem. Although recurrent fusion is almost a certainty, the increased inter-metacarpal distance following treatment typically precludes recurrent abduction of the small finger. It should be noted that in the wrist, carpal coalitions between capitate and hamate may also be observed; however, these rarely require treatment [6, 9, 12–14].

Symphalangism

Holten et al. demonstrated the presence of ectopic cartilage deposits in periarticular tissues and flexor tendons on pathology specimens from the hands of patients with Apert syndrome [6]. They proposed that the ectopic cartilage represents abnormal differentiation of the mesenchymal elements during limb development, leading to the formation of cartilage and, ultimately, bone instead of normal periarticular tissues. This ectopic cartilage eventually calcifies and is responsible for the nearly ubiquitous loss of interphalangeal joint motion and synostoses observed in patients with Apert syndrome. The metacarpal joints (MP) are mobile to varying degrees, with the range of motion differing between patients and even between digits. The lack of active movement in the interphalangeal joints (symphalangism) means that the total active movement of the finger is equivalent to the movement of the metacarpophalangeal joints [16–18]. In some patients, the distal interphalangeal (DIP) joint of the small finger may also retain mobility. In fact, thumb and small finger pinch is a commonly preferred pincer grasp in younger patients with Apert syndrome. Older children and adults often have a "favorite" one or two fingers, usually correlating with MP range of motion [15].

Physeal Plates

In addition to abnormal osseous configurations in the hand, the epiphyseal plates within the bones of the hand may also have abnormal shapes. Partial closure of the epiphyseal plate or bracketed epiphyses can be observed and may lead to clinodactyly with growth (Fig. 31.2b). Moreover, bone growth within the hands of children with Apert syndrome seems to be slower than unaffected patients, and early physeal closure or simply lack of growth potential invariably leads to diminished digit length.

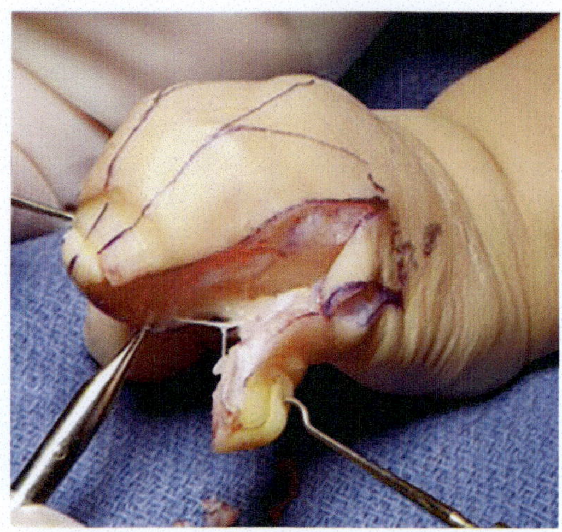

Fig. 31.3 Digital separation of the fourth webspace. Note the distal digital arterial bifurcation

Artery/Nerve

Variations in arterial branching patterns are common in Apert hands [16]. During digital separation, distal intercommunicating branches between adjacent digital arteries can be observed (Fig. 31.3). Any question as to the safety of dividing these branches can be answered by using a microvascular clamp and temporarily occluding these branches while lowering the tourniquet. Likewise, distal arterial bifurcations may also be observed and should be anticipated in flap design for commissure construction during syndactyly release. Similar situations can occur with the digital nerves; however, intraneural neurolysis can be performed such that distal neural bifurcations are rarely limiting to webspace creation. Despite the rather extensive dissection required to reconstruct the Apert hand, significant neurovascular injury is rare in experienced centers, and long-term sensory evaluations in these patients show excellent sensory function [15]. In an unpublished study out of Paris, among 84 patients with over 600 webs released, only one patient experienced distal necrosis (S. Guero, unpublished data, presented at the Workshop of the Institut

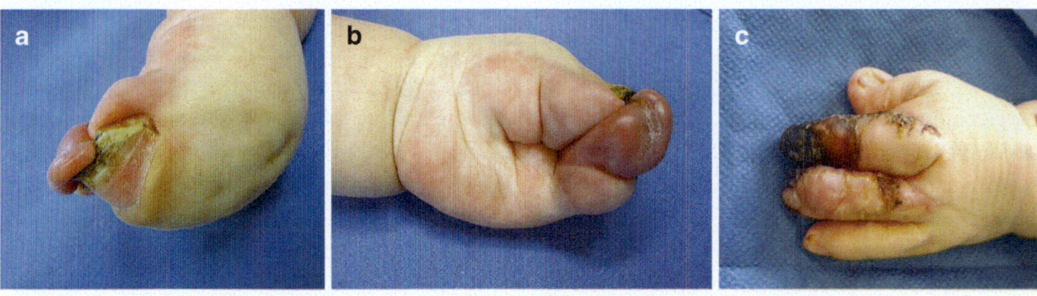

Fig. 31.4 Patient with Type III hand pre- (**a**, **b**) and postoperatively (**c**) with distal necrosis

Français de l'Institut de la Main on Syndactyly, Paris, France, December 2010; Fig. 31.4).

Tendon

Anomalies of the flexor and extensor tendons along with retinacular structures are invariably present. Flexor tendons show shortening, paired with an abnormal trajectory and bony insertion. For example, the abductor pollicis brevis (APB) has an aberrant insertion on the distal phalanx of the thumb, which is deviated radially. Unique anomalies may also be observed on the extensor side of the hand, where the extensor apparatus may be conjoined across digits. Given the absence of any interphalangeal movement, tendon reconstruction is rarely of any benefit in reconstructing the Apert hand. One exception advocated by some authors is the early release of the APB tendon, which may yield improved posture of the thumb (Fig. 31.5).

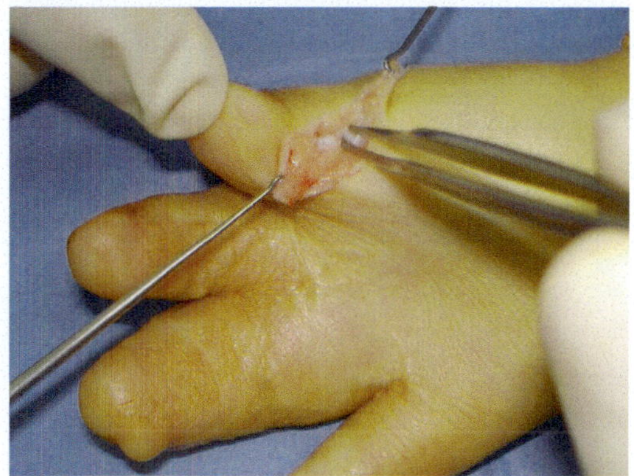

Fig. 31.5 Division of the distal insertion of the abductor pollicis brevis (APB) on the distal phalanx

Proximal Upper Extremity

Although the literature dealing with hand differences is sparse, there is even less information regarding abnormalities of the more proximal portions of the upper limb. Kasser and Upton suggested that the reasons for this are: [12]

1. More significant abnormalities in the hand and wrist.
2. No surgical treatment suggested for the shoulder or elbow differences.
3. Rarity of the condition.

Cuthbert first drew attention to the prominence of the acromial process with associated deformity of the humeral head and glenoid [17]. Kasser and Upton also demonstrated that the mobility of the glenohumeral joint in these patients was never standard, and that it worsened progressively with age. Abduction and forward flexion were restricted in all patients, while external rotation was more restricted than internal rotation. The most notable radiographic findings were glenoid dysplasia, an overgrowth of the greater tuberosity, prominence of the acromion, and inferior subluxation. Clinical findings at the elbow were less uniform. Some patients had extension restrictions, while others had limited flexion. Pronation and supination may be limited, and in rare cases, ankylosis may be present. The most common radiographic findings were hypoplasia of the capitulum, as well as deformities in the radial head. Unlike the shoulder, elbow function did not diminish over time in this study [12].

Wood et al. followed nine patients treated over 20 years [18]. They found radiographic abnormalities in eight shoulders: flattening and elongation of the glenoid fossa, flattening and elongation of the humeral head with loss of the neck, prominence of the greater tuberosity, prominence of the acromion process, subluxation of the humeral head, and secondary arthropathy. Clinically, limitation of shoulder abduction was observed, with progressive decrease in mobility of the glenohumeral joint with age. In the elbow, abnormalities were found involving the radial portion of the capitulum, while sparing the trochlea and olecranon. Five of the nine patients had radial head subluxation. Three of the nine children had elbow flexion contracture, with extension restriction [18].

In a study with nine patients aged 9 years or older, Murnaghan et al. also observed limited forward flexion and abduction of the shoulder in all patients, while extension, internal rotation, and external rotation were minimally affected. The radiographic findings paralleled those of Kasser and Upton, who also observed medial hypoplasia of the humeral head [19].

Classification of Hand Differences

Anomalies of the hand are familiar to the clinicians who treat patients with Apert syndrome. Upton has categorized the complex hand differences seen in these patients into three types based on thumb involvement, palmar concavity, and

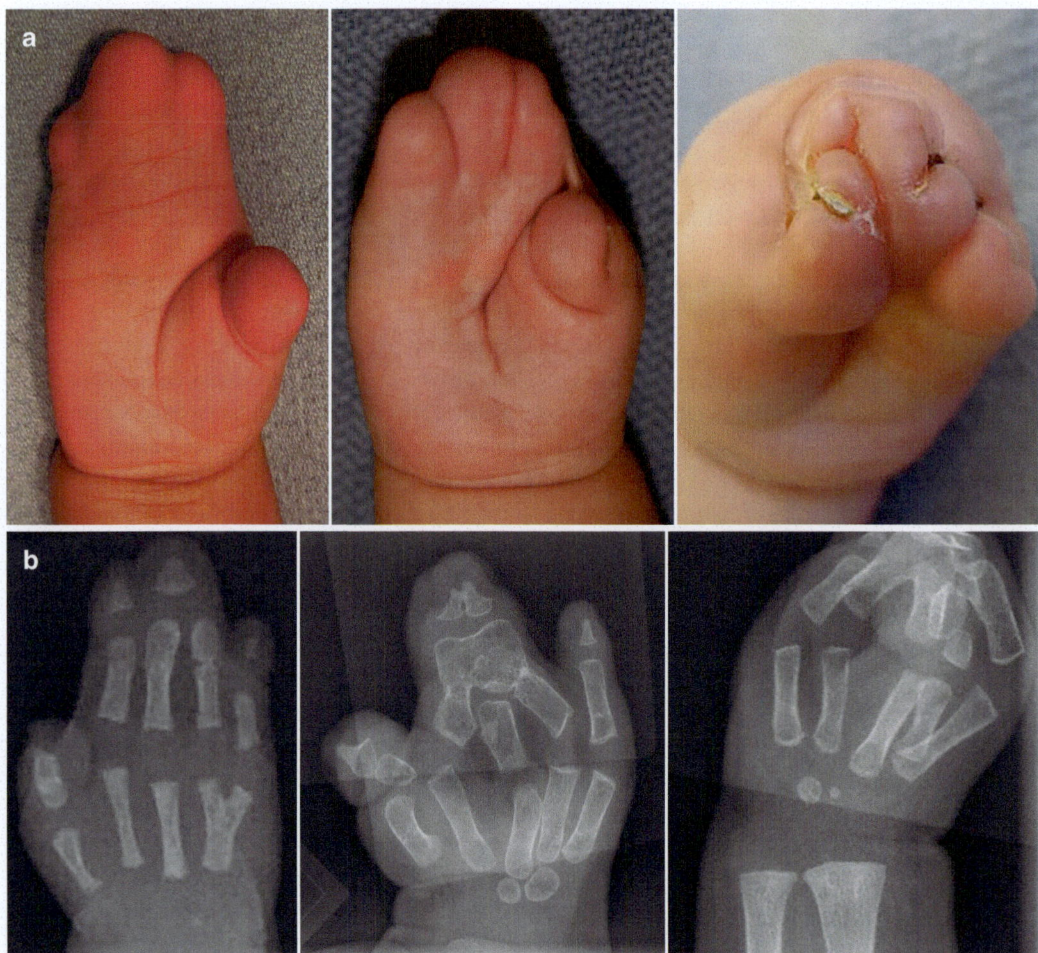

Fig. 31.6 (**a**, **b**) Representative images and radiographs of the Upton classification of the Apert hand: Type I, Type II, Type III, respectively

complexity of the phalangeal synostoses (Fig. 31.6a, b). Regardless of type, all Apert hands share the following common features: complex syndactyly involving digits that are short and lack normal interphalangeal joint motion and exhibit radial deviation of the thumb. Most patients present with identical types bilaterally, with relatively minor differences between sides. However, asymmetric syndactyly types can occasionally be observed [5, 13].

Type I

Described as a spade or obstetrician hand, the Type I hand is regarded as the least severe and usually the most straightforward to correct. The thumb is free, although the first webspace may appear shallow. The fingers align in a single plane, and the synonychia may be incomplete. The fourth webspace may have an incomplete syndactyly, and some limited interphalangeal motion may be present in the small finger [20].

Type II

Often referred to as a mitten or spoon hand, these hands present with soft-tissue syndactyly of variable extent between the thumb and index finger. The fingers adopt a concave palmar posture, with a more complex fusion of the distal phalangeal elements of the fingers.

Type III

The hoof or rosebud hand is the most severe form and the most challenging to correct. Patients with this type have a complete syndactyly of the thumb and index finger, along with complex pansyndactyly of the other digits that share a single elongated nail plate. The thumb and small finger are in close proximity, creating a palmar crevice.

In general, the range of motion decreases the higher the Upton subtype [15]. Similarly, the extent and complexity of the phalangeal synostoses tend to increase with Upton type, as well. Although this can augment the degree of difficulty with digital separation and possibly produce poorer aesthetic results, limited long-term outcome data do not demonstrate a significant difference in patient- or parent-reported outcomes.

Preoperative Evaluation

Discussions regarding surgical treatment of the Apert hand may begin before birth. Given the staged nature of the reconstructive plan and the complexities of the condition and treatment, multiple conversations with the family before any surgical intervention are beneficial. Although the differences in the appearance and function of the hand should be fully explained, it is important not to dwell only on the limitations. Parents should be made aware of the positive long-term patient-reported functional outcomes, and the opportunities to create an aesthetic hand with five digits in almost all cases. Children with Apert syndrome can engage in sports, play musical instruments, and become fully independent like their unaffected peers. The role of the hand surgeon is to facilitate these activities with both surgical and non-surgical treatment.

Imaging Modalities

Although the Upton type can easily be determined by physical examination, plain radiographs are also important for surgical planning. In particular, the number of metacarpal rays should be determined, as only four may be present on rare occasions (Fig. 31.6b). Similarly, if a deficiency in the complement of the distal phalangeal bone is noted, bone grafting may be used during the initial stage to enable the subsequent release(s) to yield the appropriate number and size of fingertips and nails. The extent of proximal phalangeal or metacarpal synostosis should be noted, as this may portend a more challenging syndactyly release or late angular deformities to address. Although more advanced forms of imaging such as computed tomography and angiography have been described, they are rarely necessary [6, 16, 20–23].

Care Coordination

All members of the team caring for families of a child with Apert syndrome should recognize the overwhelming number of doctor visits, procedures, and tests that occur during the first 3 years of life. Fortunately, care for the Apert hand is rarely, if ever, urgent, let alone emergent. While a broad goal for children with Apert syndrome is to complete the syndactyly releases by the age of three, it should be stated that no long-term negative sequelae have been reported for children who have had their syndactyly releases later in childhood [15, 20, 24]. For children with Apert syndrome who have significant medical comorbidities that demand urgent intervention or time to resolve, or for those who are somewhat delayed in growth, additional time may be taken before the hand care sequence begins. Ideally, the family should be closely supported by a craniofacial coordinator who works with the hand surgeon as well as the other members of the team to schedule surgery when the patient and family are ready.

Surgical Treatment

Timing and Sequence of Interventions

The timing and sequence of surgical interventions in Apert syndrome are influenced by the size and health status of the patient, severity of the hand deformity, and parental and surgeon goals. Consensus overviews on surgical management of the Apert hand from birth to skeletal maturity have been published [7–9, 20, 24]. Generally, it is reasonable to begin the operative sequence for digit separation around one year of age, or at a bodyweight of 10 kilograms. For patients with Type III hands, the initial syndactyly release may begin slightly earlier [9]. Before syndactyly release, some Type III, and rarely Type II, hand patients may experience maceration of the fingertips or ingrown nail plates, leading to recurrent episodes of soft tissue infection or inflammation. These episodes can irritate all involved but can usually be managed outside the operating room with aggressive nail trimming, hand hygiene, and oral antibiotics. Affected patients may also begin syndactyly release somewhat earlier than average to stop these episodes.

Separation of the digits occurs in either two or three stages, separated by at least 4 months. This time period allows tissue equilibrium at both the hand and skin graft donor sites. All Type I hands and nearly all Type II hands can be fully separated to yield five digits in two stages [9]. Optimal management of the Type III hand has been debated in the literature. Some prefer to release the first and third webspaces during the first stage, and the second and fourth webspaces in the second stage. This approach uses only two stages, similar to Type I and Type II hand reconstruction [7, 20].

An alternative approach has been proposed using three stages for Type III hands, prioritizing the border digits during the initial stage [7, 20]. This operation includes concurrent limited osteotomies of the central three-digit coalition during the first stage, to realign the fingers into a single plane. The advantages of this approach are more accurate localization of the second and third webspaces, equitable distribution of the glabrous skin, and a greatly facilitated total reconstruction with excellent aesthetic results. The primary disadvantage of this approach is the need for an additional general anesthetic. Total anesthesia time for these operations can be limited, using a two-surgeon approach to address the right and left sides simultaneously, decreasing total anesthesia time substantially.

Although most of the attention in Apert hand surgery is focused on syndactyly release, it is important to remember that additional smaller procedures can be performed later in development to improve form and function. For example, surgeons can address angular and length deficiencies in the thumb as the child approaches school age [7, 8, 20]. In addition, angular deformities may manifest or worsen during periods of rapid growth. Corrective osteotomies are well-tolerated and heal reliably to correct these differences. Fingertip or nail issues, web creep, or other skin concerns may also be sources of irritation and are easy to address. Ideally, a number of these adjunctive procedures can be combined in older patients to minimize trips to the operating room and downtime for recovery.

Specific Surgical Procedures

Syndactyly Release

As with any syndactyly release, there are multiple techniques, flap designs, donor sites, and dressing types that can yield favorable outcomes. One strategy utilizes a technique advocated by Upton [5]. Unless the patient is older, a bilateral two-surgeon approach is used. Once the anesthesia team has obtained adequate intravenous (IV) access and control of the airway, the eyes are protected with lubricant and adhesive dressings, given the increased risk of corneal exposure and desiccation in children with Apert syndrome. An underbody warming blanket and appropriate padding are placed beneath the patient. The arms are abducted carefully to accommodate differences in shoulder mobility. Both upper extremities are prepped from fingertips to axilla, along with the lower abdomen, and sterile drapes are applied. IV antibiotics are given, and steroids such as dexamethasone can be used to minimize postoperative airway reactivity and swelling.

The metacarpal–phalangeal (MP) joints of the syndactylized digits are identified by their characteristic dimples. Proximally based triangular flaps extend from the MP joints on the dorsal side, with corresponding triangular flaps on the palmar surface (Fig. 31.7). The length of these flaps can vary depending on the anticipated depth of the web, but the use of bidirectional flaps allows a margin of error in case of distal vascular bifurcation or miscalculation in flap length. Some authors will use dorsally based flaps, such as the Omega flap (Fig. 31.8). For Type I hands, others will perform a Trident flap without skin grafting [25].

The absence of interphalangeal motion obviates the need for the traditional zig-zag palmar incision and allows for a straight line volar and dorsal release to be used. This approach also favors patients with significant differences in pigment between the palmar and dorsal sides of the digit. The downside of this approach is the increased amount of skin graft needed as compared to zig-zag incisions advocated by others. Folds in the nail plate serve as a guide to distal phalangeal boundaries. However, excess nail plate and sterile and germinal matrix should be excised to achieve fingertips and nails of roughly equal size across the fingers. Another useful technique that may be used to improve fingertip appearance is the use of double pulp flaps described by Lundkvist and Barfred and modified by Buck-Gramcko [26, 27] (Fig. 31.9).

Once the markings are made, the limbs are exsanguinated, and the operation proceeds under

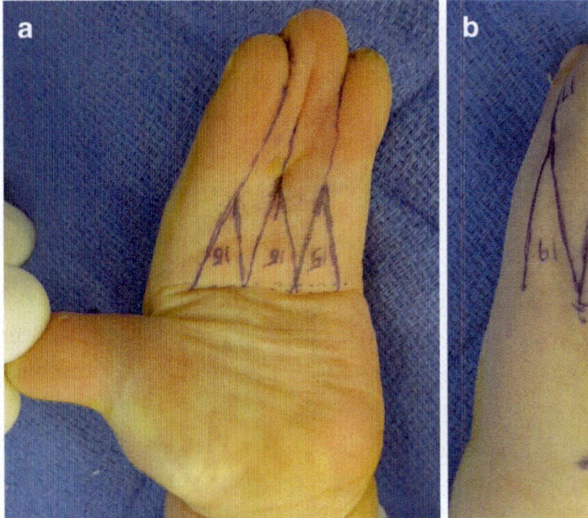

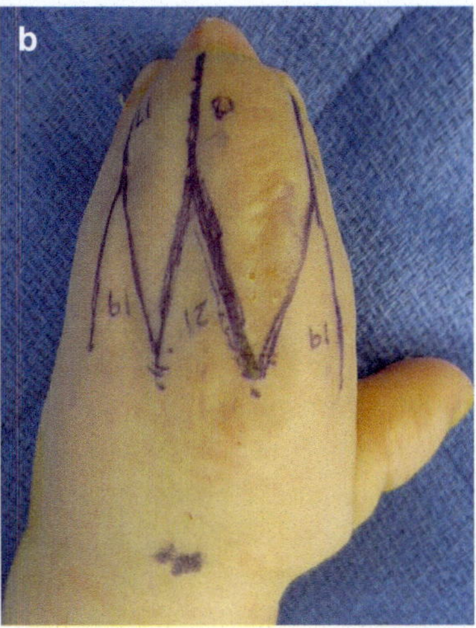

Fig. 31.7 Proximally based triangular flaps on the (**a**) palmar and (**b**) dorsal surface of the hand are marked based on the metacarpal–phalangeal (MP) joints

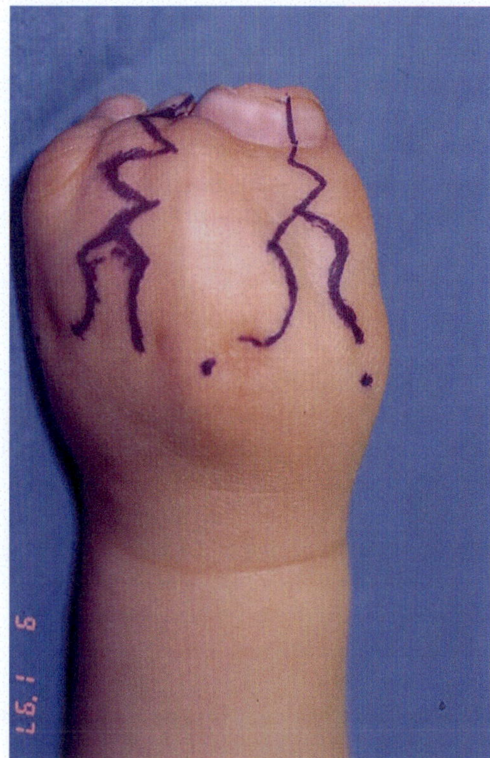

Fig. 31.8 Design of the Omega flaps

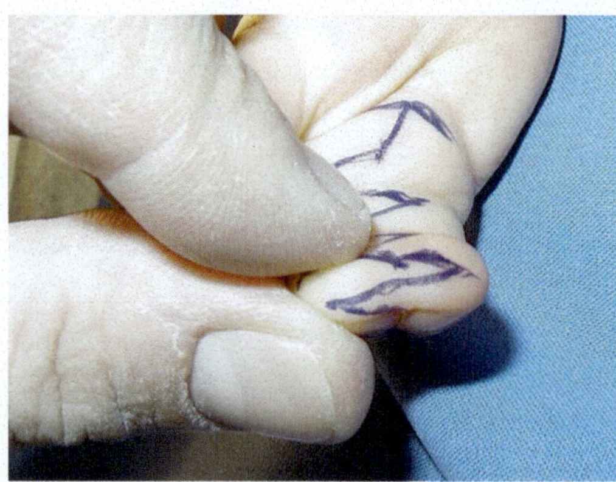

Fig. 31.9 Design of the zig-zag double pulp flaps

tourniquet control. The skin is divided with a 15-blade, and the dorsal and palmar flaps are elevated with a cuff of subjacent fat. Small crossing veins or bleeding vessels are controlled with bipolar cautery. The nail plate is divided with straight iris scissors, and the straight-line dorsal incision is continued through the germinal and

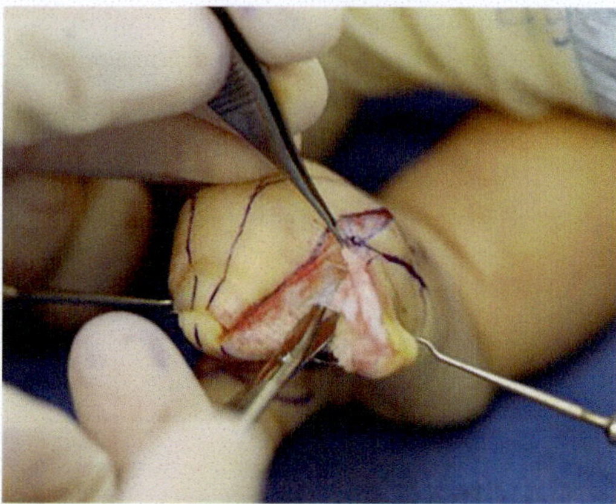

Fig. 31.10 Retrograde dissection following osteotomy

sterile matrix. From the dorsal side, the skin and subcutaneous tissues are elevated off the conjoined extensor paratenon. Once the proximal extent of the phalangeal synostosis has been localized, a straight-line incision through the extensor apparatus is carried down from the fingertip to this point. Care should be taken to create a line that divides the phalangeal bone equally between the two digits. A 2 millimeter (mm) or 4 mm straight osteotome and small mallet are then used to complete the osteotomy. Single hook retractors can be utilized to abduct the digits as the retrograde dissections begin. Spreading fine scissors above and below the fibrous ligamentous connections between the digits facilitates visualization of the neurovascular structures (Fig. 31.10). Crossing vascular branches are fairly common, and meticulous dissection of the digital neurovascular structures down to the bifurcation is essential. As mentioned earlier in the chapter, when in doubt, a 1 mm vascular clamp can be applied to a branch and tourniquet released to determine whether a branch is essential for adequate distal perfusion.

With completion of the neurovascular dissection, the dorsal flap is transposed palmarly and the palmar flap dorsally. The commissure is established with a series of interflap 6-0 absorbable sutures. Templates are made of the raw surfaces of both digits and saved for later use. Once all syndactylies have been completed and templates made, the tourniquets are released and moist gauze is placed on the open wounds while adequate perfusion is assured.

When larger quantities of skin are required, the lower abdominal skin fold is an excellent and abundant source for full-thickness skin grafts (Fig. 31.11) [7, 8, 20, 28]. A curvilinear line from one anterior superior iliac spine to the other is drawn and bisected in the midline. With some gentle cephalad traction on the abdominal skin, all templates from the right hand are arranged along this line to the right of the midline, while the same is done on the left. The resulting pattern is smoothed out into a roughly lenticular shape using a surgical marker. The area is infiltrated with a dilute epinephrine containing local anesthetic, and the graft is harvested with 15 blades, defatted, and banked for later use. Generous undermining deep to Scarpa's fascia and a meticulous layered closure of 4-0 and 5-0 Monocryl yields excellent aesthetic results. Dermabond, Steri-Strips, Telfa, and Tegaderm are used to dress the wound. Some authors correctly point out that if zig-zag incisions are used, much less graft is required. In these instances, the upper limb at the wrist, elbow, or upper arm can yield sufficient graft material with an excellent color match and limited hair follicles. Scarring of course can be variable, and the upper extremity donor site may be more visible than the lower abdomen.

Once hemostasis has been assured at the hand with bipolar cautery, the wounds are fully covered with the harvested skin graft using interrupted and running fine absorbable suture (Fig. 31.12). Although others have advocated for only partially covering the wounds with skin graft, since secondary contracture is of little concern in Apert digits, we have observed more con-

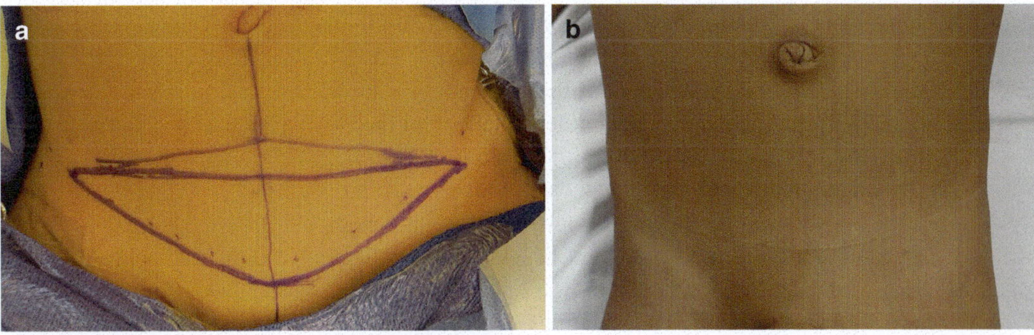

Fig. 31.11 Abdominal donor site for full-thickness skin grafts. (**a**) Pre- and (**b**) postoperative view

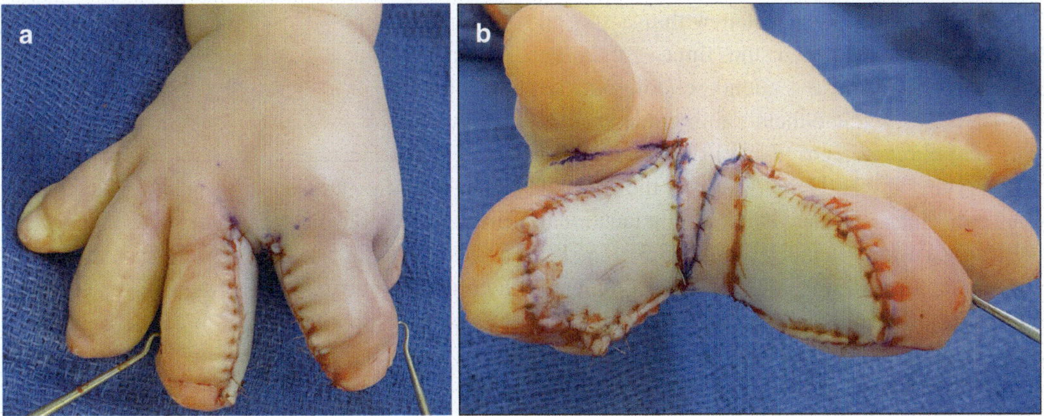

Fig. 31.12 (**a**, **b**) Open wounds are fully covered with skin grafts

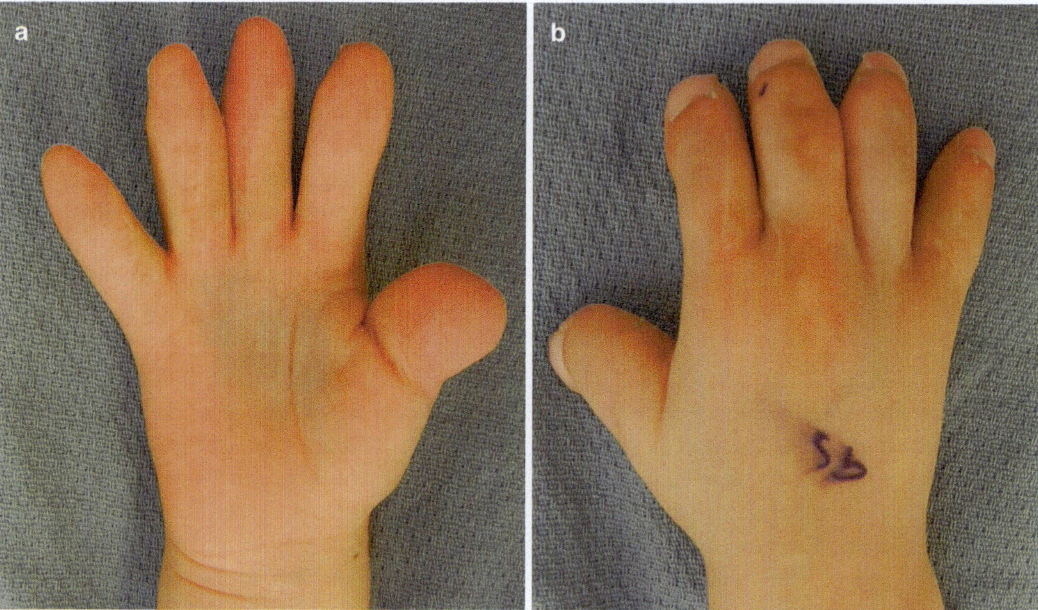

Fig. 31.13 (**a**, **b**) Postoperative appearance following two-stage release with full-thickness skin grafting

sistent aesthetic results with full coverage (Fig. 31.13) [28]. In addition, closed wounds obviate the need for painful and emotionally taxing dressing changes postoperatively. The hands are dressed with xeroform or an equivalent nonadherent dressing, moist gauze, surgical cotton, dry gauze, 2″ Kling wrap, 2″ Webril, and a full arm fiberglass cast, flexed at least 90 degrees at the elbow.

First Webspace Release

Syndactyly release of the first webspace deserves special mention. For partial, soft tissue syndactyly, a four-flap z-plasty works very well [29]. In addition to the skin release, this approach allows the surgeon to release the fascia investing the thenar musculature and abduct the first metacarpal prior to flap interdigitation and inset.

For Type III hands, there is a complete and complex syndactyly involving the first webspace [5]. In lieu of the opposing triangular flaps, a proximally based large dorsal flap is designed with its apex at the junction of the thumb and index fingertips (Fig. 31.14). A straight-line palmar incision may be designed into which this flap will be advanced—in essence, a Y to V advancement flap. Once the dorsal flap has been elevated, the straight-line release is performed in stages to allow for adjustments in its trajectory in creating the deepest and most functional first webspace [20, 24]. Templates are made on the bare areas of the thumb and index fingers as described above.

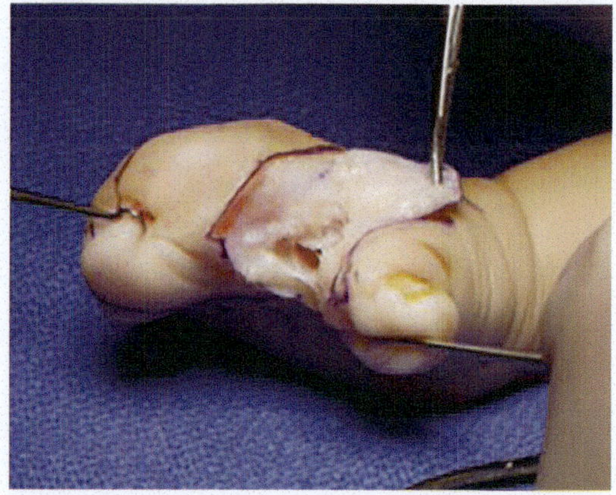

Fig. 31.14 A proximally based large dorsal flap is used for commissure creation within the first webspace of Type III hands

Alternate approaches to the first webspace in some Type II and Type III hands utilize a dorsal rotation-advancement flap described by Buck-Gramcko [30]. This can be modified by extending it on the dorsal-radial border. In some instances, the flap can be inset to avoid the need for skin grafting. For complex cases, groin flaps, forearm flaps, or microsurgical flaps have been reported, though in our experience, they are rarely, if ever, needed.

Beyond Syndactyly Release

Central Coalition Osteotomy for Type III Hands

For Upton Type III hands, a central coalition osteotomy at the first stage release (where first and fourth webspaces are released) may facilitate subsequent syndactyly release procedures [31]. The purpose of this maneuver is to flatten the central digits that are sometimes severely curved palmar-concave in the axial plane (Fig. 31.15). An incision in the hyponychium is made, exposing the distal phalanges (Fig. 31.15a). Longitudinal osteotomies are made in a retrograde fashion to release the bony union between the index, middle, and ring fingers (Fig. 31.15b). Once mobile, the palmar concavity is flattened, and the digits are stabilized with one or two transverse pins (Fig. 31.16). Release of the first and fourth webspaces in the same operation provides easy access for pin placement. The pin(s) are removed at 3–4 weeks once the cast is

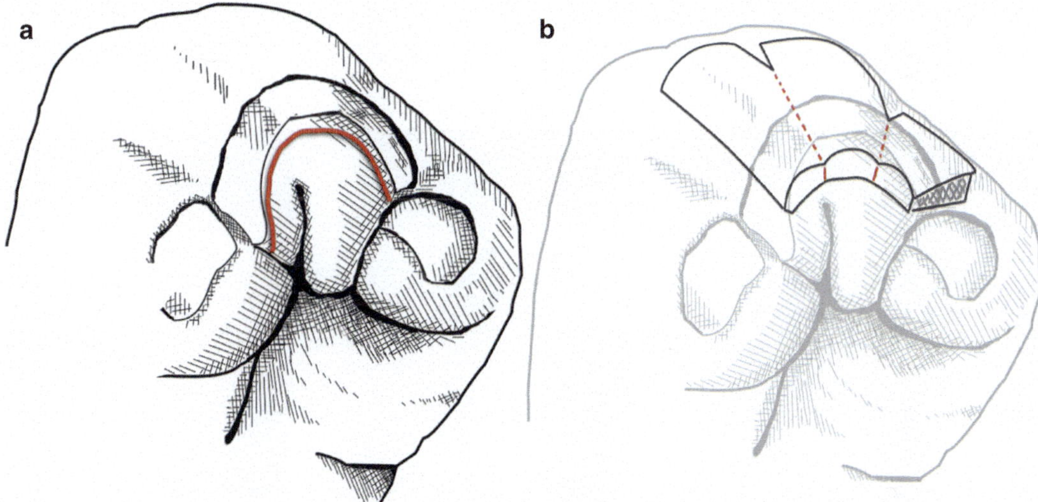

Fig. 31.15 (**a**) Central digits in the Type III hand with palmar-concave posture. (**b**) Longitudinal retrograde osteotomies may be used to realign central digital coalition, greatly facilitating subsequent digital releases. (This figure was adapted with permission from Theman TA, Upton J, Taghinia AH, Firriolo JM, Nuzzi LC, Labow BI. Central Coalition Osteotomy of Phalangeal Synostoses in the Management of the Type III Apert Hand. *J Hand Surg Am.* 2018 Nov;43 (11):1042.e1–1042.e8. © Elsevier)

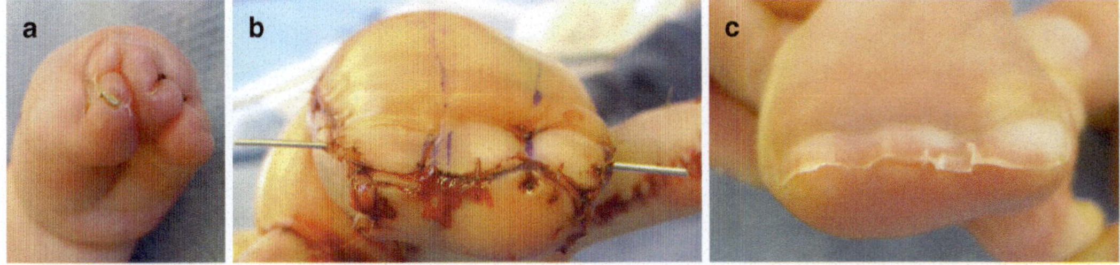

Fig. 31.16 (**a**) Type III hand prior to central coalition osteotomy. (**b**) Pins are used to stabilize the flattened digits. (**c**) Type III hand after central coalition osteotomy, with central digits now in a single plane

removed. This procedure recruits additional palmar skin and flattens the palm to make subsequent syndactyly release procedures easier. Cadaveric bone grafts may be used in between the osteotomies to augment deficient phalanges if needed (see section "Phalangeal augmentation" below).

The Thumb: 2 Approaches

The Apert thumb is usually short and radially deviated with a wide and short nail. As mentioned earlier, some authors advocate for early release of the APB tendon to limit the deforming force on the thumb during growth. Even with this approach, some degree of residual clinodactyly often remains. A longer, straighter thumb provides better function by allowing improved opposition with other digits that are usually short, stiff, and limited in range, as they articulate only at the metacarpophalangeal joints [20, 29]. The typical age for intervention is after school age when the phalanges are large enough to minimize technical margin of error. Two options are available: osteotomy with (or without) bone grafting, and distraction lengthening (Fig. 31.17) [9, 32].

The first option is commonly reserved for those with adequate length and mild-to-moderate deviation. In one stage, via a radial midlateral approach, the proximal phalanx is divided, and an opening wedge osteotomy is performed, filling the gap with cadaveric bone chips. The construct is secured with one or two pins and allowed to heal bound by a cast for 4 weeks. Previous approaches included using an iliac crest bone graft and z-plasty for soft tissue replacement. Neither has proven necessary, and the donor site

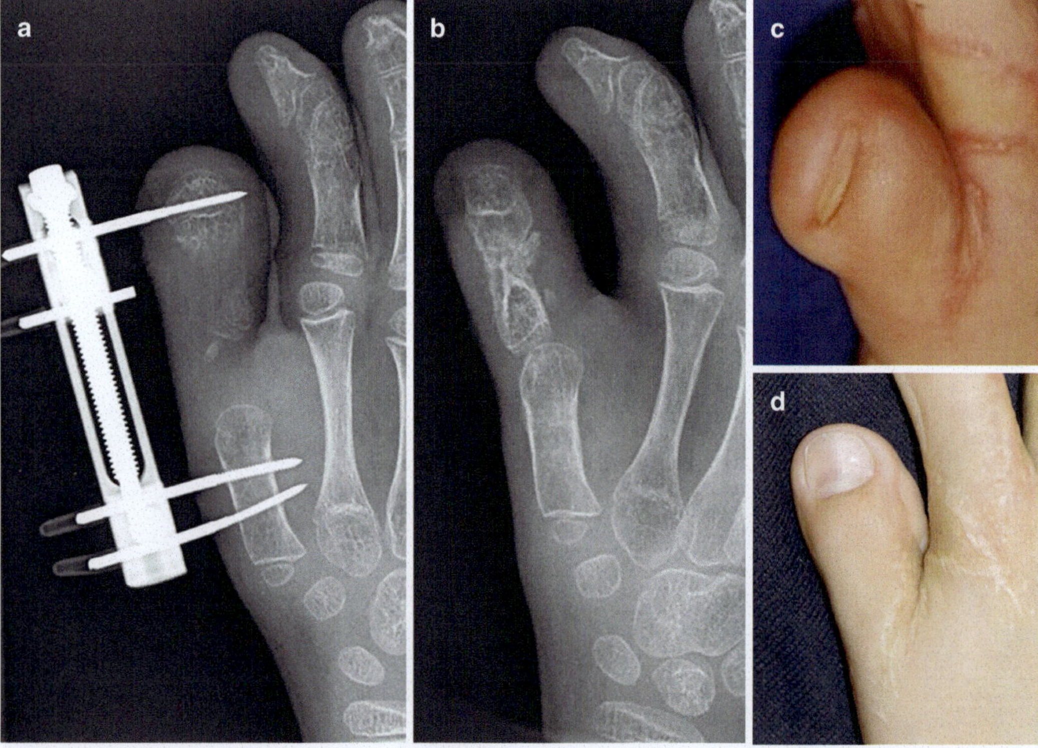

Fig. 31.17 (**a**) Distraction lengthening of Type II thumb. (**b**) Post-distraction lengthening of Type II thumb. (**c**) Type II thumb prior to distraction lengthening. (**d**) Type II thumb post-distraction lengthening. (Panels **a–c** adapted with permission from Upton J et al. Distraction Lengthening of the Apert Thumb. *Plast Reconstr Surg.* 2022 Apr 1;149 (4):691e–699e. https://pubmed.ncbi.nlm.nih.gov/35157629/ © Wolters Kluwer. Panel D adapted with permission from Boston Children's Hospital)

morbidity of pain and injury to the physis may not justify this approach.

The second option is reserved for thumbs that are shorter with more severe deviation. A uniplanar distractor, applied on the thumb's radial side, is placed, and distraction performed at about ½ to 1 mm per day. A radial midlateral approach is employed. There is often only room for one distal pin, which is placed in the distal aspect of the proximal phalanx, with two proximal pins in the metacarpal. Several centimeters of lengthening can be achieved, and distal placement can allow the nail to lengthen as well. The bone defect can be filled with graft in a second stage (Wagner technique), or allowed to fill by itself [32].

Phalangeal Augmentation

Narrow, coalesced phalanges can be augmented to provide enough subsequent width for separation. The majority of hands have five full rays and can be separated to provide five full digits. In rare cases, however, phalanges may be fused into one thin bone, and separation may result in digits that are too thin to function well. When the distal and middle phalanges are involved, especially of the central digits, these can be augmented with bone grafts to increase transverse width (Fig. 31.18). This procedure is akin to lengthening, except in the coronal plane. In the first syndactyly release operation, a hyponychial incision can expose the distal phalanges. A retrograde osteotomy, similar to the one performed for central coalition release, creates space between two proposed digits that can then be filled with cadaveric bone chips and secured with a transverse pin. A gap is created, widened, and eventually fills with enough native bone to allow separation into two distinct rays.

Abduction Deformity

There is a high incidence of metacarpal synostosis in patients with Apert syndrome [20]. Various degrees of synostosis can occur including Y or U shaped [8, 9, 13, 20]. The difference causes ulnar deviation of the small finger. It is important to remedy this deviation, as the small finger is typically the best functional digit in the Apert hand. The treatment resembles the release of metacarpal synostosis for non-syndromic differences. A dorsal approach, retracting the extensor tendons, exposes the synostosis, which is then divided longitudinally. A gap is created between the released metacarpals that is filled with bone graft–autogenous or (more typically) cadaveric (Fig. 31.19). Transverse pins secure the construct for several weeks bound by a cast. By increasing the intermetacarpal distance alone, significant abduction deformities of the small finger can be dramatically improved without any additional work at the phalangeal level (Fig. 31.20).

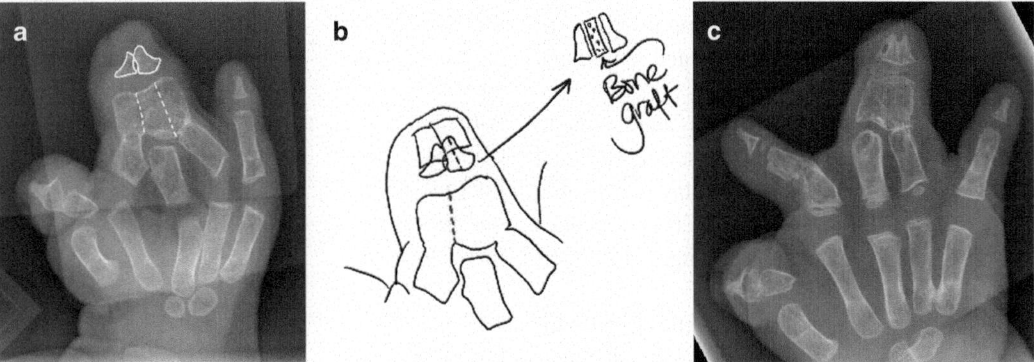

Fig. 31.18 (**a**) Limited distal phalangeal bone for three digits. (**b**) Bone graft insertion to increase transverse width. (**c**) Results after bone graft has healed and after release of index finger and sufficient distal phalangeal bone for remaining two digits. (Panels **a** and **c** adapted with permission from Boston Children's Hospital. Panel **b** created (and reused with permission) by Dr. Amir Taghinia at Boston Children's Hospital)

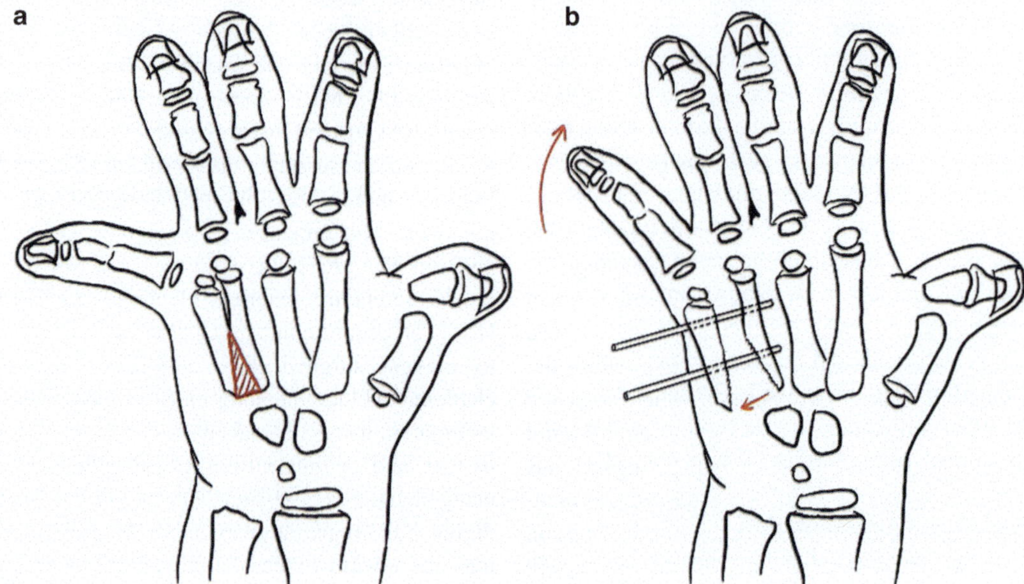

Fig. 31.19 (**a**) Longitudinal osteotomy with proximal ostectomy of the fourth and fifth metacarpal synostosis. (**b**) Clockwise rotation of the abducted small finger occurs immediately, gap between metacarpals filled with cadaveric or autogenous soft-tissue or bone graft and fixed with transverse k-wires. Although synostosis always recurs over time, the added palmar width is sufficient to prevent recurrent abduction deformity. (Panels **a** and **b** created (and reused with permission) by Dr. Amir Taghinia at Boston Children's Hospital)

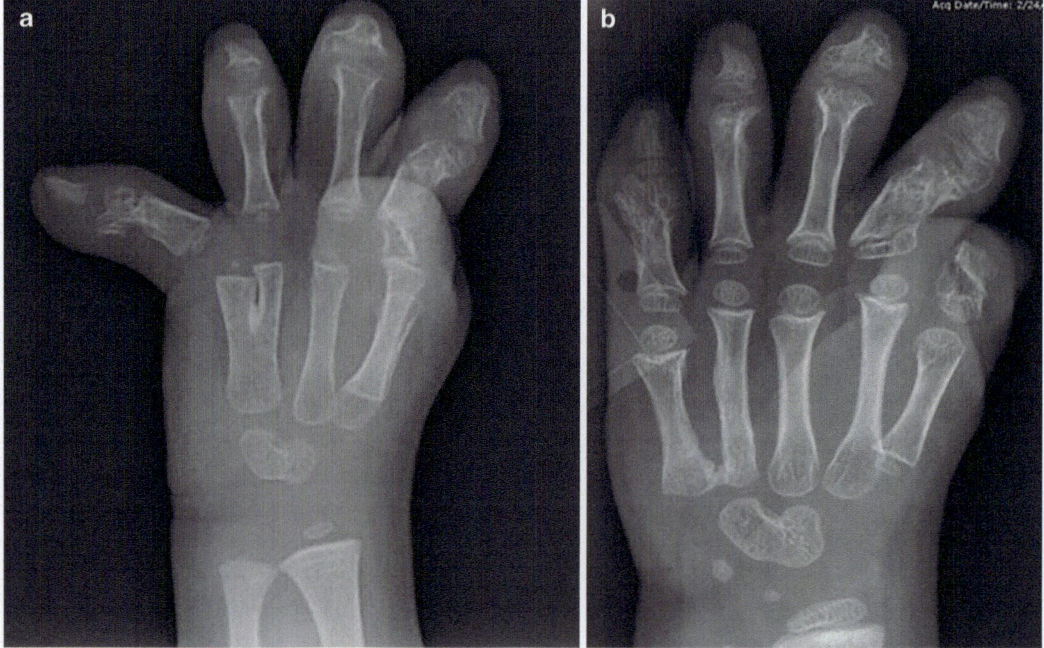

Fig. 31.20 (**a**) Radiographs demonstrating small finger ulnar deviation abduction deformity following release in Type III hand. (**b**) Deviation corrected following metacarpal synostosis release and interposition arthroplasty. (Panels **a** and **b** adapted with permission from Boston Children's Hospital)

Postoperative Care

Patients with Apert syndrome frequently present with choanal stenosis or atresia, sleep apnea, or other conditions that warrant 1:1 nursing and careful monitoring for apnea or oxygen desaturation events during the early postoperative period. At our institution, this is done in the intensive care unit (ICU). While almost all infants are transferred to the ICU after the first-stage release, this may not be necessary for subsequent operations. Besides monitoring, adequate pain control and assuring sufficient oral nutritional intake are the primary goals of care. Most patients spend one night in the hospital and are discharged home the following day.

Very few patients require opioid analgesia beyond the first postoperative day. Acetaminophen and ibuprofen are used as needed. Parents are encouraged to allow their children to engage in activities similar to what they were doing preoperatively. The abdominal donor dressing is wiped clean with diaper changes until it lifts off. The Steri-Strips similarly are allowed to lift off on their own.

After 3 weeks, the casts are removed, and bathing is encouraged to allow for dried blood and suture material to be washed away. Dry skin is managed with moisturizer. Use of the upper extremities is encouraged with play. Most of our patients are already engaged in some form of early intervention and physical therapy before surgery. This can be renewed for the upper extremity, as well, once the casts have been removed.

Outcomes

There is very little information regarding long-term functional outcomes. A recent study of adult patients with Apert syndrome assessed health-related quality of life outcomes using the 36-Item Short Form Survey (SF-36) and DASH validated instruments [15]. Additional outcomes were examined via a semi-structured interview, the Jebsen hand function test, and through traditional measures of hand function such as pinch strength, grip strength, range of motion, and sensation. Hand Types I, II, and III were relatively evenly distributed among the 22 patients in this study. SF-36 results were slightly (<10%) higher for patients with Apert syndrome compared to population norms. However, the average Disabilities of the Arm, Shoulder and Hand (DASH) score for patients with Apert syndrome was 17 (population norm is 10, higher is worse). Seventeen patients had completed high school, four had completed undergraduate programs, eight had driver's licenses, and four were working towards them. Several patients had competed in the Special Olympics. Patients described multiple friends and relationships, and two patients had children. Few patients described social anxieties.

Functional outcomes revealed that the patients with Apert syndrome performed 43–83% slower in timed tests of most tasks (page turning, simulated feeding, and stacking checkers) than individuals without Apert syndrome. Range of motion of the metacarpophalangeal (MCP) joints (only functional joint) ranged between 20 and 65 degrees, worsening with increasing hand type. Most patients had one or two digits that opposed against the thumb.

Overall, patients with Apert syndrome displayed more favorable health-related quality of life outcomes than their unaffected peers, but less favorable functional upper extremity outcomes [15].

Patient/Parent-Reported Outcomes

Limited information exists on patient/parent-reported outcomes for younger children with Apert syndrome. This is partly due to difficulty in standardizing functional outcomes across different age groups. Additionally, the rare nature of Apert syndrome results in studies with very small sizes and limited generalizability.

Some of the authors contributed to a recent (unpublished) validated survey study of parents (proxy) of children with Apert syndrome that was conducted to determine health-related quality of life and functioning of children with this condition. The parent-proxy PROMIS validated instrument was used to survey parents of 40 children with Apert syndrome between the ages of 5 and 17 years. Early results indicate that upper extremity function is highly correlated to cognitive function in children with Apert syndrome. Parent-reported anxiety and psychological well-being outcomes for their children with Apert syndrome were lower than expected based on the adult study previously mentioned. These results may indicate that either the parents' views of their children's well-being and functioning are biased or that the adult study was subject to selection bias (only those with better overall functioning participated). Regardless, it is imperative to consider the parents' perspective of their children's well-being, as parents drive treatment for their children during the early stages of their lives.

Conclusion

In sum, the surgical treatment of the Apert hand should be viewed as an integral component of care for these patients. Optimal results require a multidisciplinary approach characterized by an intentional, well-planned staged reconstruction. Comprehensive preoperative evaluation, meticulous surgical technique, and vigilant long-term monitoring can yield excellent aesthetic and functional results. In addition to syndactyly release early in life, adjunct procedures exist that may benefit patients and should be familiar to surgeons who treat Apert hands. Family-centered care with problem-based treatment recommendations allows for individualized care that can minimize stress on patients with Apert syndrome and their parents alike. Ongoing studies focused on long-term outcomes will empower individuals and families affected by Apert syndrome as they navigate a path towards enhanced health, resilience, and well-being.

References

1. Apert M. De l'acrocephalosyndactylie. Bull Mem Soc Med Hop Paris. 1906;23:1310–3.
2. Freiman A, Tessler O, Barankin B. Apert syndrome. Int J Dermatol. 2006;45(11):1341–3.
3. Hoover GH, Flatt AE, Weiss MW. The hand and Apert's syndrome. J Bone Joint Surg Am. 1970;52(5):878–95.
4. Barot LR, Caplan HS. Early surgical intervention in Apert's syndactyly. Plast Reconstr Surg. 1986;77(2):282–7.
5. Upton J. Apert syndrome. Classification and pathologic anatomy of limb anomalies. Clin Plast Surg. 1991;18(2):321–55.
6. Holten IW, Smith AW, Bourne AJ, David DJ. The Apert syndrome hand: pathologic anatomy and clinical manifestations. Plast Reconstr Surg. 1997;99(6):1681–7.
7. Fearon JA. Treatment of the hands and feet in Apert syndrome: an evolution in management. Plast Reconstr Surg. 2003;112(1):1–19.
8. Guero S, Vassia L, Renier D, Glorion C. Surgical management of the hand in Apert syndrome. Handchir Mikrochir Plast Chir. 2004;36(2–3):179–85.
9. Raposo-Amaral CE, Denadai R, Furlan P, Raposo-Amaral CA. Treatment of Apert hand syndrome: strategies for achieving a five-digit hand. Plast Reconstr Surg. 2018;142(4):972–82.
10. Dao KD, Shin AY, Kelley S, Wood VE. Synostosis of the ring-small finger metacarpal in Apert acrosyndactyly hands: incidence and treatment. J Pediatr Orthop. 2001;21(4):502–7.
11. Upton J, Khouri KS. Resection of 4th–5th metacarpal synostosis and fascial interposition for creation of a functional grip/pinch in the Apert hand. Plast Reconstr Surg. 2024;155(2):309–14.
12. Kasser J, Upton J. The shoulder, elbow, and forearm in Apert syndrome. Clin Plast Surg. 1991;18(2):381–9.
13. Garagnani L, Smith GD. Chapter 14: syndromes associated with syndactyly. In: The pediatric upper extremity. New York: Springer; 2015. p. 297–324.
14. França Bisneto EN. Congenital deformities of the upper limbs. Part II: failure of formation and duplications. Rev Bras Ortop. 2013;48(1):3–10.
15. Taghinia AH, Yorlets RR, Doyle M, Labow BI, Upton J. Long-term functional upper-extremity outcomes in adults with Apert syndrome. Plast Reconstr Surg. 2019;143(4):1136–45.
16. Harvey I, Brown S, Ayres O, Proudman T. The Apert hand–angiographic planning of a single-stage, 5-digit release for all classes of deformity. J Hand Surg Am. 2012;37(1):152–8.
17. Cuthbert R. Acrocephalosyndactyly with case report illustrating some of the radiological features. Glasgow Med J. 1954;35(12):349–56.
18. Wood VE, Sauser DD, O'Hara RC. The shoulder and elbow in Apert's syndrome. J Pediatr Orthop. 1995;15(5):648–51.
19. Murnaghan LM, Thurgur CH, Forster BB, Sawatzky BJ, Hawkins R, Tredwell SJ. A clinicoradiologic study of the shoulder in Apert syndrome. J Pediatr Orthop. 2007;27(7):838–43.

20. Pettitt DA, Arshad Z, Mishra A, McArthur P. Apert syndrome: a consensus on the management of Apert hands. J Craniomaxillofac Surg. 2017;45(2):223–31.
21. Salazard B, Casanova D. La main du syndrome d'Apert: stratégie thérapeutique [The Apert's syndrome hand: therapeutic management]. Chir Main. 2008;27(Suppl 1):S115–20.
22. Kracoff SL. Radiographic characteristics of the hand in Apert syndrome. J Hand Surg Asian Pac. 2020;25(1):82–6.
23. Van Heest AE, House JH, Reckling WC. Two-stage reconstruction of apert acrosyndactyly. J Hand Surg Am. 1997;22(2):315–22.
24. Zucker RM, Cleland HJ, Haswell T. Syndactyly correction of the hand in Apert syndrome. Clin Plast Surg. 1991;18(2):357–64.
25. Guero S. Release of partial syndactyly using a trident flap without skin grafting. J Hand Surg Eur. 2020;45(2):181–6.
26. Lundkvist L, Barfred T. A double pulp flap technique for creating nail-folds in syndactyly release. J Hand Surg Br. 1991;16(1):32–4.
27. Golash A, Watson JS. Nail fold creation in complete syndactyly using Buck-Gramcko pulp flaps. J Hand Surg Br. 2000;25(1):11–4.
28. Chang J, Danton TK, Ladd AL, Hentz VR. Reconstruction of the hand in Apert syndrome: a simplified approach. Plast Reconstr Surg. 2002;109(2):465–71.
29. Foucher G, Medina J, Navarro R, Pajardi G. Apport d'une nouvelle plastie à la reconstruction de la première commissure dans les malformations congénitales. A propos d'une série de 54 patients [Value of a new first web space reconstruction in congenital hand deformities. A study of 54 patients]. Chir Main. 2000;19(3):152–60.
30. Buck-Gramcko D. Congenital malformations. New York: Thieme Medical Publishers Inc.; 1988.
31. Theman TA, Upton J, Taghinia AH, Firriolo JM, Nuzzi LC, Labow BI. Central coalition osteotomy of phalangeal synostoses in the management of the Type III Apert hand. J Hand Surg Am. 2018;43(11):1042.e1–8.
32. Upton J, McNamara CT, Ali B, Nuzzi LC, Taghinia AH, Labow BI. Distraction lengthening of the Apert thumb. Plast Reconstr Surg. 2022;149(4):691e–9e.

Management of the Apert Foot

32

Stéphane Guero

A foot is not a hand. Foot deformities in Apert syndrome share similar features with those of the hand, but evolution with growth and the functional outcomes are dramatically different.

Few articles in the literature are devoted to the Apert foot. However, the difficulties of wearing shoes and the pain and stiffness of walking are daily concerns for some children and their families. In this chapter, we will review the tissue disturbances, point out the differences between the hand and the foot, and analyze the functional consequences and some clues for helping and treating these children.

Pathologic Anatomy

The foot shares many features described in the chapter on hand anomalies. However, we will report specific deformities of the forefoot and the tarsal bones. Firstly, it is the consequence of the embryology. The lower limb formation occurs later than the upper limb. Morphogenes are different. For example, *TBX5* is expressed in the upper limb bud and not in the lower limb bud, while *TBX6* and *PITX1* are partly responsible for the patterning of the lower limb. Interactions with the mutations of *FGRF2* in Apert syndrome are probably modified. Lastly, the function of the hand is prehension, while the foot's function is locomotion, with many consequences during growth.

Bone

Synostosis can be present without correlating with the Blauth and Von Torne [1] classification type. As for the hand, they are usually not seen at birth but appear during childhood. When reviewing 22 patients, we found 10 patients with a synostosis between the fourth and fifth metatarsal bones (M4–M5), and this is likely an underestimate since some children were still young at review. Eight patients had a bilateral synostosis between the first and second metatarsal bones (M1–M2), six were partial (Fig. 32.5a, b), two had a complete fusion, and one child had a unilateral presentation.

Symphalangism is underestimated. All our patients had a fusion of the intermediate and distal phalanges. Proximal phalanges are well developed, and metatarsophalangeal joints (MTP joints) are mobile [2] but tend to be not functional with a progressive plantar subluxation of the central rays. The hallux has been described as a delta-shaped proximal phalanx, but it is a transitory feature (Fig. 32.6a–c). In older children, the proximal and distal phalanges of the great toe are fused, and the growth of the first ray is impaired. On the contrary, the third metatarsal bone has relatively excessive

S. Guero (✉)
Institut de la Main, Paris, France

Hôpital Necker-Enfants malades, Université Paris Centre, Paris, France

J. G. Meara et al. (eds.), *Apert Syndrome*, https://doi.org/10.1007/978-3-032-12551-4_32

growth and commonly fuses proximally with the lateral cuneiform (Fig. 32.5a, b).

Extra bones are common. Radiologic examination reveals a specific feature on feet, absent in hands. Some abnormal ossifications can be found on the base of the fifth metacarpal and, in a few cases, on the first ray. Three patients out of 22 had a true duplication of the great toe, which is never reported in hands.

The great toe is broad. Many distal phalanges of the hallux are broad, and some demonstrate a distal and incomplete duplication. This is unsurprising since this feature is frequently associated with a proximal "delta" phalanx in hands. Indeed, in early ages, the proximal phalanx of the great toe is triangular, with a bracketed epiphysis on the medial side. This typical feature of the delta phalanx is much more frequent in the foot than in the hand.

Joints have variable fusions of the tarsal bones that occur during childhood. At birth, the ankle and the tarsal joints are supple. In severe cases, with age, they become stiffer. The midfoot and hindfoot progress to characteristic fusion in a supinated position.

Growth perturbation shortens the first ray. The physeal plate on the first metatarsal bone is primitively functional but can close prematurely. The proximal phalanx of the hallux rarely shows a normal growing plate. In most cases, it has a triangular shape with a bracketed epiphysis, with a more typical aspect of delta phalanx than in the Apert thumb. The great toe is increasingly in varus [2] and stops its growth when the proximal and distal phalanx fuse. It is unclear why the third metacarpal bone demonstrates a relative overgrowth compared to the adjacent metacarpal bones, leading to a fusion with the lateral cuneiform. One explanation could be the association of a synostosis with the two first metatarsal bones.

Skin

Hyperkeratosis is common. Plantar callosities are the consequence of focal hyper-pressures. With time, numbness evolves to chronic pain during footwear.

Most syndactyly is complete and complex in type 3, but, unlike the hand, there is a distal fusion of the phalanges in the foot. Cohen and Kreiborg [3] studied 37 pairs of Apert feet and classified them according to Blauth and von Torne [1]. Type 1 is fusion of toes 2–4, with toes 1 and 5 left separate. Type 1 feet account for 27% of their series. Type 2 feet show fusion of toes 2–5, with 1 separate, and account for 19% of their series. In type 2 separation of the 5th toe may be seen, but the separation will only occur on the plantar surface. Type 3 shows fusion of all toes. Type 3 was found in 54% of their series.

Toenails

Toenails are usually well segmented, but fusions can be observed in severe forms (Figs. 32.1 and 32.3). Nails on the feet can be a daily problem [4]. Parents should take great care of the nails and learn to use antiseptic solutions in case of inflammation. In recurrent infections, the only solution was separation of the toes.

Tendons

The Abductor Hallucis, homologous of the Abductor Pollicis Brevis on the thumb, is inserted distally on the base of the distal phalanx and participates in the medial deviation of the great toe. Extrinsic flexor and extensor tendons are present but not functional.

Classification

As for the hand, based on his classification of radiographic findings, Upton divided patients into two groups [5]. Group I patients present the first metatarsal and cuneiform bones well segmented at birth but an abnormal proximal phalanx of the great toe, causing a medial deviation and a resultant wide distal phalanx. Even though the first ray becomes shorter with growth, the relative stability of the first metatarsal causes no significant walking impairment. Group II patients are more symptomatic, showing a radical medial deviation of the first toe and restricted development associated to a proximal duplication of the first short metatarsal fused with the navicular bone and a common synostosis of the first and second metatarsal. Another useful classification of Apert feet, based on the number of toes involved in syndactyly, is described by Blauth and von Torne [1]. In type I, the three middle toes are fused (Fig. 32.1). In type II, only the great toe is free, with the forefoot in a relatively supinated position (Fig. 32.2). In type III, the most common pattern of their series, there is a complete fusion of the five digits with the first toe hyperextended (Figs. 32.3 and 32.4). Types on foot are grossly correlated with the type on hand, but it is not always the rule [5]. Some patients have a less severe type on the foot than on hands. For example, some have a type 2 on the hands and have a type 1 on the feet, a type 3 on the hands and a type 2 on the feet (Figs. 32.5 and 32.6).

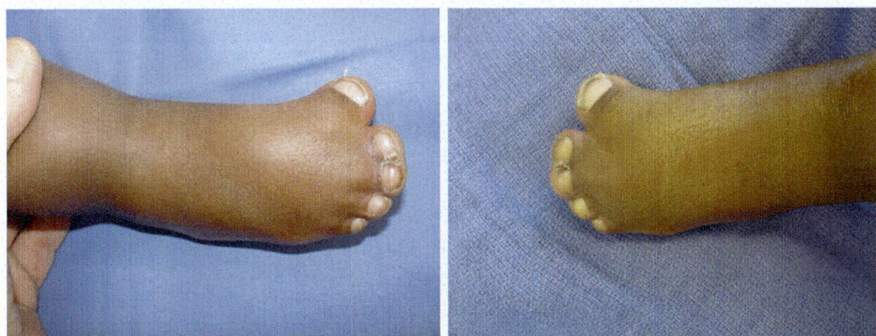

Fig. 32.1 Type 1. All toes and nails are separated, except the second and third

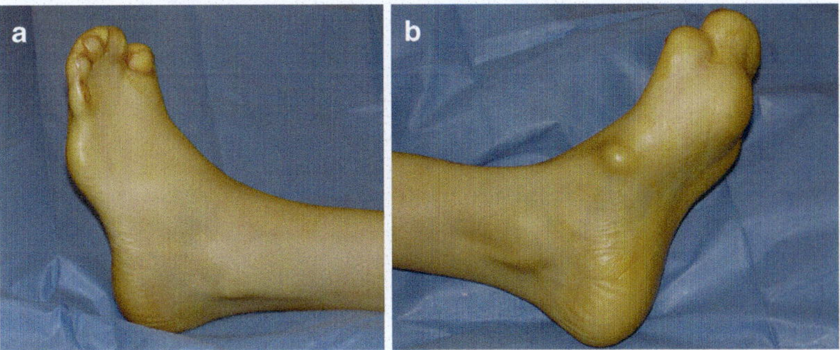

Fig. 32.2 Type 2. (**a**) Toes 2–5 are fused; the foot is in a supinated position. (**b**) Note the extra bone on the base of the metatarsal 1 and the convex forefoot due to the plantar subluxation of the heads of metatarsal 2 and 3

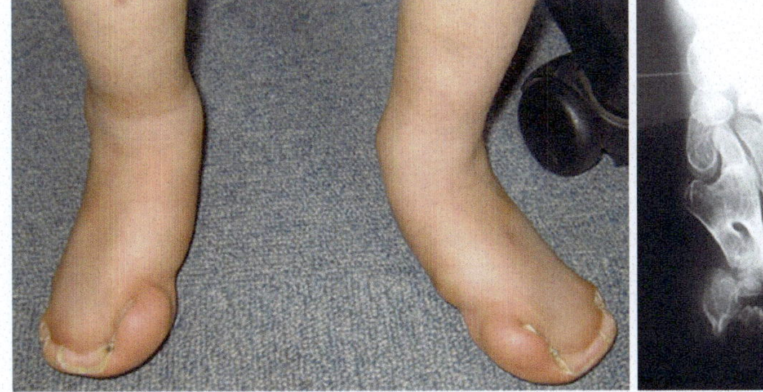
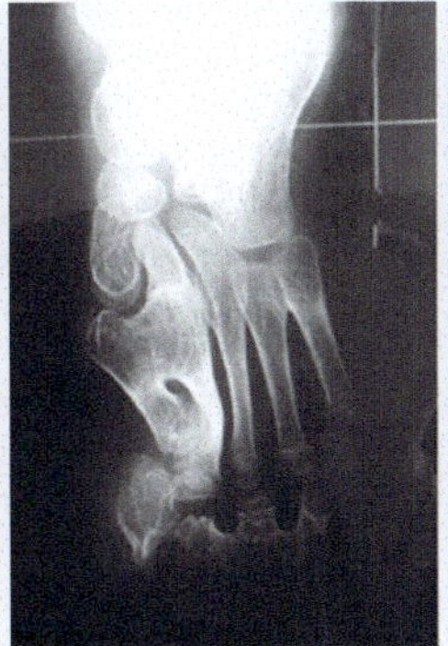
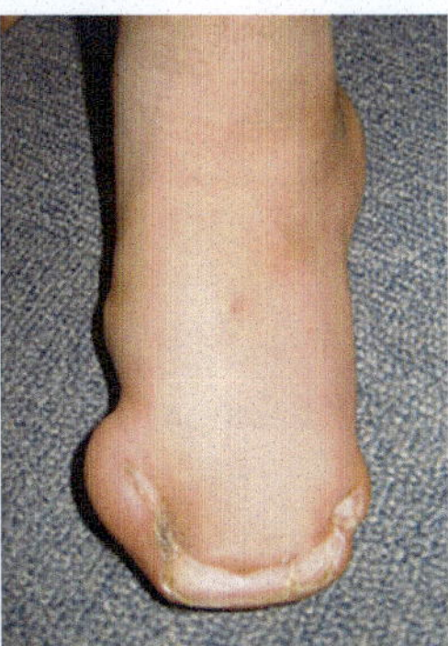

Fig. 32.3 Type 3 with fusion of M1 & M2, fusion between the bases of M2 and M3 with the cuneiform. Note the very unusual fusion of the proximal phalanges. Feet are in a supine position with hyperextension of the great toes

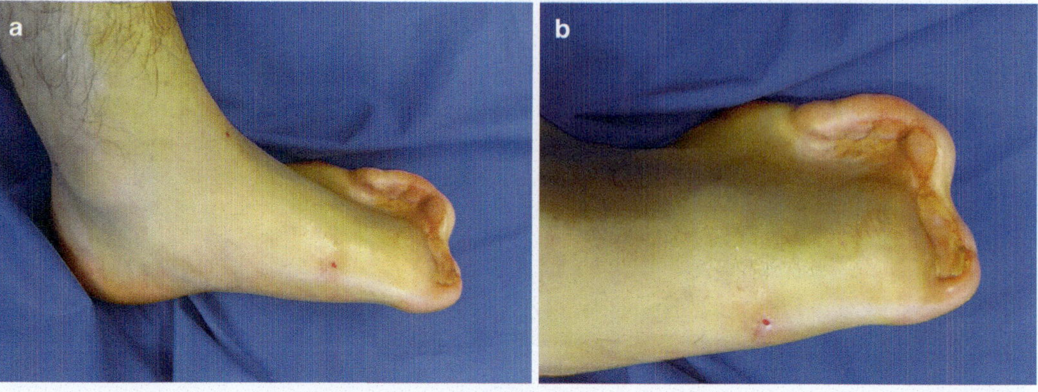

Fig. 32.4 (**a**, **b**) Another Type 3 with good alignment of the first ray but with a severe hyperextension of the 2–5 toes

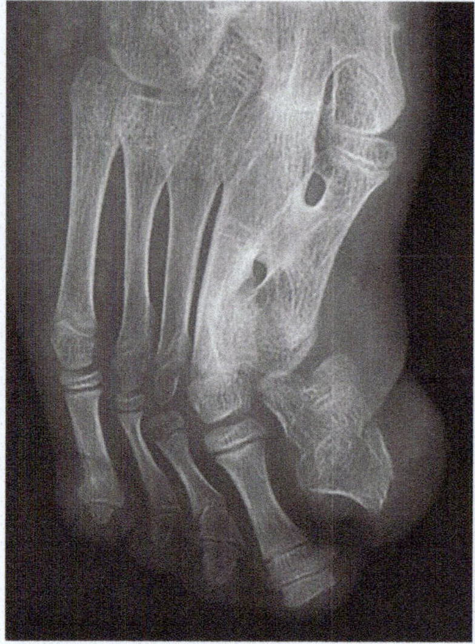

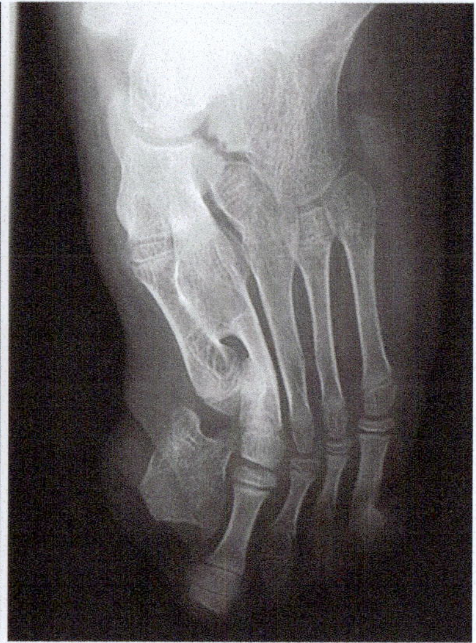

Fig. 32.5 Complex fusions on both feet. Synostosis of the first and second metatarsal bones in the base of the left foot, in the middle of M1 & M2 on the right foot. Note the fusion of the base of M2 with the central cuneiform and the fusion of M3 with the lateral cuneiform

Imaging

It is a critical step in analyzing these combined deformities. Plan X-rays can be sufficient for type 1. In complex cases, we recommend computed tomography (CT) scans with three-dimensional (3D) reconstruction to address the complex fusions and deviations of the feet. This three-dimensional imaging is the key to surgical management [6].

Functional Consequences

All the anomalies described previously are not static. They worsen with age, as growth will impair the morphology of the feet. Anderson et al. [7] reviewed specifically the foot anomalies on 43 children with Apert. The study concludes that there are widespread anomalies of the feet, with defects including both predictable dysmorphic changes and progressive fusions of the skeletal components during skeletal maturity. These fusions and their effect on growth produce increasing deformity during childhood. The clinical significance of the anomalies is that walking is often delayed, and the increasing deformity results in difficulty obtaining footwear.

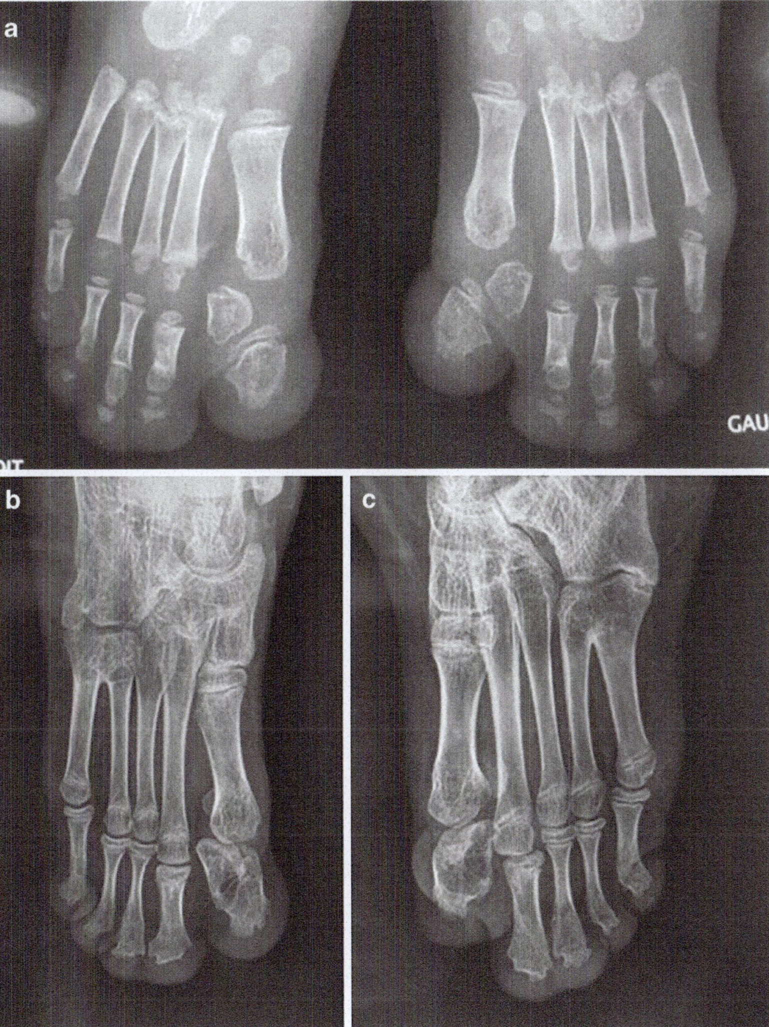

Fig. 32.6 (a–c) Modification with growth: Note the fusion of the two phalanx of the great toe, the fusion of all phalanges in toes 2–5. The fusion of the base of M3 with the lateral cuneiform and the synostoses between the bases of M4 and M5, not present at birth

Goals of the Treatment

It is impossible to reconstruct a normal foot in such complex malformations. A surgeon can address problems with footwear and gait disturbances that may limit daily activities. Parents should be informed that treatment reduces pain and infections. However, there is no solution for the progressive stiffness of the hindfoot.

Avoid Pain

- Allow shoe-wearing. The Apert foot is the worst foot for usual shoes. The width of the foot is abnormal due to extra bones or deviation of the first ray in varus. The forefoot is convex plantarly, and toes tend to be in recurvatum. Custom-made shoes are necessary but not always sufficient. Correction of the varus and all the spots of conflicts on the medial and lateral border will reduce the width. If necessary, syndactyly release will give more independence to toes and put them more plantar.
- Preserve a painless weight bearing. The convex forefoot is mainly due to an excessive plantar flexion of the second metatarsal bone. The head of M2 is under hyper-pressure and, by reaction, a callosity forms, increasing pain. Conservative treatment will use insoles

and orthopedic shoes. Surgery consists in corrective osteotomies to flatten the plantar sole and rebalance the weight on all metatarsal heads [8].

Avoid Infection

- This means an educational program for the families. They need to take care of the ingrown nails. In some cases, we should consider a syndactyly release to eliminate conflicts between nails.

Treatment

Although there is literature on treating syndactyly of the hands and feet for patients with Apert syndrome, only a few authors have focused on treating plantar metatarsal subluxation. This malformation may result from a weight shift, usually on the second metatarsal head during child growth due to a progressive shortening of the first ray. The forefoot is, therefore, characterized by a convex plantar surface, with the development of acute pain during full weight-bearing and plantar hyperkeratosis and callosities (Fig. 32.1a, b). This condition leads to functional impairment, requiring patients to wear specially designed orthopedic shoes.

Conservative Treatment

Apert children rarely wear store-bought shoes. The first step in the treatment is to make custom-made shoes. It allows the child to have a painless gait, without any conflict between the toes and the shoe. These shoes now have modern shapes and are well accepted by children and parents alike. Most of these shoes are enough for the well-being of the child. In our series of 81 children, 2/3 live normally with custom-made shoes. On the other hand, those who have been treated with orthopedic shoes and continue to suffer will be referred for surgery.

Surgery

Indications and Timing

Surgery on the feet can be delayed. There are no early functional impairments. In a young child, the ankle, the hindfoot, and the forefoot are supple. The craniofacial surgery and the hand surgery will come first. The rule is to treat conservatively with made-to-measure shoes, and when the weight-bearing or the shoe-fitting becomes difficult, we consider surgery on the feet. This was necessary in one-third of our patients, 22/74, sometimes very young children. The average age at surgery was 9 years (range 2–16 years). Fearon was performing osteotomies between the ages of 9 and 12 [9]. Tarsal fusions and other coalitions have to be corrected on an individual basis. Plantar pressure measurements using pedobarography are of great interest in documenting biomechanical foot development and abnormalities during growth and in helping with indication setting.

Techniques

Extra-bones removal is fast and easy. It is indicated when a conflict with the shoes makes the shoe-wearing painful. Treatment of the hallux varus is much more difficult. Sometimes, the medial deviation is treated by a closing wedge or a reverse-wedge osteotomy. Removing a supernumerary ray interposed between M1 and M2 can help the first ray realignment [10]. Realignment of the first ray can be more complex in the case of synostosis of M1–M2, with a special mention of the medial subluxation of the tarsometatarsal joint. Parents are aware that correcting the first ray cannot be optimal but will improve the realization of the orthopedic shoes. For Calis et al. [11], correction of brachymetatarsia and medial angulation of the great toe can be done by distraction osteogenesis. They report satisfactory results with minor complications but with 36% of early union that required reoperation. This fast bone healing is a landmark of the Apert syndrome, also reported in hand surgery during distraction of the thumb.

Syndactyly release, if indicated, does not differ from the techniques used in hands. As for hands, we use a dorsal omega flap. The flaps should be calculated longer and narrower than in hands. The debate for zigzag incision versus straight lines [9] is useless in foot, since there is a small distance between the central flap and the base of the nail. A straight line is the usual option on toes. The defects are smaller in the toes than in the fingers. A full-thickness skin graft is harvested. The best donor site, in our experience, is the medial or lateral infra-malleolar skin. The color matching is perfect, and the donor site is in the same surgical area. One plantar intermetatarsal perforator flap for the first web has been reported, providing a large first web without skin grafting [12].

More specific to the foot is the surgical treatment of the convex forefoot. We want to emphasize a simple and fast procedure that constantly gives us good and stable results [13]. It is an oblique osteotomy described by Helal [14], performed on M2, and sometimes on M3. With an accurate preoperative study of 3D images, the correct number of osteotomies and synostoses removal, which might affect the operation result, can be planned. All procedures were carried out as day surgery, under general anesthesia and tourniquet. Operative time ranges between 15 and 25 min, with no need for patient hospitalization. Nurses were required to assess pain during the immediate postoperative hours, while parents had to monitor and report their child's pain at home for the following 3 weeks.

An X-ray was taken 3 weeks postoperatively to evaluate bone healing. In the procedure, a longitudinal incision, from 2 to 4 cm in length, is performed on the dorsum of the foot, usually over the second metatarsal bone, to expose the metatarsal shaft. After identifying the metatarsal head and neck, two Hohmann retractors are placed proximal to the articular capsule, at each side of the bone, to expose the surface well and protect the surrounding structures. According to the dimension of the bone, a chisel is used to carry out the osteotomy, in an oblique direction, from dorsal–proximal to plantar–distal, with an angulation of at least 30 degrees (Fig. 32.7a–c). We do not use any specific measuring device; therefore, the angles of osteotomies are slightly different from one patient to another. It is important to cut as obliquely as possible to create a wide contact surface between the two bone stumps, promoting bone consolidation and fixation of the proximal edge of the plantar capsule. The metatarsal head will naturally be lifted and displaced backward.

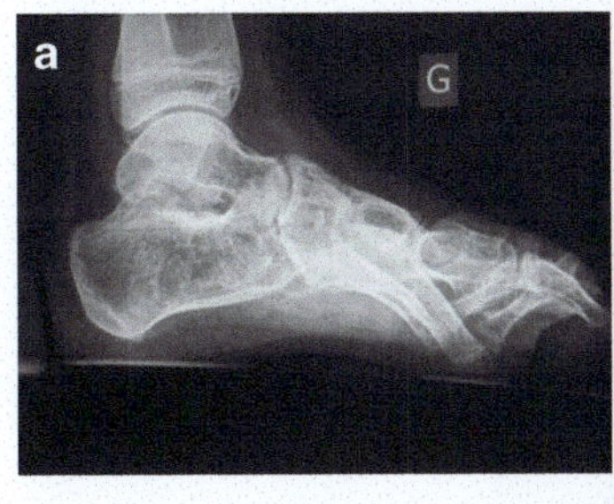

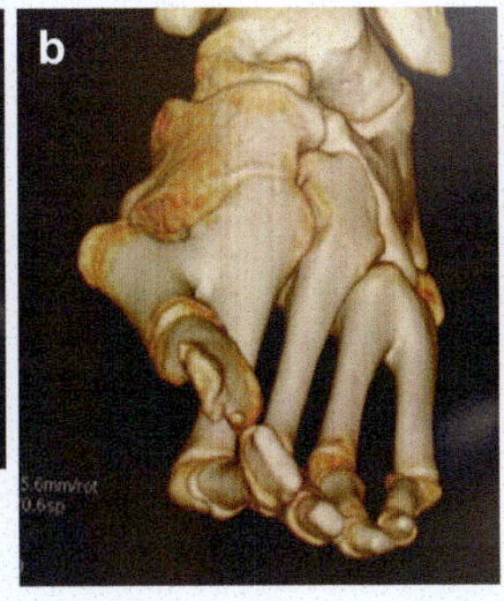

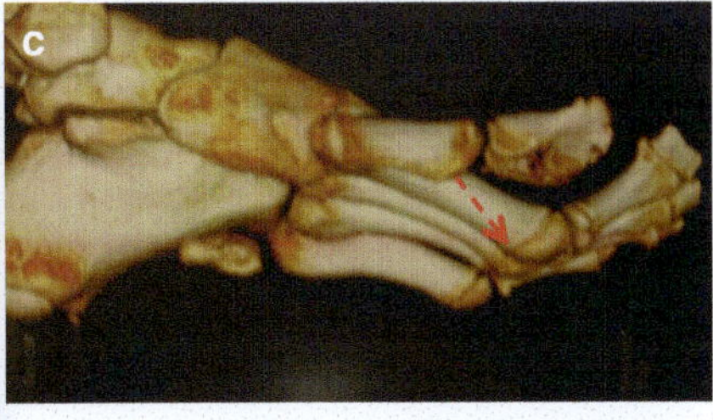

Fig. 32.7 (**a**) Lateral X-ray showing the plantar tilt of the metatarsal 2, (**b**) better documented on the 3D CT scan. (**c**) Dot line (in red) showing the direction of the osteotomy, from dorsal-proximal to plantar distal, ending just before the metatarsal head

Rongeurs are then used to cut out the sharp edges of the bone, and the skin is closed (Fig. 32.8a–c). No pinning or bone fixation is needed. We then perform an overcorrecting bandage, leaving a rolled-up gauze on the foot's plantar surface to keep the bone's two edges in place (Fig. 32.9a–c). No cast is recommended. The patient is allowed to wear full weight-bearing shoes for just 24 h postoperatively with normal shoes. In case of pain, we usually prescribe paracetamol three times a day at hospital discharge. No physiotherapy is needed (Fig. 32.10).

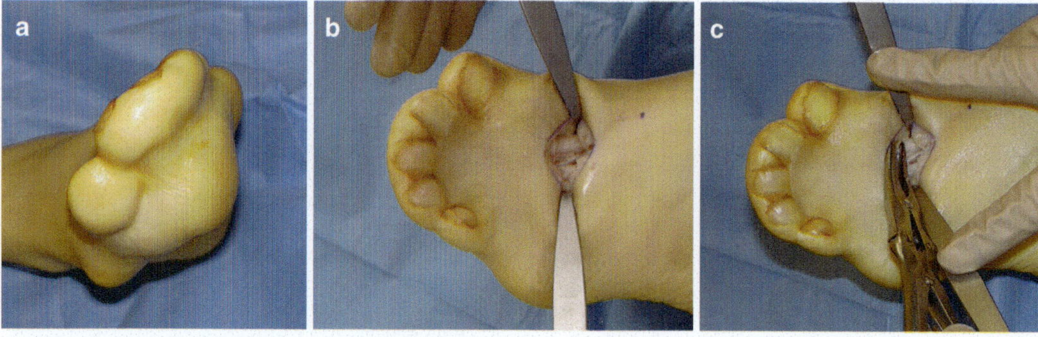

Fig. 32.8 (**a**) Convex forefoot due to the subluxation of metatarsal 2 & 3 (**b**) exposition through a single dorsal incision of the diaphysis of M2 & M3 (**c**) Sharp edges of the bones are cut out with a rongeur after the osteotomy made with a chisel

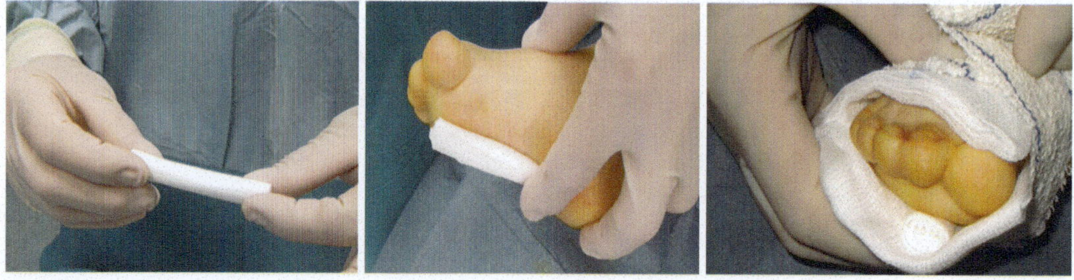

Fig. 32.9 Overcorrecting bandage leaving a rolled-up gauze on the plantar surface of the metatarsal 2 to lift the metatarsal head. Full weight bearing is allowed just 24 h postoperatively

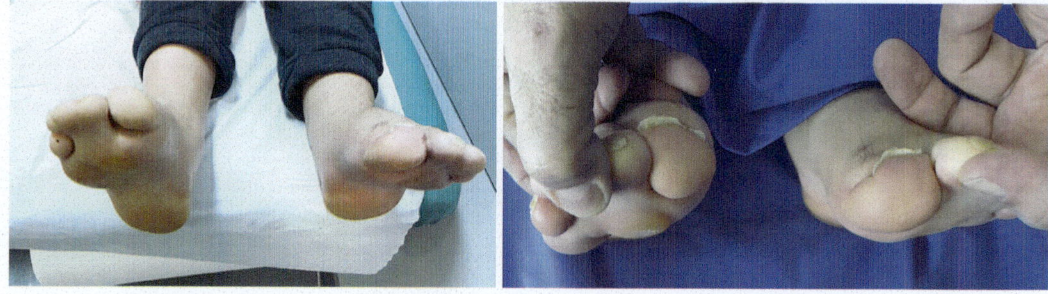

Fig. 32.10 Results after a Helal osteotomy on the left foot. The plantar callosity has regressed. On the right foot, not yet operated, the hyperkeratosis beneath the head of M2 is still present

Conclusion

The Apert foot is stiff and tends to be painful without care. Stiffness is ineluctable, but pain can be avoided with orthopedic and surgical treatment, significantly improving the quality of life of the children. We do not recommend separation of all foot syndactyly. It is indicated for functional reasons in some specific cases [10], but we do not want to add more procedures in those children. If separation is wished for cosmetic reasons, it should be the patient's choice.

References

1. Blauth W, von Torne O. "Apert's foot" (in acrocephalosyndactyly) (author's transl). Z Orthop Ihre Grenzgeb. 1978;116(1):1–6.
2. Mah J, Kasser J, Upton J. The foot in Apert syndrome. Clin Plast Surg. 1991;18(2):391–7.
3. Cohen MM Jr, Kreiborg S. Hands and feet in the Apert syndrome. Am J Med Genet. 1995;57(1):82–96.
4. Kim JS, Block LM, Zhu X, Davit AJ. Management of Paronychia in patients with Apert syndrome. Tech Hand Up Extrem Surg. 2020;25(1):30–4.
5. Upton J. Apert syndrome. Classification and pathologic anatomy of limb anomalies. Clin Plast Surg. 1991;18(2):321–55.
6. Collins ED, Marsh JL, Vannier MW, Gilula LA. Spatial dysmorphology of the foot in Apert syndrome: three-dimensional computed tomography. Cleft Palate Craniofac J. 1995;32(3):255–61; discussion 62.
7. Anderson PJ, Hall CM, Evans RD, Hayward RD, Jones BM. The feet in Apert's syndrome. J Pediatr Orthop. 1999;19(4):504–7.
8. Grayhack JJ, Wedge JH. Anatomy and management of the leg and foot in Apert syndrome. Clin Plast Surg. 1991;18(2):399–405.
9. Fearon JA. Treatment of the hands and feet in Apert syndrome: an evolution in management. Plast Reconstr Surg. 2003;112(1):1–12; discussion 3–9.
10. Stauffer A, Farr S. Is the Apert foot an overlooked aspect of this rare genetic disease? Clinical findings and treatment options for foot deformities in Apert syndrome. BMC Musculoskelet Disord. 2020;21(1):788.
11. Calis M, Oznur A, Ekin O, Vargel I. Correction of Brachymetatarsia and medial angulation of the great toe of Apert foot by distraction osteogenesis: a review of 7 years of experience. J Pediatr Orthop. 2016;36(6):582–8.
12. Soldado F, Prieto-Mere JA, Cherqaoui A, Diaz Gallardo P, Knorr J, Corona P. Plantar intermetatarsal perforator flap for first web skin-graftless syndactyly release: anatomical study and clinical application. Microsurgery. 2024;44(2):e31151.
13. Casula I, Guero S. Helal metatarsal osteotomy in Apert foot. J Pediatr Orthop. 2021;41(1):56–60.
14. Helal B. Metatarsal osteotomy for metatarsalgia. J Bone Joint Surg Br. 1975;57(2):187–92.

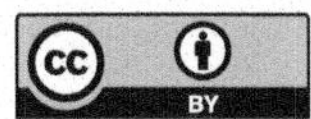

Part III

Patient, Family, and Community

33 Neurocognitive Implications, Etiological Mechanisms, and Clinical Care Recommendations

Annette C. Da Costa and Kathleen A. Kapp-Simon

Introduction

Apert syndrome is a rare craniosynostosis syndrome, with incidence estimates ranging from 1:50,000 [1] to 1:160,000 [2] live births. Autosomal dominant inheritance is the primary mode of transmission due to a mutation in fibroblast growth factor receptor 2 gene (FGFR2), although most cases are sporadic mutations. Apert syndrome is phenotypically characterized by bicoronal craniosynostosis, facial dysmorphology (particularly high prominent forehead, mid-facial hypoplasia, hypertelorism, and proptosis), hand and foot syndactyly, and vision and hearing deficits. Developmentally, Apert syndrome is associated with a high incidence of neurocognitive and language impairment [3–7].

This chapter examines the neurocognitive sequelae of Apert syndrome. We begin by reviewing the current scientific literature on neurocognitive functioning and adaptive behavior in individuals with Apert syndrome. Then, we discuss hypothesized etiological mechanisms underlying their neurocognitive development. Finally, we present a template for clinical management and future research protocols investigating the cognitive and behavioral development in individuals with Apert syndrome.

Neurocognitive Functioning in Apert Syndrome

Historically, Apert syndrome has been regarded as synonymous with intellectual disability (Magnan and Galippe, 1892 [8] cited by Renier et al. [9]). Standardized assessment of cognitive ability, however, was rare in early literature, with objective data on intellectual functioning reported on only 58 children before 1990 [10–13]. Most early data on cognitive functioning were derived from case studies and anecdotal evidence [14–16]. Intellectual disability is a major feature in most of those reports. In those early years, parents of children with Apert syndrome were counseled that their child was likely to have severe intellectual impairment and that institutional care would be the best course of action [17]. In contrast to most of the early writing on Apert syndrome, recent research, employing more empirically based assessment methods, suggests more variability in cognitive and functional outcomes for individuals with Apert syndrome. That is, while individuals with Apert syndrome may be at increased risk for intellec-

A. C. Da Costa (✉)
The Royal Children's Hospital, Melbourne, VIC, Australia

Murdoch Children's Research Institute, Melbourne, VIC, Australia
e-mail: annette.dacosta@rch.org.au

K. A. Kapp-Simon
Shriner's Children's Hospital Chicago, Chicago, IL, USA

University of Illinois at Chicago, Chicago, IL, USA

J. G. Meara et al. (eds.), *Apert Syndrome*, https://doi.org/10.1007/978-3-032-12551-4_33

tual disability, there is considerable evidence that many do not have intellectual disability and lead independent lives [6, 18, 19].

Defining Intellectual Developmental Disorder

Intellectual ability is broadly defined as encompassing skills in reasoning, problem-solving, planning, abstract thinking, judgment, and academic and experiential learning. Deficits in cognitive function often lead to impairments in adaptive functioning, such as personal care, social communication, academic progress, employment, and independence in domestic duties and financial management tasks.

The Diagnostic and Statistical Manual of Mental Disorders, Fifth Edition, Text Revision (DSM-5 TR) [20] defines intellectual developmental disorder (IDD) as the following:

> The essential features of intellectual developmental disorder (intellectual disability) are deficits in general mental abilities (Criterion A) and impairment in everyday adaptive functioning in comparison to an individual's age-, gender-, and socioculturally matched peers (Criterion B). Onset is during the developmental period (Criterion C). The diagnosis of intellectual developmental disorder is based on both clinical assessment and standardized testing of intellectual functions, standardized neuropsychological tests, and standardized tests of adaptive functioning. (Pg. 38)

Thus, the presence of significant intellectual and adaptive functioning deficits is required to meet criteria for intellectual developmental disorder (IDD). Further, the diagnosis must be based on both clinical assessment and standardized testing of *each of these* domains of functioning, with IDD defined as a score approximately two standard deviations (SD) below the mean.

The most widely accepted measures of intelligence are the Wechsler Intelligence Scales, which provide age-standardized evaluation of intellectual functioning from early childhood to adulthood (2:6 years to 90:11 years). The Bayley Scales of Infant and Toddler Development [21] have been used most frequently to assess development and currently allow for the assessment of children from 16 days of age to 42 months. The Vineland Adaptive Behavior Scale [22] is a well-validated tool for evaluating adaptive living skills and is utilized in the diagnosis of IDD.

For most currently administered intelligence and adaptive behavior tests, with a mean (M) of 100 and a standard deviation (SD) of 15, a score below 70 is consistent with IDD, although diagnoses are ultimately made based on clinical judgment. In the literature reviewed for this chapter, scores for intellectual ability are typically reported as a developmental quotient (DQ) for children under 3 years of age and as an intelligence quotient (IQ) for older children, while adaptive behavior scores are reported as a general or adaptive behavior composite (GAC).

IDD Severity Classification

In the DSM-5-TR [20], IDD is classified into four severity levels, determined primarily by the degree of independence achieved. Deficient adaptive behavior is generally defined as a score of less than 70 on measures of global adaptive functioning or in one of the areas of conceptual, social, or practical skills [23]. Table 33.1 summarizes IDD severity by its effects on cognition, education, social engagement, practical skills, and employment.

Intellectual Ability in Individuals with Apert Syndrome

For this chapter, we searched Pub Med, Psych Info, and Google Scholar databases for eligible studies using a combination of the search terms Apert syndrome with keywords of intelligence, mental development, cognition and neurodevelopment, repeated with acrocephalosyndactyly as a broader inclusive term to encompass Apert syndrome. Primary inclusion criteria were that objective cognitive assessment data were provided and that such data could be sub-classified according to intellectual level. From this search, 17 published studies met inclusion criteria. Unpublished data on 25 individuals with Apert

Table 33.1 Severity levels for intellectual developmental disorder

	Mild (GAC 50–69)	Moderate (GAC 35–49)	Severe (GAC 20–34)	Profound (GAC ≤ 19)
Cognitive	Weaknesses in reasoning, problem-solving, abstract thinking, planning, and functional use of academic skills	Markedly weak language development, problem solving and conceptual skills	Limited attainment of conceptual skills including written, language, money, numbers, and time management	May learn simple matching and sorting skills. Limited or no understanding of symbolic processes
Educational	Slow mastery of academic skills. Requires specialist classroom or classroom aide	Impaired acquisition of academic skills, with limited ability to apply independently. Specialized classroom required	Unlikely to acquire academic skills. Specialized classroom prioritizing activities of daily living and personal safety	Unlikely to acquire academic skills. Specialized classroom focused on ADLs
Social	Immature social skills and social judgement. Possible emotional lability and gullibility	Generally, uses spoken language; has capacity to form close family relationships and potential friendships. Significant difficulty with social judgement and interpretation of social cues	Language limited to single words or phrases. Can establish relationships with family and close acquaintances	Limited understanding of speech and gesture. Primarily communicates nonverbally. Responds to known individuals
Practical	May manage personal care. Support may be needed for other ADLs.[a] Individuals typically need assistance with important decisions and raising children	Can learn personal care with repetition and reminders, but requires supervision for most ADLs[a]	Requires close supervision for all ADLs[a]	Dependent on others for all ADLs including dressing, eating, elimination, health, safety. May enjoy music, watching TV, or being outside. Often have concomitant physical impairments that limit activities
Employment	Low-level qualification roles	Jobs with limited conceptual and communication skills	Sheltered workshop with close supervision	For some, sheltered workshop with close supervision

[a]*ADL* Activities of daily living: Personal care, domestic duties, community integration and financial management

syndrome obtained from one of the authors [24] were also included. Taken together, a total of 403 individuals with Apert syndrome were identified. Of this number, however, there was likely overlap of participants in studies conducted by the same group of researchers. Specifically, Sarimski [4] stated that all of their sample of 25 subjects were recruited from their sample of 41 participants in their previously published study [3]. Subjects in the Fernandes et al. [25] and Maximino et al. [7] studies overlap with those of Yacubian-Fernandes et al.'s [26] sample based on the descriptive and DQ/IQ data reported. The subjects from Renier et al. [9] and Lejeunie et al. [1] came from the same center and likely overlap. Our overall estimate of final sample size is 324 unique individuals from 14 studies [1, 3, 5, 6, 10–13, 18, 24, 27–30].

Eleven of the fourteen studies provided information about the ratio of potential to enrolled subjects. Based on their reports, individuals with DQ/IQ data represented approximately 67% of potential subjects. Primary exclusion criteria of these studies were lack of available DQ/IQ data, declined study participation, loss to follow-up, and/ or failure to meet other designated study criteria.

The 14 studies with probable unique individuals included sample sizes from 3 to 97 participants, with over a third having ten or fewer individuals. Participant ages ranged from infancy to 37 years old. With the exception of Fearon and Podner [6], all studies employed standardized measures of intellectual functioning to obtain DQ/IQ scores. Fearon and Podner [6] employed a quasi-experimental methodological approach for classification, whereby information from behavioral observation, parental feedback, school performance, and available standardized test data were utilized to determine intellectual level. They stratified their study data into categories of "normal" to mild delay (32%), moderate delay (43%), and profound delay (22%). However, they did not define these terms, making each category's characteristics unclear. For the purposes of this review, we classified individuals categorized as having moderate or profound delay in the IDD range.

From the available literature, it is challenging to precisely define the intellectual attributes of individuals with Apert syndrome. Although all studies with standardized DQ/IQ data provided some classification information, the categorization systems applied have varied. In addition, the most recent diagnostic systems, the DSM-5-TR [20] and the International Classification of Diseases-10th revision (ICD-10) [31] do not provide boundaries for intellectual functioning. Therefore, to compare the available IQ data, we utilized the classification system of the Diagnostic and Statistical Manual of Mental Disorders, Fourth Edition, Text Revision (DSM-IV-TR) [32] which has been historically used in most systems for categorizing levels of intellectual functioning.

Following the DSM-IV-TR [32] convention, we classified intellectual data into the broad ranges of IDD (DQ/IQ < 70), Borderline (DQ/IQ 70–84), and Average (DQ/IQ ≥ 85) (Table 33.2). We could stratify full subject data for 8 of the 14 studies [1, 3, 5, 10, 11, 24, 26, 30] into these intellectual sub-categories. The remaining six studies [6, 11–13, 18, 29] provided data in one or two of the sub-categories, but not all three. Hence, two studies provided information only on individuals who achieved average scores (DQ/IQ ≥ 85) [12, 29] and three provided sufficient information to classify individuals who were intellectually impaired (IQ < 70) [6, 13, 18]. From the final study by Noetzel et al. [11], we were able to correctly categorize two of the three subjects in the intellectually impaired level. Table 33.2 details the sample characteristics by intellectual category from each study.

Using the DSM-IV-TR [32] classification system, 12 of the 14 studies with a total of 293 participants provided sufficient information to categorize scores in the IDD range (DQ/IQ < 70 or, in the case of Fearon & Podner [6], moderate-to-profound delay). Of these 293 individuals, 52.6% (154/293) had global scores in the IDD range [1, 3, 5, 6, 10, 11, 13, 18, 24, 26, 28, 30]. Nine of the fourteen studies, comprising 139 participants, provided sufficient detail on intellectual level to identify individuals with scores in the Borderline range (DQ/IQ 70–84), with 33.8% (47/139) meeting this criterion [1, 3, 5, 10, 11, 24, 26, 28, 30]. Eleven of the fourteen studies, comprising a total of 170 participants, provided sufficient information for classification of subjects within the average range (DQ/IQ ≥ 85) with 22.4% (38/170) fulfilling this criterion [1, 3, 5, 10–12, 24, 26, 28–30].

Neuropsychological Findings

Few studies have examined neuropsychological outcomes in individuals with Apert syndrome beyond DQ/IQ scores. This lack of available data is critical, since neuropsychological issues related to specific cognitive processes, such as attention and executive functioning, auditory and visual processing (including short-term and working memory), long-term memory, and higher-order verbal and nonverbal reasoning skills, are important for an individual's functioning and adjustment.

We identified seven studies that provided objective information about neuropsychological

Table 33.2 Distribution of developmental and/or intellectual quotients (DQ/IQ) for individuals with Apert syndrome

Authors	*n*	Age range (Yrs.)	DQ/IQ range*			M (SD)
Papers with likely unique subjects			**< 70** ***n* (%)**	**70–84** ***n* (%)**	**≥ 85** ***n* (%)**	
Freeman & Borkowf [10]	3	NR	2 (67)	0 (0)	1 (33)	74.3 (12.7)
Noetzel et al. [11][a]	2	NR	0 (0)	1 (33)	1 (33)	NR
Lefebvre et al. [12]	25	0.08–15	NR	NR	2 (8)	63 (NR)
Patton et al. [13]	29	8–35	15 (52)	NR	NR	NR
Sarimski [3][b]	41	0.1 to >6	16 (39)	16 (39)	9 (22)	NR
Lajeunie et al. [1][c]	24	NR	15 (63)	5 (21)	4 (17)	64 (22.7)
Shipster et al. [5][d]	7 [10]	5-6 [5–6]	0 (0) [2 (20)]	1 (14) [1 (10)]	6 (86) [7 (70)]	94 (11.7) [85 (19.0)]
Yacubian-Fernandes et al. [27][e]	18	1–27	4 (22)	11 (61)	3 (17)	74 (16.1)
Da Costa et al. [28]	3	7–16	1 (33)	1 (33)	1 (33)	70 (25.1)
Fearon & Podner [6][f]	97	NR	65 (67)	NR	NR	NR
Maliepaard et al. [29]	6	6–13	NR	NR	2 (33)	77 (13.3)
David et al. [18]	28	6–10	16 (57)	NR	NR	NR
Tomita et al. [30][g]	13	5–7	3 (23)	7 (54)	3 (23)	79 (14.0)
Kapp-Simon [24]	25	1–16, 37	15 (60)	5 (20)	5 (20)	65 (17.6)
Totals	**324**	**0.1–37**	**154/293[h]** **(52.6)**	**47/139[h]** **(33.8)**	**38/170[h]** **(22.4)**	
Papers with likely duplication of subjects						
Renier et al. [9][c]	38	3–28	26 (68)	NR	NR	62 (NR)
Sarimski [4][b]	25	5–17	8 (32)	11 (44)	6 (24)	NR
Fernandes et al. [25][e]	8	7–26	2 (25)	4 (50)	2 (25)	76 (17.4)
Maximino et al. [7][e]	8	12–26	2 (25)	5 (62.5)	1 (12.5)	74 (16.3)
Totals for all subjects	**403**	**0.1–37**	**192/372[h]** **(51.6)**	**67/180[h]** **(37.2)**	**47/211[h]** **(22.3)**	

Abbreviations: *Yrs.* years, *M* mean, *SD* standard deviation, *NR* Not reported

*Note: All studies did not report number of individuals who fit each IQ classification. Sometimes different classifications were used, classifications were combined (borderline/mild/normal), or subjects fitting only one of the categories were identified (e.g., children with significant intellectual disability)

[a]Authors reported scores as average (90–109) $n = 1$; low average (80–89) $n = 1$; borderline (70–79) $n = 1$; intellectual disability (≤69) $n = 0$; only the average and borderline scores are included here

[b]Some overlap of subjects. Classifications based on parent ratings, which were found to be reliably correlated with the 16 children for whom objective data was available (reported in Sarimski [3])

[c]Possible overlap of subjects as they came from the same Center

[d]Three of ten children were unable to complete the cognitive assessment. Two of the three had receptive and expressive language scores <70; the third had receptive language = 86 and expressive language = 60. Nonverbal Quotient was not significantly different from General Cognitive Ability score. Numbers in parentheses represent stratification using receptive language scores for 3 children without a DQ/IQ score

[e]All subjects in the Maximino et al. [7] and Fernandes et al. [25] samples are also included in Yacubian-Fernandes study sample [27]

[f]Information on psychological testing was not presented. Authors state: "All patients were categorized according to their developmental level based on a compilation of metrics, including observation, parental feedback, testing scores, and school level and performance" (Pg. 133). Subjects were stratified into three levels of development: level A, 32% (normal to mild delay), level B, 43% (moderate delay), and level C 22% (profound delay). Mild, moderate and profound delay were not defined. Estimate is based on those classified as moderate to profound delay

[g]This is a longitudinal study. The scores from the last assessment are used in this table

[h]The denominator for these calculations is the total number of subjects in the studies that included the corresponding category of intellectual development

functioning in Apert syndrome beyond global DQ/IQ scores, albeit with limited sample sizes. Da Costa et al. [33] described broader neuropsychological function in two children with Apert syndrome. The studies by Shipster et al. [5] and Maximino et al. [7] provided information on cognition and language development. Attentional regulation was addressed in the studies of Sarimski [4], Shipster et al. [5] and Fearon and Podner [6]. Finally, Hilton [34] examined academic attainment, specifically mathematical ability.

Da Costa et al. [33] provided neuropsychological data on two children with differing cognitive profiles. One child (aged 7 years) presented with a history of global developmental delay and met criteria for moderate IDD based on performance on standardized measures of nonverbal intelligence (Leiter-R, selected due to the child's predominant nonverbal status) and adaptive functioning (Vineland Adaptive Behavior Scales). This child could follow simple, rote commands; however, communication occurred primarily through facial expression and gesture. This child also showed impairments in gross motor development (delayed walking with poor coordination), fine motor delays secondary to hand syndactyly, and significant impairment in personal, domestic, and community living skills.

The second individual was a 14-year-old male of average intellectual ability (Full Scale IQ = 94 on the age-standardized version of the Wechsler Intelligence Scales). This child attended a mainstream educational program with the support of an integration aide, partly to address behavioral challenges impacting interactions with teachers and peers. Although the individual's overall intelligence was within the average range, comprehensive neuropsychological testing identified several areas of specific cognitive and behavioral concern. Specifically, the child's ability to process information was slower than average, due to a combination of slowed eye-hand coordination and mental processing speed. While academic, language, and memory skills were generally intact, the child had significant difficulty with tasks related to executive functioning. This included impairments in cognitive regulation, such as attention, working memory, planning, and organizational skills, and difficulties with behavioral regulation, including inhibitory control. Da Costa concluded that the profile of cognitive and behavioral deficits seen for this child was consistent with dysfunction of anterior brain regions.

Two papers have addressed both cognitive function and language skills in individuals with Apert syndrome [5, 7]. In their sample of ten children with Apert syndrome aged 4:11 to 5:11 years, Shipster et al. [5] used the British Abilities Scales II (BAS) [35] to assess General Cognitive Abilities (GCA) and Nonverbal Functioning (NVF), and the Clinical Evaluation of Language Fundamentals-PreSchool (CELF) [36] and parental interview using the Preschool Language Scale-3 (PLS-3) [37] to assess language skills. Scores were not obtained for three children on the BAS GCA, two on the BAS NVS, four on the CELF receptive and expressive scales, and five on the PLS-3 expressive scale. The authors reported that these missing scores occurred because the children lacked the language ability and/or attentional skills required for task completion. For children able to complete the test, average [standard score (SS) $\geq$ 85] GCA scores were obtained for six of seven children and average NVF scores were obtained for all eight children. In contrast, expressive language was assessed to be significantly impaired in eight of ten children (all 8 received expressive SS $\leq$ 71 on the CELF or PLS-3). Five of ten children obtained receptive language scores in the average range ($\geq$ 85). Overall, 80% of the sample met criteria for severe language impairment (SS $\leq$ 71) for either expressive only (40%), or both expressive and receptive (40%) ability.

Maximino et al. [7] reported on intelligence (IQ) scores, behavioral observations of language, objective measures of vocabulary and receptive language, and school achievement data on eight individuals aged 12–26 years. One individual exhibited an IQ in the average range (SS = 104) as well as reportedly well-developed receptive and expressive language abilities and high school performance (school achievement categories were listed as low, medium, and high without clarification of the level of performance indicated by each term). Based on a combination of objective testing and observational data, five of the seven individuals with IQ scores ≤85 showed deficits in expressive vocabulary development. Language comprehension was generally stronger, with four of seven individuals demonstrating abilities within normal limits. Regarding academic skills, all seven subjects with IQs ≤ 85 were reported to obtain scores within the low range for reading, arithmetic, and writing.

An increased incidence of attention problems in children with Apert syndrome has been identified from parental report, based on standardized questionnaires [4, 29]. Sarimski [4] reported that 40% (n = 25) of their school-aged sample scored above the 95th percentile for attentional problems on the parent-reported Child Behavior Checklist [38]. Using the same measure, Maliepaard et al. [29] reported a mean T-score above the 95th percentile (M = 67.7, SD = 11.6) for attention problems in six of six individuals with Apert syndrome. Follow-up of these six individuals using the Diagnostic Interview Schedule for Children revealed that most met criteria for attention-deficit/hyperactivity disorder (ADHD), Predominantly Inattentive Type. Shipster et al. [5] used a non-standardized descriptive observational measure to rate attention in ten children aged 4- to 6-years, and reported that nine of their sample exhibited significant attention problems during the assessment process. Fearon and Podner [6] noted that "many" of the children in their sample were diagnosed with ADHD.

Hilton [34] assessed auditory short-term and working memory capacity (digit recall forward and backwards) and visual–spatial immediate memory span (block recall) in ten children aged 4 to 11 years. Using digits backwards as a proxy for cognitive development [39], overall six of the ten children either could not complete the task (3 of 6) or received a SS ≤ 85 (3 of the 6). The remaining four children obtained a SS >100. Rote memory and visuospatial memory (70% with SS >100) were better developed. Sarimski [40] reported memory challenges in five of nine children between the ages of 2:5 and 12:3 years of age based on performance on the Memory Scale of the McCarthy Scales of Children's Abilities [41], the Number Recall subtest of the Wechsler Intelligence Scales [42], or the Sequential Abilities scale of the Kaufman Assessment Battery for Children [43].

Academic difficulties, particularly in mathematics, have been reported in Apert syndrome samples. Fearon and Podner [6] noted a particular weakness in mathematics skills in their sample, while Sarimski [40] identified significant impairments in mathematics in four of nine children aged 2–12 years. Hilton [34] provided the first longitudinal study of math-related skills in ten children, aged 4–11 years. A case study approach was employed to assess auditory and visual–spatial short-term and working memory capacity, the development of finger gnosis, and arithmetic skills. Regarding math performance, mathematical reasoning (M = 81.7, SD = 16.2) and numerical operations (M = 79.6, SD = 18.5) were assessed. Overall, 40% (4/10) of the children were significantly delayed (SS < 70) in one of the two areas (20%) or both areas (20%). Four other children had scores that were deemed low enough to put them at risk of math failure (SS between 70 and 85). The author made the point that finger counting is an important correlate of later verbal counting and arithmetic understanding, but that children with Apert syndrome do not generally use this strategy spontaneously, likely due to delayed development of finger gnosis. Thus, it was recommended that specific instruction in strategies to develop finger gnosis, finger counting, and fine motor skills be incorporated into the education plan for young children with Apert syndrome as soon as possible after syndactyly release.

Adaptive Behavior

Data specific to adaptive functioning for individuals with Apert syndrome is limited. With the exception of the child with IDD in Da Costa et al.'s [33] case study, none of the studies characterizing IQ/DQ offer standardized data on adaptive behavior for individuals with Apert syndrome. Fearon and Podner's [6] categories, while not standardized, did seem to consider adaptive functioning. Their ratings were based on parental feedback, observations of independent functioning, academic progress reports, and, where available, standardized test results. Using these criteria, they estimated that 65 of 97 (67%) individuals were characterized as having moderate-to-profound delays.

Four other studies provided insights into adaptive functioning, focusing on education, employment, and independence [13, 18, 19, 44] (Table 33.3). Together, outcomes for 89 individuals were reported, with the majority (n = 75) being adults (age ≥ 18 years). These 89 individuals represented about 54% of the 166 subjects who met criteria for inclusion in the four studies; exclusion criteria were not consistently defined, although descriptions included participants who had inconsistent treatment or incomplete treatment protocols, lost to follow-up, or deceased. Thus, the sample data provided may represent a bias towards those with sufficient family support to complete treatment, those satisfied with the treatment protocols of a particular center, or other unexplained factors.

Information about educational placement was available for 68.5% (61/89) of the individuals with Apert syndrome across these four studies (Table 33.3). Of these, approximately 41% (25/61) had attended a mainstream school setting with some type of support services in place (e.g., an education aide or pull-out services for one or more academic areas). More than half of the individuals (33/61) were educated within a special education classroom. Of the three remaining individuals, two did not attend school, and the other did not complete their eighth grade year.

Eighty-three percent (74/89) of the individuals were at least 18 years of age at the time of study, offering some insight on adult educational and employment outcomes (Table 33.3) [13, 18, 19, 44]. Among these, 70.3% (52/74) completed 12 years of schooling, either with or without a completion degree. Of the 52 who had completed 12 years of schooling, 51.9% (27/52) had gone on for post-high-school vocational or college education. Forty-two percent (31/74) were gainfully employed in mainstream jobs; 5% (4/74) worked in sheltered workshops; and 20% (15/74) had no gainful employment (Table 33.3).

Limited information was available regarding psychological well-being, social relationships, and adult independence in the studies reviewed [13, 18, 19, 44]. In the studies where this was assessed, 55% (33/60) of participants self-reported satisfactory social relationships, while 35% (18/52) reported depressive symptoms. Most individuals were not involved in a relationship with a significant other (90%, 54/60). Only one study, by Tovetjärn and colleagues [19], reported on living arrangements, with 54% (13/24) of subjects living with their parents (Table 33.3).

Patton et al. [13] provided information on intellectual functioning, education, and employment status in their study sample. They found that 52% (15/29) met criteria for IDD and all 15 attended a special education setting (one at a School for the Deaf, the remaining in a school for children with IDD). Of the 48% (14/29) of individuals with an IQ > 70, 36% (5/14) were in a specialist school (one each for physical and visual disability and three in a school for children with IDD). The remaining nine individuals attended a mainstream classroom with support. Seven of the nine individuals attending a mainstream school were identified as "school leavers"; however, only three of the seven school leavers had passed any CSE (Certificate of Secondary Education) exams. Of the 14 individuals who were ≥ 18 years at the time of the study review, four were in full-time employment, two were in continuing education, and one worked in a sheltered workshop. The remaining seven had diagnoses of IDD. One of these had severe IDD and was residing in a psychiatric institution. No additional information was provided for the remaining six individuals with IDD.

Table 33.3 Education, employment, and psychological well-being in adults with Apert syndrome

	Patton et al. [13]	Allam et al. [44]	Tovetjärn et al. [19]	David et al. [18]	Total
Subject pool	N[a] (%)	N[a] (%)	N[a] (%)	N[a] (%)	N[a] (%)
Total Meeting Criteria for study	36 (100)	24 (100)	33 (100)	73 (100)	**166 (100)**
Deceased	4/36 (11.1)	0	5/33 (15.2)	3/73 (4.1)	**12/166 (7.2)**
Provided data	29/36 (80.5)	8 (33.3)	24/33 (72.7)	28/73 (38.4)	**89/166 (53.6)**
Mean age (range)	19.25 yrs (8, 10–36)	30.4 yrs (23–42)	29.5 yrs (19–50)	18.5 yrs (not reported)	**24.4 (8–49)**
Education setting: Total N[a]	**29 (100)**	**8 (100)**	**24 (100)**	**28 (100)**	**89 (100)**
Mainstream w Support	9/29 (31.0)	5/8 (62.5)	Unknown	11/28 (39.3)	**25/61 (41.0)**
Special Education	20/29 (69.0)	3/8 (37.5)	3/24 (12.5)	7/28 (25.0)	**33/61 (37.1)**
None or Elementary	0	0	1/24 (4.2)	2/28 (7.1)	**3/61 (4.9)**
No information about educational setting	0	0	20/24 (83.3)	8/28 (33.3)	**28/89 (31.5)**
Subjects > 18 years	**14 (48.3)**	**8 (100)**	**24 (100)**	**28 (100)**	**74 (83.1)**
High School Completed with or without degree	7/14 (50.0)	8/8 (100)	19/24 (79.2)	18/28 (64.3)	**52/74 (70.3)**
Vocational/College with or without degree	3/7 (42.9)	3/8 (12.5)	8/19 (42.1))	8/18 (28.6)	**22/52 (42.3)**
Schooling terminated due to IDD	7/14 (50.0)	0	1/24 (4.2)	2/28 (7.1)	**10/74(13.5)**
No Information	0	0	4/24 (16.7)	8/28 (28.6)	**12/74 (16.2)**
Employment					
Full Time Education	2/14 (14.3)	0	8/24 (33.3)	12/28 (42.9)	**22/74 (29.7)**
Employed	4/14 (28.6)	3/8 (37.5)	14/24 (58.3)	10/28 (41.7)	**31/74 (41.9)**
Unemployed	7/14 (50)	5/8 (62.5)	0	3/28 (12.5)	**15/74 (20.3)**
Sheltered Workshop	1/14 (7.1)	0	0	3/28 (12.5)	**4/74 (5.4)**
No Information	0	0	2 (8.3)	0	**2/74 (2.7)**
Psychological well-being		**8**	**24**	**28**	**60 (81.1)**
Friendship Group 2+	Not assessed	7 (87.5)	11 (45.8)	15 (53.6)	**33/60 (55.0)**
Isolated	Not assessed	1 (12.5)	5 (20.8)	6 (21.4)	**12/60 (20)**
Depression	Not assessed	Not assessed	17 (73.9)	1 (3.6)	**18/52 (34.6)**
No Information	14 (100)	0	8 (33.3)	7 (25.0)	**29/74 (39.2)**
Relationships		**8**	**24**	**28**	**60/74 (81.6)**
Married or partnered	Not assessed	2/8 (25)	1/24 (4.2)	2/24 (7.1)	**5/60 (8.3)**
Single	Not assessed	6/8 (75)	22/24 (91.6)	26/24 (92.9)	**54/60 (90.0)**
No information	14 (100)	0	1/24 (4.2)	0	**1/60 (1.7)**
Living arrangement			**24**		**24/74 (32.4)**
With Parents	Not assessed	Not assessed	13 (54.2)	Not assessed	**13/24 (54.2)**
Apartment	Not assessed	Not assessed	10 (41.7)	Not assessed	**10/24 (41.7)**
Care Center	Not assessed	Not assessed	1 (4.2)	Not assessed	**1/24 (4.2)**
No Information	14/14 (100)	8/8 (100)	0	28/28 (100)	**49/74 (66.2)**

[a]Denominators are based on total number of subjects with data in that category

Neurocognitive and Behavioral Concerns

Emotional, behavioral, attentional, and social problems have been reported with high frequency in individuals with Apert syndrome [5, 6, 12, 29, 45–47]. Two studies reported that these problems occurred with greater frequency in individuals with craniosynostosis, including Apert syndrome, with IQ scores <85 compared to those of average or higher IQ [29, 45]. This finding is not specific to Apert syndrome; in general, individuals with

IDD have higher incidences of comorbid ADHD and other emotional and behavioral disorders [48–51]. Children presenting with comorbid IDD and ADHD in the general population are also more likely to exhibit symptoms of externalizing problems including oppositional behaviors and conduct problems [52]. Given these findings, individuals with Apert syndrome who also present with a diagnosis of mild to borderline IDD should be carefully screened for behavioral and emotional problems, as these difficulties can meaningfully impact one's day-to-day functioning and quality of life.

Summary of Neurocognitive and Adaptive Functioning

From these findings, it is evident that a diagnosis of Apert syndrome is not necessarily synonymous with a diagnosis of IDD. In the reviewed studies, intellectual functioning in more than 20% of individuals with Apert syndrome fell within the average range (DQ/IQ > 85). Nonetheless, this review is consistent with other authors' conclusions that individuals with Apert syndrome are at increased risk of developing IDD, with an estimated 54% of individuals falling in the IDD range (DQ/IQ < 70) compared to 2.2% in normative population averages.

With few exceptions, cognitive impairment in Apert syndrome has been determined based on composite DQ/IQ scores. A limited number of studies have included information on more specialized cognitive processes, such as verbal and nonverbal reasoning, auditory and visual information processing skills, long-term memory, attention, and executive function. Most individuals with Apert syndrome were found to have deficits in one or more of these areas, even for individuals with average intellectual abilities.

An important consideration from these conclusions is the lack of available data on hearing loss related to neurodevelopment in Apert syndrome. There is considerable evidence of significant hearing impairment in individuals with Apert syndrome that persists into adulthood [19, 53–55]. None of the reviewed studies investigated the impact of hearing loss on cognitive, language, or adaptive functioning; however, Maximino et al. [7] excluded individuals with any hearing impairment (number excluded not reported), and Shipster et al. [5] acknowledged that all ten of the children in their study had ongoing mild-to-moderate hearing loss treated with grommets or hearing aids. The impact of hearing loss as an additional risk factor for deficits in neurocognitive development needs further investigation. At a minimum, hearing status at the time of evaluation as well as history of hearing loss should be reported when investigating neurocognitive outcomes in this high-risk population.

Similarly, the available studies do not investigate the impact of visual impairments on cognitive functioning of individuals with Apert syndrome. Visual impairments occur at a high rate in individuals with Apert syndrome, with de Jong et al. [55] reporting that 76% ($n = 29$) individuals presented with refractive errors and 93% presented with strabismus. The literature on cognitive functioning and strabismus in individuals without Apert syndrome suggests that perceptual reasoning, fine motor skills, and visual perceptual skills may be decreased [56, 57], though some studies report compensation as children age [58]. Strabismus has also been associated with atrophy of gray and white matter volume [59], potentially exacerbating developmental concerns. For these reasons, visual status should be considered when discussing neurocognitive outcomes for individuals with Apert syndrome.

Most available literature on adaptive functioning comes from four studies [13, 18, 19, 44]. These studies have focused primarily on adult outcomes in individuals who have been long-term participants in clinical care. Findings indicate that most individuals with Apert syndrome attend a formal educational program, with almost 60% completing 12 years of schooling, with or without a degree. Most individuals required specialized support either within the mainstream classroom or in a specialized classroom. Nearly a third of individuals went on to undertake vocational or post-secondary education (30%). Sixty percent of adult individuals no longer in school had attained independent employment. When assessed, most individuals were not in a romantic relationship, but more than half reported having a friendship group of at least two people.

There is limited information on the adaptive functioning of children and adolescents with Apert syndrome. For instance, the degree to which independent walking, dressing, and toileting are delayed in children with Apert syndrome remains unclear. Additionally, there is insufficient data on how children with Apert syndrome engage in social activities. While hand and foot syndactyly likely affect self-care independence given the impacts on motor functioning, research in this area is scarce. Hilton's [34] study highlighted the impact of hand syndactyly on the development of mathematical skills, but this represents only a single study. More comprehensive information is required to effectively educate parents and teachers on how to best support children with Apert syndrome in developing adaptive skills.

Slightly more than a third of the individuals in our review obtained IQ scores in the borderline range (IQ 70–84), more than double population estimates of 12–14%. We have kept this category in our review, even though it is not well-defined in current diagnostic systems, the DSM-5-TR [20] and the International Classification of Diseases-10th revision (ICD-10) [60], because individuals with borderline intellectual ability and related adaptive behavior difficulties may still need increased support. Even without a diagnosis of Apert syndrome, individuals in the borderline range for intellectual abilities are at greater risk of social, behavioral, and academic difficulties [61–64]. However, because borderline intellectual disability is not a distinct clinical diagnosis, support services in schools and society as a whole are limited. This lack of services may be related to increased difficulties for individuals with borderline intellectual functioning in adult functioning (e.g., housing, managing finances, drug abuse, legal problems, social isolation), compared to individuals without IDD [63]. Given this increased risk, individuals with both borderline intellectual functioning and Apert syndrome should be monitored closely by their healthcare providers to ensure that they are receiving necessary services, including educational support and mental health services when needed. Additionally, borderline intellectual functioning may not be recognized in some individuals with Apert syndrome. In that case, they may not receive the support they need to participate meaningfully in medical decision-making as they age.

Many of the older individuals included in this review were born and treated in the 1970s and 1980s. Newer treatment approaches and more aggressive educational interventions may help individuals achieve higher cognitive and educational levels. For example, Fearon and Podner [6] report that 67% of the individuals treated consistently in their Center from birth demonstrated typical development or only mild developmental delay. As such, ongoing research on long-term outcomes for individuals with Apert syndrome will be necessary to better understand the neurodevelopmental course in the context of medical intervention and to identify more specific areas of neurocognitive development that would benefit from support.

Predictors and Correlates of Neurocognitive Impairment in Apert Syndrome

The etiological mechanisms underlying the common neurocognitive impairments in Apert syndrome, with accompanying implications for adaptive living skills, educational and vocational outcomes, and psychosocial development, likely reflect a complex interplay of multiple factors. In the following sections, we address the primary predictive and correlative determinants of neurocognitive outcome in Apert syndrome identified from the empirical literature, specifically (1) expression of gene mutations, including implications for central nervous system (CNS) formation and development, (2) CNS growth disturbances, (3) treatment considerations, and (4) psychosocial and environmental factors. We also present the literature on the associations between neurocognitive function and these etiological risk factors.

Genetic Mutations and Central Nervous System Development

There is convincing evidence for the role of CNS development and maldevelopment secondary to the expression of gene mutations in Apert syndrome, with implications for neurocognitive function. Many craniosynostosis disorders originate in specific embryological processes, including brain patterning, fusion of the tissues in the face, and bone differentiation in the skull vault [65]. In Apert syndrome, one of two specific missense mutations of fibroblast growth factor receptor 2 gene (FGFR2) has been identified in most cases; referred to as S252W and P253R. FGFR2 expression affects the skeletal structure as well as the brain and has been implicated for its contribution to CNS development in humans and animals [66–68].

Regarding specific mechanisms, the FGFR2 gene interacts with the L1 cell adhesion molecule gene (L1CAM) gene. L1CAM plays a critical role in the development of the central nervous system, including regulation of axonal outgrowth, formation of the ventricular system, and myelination [69]. Disruptions caused by the L1CAM gene have been linked to maldevelopment of brain white matter structures [69, 70] and neurodevelopmental disorders [71]. White matter structures, such as the corpus callosum, are essential fibrous tracts that connect different brain regions and are pivotal in supporting cognitive, visual, motor, behavioral, and emotional functioning. White matter changes are among the most frequently occurring CNS anomalies in Apert syndrome. The role of the FGFR2 and L1CAM interaction accordingly plays a plausible role in the etiology of both the CNS anomalies and neurodevelopmental challenges in Apert syndrome.

Of the primary brain abnormalities in individuals with Apert syndrome, non-progressive ventriculomegaly occurs with the highest incidence [72–75]. The white matter malformations most commonly identified in Apert syndrome include corpus callosum agenesis, absence or hypoplasia of the septum pellucidum, and malformations of the cingulate gyrus [6, 72, 75–78]. Hippocampal hypoplasia or dysplasia is also reported [72, 79].

Neurocognitive Correlates of Gene Mutations in Apert Syndrome

Studies investigating the relationship between FGFR2 gene mutations and neurocognitive function are limited. Of those conducted, authors have speculated [1, 6, 25] that cognitive function may vary according to the specific FGFR2 mutation subtype. However, these authors have reached differing conclusions.

Lejeune et al. [1] reported on the cognitive profiles of 24 individuals with Apert syndrome, 15 with the S252W mutation and nine with the P253R mutation. They found that rates of intellectual impairment were significantly higher in those with the P253R mutation. In contrast, Fernandes et al. [25] reported that the one individual (out of 7) with the P253R mutation in their study was of average intelligence (IQ = 108), while the mean IQ of the six individuals with the S252W deletion fell within the range of intellectual disability (mean IQ = 67.2; range = 47–78). Finally, in their sample of 17 individuals with the S252W mutation and 16 with the P253R mutation, Fearon and Podner [6] found no significant differences in cognitive function according to mutation subtype.

Notably, these findings suggest wide cognitive variability in individuals with Apert syndrome with the FGFR2 mutation, with no conclusive evidence for those deemed at greater risk according to specific subtype. While this may in part be due to the small sample sizes, other etiological mechanisms should be considered in understanding the basis of the observed neurocognitive deficits in Apert syndrome. These include the presence and severity of brain anomalies, medical risk factors, and psychosocial variables. Future research addressing the interactional role of the FGFR2-L1CAM alongside cognitive data may be an important area of inquiry.

Neurocognitive Correlates of CNS Anomalies in Apert Syndrome

The cognitive implications of the frequently occurring CNS anomalies in Apert syndrome remain unclear. Few studies have presented combined cognitive and neuroimaging data. Of those available, the breadth of cognitive testing utilized has been restricted, and varied and inconclusive results are reported.

Murovic et al. [80] assessed intellectual functioning in 15 individuals with Apert syndrome who exhibited an average IQ in the range of borderline intelligence (IQ = 72.5). No correlation between IQ and ventricular size was identified. Renier et al. [9] found that individuals with septal defects were more likely to have an IQ below 70, falling significantly lower than those with a normal septum pellucidum. They identified no relationship between IQ scores and the presence of corpus callosum anomalies and ventriculomegaly. Additionally, the relationship in IQ scores between individuals with no brain malformation (50%) and those with at least one brain malformation (23%) was nonsignificant.

Yacubian-Fernandez et al. [26] reported a nonsignificant relationship between IQ scores and presence or absence of structural brain malformations (ventriculomegaly, malformations of the corpus callosum and/or the septum pellucidum, and arachnoid cysts), in their sample of 18 individuals with Apert syndrome. Brain structure was reported as normal for 8 of the 18 individuals, with IQ scores ranging from borderline to average (IQ ranged from 70 to 104). One individual with isolated hypoplasia of the corpus callosum had an IQ score of 85 (lower end of average); two individuals with isolated hypoplasia of the septum pellucidum presented with IQ scores in the IDD range (IQs = 47 and 56). The remaining seven individuals had two or more brain malformations, and IQ scores ranging from the IDD to average ranges (IQs ranged from 45 to 108).

Fearon and Podner [6] also reported no association between white matter deficits and cognition. However, developmental level was primarily determined through qualitative means (e.g., observation, parental feedback, and school level and performance).

The interpretative significance of study findings on brain malformations and cognitive development that has been reported is compromised by the small sample sizes available and the reliance upon global IQ as a marker of cognitive function. The influence of moderating variables, such as environmental and psychosocial vulnerabilities, should also be considered.

Based on currently available data, there is no clear evidence for a causal relationship between primary brain malformation and cognitive development in individuals with Apert syndrome. This may be in part due to the restricted range of cognitive measures employed in available studies. Evidence from other clinical populations, however, suggests a wide array of potential cognitive deficits in individuals with primary brain malformation. Broadly, researchers have identified associations between brain white matter integrity and cognitive development, such as attention, impulsivity, risk-taking, memory, and cognitive flexibility [81–83]. Regarding the common CNS anomalies in Apert syndrome, partial or complete agenesis of the corpus callosum has been associated with impairments in cognitive status, language, motor control, and coordination [84]. Isolated fetal ventriculomegaly has been associated with autism spectrum disorder traits, difficulties in sustained attention and working memory, and sensation-seeking behaviors [85]. Hydrocephalus has been identified to have long-term effects on white matter development and brain network connectivity, and cognitively, associated with deficits in nonverbal intelligence, attention, working memory, and broader executive function [86, 87]. Data on the cognitive correlates of septum pellucidum anomalies, however, appears inconclusive, with some authors citing increased cognitive risk [88] and others finding no relationship with cognitive, emotional, or behavioral problems [89].

Regarding future research, analyzing data from advanced neuroimaging techniques that permit evaluation of white matter integrity at the microstructural level, such as magnetic resonance imaging (MRI) with diffusion tensor imaging (DTI) sequencing, alongside comprehensive standardized neurocognitive assessment data, would help clarify the relationship between CNS function and neurocognition and behavior in individuals with Apert syndrome.

Timing of Onset of CNS Growth Disturbances: Theoretical Perspectives

Brain development is a protracted process in humans, commencing in the third gestational week and continuing into early adulthood [90]. Throughout this time, macrostructural and microstructural changes take place to reshape the brain's structural networks and optimize adaptability to manage sophisticated cognitive and functional demands. The most rapid brain growth occurs prenatally and is principally concerned with gross structural formation [91]. Postnatal development is primarily associated with elaboration of the CNS, involving rapid synaptogenesis, dendritic development, and myelination.

Both prenatal and postnatal development are characterized by expanding cortical connectivity, linked to increases in the number and size of cortical regions [92]. There is an increase in cortico-cortical connections, leading to the formation of distributed neural networks [93] which underpin the complexity of human behavior. In addition to CNS growth, throughout infancy and childhood, neurodevelopmental processes respond to genetic and environmental cues to create efficient networks that subserve motor, visual, behavioral, cognitive and emotional function [94]. This highlights the complex interaction between brain development, genetics, and environmental factors such as psychosocial status on neurodevelopmental outcomes in the general population and clinical samples.

Critical Periods in CNS Development

Intrinsic to the maturation of the CNS is the notion of critical or "sensitive" periods, which represent "windows of opportunity" that are important for the major progression and consolidation of key behavioral functions. These intervals are critical to the acquisition of subsequent skills and the establishment of interconnectivity with other systems. Critical periods occur at various times from the prenatal period to early adulthood. The brain is deemed at heightened vulnerability during these times, with disruption to rapidly developing neuronal networks impacting the final outcome of the CNS [95, 96]. Children who incur disturbances to brain development during the prenatal period or first year of life are deemed most vulnerable and show the most significant impairment [97, 98].

Structural Formation

Interruptions to brain development during the prenatal period, including via the mechanism of genetic aberration, is likely to have a significant impact upon cerebral development [90]. The high incidence and nature of white matter cortical malformations in Apert syndrome are consistent with brain structures commonly compromised by disturbances to brain development due to genetic aberration and other forms of prenatal disturbances to CNS development. This again highlights the primary role of the expression of gene mutations on white matter integrity and associated neurocognitive outcomes in individuals with Apert syndrome and other genetically determined craniosynostosis disorders.

Synostosis Progression

In addition to the nature of cerebral malformations, genetic mutations likely dictate the timing of onset of craniosynostosis and the progressive abnormal osseous growth patterns in Apert syndrome and other forms of syndromic craniosynostosis disorders. Skull and CNS growth are intricately related, with abnormal skull growth corresponding to significant implications for the developmental course of the maturing CNS. Brain growth compression in the sites of sutural fusion and abnormally redirected, compensatory growth to accommodate the rapidly growing brain can have implications at both the macro and microstructural level. Importantly, the pathophysiological mechanism of craniosynostosis occurs for an extended period of time pre and postnatally, which corresponds to a period of significant CNS development. From a timing perspective, this can disrupt the tightly defined, sequentially organized process of cerebral maturation, leading to deviant CNS formation patterns, with corresponding cognitive sequelae.

Timing of Surgical Intervention

Historically, the risk to the developing brain by the mechanisms of synostosis has dictated mainstay treatment protocols, with cranial vault reconstruction recommended to be performed no later than the first year of life [99] to mitigate the risk of brain compromise. Renier and colleagues [9, 99] provided the first data in support of early surgical correction to increase skull volume in Apert syndrome. They reported that infants who underwent the surgical procedure prior to 12 months of age were more likely to obtain an IQ score > 70 on standardized assessment after 3 years of age, compared with those who received an operation later in life. In contrast, other researchers have not found a relationship between age at surgery and neurocognitive outcomes for individuals with the syndrome [6, 26, 30, 40].

Intracranial Pressure

Raised intracranial pressure (ICP) occurs with significant frequency in syndromic craniosynostoses and occurs in as many as 83% of individuals with Apert syndrome if left untreated [100]. Causative mechanisms for elevated ICP vary and include abnormal intracranial venous drainage [101, 102], hydrocephalus [103, 104], and airway obstruction [100, 105]. While remaining a controversial area, authors have hypothesized a causal relationship between elevated ICP and neurocognitive function in craniosynostosis disorders, contending that the condition can exert significant stress on the brain, with consequent risk to cognitive function [103, 106, 107].

Regarding the known implications of these mechanisms of raised ICP, hydrocephalus, which occurs with incidence rates ranging from approximately 7–12% in Apert syndrome samples [9, 72, 74, 80, 100], is a likely contributor to neurocognitive dysfunction for some individuals with Apert syndrome. The neurocognitive risk has been demonstrated by evidence from other clinical populations showing a broadly typified pattern of cognitive impairments, particularly deficits in working memory, attention, and spatial abilities [86].

The premise that elevations in ICP is responsible for the common neurocognitive compromise in Apert syndrome has been difficult to support conclusively. In their review of the literature on the relationship between intracranial hypertension and cognitive and behavioral function in Apert syndrome, Doerga et al. [46] concluded that findings support the theory that the behavioral problems and lowered mental capabilities are inherent to the syndrome, and not a consequence of ICP. Based on the available evidence, it appears that other mechanisms, particularly genetic aberrations, may play a more significant role in the cognitive impairments in individuals with Apert syndrome.

Obstructive Sleep Apnea

Obstructive sleep apnea (OSA) is a complication of airway obstruction. It occurs with high frequency in individuals with Apert syndrome, with estimated occurrence rates ranging from 49.8 (n = 19) [108] to 80.6% (n = 31) [109] OSA has been associated with a consistent pattern of deficits in cognition, particularly in attention, episodic memory, and executive function [108, 110]. Bannink et al. [108] conducted the only known study addressing the relationship between OSA and behavioral function in Apert syndrome. From parental ratings on standardized questionnaires, they identified a significant association between severity of OSA and total problem behaviors in their sample. The implications of these findings are unclear. Evidence from other studies indicates some improvement in cognition following medical intervention for OSA [111, 112] which may suggest these impacts upon cognition are not necessarily permanent, nor a primary cause of neurocognitive impairment in Apert syndrome. Other comorbidities, such as CNS anomalies, appear to be a more plausible explanation. However, further research is needed to determine the extent to which OSA is a factor in both the nature and severity of cognitive impairments evident in children with Apert syndrome. Early cranial vault expansion may decrease the incidence of OSA in individuals with Apert syndrome [100].

Treatment Considerations

Surgical Intervention

The mainstay management of Apert syndrome typically involves a significant number of surgical interventions, with the rationale being primarily functional in nature. This includes mitigation or treatment of raised ICP, management of airway compromise, decreasing the risk of visual impairment (particularly exophthalmos), and correction of hand and foot syndactyly.

Particularly in Apert syndrome, treatment of craniosynostosis requires major cranial vault surgery, which involves manipulation of the cranium and its underlying contents. This procedure carries all the inherent risks of craniofacial and neurosurgical procedures. Typically, more than one such procedure is required [6, 9, 113]. For example, in their sample of 94 individuals with Apert syndrome, Breik et al. (2016) [113] reported that 130 transcranial procedures (e.g., bifronto-orbital advancement) were performed and 70% of the individuals underwent at least two such procedures.

Postoperative complications following cranial vault expansion surgery include development of cerebral spinal fluid leak, hindbrain herniation, and infection [6, 113, 114]. In their review of treatment for 135 individuals with Apert syndrome, Fearon and Podner [6] reported six infections from a total of 266 cranial vault remodeling procedures (2.3%) and six infections in 92 midface advancement procedures (6.5%), which required an additional operative procedure. Breik et al. [113] reported complications in 18% of 130 procedures with the most common being CSF leaks and acute hydrocephalus.

Anesthesia Risk

Research addressing the relationship between anesthesia exposure during infancy and early childhood and cognitive outcomes in later years has yielded inconsistent findings. There is limited evidence that exposure to anesthesia prior to 3 years of age (particularly multiple exposures) is associated with poorer cognitive and behavioral outcomes at later ages [115–118]. However, in their review, Ing and Bellinger [119] concluded that early anesthesia exposure increased the risk of attention problems, but not intelligence or academic achievement. Similarly, Pennings et al. [118] reported that prolonged prior exposure to anesthesia may affect cognitive skills related to executive functioning, such as selective attention, and mental speech and information processing speed in adults. The only research examining association of anesthesia exposure to later neurodevelopmental outcomes in children with craniosynostosis comes from the Infant and Child Learning Project, investigating impact of single suture craniosynostosis on neurodevelopment across the same group of children from infancy to early elementary school [120, 121]. At 3 years of age, the combination of longer surgeries and longer exposure to inhaled anesthesia was associated with poorer outcomes in cognition, language, and motor development. At 7 years of age, a relationship between cognition and both age at surgery and length of anesthesia exposure was identified. Infants who were younger at initial surgery and had shorter anesthesia exposure had better cognitive, language, memory, and achievement scores at the age of 7 years than those who were older at initial surgery and had longer anesthesia exposure. However, these results were confounded by family socioeconomic status (SES), in that infants who were older at the time of surgery tended to come from lower SES households.

Since SES is a known confound of neurodevelopment [122, 123], it may be that the lower neurodevelopmental scores were secondary to SES rather than either anesthesia exposure or age at surgery.

Psychosocial Factors

Researchers have identified the critical role of family support for improved psychosocial outcomes, including better cognitive development in children with Apert syndrome [9, 18, 27]. Renier et al. [9] reported that a supportive family environment, along with early cranial surgery and normal brain structure, was critical for typical cognitive development in individuals with Apert syndrome. Yacubian-Fernandez et al. [26] identified the family environment, including parental education, as the only factor associated with cognitive and behavioral outcomes. Interestingly, they did not find that cognitive development was related to the presence of brain malformation nor age at time of initial operation, as other authors have contended. Family status, particularly parental educational background and financial resources, has also consistently been associated with better cognitive outcomes in individuals with and without craniosynostosis [82, 122–125]. While craniofacial teams cannot plausibly change family SES, they can offer families information and support to minimize the stress on the family system and enhance families' capacity for providing a supportive environment [126].

Summary of Predictors and Correlates of Neurocognitive Impairment in Apert Syndrome

Individuals with Apert syndrome are at heightened risk of neurocognitive impairment, including IDD. The most robust evidence regarding etiological mechanisms underlying neurocognitive deficit in this condition relates to gene expressivity and its' role in central nervous system development. Other potential risk factors affecting neurocognitive outcome include the necessity for numerous surgical procedures and related risks (e.g., anesthesia exposure), raised ICP, the timing of CNS growth disturbances due to genetic aberration upon the course of cerebral development, and psychosocial and environmental influences.

A dominant theme from our review of literature concerning the relationship between etiological mechanisms and neurocognitive function in Apert syndrome is the scarcity of available studies and inconsistency among their findings. Relatedly, many such studies have small sample sizes, which makes reliable statistical analysis difficult, and limits meaningful conclusions. An additional inherent problem has been the absence of systematic neuropsychological testing employing standardized measures.

Future Research Directions

There is an urgent need for high-quality research in Apert syndrome on the neurocognitive and adaptive behavior of individuals and etiological mechanisms for impairment. Many studies addressing the neurocognitive phenotype of Apert syndrome have employed aggregate measures, such as global IQ, to quantify neurocognitive outcome. It is essential, however, to evaluate specific cognitive skills, such as attention and memory, to understand the unique strengths and weaknesses of affected individuals and, accordingly, develop therapeutic interventions with specificity and precision. This is important since these skills, particularly later-maturing abilities such as attention and executive function, have a critical influence upon general adaptive living skills, education, vocational, and social outcomes.

We provide a template of recommended, well-validated measures of neurocognitive and adaptive behavioral function for both clinical management and research purposes in the assessment of individuals with Apert syndrome (see Table 33.4). Recommended tools include the Bayley Scales of Infant and Toddler Development [21] for the assessment of infant neurodevelopment. The Ages and Stages Questionnaire [127]

Table 33.4 Potential measures and timeline for standardized data collection for research

Professional assessment	What is assessed	Suggested age of administration for research
Bayley-4 [21]	Cognition, motor, language, socio-emotional, and adaptive behavior	Before cranial surgery, 12–18 months after surgery If no cranial surgery, 1 and 3 yrs
WPPSI-IV [129]	Verbal comprehension, fluid reasoning, visual-spatial processing, working memory, and processing speed	Age 5 ± 1 yr
WISC-V [130]	Verbal comprehension, fluid reasoning, visual-spatial processing, working memory, and processing speed	Age 8 ± 1 yr
WAIS-V [134]	Verbal comprehension, fluid reasoning, visual-spatial processing, working memory, and processing speed	At least once after age 16
WIAT-4 [138]	Measures academic skills in reading, writing, speaking, listening, and math	5, 8, 12 and once after 16 yrs
D-KEFS [136]	Measures visual-motor sequencing, verbal fluency, design fluency, ability to inhibit responses, concept formation and problem solving, ability to formulate questions, verbal reasoning	8 and 12 yrs
Parent / Caregiver Measures		
Vineland-3 [22]	Measures adaptive skills in communication, daily living skills, socialization, and motor skills	1, 2, 3, 8, 12, 16 yrs; At least once in the 20s, 30s, 40s*
ASEBA [38]	*Internalizing problems:* Anxiety, Depression, Somatic; *Externalizing problems:* Rule-breaking, Aggression; *Social, thought, attention problems;* *DSM-Related Scales* Affective, anxiety, somatic, ADHD, oppositional defiant, conduct problems	18 mos, 3 yrs, 5, 8, 12, 17 yrs At least once in the 20s, 30s 40s*
BRIEF-2 [137]	Measures executive functioning: Inhibit, self-monitor, shift, emotional control, working memory, and organization of materials	5, 8, and 12 yrs
CCC-2 [139]	Measures language development (vocabulary, comprehension); pragmatic communication skills; and structural language problems	5, 8, and 12 yrs

Bayley-4: Bayley Scales of Infant and Toddler Development, Fourth Edition [21]; WPPSI-IV: Wechsler Preschool and Primary Scale of Intelligence- 4th Edition [129]; WISC-V: Wechsler Intelligence Scale for Children-Fifth Edition [130]; WAIS-V: Wechsler Adult Intelligence Scale-Fifth Edition [134]; WIAT-4: Wechsler Individual Achievement Test-Fourth Edition [138]; D-KEFS: Delis-Kaplan Executive Function System [136]; Vineland-3: Vineland Adaptive Behavior Scales-Third Edition [22]; The Achenbach System of Empirically Based Assessment (ASEBA) [38]; BRIEF-2: Behavior Rating Inventory of Executive Function-Second Edition [137]; CCC-2: Children's Communication Checklist-2 [139]

*Unless individual with Apert syndrome is under guardianship of another responsible adult, completion requires consent of individual with Apert syndrome

serves as a helpful clinical screening tool for assessing infant and early childhood development; however, it is more effective at detecting severe delay than mild or moderate delay [128] and thus may not achieve sensitivities required for clinical epidemiological research purposes. The Wechsler Intelligence Scales [42, 129–134] are the gold-standard, widely employed measure of intellectual function, applicable from age 2:6 years to late adulthood. In cases where individuals exhibit substantial cognitive impairment, the Leiter International Performance Scale [135], which employs nonverbal assessment methods, may be used as an alternative to the Wechsler

Intelligence Scales. The Delis-Kaplan Executive Function System [136] and Behavior Rating Inventory of Executive Function [137] provide measures of executive function. The Vineland Adaptive Behavior Scales [22] provide comprehensive information about adaptive level.

Regarding the etiology of neurocognitive impairment in Apert syndrome, future research should integrate genetic testing and neuroimaging data to determine the impact of genetic and neurobiological markers upon neurocognition. The role of the FGFR2-L1CAM interaction on neurodevelopment is an important line of further research inquiry in this regard. Early studies examining the relationship between central nervous system development and neurocognition in Apert syndrome have predominantly employed gross structural neuroanatomical measures. Advancements in neuroimaging techniques, including diffusion tensor imaging (DTI), now offer detailed insights into anatomical structure, as well as brain connectivity at the microstructural level. This enables examination of the relationship between CNS integrity and neurocognitive variables with greater depth and precision than conventional imaging techniques alone. The role of moderating risk variables, such as medical and psychosocial factors, should also be examined in conjunction with neurocognitive, genetic, and neuroimaging data.

Given the rarity of Apert syndrome, establishing craniofacial team consortiums to systematically collect relevant genetic, neuroanatomical, neurocognitive, and adaptive behavioral data following a unified protocol on a longitudinal basis is imperative toward accomplishing these recommended research objectives. At a translational level, this would most importantly contribute to the development of accurate and timely clinical care protocols for the management of individuals with Apert syndrome.

References

1. Lajeunie E, Cameron R, El Ghouzzi V, de Parseval N, Journeau P, Gonzales M, et al. Clinical variability in patients with Apert's syndrome. J Neurosurg. 1999;90(3):443–7.
2. Wenger TL, Hing AV, Evans KN. Apert Syndrome. In: Adam MP, Feldman J, Mirzaa GM, Pagon RA, Wallace SE, Amemiya A, editors. GeneReviews(®). Seattle (WA): University of Washington, Seattle. Copyright © 1993–2025, University of Washington, Seattle. GeneReviews is a registered trademark of the University of Washington, Seattle. All rights reserved; 1993.
3. Sarimski K. Children with Apert syndrome: behavioural problems and family stress. Dev Med Child Neurol. 1998;40(1):44–9.
4. Sarimski K. Social adjustment of children with a severe craniofacial anomaly (Apert syndrome). Child Care Health Dev. 2001;27(6):583–90.
5. Shipster C, Hearst D, Dockrell JE, Kilby E, Hayward R. Speech and language skills and cognitive functioning in children with Apert syndrome: a pilot study. Int J Lang Commun Disord. 2002;37(3):325–43.
6. Fearon JA, Podner C. Apert syndrome: evaluation of a treatment algorithm. Plast Reconstr Surg. 2013;131(1):132–42.
7. Maximino LP, Ducati LG, Abramides DVM, Corrêa CC, Garcia PF, Fernandes AY. Syndromic craniosynostosis: neuropsycholinguistic abilities and imaging analysis of the central nervous system. Arq Neuropsiquiatr. 2017;75(12):862–8.
8. Magnan V, Galippe V. Accumulation de stigmates physique chez un débile. Brachycéphalie, plagiocéphalie, acrocéphalie, asymétrie faciale, atrésie buccale, syndactylie des quatre xtrémités. Compte-rendus Hebdomadaires des Séances et Mémoires de la Société de Biologie. 1892;4:277–87; 1982;4.
9. Renier D, Arnaud E, Cinalli G, Sebag G, Zerah M, Marchac D. Prognosis for mental function in Apert's syndrome. J Neurosurg. 1996;85(1):66–72.
10. Freeman JM, Borkowf S. Craniostenosis. Review of the literature and report of thirty-four cases. Pediatrics. 1962;30:57–70.
11. Noetzel MJ, Marsh JL, Palkes H, Gado M. Hydrocephalus and mental retardation in craniosynostosis. J Pediatr. 1985;107(6):885–92.
12. Lefebvre A, Travis F, Arndt EM, Munro IR. A psychiatric profile before and after reconstructive surgery in children with Apert's syndrome. Br J Plast Surg. 1986;39(4):510–3.
13. Patton MA, Goodship J, Hayward R, Lansdown R. Intellectual development in Apert's syndrome: a long term follow up of 29 patients. J Med Genet. 1988;25(3):164–7.
14. Cohn MS, Mahon MJ. Apert's syndrome (acrocephalosyndactyly) in a patient with hyperhidrosis. Cutis. 1993;52(4):205–8.
15. McNaughton PZ, Rodman OG. Apert's syndrome. Cutis. 1980;25(5):538–40.
16. Roberts KB, Hall JG. Apert's acrocephalosyndactyly in mother and daughter: cleft palate in the mother. Birth Defects Orig Artic Ser. 1971;7(7):262–4.
17. Galli ML. Letter: Apert syndrome does not equal mental retardation. J Pediatr. 1976;89(4):691.

18. David DJ, Anderson P, Flapper W, Syme-Grant J, Santoreneos S, Moore M. Apert syndrome: outcomes from the Australian craniofacial unit's birth to maturity management protocol. J Craniofac Surg. 2016;27(5):1125–34.
19. Tovetjärn R, Tarnow P, Maltese G, Fischer S, Sahlin PE, Kölby L. Children with Apert syndrome as adults: a follow-up study of 28 Scandinavian patients. Plast Reconstr Surg. 2012;130(4):572e–6e.
20. Association AP. Diagnostic and statistical manual of mental disorders (5th ed., text rev.). 2022.
21. Bayley N, Aylward. P. Bayley scales of infant and toddler development. 4th ed. Bloomingdale: Pearson; 2019.
22. Sparrow S, Ciccheti DV, Saulnier CA. Vineland adaptive behavior scales, third edition (Vineland-3). Bloomington: NCS Pearson; 2016.
23. Platt JM, Keyes KM, McLaughlin KA, Kaufman AS. Intellectual disability and mental disorders in a US population representative sample of adolescents. Psychol Med. 2019;49(6):952–61.
24. Kapp-Simon KA. Unpublished data.
25. Fernandes MB, Maximino LP, Perosa GB, Abramides DV, Passos-Bueno MR, Yacubian-Fernandes A. Apert and Crouzon syndromes-cognitive development, brain abnormalities, and molecular aspects. Am J Med Genet A. 2016;170(6):1532–7.
26. Yacubian-Fernandes A, Palhares A, Giglio A, Gabarra RC, Zanini S, Portela L, et al. Apert syndrome: factors involved in the cognitive development. Arq Neuropsiquiatr. 2005;63(4):963–8.
27. Yacubian-Fernandes A, Palhares A, Giglio A, Gabarra RC, Zanini S, Portela L, et al. Apert syndrome: analysis of associated brain malformations and conformational changes determined by surgical treatment. J Neuroradiol. 2004;31(2):116–22.
28. Da Costa AC, Walters I, Savarirayan R, Anderson VA, Wrennall JA, Meara JG. Intellectual outcomes in children and adolescents with syndromic and nonsyndromic craniosynostosis. Plast Reconstr Surg. 2006;118(1):175–81; discussion 82–3.
29. Maliepaard M, Mathijssen IM, Oosterlaan J, Okkerse JM. Intellectual, behavioral, and emotional functioning in children with syndromic craniosynostosis. Pediatrics. 2014;133(6):e1608–15.
30. Tomita S, Miyawaki T, Nonaka Y, Sakai S, Nishimura R. Surgical strategy for Apert syndrome: retrospective study of developmental quotient and three-dimensional computerized tomography. Congenit Anom (Kyoto). 2017;57(4):104–8.
31. Organization WH. The ICD-10 classification of mental and behavioural disorders: diagnostic criteria for research. Geneva: World Health Organization; 1993.
32. Association AP. Diagnostic and statistical manual of mental disorders (4th ed., text rev.). Washington, DC, 2000.
33. Da Costa AC, Savarirayan R, Wrennall JA, Walters I, Gardiner N, Tucker A, et al. Neuropsychological diversity in Apert syndrome: a comparison of cognitive profiles. Ann Plast Surg. 2005;54(4):450–5.
34. Hilton C. A longitudinal study of the role of fingers in the development of early number and arithmetic skills in children with Apert syndrome. J Anat. 2024;245(6):914–29.
35. Elliot CD, Smith P, McCulloch K. The British ability scales II. Windsor: NFER Nelson; 1997.
36. Wiig EH, Secord WA, Semel EM. Clinical evaluation of language fundamentals – preschool. San Antonio: The Psychological Corporation; 1992.
37. Zimmerman IL, Steiner VG, Pond RE. Preschool language Scale-3. San Antonio: The Psychological Corporation; 1992.
38. Achenbach TM. The Achenbach system of empirically based Assessement (ASEBA): development, findings, theory, and applications. Burlington: University of Vermont, Research Center for Children, Youth, & Families; 2009.
39. Gathercole SE, Alloway TP. Practitioner review: short-term and working memory impairments in neurodevelopmental disorders: diagnosis and remedial support. J Child Psychol Psychiatry. 2006;47(1):4–15.
40. Sarimski K. Cognitive functioning of young children with Apert's syndrome. Genet Couns. 1997;8(4):317–22.
41. McCarthy D. Manual for the McCarthy scales of children's abilities. New York: Psychological Corporation; 1972.
42. Wechsler D. Wechsler intelligence scale for children—revised. San Antonio: The Psychological Corporation; 1974.
43. Kaufman AS, Kaufman NL. Kaufman assessment battery for children. Circle Pines, MN: American Guidance Service; 1983.
44. Allam KA, Wan DC, Khwanngern K, Kawamoto HK, Tanna N, Perry A, et al. Treatment of apert syndrome: a long-term follow-up study. Plast Reconstr Surg. 2011;127(4):1601–11.
45. van der Vlugt JJB, van der Meulen J, Creemers HE, Willemse SP, Lequin ML, Okkerse JME. The risk of psychopathology in children with craniosynostosis. Plast Reconstr Surg. 2009;124(6):2054–60.
46. Doerga PN, Rijken BFM, Bredero-Boelhouwer H, Joosten KFM, Neuteboom RF, Tasker RC, et al. Neurological deficits are present in syndromic craniosynostosis patients with and without tonsillar herniation. Eur J Paediatr Neurol. 2020;28:120–5.
47. Stock NM, Costa B, Wilkinson-Bell K, Culshaw L, Kearney A, Edwards W. Psychological and physical health outcomes in adults with craniosynostosis. Cleft Palate Craniofac J. 2023;60(3):257–67.
48. Voigt RG, Barbaresi WJ, Colligan RC, Weaver AL, Katusic SK. Developmental dissociation, deviance, and delay: occurrence of attention-deficit-hyperactivity disorder in individuals with and without borderline-to-mild intellectual disability. Dev Med Child Neurol. 2006;48(10):831–5.

49. Einfeld SL, Ellis LA, Emerson E. Comorbidity of intellectual disability and mental disorder in children and adolescents: a systematic review. J Intellect Develop Disabil. 2011;36(2):137–43.
50. Buckley N, Glasson EJ, Chen W, Epstein A, Leonard H, Skoss R, et al. Prevalence estimates of mental health problems in children and adolescents with intellectual disability: a systematic review and meta-analysis. Aust N Z J Psychiatry. 2020;54(10):970–84.
51. Mahony BW, Tu D, Rau S, Liu S, Lalonde FM, Alexander-Bloch AF, et al. IQ modulates coupling between diverse dimensions of psychopathology in children and adolescents. J Am Acad Child Adolesc Psychiatry. 2023;62(1):59–73.
52. Ahuja A, Martin J, Langley K, Thapar A. Intellectual disability in children with attention deficit hyperactivity disorder. J Pediatr. 2013;163(3):890–5.e1.
53. Gould HJ, Caldarelli DD. Hearing and otopathology in Apert syndrome. Arch Otolaryngol. 1982;108(6):347–9.
54. Rajenderkumar D, Bamiou DE, Sirimanna T. Audiological profile in Apert syndrome. Arch Dis Child. 2005;90(6):592–3.
55. de Jong T, Bannink N, Bredero-Boelhouwer HH, van Veelen ML, Bartels MC, Hoeve LJ, et al. Long-term functional outcome in 167 patients with syndromic craniosynostosis; defining a syndrome-specific risk profile. J Plast Reconstr Aesthet Surg. 2010;63(10):1635–41.
56. Webber AL, Wood JM, Gole GA, Brown B. The effect of amblyopia on fine motor skills in children. Invest Ophthalmol Vis Sci. 2008;49(2):594–603.
57. Sun CK, Tseng PT, Wu CK, Li DJ, Chen TY, Stubbs B, et al. Therapeutic effects of methylphenidate for attention-deficit/hyperactivity disorder in children with borderline intellectual functioning or intellectual disability: a systematic review and meta-analysis. Sci Rep. 2019;9(1):15908.
58. Ibrahimi D, Mendiola-Santibañez JD, Gkaros AP. Analysis of the potential impact of strabismus with and without amblyopia on visual-perceptual and visual-motor skills evaluated using TVPS-3 and VMI-6 tests. J Optom. 2021;14(2):166–75.
59. Ouyang J, Yang L, Huang X, Zhong YL, Hu PH, Zhang Y, et al. The atrophy of white and gray matter volume in patients with comitant strabismus: evidence from a voxel-based morphometry study. Mol Med Rep. 2017;16(3):3276–82.
60. (WHO) WHO. International Classification of Diseases, Eleventh Revision (ICD-11). 2019/2021.
61. Gigi K, Werbeloff N, Goldberg S, Portuguese S, Reichenberg A, Fruchter E, et al. Borderline intellectual functioning is associated with poor social functioning, increased rates of psychiatric diagnosis and drug use--a cross sectional population based study. Eur Neuropsychopharmacol. 2014;24(11):1793–7.
62. Peltopuro M, Ahonen T, Kaartinen J, Seppälä H, Närhi V. Borderline intellectual functioning: a systematic literature review. Intellect Dev Disabil. 2014;52(6):419–43.
63. Nouwens PJG, Lucas R, Smulders NBM, Embregts P, van Nieuwenhuizen C. Identifying classes of persons with mild intellectual disability or borderline intellectual functioning: a latent class analysis. BMC Psychiatry. 2017;17(1):257.
64. Pulina F, Lanfranchi S, Henry L, Vianello R. Intellectual profile in school-aged children with borderline intellectual functioning. Res Dev Disabil. 2019;95:103498.
65. Wilkie AO, Morriss-Kay GM. Genetics of craniofacial development and malformation. Nat Rev Genet. 2001;2(6):458–68. https://doi.org/10.1038/35076601.
66. Dono R, Texido G, Dussel R, Ehmke H, Zeller R. Impaired cerebral cortex development and blood pressure regulation in FGF-2-deficient mice. EMBO J. 1998;17(15):4213–25.
67. Vaccarino FM, Schwartz ML, Raballo R, Rhee J, Lyn-Cook R. Fibroblast growth factor signaling regulates growth and morphogenesis at multiple steps during brain development. Curr Top Dev Biol. 1999;46:179–200.
68. Gremo F, Presta M. Role of fibroblast growth factor-2 in human brain: a focus on development. Int J Dev Neurosci. 2000;18(2–3):271–9.
69. Linneberg C, Toft CLF, Kjaer-Sorensen K, Laursen LS. L1cam-mediated developmental processes of the nervous system are differentially regulated by proteolytic processing. Sci Rep. 2019;9(1):3716.
70. Ahmed RR, Medhat AM, Hamdy GM, Effat LKE, Abdel-Hamid MS, Abdel-Salam GMH. X-linked hydrocephalus with new L1CAM pathogenic variants: review of the most prevalent molecular and phenotypic features. Mol Syndromol. 2023;14(4):283–92.
71. Christaller WA, Vos Y, Gebre-Medhin S, Hofstra RM, Schäfer MK. L1 syndrome diagnosis complemented with functional analysis of L1CAM variants located to the two N-terminal Ig-like domains. Clin Genet. 2017;91(1):115–20.
72. Cohen MM Jr, Kreiborg S. The central nervous system in the Apert syndrome. Am J Med Genet. 1990;35(1):36–45.
73. Cinalli G, Sainte-Rose C, Kollar EM, Zerah M, Brunelle F, Chumas P, et al. Hydrocephalus and craniosynostosis. J Neurosurg. 1998;88(2):209–14.
74. Hanieh A, David DJ. Apert's syndrome. Childs Nerv Syst. 1993;9(5):289–91.
75. Breik O, Mahindu A, Moore MH, Molloy CJ, Santoreneos S, David DJ. Central nervous system and cervical spine abnormalities in Apert syndrome. Childs Nerv Syst. 2016;32(5):833–8.
76. Florisson JM, Dudink J, Koning IV, Hop WC, van Veelen ML, Mathijssen IM, et al. Assessment of white matter microstructural integrity in children with syndromic craniosynostosis: a diffusion-tensor imaging study. Radiology. 2011;261(2):534–41.

77. Rijken BF, Leemans A, Lucas Y, van Montfort K, Mathijssen IM, Lequin MH. Diffusion tensor imaging and fiber tractography in children with craniosynostosis syndromes. AJNR Am J Neuroradiol. 2015;36(8):1558–64.
78. Munarriz PM, Pascual B, Castaño-Leon AM, García-Recuero I, Redondo M, de Aragón AM, et al. Apert syndrome: cranial procedures and brain malformations in a series of patients. Surg Neurol Int. 2020;11:361.
79. Tokumaru AM, Barkovich AJ, Ciricillo SF, Edwards MS. Skull base and calvarial deformities: association with intracranial changes in craniofacial syndromes. AJNR Am J Neuroradiol. 1996;17(4):619–30.
80. Murovic JA, Posnick JC, Drake JM, Humphreys RP, Hoffman HJ, Hendricks EB. Hydrocephalus in Apert syndrome: a retrospective review. Pediatr Neurosurg. 1993;19(3):151–5.
81. Lebel C, Deoni S. The development of brain white matter microstructure. NeuroImage. 2018;182:207–18.
82. Dai X, Hadjipantelis P, Wang JL, Deoni SCL, Müller HG. Longitudinal associations between white matter maturation and cognitive development across early childhood. Hum Brain Mapp. 2019;40(14):4130–45.
83. Goddings AL, Roalf D, Lebel C, Tamnes CK. Development of white matter microstructure and executive functions during childhood and adolescence: a review of diffusion MRI studies. Dev Cogn Neurosci. 2021;51:101008.
84. D'Antonio F, Pagani G, Familiari A, Khalil A, Sagies TL, Malinger G, et al. Outcomes associated with isolated agenesis of the corpus callosum: a meta-analysis. Pediatrics. 2016;138(3):e20160445.
85. Kyriakopoulou V, Davidson A, Chew A, Gupta N, Arichi T, Nosarti C, et al. Characterisation of ASD traits among a cohort of children with isolated fetal ventriculomegaly. Nat Commun. 2023;14(1):1550.
86. Zaksaite T, Loveday C, Edginton T, Spiers HJ, Smith AD. Hydrocephalus: a neuropsychological and theoretical primer. Cortex. 2023;160:67–99.
87. Adam R, Ghahari D, Morton JB, Eagleson R, de Ribaupierre S. Brain network connectivity and executive function in children with infantile hydrocephalus. Brain Connect. 2022;12(9):784–98.
88. Bodensteiner JB, Schaefer GB, Craft JM. Cavum septi pellucidi and cavum vergae in normal and developmentally delayed populations. J Child Neurol. 1998;13(3):120–1.
89. Dremmen MHG, Bouhuis RH, Blanken LME, Muetzel RL, Vernooij MW, El Marroun H, et al. Cavum septum pellucidum in the general pediatric population and its relation to surrounding brain structure volumes, cognitive function, and emotional or behavioral problems. AJNR Am J Neuroradiol. 2019;40(2):340–6.
90. Anderson V, Spencer-Smith M, Wood A. Do children really recover better? Neurobehavioural plasticity after early brain insult. Brain. 2011;134(Pt 8):2197–221.
91. Casey BJ, Giedd JN, Thomas KM. Structural and functional brain development and its relation to cognitive development. Biol Psychol. 2000;54(1–3):241–57.
92. Rakic P. Specification of cerebral cortical areas. Science. 1988;241(4862):170–6.
93. Selemon LD, Goldman-Rakic PS. Common cortical and subcortical targets of the dorsolateral prefrontal and posterior parietal cortices in the rhesus monkey: evidence for a distributed neural network subserving spatially guided behavior. J Neurosci. 1988;8(11):4049–68.
94. Deoni SC, O'Muircheartaigh J, Elison JT, Walker L, Doernberg E, Waskiewicz N, et al. White matter maturation profiles through early childhood predict general cognitive ability. Brain Struct Funct. 2016;221(2):1189–203.
95. Anderson V, Pentland L. Residual attention deficits following childhood head injury: implications for ongoing development. Neuropsychol Rehabil. 1998;8(3):283–300.
96. Gogtay N, Giedd JN, Lusk L, Hayashi KM, Greenstein D, Vaituzis AC, et al. Dynamic mapping of human cortical development during childhood through early adulthood. Proc Natl Acad Sci USA. 2004;101(21):8174–9.
97. Anderson V, Bond L, Catroppa C, Grimwood K, Keir E, Nolan T. Childhood bacterial meningitis: impact of age at illness and acute medical complications on long term outcome. J Int Neuropsychol Soc. 1997;3(2):147–58.
98. Duchowny M, Jayakar P, Harvey AS, Resnick T, Alvarez L, Dean P, et al. Language cortex representation: effects of developmental versus acquired pathology. Ann Neurol. 1996;40(1):31–8.
99. Renier D, Sainte-Rose C, Marchac D, Hirsch JF. Intracranial pressure in craniostenosis renJ. Neurosurg. 1982;57(3):370–7.
100. Marucci DD, Dunaway DJ, Jones BM, Hayward RD. Raised intracranial pressure in Apert syndrome. Plast Reconstr Surg. 2008;122(4):1162–8.
101. Taylor WJ, Hayward RD, Lasjaunias P, Britto JA, Thompson DN, Jones BM, et al. Enigma of raised intracranial pressure in patients with complex craniosynostosis: the role of abnormal intracranial venous drainage. J Neurosurg. 2001;94(3):377–85.
102. Hayward R. Venous hypertension and craniosynostosis. Childs Nerv Syst. 2005;21(10):880–8.
103. Renier D, Lajeunie E, Arnaud E, Marchac D. Management of craniosynostoses. Childs Nerv Syst. 2000;16(10–11):645–58.
104. Collmann H, Sörensen N, Krauss J. Hydrocephalus in craniosynostosis: a review. Childs Nerv Syst. 2005;21(10):902–12.
105. Gonsalez S, Hayward R, Jones B, Lane R. Upper airway obstruction and raised intracranial pressure

in children with craniosynostosis. Eur Respir J. 1997;10(2):367–75.
106. Hayward R, Britto J, Dunaway D, Jeelani O. Connecting raised intracranial pressure and cognitive delay in craniosynostosis: many assumptions, little evidence. J Neurosurg Pediatr. 2016;18(2):242–50.
107. Mathijssen I, de Goederen R, Versnel SL, Joosten KFM, van Veelen MC, Tasker RC. Letter to the Editor. Raised intracranial pressure and cognitive delay in craniosynostosis. J Neurosurg Pediatr. 2017;20(5):498–502.
108. Bannink N, Maliepaard M, Raat H, Joosten KF, Mathijssen IM. Obstructive sleep apnea-specific quality of life and behavioral problems in children with syndromic craniosynostosis. J Dev Behav Pediatr. 2011;32(3):233–8.
109. Inverso G, Brustowicz KA, Katz E, Padwa BL. The prevalence of obstructive sleep apnea in symptomatic patients with syndromic craniosynostosis. Int J Oral Maxillofac Surg. 2016;45(2):167–9.
110. Bucks RS, Olaithe M, Rosenzweig I, Morrell MJ. Reviewing the relationship between OSA and cognition: where do we go from here? Respirology. 2017;22(7):1253–61.
111. Dillon JE, Blunden S, Ruzicka DL, Guire KE, Champine D, Weatherly RA, et al. DSM-IV diagnoses and obstructive sleep apnea in children before and 1 year after adenotonsillectomy. J Am Acad Child Adolesc Psychiatry. 2007;46(11):1425–36.
112. Chervin RD, Ruzicka DL, Giordani BJ, Weatherly RA, Dillon JE, Hodges EK, et al. Sleep-disordered breathing, behavior, and cognition in children before and after adenotonsillectomy. Pediatrics. 2006;117(4):e769–78.
113. Breik O, Mahindu A, Moore MH, Molloy CJ, Santoreneos S, David DJ. Apert syndrome: surgical outcomes and perspectives. J Craniomaxillofac Surg. 2016;44(9):1238–45.
114. Thompson DN, Jones BM, Harkness W, Gonsalez S, Hayward RD. Consequences of cranial vault expansion surgery for craniosynostosis. Pediatr Neurosurg. 1997;26(6):296–303.
115. Zhang H, Du L, Du Z, Jiang H, Han D, Li Q. Association between childhood exposure to single general anesthesia and neurodevelopment: a systematic review and meta-analysis of cohort study. J Anesth. 2015;29(5):749–57.
116. Jia X, Tan S, Qin Y, Wei Y, Jiang Y, Pan S, et al. Experiencing anesthesia and surgery early in life impairs cognitive and behavioral development. Front Neurosci. 2024;18:1406172.
117. Cornelissen L, Coffman S, Kim I, Underwood E, Tao A, Maloney MG, et al. Neurodevelopment at 10 months and 2-3 years old after early and prolonged anaesthesia in infancy: General Anaesthesia & Brain Activity study (GABA) secondary analysis. BJA Open. 2025;14:100383.
118. Pennings CH, Van Boxtel M, De Korte-De Boer D, Buhre W, Vossen CJ. Anaesthesia as a risk factor for long-term cognitive decline: results of the prospective MAAS cohort study. Eur J Anaesthesiol. 2025;42(5):468–77.
119. Ing C, Bellinger DC. Long-term cognitive and behavioral outcomes following early exposure to general anesthetics. Curr Opin Anaesthesiol. 2022;35(4):442–7.
120. Naumann HL, Haberkern CM, Pietila KE, Birgfeld CB, Starr JR, Kapp-Simon KA, et al. Duration of exposure to cranial vault surgery: associations with neurodevelopment among children with single-suture craniosynostosis. Paediatr Anaesth. 2012;22(11):1053–61.
121. Kapp-Simon K, Wallace ER, Collett BR, et al. Surgery age, anesthesia exposure, and neurodevelopment in children with single-suture craniosynostosis. 73rd Annual Meeting of the American Cleft Palate-Craniofacial Association; April 8; Atlanta, GA, 2016.
122. Bradley RH, Corwyn RF. Socioeconomic status and child development. Annu Rev Psychol. 2002;53:371–99.
123. Alex AM, Aguate F, Botteron K, Buss C, Chong YS, Dager SR, et al. A global multicohort study to map subcortical brain development and cognition in infancy and early childhood. Nat Neurosci. 2024;27(1):176–86.
124. Duncan GJ, Magnuson K. Socioeconomic status and cognitive functioning: moving from correlation to causation. Wiley Interdiscip Rev Cogn Sci. 2012;3(3):377–86.
125. Gray KE, Kapp-Simon KA, Starr JR, Collett BR, Wallace ER, Speltz ML. Predicting developmental delay in a longitudinal cohort of preschool children with single-suture craniosynostosis: is neurobehavioral assessment important? Dev Med Child Neurol. 2015;57(5):456–62.
126. Stock NM, Marik P, Magee L, Aspinall CL, Garcia L, Crerand C, et al. Facilitating positive psychosocial outcomes in craniofacial team care: strategies for medical providers. Cleft Palate Craniofac J. 2020;57(3):333–43.
127. Squires J, Bricker D. Ages and stages questionnaire (ASQ): a parent completed child monitoring system. 3rd ed. Brooks Publishing Company; 2009.
128. Duggan C, Irvine AD, OBH J, Kiely ME, Murray DM. ASQ-3 and BSID-III's concurrent validity and predictive ability of cognitive outcome at 5 years. Pediatr Res. 2023;94(4):1465–71.
129. Wechsler D. Wechsler preschool and primary scale of intelligence. 4th ed. Bloomington: Pearson; 2012.
130. Wechsler D. Wechsler intelligence scale for children. 5th ed. Bloomington: The Psychological Corporation; 2014.

131. Wechsler D. Wechsler adult intelligence scale. 4th ed. San Antonio: Pearson; 2008.
132. Wechsler D. The Wechsler intelligence scale for children. 3rd ed. San Antonio: The Psychological Corporation; 1991.
133. Wechsler D. The Wechsler intelligence scale for children. 4th ed. San Antonio: The Psychological Corporation; 2003.
134. Wechsler D. Wechsler adult intelligence scale. 5th ed. Pearson Assessments; 2024.
135. Roid G, Miller LJ, Pomplun M, Koch C. Leiter-3: nonverbal cognitive and neuropsychological assessment. Wood Dale: Stoelting ewCompany; 2013.
136. Delis DC, Kaplan E, Kramer JH. Delis-Kaplan Executive Function System (DKEFS). San Antonio: Psychological Corporation; 2001.
137. Gioia GA, Isquth PK, Guy SC, Kenworthy L. Behavior rating inventory of executive function, second edition professional manual. Lutz, FL: PAR; 2015.
138. Pearson N. Wechsler individual achievement test, fourth edition (WIAT-4). 2020.
139. Bishop N. The children's communication checklist-2. Pearson Assessments; 2006.

34 Social and Psychological Impacts and Recommendations

Nicola M. Stock, Matthew L. Speltz,
and Kathleen A. Kapp-Simon

Background

Craniosynostosis is defined by the premature fusion of one or more skull sutures. This condition becomes visibly apparent for most individuals in the first few months of life. Skull shape is affected by the restricted growth of bony tissue perpendicular to the fused suture, as well as compensatory growth in unfused bony tissue.

Among the genetic syndromes characterized by multiple suture fusions, Apert syndrome is the most common, accounting for nearly half of all syndromic synostoses [1]. Nevertheless, Apert syndrome remains a rare condition, with population-based incidence estimates ranging from 1:50,000 [2] to 1:160,000 births [3].

Apert syndrome has a relatively distinct morphological phenotype characterized by bicoronal craniosynostosis, an altered facial appearance (mid-facial hypoplasia, hypertelorism and proptosis), and limb differences, primarily syndactyly [4]. Genetically, most cases of Apert syndrome are sporadic, although autosomal dominant inheritance has been reported [5]. In nearly all individuals with Apert syndrome, one of two specific missense mutations of the fibroblast growth factor receptor 2 gene (FGFR2) has been found [2, 6–8]. These "point mutations" are adjacent amino acid substitutions designated as S252W and P253R [6].

In early life, medical management of children with Apert syndrome is primarily focused on surgery to address the fused coronal sutures, midfacial hypoplasia, and syndactyly. The typical child with AS will have experienced about 10 major surgeries before they reach the early elementary school years [7, 9]. In addition to surgical procedures, other healthcare specialists and services may come into play depending on individual variation in morphology and its functional consequences. Examples include hearing and vision impairments secondary to craniosynostosis, limited fine and gross motor abilities related to the severity of syndactyly, and speech and language problems due to structural malformations or secondary to hearing impairment [9].

Neurodevelopmental and Behavioral Characteristics of Apert Syndrome

Individuals with Apert syndrome are at high risk for learning challenges, including intellectual developmental disorder (IDD). Some of the adap-

N. M. Stock (✉)
Centre for Appearance Research, University of the West of England, Bristol, UK
e-mail: Nicola2.Stock@uwe.ac.uk

M. L. Speltz
Department of Psychiatry and Behavioral Sciences, University of Washington, Seattle, WA, USA

K. A. Kapp-Simon
Shriners Children's Hospital, Chicago, IL, USA

University of Illinois, Chicago, IL, USA

J. G. Meara et al. (eds.), *Apert Syndrome*, https://doi.org/10.1007/978-3-032-12551-4_34

tive challenges faced by individuals with IDD include delayed mastery of self-help skills and difficulties understanding rules, learning from mistakes, and postponing a desired behavior if circumstances demand it [10]. Children with Apert syndrome may also have difficulty adjusting their emotions to the demands of the environment [11]. These challenges may present in the form of externalizing or "under-controlled" behaviors (such as aggression, self-harm, immaturity, and non-compliance) and/or internalizing or "over-controlled" behaviors (such as shyness, withdrawal, anxiety, and avoidance) [12–15]. Individuals with Apert syndrome may also exhibit behaviors categorized as overfriendly, overactive/hyperactive, or restless [11]. Difficulties with persistence, focus, and/or attention are frequently mentioned in conjunction with research on Apert syndrome [7, 15–18].

Significant behavior problems may be more prevalent among children with Apert syndrome who have more severe developmental concerns or IDD than those without these additional risks. This is supported by several studies in which children with syndromic craniosynostosis, who presented with mild to severe IDD, displayed more internalizing, externalizing, and attention problems than children with higher intellectual abilities [11, 13, 15]. Increased behavior problems, in addition to sleep disturbance, are also reported for children with Apert syndrome who present with obstructive sleep apnea [14].

Importantly, an individual's functioning may also be impacted by skeletal and sensory differences associated with Apert syndrome. The dysmorphic skeletal changes and progressive fusion of multiple bony structures associated with Apert syndrome [19, 20] may affect the individual's ability to walk and use their hands, engage in self-help and play, and participate in educational or athletic activities [17, 19, 21, 22]. Children with Apert syndrome are also at high risk of visual problems, particularly strabismus and refractive errors, as well as hearing loss [23]. Vision problems, particularly the lack of convergence, may increase the difficulty that others have in determining where children with Apert syndrome are looking, resulting in a perception of abnormal eye contact [11]. Visual challenges and hearing loss have been linked to behavioral problems, particularly anxiety and attention problems, in the general population and may be relevant for children with Apert syndrome [24–28].

As a result of these challenges, children with Apert syndrome almost universally require supportive services in school [18]. These services typically include speech and language therapy, occupational and physical therapy, and, for some, vision and hearing support. Children with Apert syndrome and IDD may require more intensive school supports, such as placement in a special education classroom.

The Psychosocial Impact of Apert Syndrome on the Individual

Throughout the lifespan, the various characteristics of Apert syndrome can have a profound impact on many aspects of the individual's social and psychological well-being. Children typically become more self-aware around 5 years of age, and this is often when those with Apert syndrome begin to understand they are "different." [29] Peers may ask questions about or comment on their appearance, speech differences, or hearing needs, which can come as a shock to the child if they have never had to respond to these reactions before [30]. Even well-meaning peers may try to "take care of" children who look different rather than engaging them in developmentally appropriate play [30]. In some cases, teasing and bullying or active social exclusion may become a cause for concern [18, 31]. Not being treated equally among peers may impact self-confidence and self-perception related to social acceptance and worth [32–34]. Parents, family members, and teachers may be unsure how to speak to the child about their differences and may worry they will incite further problems if the issue is raised [29]. Concurrently, those with Apert syndrome may experience difficulties in participating appropriately in family, school, and community activities due to the impacts of the condition on neurodevelopment and communication [12, 18]. Social proficiency has been identified as a common obstacle for individuals with Apert syndrome, particularly those with learning challenges [11].

Connecting with peers, establishing friendships, and finding a sense of belonging may therefore pose a more significant challenge for individuals with Apert syndrome.

> *Going out was difficult when I was younger because people look at me (...). It feels stressful and uncomfortable because you know someone's looking at you and you just don't want them to.*
> —young person with Apert syndrome; in Netherton et al., 2023.

During the school years, a child's learning and school engagement may be impacted by a teacher's lack of knowledge about the condition or by inconsistent implementation of the necessary educational accommodations [35]. Teachers may also underestimate the child's abilities, resulting in limited educational opportunities [30]. Further, hospital appointments, medical interventions, and other necessary support services may result in repeated school absences [36].

Medical treatment to "correct" the form and function of the head, face, and other parts of the body may also implicitly or directly emphasize to the child that they are different [30, 37]. Surgical interventions in particular can be extremely stressful for children, especially if long recovery periods are necessary and/or changes to facial appearance occur [38]. Medical traumatic stress has been reported among individuals who experience frequent and/or significant medical events, including those in the craniofacial population [39]. To mitigate this, young people have expressed a desire to be included in treatment decisions. Yet, guidelines for shared decision-making are not always followed, particularly if the young person has compromised learning and memory skills [40, 41].

> *When they [operated on] my head I thought "I'm not going to survive this" (...). When I came round from the oxygen I was happy (...), because I knew I was alive.*
> —young person with Apert syndrome; in Netherton et al., 2023.

As the individual grows older, key time points may bring specific challenges. This can include transitions to different educational settings and the move from child to adult health services [30, 42]. Navigating treatment decisions and accessing appropriate and timely care can be especially difficult in the context of living with a rare condition [43]. Gaining meaningful employment may also pose a significant challenge for individuals with Apert syndrome, due to discrimination and/or a lack of adequate workplace support [44], and individuals with Apert syndrome may be less likely to live independently [45]. Adults with a range of craniofacial conditions, including Apert syndrome, commonly report concerns about sexual intimacy and increased anxiety about romantic relationships [44–46]. Starting a family may also evoke some distress due to the genetic recurrence risk [47].

> *I have qualifications and experience but feel I am not being employed due to my disability... I have found it very stressful and have wanted to give up.*
> —young adult with craniosynostosis; in Stock et al., 2023.

Together, these experiences can affect the individual's identity formation and self-esteem [31]. Elevated levels of anxiety have been observed in a significant minority of adults with craniofacial conditions such as Apert syndrome, alongside some evidence of depressive symptoms and impacted quality of life [12, 14, 44, 46]. Despite the numerous challenges, many positive outcomes have also been recorded among individuals with craniofacial conditions, including self-acceptance, resiliency, and personal growth [48, 49]. With appropriate support in place, individuals with Apert syndrome have the opportunity to lead rich and satisfying lives [50].

The Psychosocial Impact of Apert Syndrome on Caregivers and Families

Apert syndrome can strongly impact the lives of caregivers and the wider family unit, as well as the individuals themselves. The birth of any child with significant medical and/or developmental needs poses a range of psychological and social challenges for new parents [51, 52]. In addition to taking care of a newborn, parents must adjust to the news of their child's diagnosis and the long-term treatment pathway ahead [53]. For parents of a child with a rare condition, such as Apert syndrome, the diagnostic experience itself may bring uncertainty, due to a lack of knowledge of the condition among health professionals [54, 55]. This can lead to a delay in the diagnosis and/or referral to a specialist team, as well as a lack of reliable information about the prognosis and/or treatment plan once the diagnosis is given [35, 54].

> *It took six months before we had a diagnosis. That was the worst period of time for us, not knowing what it was. It didn't feel safe not to know.*
> —parent of a child with a rare craniofacial condition; in Feragen et al., 2020.

Parents may experience a range of emotional reactions to their child's diagnosis, including shock, guilt, grief, and despair. They may also feel abandoned by health professionals, distressed by what they find through their independent information-seeking, and fearful of the future [35]. During these early days and months, it is common for parents to lose confidence in the healthcare system and to feel frustrated that their concerns are not being heard [54].

Once associated with a specialist craniofacial team, healthcare satisfaction among parents tends to increase, with families valuing health professionals' knowledge and technical competence [53, 54]. Yet, some dissatisfaction with certain aspects of care remains, including coordination within and between specialist and local services, associated financial and logistical burdens, and the complexity of treatment decision-making [53]. Parents often adopt the roles of coordinator, advocate, and expert regarding their child's care, and make significant changes to their daily lives to meet these responsibilities [30, 54, 55]. Long-term treatment can involve peaks and troughs, fluctuating between periods of stability and periods of intensive medical treatment [35]. Some parents have described symptoms of post-traumatic stress as a response to their child's medical care, particularly following surgical intervention or life-threatening medical situations [56].

> *For the first two years of [my son's] life we virtually lived [at the hospital]. It's mentally draining… It does take up a big part of your life.*
> —parent of a child with Apert syndrome; in Netherton et al., 2023.

These demands can place additional pressure on family life, which may incite conflict between spouses/partners, and negatively impact other family members [14, 30, 55]. The behavioral and communication difficulties associated with Apert syndrome can also complicate and challenge familial relationships and negatively affect parental well-being [11, 57]. Outside the home, parents must frequently cope with staring, comments, and questions from members of the public, which can be offensive and distressing, even when well-intended [30, 58].

Parents may worry for their child about actual or anticipated teasing and bullying and go to great lengths to shield or defend their child against misconceptions and difficult social reactions [54, 59]. A lack of societal awareness of rare conditions can also result in difficulties accessing social benefits and appropriate educational accommodations [59].

> *We've seen the way people react to [our daughter's] appearance and make judgments… That really infuriates me.*
> —parent of a child with Apert syndrome; in Netherton et al., 2023.

Caring for a child with additional needs requires caregivers to continually adjust to the demands of their child's condition and interact with multiple systems of care to ensure these needs are met [35]. As a result, caregivers may experience significantly greater levels of stress, anxiety, and depression, as well as poorer physical health than parents of unaffected children [14, 55, 60, 61]. Yet, many parents also demonstrate a wide range of effective coping strategies and resiliency throughout their child's journey in response to repeated stressful situations [53]. Maintaining hope and optimism, engaging in social and peer support, and taking an active role in treatment plans have all been shown to protect parents from psychological distress [53]. When caregivers can successfully navigate the demands placed on them, personal growth, including greater inner strength and parental self-efficacy, is likely to follow [62].

> *You learn a lot about yourself… The experience of being so low and then…to rise again… I believe I am a strong person, that I have managed this… That I survived.*
> —parent of a child with a rare craniofacial condition; in Feragen et al., 2020.

Clinical Implications and Interventions

Given the wide range of impacts of Apert syndrome on the psychosocial well-being of individuals and their families, recent clinical guidelines [63, 64] have included specialized psychosocial services as an integral part of comprehensive care. Psychologists can work across the lifespan of affected individuals and their families to provide support for new parents, address behavioral, social, and emotional concerns, work with schools and other local services, and help patients and families to make informed medical decisions [65]. Yet, many countries worldwide still lack the resources to provide this level of psychological input. Even in those countries with a high level of resources, evidence to support specific interventions to prevent and address common problems among those affected by craniofacial conditions remains relatively scarce [66, 67]. The interventions with the most supporting evidence have typically targeted appearance-related anxiety and/or social anxiety and are based on cognitive behavioral therapy (CBT) and social skills training [68, 69]. One example is the online interactive Face IT program, originally developed for adults [70] and later redesigned for young people (YP Face IT) [71]. Both programs are examples of online self-help, although supervision by a trained clinician may also be recommended. YP Face IT has recently been adapted and translated for use in Norway and the Netherlands.

Another intervention that has shown initial promise in the craniofacial field is the Promoting Resilience In Stress Management (PRISM) program, a brief, skills-based program designed to enhance perceived resilience and mitigate psychological distress in adolescents and young adults with serious illness and their families [72, 73]. The caregiver version of the PRISM intervention was piloted with English-speaking caregivers of children with craniofacial conditions in the United States and demonstrated 100% acceptability among those who took part [74]. Further trials of this intervention are forthcoming.

More general interventions that have demonstrated value in the craniofacial field include the delivery of psychoeducation. This often comes in the form of an information booklet [75–77], designed to inform patients and their families about the condition and its treatment, and address common psychosocial concerns, or in a short film format [78]. Psychoeducation can also be offered informally, such as by a clinical nurse specialist following a diagnosis [79]. Formal or informal peer support is also recognized as a useful mechanism for connecting people with similar life experiences. This may be delivered remotely or in person through a support group, event, podcast, or residential camp. Connecting families and individuals to local/international support organizations and groups can encourage community and increase self-esteem and perceptions of social acceptance [80–83] (Table 34.1).

Regardless of primary discipline, health providers can also consider implementing various strategies to facilitate psychosocial well-being during routine care. For example, all team members can ensure they speak to the family as soon as possible after a diagnosis, provide reliable and consistent information in different formats, demonstrate empathy, reassure the family the condition is not their fault, and explain that the emotions they are experiencing represent an understandable reaction to a challenging situation [68, 84]. Health providers can also help individuals and families to practice confident communication to cope with other people's reactions and involve them in treatment decisions [84]. Avoiding terminology with negative connotations can also help to reduce the stigma and distress felt by individuals and families (e.g., say "diagnosis" instead of "defect," and "surgery" instead of "repair") [84]. The integration of routine screening for psychosocial distress among patients and their caregivers is one approach to identifying those at risk and a way to focus limited resources on those who most need support (see Table 34.2). In particular, the authors recommend using the PedsQL Family Impact module to assess caregiver well-being, the CBCL to measure child development, and the PROMIS measures to assess patient well-being.

Table 34.1 Psychosocial resources

Resource	Target audience	Source
Booklet: Managing a Diagnosis of Craniosynostosis	Parents/families	www.headlines.org.uk/for-parents
Booklet: Surgery for Craniosynostosis	Parents/families	www.headlines.org.uk/for-parents
Born a Hero Foundation	Parents/families	www.bornahero.org
Films: Living with Craniosynostosis in Adulthood	Young people/adults	www.headlines.org.uk/for-adults
Booklet: Living with Craniosynostosis in Adulthood	Young people/adults	www.headlines.org.uk/for-adults
MyFace, MyStory podcast hosted by MyFace	Craniofacial community	www.myface.org/mystory
Educational Resources from the American Cleft Palate-Craniofacial Association	Parents/families/young people/adults	www.acpacares.org/resource/educational-materials
Video Library from the Children's Craniofacial Association	Craniofacial community	www.youtube.com/@ChildrensCraniofacia
Advice and Guidance from Changing Faces	Visible difference community	www.changingfaces.org.uk/advice-guidance
Psychosocial Strategies for Medical Providers	Medical providers	www.pubmed.ncbi.nlm.nih.gov/31446785

Table 34.2 Potential measures and timeline for psychosocial screening

Instrument	Languages available (cost)	Items scales	Reporter	Focus of instrument	Suggested frequency of administration
PedsQL familyimpact[a] [87]	60+ (free for clinic use)	3–6 items per scale 10 scales	Parent	Family functioning, parental health-related quality of life	Initial visit, Ages 2, 5, 8, 10, 15, 18
PAT-CV[a] [89]	English (annual fee)	8–20 items per scale 8 scales	Parent or caregiver	Family functioning and resources, child, sibling problems, craniofacial specific concerns	Initial visit, Ages 2, 5, 8, 10, 15, 18
PROMIS[b]	English, Spanish, other languages available (free, except for translations)	4–8 items per short-form scale; multiple scales to choose from	Parent or caregiver. Self-report	*Recommend short-form scales:* anxiety, depression, social functioning, cognitive *Self-report only*: stigma	Parent/caregiver: annually, 3–18 yrs. Self-report: annually, 8 years to adult
CBCL/YSR ASEBA[b] [85]	90+ (low cost after initial investment for computer scoring; hand scoring possible)	8–18 items per scale 3 competence scales 8 syndrome scales 5–6 DSM-related scales scored from same item bank	Parent or caregiver. Self-report	*Adaptive behavior:* activities, social, school *Internalizing problems:* anxiety, depression, somatic. *Externalizing problems:* rule-breaking, aggression. *Social, thought, attention problems.* *DSM-related scales* Affective, anxiety, somatic, ADHD, oppositional defiant, conduct problems	Parent/caregiver: annually, 18 months to adult Self-report: annually, 11 years to adult

(continued)

Table 34.2 (continued)

Instrument	Languages available (cost)	Items scales	Reporter	Focus of instrument	Suggested frequency of administration
Strengths and difficulties[b] [86]	80+ (free)	5 items per scale 5 scales	Parent or caregiver. Self-report	Emotional symptoms, conduct problems, hyperactivity, peer-related behavioral problems, and prosocial behavior	Parent/caregiver: annually 4–17 years Self-report: annually, 11 years to adult
FACE-Q [88]	English, some scales in up to 22 languages (free)	6–12 items per scale 27 scales to choose from	Self-report	Appearance, health-related quality of life, facial function, adverse effects	Selected scales as part of a clinic visit to determine patient concerns or pre–/post- surgery

Note: *ASEBA* Achenbach System of Empirically Based Assessment, *CBCL/YSR* Child Behavior Checklist/Youth Self-Report, *PedsQL* Pediatric Quality of Life, *PROMIS* Patient-Reported Outcomes Measurement Information System (http://www.healthmeasures.net/search-view-measure)
[a]Choose 1 of these measures; [b]Choose 1 of these measurement systems

The Utility of a Behavioral Phenotype for Apert Syndrome

To better articulate the psychosocial functioning of individuals with genetic syndromes, it is important not only to consider morphology (or physical phenotype) but also the possibility of a distinctive "behavioral phenotype." This term typically refers to a constellation of observed behaviors and/or inferred internal processes that occur more often in people with a specific genetic syndrome than those without that syndrome [90]. The potential range of phenotypic behaviors and internal events is far-reaching, including neuropsychological strengths and weaknesses (e.g., intelligence, learning and memory), temperament and personality, behavioral adjustment and socialization, and self-perception (i.e., how individuals view their physical and mental attributes and how this may affect thoughts and feelings) [32]. Well-known behavioral phenotypes with potential relevance for Apert syndrome are those associated with IDD and certain morphological anomalies such as those seen in Down, Williams, Angelman, and Prader–Willi syndromes [91, 92].

Behavioral phenotypes can lead to some degree of stereotyping and risk of self-fulfilling "prophecies," [93] but clinicians and researchers have largely pointed to their heuristic and clinical value [90, 93]. Behavioral phenotypes bring an enhanced focus on the possibility of genotype–phenotype interactions, interactions that could potentially uncover the genetic origins, and pathophysiology of certain neurobehavioral disorders. For example, as noted earlier in the chapter, most individuals with Apert syndrome have one of two specific missense mutations of the FGFR2 gene. Clinical observations have suggested that there may be both morphological and behavioral differences associated with this genetic distinction [2]. In craniofacial programs that routinely collect infancy genetic data, this could be an easily testable hypothesis with the longitudinal use of standardized behavior checklists.

Another advantage of a behavioral phenotypic framework is the provision of anticipatory guidance for clinicians, educators, and families about intervention targets. For example, the behavioral phenotype associated with Williams syndrome is characterized by an abnormally low level of stranger anxiety that elevates the risk of social exploitation [94]. This well-studied trait has led to effective teaching interventions to foster the use of appropriate stranger evaluation skills [95]. Many other examples of psychosocial assessment and intervention strategies can be found based on the known or hypothesized behavioral phenotypes of genetic syndromes [96–98]. However, comparable data regarding heritable forms of craniosynostosis, including Apert syndrome, are currently lacking.

Directions for Future Research in Apert Syndrome

Studies of the psychological characteristics and impacts of Apert syndrome remain scarce. The studies that have been conducted are often limited by small samples and ascertainment bias, in addition to a preponderance of cross-sectional studies using inconsistent methods and measures. These methodological challenges are due in part to the low incidence and prevalence of Apert syndrome. Multi-center and multi-country studies with longitudinal designs are ultimately needed to increase sample sizes and opportunities for repeated assessments of the same individuals over time and across critical developmental stages [99]. Consensus among investigators on outcome measures with both research and clinical utility is required to compare findings across studies [99]. Considered approaches to data collection that ensure the inclusion of children with complicated clinical presentations and significantly compromised learning abilities are also necessary to understand the full spectrum of the condition and to target resources for those at the highest risk. Specifically, longitudinal studies that begin in infancy and provide detailed information about early development, attachment relationships, and family coping during the first years of life would be beneficial [100]. Routine use of an early developmental screener such as the Ages and Stages Questionnaires [101] would provide important clinical information about areas of risk and contribute to the evidence base. From age 2, measures of social and behavioral adjustment using the Child Behavior Checklist [85] and adaptive behavior using the Adaptive Behavior Assessment System [102] (third edition) would allow for repeated assessments of adjustment and adaptive behavior across the lifespan (Table 34.3).

In addition to using more ambitious study designs, qualitative approaches can offer complementary insight into the unmet needs of individuals and family members, potentially leading to the formulation of novel hypotheses for subsequent quantitative studies and clinical trials. Person-oriented (vs. variable-focused) data collection and analytic methods (such as cluster analysis and latent profile analysis) also allow for the examination of individual risk profiles [103], which may be better suited to rare conditions than traditional inferential research and related statistical analyses. This approach could eventually lead to the predictive modeling of high-risk versus low-risk individuals with Apert syndrome and help us distinguish between optimal and poor psychosocial functioning. Qualitative and

Table 34.3 Potential measures and timeline for standardized data collection for research

Instrument	Reporter	Suggested frequency of administration for research
ASQ	Parent or caregiver	Before cranial surgery, 6 months after surgery, 4 years
CBCL 1.5–5	Parent or caregiver, teacher	2–3, 5 years
CBCL 6–18	Parent or caregiver	7–8, 10, 15, 17 years
ABCL 19–59	Parent or caregiver	At least once in the 20s, 30s, 40s*
Vineland-3	Parent or caregiver	2–3, 5, 8, 12, 16 years At least once in the 20s, 30s, 40s*
PROMIS	Self-report	8, 10 years
YSR	Self-report	12, 15, 17 years
ASR 18–59	Self-report	At least once in the 20s, 30s, 40s

Note: *ASQ* Ages and Stages Questionnaire, *CBCL* Child Behavior Checklist, *ABCL* Adult Behavior Checklist, *PROMIS* Patient-Reported Outcomes Measurement Information System, *YSR* Youth Self-Report, *ASR* Adult Self-Report
*Unless the individual with Apert syndrome is under guardianship of another adult, completion requires consent of the individual with Apert syndrome

individual-focused approaches could also help to generate hypotheses about a behavioral phenotype for Apert syndrome.

More broadly, including coping, resiliency, and growth alongside challenges would provide a more rounded view of psychosocial adjustment [99]. Further, an emphasis on "cross-condition" analyses may be beneficial in pursuing a more comprehensive understanding of Apert syndrome. This may include drawing on knowledge from other craniofacial conditions, rare conditions and genetic syndromes, and other conditions affecting appearance, as well as chronic medical illnesses and neurodevelopmental disabilities. Ultimately, a more substantial evidence base is essential if we are to establish a clear pathway for psychosocial intervention and optimize psychological health in this complex and underserved population.

Conclusions

This chapter has outlined the physical, neurodevelopmental, and behavioral aspects of Apert syndrome, and described the known psychosocial impacts of the condition and its treatment. The authors encourage health providers to consider implementing the recommended strategies into routine practice, in addition to using screening tools and specific evidence-based psychosocial interventions where feasible. Researchers are encouraged to consider the utility of a behavioral phenotype to guide clinical practice, and to pursue a strengthened evidence base to inform optimal person-centered care.

References

1. Boulet SL, Rasmussen SA, Honein MA. A population-based study of craniosynostosis in metropolitan Atlanta, 1989–2003. Am J Med Genet. 2008;146A(8):984–91. https://doi.org/10.1002/ajmg.a.32208.
2. Lajeunie E, Cameron R, El Ghouzzi V, de Parseval N, Journeau P, Gonzales M, Delezoide AL, Bonaventure J, Le Merrer M, Renier D. Clinical variability in patients with Apert's syndrome. J Neurosurg. 1999;90(3):443–7. https://doi.org/10.3171/jns.1999.90.3.0443.
3. Wenger TL, Hing AV, Evans KN. Apert Syndrome. In: GeneReviews. Seattle: University of Washington; 2019. PMID: 31145570.
4. Varlas VN, Epistatu D, Varlas RG. Emphasis on early prenatal diagnosis and perinatal outcomes analysis of Apert syndrome. Diagnostics. 2024;14(14):1480. https://doi.org/10.3390/diagnostics14141480.
5. OMIM (Online Mendelian Inheritance in Man). 2024. Available at: https://www.omim.org/entry/101200?search=Aperts%20Syndrome&highlight=%28syndrome%7Csyndromic%29%2Capert.
6. Wilkie AO, Slaney SF, Oldridge M, Poole MD, Ashworth GJ, Hockley AD, Hayward RD, David DJ, Pulleyn LJ, Rutland P, et al. Apert syndrome results from localized mutations of FGFR2 and is allelic with Crouzon syndrome. Nat Genet. 1995;9(2):165–72. https://doi.org/10.1038/ng0295-165.
7. Fearon JA, Podner C. Apert syndrome: evaluation of a treatment algorithm. Plast Reconstr Surg. 2013;131(1):132–42. https://doi.org/10.1097/PRS.0b013e3182729f42.
8. Liu C, Cui Y, Luan J, Zhou X, Han J. The molecular and cellular basis of Apert syndrome. Intractable Rare Dis Res. 2013;2:115–22. https://doi.org/10.5582/irdr.2013.v2.4.115.
9. Hilton C. An exploration of the cognitive, physical and psychosocial development of children with Apert syndrome. Int J Disabil Dev Edu. 2017;64(2):198–210. https://doi.org/10.1080/1034912X.2016.1194379.
10. ACPA (American Cleft Palate-Craniofacial Association). Help with social situations. 2018. Available at: https://acpacares.org/wp-content/uploads/2023/01/Social-Situations_2018-factsheet_web-1.pdf.
11. Sarimski K. Children with Apert syndrome: behavioural problems and family stress. Dev Med Child Neurol. 1998;40(1):44–9. https://doi.org/10.1111/j.1469-8749.1998.tb15355.x.
12. Sarimski K. Social adjustment of children with a severe craniofacial anomaly (Apert syndrome). Child Care Health Dev. 2001;27(6):583–90. https://doi.org/10.1046/j.1365-2214.2001.00224.x.
13. van der Vlugt JJB, van der Meulen JJNM, Creemers HE, Willemse SP, Lequin ML, Okkerse JME. The risk of psychopathology in children with craniosynostosis. Plast Reconstr Surg. 2009;124(6):2054–60. https://doi.org/10.1097/PRS.0b013e3181bcf2dc.
14. Bannink N, Maliepaard M, Raat H, Joosten KF, Mathijssen IM. Health-related quality of life in children and adolescents with syndromic craniosynostosis. J Plast Reconstr Aesthet Surg. 2010;63(12):1972–81. https://doi.org/10.1016/j.bjps.2010.01.036.
15. Maliepaard M, Mathijssen IM, Oosterlaan J, Okkerse JM. Intellectual, behavioral, and emotional functioning in children with syndromic craniosynos-

tosis. Pediatrics. 2014;133(6):e1608–15. https://doi.org/10.1542/peds.2013-3077.
16. Lefebvre A, Travis F, Arndt EM, Munro IR. A psychiatric profile before and after reconstructive surgery in children with Apert's syndrome. Br J Plast Surg. 1986;39(4):510–3. https://doi.org/10.1016/0007-1226(86)90122-0.
17. Doerga PN, Rijken BFM, Bredero-Boelhouwer H, Joosten KFM, Neuteboom RF, Tasker RC, Dremmen MHG, Lequin MH, van Veelen MLC, Mathijssen IMJ. Neurological deficits are present in syndromic craniosynostosis patients with and without tonsillar herniation. Eur J Paediatr Neurol. 2020;28:120–5. https://doi.org/10.1016/j.ejpn.2020.06.018.
18. Shipster C, Hearst D, Dockrell JE, Kilby E, Hayward R. Speech and language skills and cognitive functioning in children with Apert syndrome: a pilot study. Int J Lang Commun Disord. 2002;37(3):325–43. https://doi.org/10.1080/13682820210138816.
19. Fearon JA. Treatment of the hands and feet in Apert syndrome: an evolution in management. Plast Reconstr Surg. 2003;112(1):1–19. https://doi.org/10.1097/01.PRS.0000065908.60382.17.
20. Stauffer A, Farr S. Is the Apert foot an overlooked aspect of this rare genetic disease? Clinical findings and treatment options for foot deformities in Apert syndrome. BMC Musculoskelet Disord. 2020;21(1):788. https://doi.org/10.1186/s12891-020-03812-2.
21. Mason WH, Wymore M, Berger E. Foot deformities in Apert's syndrome. Review of the literature and case reports. J Am Podiatr Med Assoc. 1990;80(10):540–4. https://doi.org/10.7547/87507315-80-10-540.
22. Hilton C. A longitudinal study of the role of fingers in the development of early number and arithmetic skills in children with Apert syndrome. J Anat. 2024; online ahead of print. https://doi.org/10.1111/joa.14111.
23. Rostamzad P, Arslan ZF, Mathijssen IMJ, Koudstaal MJ, Pleumeekers MM, Versnel SL, Loudon SE. Prevalence of ocular anomalies in craniosynostosis: a systematic review and meta-analysis. J Clin Med. 2022;11(4):1060. https://doi.org/10.3390/jcm11041060.
24. le Clercq CMP, Labuschagne LJE, Franken MJP, de Jong RJB, Luijk MPCM, Jansen PW, van der Schroeff MP. Association of slight to mild hearing loss with behavioral problems and school performance in children. JAMA Otolaryngol Head Neck Surg. 2020;146(2):113–20. https://doi.org/10.1001/jamaoto.2019.3585.
25. Stevenson J, Kreppner J, Pimperton H, Worsfold S, Kennedy C. Emotional and behavioural difficulties in children and adolescents with hearing impairment: a systematic review and meta-analysis. Eur Child Adolesc Psychiatry. 2015;24(5):477–96. https://doi.org/10.1007/s00787-015-0697-1.
26. Lee YH, Repka MX, Borlik MF, Velez FG, Perez C, Yu F, Coleman AL, Pineles SL. Association of strabismus with mood disorders, schizophrenia, and anxiety disorders among children. JAMA Ophthalmol. 2022;140(4):373–81. https://doi.org/10.1001/jamaophthalmol.2022.0137.
27. Ong JJ, Smith L, Shepherd DA, Xu J, Roberts G, Sung V. Emotional behavioral outcomes of children with unilateral and mild hearing loss. Front Pediatr. 2023;11:1209736. https://doi.org/10.3389/fped.2023.1209736.
28. Huang TL, Pineles SL. Strabismus and pediatric psychiatric illness: a literature review. Children (Basel). 2023;10(4):607. https://doi.org/10.3390/children10040607.
29. Feragen KJB, Myhre A, Stock NM. "Will you still feel beautiful when you find out you are different?": parents' experiences, reflections, and appearance-focused conversations about their child's visible difference. Qual Health Res. 2022;32(1):3–15. https://doi.org/10.1177/10497323211039205.
30. Netherton J, Horton J, Stock NM, Shaw R, Noons P, Evans MJ. Psychological adjustment in Apert syndrome: parent and young person perspectives. Cleft Palate Craniofac J. 2023;60(4):461–73. https://doi.org/10.1177/10556656211069817.
31. Johns AL, Stock NM, Costa B, Feragen KB, Crerand CE. Psychosocial and health-related experiences of individuals with microtia and craniofacial microsomia and their families: narrative review over 2 decades. Cleft Palate Craniofac J. 2023;60(9):1090–112. https://doi.org/10.1177/10556656221091699.
32. Kapp-Simon KA, Simon DJ, Kristovich S. Self-perception, social skills, adjustment, and inhibition in young adolescents with craniofacial anomalies. Cleft Palate Craniofac J. 1992;29:352–6. https://doi.org/10.1597/1545-1569_1992_029_0352_spssaa_2.3.co_2.
33. Pope AW, Ward J. Self-perceived facial appearance and psychosocial adjustment in preadolescents with craniofacial anomalies. Cleft Palate Craniofac J. 1997;34(5):396–401.
34. Feragen KB, Stock NM. A longitudinal study of 340 young people with or without a visible difference: the impact of teasing on self-perceptions of appearance and depressive symptoms. Body Image. 2016;16:133–42.
35. Stock NM, Costa B, Parnell J, Johns AL, Crerand CE, Feragen KB, Stueckle LP, Mills A, Magee L, Hotton M, Tumblin M, Schefer A, Drake AF, Heike CL. A conceptual thematic framework of psychological adjustment in caregivers of children with craniofacial microsomia. Cleft Palate Craniofac J. 2024; online ahead of print. https://doi.org/10.1177/10556656241124528.
36. Fitzsimons K, Deacon SA, Copley LP, Park MH, Medina J, van der Meulen JH. School absence and achievement in children with isolated orofacial clefts. Arch Dis Childhood. 2021;106(2):154–9. https://doi.org/10.1136/archdischild-2020-319123.

37. Myhre A, Agai M, Dundas I, Feragen KB. "All Eyes on Me": a qualitative study of parent and patient experiences of multidisciplinary care in craniofacial conditions. Cleft Palate Craniofac J. 2019;56(9):1187–94. https://doi.org/10.1177/1055665619842730.
38. Myhre A, Rabu M, Feragen KB. The need to belong: subjective experiences of living with craniofacial conditions and undergoing appearance-altering surgery. Body Image. 2021;38:334–45. https://doi.org/10.1016/j.bodyim.2021.05.008.
39. Crerand CE, Feragen KB, Johns AL, Umbaugh H, McClinchie M, Drake AF, Heike CL, Yi-Frazier JP, Stock NM. Pediatric medical traumatic stress in individuals with craniofacial conditions. ASHA Perspect SIG 5. 2024;9(3):570–81. https://doi.org/10.1044/2024_PERSP-23-00236.
40. Bates A, Forrester-Jones R, McCarthy M. Specialist hospital treatment and care as reported by children with intellectual disabilities and a cleft lip and/or palate, their parents and healthcare professionals. J Appl Res Intellec Disabil. 2020;33(2):283–95. https://doi.org/10.1111/jar.12672.
41. Kapp-Simon KA, Edwards T, Ruta C, Bellucci CC, Aspinall CL, Strauss RP, Topolski TD, Rumsey NJ, Patrick DL. Shared surgical decision making and youth resilience correlates of satisfaction with clinical outcomes. J Craniofac Surg. 2015;26(5):1574–80. https://doi.org/10.1097/SCS.0000000000001892.
42. McWilliams D, Thornton M, Hotton M, Swan MC, Stock NM. "It's On Your Shoulders Now" transitioning from child-to-adult UK Cleft Lip/Palate Services: an exploration of young adults' narratives. Cleft Palate Craniofac J. 2024; online ahead of print. https://doi.org/10.1177/10556656241236006.
43. von der Lippe C, Diesen PS, Feragen KB. Living with a rare disorder: a systematic review of the qualitative literature. Mol Genet Genomic Med. 2017;5(6):758–73. https://doi.org/10.1002/mgg3.315.
44. Stock NM, Costa B, Wilkinson-Bell K, Culshaw L, Kearney A, Edwards W. Psychological and physical health outcomes in adults with craniosynostosis. Cleft Palate Craniofac J. 2023;60(3):257–67. https://doi.org/10.1177/10556656211059966.
45. Tovetjärn R, Tarnow P, Maltese G, Fischer S, Sahlin PE, Kölby L. Children with Apert syndrome as adults: a follow-up study of 28 Scandinavian patients. Plast Reconstr Surg. 2012;130(4):572e–6e. https://doi.org/10.1097/PRS.0b013e318262f355.
46. Roberts RM, Mathias JL. Predictors of mental health in adults with congenital craniofacial conditions attending the Australian craniofacial unit. Cleft Palate Craniofac J. 2013;50(4):414–23. https://doi.org/10.1597/11-105.
47. McAllister M, Davies L, Payne K, Nicholls S, Donnai D, MacLeod R. The emotional effects of genetic diseases: implications for clinical genetics. Am J Med Genet. 2007;143A:2651–61. https://doi.org/10.1002/ajmg.a.32013.
48. Beaune L, Forrest CR, Keith T. Adolescents' perspectives on living and growing up with Treacher Collins syndrome: a qualitative study. Cleft Palate Craniofac J. 2004;41(4):343–50. https://doi.org/10.1597/02-158.1.
49. Stock NM, Feragen KB, Rumsey N. Adults' narratives of growing up with a cleft lip and/or palate: factors associated with psychological adjustment. Cleft Palate Craniofac J. 2016;53(2):222–39. https://doi.org/10.1597/14-269.
50. Strauss RP. "Only skin deep": health, resilience, and craniofacial care. Cleft Palate Craniofac J. 2001;38(3):226–30. https://doi.org/10.1597/1545-1569_2001_038_0226_osdhra_2.0.co_2.
51. Cousino MK, Hazen RA. Parenting stress among caregivers of children with chronic illness: a systematic review. J Pediatr Psychol. 2013;38(8):809–28. https://doi.org/10.1093/jpepsy/jst049.
52. Masefield SC, Prady SL, Sheldon TA, Small N, Jarvis S, Pickett KE. The caregiver health effects of caring for young children with developmental disabilities: a meta-analysis. Matern Child Health J. 2020;24(5):561–74. https://doi.org/10.1007/s10995-020-02896-5.
53. Stock NM, Blaso D, Hotton M. Caring for a child with a cleft lip and/or palate: a narrative review. Cleft Palate Craniofac J. 2024; online ahead of print. https://doi.org/10.1177/10556656241280071.
54. von der Lippe C, Neteland I, Feragen KB. Children with a rare congenital genetic disorder: a systematic review of parent experiences. Orphanet J Rare Dis. 2022;17(1):375. https://doi.org/10.1186/s13023-022-02525-0.
55. Costa B, Edwards W, Wilkinson-Bell K, Stock NM. Raising a child with craniosynostosis: psychosocial adjustment in caregivers. Cleft Palate Craniofac J. 2023;60(10):1284–97. https://doi.org/10.1177/10556656221102043.
56. Feragen KB, Stock NM, Myhre A, Due-Tonnessen BJ. Medical stress reactions and personal growth in parents of children with a rare craniofacial condition. Cleft Palate Craniofac J. 2020;57(2):228–37. https://doi.org/10.1177/1055665619869146.
57. Feragen KB, Stock NM. Psychological adjustment to craniofacial conditions (excluding oral clefts): a review of the literature. Psychol Health. 2017;32(3):253–88. https://doi.org/10.1080/08870446.2016.1247838.
58. Zeytinoğlu Saydam S, Çüçülayef MA, Doğan TN, Crerand CE, Özek M. Social experiences of Turkish parents raising a child with Apert syndrome: a qualitative study. Cleft Palate Craniofac J. 2021;58(3):354–61. https://doi.org/10.1177/1055665620944761.
59. Klein T, Pope AW, Getahun E, Thompson J. Mothers' reflections on raising a child with a craniofacial anomaly. Cleft Palate Craniofac J. 2006;43(5):590–7. https://doi.org/10.1597/05-117.

60. Cohn LN, Pechlivanoglou P, Lee Y, Mahant S, Orkin J, Marson A, Cohen E. Health outcomes of parents of children with chronic illness: a systematic review and meta-analysis. J Pediatr. 2020;218:166–177.e2.
61. Bayer ND, Wang H, Yu JA, Kuo DZ, Halterman JS, Li Y. A national mental health profile of parents of children with medical complexity. Pediatrics. 2021;148(2):e2020023358.
62. Walsh F. Family resilience: a developmental systems framework. Eur J Dev Psychol. 2016;13:1–12.
63. ACPA (American Cleft Palate-Craniofacial Association). Parameters for evaluation and treatment of patients with cleft lip/palate or other craniofacial differences. Cleft Palate Craniofac J. 2018;55(1):137–56. https://doi.org/10.1177/1055665617739564.
64. Mathijssen IMJ. Updated guideline on treatment and management of craniosynostosis. J Craniofac Surg. 2020;4(32):371–450. https://doi.org/10.1097/SCS.0000000000007035.
65. Hotton M, Cropper J, Rundle J, Crawford R. The role of the clinical psychologist within a cleft service. Br Dent J. 2023;234:887–91. https://doi.org/10.1038/s41415-023-5952-0.
66. Norman A, Persson M, Stock NM, Rumsey N, Sandy J, Waylen A, Edwards Z, Hammond V, Partridge L, Ness A. The effectiveness of psychosocial intervention for individuals with cleft lip and/or palate. Cleft Palate Craniofac J. 2015;52(3):301–10. https://doi.org/10.1597/13-276.
67. Waite E, Jenkinson E, Kershaw S, Guest E. Psychosocial interventions for children and young people with visible differences resulting from appearance-altering conditions, injury, or treatment effects: an updated systematic review. J Pediatric Psychol. 2024;49(1):77–88. https://doi.org/10.1093/jpepsy/jsad080.
68. Kapp-Simon KA. Psychological interventions for the adolescent with cleft lip and palate. Cleft Palate Craniofac J. 1995;32(2):104–8. https://doi.org/10.1597/1545-1569_1995_032_0104_piftaw_2.3.co_2.
69. Clarke A, Thompson A, Jenkinson E, Rumsey N, Newell R. CBT for appearance anxiety: psychosocial interventions for anxiety due to visible difference. London: John Wiley & Sons, Ltd; 2013.
70. Bessell A, Brough V, Clarke A, Harcourt D, Moss TP, Rumsey N. Evaluation of the effectiveness of Face IT: a computer-based psychosocial intervention for disfigurement-related distress. Psychol Health Med. 2012;17(5):565–77. https://doi.org/10.1080/13548506.2011.647701.
71. Williamson H, Hamlet C, White P, Marques EMR, Cadogan J, Perera R, Rumsey N, Hayward L, Harcourt D. Study protocol of the YP Face IT feasibility study: comparing an online psychosocial intervention versus treatment as usual for adolescents distressed by appearance-altering conditions/injuries. BMJ Open. 2016;6:e012423. https://doi.org/10.1136/bmjopen-2016-012423.
72. Rosenberg AR, Yi-Frazier JP, Eaton L, et al. Promoting resilience in stress management: a pilot study of a novel resilience-promoting intervention for adolescents and young adults with serious illness. J Pediatr Psychol. 2015;40(9):992–9. https://doi.org/10.1093/jpepsy/jsv004.
73. Yi-Frazier JP, Fladeboe K, Klein V, et al. Promoting resilience in stress management for parents (PRISM-P): an intervention for caregivers of youth with serious illness. Fam Syst Health. 2017;35(3):341. https://doi.org/10.1037/fsh0000281.
74. Fladeboe KM, Stock NM, Heike CL, Evans KN, Junkins C, Stueckle L, O'Daffer A, Rosenberg AR, Yi-Frazier JP. Feasibility and acceptability of the promoting resilience in stress management-parent (PRISM-P) intervention for caregivers of children with craniofacial conditions. Cleft Palate Craniofac J. 2024;61(7):1125–33. https://doi.org/10.1177/10556656231157449.
75. Pidgeon TE, Blore CD, Webb Y, Horton J, Evans M. A patient information leaflet reduces parental anxiety before their child's first craniofacial multidisciplinary outpatient appointment. J Craniofac Surg. 2017;28(7):1772–6. https://doi.org/10.1097/SCS.0000000000003955.
76. Millgard M, Myhre A, Due-Tonnessen BJ, Feragen KB. Parents' Perception of the benefit of receiving a patient information leaflet prior to attending a craniofacial multidisciplinary team appointment. Cleft Palate Craniofac J. 2023; online ahead of print. https://doi.org/10.1177/10556656231219579.
77. Stock NM, Kearney A, Horton J, Pearse L, O'Driscoll M, Murfett L, Hilton C, Pearse K, Wilkinson-Bell K. A booklet to promote psychological health in new families affected by craniosynostosis. J Craniofac Surg. 2022;33(6):1670–3. https://doi.org/10.1097/SCS.0000000000008454.
78. Stock NM, Costa B, Bannister W, Ashby C, Matthews N, Hebden L, Melles L, Hilton-Webb Z, Smith S, Kane K, Carter L, Kearney A, Piggott K, Russell C, Wilkinson-Bell K. "When I was Younger, My Story Belonged to Everyone Else": co-production of resources for adults living with craniosynostosis. Cleft Palate Craniofac J. 2024; online ahead of print. https://doi.org/10.1177/10556656241236580.
79. Searle A, Neville P, Ryan S, Waylen A. The role of the clinical nurse specialist from the perspective of parents of children born with cleft lip and/or palate in the United Kingdom: a qualitative study. Clin Nurse Spec. 2018;32(3):121–8. https://doi.org/10.1097/NUR.0000000000000371.
80. Stock NM, Guest E, Stoneman K, Ridley M, Evans C, LeRoy C, Anwar H, McCarthy G,

Cunniffe C, Rumsey N. The contribution of a charitable organization to regional cleft lip and palate services in England and Scotland. Cleft Palate Craniofac J. 2020;57(1):14–20. https://doi.org/10.1177/1055665619862727.
81. Dawson S, Devine MA. The effect of a residential camp experience on self-esteem and social acceptance of youth with craniofacial differences. Ther Recreat J. 2010;44(2):105–20.
82. Bogart K, Hemmesch A. Benefits of support conferences for parents of and people with Moebius syndrome. Stigma Health. 2015;1(2):109–21. https://doi.org/10.1037/sah0000018.
83. Ardouin K, Davis N, Stock NM. Expanding support services for adults born with cleft lip and/or palate in the United Kingdom: an exploratory evaluation of the cleft lip and palate association adult services programme. Cleft Palate Craniofac J. 2022;59(4_suppl2):S48–56. https://doi.org/10.1177/10556656211025415.
84. Stock NM, Marik P, Magee L, Aspinall CL, Garcia L, Crerand CE, Johns AL. Facilitating positive psychosocial outcomes in craniofacial team care: strategies for medical providers. Cleft Palate Craniofac J. 2020;57(3):333–43. https://doi.org/10.1177/1055665619868052.
85. Achenbach TM. The Achenbach System of Empirically Based Assessment (ASEBA): development, findings, theory, and applications. Burlington, VT: University of Vermont Research Center for Children, Youth & Families; 2009. Available at: http://www.aseba.org.
86. Goodman R. The strengths and difficulties questionnaire. 2001. Available at: https://www.sdqinfo.org/a0.html.
87. Varni JW. Pediatric Quality of Life measures. Available at: https://eprovide.mapi-trust.org/instruments/pediatric-quality-of-life-inventory.
88. Klassen A, Wong K. FACE-Q Available at: https://qportfolio.org/face-q/craniofacial.
89. Crerand CE, Kapa HM, Litteral J, Pearson GD, Eastman K, Kirschner RE. Identifying psychosocial risk factors among families of children with craniofacial conditions: validation of the psychosocial assessment tool-craniofacial version. Cleft Palate Craniofac J. 2018;55(4):536–45. https://doi.org/10.1177/1055665617748010. Available at: https://www.psychosocialassessmenttool.org.
90. Waite J, Heald M, Wilde L, Woodcock K, Welham A, Adams D, Oliver C. The importance of understanding the behavioural phenotypes of genetic syndromes associated with intellectual disability. Paediatr Child Health. 2014;24(10):468–72. https://doi.org/10.1016/j.paed.2014.05.002.
91. Cassidy SB, Morris CA. Behavioral phenotypes in genetic syndromes: genetic clues to human behavior. Adv Pediatr Infect Dis. 2002;49:59–86.
92. Moldavsky M, Lev D, Lerman-Sagie T. Behavioral phenotypes of genetic syndromes: a reference guide for psychiatrists. J Am Acad Child Adol Psychiatr. 2001;40(7):749–61. https://doi.org/10.1097/00004583-200107000-00009.
93. O'Brien G. Behavioural phenotypes. J Res Soc Med. 2000;93(12):618–20. https://doi.org/10.1177/014107680009301204.
94. Riby DM, Kirk H, Hanley M, Riby LM. Stranger danger. J Intellect Disabil Res. 2014;58:572–82. https://doi.org/10.1111/jir.12055.
95. Fisher MH. Evaluation of a stranger safety training programme for adults with Williams syndrome. J Intellect Disabil Res. 2014;58(10):903–14. https://doi.org/10.1111/jir.12108.
96. Feeley KM, Jones EA. Addressing challenging behaviour in children with Down syndrome: the use of applied behaviour analysis for assessment and intervention. Downs Syndr Res Pract. 2006;11(2):64–77. https://doi.org/10.3104/perspectives.316.
97. Ho AY, Dimitropoulos A. Clinical management of behavioral characteristics of Prader-Willi syndrome. Neuropsychiatr Dis Treat. 2010;6:107–18. https://doi.org/10.2147/ndt.s5560.
98. Thom RP. Psychiatric and behavioral manifestations of Williams syndrome. Curr Opin Psychiatry. 2024;37(2):65–70. https://doi.org/10.1097/YCO.0000000000000914.
99. Stock NM, Feragen KB, Rumsey N. Toward a conceptual and methodological shift in craniofacial research. Cleft Palate Craniofac J. 2018;55(1):105–11. https://doi.org/10.1177/1055665617721925.
100. Speltz ML, Galbreath H, Greenberg MT. A developmental framework for psychosocial research on young children with craniofacial anomalies. In: Eder RA, editor. Craniofacial anomalies. New York: Springer; 1995.
101. Squires J, Bricker D. Ages and Stages Questionnaire (ASQ): a parent completed child monitoring system. 3rd ed. Brooks Publishing Company; 2009.
102. Harrison PL, Oakland T. Adaptive behavior assessment system (Third Edition). 2015. Available at: https://link.springer.com/referenceworkentry/10.1007/978-3-319-57111-9_1506.
103. Gartstein MA, Prokasky A, Bell MA, Calkins S, Bridgett DJ, Braungart-Rieker J, Leerkes E, Cheatham CL, Eiden RD, Mize KD, Jones NA, Mireault G, Seamon E. Latent profile and cluster analysis of infant temperament: comparisons across person-centered approaches. Dev Psychol. 2017;53(10):1811–25. https://doi.org/10.1037/dev0000382.

35 Living with Apert Syndrome: Patient Perspectives

Madelyn Mulreaney, Alicia Potter, and Dionna Santucci

Introduction

In this chapter, individuals with Apert syndrome share their diverse experiences and perspectives on life with the rare diagnosis. The authors interviewed eight people with Apert syndrome who have lived in eight different countries and range in age from 18 to 57. The interviews took place from October 2024 to April 2025 and are lightly edited for clarity and length.

Interview participants were identified through either digital media coverage or referrals from surgeons affiliated with this textbook. Patients referred by our editors or contributors were assured they could speak openly about their experiences with affiliated hospitals and doctors, without affecting their care or relationship with the medical team.

Though informed by qualitative research, this chapter takes a journalistic approach. Each of its four main sections begins with accounts from the individual's childhood, followed by topics such as medical treatment, education, and family life. Long-form interview excerpts preserve the individuals' voices. In their own words, the people with Apert syndrome share their struggles and joys, offering ways to increase understanding and improve care. Shorter profiles presented in this chapter feature excerpts from interviews conducted with an interpreter.

Particularly noteworthy may be content that explores the challenges of transitioning to adult healthcare and the desire to defy expectations and misjudgments. Almost all the narratives underscore the critical role of allies and advocates, whether a parent, teacher, or sibling. Taken together, the interviews drive home an essential insight: while people with Apert syndrome may share common experiences, they are highly unique individuals who regard their diagnosis as only one part of their identities.

As authors without craniofacial or other appearance differences, we recognize that our criteria for selecting interview excerpts are not informed by lived experience and may reflect biases. To help mitigate this possibility, the individuals reviewed their sections before publication. In addition, we did not redact language that could be considered offensive or atypical for an academic text, including profanity, slang, or slurs. We chose to keep such content to avoid misrepresenting the people interviewed and to retain the authenticity of their responses. As a result, the interviews fully express the individual's perspective on life with a rare diagnosis—one that notably causes visible differences and requires intensive, years-long medical care.

M. Mulreaney · A. Potter (✉) · D. Santucci
Department of Plastic and Oral Surgery,
Boston Children's Hospital, Boston, MA, USA
e-mail: Alicia.Potter@childrens.harvard.edu

J. G. Meara et al. (eds.), *Apert Syndrome*, https://doi.org/10.1007/978-3-032-12551-4_35

Angelica and Marco Garcia

City of Manila, Philippines
Guadalajara, Mexico
Salt Lake City, Utah, United States

Angelica Garcia was born in Manila, the Philippines, in 1992. When she was 9, she and her family moved to Orange County, California. She later attended college at Brigham Young University-Idaho. Marco Garcia was born in Guadalajara, Mexico, in 1982. At age 10, he moved with his family to Southern Texas, going on to study at the University of Texas at Brownsville. Angelica and Marco met on Facebook in 2016 and have been married for the last eight years (Fig. 35.1). They now live in Salt Lake City, Utah, with their 5-year-old daughter Mina, who also has Apert syndrome. Marco works as a home health aide and support staff member for a nonprofit organization that provides transitional assistance to individuals with barriers to employment. Angelica is a thrift store associate at Deseret Industries and serves on the Head Start Advantage Policy Council at Mina's preschool.

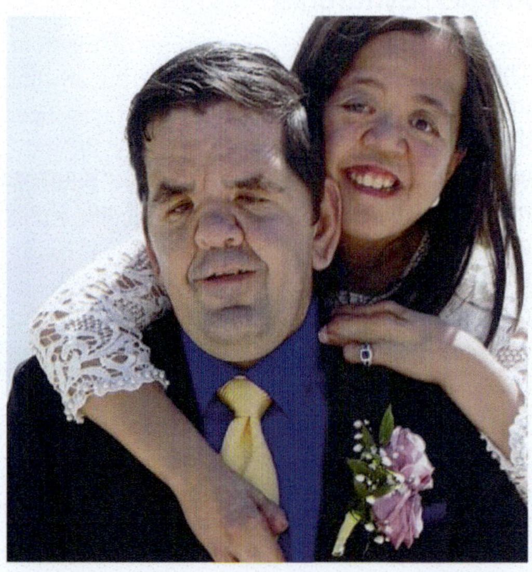

Fig. 35.1 Marco and Angelica on their wedding day

Early Lives

Angelica: When I was born, there was the theory that I would not live long. But I was blessed to be born into the family that I was, because my great-uncle is a doctor. He's a pediatrician, and so I had a very stable, secure, and helpful doctor. My great-uncle knew a surgeon who could operate on my hands and was able to set it up. When I was 6 years old, I had surgery to separate my pinkies and thumbs.

After preschool, my mother tried to enroll me in my older sister's Catholic private school. And they said, "Your daughter doesn't belong here. Your daughter belongs in a mental institution, because she has Apert syndrome." My mother, through her tears, spoke up for herself and said, "My daughter is very, very smart. She can do things. She can learn." But it didn't work out going to that school. We then applied for me to go to kindergarten at this other private Catholic school, St. Joseph's College. The principal felt empathy for me, and she gave me a chance. I was able to attend kindergarten (Fig. 35.2) through, I want to say, fifth grade. The rest of the St. Joseph's experience was very positive. I had my true friends, my inner circle.

Marco: Did I know that I grew up with a disability? I did. But until third grade I didn't know what it was called. I asked my mom, and she was like, "Well, they did tell me in the hospital, but I never told you because of the way that I treated you." I grew up with four brothers and obviously my parents. And one thing that I loved about growing up in my family was that they never really talked about Apert syndrome.

My brothers would say, "Hey, Marco! We ride bikes. You're going to ride a bike." Or "We play sports, you play sports." The same with my cousins. "We're going to go run, let's go run!" I'm very athletic, and I do what I can and I'm content with that. But my brothers and cousins were like, "We're not going to feel sorry for you, because we know what you can do. We know what you're capable of."

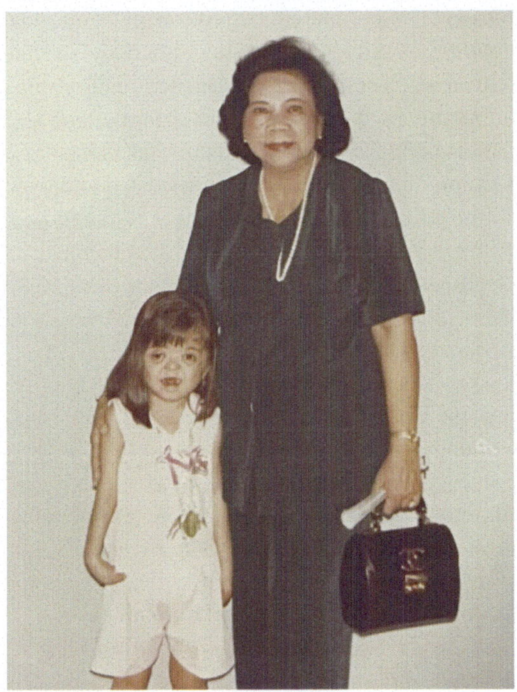

Fig. 35.2 Angelica at her kindergarten graduation with her late grandmother, Lory

Angelica: My American education started in third grade, though I was pretty sure that I had done third grade in the Philippines. My elementary school was so much fun! My class had a "Welcome, Angelica!" morning. They literally had that written in their agenda. My two classmates—both of whom I'm still friends with to this day—took me on a tour of the elementary school campus. And there was this lunch lady. She came up to me and said, "Angelica, my name is Sally. I just wanted you to know, first of all, welcome. And, second of all, if you need me to open anything, please feel free to ask me, and I will open it for you every single time." Obviously, that not only made my day but my elementary school experience.

Middle school was fun too. My first sixth-grade dance was then, and I was so excited. I don't know why, but I was making funny faces, and they photographed my face like that and put it in the yearbook. But I thought, Okay, it's just a sixth-grade kind of thing. I was laughing at it.

Moving to the United States

Marco: My mother is a certified teacher in a foreign language, and that language is English. What really ticked her off when we got to the United States was that my school placed me in special [education]. They said we can't place him in second-grade or third-grade general ed because, in a word, he's "retarded." *[Ed. Note: Marco's mother later succeeds in overturning the placement.]* Once that happened, my actual scholastic school year started. I had a better IEP (Individualized Education Program) and more understanding teachers.

There was some harsh bullying, though. Fifth-graders, being loud, would be like, "Hey, guys, look at Marco!" I'd be like, Why is everybody laughing at me? But I survived it. I don't look back on it. Eventually, I played sports in middle and high school, graduating at 19.

Defying Expectations

Angelica: My IEP case carrier in high school made assumptions about my future. He was like, "We're going to have you graduate not with a high school diploma but a secondary certificate and have you go to two years of community college." I know there's nothing wrong with that, but I felt like he was putting me in a box. I was like, No, I want to go to college. I want to do the traditional high school junior, senior experiences, and then graduate with a diploma and go to college. So at the end of my sophomore year, going into junior year, I turned 18 and I was an adult. I took over my IEP. I said, We're going to take impressive and rigorous classes during the last two years of high school! I got all the credits I needed and graduated with a diploma, and right off the bat, I got my college acceptance to Brigham Young University-Idaho.

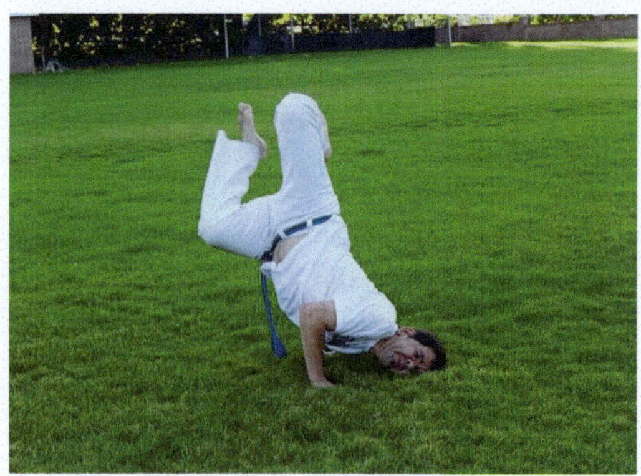

Fig. 35.3 Marco practicing a capoeira move

Marco: I started practicing the Brazilian martial art capoeira as a college student back in Texas. When I first began, it was like, Can he do it? I was like, Can I try? When I moved here [in 2012], I already knew enough moves to get my third belt. My teacher was even surprised. Now sometimes I teach beginners the basic moves. I tell the other students, "No mercy!" before we start, because I don't want that. I'm on my fourth belt (Fig. 35.3).

I take it very tragically that some of the drivers [at my workplace], if they don't know me, think I live in the group home where I work. Or when they drop me off, they see an older lady or somebody much older, and they're like, "Okay, Marco, there's your mom waiting for you!" It's my neighbor. My neighbor will be like, "Wait, what? You called me his mom?" I've told them repeatedly, I live here, I work *there.* Not the other way around.

Because people see me with the disability that I have, they don't think I can stand up for myself. And that's been the case since, I want to say, fifth grade.

How They Met

Marco: I don't friend people on Facebook unless I know them. But I saw Angie and thought, She's cute.

Angelica: We became Facebook friends in June 2016.

Marco: From June to August—it took me that long to write a post about somebody special and ask her for a long-distance relationship. At this point, she lived in California, and she was studying at BYU-Idaho and in her last semester. So we dated—cyber-dated and over the phone. But in January, she was like, If you want to continue this, we've got to meet in person to make sure we're not catfishing.

Angelica: Do it the right way.

Marco: Do it the right way. So on January 11 or the day before, we were talking late at night.

Angelica: It was the night before the opening social for the Political Affairs Society, an organization I was in at my college. We were about to host a breakfast-for-dinner event.

Marco: And she's like, Crap, we don't have a griddle. So here I am with the love of my life. We hung up around eleven o'clock. I ran to Walmart, back when it was open to two, three, four in the morning. I get a griddle. Then I caught the bus that morning from Salt Lake City to Rexburg. *[Ed. Note: BYU-Idaho is in Rexburg, Idaho, 240 miles away.]*

When we hit Idaho Falls, it was white [with snow] and really cold. We were going slow because the roads were icy. There weren't that many passengers, so I told the bus driver our love story. And he was like, You're bringing a griddle from Salt Lake City to Rexburg just because your girlfriend needs one? I said yeah. The bus driver was like, That's true love.

Angelica: It was around 35 degrees. But I was numb with happiness and in awe that we were finally doing this. There was that tingly feeling of I'm finally meeting this guy! This guy who I said "I love you" to on New Year's Eve. I was in awe but not necessarily in disbelief—more contentment. Marco got off the bus and he kissed me. I was like, Wow! Wow! We're meeting and we've kissed! And, yes, he has a griddle. That night, we went to the opening social and essentially had our first date.

Seeing the Spectrum

Angelica: The one thing that we can say that is crucial is there is a spectrum of people with Apert syndrome—from the people with Apert syndrome who are low-functioning to the people with Apert syndrome who are high-functioning. We'd like to emphasize that the differences matter and are beautiful, and everyone matters, while being realistic about what everyone can do. There's a huge diversity within the Apert syndrome community—personal, economic, and cultural—and different kinds of beliefs and upbringings. We are not all the same. We are not all like cookie-cutter molding. I think that's important to highlight, because I feel like there is a societal stigma that since we all have the same syndrome, we are all basically the same. Marco and I are married, we have the same syndrome, and we're made for each other. But there are as many distinct opposites in us as there are similarities.

I wish people, like parents, would be more actively engaged and proactive to realistically help their child plan for their life. It's possible for higher-functioning people with Apert syndrome to think not only about the present but also their future. It's okay to be taken care of in a group home, but it's also beautiful to be able to live as independently as we can (Fig. 35.4).

Marco: For me, it goes back to one of my favorite movies: "Coach Carter," a basketball movie with a kid who's Hispanic. He asks, "What is our deepest fear?" He says it's not that people fear they are inadequate. It's that they fear they are powerful beyond measure. I like that quote because it's like life. It speaks to people with Apert syndrome who want to grow. It's a better way to look at it.

To read about Angelica and Marco's parenting experiences and advocacy work, see Chap. 36: *Caring for a Child with Apert Syndrome: Family Perspectives, Advocacy, and Support.*

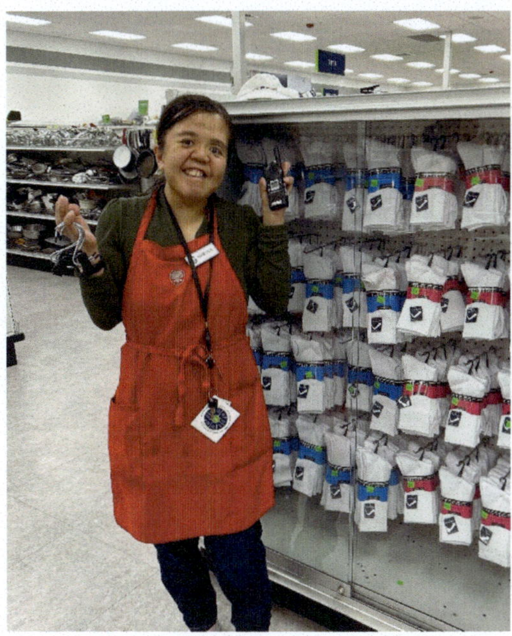

Fig. 35.4 Angelica working the New Value case at her local Deseret Industries thrift store

Mebin
Age: 18
Kerala, India

My parents told me that they were unaware about my condition 'til after my birth. The diagnosis of Apert syndrome was made later. My growth milestones were delayed, as I started walking at 2 years of age. Speech was delayed, too, and was difficult as I had a cleft palate, but after the first surgery my speech improved. Because of my fused fingers, I used to use both hands for writing and drawing. Over years after multiple finger surgeries, I started primary school [two years late] at 7 years [old]. All the teachers in school were very supportive, and they encouraged my parents to admit me in normal school instead [of] special needs school. But probably due to my appearance and way I spoke, I did not have many friends growing up.

(continued)

The happiest moment in my life was when I passed tenth grade with good marks, and my fight against odds to achieve the merit was published in the newspaper. Currently, I'm in eleventh standard of higher secondary school. I live with my parents and brothers. I love watching TV dramas and cycling. I'm still exploring my interests to pursue my higher education after finishing school.

Commentary from Mebin's father: I counsel parents of children with Apert syndrome. A primary problem in our country is parents abandon syndromic children. We know a family from our village who has a syndromic kid. Even after explaining multiple times and sharing our experiences, we could not get them to care for the child.

This interview was conducted with the assistance of Pramod Subash, BDS, MDS, Chief of Cranio-Maxillofacial Surgery at Amrita Hospital, Kochi.

Kaddy Thomas

Clevedon, England, United Kingdom

Kaddy Thomas was born in Birmingham, England, and spent the early years of her life living in Sunfield Children's Home, a school and home for children with complex learning and behavioral needs. At age 9, she was placed in a residential children's home under the care of Birmingham Social Services until she was 17 years old. She received medical care at Birmingham Children's Hospital before transferring to Great Ormond Street Hospital. Now 57, Kaddy is a single mother who lives with her 19-year-old son Elijah in Clevedon, England. Elijah also has Apert syndrome. For over a decade, Kaddy has worked as the manager for Elijah's care team. Additionally, she is the founder of Elijah's Hope and Carers Collective, nonprofit organizations that provide advice, support, and education for families and individuals affected by Apert syndrome (Fig. 35.5). In 2025, Kaddy was named "Community Hero" in *Woman & Home* magazine's Amazing Women Awards for her contributions to improving resources and community for unpaid caregivers.

Early Years

Kaddy: I was born in Birmingham, but my family heritage is African, from Gambia, and my mother was 22 when she had me. She didn't know that she was going to have a child with Apert syndrome. Back in 1968, I guess the healthcare professionals' knowledge of Apert syndrome was very limited. So, not only did my mother obviously have a baby who had Apert syndrome, but she was also told that I was going to be—they used the words "severely retarded." Now, we use "severe learning disabilities" over here. I think the prospect of bringing up a child who was going to have physical disabilities and who was going to be "mentally retarded" was too much

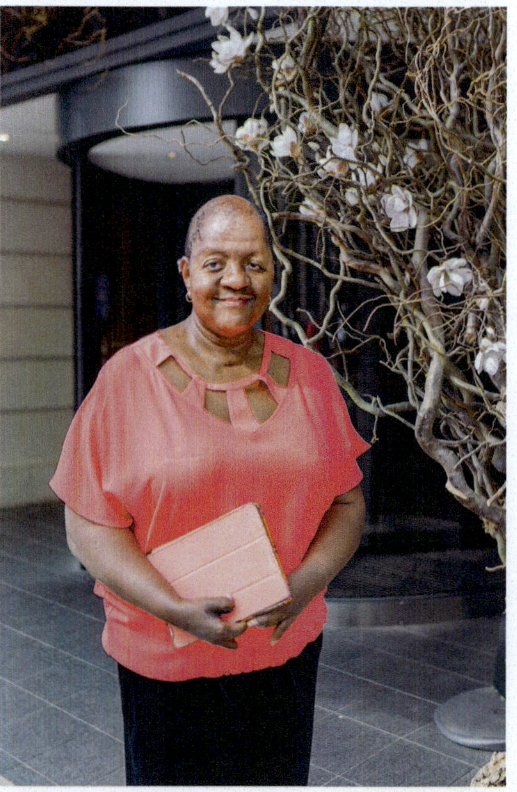

Fig. 35.5 Kaddy is the founder of two nonprofits. *Photo: AKP Branding Stories*

for my mother, who only had a brother to support her. I guess after a year, it was too much for her to bear, so she abandoned me.

As I was growing up, they discovered that mentally, I was bright, intelligent, and that Sunfield Children's Home was not the place for me to be, although it was all I'd ever known. So when I moved out of that environment into a residential children's home in Birmingham, it was a bit alien to me.

In terms of what happened to my mother, I'm not quite sure.

Growing Up in Residential Care

Kaddy: How I describe being brought up in care is that you get fed, you get watered, you get clothes on your back, you get a roof over your head, but you don't get that love and security that you would ordinarily get if you were raised in a family. So I guess I grew up quite, well, really insecure. Always longed to be loved and accepted. Yeah, just that longing to be loved by people. What I also experienced was that people would come and go out of my life, so you would kind of build a relationship with a member of staff, and then they would leave without any warning.

When you're brought up in care, you don't know where your family come from, or you don't know where you've come from. You kind of have no sense of identity. Obviously, you can see I'm Black, but culturally, I don't identify as Black, because I was brought up in residential care, which was predominantly white. You don't get cultured, and you don't get your history. You don't get your heritage.

On Surgery

Kaddy: I had various surgeries as a child and as a young person. In fact, I had two surgeries on my left hand, where they separated the digits. But, functionality-wise, it didn't make any difference how I use it—in fact, I'm right-handed—and the aftercare was really painful. I also had surgery on my skull. I had surgery on my feet because I wanted to separate my toes. But I think when [the doctors] went in there, they were like, "This is going to be a bit more complicated than we anticipated." So they just put pins in my feet, which I've still got in to this day. Then, when I was about 13, I had surgery on my skull. They cut open my skull from ear to ear, built up my forehead, and built up my cheekbones. That was major surgery. I was in intensive care for a period of time. I had a tracheostomy for a bit. My jaw was wired as well, so I just had to live on a liquid diet for six weeks. That wasn't pleasant, because I loved food.

Defying Expectations

Kaddy: I think one of the main challenges when it comes to visible, different disabilities is that people look at you and make a judgment—and maybe it's not an obvious judgment. Like, when I was growing up, I can't ever remember being [overtly] judged or treated any differently, and that's probably partly because I'm quite outgoing anyway, and I probably would have challenged the status quo. I would have challenged anybody.

I had really good relationships as I was growing up because I was very sociable and chatty. I like fun. But as a young person, I think because I spent six years at Sunfield Children's Home, there was that thing within me that always felt like I needed to show people that I'm actually quite an intelligent young lady. That I've got the faculties all together, and whilst I might look a little bit different, you know, actually I'm not.

I think a lot of [my resiliency] came from within. When you're in residential care, relationships are very fleeting. You haven't really got a role model. Well, you kind of look at some of the staff that are caring for you, but there's no real role model. And I adopted this "I can't rely on anybody else" attitude. Nobody else is ever going to help me. I still, to a certain extent, have this independent mindset of, "Actually, there's just me." I don't think I was consciously aware of that as I was growing up, but that was definitely the mindset that I had throughout my childhood. And I think that kind of stemmed from that whole, you know, you build a relationship with somebody, and then they leave, or they die, basically. So it's kind of like, well, if I get attached to somebody, then they're not going to stay around long enough for me to...yeah.

Entering the Workforce

Kaddy: When I left school, I did a youth training scheme, because I wanted to become a cook. I worked in an orthopedic hospital for a period of time, learning the ropes on working in the kitchen. Then at 17, I went, "You know what? I'm ready for independence." So I declared myself homeless—although [technically] I wasn't—and ended up in a high-rise flat in Birmingham. And then I spent a year kind of not making great decisions.

I worked for a Quaker college as an assistant cook, and then I became a waitress. I started catering in college to become a qualified chef, but when I started out in the restaurants, went into the kitchens, I realized that I hated being in there. So I lasted in the kitchens for two days. I went back out to the restaurants, became a qualified waitress, finished college, then I started working for a homeless organization called Saint Basil's. Absolutely loved that. I worked for the organization for a total of probably about 11 years but worked directly with homeless young people for five years. Then I moved into the head office and was a receptionist administrator for another five years.

Transitioning from Pediatric to Adult Care

Kaddy: I feel like I just got left [after I turned 18]. You have all this experience of being under one hospital, and then you reach an age where they can't treat you anymore. And you're kind of just left. Even when I went back and saw the adult Apert syndrome team, because I didn't need any surgery, it was almost like, "What do you want us to do with you?" But I've got Apert syndrome. I'm always going to have Apert syndrome. I want to be under the care of a craniofacial team just in case, I don't know, to be reviewed and monitored.

Because things change as you grow up, and I've certainly noticed a change within my own life.

I've discovered in my mature age as somebody with Apert syndrome, it almost gets more complicated.

So I'm a bit peeved, if you like, with the adult craniofacial team from my experiences of [how they] looked after me. Because when you've got a rare disease, you're always going to have it. I think, you know, whilst you might not need surgery, there is something about understanding what's going on with your body and how it's going to affect you. And if you *did* need surgery, or if you had a particular problem with an area of your body in relation to Apert syndrome, to have somebody that you can pick up the phone and say, "Can I make an appointment?" would be really beneficial.

Advice for Medical Professionals

Kaddy: Another thing is: we're human. We're human beings with feelings and emotions. It's having that in-depth knowledge of what Apert syndrome is and that it affects each and every one of us differently. There's no two [identical] patients with Apert syndrome. There's no two people in the world that have the same experiences (Fig. 35.6). We're all affected by the condition differently.

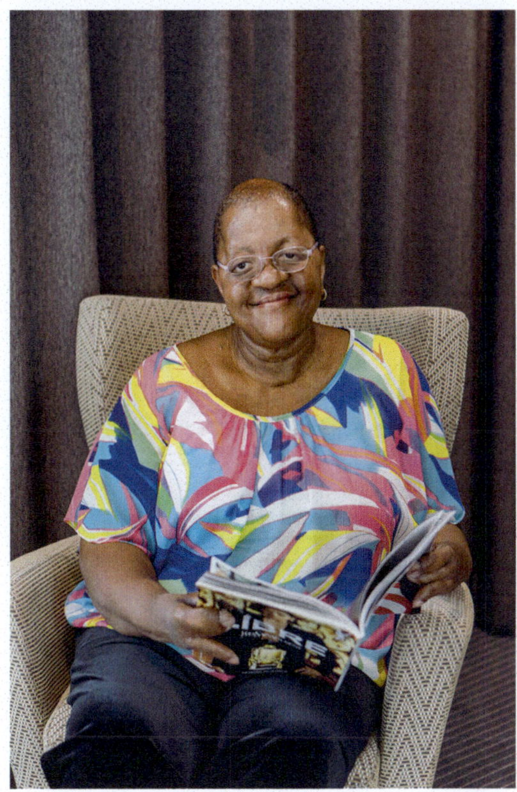

Fig. 35.6 Kaddy in 2023. *Photo: AKP Branding Stories*

To read about Kaddy's parenting experiences and advocacy work, see Chap. 36: *Caring for a Child with Apert Syndrome: Family Perspectives, Advocacy, and Support.*

Nohaila
Age: 20
Paris, France

I was born in Morocco and then I went to France. I was going back and forth, and I was operated on several times. In Morocco, [I felt as if] I'm the only one, the only one who has [Apert syndrome]. People would say, Oh, look at her. Look how she speaks. Look at her face. Look at her mouth. But in France, I did see other people. I saw another person like this, and I saw someone without hands or feet.

(continued)

I was ashamed before, but I'm not anymore. I work in a kitchen, in the restaurant field. I like spending time in the kitchen cooking, especially baked goods. Baking and cooking—those are my passions since I was little.

This interview was conducted with the help of an interpreter.

Vivi Zhang

Schenectady, New York, United States

Vivi Zhang, 30, lives with her family in Schenectady, New York (Fig. 35.7). After being diagnosed with Apert syndrome at birth, she underwent multiple surgeries at Boston Children's Hospital. In 2019, Vivi graduated with a B.A. in English from the University at Albany. She has written about her experiences with Apert syndrome on "The Mighty," an online community that publishes essays and articles by people living with health diagnoses and disabilities.

Early Life

Vivi: There were a bunch of cliques and groups in elementary school (Fig. 35.8). I didn't really have many friends or a close companion that I could sit down and have a deep conversation with, as much as you could do that as a child!

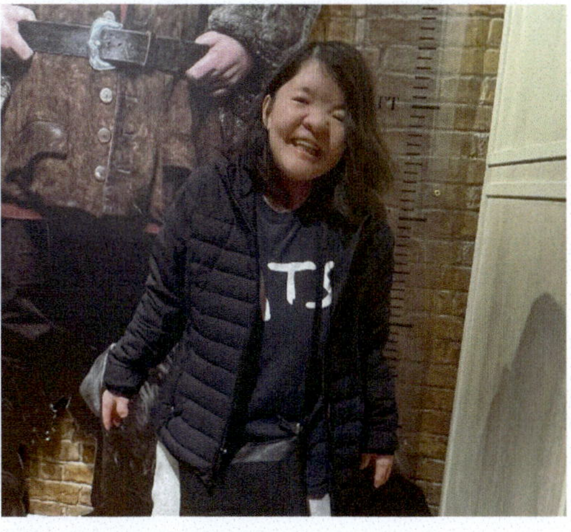

Fig. 35.7 Vivi, age 29

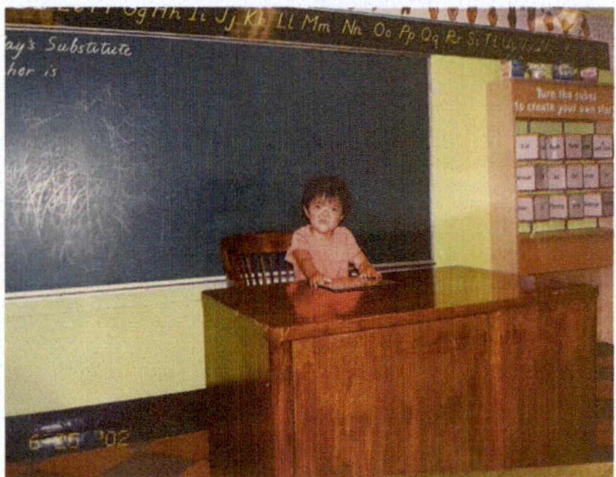

Fig. 35.8 Vivi at school, age 6

To share secrets, trust. I didn't have that companionship. I was mostly alone. I lingered in the background, and I was pretty lonely. My mom likes to say it was also because of emotional maturity. The other kids were a bit more sophisticated. I was still a little kid, doing kiddie stuff. I wasn't at the same level as them. There was an imbalance.

[The other kids] didn't express it verbally, but I could feel internally that in their minds they had misconceptions. Everyone has misconceptions about people who are different. But that's stressful. I remember kids, like little kids, would stare at my face because they saw it as different and strange.

But in fifth grade, one of my surgeries was scheduled during September. I had to repeat fifth grade and not go on to the middle school. I would be missing a lot of school, and it would be hard to catch up, especially going into a new school. So when I repeated fifth grade, I met a lot of new people. It was mostly because the teacher mentioned why I was there. I felt that circle of friends. I had more friends in that class than I did before. That changed my social life.

I remember I had a close relationship with my elementary school music teacher. She believed in me. She knew what I was going through, and she didn't hold that against me. She knew I was something special, even beyond my disability. She always had faith in me, and she was always in my corner. She saw me as someone.

On Surgery

Vivi: Honestly, it was all sort of scary and intimidating. But I think the thing that I was most concerned about was going under anesthesia. That was the part that I was most not looking forward to, because it was very stressful. I don't know how I braced myself. When I was younger, the surgeons always had either my mom or dad come with me to the OR, and then once I was asleep, my parents would leave. Having them brought some comfort, even though I was still sobbing. They stopped coming in when I got older. By then, I learned to brace myself, take a breath, and just be calm.

A consistent, supportive healthcare team is essential. To always have them on your side. My doctors never talked down to me. They treated me on the same level. [The surgical care for Apert syndrome] takes years, but so long as you have the endurance—the emotional endurance—the hard climb will be worth the effort (Fig. 35.9).

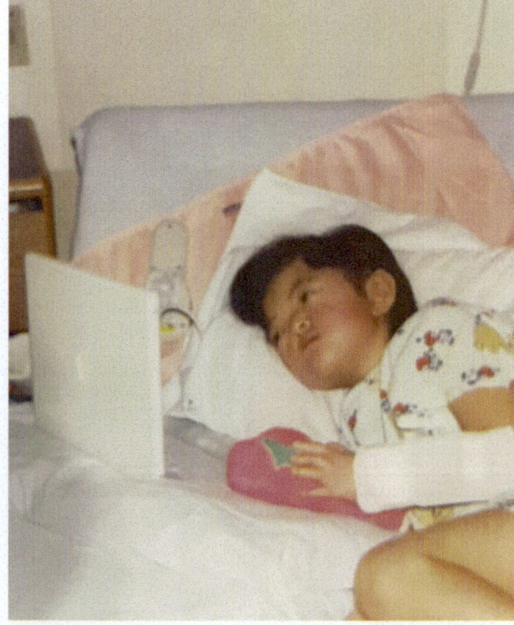

Fig. 35.9 Vivi, age 8, in the hospital recovering from hand surgery

Becoming an Adult

Vivi: Going to college changed me. It taught me a lot about myself. It definitely was a different and interesting experience. There was acceptance, then welcoming. It felt very much like a camaraderie.

Sometimes now I feel like [my relationship with Apert syndrome] is at a standstill. It's not changing. It stands still. Sometimes I don't recognize that I have it, because I am just like any other normal person. I like to write. I like to go out with my dog (Fig. 35.10). I like to read. Listen to music.

Transitioning to adult medical care was something that I kind of did on my own. It was hard to find, especially my dental care. I've been unemployed, and I'm still trying to find a job. That's not easy. I'm off my parents' insurance, and even so, they're both retired. I am mostly paying out of pocket.

Telling Her Side

Vivi: I was in middle school when I fell in love with writing, around 12 or 13 years old. I wasn't writing personal narratives at the time, mostly fiction stuff, but I've been writing ever since. I first discovered "The Mighty" on Facebook. I saw that it had a lot of articles about different types of disabilities and needs that are always talked about, like diabetes and autism and Down syndrome. No one talks as much about Apert syndrome, because it's not as known. [My desire to write about myself] also stems from my mom, who had written a book about me and my experience with Apert syndrome. It was published in China and is in Chinese. I was like, No one here can read it! I can barely read it. I wanted to go off that and tell my side. It makes people I know, people I would know, want to hear about Apert syndrome. They can learn and educate themselves and then be informed, maybe inspired.

My family and friends were surprised and in awe. They had praise. Some of my friends shared my articles on their Facebook pages to spread it. They were very supportive and proud. There was also a strong response [from strangers commenting on the essays]. It was refreshing compared to back when I was younger. I had a YouTube channel, and I would post videos of myself, and some of those comments weren't as nice and funny. It was a big change, and I was pleased to see the reversal. It's my most personal writing. I definitely see my writing as a form of activism. It's a way of sharing my experience, and my experience with Apert syndrome. Hopefully, it will move people emotionally, stir something in them. My motive for writing those articles was to help people see me. Apert syndrome is a part of me, but it's not all of me (Fig. 35.11). It's just one part of everything else.

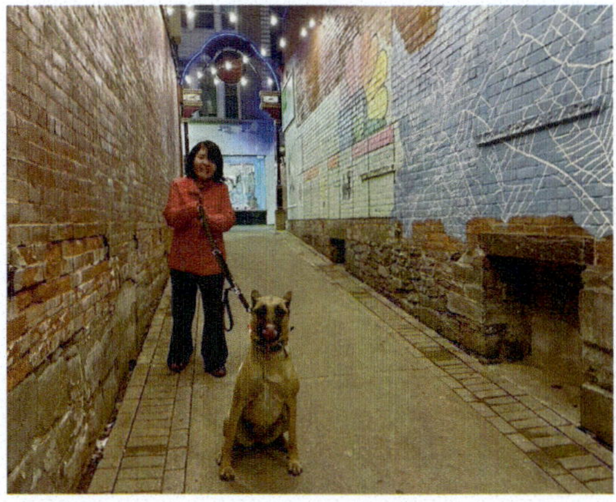

Fig. 35.10 Vivi walking her dog, Maggie

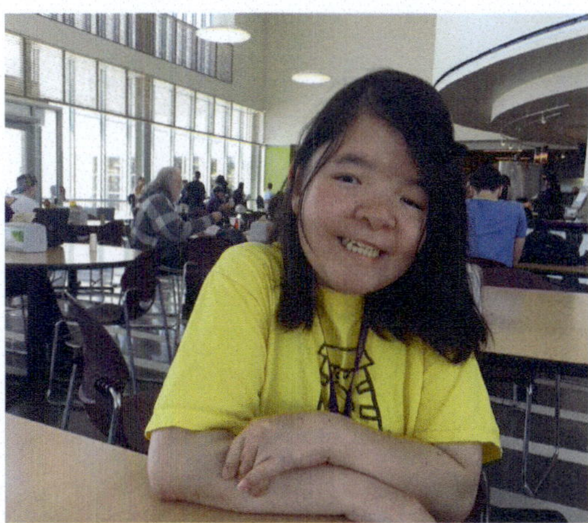

Fig. 35.11 Vivi, age 20, on campus at the University at Albany

Apert syndrome is not the end of the world. It's not contagious, and it's not a curse. But when I say it's not a curse, it's not a complete blessing. It's in the middle.

Josemon
Age: 21
Kedamoru, Kerala, India

I was born at Kedamoru, a village in Kerala, India. When I was 9 years old, we visited a dentist for the correction of my teeth who advised us to visit Amrita Hospital [to receive a diagnosis and treatment for Apert syndrome].

I was at a residential school 'til tenth standard where I made few friends. Even though my school was not a special school, it had other kids with disabilities. So, I never had any negative experiences [there]. I'm currently in eleventh standard, though I couldn't attend school for a few years due to surgeries. In my free time, I enjoy watching action movies on television. I also help my dad [who has Apert syndrome] with farming, and after completing my twelfth standard, I plan to continue with farming. I'm also planning to enroll in driving classes soon, and I'm looking forward to traveling as well.

This interview was conducted with the assistance of Pramod Subash, BDS, MDS, Chief of Cranio-Maxillofacial Surgery at Amrita Hospital, Kochi.

Luca Paolacci

Rome, Lazio, Italy
Boston, Massachusetts, United States

Luca Paolacci was born in Rome, Lazio, Italy, where he was diagnosed with Apert syndrome. At 2 years old, Luca and his family relocated to the United States to continue his care at Boston Children's Hospital. Luca grew up in an athletic family that introduced him to many sports at a young age. Now 26, Luca divides his time between the Boston area and Rome (Fig. 35.12). He works part-time as a data analyst at an engineering company, and he is also pursuing a bachelor's degree in engineering through The Open University. He plays tennis and rugby in his free time and recently took up sailing.

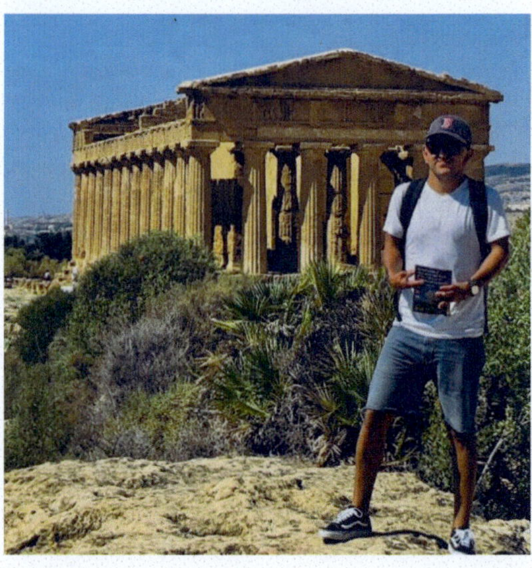

Fig. 35.12 Luca, age 25, at the ruins of the Temple of Concordia, Agrigento, Sicily, Italy

Early Life

Luca: When I was born, the doctor simply showed me to my mom and said, "Here's your baby!" He told her that maybe there were things to be corrected down the line. But he said that there are some very good specialists here in Italy. Otherwise, if you would prefer to be followed by the Boston surgeons, then you were perfectly within your right to do so. Immediately afterward, I was tested, and it came out with a diagnosis for Apert syndrome. When I was maybe a year old, possibly 2, they decided to undergo that treatment because they noticed severe syndactyly in my feet and hands.

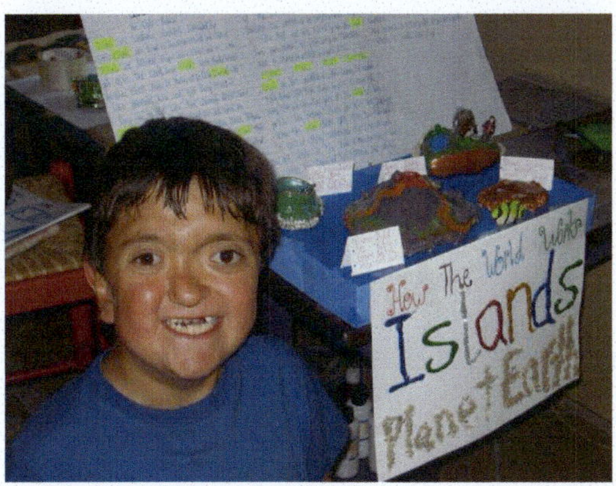

Fig. 35.13 Luca, age 8, proudly sharing a school project with his classmates

So after this, I began this back and forth between Italy and Boston. There were surgeons in Liguria, in the north of Italy, who followed my case and who helped in correcting this. That resulted in the involuntary amputation of index and middle finger on my right hand. Due to the complex nature of syndactyly, unfortunately, sometimes these limbs must be sacrificed for the rest of them to survive.

I have hazy recollections of making the definitive move [to Boston]. But the overall procedures when I was a little older were generally straightforward, because the surgeons were very relaxed, very tranquil, and they always had a very clear series of steps to undertake each procedure. For me, it just signified a slight modification in my day-to-day life (Fig. 35.13). I didn't even realize until shortly down the line that I even had Apert syndrome. I just thought that I had a few things that needed to be corrected, because I wasn't even taught to have that [label].

On Surgery

Luca: The focus of each surgery was, Is your child going to be functional? We don't care about the aesthetic. Is he going to be functional? Does he have problems walking? Okay, let's tackle that area. For example, when I was maybe 8, my surgeon had me come to the hallway outside his office before an operation. He had me walk up and down the hallway and then he had me jog up and down. He was like, "Well, you're actually performing better than I thought, and you're running pretty fast, so when we work on your feet, we're going to take away what's stopping you from running even faster." As a result, it made my quality of life much better, since wearing shoes—which is a normally not-so-much thought of part of our life—just became even more comfortable and pleasurable. I could say to myself, Okay, shoes slip in and I can walk comfortably, no need to stop and massage my foot, the balls of my feet, because of tension or pain.

The main concept [is that] as you grow into adulthood, various changes occur, not only in your stature or your body dimensions but also in your fine motor skills, coordination, dexterity, and comfort. I believe it was my plastic surgeon who once advised me to put off some of my operations. He said, you're still in the process of growing, so you don't know how your bones are going to look once you reach adulthood. [He said] the best bet you can possibly have is to let your bones grow and later down the line, just tweak them here and there to suit your functional needs. If you see that you cannot really function as effectively as you would have with a corrective surgery, then perhaps that would be the best course of action.

An Active Family

Luca: I'm the youngest of three [children]. Both of my siblings are more than a decade older than me. My sister is 14 years older; my brother is 11 years. So growing up, I was often the little brother seated backstage at a ballet performance. I was immersed in different environments from an early age.

My parents were the main influencers behind encouraging me to play sports (Fig. 35.14). My father played soccer when he

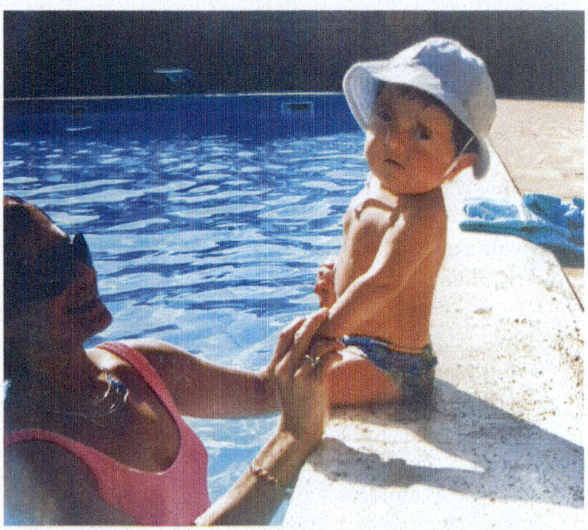

Fig. 35.14 Seven-month-old Luca getting ready to join his mom in the pool

was younger, and he also coached soccer for a while. He encouraged me to try a little bit of that, since it is a very popular sport in both the United States and Italy. My mom used to horseback ride, and she played field hockey in high school and college, so had a lot of diverse sports on her side. She also encouraged me to play tennis. My maternal grandfather was a passionate skier, so we used to go up to New Hampshire frequently.

My sister was a professional classical ballerina. She would always have me come backstage with other dancers and introduce me simply as her brother. The other dancers were happy to have me around, and I was later able to participate in a ballet workshop every now and then with differently abled kids. We would be shadowed by dancers from the company who would teach us those little jumps or deep movements and a bit of coordination.

My brother was more into combat sports, particularly martial arts like Muay Thai, boxing, as well as soccer, and he would take me out to watch his matches, so I had that integration into sports since I was tiny.

I'm still playing rugby. Still playing tennis. And this year, I decided to try out sailing. So sort of broadening the general area of expertise.

On and Off the Field

Luca: I was active in a lot of senses, and that's one of the reasons why I was able to integrate very well into society as not only a differently abled human being but just as a person in general, because that's sort of the environment I was brought up in.

My motivation for participating in sports was directly related to living with Apert syndrome. My mother believed it was not a question of what you looked like and what sort of conditions you were diagnosed with. If there is nothing separating you from achieving what these other kids are achieving, by all means, go ahead. And this was more for the fine-tuning of my motor skills, to be able to apply myself in different scenarios that involve different levels of dexterity, different levels of precision. That was a driving force behind not only sports but what led from sports to everyday life.

It also taught other kids to appreciate the unique skills I brought to the team. They saw a shorter kid with crooked fingers and small feet, and a couple of times, people said, "Can you actually run like the other kids? Can you actually pass a ball like the other kids or handle a tennis racquet?" And so I said, "Look, watch me, and you be the judge of what you see." Afterwards, they were like, "Oh, that is a different technique or style of holding the racquet, but if it works for you and you're able to succeed in that way, then by all means come join our team" (Fig. 35.15).

Nowadays you might get the mentality that you'll have people who look different in a different category and sometimes they're encouraged from childhood, sometimes from their own parents, to be in that separate category, with people like themselves. So don't go play with the quote-unquote "normal" kids, go play with the other kids who have Down syndrome, or the other kids who have Apert syndrome.

It's a very debated topic—to be separate in sports instead of together. I believe that they

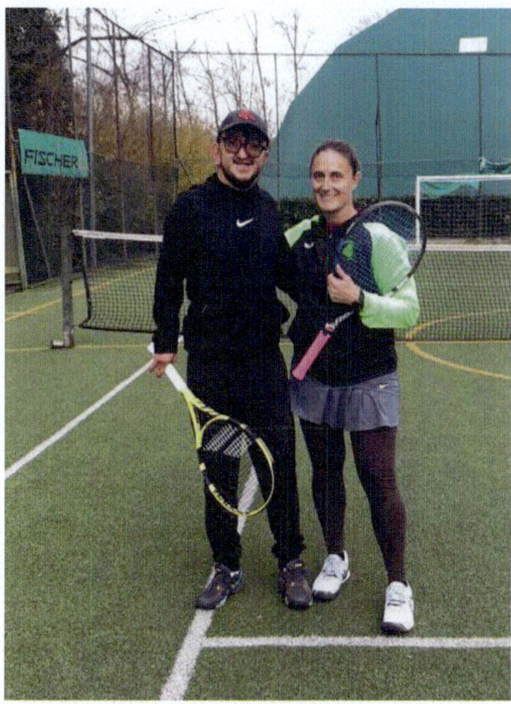

Fig. 35.15 Luca, age 25, and his tennis coach

should be playing together unless there's a compelling reason not to. I've even seen kids with one leg wrestle kids with two legs and flip them over. Kids with one arm play rugby at the college level with other guys with two arms. My opinion is that there should be no boundaries. That's just the way that I feel about it.

Defying Expectations

Luca: I never had people assume that I wasn't capable intellectually, because I studied at the same pace, turned in the same assignments, and the scores spoke for themselves. The main thing for me was I'd have the odd person come up to me and say, "Uh, don't you need a prosthetic to pick up a ball?" It was assumed that I might not run (Fig. 35.16). That was something that followed me around, because you didn't necessarily get shunned, but you would feel sort of tension if people saw [me] in the weight room, lifting weights. If someone walked by, they might look at me funny,

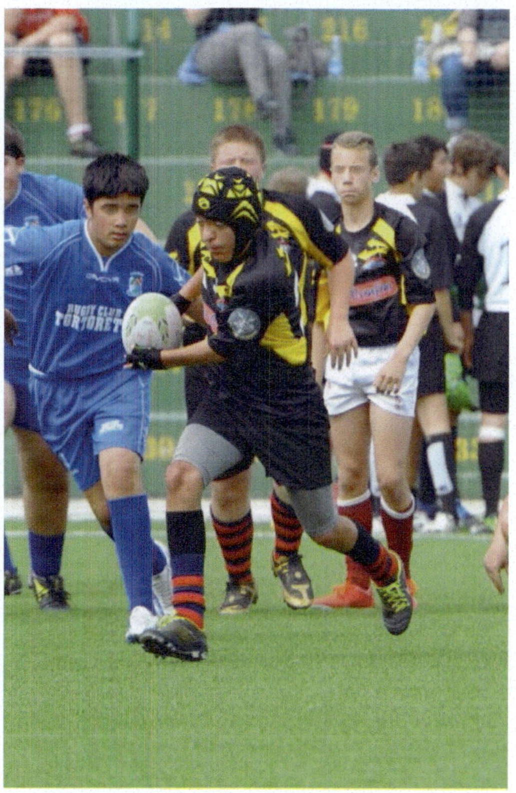

Fig. 35.16 Luca, age 14, competing in a rugby match

because why is a kid with three fingers lifting those dumbbells? If it's not harming me, then it shouldn't bother anyone else.

My mom wasn't overly feisty, but she would definitely defend me when the time came. She would also push me forward, encourage me, and say, "No, Luke, why should you not play that sport or that activity just because it's risky?" To the point where she even encouraged me to do canyoning, which is a form of rock-climbing, swinging through gorges, and you have to jump to neighboring gorges. It's been sort of funny, because the moral of story is: if you have to engineer different ways in order to accomplish a task, then, yeah, you do it. It might mean that you have to scale a rockface with just the tips of your toes or your fingers, while other people are doing it with their hands. But you'll get there in the end. Sometimes, you just take a slightly different route.

Conclusion

This chapter represents a sampling of individuals' experiences with Apert syndrome. There are members of the Apert community whom we did not include due to limits of time and space, most notably, individuals with other intersectional identities, adopted children, and patients from additional geographic regions. Still, the stories gathered share common experiences and perspectives, even descriptions and language.

Key similarities touch upon healthcare, social connections, and personal growth. Patients with Apert syndrome reported positive medical experiences when providers treated them as informed partners in their healthcare. Beyond the clinical setting, however, childhood was sometimes marked by feelings of loneliness and isolation—not only from outright bullying but also from the sense that others judged, and misjudged, them based on their appearance. Yet the individuals traced moments of courage, self-discovery, and perseverance to the acceptance and kindness they received from family, school, and social circles. By seeking out new experiences and challenging assumptions, many gained a sense of fulfillment and a clearer understanding that they are much more than their diagnosis.

In this way, the interviews highlight a need to acknowledge the individuality of people in the Apert community. From Vivi Zhang's desire to write her truth to Angelica and Marco Garcia's path to marriage and a family, we hope that the lives portrayed foster greater empathy and understanding, ultimately leading to more compassionate and holistic care.

We offer our most sincere thank-you to the individuals who shared their time with us. We are grateful for their generosity, insights, and openness, especially their willingness to revisit sometimes difficult and painful experiences.

Resources by Patients, for Patients

Apert International (Apert USA): This Facebook group is exclusive to patients with Apert syndrome and their parents and serves as an international resource for support, information, and community.

https://www.facebook.com/groups/apertusa/

Children's Craniofacial Association: Offers support for individuals and families affected by craniofacial differences through education and empowerment. Hannah Brown wrote this blog post to discuss her life and recent milestones as a person born with Apert syndrome.

https://ccakids.org/

Elijah's Hope: This nonprofit is specifically focused on improving the physical and psychological health of individuals with Apert syndrome.

https://www.carers-collective.co.uk/elijahs-hope

Five Star Adaptive: A journalist and disability rights activist runs this website which vets and lists tools, technology, and products useful for easing the daily routines and care of individuals with a disability.

https://fivestaradaptive.com/

MyFace: An online resource that offers support, community, and online resources for adults and children with facial differences. Dina Zuckerberg, who has Apert syndrome, hosts its "myFace, myStory" podcast. This episode features a conversation among three lifelong friends who were all born with Apert syndrome.

https://www.myface.org/

The Mighty: Patients and relatives blog first-hand accounts of their experiences. Writer Vivi Zhang has posted essays reflecting on varying facets of her life as a person with Apert syndrome.

(continued)

https://themighty.com/

TikTok—MouseketeerJonathan: Jonathan documents his life as a person with Apert syndrome, showing how he navigates and thrives in the world around him.

https://www.tiktok.com/@mouseketeerjonathan

References

1. Angie and Marco Garcia Speak At Neil Armstrong Academy in UT. CCAKidsBlog, 4 December 2018. https://www.ccakidsblog.org/2018/12/wonderwednesday-angie-and-marco-garcia.html Accessed 13 Nov 2024.
2. "Beyond 'Difficult.'" n.d. CareTalk. https://www.caretalk.co.uk/opinion/beyond-difficult/ Accessed 16 Oct 2024.
3. Boston Children's Hospital patient defying the odds after 22 years of treatment for rare illness. WHDH Boston. 26 December 2022. https://whdh.com/news/boston-childrens-hospital-patient-defying-the-odds-after-22-years-of-treatment-for-rare-illness/ Accessed 14 Nov 2024.
4. Carers Collective. n.d. https://www.carers-collective.co.uk/meet-our-founder-kaddy Accessed 16 Oct 2024.
5. Coughlan E. "I was abandoned by my mother as a baby over my rare genetic condition - then my life was turned upside down again after my son became brain damaged at 18 months old." Daily Mail. 6 June 2023. https://www.dailymail.co.uk/femail/article-12164841/I-abandoned-mother-rare-genetic-condition-baby-brain-damaged.html Accessed 16 Oct 2024.
6. Garcia A, Garcia M. Personal interview. 28 February 2025, virtual.
7. Garcia A, Garcia M. Personal interview. 14 November 2024, virtual.
8. Garcia A, Garcia M. Personal interview. 21 November 2024, virtual.
9. Josemon. Personal interview. April 2025.
10. "Kaddy Thomas Talks About Finding Out Her Son Had Brain Damage." Daily Mail. 6 June 2023. https://www.dailymail.co.uk/video/reallife/video-2954041/Video-Kaddy-Thomas-talks-finding-son-Eijah-brain-damage.html Accessed 16 Oct 2024.
11. Louisiana Students Read Wonder and Skype with "Real-Life Auggies" CCAKidsBlog, 7 November 2017. https://www.ccakidsblog.org/2017/11/wonderwednesday-louisiana-students-read.html Accessed 13 Nov 2024.
12. Mebin. Personal interview. April 2025.
13. Nohaila. Personal interview. 16 December 2024, virtual.
14. Paradis K. "Pieces at work: Luca's experience with Apert syndrome." Boston Children's Hospital. 13 February 2023. https://answers.childrenshospital.org/luca-apert/ Accessed 14 Nov 2024.
15. Park Y. "Vivi Zhang: a fruit loop among cheerios." 19 April 2016. https://ekdbs0503.wordpress.com/2016/04/19/vivi-zhang-a-fruit-loop-among-cheerios/ Accessed 31 Oct 2024.
16. Paolacci L. Personal interview. 15 November 2024, virtual.
17. Paolacci L. Personal interview. 24 January 2024, virtual.
18. Sved R. "The Power of Storytelling Resonates!" Kaddy Thomas on Harnessing Experience and Passion to Create Authentic Change. 3rd Sector Mission Control. 14 November 2024. https://www.3rdsectormissioncontrol.co.uk/the-power-of-storytelling-resonates-kaddy-thomas-on-harnessing-experience-and-passion-to-create-authentic-change/ Accessed 16 Oct 2024.
19. Thomas K. Personal interview. 18 October 2024, virtual.
20. Thomas K. "I became a full-time carer for my son after surgery left him with brain damage" Metro. 26 June 2022. https://metro.co.uk/2022/06/26/i-became-a-carer-for-my-son-after-surgery-left-him-with-brain-damage-16844337/ Accessed 16 Oct 2024.
21. Zhang V. Personal interview. 1 November 2024, virtual.
22. Zhang V. "To the little girl with Apert syndrome who feels like she's all alone." The Mighty. 12 September 2024. https://themighty.com/topic/apert-syndrome/t0-the-little-girl-with-apert-syndrome-who-feels-like-shes-all-alone/ Accessed 31 Oct 2024.
23. Zhang V. "5 Important Things I Learned From Having Apert Syndrome." The Mighty. 12 September 2024. https://themighty.com/topic/apert-syndrome/5-important-things-ive-learned-from-having-apert-syndrome/ Accessed 31 Oct 2024.
24. Zhang V. "A personal playlist for tough times with Apert syndrome." The Odyssey. 15 August 2017. https://www.theodysseyonline.com/personal-playlist-tough-times-apert-syndrome# Accessed 31 Oct 2024.

36 Caring for a Child with Apert Syndrome: Family Perspectives, Advocacy, and Support

Alicia Potter, Madelyn Mulreaney, and Dionna Santucci

Introduction

This chapter aims to capture a meaningful microcosm of families' experiences with Apert syndrome. The authors interviewed eight parents who had cared for children with Apert syndrome in four different countries. The children now range in age from 5 to 33 years old. Three of the parents also have Apert syndrome. The interviews took place from October 2024 to March 2025 and are lightly edited for clarity and length.

Interview participants were identified through either digital media coverage or referrals from surgeons affiliated with this textbook. Parents referred by our editors or contributors were assured they could speak openly about their experiences with affiliated hospitals and doctors, without affecting their child's care or relationship with the medical team.

Though informed by qualitative research, this chapter takes a journalistic approach. Each of its five sections begins with an account of the child's first hours and days, followed by the family's story—a descriptive introduction to the child, social and medical challenges, and advocacy work. Long-form interview excerpts preserve the parents' voices. In their own words, the families share their struggles and joys, offering ways to increase understanding and improve care. The narratives also highlight their pioneering efforts to educate others and create communities of connection and support. Above all, this chapter seeks to show how these parents see their children: as whole, complex, and deeply loved individuals, undefined by their rare diagnosis.

As authors without craniofacial or other appearance differences, we recognize that our criteria for selecting interview excerpts are not informed by lived experience and may reflect biases. To help mitigate this possibility, the families reviewed their sections before publication. In addition, we did not redact language that could be considered offensive or atypical for an academic text, including profanity, slang, or slurs. This was done to represent the people interviewed and their responses accurately. As a result, the interviews fully express the individual's perspective on life with a child with a rare diagnosis—one that notably causes visible differences and requires intensive, years-long medical care.

Rabia Aziz

Karachi, Pakistan

Rabia Aziz lives with her husband and three children in Karachi, Pakistan. In 2013, she gave birth to her second child, Aaliya, who has Apert syndrome. Now 13 years old, Aaliya traveled to the

A. Potter (✉) · M. Mulreaney · D. Santucci
Department of Plastic and Oral Surgery, Boston Children's Hospital, Boston, MA, USA
e-mail: Alicia.Potter@childrens.harvard.edu

J. G. Meara et al. (eds.), *Apert Syndrome*, https://doi.org/10.1007/978-3-032-12551-4_36

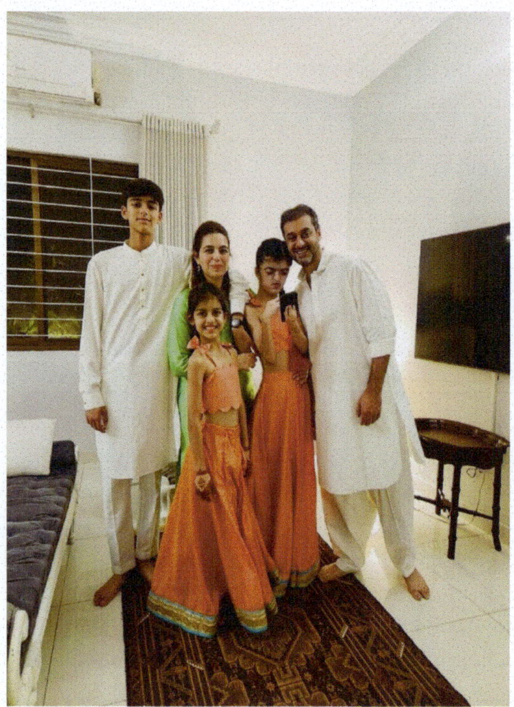

Fig. 36.1 Aaliya, age 12, celebrating Eid with her family

United States at 9 months to undergo multiple procedures at Medical City Children's Hospital in Dallas, Texas. Shortly after Aaliya's birth, Rabia founded Special Needs Pakistan, a Facebook group that currently has over 26,000 followers. In addition, she has shared the story of her daughter's early medical care in the TEDx Talk "Raising Aaliya, Rising Above" (Fig. 36.1).

Aaliya's Birth

Rabia As the gynecologist took the baby out, I heard a deafening whisper in the [operating theater] as if the nurses were in disbelief. One of the nurses asked me, "Would you like to see the baby?" And the gynecologist stepped in, and she said, "Of course, she wants to see the baby. She waited so long for this." By this time, I didn't know what was going on. It was very overwhelming. They'd wrapped the baby in a green cloth and showed me only her face, which was just so beautiful and pink. She was taken to be monitored and checked out. In recovery, the gynecologist, my main surgeon, came up to me, and she said, "Well, Rabia, you're good, you're stable, but the baby has been born without fingers, and she has webbed feet." And I was like, "Okay, well, is that all?"

Little did I know that not having fingers was the least of my worries. They were thinking that it could be craniofacial, and most of the fellows and residents had only seen one page about babies with Apert syndrome. There was no literature in terms of having case studies or having children at the hospital with that particular syndrome. A couple of hours in, I requested to be wheeled into the neonatal intensive care unit (NICU), and once I saw the baby in the incubator, everything else was history. I put my hands through the glove, and with her fingerless palm, she just grabbed it. And that was our first union. I took her out of that glass box and gave her first nursing.

I had to be kept in the hospital for about a day. They said, "We can't keep the baby because she's healthy. She's nursing, She's absolutely fine. You need to just take her home and give her a lot of love." And so that was the point—the turning point—where I just didn't understand. What does it mean when you say take the baby home and give her a lot of love? What's going to happen to her head? What's going to happen to her hands? It's like, oh my God, let me start. Let me start researching.

Culture of Shame and Stigma

Rabia Living in a culture that is predominantly based on shame and stigma, bringing children into this world does not permit you to avoid the shame and stigma. And it started from home. My loved ones and supporters contemplated what it could have been or what I had done: "You shouldn't have eaten too much chicken that was processed," or "It was that indulgence that you had with alcohol" or "You party too much," which I didn't. The reactions [from other women] were very, very morbid. They were like, "You're going to go directly into heaven. You've given birth to an angel." Or it's like, "All your sins have been forgiven," or "Look at it this way: it can't get any worse."

A term which was used constantly was, "Oh, *Bechari*!" You know the amount of pity and dreadful sympathy that I had to hear on behalf of my child? "How is she going to get married now?" Because obviously, in South Asian communities, the first and the last thing one thinks about is marriage. You have to be groomed to be a good bride. "What's going to be her life now?" And I was like, "You know what? I'm going to worry about how she's going to be able to feed herself before I can even dive into those things."

There were moments when I would take my son to the playground, and I'd become so numb that there were tears streaming down my face which I couldn't even feel. But the numbness gave me clarity into how to not only face those reactions, but how I wanted to really, really introduce Aaliya into this world. When I asked my husband Ashail how will we introduce Aaliya, he said, "We will tell it as it is." And that was not through a pitiful eye. It was through a proud eye—really, really putting her out there saying, "Hey, this is me. Take it or leave it. I'm not asking you to be beside me. I've got a cool tribe with me." I started powering up for that (Fig. 36.2).

Introducing Aaliya

Rabia Aaliya is headstrong. She has this beautiful, contagious smile. She has this sparkle in her eyes. She's tall. She's almost reaching my chin. And she knows what she wants. She communicates through music, because she still is very non-verbal. She loves Bollywood music. The sad days have the sad songs, and the lonely days have the lonely songs. And when we are at the hospital, which is her comfort zone, or at the beach, which is her favorite place in the world, it is all laughter, giggles, and upbeat music.

She loves shorts and soft clothes. She has a way of saying, "No, I will not wear this." She will put it aside. She loves being groomed and taken care of. She has pride in the way she is groomed. If she doesn't like something, she'll be vocal about it and put her hand forward. She's very, very aware of her body and her presence. And she is social. She knows her siblings. They love her, and she loves her family around her (Fig. 36.3).

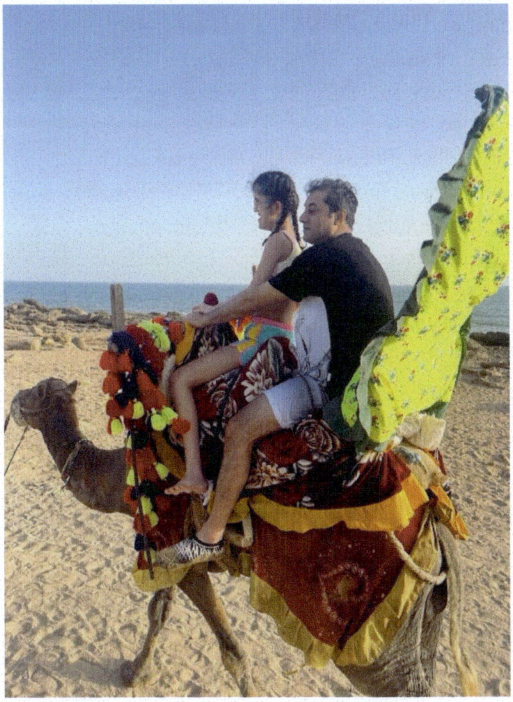

Fig. 36.2 Aaliya's first camel ride, age 12, with her father

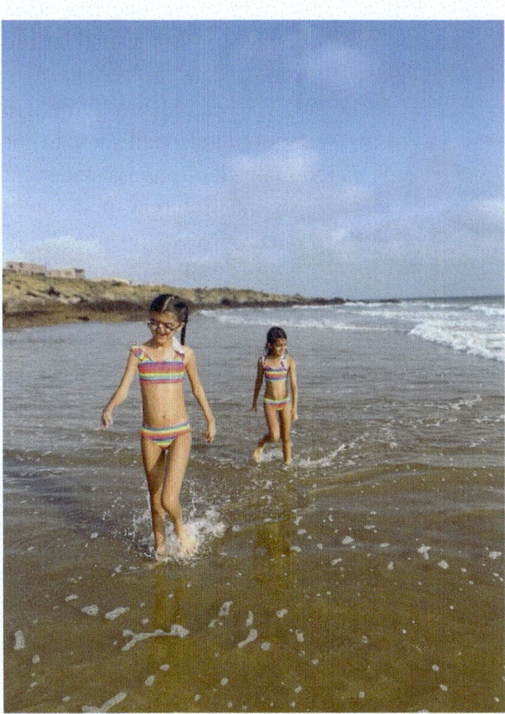

Fig. 36.3 Aaliya, age 10, enjoying the beach with her sister Alayna

Early Sibling Response

Rabia Raising children around Aaliya was the tougher bit, which taught me a lot. Aaliya has a brother who's three and a half years older, and she has a sister who's three and a half years younger. It would break my heart when other children would call her "Frankenstein" or "monster." I still remember my son was in kindergarten when Aaliya was born, and the kinds of things that he had to hear were, "He has a sister who's Frankenstein." "Halloween is coming up. Can you bring your sister?" Those were really hurtful. And by grade three, he told me, "Ma, don't bring Aaliya." I said, "You know what? If you're not going to love her, and if you're not going to accept her, nobody will." So I think for me, it was not just having Aaliya accept herself. It was having her own accept her unconditionally, so that the world could accept her.

No Systems of Care

Rabia Back in 2013, there were no multidisciplinary teams. I had to sit through consulting clinics for hours on end. There was no such appointment system. So I had to rush to pediatric cardiology in the morning, and then run to the plastic surgeon in the evening. There were no integrated services.

Nobody was telling me what to do or who the expert was. And so, [on the] sixth day of birth, I had my child at the pediatric orthopedics table where [the surgeon] told me, "Why did you not abort this child?" And the conversation was, "She has so many anomalies, and you should have gotten rid of her." And I said, "You know what? I'm really, really thankful for your conversation and your advice, but currently she's on your examination table, so please tell me what you can do." Those are the kind of experiences I had, and I was informed, educated, privileged, and resourceful. So you can well imagine if somebody doesn't have those four [qualities] and time and money, what would they do? They wouldn't be anywhere. They would just take the child home and give them whatever care they can.

I was doing it all by Googling. There were mums in Australia, mums in United Kingdom, mums in the United States, mums in India, mums all over globally, who were giving their two bits of learned things [online]. I was able to take that back to the healthcare system and demand, "Look, I know this is possible. So can you give me an insight? How are we going to do an MRI (Magnetic Resonance Imaging)? This is the way it was done in the United States, so can we do it the same way here?" And when I was taking all that information back and being a bossy mom, I was able to push through the chaos and the madness.

Leaving Karachi for Dallas

Rabia I sent an email to Dr. Fearon. *[Ed. Note: Jeffrey A. Fearon, MD, Craniofacial Center, Medical City Children's Hospital, Dallas, Texas]* And he responded to me within seven or eight hours. He sent me a lovely email. The first thing he said was congratulations and how are you doing? In the past five months, I had not been asked how I was, because I was just functioning. And so to be asked how I was just did something for me. We exchanged a whole load of emails. He gave me a plan of action. And that started rolling the ball. By seven months of birth, we were applying for our US visa. And by the ninth month of Aaliya's birth, we were headed to Dallas (Fig. 36.4).

What I really admired about having my child go through the surgeries in the United States was how I was guided and counseled through the procedures. It's something that does not happen in my part of the world where maybe now adult procedures may be walked through. But in terms of procedures in pediatric care, caregivers are looked down upon as people who wouldn't understand, or individuals who have no knowledge, as opposed to really, really taking them through the whole lowdown. "Step one will be this. Step two will be this. You need to get this blood work done.

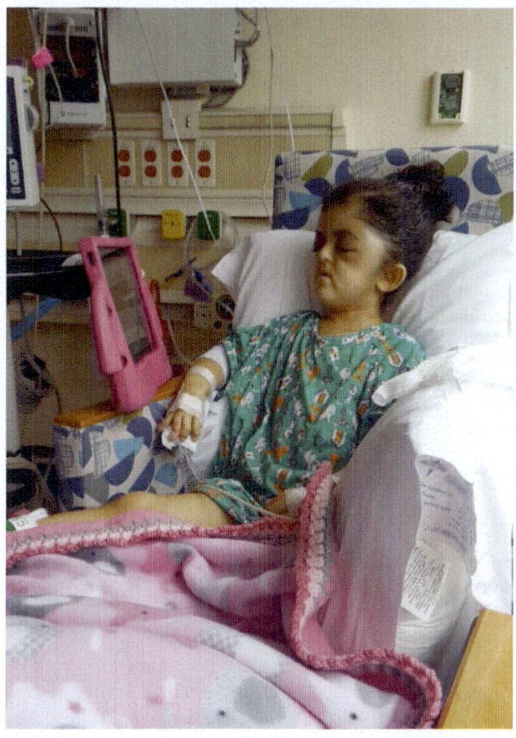

Fig. 36.4 Aaliya, age 4, in the pediatric intensive care unit (PICU) after an 11-hour surgery

This blood work will be done 12 hours before this needs to be done." Guidance and counseling are two things that can make or break the entire journey.

A Viral Question

Rabia Coming from a Third World country, we struggle with education and awareness. So when I started asking questions, it was like, Why are you asking all these questions? Why are you asking about a child? A child who is born differently has to be treated differently. And so when I started blogging every day within the first few days of Aaliya's birth, I wasn't just documenting her life. I was documenting other lives around her, other resources around her, free resources that came up, unavailed resources that came up, what kind of therapists are around. People did not know the difference between occupational and speech and what the audiology department can do. I started documenting what the government does for welfare or special needs.

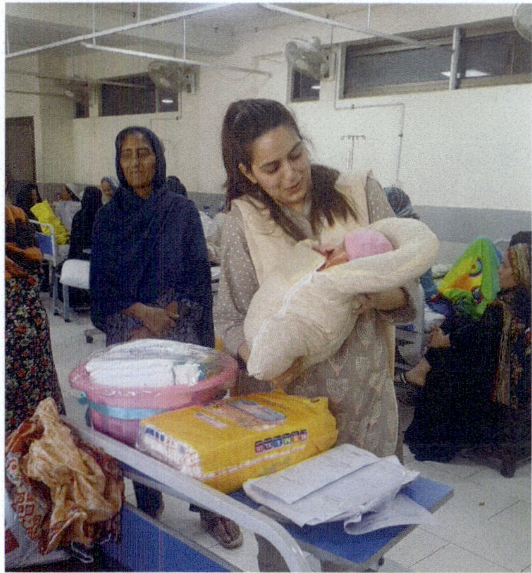

Fig. 36.5 Rabia in 2024 working at a local hospital to raise awareness for babies born with different abilities by providing counseling and psychoeducation to their caregivers

So about five months into her birth, it's like, well, you're writing all the time. Why don't you put all of this in one place? And that's how Special Needs Pakistan was born. My parents, siblings, strangers across the world became my support system. Some whom I had never met (Fig. 36.5). "How are you doing?" became a viral question throughout the community groups that I run. We're going to talk about the child anyway, but *how are you?* And that completely changes the way the person feels about themselves, whether it's a mum or dad or caregiver.

Advice to Other Families

Rabia There will be a lot of challenges. There will be a lot of difficulties. But let your child be the child that they need to be, not what you want them to be. I had thought my Aaliya would be a dancer. Would go to an Ivy League. But she spends her day being calm and happy. Take yourself out of your child's equation. Step out of it.

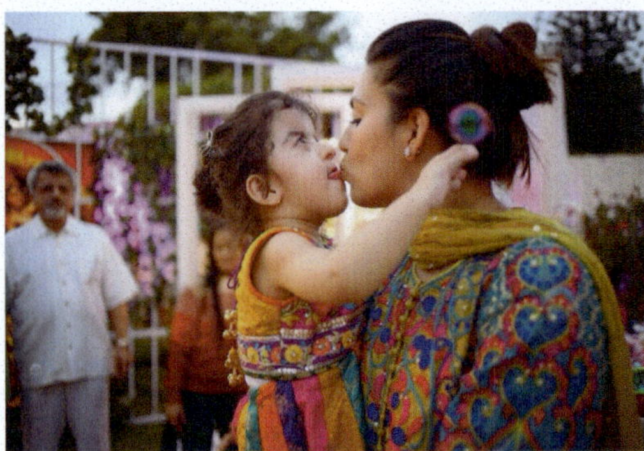

Fig. 36.6 Aaliya and Rabia at Aaliya's Bollywood-themed third birthday party

You're there to facilitate for them, you're there to take care of them, but you're not there to walk in their shoes while they go through this journey. Their journey is their journey, and our journey as a caregiver is ours. And it's a tough one. Be graceful and take care of yourself. Because if you take care of yourself, you'll be able to take care of your child (Fig. 36.6).

Angelica and Marco Garcia

Salt Lake City, Utah, United States

Married for eight years, Angelica and Marco Garcia met through Facebook. They both have Apert syndrome and live in Salt Lake City, Utah. In 2017, Angelica gave birth at 28 weeks to R.J., a baby boy with Apert syndrome who lived for one day. Today, the Garcias are parents to 5-year-old Mina, who was born with Apert syndrome at 36 weeks in 2020. Angelica and Marco are active in "The Wonder Project," a US-based program inspired by R.J. Palacio's novel *Wonder*. The initiative educates schoolchildren about craniofacial differences, with an emphasis on empathy and anti-bullying (Fig. 36.7).

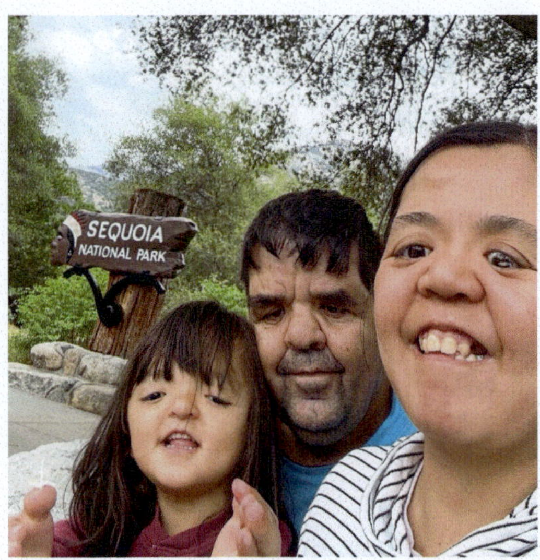

Fig. 36.7 Mina, Marco, and Angelica on a family trip in 2025

A Second Pregnancy

Angelica We were going to family therapy since we were still grieving R.J. I did an EMDR [exercise] with our therapist. I remember the most powerful feeling was painting [the experience of loss] as a picture. I envisioned I was ready to come out of the storm of sadness and grief and darkness and into the rainbow—to bask in the rainbow. So when I found out that I was pregnant with Mina, it felt like it was meant to be. And I was happy, of course! It felt like all of the things that were surrounding me were good, even though there was a sad, difficult previous experience, being R.J.

Marco That experience [of losing R.J.] shook me very hard. I was 37, and I never thought that at that age that I was going to have to bury my kid. We are religious, so when Angie became pregnant again, I prayed. I was like, God, if you don't do it for me, do it for Angie, because I knew how much it meant to her to be a mom. Even though we were officially parents, [we wanted] to be hands-on and see our roots grow.

Angelica We consulted with my doctor and a geneticist. And after the first ultrasound, we all felt that, oh, this is a healthy baby. The baby has Apert like us, but if you look at the first few ultrasounds of R.J. and then of Mina, there are contrasts, differences. Mina was this perfectly healthy baby.

Marco She was going to make it.

Mina's Birth

Angelica I basically took control of this labor and delivery. For example, I did not wear a hospital gown. I wore one of my very loose, relaxed dresses. I wanted to feel pretty. I wanted to feel glamorous. I wanted to feel like I was in control, even though it was the first months of the pandemic. Right before the pushing began, I accidentally pressed the button that administered more medicine for my epidural. I pressed it twice. So by the time that I had to push Mina out, I was so relaxed. I felt like I was in a spa. It was like the most wonderful thing: my dress, my glamour feeling, everything added together. It was the most serene, most tranquil, and I'm pretty sure, most spa-like delivery ever. Mina came out and she cried and we cried. We cried because she was crying. Because R.J. didn't cry.

They wheeled Mina down to the NICU, but it was not as urgent [as with R.J.]. With Mina, it was more like the party bus. Everyone was following Mina to the NICU. Marco got to spend her first moments with her, and I'm glad he had that. He also had that with R.J. As soon as I got cleaned up, I went to the NICU to meet our miracle child. She was breathing. I stroked her. I touched her. I gently laid my hands on her, and she woke up and she cried again. It was the best sound ever (Fig. 36.8).

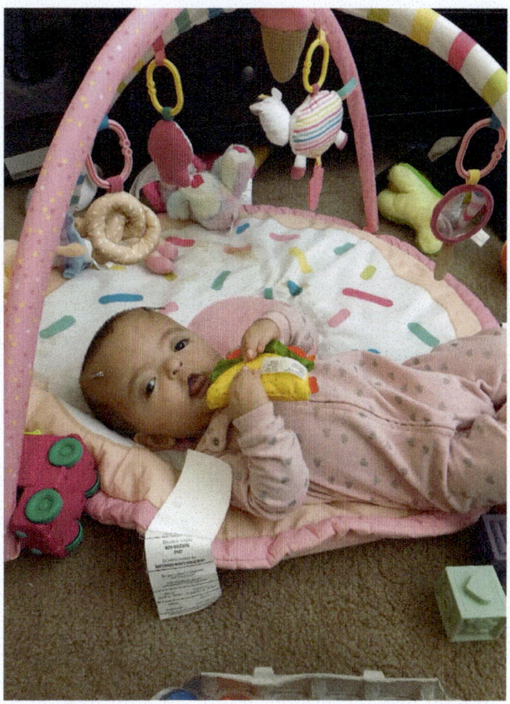

Fig. 36.8 Mina at 10 months old after cranial vault distraction surgery

Introducing Mina

Marco We feel bad for our neighbors downstairs, because Mina loves to run and jump. I call her my "Mini Me." Put her on a trampoline, and she plays for hours. She loves coloring. She loves building with Magna-Tiles. She takes the spotlight. She leads the class. At church, she's got her little posse. She's the perfect combination of me and Angie: she's outgoing and running around like me, but sensitive like Angie. On the playground, she'll slide down the open slide but hesitates on the one with the tunnel.

Angelica Mina is a piece of art. A majestic masterpiece. She's caring and funny. She's super sassy. This year, she's become much more aware of emotions, both hers and people around her. Her empathy has really grown. If she sees a classmate crying, she runs to them and says, "What's wrong?" She tries to comfort them. She's one of the most beautiful souls I've ever known. She's already her own person.

Parenting from Lived Experience

Marco Doctors sometimes underestimate how much knowledge we have about our own conditions. Me and Angie obviously have one Apert gene and one good gene each. R.J. unfortunately got both of the Apert genes, and so that's what made his Apert more severe. We knew what we were walking into when we became parents, and that the outcome might be hard.

Angelica In the NICU after Mina was born, everyone was totally keeping us in the loop and trying to teach us, educate us. But they didn't know about the Dr. Brown's bottles and how they're the gold standard for every baby with Apert syndrome. I knew. At one point, I said, "Hey, when I was born, my dad was holding me in a way that his elbow was raised and my head was elevated." They really listened to us. They said let's find ways to feed Mina while she's elevated.

Marco We know that our experiences are going to be Mina's experiences. It's like a foreshadowing of our past lives, but some things are better. We're at a playground now, and I haven't heard any name-calling from the other kids. No one is asking, "What's wrong with you?" or "Mom, what's wrong with her?"

Angelica We have friends with Apert syndrome who don't want to have babies, because they don't want to put them through the suffering of surgeries and medical interventions. They don't want to put them through the bullying. They want to prevent children with Apert from experiencing the brutal harshness of society. I get that, and I respect that. All of that is truth. At the same time, it depends on your own personal experience, which is always validated. We don't expect Mina's journey to be a copycat triplicate of ours (Fig. 36.9). But so far, our experiences have been wonderful.

Marco We just try our best. Being a parent after a tragic loss is hard, but it's not impossible.

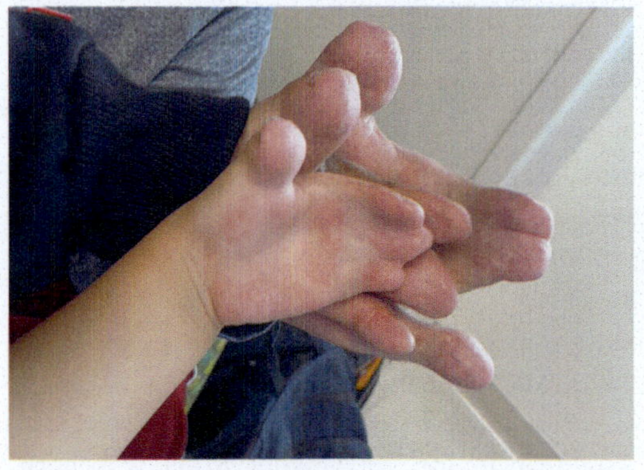

Fig. 36.9 The Garcia family's self-portrait of their hands

Visiting Schools Together

Angelica I started visiting schools because I wanted to do it for my son, like if he had made it, if he had gone to school. Now we're doing it for our daughter. We want to strengthen the bridge of awareness and communication and of human social interaction, so that by the time that Mina goes to school, she will love kindergarten through middle school, right where bullying runs rampant. By then, more people will be more aware and less harsh when it comes to people and kids with differences.

We do a Q&A forum, because we found that at first the kids, especially the sixth-graders, are a little shy, like, "Whoa! These people!" One kid asked, "Are you an Apple or Android person?" And I'm like, "We're Apple iPhone people," and then the lightbulb will go on in their head: I have an iPhone too! And the more questions they ask, and the more we answer them, the more they're like, "Oh my gosh, I love that too!" We can jump, we can dance. Marco can do martial arts. We're building connections (Fig. 36.10).

Marco A high school invited us to talk, and we answered their questions, which were a little deeper. A couple of months later we were shopping at Christmas, and some people started looking at us. But it went back to we went to their school to talk about one thing, and then we were doing our shopping. I think they thought it was

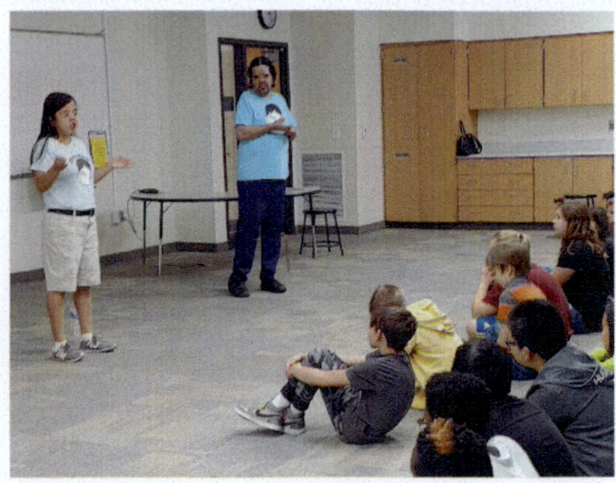

Fig. 36.10 Angelica and Marco speaking at Neil Armstrong Academy in West Valley, Utah

cool to see us at the store and doing our own thing like their parents. That's where I see the fruits of our labor. They see us on the street, and they're like, "Hey, you came to my school, right? Hey, man!"

Angelica And we're not scary anymore. We're not unapproachable. In that moment of connection, it kind of goes beyond the whole educating kids about us as people with facial differences. Like even though our hands and our faces look different, we're not monsters. We also touch a little bit on bullying, because that is connected. I basically encourage the kids like, everyone's going through something, and it can go into adulthood.

Marco I try to motivate younger people, like "Hey, if I could play basketball, you could play." I see myself as an advocate. It's a part of my life: I'm going to help you. I'm not going to do it for you, but we're going to do this together.

> To read about Angelica's and Marco's experiences growing up with Apert syndrome, see Chap. 35: *Living with Apert Syndrome: Patient Perspectives*.

Kaddy Thomas

Clevedon, England, United Kingdom

Kaddy Thomas is a single mother who lives with her 19-year-old son Elijah in Clevedon, England. Both Kaddy and Elijah have Apert syndrome. When Elijah was 18 months old, he developed an infection related to one of his craniofacial surgeries that resulted in a lifelong brain injury and complex care needs. For the past decade, Kaddy has worked full-time without pay as the manager for Elijah's care team. In 2013, Kaddy founded Elijah's Hope, a Community Interest Company that provides advice, support, and education for individuals and families affected by Apert syndrome. Additionally, Kaddy is the founder of Carers Collective, a nonprofit that hosts a six-week virtual training program with solutions-based coaching to help caregivers build resilience and well-being.

Elijah's Birth

Kaddy Before I became pregnant, I went and saw a genetics consultant who took some blood and said that I had the gene. So there was a 50-50 chance that my child would possibly have Apert syndrome. When I became pregnant, the first thing I did was call up the genetics consultant. When they told me some of the tests that they go through to establish whether your child has got Apert or not, and some of those tests had the risk of miscarriage—miscarriage!—I was like, There's no way I'm having that test. If my baby's got Apert, then so be it. I'm not going to get rid of it just because it's got Apert syndrome.

Throughout the whole of my pregnancy, I probably had more scans than the average mother out there, and it was halfway through my pregnancy that [the doctors] went, "Oh, there's something! We've detected something, but we don't quite know what." And I'm a detailed woman when it comes to information, particularly about me. So I was like, well, I can't deal with it if there's something not quite right here. I need to know what. I went and got a private 4D scan, and within seconds of them scanning me, they said, "Yep, he's got Apert syndrome."

I was really happy about having a baby, absolutely over the moon when Elijah came. It's kind of like the first time in my life that I've ever experienced having blood-related family. It was just one of those experiences where you go, Wow, I'm a mother, and, you know, I'm related to him (Fig. 36.11).

I had loads of questions, because I was a single parent. The father of my child didn't want to know [Elijah], so I didn't have him to support me. I didn't have his family to support me either. The Church's attitude was, well, you've made your bed, you're going to lie in it. I might have had a

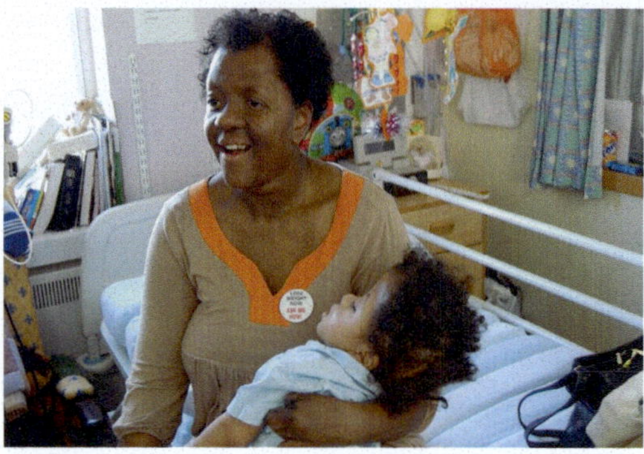

Fig. 36.11 Kaddy and Elijah at Birmingham Children's Hospital in 2008

child out of wedlock, but I did not ask for this. So I was very much on my own.

I think the assumption was because I had Apert syndrome, that I didn't need any support now that I got a child with the same condition. But I said, I'm a new mother. Just getting my head around having a little person to look after is big enough for me to handle. I don't want to have to then think about navigating the whole Apert surgery journey.

Introducing Elijah

Kaddy I'm always amazed how parents will introduce their child as a condition. I like to introduce Elijah as a young man who's now 19. He's a real flirt. Loves women with blonde hair, big boobs. He loves the great outdoors. He's really into sport, football, rugby—particularly ladies' football. He's a real character, despite what he's been through. He's got quite a warped, dry sense of humor. He loves watching films, skateboarding, "MasterChef Australia." He absolutely loves slapstick comedy. He loves listening to gossip. He's got an eye gaze, and he's very good at saying, "I don't want to talk." [He's a] very decisive young man who knows what he wants to do.

He loves me. Loves the water and loves swimming. He loves music. He's got a really wide range of taste when it comes to music. When he was younger, it was classical. Now it's quite varied. He's delightful, amazing, courageous, brave, strong. No matter what is thrown at him, he springs back from it. He's just incredible, and I'm proud of him. Yeah, he's a real character (Fig. 36.12).

Becoming More Vocal

Kaddy Prior to Elijah becoming brain injured, he was born with Apert syndrome, a cleft on his soft palate, and a heart murmur. That was all he was born with. When Elijah became brain injured, I became very angry, bitter, really quite well traumatized. It was a very traumatizing experience. I would explode at any given moment, at any given thing. I used to say to the nurses on the ward, "I don't expect you to like being the brunt of my frustration, but this is not a normal situation." And I think after brain injury, I became more vocal and a lot more assertive, and a lot more confident to voice my concerns and worries. If I felt the need to repeat the message numerous times until I was heard, that's what I would do.

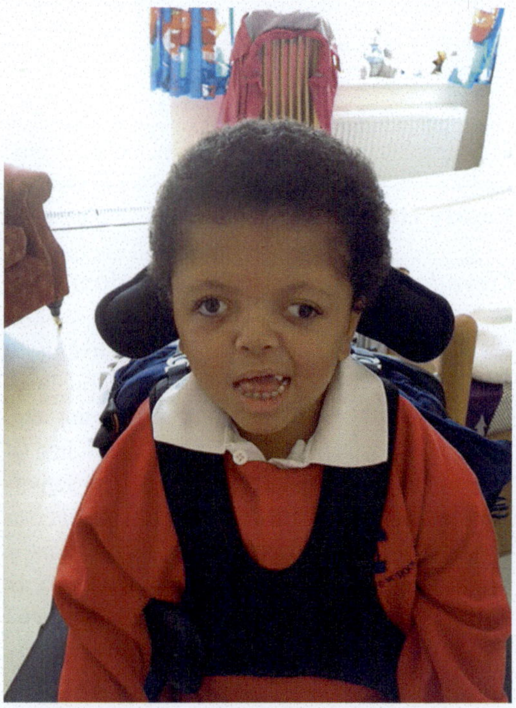

Fig. 36.12 Elijah, age 8, about to head to school

You kind of look at healthcare professionals and doctors thinking, well, they've got all the knowledge, they know best. But now I'll argue with anyone. I don't care who you are, whether you're head of craniofacial surgery, head of plastic surgery. If I think there's something wrong with my young man, then I'm not moving from this place until you've sorted it out. I think as a parent, if doctors are not hearing what you're saying, you just need to keep on and on. When you start swearing or shouting, though, your message gets lost, so you have to communicate in a really calm, considered manner. But that's only come through experience. Who knows their child better than their parent, yeah? So if a healthcare professional is not listening to a parent, then there's something wrong there.

Trauma in Many Layers

Kaddy For me, parent trauma is multifaceted, depending on the experience that we either observe with our child or our loved one. Or it's how we've been treated—and continuously get treated, in my view—because, you know, I've been through hell and back.

Trauma comes in many layers. I found it traumatic when I stood at the end of my child's bedside and I saw him struggling and gasping for breath, and the nurse that was on shift at that particular time was just trying to manage him. But I've also seen when he's been in hospital, and he's got a whole team around him trying to, you know, [save] him. I've also seen it where his head's leaking cerebral fluid, and I'm not being heard or listened to, and then it's just left until it's too late, and then [the doctors] are like, we're still going to not be straight with you.

It's kind of like that thing where people don't even ask you, "How is this affecting you?" It's that at no point does anybody say, "If we could do things differently again, how would you want to be treated?" It's almost like trauma is piled onto trauma, because before you've even got recovered from that trauma, something else happens. Bang! You're not listened to, or you're disrespected, or you're undermined.

Setting Up Elijah's Hope

Kaddy I think there's thousands of carers out there who get battered by the system—or, we call it "the system," but the system is made up of human beings. Let's have it, right? You get absolutely battered, slaughtered, persecuted, and just don't recover from that. And, then, there's somebody like me who gets battered, but then goes, I'm not staying down. I'm going to rise from this. I'm going to learn from it. Because what I say is: shit happens to us all. The reality is, we have decided that once we've recovered from whatever has affected us, it's not going to affect where we're going.

I set up Elijah's Hope to empower parents to have a voice and not be scared of social workers or doctors. But then, it kind of turned into a bit of an Apert awareness-raising organization. So I wrote blogs on Apert syndrome, connected with the Apert online community. It's kind of like that whole, you know, educating, empowering, resourcing dialogue and being able to make decisions without living in fear that social services are going to hit you with a red brick.

Creating Carers Collective

Kaddy Three years into care managing, I didn't get any support. I didn't have a line manager. There was no training. And there was no personal development plan, no regular supervision. Being the woman I am, I went out and got me a coach. Absolute game changer. I'm a manager that is more assertive, certainly more confident. I delegate a lot more. I take no shit. I take no prisoners. Being coached really has developed me as a manager and as a person, so my thought process was: well, how many carers out there are doing what I do, managing, liaising, facilitating, planning, having to think strategically, having to communicate with multiple professionals? I just thought, right, let's set up Carers Collective.

What I like to do when I'm listening to other carers is help or support them in being able to communicate and advocate more effectively for

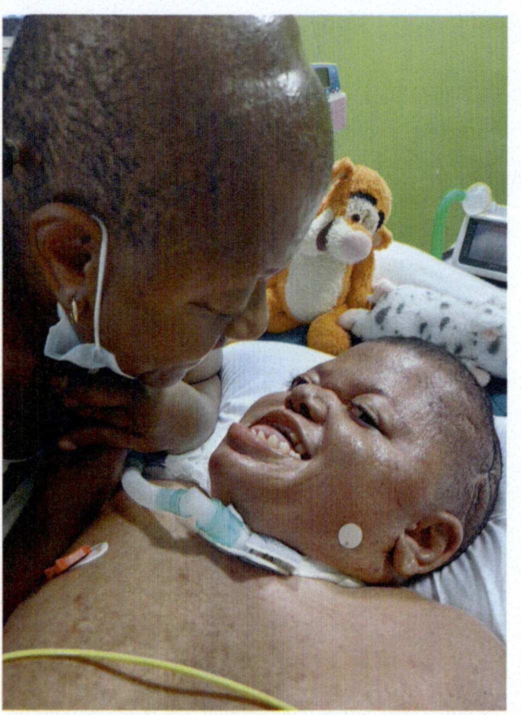

Fig. 36.13 Kaddy and Elijah at Birmingham Children's Hospital in 2023

their loved ones. And I like it when a carer comes to me in one way—be it burnt out, fatigued, frustrated—and then by the end of a six-week period, or be over a course of time of building a relationship with them, there's change in them for the good. Because it's like that ripple effect is it, isn't it? If we're not well, then it has an immediate effect on our child or young person, on our husband, on our wife. So, if we're well, then that has an immediate effect on the person that we're caring for, but it also has a larger ripple effect of the wider family and community (Fig. 36.13).

To read about Kaddy's experiences growing up with Apert syndrome, see Chap. 35: "*Living with Apert Syndrome: Patient Perspectives*."

Natalia and Igor

Brazil

Natalia and Igor live in Brazil with their three children, including their 8-year-old son João, who has Apert syndrome. Shortly after João was born, the family moved from Brazil to the United States for two years so that he could undergo multiple surgeries. The parents are now advocating for change at the federal and systems levels in Brazil to enhance care and raise awareness for Apert syndrome. Their current efforts focus on educating parents, doctors, and hospitals about the need for better information on Apert syndrome and its treatment protocols, as well as advocating for improved access to time-sensitive surgeries. Teaming with doctors in the United States, France, and Brazil, they have also organized the first international symposium on craniosynostosis in Brazil. The family collaborates on some initiatives with the Brazilian Association of Apert Syndrome (Fig. 36.14).

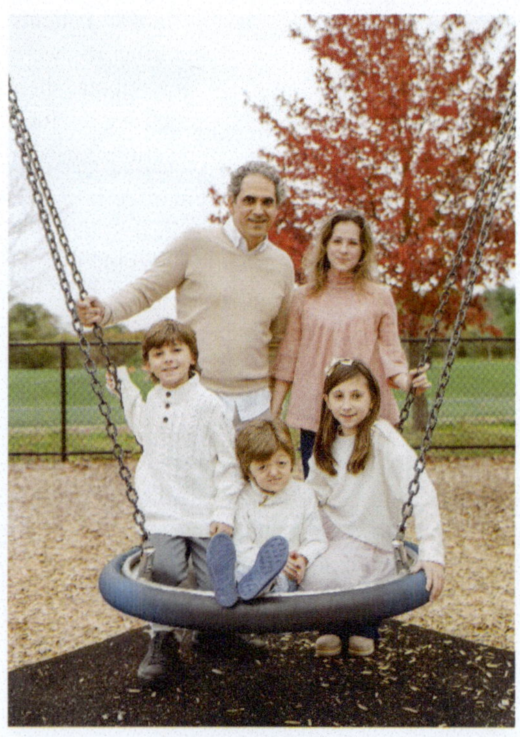

Fig. 36.14 A family portrait from 2021

João's Birth

Natalia On the day João was born, it was an unexpected situation. We could only see that he had a syndrome, and they didn't know what it was. He was born with webbed fingers and toes and a different shaped head. I could see that they didn't want to show him to me. I said, "Can I see him?" They didn't know exactly what to tell me. I saw that something was going on, but I had no idea what.

In the end, they showed him to me, but he was all wrapped. They told me, "He has a problem breathing a little bit, so we'll just take him to the [intensive care unit]." I asked, "Is there something wrong?" So they started saying, "Yes, we don't know exactly what it is, but we will. We will need some time to understand."

A Lack of Information

Igor It was difficult to get information that we could trust and that would allow us to feel comfortable about deciding on treatment. For the first ten to fifteen days, we were very anxious. We had different information from different doctors, and it was not connected.

Natalia We felt helpless. We wanted to educate ourselves, but much of the information on the Internet was very old, like from the '70s. It seemed as if they took from the worst cases and put them on the Internet. So initially, it was hard for us to know what to do. We learned that João needed this big surgery around his fourth month. He would need to have his head opened in a surgery with blood transfusion. But it was terrifying for us to hear that our newborn baby would have to go through this.

Family Support

Natalia We were very lucky to have family and friends who helped us. They asked everybody to learn if there were other ways of doing this. They were going to the Internet, asking doctors and our network in the United States. They found the website of an informative US children's hospital. It wasn't easy to find, but it was where we started to understand the different treatment milestones at different ages.

Igor We had a second opinion with the doctors in the US hospital, and they had information for thirteen years of treatment. We found that more reliable, and we saw a video with a neurosurgeon showing the procedure. There was no need for a blood transfusion. We felt more comfortable about doing this in the United States. We made the decision to move there (Fig. 36.15).

Waiting for Milestones Miles Away

Igor We had to quit jobs to go to the United States. We were not 100% sure, but we felt we should do the best for João. There was a picture that Natalia chose to place on the door of the hospital where João was born, and it was of a big balloon carrying away a house. It was the feeling that João had come to bring us to a new journey. I took this picture under my arm, and we left our apartment.

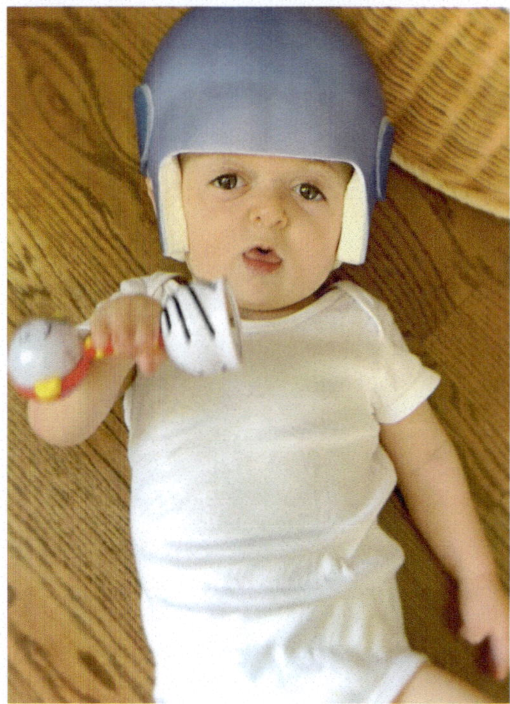

Fig. 36.15 João at 5 months old wearing a helmet after cranial surgery

Natalia It took us a while to understand how Apert affected João. It was step by step. João did the development milestones for babies well. But as soon as he achieved crawling, I would say, Oh my God, oh yeah, he can crawl! Okay, let's go for the next one. Then he can walk. Perfect, let's go for the next one.

His vision was delayed, and we thought he might be blind. Our ophthalmologist in the United States said that we couldn't tell for sure until he reaches 6 months. So we had to wait. Around 7 or 8 months, we finally understood that João could see. And it was a big celebration. [His doctors] kept saying that we could only understand how he would cognitively develop in his third, fourth year. They said you will know by how he interacts. Once again, we had to wait. It was always worrisome for us if he would be able to do everything. It took years for us to really say, okay, everything is fine. It was a time in which we had to exercise patience and faith.

Introducing João

Igor João is very smart. He's a good student in class. At home, we keep calling him to do his duties, and he doesn't listen. Once, we asked his teachers, Do you think that João hears well? One of the teachers said, "I will pay attention." [She then reported], "Every time I tell him, 'João, you have five minutes to finish your homework, he just sits down. He doesn't ask what he needs to do, and he does everything right, while some of his friends keep asking, 'What should I do?'" So that's how we learned João hears well! He has a great sense of humor. A lot of charm. He likes to tease. He talks with everyone. He's curious. He likes to read and to play with technology, you know, games.

Natalia João is very ironic. How do you say in English *moleque?* He's very independent, which gave us some confidence. He was always eager to do everything by himself. He plays soccer. He has friends and a social life. He is bullied, but he defends himself well. It's part of his life. He's fearless. We like to say that Apert syndrome is just a detail in our son's life (Fig. 36.16).

Starting with Baby Steps

Natalia When João was around 3 or 4 years old, we looked back and felt we had access to so many good things for him—the right timing for his surgeries, the support of our families, the means to go to the United States for two years. We felt so lucky and grateful. That's when we started thinking, We have to give back. We have to improve the way this community accesses information. We have to do something.

We felt like maybe we could start doing little things that could be big. We began by asking to translate the US hospital's website, the same page that we saw when João was born, because they had really helpful material, but it was in English. We speak English, but it was still hard for us because of all the medical terms, and in the first month,

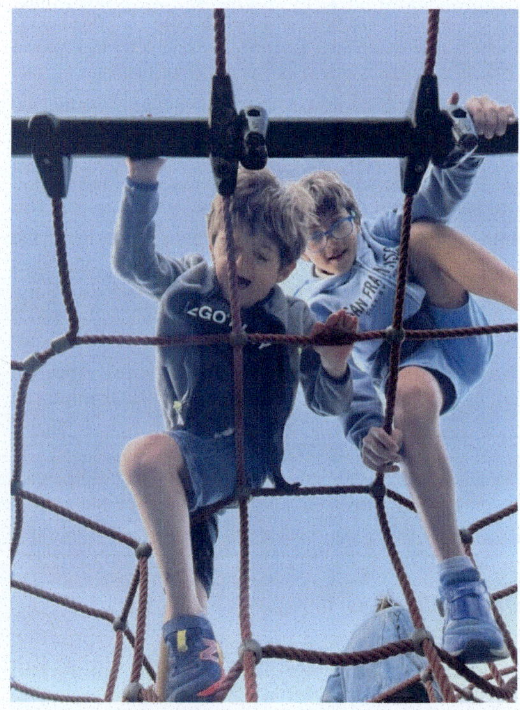

Fig. 36.16 João, age 7, and his brother at the playground

your head is not working well with a newborn. We were wondering if we could translate this into Portuguese so that other people in Brazil can access this information. So we started by doing this. It evolved to other ideas: how could we spread the information? How could we help with the research for the syndrome? We started with baby steps, but baby steps can change a lot of things.

Improving the System

Natalia The health system in Brazil is great, in theory, because everyone has access to it [for free]. But there is room for improvement. For example, there is a window for best results when we talk about craniosynostosis surgery for kids with Apert syndrome. It's in the first year. The system doesn't understand this point and postpones the procedure over others that are considered more urgent. By missing the correct timing, the risk of developmental consequences for the child rises a lot. We help to shed light on these gaps to improve them.

Igor During the International Symposium, we have worked to improve access to reliable information and access to doctors who can do the first surgery. We were trying to help other hospitals to be able to do the surgery in Brazil, because not everyone can quit their jobs and go to the United States or even to São Paulo to have the treatment. Reliable information and treatment must be more accessible for everyone. This is a huge point: it's not only having the best treatment, but the treatment must be close to the family, so that the family does not need to move. After the International Symposium, we believe that the Ministry of Health was sensible for the case and started working on improvements on the federal system level (Fig. 36.17).

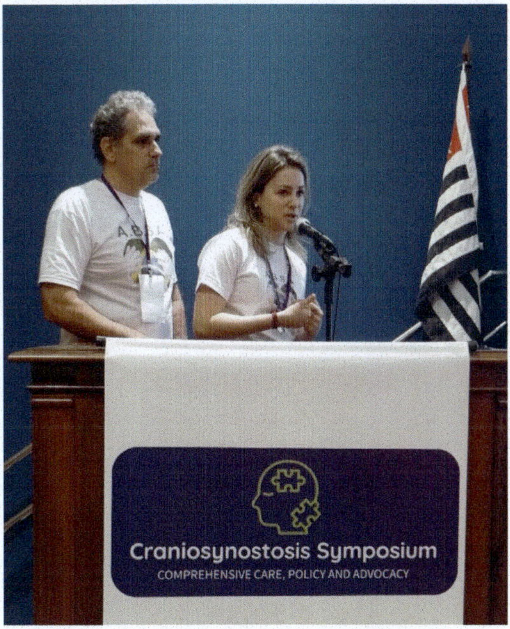

Fig. 36.17 Igor and Natalia speaking at the International Symposium of Craniosynostosis in March 2024

An Appeal to Researchers

Natalia Our feeling is that the doctors work in clusters [in medical centers and different countries]. From the parents' perspective, this doesn't make sense. But we're talking about a rare syndrome. They need to put these cases together to develop the research faster. Otherwise, it's just too slow. They need collaboration. Our desire is that at some point—and perhaps this textbook will help—doctors around the world will be able to do collaborative research for Apert and other craniofacial syndromes.

Advice to Other Families

Natalia In the first years, you really need to take it 24 hours at a time. Because you don't know how the outcome is going to be. It's like a blank page. You don't know how your kid is going to develop. So you need to celebrate—celebrate every step!

One of the doctors advised us from the beginning, "Never limit your child." And this was very important, because sometimes you have a kid with a syndrome, and you keep thinking, Oh, maybe he's not going to be able to do this or that,

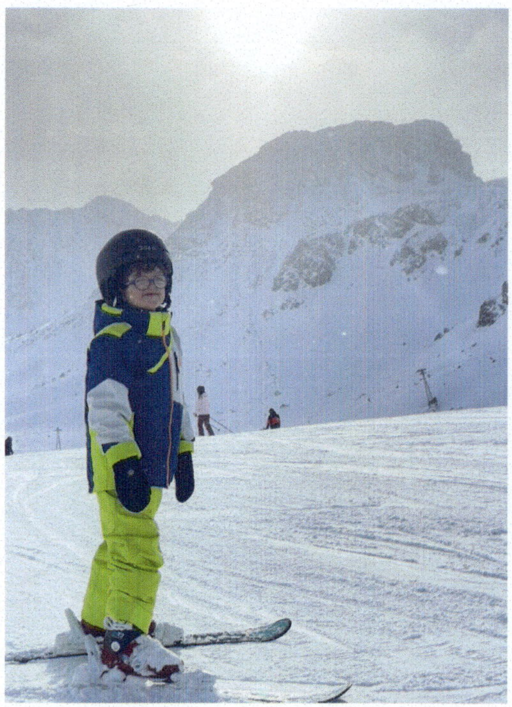

Fig. 36.18 João, age 7, on a family ski trip in Switzerland

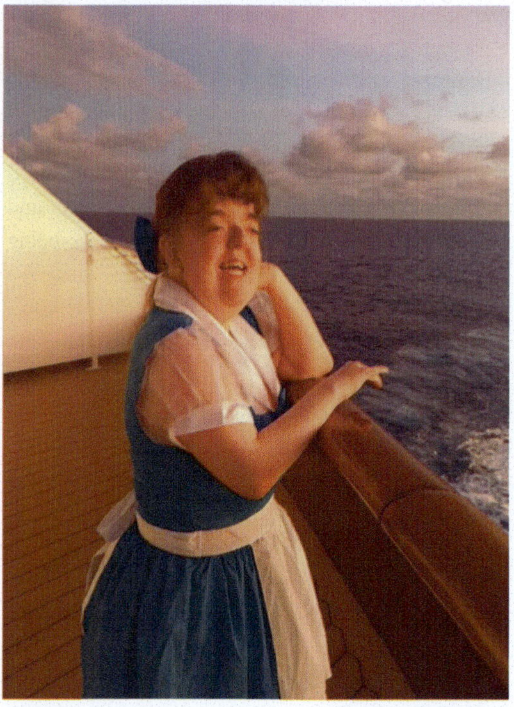

Fig. 36.19 Teeter aboard a Disney cruise in 2016

so I'm not going to expose him. But if you don't expose the child, he is never going to reach his full potential (Fig. 36.18).

Igor I think the message here for any parents is really try to stimulate the child. Because we may learn that the child doesn't have limits, and they keep improving. Apert will be, at the end, just a simple element in the life of the child.

Cathie and Don Sears

Columbia, South Carolina, United States

Cathie and Don Sears are the parents of Elizabeth "Teeter" Sears, a 33-year-old woman who has Apert syndrome. The Sears family lives in Columbia, South Carolina, where Teeter grew up receiving care at the University of SC Specialty Clinics at Richland Memorial Hospital. In 1995, Don and Cathie launched "Teeter's Page," a website providing resources and connections to families of children with Apert syndrome, as well as adults with Apert syndrome. The site grew into Apert International, Inc., currently the largest family support organization for Apert syndrome in the world. As an extension of this work, the Sears family has also organized social events and Disney cruises for the Apert community; their most recent annual gathering in Myrtle Beach, South Carolina, brought together more than 60 attendees from across the United States (Fig. 36.19).

Teeter's Birth

Cathie When Teeter was born, we had no idea, but they immediately diagnosed her with Apert syndrome. There was a neonatologist in the room with us, and she came over and she said, "You see her hands? See her feet? She has Apert syndrome." So we were lucky, even back in 1992, that they knew. They got a picture of us with her, and they immediately took her to a Level 3 care

NICU here in town. I didn't see her for three days (Fig. 36.20).

Don We did have a nurse that was on call that night. She had a craniofacial issue. She was the nurse that was there when Elizabeth was born, and she was so instrumental in helping us adjust to the critical first few hours. We just didn't know what to do. We were getting mixed messages from the doctors and everyone else, and she was the one who kind of calmed us down and said, "Look, I know it's going to be okay."

Cathie We loved her so much that Teeter's middle name is "Denise"—we named her after the nurse.

Don We were given a Xerox copy from a 1960 book called *Human Deformities*. There were two pages with some illustrations and a brief description of Apert syndrome with a very bleak outlook. That was the best that they could pull at the small rural hospital that we were at to begin with, and then we got more information from a geneticist later in the next few weeks. He was very interested in talking with us. A case just doesn't come along here often, so Teeter was kind of a celebrity in the NICU.

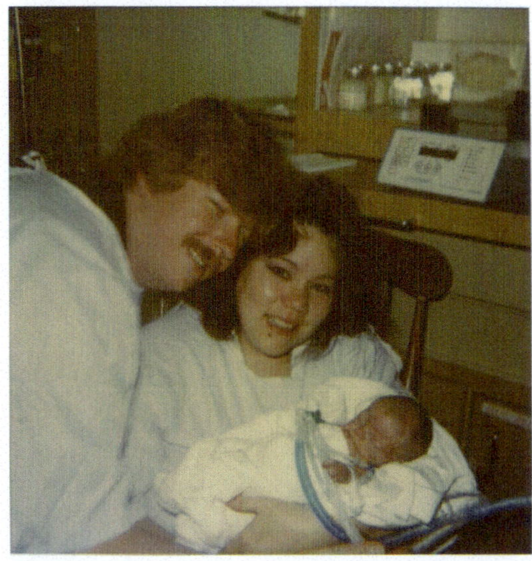

Fig. 36.20 Don and Cathie with 3-week-old Teeter in the NICU

An Empty House

Cathie Bringing Teeter home was extremely scary to me. I've got panic disorder to begin with. And, of course, all I worried about was her dying under my care. I'd never held a baby in my life. I'd never changed a diaper. I'd never fed a baby. They had to teach us in NICU.

We came home to an empty house. For most people, they come home, and there's a joyous occasion where, you know, you got a little celebration, congratulations, and all this. And there was nobody here. It was just Don and I to take care of her. The depression was pretty bad with me.

One of the things that happened when Teeter was at NICU, when we first started bottle-feeding her, is that she aspirated and she turned blue, and they ran us out of the room. They had to code her to bring her back. So, of course, every time I fed her, that's all I could think about. She didn't know how to drink, and that scared me. I got to the point where I got OCD (Obsessive Compulsive Disorder) about having to write everything down. Every time she drank something, I'd have to write down and try to figure out at the end of the day whether she'd had enough, because she wasn't putting on much weight. She was four and a half pounds when she came home. My parents got aggravated at me for having to do that, and they fussed with me about it.

I remember one of the things my mother asked me was, "What are you going to do with her?" That was one of the first questions. I don't know what she meant by that. I never really questioned her. You know, we just said we'll take her home and love her. What else can you do? I can still hear her saying that to me: "What are you going to do with her?" (Fig. 36.21).

Introducing Teeter

Cathie Teeter is into cosplay. She's into Star Wars. She gets really obsessed with certain things. She goes 100%. She loves to sew. She cuts out pieces of felt, and she sews "little people" she calls them. And right now, since she's into Star Wars, she creates little Star Wars charac-

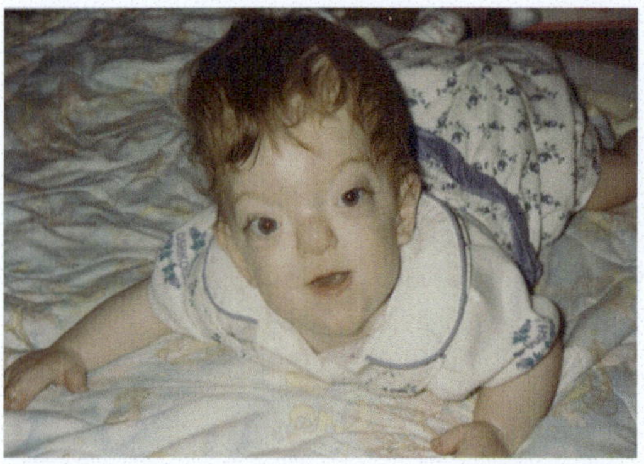

Fig. 36.21 Teeter shortly after her first birthday

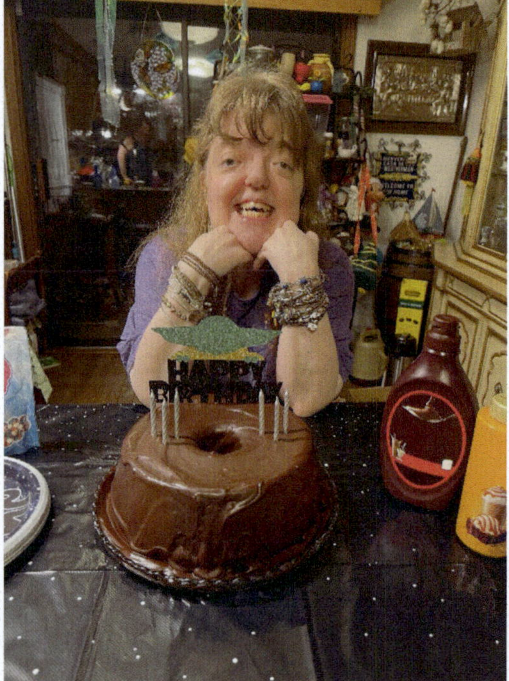

Fig. 36.22 Teeter celebrating her 33rd birthday

ters with her sewing. She loves to sing and dance. She puts on a show every day. She loves her iPhone and iPad. She loves games, painting, and drawing (Fig. 36.22).

Don She was reading on a college level when she was 10. She can read and comprehend anything you put in front of her, except maybe a math textbook. She memorizes facts, figures, birthdates. She loves the IMDb, the movie database. She'll tell you who was the producer of a movie in 1940 and when his wife's birthday was. She just memorizes all these facts and figures, and she's amazing with stuff like that. She's super, super intelligent in the way she talks and what she understands, and then she'll turn around and just be a total 10-year-old goofball. We have done our very best to bring her up with no self-esteem issues. There's nobody she doesn't like because of who they are. There are individuals she doesn't care for but not many.

Cathie People ask, "Do people stare at her whenever you go places?" We used to go out to a restaurant here in town, and every time she'd go in there, she'd say, "Hey, everybody, I'm here!" And, of course, everybody would turn around and stare and smile. We would get people looking at her because she's loud. She introduces herself as she comes in the door. But we get smiles back.

Founding a Community

Don Teeter was about 4, and we had been through all the surgeries, and we were sort of like, Okay, what's next? What are we looking for? We're looking for somebody to either commiserate or guide us. Just looking for some type of relational information with other parents and at the time the Internet was so new. If you searched for "Apert," what you came back with was the aperture settings on a camera. That's it.

I just put a little page out there [online]. I put Teeter's picture on there, and I said, if anybody else has experience, please let us know. And within a week, I had heard from a couple on the West Coast, and they had a daughter about the same age, and she was aware of a mailing list, a pen-pal type mailing list, so we wrote to them. Things finally started to look up a little bit as far as knowing other people. We were mailing videotapes back and forth across the country of our kids crawling around.

I taught myself how to write web pages, and I heard from a couple more people and said, "Send me pictures. We'll scan them in, and we'll make a little club." And as time went by, the little club grew, and we had dozens and then hundreds of people who found us and wanted to be part of it. Now it's thousands.

From Online to In-Person

Don After a few years of having this club, one of the parents, a best friend of Cathie's named Judy, prodded Cathie to come to the beach with us for a vacation. We'd go to Myrtle Beach every year.

Cathie We had the best time! So in 1999, I decided let's open this up, and I opened it up to my Listserv group, and we had 13 or 14 families come that first year. And it was amazing to actually meet other families with children with Apert, and we met a couple of adults with Apert syndrome.

Don There's a lot of solidarity between the parents and families that are impacted with any syndrome like this when they get together. It's a common bond. It just transcends what you would normally get out of a friendship.

Cathie A lot of us moms, we talk very, very deeply about things. That's one of the reasons why we don't have a lot of outsiders in my Apert International group on Facebook. It's because there are days when some parents decide we hate Apert syndrome. And it's not that they hate their child. They hate the syndrome, and we want to complain and cry and talk to our friends about how aggravated we are. And we don't want our next-door neighbor reading that. We don't want our parents reading that. We want other parents who understand. And the next day, things lighten up, and we feel a little bit better, and that's one of the reasons why I keep my group private.

Don What happened is the parents that we trained, trained others, [who] trained others, [who] trained others. So the parents of the 6-year-olds are now bringing along the parents of the 3-year-olds who are bringing along the parents of the newborns. I wish I could take credit for planning all this out, but I didn't. I started it all with a single page, because we were looking for somebody else in the world who could relate to us. We were very fortunate that it caught on, and we were able to connect with other people like ourselves.

Advice to Other Families

Don It's not that we try to avoid the subject [of Apert syndrome with Teeter]. It's just we didn't feel like it was necessary to point it out and explain something that she hadn't asked about. And then as she grew up, we started having these events and meeting more and more kids with Apert syndrome and adults with Apert syndrome. To her, that's her normal. She understands that she's different, but she doesn't dwell on it.

Cathie She'll say something, like, "My thumbs are backwards," and I'll say, "Yeah, they are. That's cool." She asked me once, "You think in a past life I had toes?" I said, "You probably did."

Don We learned from the adults who had Apert syndrome who were able to relate to us and give us some guidance. We were able to talk to them on an adult level and say, "How do you really feel? How is this affecting you? And what should we do differently?" And they were able to guide us and tell us, you know, that there are days when I just don't want to look in the mirror, and it's awful, and there are other days when it's okay. They said just do what you're doing, because Teeter's great. Teeter's doing fantastic. As long as she looks in the mirror every day and likes who she sees, we're not changing anything.

That's the advice that I would give to any parent with any child. Not just Apert syndrome. If they like who they are, then you don't need to mess with that, because isn't that kind of like the goal of everybody? To love yourself? And you've got to do your best to get there.

Cathie Raise your child like any other child.

Don We get so focused on the physical that a lot of times the emotional, the spiritual, the psychological, is not as focused on as the physical is. Teeter's got blonde hair and fused toes and something called Apert syndrome, and she's got a goofy smile and great personality. But she's not Teeter with Apert syndrome. She's Teeter (Fig. 36.23).

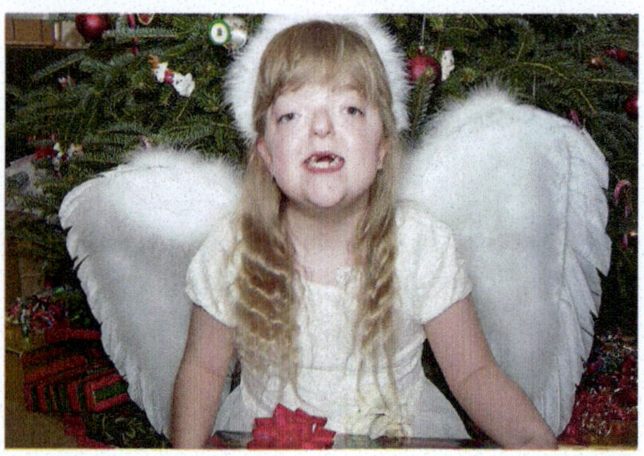

Fig. 36.23 Teeter at Christmas, age 7

No Better Child

Cathie I wouldn't change her. It's been a great life with her for 33 years. I mean, there's been some sad points for surgeries and stuff like that. But we couldn't have asked for a better child. If I could go back and have a regular child who doesn't have Apert syndrome, I don't think I would.

Don My God! How boring would that be? For whatever way we were chosen, we were chosen correctly.

Conclusion

This chapter represents a sampling of caregivers' experiences with Apert syndrome. There are members of the Apert community whom we did not include due to limits of time and space, most notably, families with adopted children; siblings; and caregivers from additional geographic regions. Still, the stories gathered share common experiences and perspectives. Families described similar feelings of confusion, uncertainty, and trauma surrounding an Apert diagnosis at birth, as well as around surgical treatments. All of the caregivers expressed a fierce, unwavering love for their child with Apert syndrome—a source of resilience, strength, and tangible joy. They also emphasized that Apert syndrome was only a part of their child's identity. In this way, the interviews highlight a need to acknowledge the individuality of caregivers and children in the Apert community.

Advocacy efforts and support networks have grown out of gaps in care for Apert families. These initiatives range from close-knit online communities and popular social events to national and international collaborations. All serve as grassroots sources of strength, knowledge, and belonging. From Rabia Aziz's embrace of "How are you?" to Kaddy Thomas' efforts to heal caregiver trauma, the experiences described offer ideas and actions to consider as part of holistic care for this community.

We offer our most sincere thank-you to the families who shared their time with us. We are grateful for their generosity, insights, and openness, especially their willingness to revisit sometimes difficult and painful experiences.

Resources by Caregivers and Families, for Caregivers and Families

Apert International (Apert USA): This Facebook group is exclusive to patients with Apert syndrome and their parents and serves as an international resource for those looking for support, information, and community.

https://www.facebook.com/groups/apertusa/

Apert International, Inc.: This 501(c)(3) nonprofit foundation provides education and information to the general public about Apert syndrome, as well as direct financial and emotional assistance based on need to families affected by Apert syndrome.

https://www.apert-international.org/

BabyFace: A Story of Heart and Bones by Jeanne McDermott: A science journalist chronicles the first years of raising her son with Apert syndrome in this memoir.

Brazilian Association of Apert Syndrome: Formed by mothers of children with Apert syndrome, this organization works to spread awareness of the condition while offering support for patients and their families.

(continued)

https://journals.lww.com/jcraniofacial-surgery/citation/2018/09000/founding_of_the_brazilian_association_of_apert.75.aspx

Carers Collective: An online six-week course dedicated to helping caregivers learn how to better care for their loved ones as well as themselves.

https://www.carers-collective.co.uk/

Children's Craniofacial Association: Offers support for individuals and families affected by craniofacial differences through education and empowerment. A poem written by the brother of a boy with Apert syndrome sheds light on the parental and sibling experience.

https://ccakids.org/

Elijah's Hope: This nonprofit is focused on improving the physical and psychological health of individuals with Apert syndrome.

https://www.carers-collective.co.uk/elijahs-hope

Five Star Adaptive: A journalist and disability rights activist runs this website which vets and lists tools, technology, and products useful for easing the daily routines and care of individuals with disabilities.

https://fivestaradaptive.com

Instagram—Talia Oatway: A social media influencer advocates for understanding Apert syndrome by posting what goes into caring for and supporting her son, Oakley.

https://www.instagram.com/talia.oatway/?hl=en

Special Needs Pakistan: An online support group offering a network of resources for parents, siblings, families, and friends of individuals with disabilities in Pakistan.

https://www.facebook.com/groups/685128974913634/

Teeter's Page: Educates the public and advocates for families of children with Apert syndrome. The site keeps a list of written works about Apert syndrome, while another section spotlights individuals with Apert syndrome around the world.

https://www.apert.org/

The Mighty: Patients and relatives blog first-hand accounts of their experiences. Author and mother Jeannie Ewing writes about her daughter's Apert diagnosis and the challenges that come with it.

https://themighty.com/

TikTok—Acacia Beach: A mother documents life with her daughter with Apert syndrome. She answers the Internet's questions with in-depth responses and highlights her daughter's triumphs.

https://www.tiktok.com/@acaciabeach

References

1. Angie and Marco Garcia Speak At Neil Armstrong Academy in UT (2018) CCAKidsBlog, 4 December. https://www.ccakidsblog.org/2018/12/wonderwednesday-angie-and-marco-garcia.html. Accessed 13 Nov 2024.
2. Aziz R. 2024. Personal interview. 10 October, virtual.
3. Aziz R. "Raising Aaliya, Rising Above." Record. Video. TEDx Talk; 2014. https://www.youtube.com/watch?v=uoPiQTMj7as
4. Beyond 'Difficult' (n.d.) CareTalk. https://www.caretalk.co.uk/opinion/beyond-difficult/. Accessed 16 Oct 2024.
5. Carers Collective (n.d.). https://www.carers-collective.co.uk/meet-our-founder-kaddy Accessed 16 Oct 2024.
6. Coughlan E. (2023) "I was abandoned by my mother as a baby over my rare genetic condition—then my life was turned upside down again after my son became brain damaged at 18 months old." *Daily Mail.* 6 June. https://www.dailymail.co.uk/femail/article-12164841/I-abandoned-mother-rare-genetic-condition-baby-brain-damaged.html. Accessed 16 Oct 2024.
7. Garcia A, Garcia M. Personal interview. 28 February, virtual; 2025.
8. Garcia A, Garcia M. Personal interview. 21 November, virtual; 2024.

9. Garcia A, Garcia M. 2024. Personal interview. 14 November, virtual.
10. Igor and Natalia. 2025. Personal interview. 21 March, virtual.
11. "Kaddy Thomas Talks About Finding Out Her Son Had Brain Damage" (2023) Daily Mail. 6 June.
12. https://www.dailymail.co.uk/video/reallife/video-2954041/Video-Kaddy-Thomas-talks-finding-son-Eijah-brain-damage.html
13. Louisiana Students Read Wonder and Skype with "Real-Life Auggies" (2017) CCAKidsBlog, 7 November. https://www.ccakidsblog.org/2017/11/wonderwednesday-louisiana-students-read.html. Accessed 13 Nov 2024.
14. Sears C., Sears D. 2024. Personal interview. 25 October, virtual.
15. Sears D, Cathie. (n.d.) "Teeter's Page." *Apert* International. https://www.apert.org/. Accessed 24 Oct 2024.
16. Sved R. (2024) "The power of storytelling resonates!" Kaddy Thomas on Harnessing Experience and Passion to Create Authentic Change. 3rd Sector Mission Control 14 November.
17. https://www.3rdsectormissioncontrol.co.uk/the-power-of-storytelling-resonates-kaddy-thomas-on-harnessing-experience-and-passion-to-create-authentic-change/. Accessed 16 Oct 2024.
18. Thomas K. 2024. Personal interview. 18 October, virtual.
19. Thomas K. (2022) "I became a full-time carer for my son after surgery left him with brain damage" Metro 26 June. https://metrocouk/2022/06/26/i--became-a-carer-for-my-son-after-surgery-left-him-with-brain-damage-16844337/. Accessed 16 Oct 2024.

37 Economic Considerations for the Treatment of Syndromic Craniosynostosis

Greta Davis, Solomon Lee, Ting-Chen Lu,
Cassio Eduardo Raposo-Amaral, John G. Meara,
and John Rose

Introduction

Apert syndrome, or acrocephalosyndactyly type I, is a congenital disorder with significant systemic effects, which in turn translate into considerable economic consequences. Patients with Apert syndrome have variable expressions of multi-suture craniosynostosis, midface retrusion, palatal abnormalities, feeding issues, dental abnormalities, ocular abnormalities, hearing loss, multi-level airway obstruction, complex syndactyly and other limb anomalies, spinal fusions, progressive synostosis, neurologic deformities, intellectual disability, cardiovascular anomalies, gastrointestinal issues, genitourinary issues, and skin changes [1]. Depending on the severity of the phenotype, these conditions can lead to considerable individual and societal costs over a patient's lifetime, not only in direct healthcare costs but also in opportunity cost and loss of productivity.

Fortunately, timely diagnosis, medical and surgical interventions, and surveillance to prevent secondary manifestations can significantly mitigate the morbidity associated with Apert syndrome [2]. The Disease Control Priorities, Third Edition, has also clearly established that many surgical procedures can be essential, cost-effective, and feasible to implement [3]. However, data regarding the economic impact of Apert syndrome are severely lacking, and it is difficult to guide resource-based clinical and policy decisions regarding craniosynostosis treatment without the associated economic data.

As of this writing, there are no studies evaluating the costs associated with comprehensive treatment of Apert syndrome, and even when the search is broadened to include all forms of craniosynostosis, there is minimal economic data available. Given the paucity of data, we have decided to focus the scope of this chapter on

G. Davis
Division of Plastic and Reconstructive Surgery, Center for Health Equity in Surgery and Anesthesia, UC San Francisco Medical Center, San Francisco, CA, USA

S. Lee
Division of Plastic and Reconstructive Surgery, UC San Francisco Medical Center, San Francisco, CA, USA

T.-C. Lu
Department of Plastic and Reconstructive Surgery and Craniofacial Research Center, Chang Gung Memorial Hospital, Linkou, Taiwan

C. E. Raposo-Amaral
Institute of Plastic and Craniofacial Surgery, SOBRAPAR Hospital, Campinas, São Paulo, Brazil

J. G. Meara
Department of Plastic and Oral Surgery, Boston Children's Hospital, Harvard Medical School, Boston, MA, USA

J. Rose (✉)
Division of Plastic and Reconstructive Surgery, Center for Health Equity in Surgery and Anesthesia, Philip R. Lee Institute for Health Policy Studies, UC San Francisco Medical Center, San Francisco, CA, USA
e-mail: John.Rose@ucsf.edu

J. G. Meara et al. (eds.), *Apert Syndrome*, https://doi.org/10.1007/978-3-032-12551-4_37

exploring the economic considerations for the treatment of craniosynostosis, using this aspect of the disease as a pathway toward understanding the larger economic implications for Apert and other craniosynostosis syndromes. This chapter thus aims to review the current state of the literature on the economic impact of syndromic craniosynostosis treatment, review the necessary elements of cost-effectiveness and cost–benefit analysis (CBA) , identify known and unknown data variables pertinent to the treatment of craniosynostosis, and outline a roadmap towards the meaningful economic analysis of craniosynostosis treatment.

Literature Review

We searched PubMed/Medline with MeSH headings "Acrocephalosyndactyly" and "Costs and Cost Analysis" from inception through March 2025. "Acrocephalosyndactyly" header includes Apert syndrome, and "Costs and Cost Analysis" includes relevant sub-headers such as "Cost-Benefit Analysis," "Cost-Effectiveness Analysis," and "Health Care Costs." The search generated two articles, neither of which were specific to Apert syndrome nor contained a formal economic analysis. MeSH terms were broadened to "Craniosynostoses" and "Costs and cost analysis." Search results, supplemented by manual review of bibliographies of retrieved studies, generated 27 articles. These were screened for relevance to the surgical treatment of craniosynostosis based on the title and abstract. Articles were included for formal review if they pertained to surgical treatment of craniosynostosis and included some cost metric (10 of 24 articles) [4–13]. Full-text reviews of articles satisfying the inclusion criteria were then performed (Fig. 37.1). Of the 10 studies included in qualitative synthesis, one article contained cost-effectiveness analysis but only regarding diagnostic strategies and one article provided a narrative summary of relative costs following intervention on Apert syndrome in a low- and middle-income countries (LMIC) setting but was specific to mandibular and midface hypoplasia [8]. No articles addressed surgical intervention of

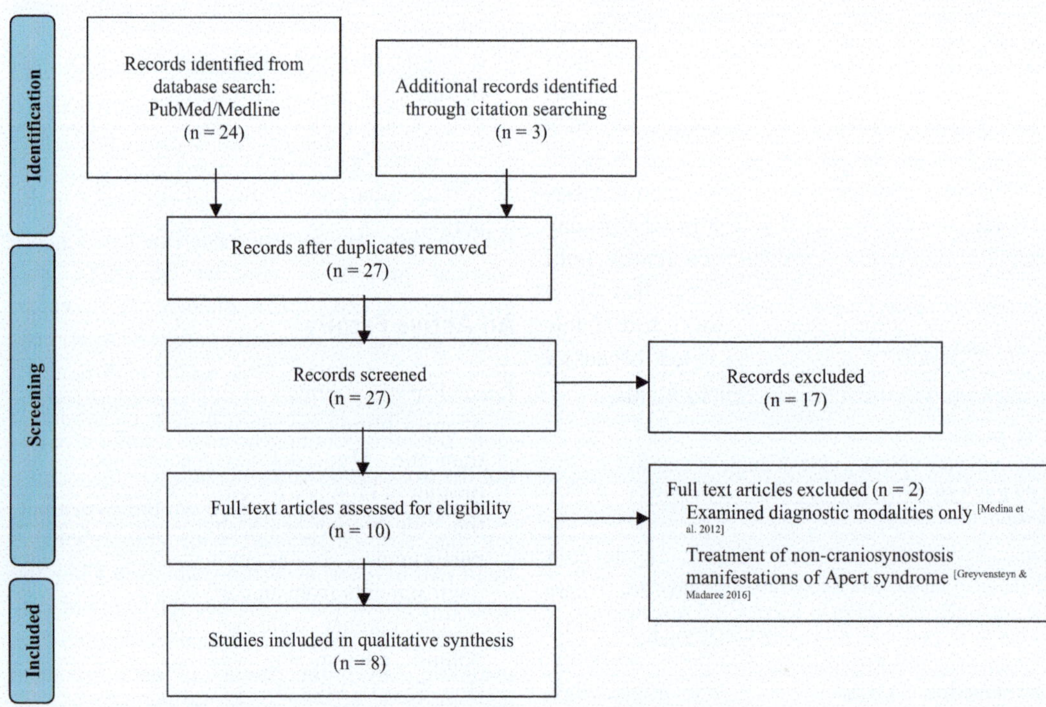

Fig. 37.1 Preferred reporting items for systematic reviews and meta-analyses (PRISMA) flowchart for systematic review

craniosynostosis alongside a formal economic methodology such as a cost-effectiveness or cost–benefit analysis. Nonetheless, existing publications provide valuable insight into reimbursement rates, which can be used to estimate economic impact in the absence of formal analyses, as discussed later in this chapter.

Cost Analysis Model Review

Given the lack of existing studies that model cost analyses for the treatment of craniosynostosis, we will briefly review the components of two widely used cost analysis models to identify where the economic data for craniosynostosis treatment is specifically needed. Cost-effectiveness analysis (CEA) is generally the primary tool for economic analysis of healthcare interventions. While used less frequently, cost–benefit analysis (CBA) is another useful tool for assessing the broader societal impact of healthcare interventions and their investment value [14].

A cost-effectiveness analysis (CEA) generates a cost-effectiveness ratio (CER) equal to the net cost divided by changes in health outcomes. Net cost is the cost of an intervention minus the averted medical and productivity costs. Changes in health outcomes are equal to outcomes with the intervention minus outcomes without the intervention. In a cost–benefit analysis (CBA), net benefit is generally conceptualized as total benefit minus the cost, a benefit-to-cost ratio, or an economic valuation of health benefits. Benefits are defined as the monetary value of health outcomes, including averted medical costs, gains in productivity, non-market items, or other monetized health improvements. Costs of illness may include direct medical costs, indirect costs, intangible costs, and opportunity costs [15].

While direct costs are more easily identifiable, quantifying indirect costs and the gradient of healthcare outcomes can be far more complex. Disability-adjusted life years (DALYs) and quality-adjusted life years (QALYs) are two workhorse metrics in healthcare economics that have attempted to quantify the comprehensive disease burden on a patient's life by incorporating both mortality and morbidity in their calculations.

DALYs are equal to the sum of years of life lost (YLL) and the years lived with disability (YLD) for a given cause, age, sex, and year. YLLs are equal to the number of deaths due to a cause (N) multiplied by the standard loss function (L) specifying years of life lost for a death, with the loss function being based on the latest frontier national projected life expectancy. YLDs are calculated as the number of incident cases for a cause (I) multiplied by the disability weight (DW) and the average duration of the disease until remission or death (L). Disability weight ranges from 0 (perfect health) to 1 (equivalent to death). Additional adjustments such as age-weighting, time discounting, and comorbidity adjustment can be added to the calculation [16].

A QALY is defined as the additional years of life gained multiplied by the health-related quality of life (HRQL) [17]. HRQL is assigned a utility weight from 0 (death) to 1 (perfect health) which is determined by five dimensions (EQ-5D): mobility, self-care, usual activities, pain/discomfort, and anxiety/depression [18].

Both DALYs and QALYs, while inverse to one another, are essentially metrics that combine mortality and morbidity from a cause into a single unit. For both measures, the mortality component is unambiguously defined (dependent on age of death), while the disability/quality of life component is subject to more variable quantification. Between the two, DALYs have become the more dominant metric used in quantifying the global disease burden.

In summary, the independent variables needed to complete a cost analysis are costs and health outcomes. Costs include direct costs (e.g., surgery, medication, supplies, diagnostic tools, surveillance), indirect costs (e.g., staff, facility overhead), and opportunity costs (e.g., loss of potential income, productivity). Health outcomes variables are disease incidence, duration and severity, mortality and life expectancy, disability weights, health-related quality of life measures, and the impact of an intervention on all those same measures pre- and post-treatment. The calculated CER can then be compared to gross domestic product (GDP) per capita to determine cost-effectiveness.

In the following sections, we review the available data for each of these variables relevant to the treatment of syndromic craniosynostosis.

Understanding the Economic Value of Surgical Interventions

Section Objective *Acknowledging the gap in available data on the cost-effectiveness of treating craniosynostosis, we present a framework for performing an economic analysis, emphasizing the relevant cost/burden domains for this treatment.*

Economic evaluations support informed decision-making by clinicians and policymakers. Specifically, cost-effective analyses enable comparison of the relative value of different surgical interventions and priority investments; this is particularly relevant in low- and middle-income country contexts which face disproportionate barriers in access to specialty surgical care. Performing an effective economic analysis in the pediatric population is challenging, due in part to an inability to predict future cognitive abilities or late-presenting diseases. As such, the evidence base for the cost-effectiveness of surgery for craniosynostosis, and especially syndromic craniosynostoses which carry variable phenotypic expression, is incomplete.

Cost-effectiveness is commonly expressed through DALYs–DALYs and the DW aspect are already defined in the prior section. Re-defining here makes the chapter seem like it was pieced together from multiple authors without proofing/merging well. The World Health Organization Choosing Interventions that are Cost-Effective (WHO-CHOICE) guidelines have historically defined the following thresholds for assessing cost-effectiveness of an intervention: an intervention is very cost-effective if it costs less than the GDP/capita per DALY averted, cost-effective if one to three times the GDP/capita per DALY averted, and not cost-effective if greater than three times the GDP/capita per DALY averted [19]. The WHO's Global Burden of Disease (GBD) studies summarize DALY and DW estimates for 288 disease states using 56,604 data sources. Yet, DALY estimates for surgically treatable conditions are limited due to the vast number of surgical diagnoses and procedures, variable complexity of treatment, and lack of corresponding DWs [22].

Although few economic analyses focus on pediatric surgical care, the orofacial cleft literature contains numerous cost-effectiveness studies that represent a global perspective and may serve as proxies for the craniosynostosis population due to shared longitudinal, multidisciplinary care models and frequent interplay from genetic and syndromic conditions. According to the GBD 2004 study, the uncorrected DW for cleft lip is 0.098 and cleft palate 0.230; after treatment, these DWs decrease to 0.016 and 0.015, respectively [20, 21]. DALYs are calculated as the sum of YLL plus YLD using these DWs [23] as discussed above. Cost-effectiveness analyses can then be performed by multiplying the facility or regional reimbursement rate for a given surgery by total number of cases performed and dividing by average DALYs averted as a result of surgery to give a CER. In the cleft literature, the average DALYs averted per patient ranges from 2.49 to 10.59, and the average CER ranges from $39 to $705 (in 2020 USD) in low- and middle-income contexts [24, 25].

While DWs for craniosynostosis have not yet been established, DWs have been assigned for various conditions associated with acrocephalosyndactyly in GBD 2021, as displayed in Box 37.1. Significant variability in DW exists between anomalies and by severity for a given congenital anomaly. Thus, assigning a range of DWs that captures the broad phenotypic manifestations of syndromic craniosynostosis is challenging. Nonetheless, strategies to reliably investigate the economic impact of craniosynostosis and its therapeutic interventions are critical.

Box 37.1 Disability weights for surgically treatable congenital anomalies according to the Global Burden of Disease studies

Definition	Disability weight
Syndactyly	
Disfigurement level 1 due to polydactyly and syndactyly (lowest severity)	0.011
Disfigurement level 2 and moderate motor impairment due to congenital limb deficiency (highest severity)	0.124
Orofacial cleft	
Disfigurement level 1 due to orofacial clefts (lowest severity)	0.011
Disfigurement level 2 and speech problems due to orofacial clefts (highest severity)	0.115
Encephalocele[a]	
Borderline intellectual disability due to encephalocele (lowest severity)	0.011
Profound intellectual disability due to encephalocele (highest severity)	0.200

Definitions and disability weights according to GBD 2021 [22]

[a]Encephalocele is not an acrocephalosyndactyly-associated diagnosis but included for reference as it is the only congenital pediatric anomaly affecting the calvarium with variable severity that is represented in GBD 2021

Economic Impact of Untreated Craniosynostosis

Section Objective *To present data behind the prevalence of craniosynostosis and the impact of lack of access to (or delays in) surgical intervention.*

Despite significant morbidity and mortality that result from untreated or late-presenting cases, craniosynostosis has not been considered an essential surgical condition, and access to surgical care remains limited outside of major academic centers. Globally, craniosynostosis affects roughly 5.9 per 10,000 live births [26], though variability exists by geographic location. Syndromic craniosynostosis represents a minority of total cases and ranges from 0.06–0.15 per 10,000 for Apert syndrome to 0.2–0.4 per 10,000 for Saethre–Chotzen syndrome [27]. To illustrate the global burden of surgery due to craniosynostosis, [26] modeled birth prevalences by continent for 2019 reported the highest projection of new cases in Asia (43,536) and Africa (25,494), and lowest in Oceania (408). Craniosynostosis is often of lower priority relative to other pediatric surgical conditions in areas where access to surgical care is most restricted. As such, a significant number of these cases go untreated.

Untreated craniosynostosis changes skull shape and restricts calvarial growth, which can result in elevated intracranial pressure that can impact vision and neurodevelopment. The cognitive development of children born with craniosynostosis is variable, and the relationship between intracranial hypertension and neurodevelopment remains an area of active research. However, studies have demonstrated challenges with psychosocial development and social inclusion among children with syndromic craniosynostosis relative to typically developing children [28–30]. The consequences of delayed treatment depend largely on the severity of intracranial volume restriction. In general, the risk of complications increases with age at the time of repair and is highest beyond 12 months of age [31, 32]; patients with acrocephalosyndactyly and associated congenital anomalies experience the greatest age-related increase in the risk of perioperative complications [31]. Delays in initial surgical consultation and subsequent repair are especially consequential as certain procedures, such as strip craniectomy, have a limited window of efficacy.

These burdens, from social stigmatization to loss of function or intellectual ability, carry economic significance and, as such, are considered in the determination of DWs by the GBD study. Further research is needed to understand the comprehensive burdens of different phenotypic expressions of syndromic craniosynostosis, including pre- and post-treatment. Due to the significant psychosocial implications of craniosynostosis, measuring the efficacy of surgical interventions using quality of life scales is equally as important as defining the financial and societal implications and should also be prioritized in future studies [33].

Econometrics for the Surgical Treatment of Craniosynostosis

Section Objective *To present the scope and lack of existing data necessary for the calculations of cost-effectiveness, cost-benefit, and economic losses with a focus on patients with syndromic conditions.*

Disability-Adjusted Life Years (DALYs)

As previously described, cost-effectiveness analyses assess the relative value of healthcare interventions and help establish priorities for investment. To address the global deficit of craniofacial care provision, especially as it relates to the treatment of craniosynostosis and prevention of neurodevelopmental sequelae, we must start by examining the availability of data for DALY estimation. DALY is calculated as follows [35]:

- $DALY_{(c,s,a,t)} = YLL_{(c,s,a,t)} + YLD_{(c,s,a,t)}$ for given cause *c*, age *a*, sex *s* and year *t*
- $YLL_{(c,s,a,t)} = N_{(c,s,a,t)} \times L_{(s,a)}$
  - $N_{(c,s,a,t)}$ is the number of deaths due to the cause *c* for the given age *a* and sex *s* in year *t*
  - $L_{(s,a)}$ is a standard loss function specifying years of life lost for a death at age *a* for sex *s*
- $YLD_{(c,s,a,t)} = I_{(c,s,a,t)} \times DW_{(c,s,a)} \times L_{(c,s,a,t)}$
  - $I_{(c,s,a,t)}$ = number of incident cases for cause *c*, age *a* and sex *s*
  - $DW_{(c,s,a)}$ = disability weight for cause *c*, age *a* and sex *s*
  - $L_{(c,s,a,t)}$ = average duration of the case until remission or death (years)

Starting with YLL, the data required to calculate the potential years lost for a population is the number of deaths secondary to craniosynostosis multiplied by the premature loss of years when comparing age of death to frontier life expectancy. The frontier life expectancy data for most populations is readily available via the United Nations (UN) World Population Prospects 2024 [36]. Mortality data for craniosynostosis are once again unavailable through the typical databases such as GBD 2021 and WHO Global Health Estimate [[22, 37, 78]; WHO GHE]. Turning to the literature, mortality data is equally wanting. Several retrospective reviews identify perioperative mortality related to surgical intervention for craniosynostosis to range from 0 to 1% [38–42]. No studies exist, however, on overall life expectancy for either untreated or treated craniosynostosis, which is necessary for the YLL calculation.

For YLD calculation, data for incidence, case duration until remission, and disability weight is required. Since craniosynostosis is a congenital deformity, incidence is equivalent to the birth prevalence. The birth prevalence for craniosynostosis is estimated to be 1:2100–2500 live births [43, 44]. Approximately 20% of craniosynostosis cases are thought to be syndromic [45]. Apert syndrome is far rarer with estimated birth prevalence ranges from 1:80,000 to 160,000 live births [46, 47].

If left untreated, the duration of the case until remission is equivalent to the life expectancy of an untreated patient, for which there are no documented studies. If successfully treated, patients should be able to reach their new baseline level of functioning within a year of recovery and maintain that throughout their lives. Complication rates after surgery range from 5 to 39%, and serious complications that require additional intervention can range from 3.5 to 21.4% [38–42, 48]. Recovering from these complications can be factored into the calculation of case duration before reaching remission.

Disability weights are perhaps the most difficult to ascertain as they are subject to value judgments. As defined by WHO, "disability is used broadly to refer to departures from optimal health in any of the important domains of health and disability weights should reflect the general population judgments about the 'healthfulness' of defined states, not any judgments of quality of life or the worth of persons or the social undesirability or stigma of health states [49]." The original descriptions for disability weight values are presented in Table 37.1.

To assign weights to craniosynostosis, we must evaluate the comprehensive functionality of a patient regarding the interest areas of recreation, education, procreation, and occupation. For our exercise, we will focus on syndromic craniosynostosis specific to Apert syndrome as intellectual ability highly varies between different syndromes. For Apert syndrome, most treated individuals have normal intellect or mild intellectual disability with some reported cases of moderate-to-severe intellectual disability [50–52]. A known risk factor for intellectual disability is delay of surgical intervention until after one year of age [1]. Thus, an approximation for intellectual functioning could be that untreated craniosynostosis will lead to moderate-to-severe intellectual disability, while treated craniosynostosis will lead to normal intellect or mild intellectual disability. Although there are no published disability weight estimates for craniosynostosis, GBD 2021 does have disability weights for "intellectual disabilities due to other chromosomal abnormalities" (Table 37.2).

Acknowledging the limited information and assumptions made in the untreated versus treated population, these disability weights could serve as soft proxies for syndromic craniosynostosis in calculating DALYs.

Cost-Effectiveness Analysis: Cost-Effectiveness Ratio (CER)

After DALYs have been established, cost-effectiveness analyses can be performed by multiplying reimbursement rate for a given surgery by total number of cases performed and dividing by average DALYs averted as a result of surgery. Unfortunately, most of the craniosynostosis literature misuses the term "cost effective," instead

Table 37.1 Definitions of disability weighting according to Murray et al [35]

Class	Description	Weight
Class 1	Limited ability to perform at least one activity in one of the following areas: Recreation, education, procreation, or occupation	0.096
Class 2	Limited ability to perform most activities in one of the following areas: Recreation, education, procreation, or occupation	0.220
Class 3	Limited ability to perform activities in two or more of the following areas: Recreation, education, procreation, or occupation	0.400
Class 4	Limited ability to perform most activities in all of the following areas: Recreation, education, procreation, or occupation	0.600
Class 5	Needs assistance with instrumental activities of daily living such as meal preparation, shopping, or housework	0.810
Class 6	Needs assistance with activities of daily living such as eating, personal hygiene, or toilet use	0.920

Table 37.2 Disability weights of intellectual disability due to other chromosomal abnormalities according to GBD 2021 [22]

Severity	Description	Mean	Low	High
Mild	Has low intelligence and is slow in learning at school. As an adult, the person can live independently, but often needs help to raise children and can only work at simple supervised jobs	0.043	0.026	0.065
Moderate	Has low intelligence and is slow in learning to speak and to do even simple tasks. As an adult, the person requires a lot of support to live independently and raise children. The person can only work at the simplest supervised jobs	0.100	0.066	0.142
Severe	Has very low intelligence and cannot speak more than a few words, needs constant supervision and help with most daily activities, and can do only the simplest tasks	0.160	0.107	0.226

applying this term in the comparison of charges for two surgical interventions and labeling the less costly as the more cost-effective treatment. This definition neglects the health economics significance of a cost-effective analysis [33].

Nonetheless, existing publications can provide information about reimbursement rates used in calculating cost-effectiveness ratios [34]. As previously mentioned, only eight peer-reviewed papers evaluated economic data related to surgical intervention for craniosynostosis. Table 37.3 summarizes their findings.

Six of the papers were related to sagittal, nonsyndromic, or single-suture craniosynostosis [5, 7, 9–12], while two papers evaluated any type of craniosynostosis [6, 13]. Seven papers compared outcomes for endoscopic versus open surgery [5–7, 9, 11–13], while one compared outcomes between high- and low-volume centers [10]. Seven papers exclusively considered costs related to surgical intervention within the first year of life [5–7, 9–12], and one considered total procedural charges at any age with subgroup analysis for patients operated under one year of age [13]. Cost was variably calculated with seven of the papers relying on hospital charges [6, 7, 9–13] and only one paper exploring actual "costs," referring to expenses incurred by the hospital system and out-of-pocket payments made by the patient [5]. This sole paper accounted for both direct and indirect costs to the patient, such as hospital overhead costs [5]. Papers varied in

Table 37.3 Summary of cost data availability in craniosynostosis literature

Authors & year	Location	Pathology	Intervention	Cost inclusion	Cost value	Currency	Inflation adjusted
Abbott et al. (2012) [5]	Boston, USA	Sagittal craniosynostosis	Endoscopic versus open repair	Medical, orthodontic, clinic, patient costs	$23,377[d] vs. $55,121[a]	USD 2009	Yes
Chan et al. (2013) [6]	Tulane, USA	Any craniosynostosis	Endoscopic versus open repair	Medical, orthodontic charges	$24,404[d] vs. $42,744[a]	USD 1998–2009	No
Vogel et al. (2014) [7]	Cincinnati, USA	Sagittal craniosynostosis	Endoscopic versus open repair	Medical, orthodontic, clinic, patient charges	$37,256[d] vs. $56,990[a]	USD 2006–2011	No
Garber et al. (2017) [9]	Utah, USA	Sagittal craniosynostosis	Endoscopic versus open repair	Medical, orthodontic charges	$21,203[d] vs. $45,078[a]	USD 2013 and prior	No
Chattha et al. (2018) [10]	HCUP database, USA	Non-syndromic craniosynostosis	Any approach (not specified)	Medical charges	$55,839[b] vs. $62,325[c]	USD 2012	Unspecified
Liles et al. (2019) [11]	Nashville, USA	Sagittal craniosynostosis	Endoscopic versus open repair	Medical, orthodontic, clinic, patient charges	$18,081[d] vs. $31,314[a]	USD 2015	Yes
Zubovic et al. (2020) [12]	St. Louis, USA	Non-sagittal single suture	Endoscopic versus open repair	Medical, orthodontic, clinic, patient charges	$50,840[d] vs. $95,588[a]	USD 2018	Yes
Kwon et al. (2025) [13]	HCUP database, USA	Any craniosynostosis	Endoscopic versus open repair	Medical charges	$66,816[d] vs. $146,271[a]	USD 2018–2021	Unspecified

[a] Open repair
[b] High volume center
[c] Low volume center
[d] Endoscopic repair

including orthotic charges, clinic charges, and patient costs. Only three papers explicitly adjusted for inflation to a single calendar year [5, 11, 12]. All papers were based on costs in the United States.

These articles highlight the extent to which economic data are lacking for syndromic craniosynostosis treatment. No paper adequately considered the complex multi-suture craniosynostosis typically associated with Apert syndrome. Nevertheless, data examining costs for open surgical repair can serve as a proxy for treatment of syndromic craniosynostosis, for which open surgical treatment is typical [13]. The available literature suggests that mean cost in the United States for open surgical management of craniosynostosis ranges between $31,314 and $146,271 in the first year of life.

While plausible as a loose estimate for costs, the aforementioned limitations make it difficult to generalize the data for analytic use outside the specific context in which it was gathered. For more accurate models, future studies should evaluate the full spectrum of costs specific to multi-suture syndromic craniosynostosis. This includes the cost of more complex open surgery with increased operative time, blood loss, complication rate, hospital stay, etc., which will likely increase the intervention costs beyond current estimates. Productivity costs associated with treatment must also be examined to define the significant losses incurred by families due to travel to academic centers where most of these surgeries are performed, resulting in additional costs for transportation, accommodation, missed wages, and more. Furthermore, future studies must begin to quantify the monetary value of future medical costs averted or productivity gained by the surgical intervention, which has not been explored in the literature. Untreated syndromic craniosynostosis can lead to intellectual disability and high economic cost. Still, the degree to which surgical intervention can mitigate that cost must be quantified for meaningful translation into a net cost calculation.

Cost–Benefit Analyses: Value of Statistical Life

The aforementioned measures (DALY and CEA) consider morbidity and mortality resulting from surgical disease. While this is paramount, it is also necessary to consider the secondary effects of untreated surgical conditions, such as their large-scale economic impact. Microeconomic studies examine the impact on individuals and households due to loss of productivity and relate loosely to the cost studies described earlier in this chapter. In contrast, macroeconomic studies inspect the wider impacts of surgical disease on society and global economies. Such analyses require a clear definition of the disease state, outcomes with and without intervention, and the economic impact of ill health at the micro- and macroeconomic levels [53, 54].

While various studies have defined the human capital gains following surgical intervention for other disease states, there are currently no publications that describe economic impact of craniosynostosis or craniofacial syndromes in these terms [55, 61]. In the broader surgical literature, studies have specifically investigated the economic impact of pediatric plastic surgery interventions at the national level [55–57] and several at regional and global levels [21, 58–60]. Collectively, these publications demonstrate the massive societal benefits of children's surgical care, particularly in low- and middle-income contexts. While societal benefits of craniosynostosis surgery remain undefined, it is noteworthy to explore the data requirements for select examples of cost–benefit frameworks to fill this gap in the literature.

One approach seeks to directly calculate the value of foregone economic productivity in the labor force secondary to a given disease state. Various modeling exercises fall under this human capital approach, including Gross National Income Per Capita, Present Value of Lifetime Earnings, and Value of Lost Output. From unique perspectives and with different assumptions, these models involve contextualizing disease in relation to an individual's potential economic contribution. They can be estimated using DALYs averted through surgical intervention, disease-specific mortality rates, labor force participation, earnings/salary data, population census age distribution, and Gross National Income (GNI) or Gross Domestic Product (GDP) per capita [55, 58, 61]. While some of these variables are readily available (i.e., GNI per country), this approach shares the challenges stemming from lack of DALY and mortality estimates for craniosynostosis and associated syndromes and disregards externalities of illness (such as the effect of illness on family members). Furthermore, these metrics have been criticized for valuing humans as machines whose only inherent value is reflected in wages earned.

Alternatively, the value of a statistical life (VSL), assigns a monetary value to changes in health risk based on individual valuation of wealth relative to small changes in risk of morbidity and mortality [58]. Fundamentally, VSL corresponds to the maximum amount of money a person is willing to pay to save one life. This "preference" or value placed on a statistical life may be "stated" in survey data or "revealed" in labor market choices. VSL can also differentiate preferences for many nonfatal health risks. For these reasons, individual valuation of a statistical life will typically be much larger than mere wages alone. VSL has grown in popularity amongst economists for its ability to reflect how individuals monetarily assign value to health and well-being; serving as a guide for policymakers to achieve societal value for money invested.

Assigning VSL for a congenital condition, particularly one with multiple clinical manifestations like Apert syndrome, is challenging due to variable phenotype severity, life expectancy, and quality of life impacts, let alone variability in individual valuation of risk reduction. The VSL calculation requires both a constant value per DALY and mortality risk [55, 56]. As previously established, no studies have defined DALYs for craniosynostosis or, more broadly, craniofacial syndromes. Estimations based on proxies, as described in the prior section, may circumvent this gap but are likely insufficient to produce reliable VSL calculations in this context.

As discussed, Apert syndrome is associated with multiple clinical manifestations. When examining the literature on each associated condition, only orofacial cleft surgery has been described using cost–benefit analysis in a globally representative fashion. Using the human capital approach, these studies describe an economic benefit of USD \$3191 to \$32,203 per primary cleft lip repair and USD \$4110 to \$87,393 per cleft palate repair [57, 59, 62]. Using a VSL approach the cumulative economic benefit for treating all incident orofacial clefts in sub-Saharan Africa is \$5.4 to \$9.7 billion USD [21]. This suggests even greater economic benefit following comprehensive treatment of the congenital manifestations of Apert syndrome when compared to orofacial clefts alone.

It is important to note once again that the economic impact of Apert syndrome is unlikely to equal the sum of each associated condition but rather represents a complex interaction that is not captured by modeling each condition in isolation. Factors such as timing of surgery further complicate these measures as, for example, syndactyly release before the development of fine motor skills has been shown to significantly impact long-term motor function and psychosocial development [63]. Due to the absence of craniosynostosis in econometrics literature and heavy reliance on proxies for estimation of economic benefit, we present the following case series to highlight global similarities and differences in managing Apert syndrome and its associated financial implications.

Global Perspectives

Section Objective *To demonstrate the variation in financing and costs from a diverse selection of centers providing care for patients with Apert syndrome.*

The financing and payment for the treatment of Apert syndrome vary widely worldwide due to differences in healthcare systems, insurance coverage, and economic factors. As discussed in the preceding sections, CEA and CBA consider the cost of an intervention relative to the GDP per capita of a country. As such, the results of these analyses may differ significantly from country to country based on differences in both the currency value assigned to surgical intervention and the overall economic status of the country. To illustrate this variability, we present a case series of the financial considerations related to the care of patients with syndromic and non-syndromic craniosynostosis in different healthcare systems. These case studies are drawn from healthcare centers treating patients with Apert syndrome to explore the role of financing mechanisms (i.e., public vs private vs charitable non-governmental organizations), barriers to access (i.e., rurality, socioeconomic status), and financial burden on patients (i.e., out of pocket expenditures). The results of the case series are described below and summarized in Table 37.4.

The ten healthcare facilities surveyed were a mixture of public and private institutions, some with university affiliations and others strictly philanthropic (Table 37.4). These facilities represented a diverse range of sociopolitical contexts, including centers in multiple continents from the following countries: Taiwan, Ethiopia, Pakistan, Brazil, Mexico, South Africa, China, Canada, and the United States. All facilities identified as tertiary referral centers for craniofacial care with specialized multidisciplinary networks in large cities. In most places, the government played a role in supporting the delivery of healthcare services for patients with Apert syndrome, either through sponsorship or public insurance, but specialty care typically incurred both direct and indirect costs beyond what public mechanisms cover. Some sites report costs predominately being covered through national health insurance (i.e., University of KwaZulu-Natal in South Africa), most reported a mixed financing between public and private insurance (i.e., Boston Children's Hospital in the United States of America), and others were almost completely out-of-pocket (i.e., Northwest General Hospital and Research Centre in Pakistan).

The survey revealed multiple financial challenges and cost-saving strategies that were tailored to each setting. Direct costs for surgery were not available from all sites but reached as much as $13,000 USD in China and $50,000 USD in Mexico. Components of surgical care that were sometimes not covered through insurance included distraction hardware, implants, orthodontics (especially those considered "cosmetic"), and three-dimensional (3D) models for planning. Direct non-medical costs and indirect costs included travel to large cities (especially for follow-up appointments and ancillary care), accommodation, lost wages from caregiving, and adaptive equipment for daily living. Out-of-pocket payments varied widely, often creating financial burden for patients and their families. In order to offset the financial burden of out-of-pocket expenses, most hospitals reported partnerships with philanthropic or nongovernmental organizations (i.e., Noordhoff Craniofacial Foundation and Taiwan Foundation for Rare Disorders at Chang Gung Memorial Hospital, BAAS and SmileTrain in Brazil, Zakat Foundation and Bait-ul-Mal at Northwest General Hospital and Research Centre in Pakistan) or raised funds on their own (i.e., SOBRAPAR and Chang Gung's Social Service Department). Cost-saving strategies included clustering surgeries at one time to eliminate redundancy, early intervention to avoid costly complications of untreated disease, implementation of cost-effective protocols for efficient care, reusing expensive distractors, managing supply chains to allow bulk purchases, and telemedicine consultation with community-based rehabilitation to reduce travel. Despite these efforts, multiple challenges remain, and most programs engage in advocacy campaigns to lobby policy-

Table 37.4 Financial considerations for treating craniosynostosis in different global contexts

FACILITY	CHANG GUNG MEMORIAL HOSPITAL *TAOYUAN, TAIWAN*	ALERT[a] COMPREHENSIVE SPECIALIZED HOSPITAL *ADDIS ABABA, ETHIOPIA*	NORTHWEST GENERAL HOSPITAL AND RESEARCH CENTRE *PESHAWAR, PAKISTAN*	SOBRAPAR[b] HOSPITAL *CAMPINAS, BRAZIL*	HOSPITAL ANGELES DEL PEDREGAL *MEXICO CITY, MEXICO*
Facility type	Private philanthropic network	Public, tertiary care facility	Private academic	Private philanthropic	Private
Healthcare payment mechanisms	National Health Insurance (NHI), a single-payer, universal healthcare system with supplementary private insurance plans	Government-allocated funding from national registry, community-based health insurance with waivers for low-income patients, and out-of-pocket (OOP) expenditures at point of care	Mixture of public and private assistance, where national Sehat Sahulat program aims for near-universal access, with coverage of some ancillary services. But public and private insurance both fall short of comprehensive care for Apert syndrome	Sistema Único de Saúde (SUS), a government-run and funded public health system. Government tax waivers and dedicated funding for surgical care delivery offset facility costs	Mixture of public and private; but national health resources available through Mexican Institute of Social Security ("IMSS") do not cover multidisciplinary care for craniosynostosis
Cost of treatment for Apert syndrome and craniosynostosis	All treatment costs, including surgery, hospitalization, and outpatient visits, are covered by NHI, with the exception of distraction hardware. Charitable funds are available to cover distractor cost for families experiencing financial hardship	Variable: Direct OOP cost to patient unknown but estimated to be a significant percentage of the GDP per capita due to long distances traveled for care, long hospitalization and need for frequent follow-up	Services for Apert and craniosynostosis are covered out-of-pocket by patients and families, supported by philanthropic support (i.e., Zakat Foundation or Bait-ul-Mal)	Reimbursement is allocated as a predetermined fee-for-service amount, which is often less than actual costs incurred by the treating facility	Fees are covered by patients or private health insurance
Challenges	Newer, costly surgical implants used for rare syndromic cases are not reimbursed by the NHI despite their important role in early vault expansion	Surgical care is concentrated primarily in the capitol city resulting in high OOP costs for travel and lodging. Currently no institutional treatment protocols for multidisciplinary care	Challenges are institutional, patient level, financial, and systemic level, including limited number of specialized centers, geographic barriers for access (from Pakistan and Afghanistan), delayed diagnosis, poverty, & lack of national registry	Incomplete implementation of SUS in rural and impoverished regions creates disparities in infrastructure, health workforce and essential resources	Fees for craniosynostosis surgery may be as high as $50,000 USD and are covered by the patient or private insurance

Cost-saving strategies	Financial support through charitable organizations, such as the Noordhoff craniofacial foundation and Taiwan Foundation for Rare Disorders, and the CGMH social service department is available to patients and families and allocated according to socioeconomic status/need	Aside from sporadic humanitarian aid, there are no systems in place to offset direct OOP costs. Facilities absorb costs that exceed government reimbursement amounts, placing extra burden on an already strained system	Some ancillary services are available in government hospitals but specialized multi-disciplinary is not routinely included. Clustering combined surgeries, streamlining hospital protocols, standardized efficient diagnostics, supply chains allowing bulk purchases. Telemedicine consultation and community-based rehabilitation, and promoting policy reforms	Support for transportation/lodging available through foundations (i.e., BAAS). Multidisciplinary care allows for clustering simultaneous procedures to reduce cost. SOBRAPAR, a private philanthropic hospital, engages in fundraising to offset differences in reimbursement amount	Multidisciplinary care allows for clustering simultaneous procedures to reduce cost. Subsequent revisionary procedures are recommended with strict indications criteria

FACILITY	**UNIVERSITY OF KWAZULU-NATAL** ***DURBAN, SOUTH AFRICA***	**PLASTIC SURGERY HOSPITAL**[c] ***BEIJING, CHINA***	**HOSPITAL FOR REHABILITATION OF CRANIOFACIAL ANOMALIES**[d] ***BAURU, BRAZIL***	**BOSTON CHILDREN'S HOSPITAL** ***BOSTON, USA***
Facility type	Public	Public	Public	Private academic
Healthcare Payment Mechanisms	Mixture of governmental health services and private insurance, where roughly 80% of population is covered within public sector	Governmental financing via China Healthcare Security covers near-universal access but with incomplete coverage for specialist care	Financing comes from the government and University[d]. There is no private insurance in public hospitals. Multidisciplinary care (including dental/speech) is coordinated on site	40% of children are covered by Medicaid in Massachusetts and 58.5% are covered by private insurance. Only 1.5% of Massachusetts children are uncovered
Cost of treatment for Apert syndrome and craniosynostosis, in general	Care for patients with Apert syndrome is included in national health service	Craniofacial reconstruction costs roughly \$6,800 USD, LeFort III RED[e] costs roughly \$13,700 USD, and syndactyly correction costs roughly \$6,500 USD, with public insurance covering 20–40%, although allocation decisions vary by province	Final budgetary items are complex, but government payment for surgical care is roughly \$730 USD. The University[d] also supports craniofacial care	In Massachusetts children with Medicaid have no out of pocket expenses. Children covered by private insurance may have OOP expenses that vary by insurer

(continued)

Table 37.4 (continued)

Challenges	Coverage of adjunctive therapies including orthodontics, distractions, and planning/models	Long-term rehabilitation and supportive care including orthodontics, speech, and hearing aids, and lifelong follow-ups for monitoring (i.e., ICP). OOP expenses include 3D models and custom orthodontics. Indirect costs include travel to large cities, accommodation, lost wages from caregiving, and adaptive equipment for daily living	Newer technologies (i.e., distractors) are in limited supply. Additionally, patients often travel from outside Sao Paulo with limited capacity for prolonged stays for ancillary care (i.e., orthodontics, speech therapy, psychology)	OOP include direct costs of copayments and deductibles. OOP also include indirect costs for travel, food, and lodging. OOP payments in Massachusetts are capped at $9,450 per year by law for individuals
Cost-saving strategies	Multidisciplinary care allows for clustering simultaneous procedures to reduce cost and redundancy	Multidisciplinary care allows for clustering simultaneous procedures, early intervention to avoid costly complications, and global collaboration to implement cost-effective protocols. Partnerships with policymakers to encourage correct categorizations and with non-governmental organizations for financial aid.	Multidisciplinary care is coordinated on site. Newer technologies (i.e., distractors) are reused. Genetics tests deferred in some cases.	Multidisciplinary care is coordinated on site and allows for efficient clinic visits with all providers present. Whole genome screening is supported thought a hospital grant. The hospital has a free care budget each year to support international patients with financial needs

[a] African Leprosy, Tuberculosis, Rehabilitation, and Training (ALERT), [b] Brazilian Society for Research and Care of Craniofacial Rehabilitation (SOBRAPAR), [c] Plastic Surgery Hospital, Chinese Academy of Medical Sciences & Peking Union Medical College, [d] University of Sao Palo, [e] Rigid External Distraction (RED)

makers to expand access and coverage for complex craniofacial care.

Economic Impacts of Technology and Innovation

Section Objective *To present novel technologies and innovations aimed at reducing the overall burden of treating craniosynostosis.*

Despite the limitations of existing cost studies and lack of actionable baseline cost data, developing strategies to mitigate drivers of economic burden is imperative. The impact of technology on healthcare economics is variable, as the introduction of more expensive equipment and diagnostic tools can directly increase treatment costs, while earlier diagnosis and intervention enabled by these tools can produce improved clinical outcomes. Regarding craniosynostosis surgery, the evolution in diagnostic and treatment paradigms over the past decade has offered promising economic benefits.

Screening Tools

Disparities related to patient, societal, and institutional factors exist in the care of children with craniosynostosis globally. Several studies have demonstrated the impact of race/ethnicity on access to timely surgical care, with nonwhite patients presenting later for initial consultation [65, 66]. Timing of presentation is particularly relevant for this patient population, as early surgical intervention has been associated with improved clinical outcomes and higher intelligence quotients in both non-syndromic and syndromic craniosynostosis [67, 68]. Low-cost, accessible mobile screening applications such as CranioSure (Madison, Wisconsin), particularly when combined with public health awareness campaigns, can facilitate early diagnosis and secondarily reduce economic burdens associated with craniosynostosis.

Hospitalization Protocols

Routine intensive care admission and conservative discharge pathways lead to unnecessary prolongation in length of hospital stay across surgical disciplines. A 2023 study examined the impact of a cranial pediatric neurosurgery Enhanced Recovery After Surgery (ERAS) protocol and noted a reduction of in-hospital costs for protocolized patients following craniosynostosis surgery [69]. Protocols that encourage direct surgical ward admission following cranial vault remodeling have also been shown to shorten length of hospitalization while reducing total healthcare costs [70–72]. However, such protocols have not been studied in patients with syndromic craniosynostosis. Additional strategies to reduce the duration or need for intensive care unit stay and total length of hospitalization have the potential to drive down costs further.

Surgical Coordination

As presented in the Brazilian case study, collaboration within a multidisciplinary team provides opportunities to combine staged procedures under a single anesthetic event. For example, scheduling index syndactyly reconstruction at the same time as cranial vault reconstruction is feasible as both procedures can be performed simultaneously. For patients with multiple congenital anomalies requiring surgical intervention, as is found in Apert syndrome, reducing the total number of visits to the operating room not only saves time and financial resources but also decreases the number of days spent in hospital, total recovery time, and overall anesthetic risk.

Treatment Paradigms

Economic analyses can drive treatment protocols toward more cost-effective approaches, yet clinical necessity can also alter treatment paradigms. In the last decade, posterior vault distraction osteogenesis (PVDO) and endoscopic strip craniectomy have increasingly been employed early as staged procedures with favorable outcomes, most notably a reduction in the need for future surgeries to address relapse due to greater volume expansion achieved with PVDO [73–75]. This is especially relevant for patients with syndromic craniosynostosis who may require earlier intervention to alleviate elevated intracranial pressure and historically undergo multiple staged procedures [76].

Expansion of Access to Surgery

Direct non-medical and indirect costs incurred by patients and their families for productivity losses, travel, and accommodation, for example, are significantly influenced by the limited availability of multidisciplinary craniofacial care teams outside of specialized academic centers. Demonstrating the cost-effectiveness of craniosynostosis surgery is an early step toward increasing investment in the training of surgeons and expansion of infrastructure to support treatment. However, urgent cross-border collaboration is essential to ensure high-quality care for patients with craniosynostosis, particularly in regions or countries lacking the necessary expertise. For example, the European Directive 2011/24/EU recognized the value of cross-border cooperation to extend specialist care to patients with rare genetic diseases, prompting the launch of numerous European Reference Networks (ERNs) to pool disease-specific expertise and resources [77]. One such network, the ERN-CRANIO, focuses on rare and/or complex craniofacial anomalies, including craniosynostosis. This represents a strategy that can be implemented in the immediate term to expand sub-specialty surgical access to global populations.

In an era of significant technological advancement and innovation in surgical care delivery, we must consider the potential economic harms and benefits for the patient, health system, and society as a whole. Identifying strategies that improve health outcomes while reducing the economic burden is prudent. While notable advancements have been made in the diagnosis and treatment of craniosynostosis, the evidence base for treating syndromic cases remains incomplete.

Conclusion

Summary of Available Data

We still lack significant data necessary for a proper cost analysis of syndromic craniosynostosis treatment. Some cost data are available but variable in quality and limited in scope. Additional evaluation specific to craniosynostosis and consideration for costs averted and productivity gained will be necessary to complete economic calculations. For health outcomes, incidence is known but mortality and life expectancy data around treated and untreated craniosynostosis are severely lacking. Average duration of the case until remission and disability weights can be approximated with some underlying assumptions, but without life expectancy data, the DALY calculation is incomplete. When these gaps in cost and health outcomes data are fulfilled, all the components for econometric analysis will be in place.

Economic Consideration for Apert Syndrome

Although we have largely focused on syndromic craniosynostosis in this chapter to narrow the scope of our economic considerations, we recognize that Apert syndrome is a complex multisystem condition of which craniosynostosis is just one part. To perform a comprehensive analysis of the economic impact of Apert syndrome, one approach would be to collect the data described in this chapter for all the phenotypic expressions of Apert syndrome including the ocular complications, midface retrusion, airway issues, and complex syndactyly among others. However, a complexity to that calculation is that the cumulative impact of the various systems involved is greater than the sum of its parts. For a patient with moderate intellectual disability and complex syndactyly, the disability weight cannot just be the sum of "moderate intellectual disability due to other chromosomal abnormalities" and "disfigurement level 2 and moderate motor impairment due to congenital limb deficiency" based on the GBD 2021 disability weights [22]. The two conditions interact with and compound each other in ways the current disability weights do not capture. The complexity is even further exacerbated for Apert syndrome, in which multiple organ systems are involved.

As such, Apert syndrome must be evaluated as a whole rather than its individual parts for the most accurate analysis. Fortunately, Apert syndrome is a clearly defined condition with a known genetic marker and relatively consistent phenotypic expression despite the involvement of multiple organ systems and variable severity. Despite the current scarcity, this uniformity makes Apert syndrome an excellent target for data collection. The greatest barrier to collecting data on Apert syndrome is its low birth prevalence.

As such, we propose three avenues for improving the current state of the science:

1. Develop national registries for Apert syndrome and other rare congenital syndromes based on their genetic markers. Because Apert syndrome is clearly identifiable, it should be relatively easy to track the cases within most hospital systems. Patients with Apert syndrome also tend to be followed frequently within healthcare systems due to their many surveillance needs, making long-term data readily available.
2. Extending national registries to regional or global scales would be the next step to overcome the narrow perspective of any single setting. In high-income countries, the data gathered for patients with Apert syndrome would likely lean heavily toward those receiving treatment. Very few cases would be available to gather data on untreated or late presentation of Apert syndrome. As for orofacial cleft data, extending the pool to low- and middle-income countries with more delayed or untreated cases would greatly expand the data necessary to formulate a comparison between treated and untreated populations for cost analysis models.
3. Lastly, existing multinational databases must further differentiate their data to capture congenital syndromes with sufficient granularity for meaningful analysis. Looking at the Institute for Health Metrics and Evaluation GBD as an example, information on Apert syndrome is likely already being captured within the 56,604 primary data sources used to generate the 2021 report, but the closest category for capturing Apert syndrome was "other congenital birth defects" without further subdivision. For every iteration of GBD, new disease categories are being introduced, with 288 diseases in the 2021 report compared to 234 in the 2019 report [22, 78]. Including craniosynostosis, and more specifically, Apert syndrome, in future iterations would provide an incredible resource of consolidated information on the disease with reasonable short-term feasibility. Advancing these data systems will ultimately enable more rigorous, comprehensive, economic analyses that can meaningfully inform clinical care and policy for Apert syndrome.

Acknowledgements The authors would like to formally acknowledge contributions of the following individuals: Nivaldo Alonso MD, Tariq Khan MBBS, Anil Madaree MD, Hellina Legesse Mamo MD FCS-ECSA, Fernando Molina MD, and Bin Song MD MPH.

References

1. Wenger TL, Hing AV, Evans KN. Apert syndrome. In: Adam MP, Feldman J, Mirzaa GM, et al., editors. GeneReviews® [Internet]. Seattle (WA): University of Washington, Seattle; 1993–2024; 2019. https://www.ncbi.nlm.nih.gov/books/NBK541728/.
2. McCarthy JG, Warren SM, Bernstein J, Burnett W, Cunningham ML, Edmond JC, Figueroa AA, Kapp-Simon KA, Labow BI, Peterson-Falzone SJ, Proctor MR, Rubin MS, Sze RW, Yemen TA, et al. Parameters of care for craniosynostosis. Cleft Palate Craniofac J. 2012;49:1S–24S.

3. Debas HT, Donkor P, Gawande A, Jamison DT, Kruk ME, Mock CN, editors. Essential surgery: disease control priorities, third edition (volume 1). Washington (DC): The International Bank for Reconstruction and Development/The World Bank; 2015. PMID: 26740991
4. Medina LS, Richardson RR, Crone K. Children with suspected craniosynostosis: a cost-effectiveness analysis of diagnostic strategies. AJR Am J Roentgenol. 2002;179(1):215–21. https://doi.org/10.2214/ajr.179.1.1790215.
5. Abbott MM, Rogers GF, Proctor MR, Busa K, Meara JG. Cost of treating sagittal synostosis in the first year of life. J Craniofac Surg. 2012;23(1):88–93. https://doi.org/10.1097/SCS.0b013e318240f965. PMID: 22337381
6. Chan JW, Stewart CL, Stalder MW, St Hilaire H, McBride L, Moses MH. Endoscope-assisted versus open repair of craniosynostosis: a comparison of perioperative cost and risk. J Craniofac Surg. 2013;24(1):170–4. https://doi.org/10.1097/SCS.0b013e3182646ab8. PMID: 23348279
7. Vogel TW, Woo AS, Kane AA, Patel KB, Naidoo SD, Smyth MD. A comparison of costs associated with endoscope-assisted craniectomy versus open cranial vault repair for infants with sagittal synostosis. J Neurosurg Pediatr. 2014;13(3):324–31. https://doi.org/10.3171/2013.12.PEDS13320. Epub 2014 Jan 10. PMID: 24410127
8. Greyvensteyn GA, Madaree A. A low-cost method of craniofacial distraction osteogenesis. J Plast Reconstr Aesthet Surg. 2016;69(3):409–16. https://doi.org/10.1016/j.bjps.2015.10.034.
9. Garber ST, Karsy M, Kestle JRW, Siddiqi F, Spanos SP, Riva-Cambrin J. Comparing outcomes and cost of 3 surgical treatments for sagittal synostosis: a retrospective study including procedure-related cost analysis. Neurosurgery. 2017;81(4):680–7. https://doi.org/10.1093/neuros/nyx209. PMID: 28449032
10. Chattha A, Bucknor A, Curiel DA, Ultee KHJ, Afshar S, Lin SJ. Treatment of Craniosynostosis: the impact of hospital surgical volume on cost, resource utilization, and outcomes. J Craniofac Surg. 2018;29(5):1233–6. https://doi.org/10.1097/SCS.0000000000004561. PMID: 29762328
11. Liles C, Dallas J, Hale AT, et al. The economic impact of open versus endoscope-assisted craniosynostosis surgery. J Neurosurg Pediatr. 2019;24(2):145–52. Published 2019 May 31. https://doi.org/10.3171/2019.4.PEDS18586.
12. Zubovic E, Lapidus JB, Skolnick GB, Naidoo SD, Smyth MD, Patel KB. Cost comparison of surgical management of nonsagittal synostosis: traditional open versus endoscope-assisted techniques. J Neurosurg Pediatr. 2020;25(4):351–60. Published 2020 Jan 10. https://doi.org/10.3171/2019.11.PEDS19515.
13. Kwon DY, Villavisanis DF, Choe A, et al. Complication rates and cost of endoscopic and open surgical approaches to management of craniosynostosis: a large, national, inpatient cohort evaluation. Cleft Palate Craniofac J. 2025; https://doi.org/10.1177/10556656251320746. PMID: 39980389
14. Brent RJ. Cost-benefit analysis versus cost-effectiveness analysis from a societal perspective in healthcare. Int J Environ Res Public Health. 2023;20(5):4637. https://doi.org/10.3390/ijerph20054637. PMID: 36901658; PMCID: PMC10001534
15. CDC. Economic Evaluation Overview. Centers for Disease Control and Prevention, Office of Policy, Performance, and Evaluation. https://www.cdc.gov/policy/polaris/economics/index.html
16. WHO methods and data sources for global burden of disease estimates 2000–2019. Global Health Estimates Technical Paper WHO/DDI/DNA/GHE/2020.3. December 2020.
17. Prieto L, Sacristán JA. Problems and solutions in calculating quality-adjusted life years (QALYs). Health Qual Life Outcomes. 2003;9(1):80. https://doi.org/10.1186/1477-7525-1-80. PMID: 14687421; PMCID: PMC317370
18. Gamst-Klaussen T, Lamu AN. Does the EQ-5D usual activities dimension measure what it intends to measure? The relative importance of work, study, housework, family or leisure activities. Qual Life Res. 2020;29(9):2553–62. https://doi.org/10.1007/s11136-020-02501-w. Epub 2020 Apr 23. PMID: 32328996; PMCID: PMC7434786
19. Bertram MY, Lauer JA, Stenberg K, Torres Edejer TT. Methods for the economic evaluation of health care interventions for priority setting in the health system: an update from WHO CHOICE. Int J Health Policy Manag. 2021;10(11):673–7. https://doi.org/10.34172/ijhpm.2020.244.
20. Mathers C, Fat DM, Boerma JT, et al. The global burden of disease: 2004 update. World Health Organiztation, 2008. Geneva.
21. Alkire B, Hughes CD, Nash K, Vincent JR, Meara JG. Potential economic benefit of cleft lip and palate repair in sub-Saharan Africa. World J Surg. 2011;35(6):1194–201. https://doi.org/10.1007/s00268-011-1055-1.
22. Global Burden of Disease Collaborative Network. Global Burden of Disease Study 2021 (GBD 2021) Disability Weights. Seattle, United States of America: Institute for Health Metrics and Evaluation (IHME), 2024.
23. Xue F, Kim DD, Cohen JT, Neumann PJ, Ollendorf DA. Using QALYs versus DALYs to measure cost-effectiveness: how much does it matter? Int J Technol Assess Health Care. 2020;36(2):96–103. https://doi.org/10.1017/S0266462320000124.
24. Hamze H, Mengiste A, Carter J. The impact and cost-effectiveness of the Amref Health Africa-Smile Train Cleft Lip and Palate Surgical Repair Programme in Eastern and Central Africa. Pan Afr Med J. 2017;28:35. https://doi.org/10.11604/pamj.2017.28.35.10344.

25. Chung KY, Ho G, Erman A, Bielecki JM, Forrest CR, Sander B. A systematic review of the cost-effectiveness of cleft Care in low- and middle-income countries: what is needed? Cleft Palate Craniofac J. 2023;60(12):1600–8. https://doi.org/10.1177/10556656221111028.
26. Shlobin NA, Baticulon RE, Ortega CA, Du L, Bonfield CM, Wray A, Forrest CR, Dewan MC. Global epidemiology of craniosynostosis: a systematic review and meta-analysis. World Neurosurg. 2022;164:413–423.e3. https://doi.org/10.1016/j.wneu.2022.05.093.
27. Katouni K, Nikolaou A, Mariolis T, Protogerou V, Chrysikos D, Theofilopoulou S, Filippou D. Syndromic craniosynostosis: a comprehensive review. Cureus. 2023;15(12):e50448. https://doi.org/10.7759/cureus.50448.
28. Arnaud E, Marchac D, Renier D. Reduction of morbidity of the frontofacial monobloc advancement in children by the use of internal distraction. Plast Reconstr Surg. 2007;120(4):1009–26. https://doi.org/10.1097/01.prs.0000278068.99643.8e.
29. de Jong T, Maliepaard M, Bannink N, Raat H, Mathijssen IMJ. Health-related problems and quality of life in patients with syndromic and complex craniosynostosis. Child's Nervous Sys. 2012;28(6):879–82. https://doi.org/10.1007/s00381-012-1681-4.
30. Maliepaard M, Mathijssen IM, Oosterlaan J, Okkerse JM. Intellectual, behavioral, and emotional functioning in children with syndromic craniosynostosis. Pediatrics. 2014;133(6):e1608–15. https://doi.org/10.1007/s00381-012-1681-4.
31. Bruce WJ, Chang V, Joyce CJ, Cobb AN, Maduekwe UI, Patel PA. Age at time of craniosynostosis repair predicts increased complication rate. Cleft Palate Craniofac J. 2018;55(5):649–54. https://doi.org/10.1177/1055665617725215.
32. Hauc SC, Junn A, Dinis J, Phillips S, Alperovich M. Disparities in craniosynostosis outcomes by race and insurance status. J Craniofac Surg. 2022;33(1):121–4. https://doi.org/10.1097/SCS.0000000000008100.
33. Thoma A, Ignacy TA. Health services research: impact of quality of life instruments on craniofacial surgery. J Craniofac Surg. 2012;23(1):283–7. https://doi.org/10.1097/SCS.0b013e318241ba7a.
34. Chaij JM, Hammond JB, Palmer SK, et al. Medicaid's cranio-cap: Medicaid reimbursement for craniosynostosis repair is not rending with the rate of inflation. J Craniofac Surg. 2025.;Online ahead of print; https://doi.org/10.1097/SCS.0000000000011165.
35. Murray CJ. Quantifying the burden of disease: the technical basis for disability-adjusted life years. Bull World Health Organ. 1994;72(3):429–45. PMID: 8062401; PMCID: PMC2486718
36. World Population Prospects. United Nations. https://population.un.org/wpp/. Accessed 1 Oct 2024.
37. Global Health Estimates. World Health Organization. https://www.who.int/data/global-health-estimates. Accessed 1 Oct 2024.
38. Jones BM, Jani P, Bingham RM, Mackersie AM, Hayward R. Complications in paediatric craniofacial surgery: an initial four year experience. Br J Plast Surg. 1992;45(3):225–31. https://doi.org/10.1016/0007-1226(92)90083-a.
39. Kirkpatrick WN, Koshy CE, Waterhouse N, Fauvel NJ, Carr RJ, Peterson DC. Paediatric transcranial surgery: a review of 114 consecutive procedures. Br J Plast Surg. 2002;55(7):561–4. https://doi.org/10.1054/bjps.2002.3923.
40. Lee HQ, Hutson JM, Wray AC, et al. Analysis of morbidity and mortality in surgical management of craniosynostosis. J Craniofac Surg. 2012;23(5):1256–61. https://doi.org/10.1097/SCS.0b013e31824e26d6.
41. McCarthy JG, Glasberg SB, Cutting CB, et al. Twenty-year experience with early surgery for craniosynostosis: I. Isolated craniofacial synostosis--results and unsolved problems. Plast Reconstr Surg. 1995;96(2):272–83. https://doi.org/10.1097/00006534-199508000-00004.
42. Poole MD. Complications in craniofacial surgery. Br J Plast Surg. 1988;41(6):608–13. https://doi.org/10.1016/0007-1226(88)90168-3.
43. Boulet SL, Rasmussen SA, Honein MA. A population-based study of craniosynostosis in metropolitan Atlanta, 1989–2003. Am J Med Genet A. 2008;146A(8):984–91. https://doi.org/10.1002/ajmg.a.32208. PMID: 18344207
44. Lajeunie E, Le Merrer M, Bonaïti-Pellie C, Marchac D, Renier D. Genetic study of nonsyndromic coronal craniosynostosis. Am J Med Genet. 1995;55(4):500–4. https://doi.org/10.1002/ajmg.1320550422. PMID: 7762595
45. Johnson D, Wilkie AO. Craniosynostosis. Eur J Hum Genet. 2011;19(4):369–76. https://doi.org/10.1038/ejhg.2010.235. Epub 2011 Jan 19. PMID: 21248745; PMCID: PMC3060331
46. Cohen MM Jr, Kreiborg S, Lammer EJ, Cordero JF, Mastroiacovo P, Erickson JD, Roeper P, Martínez-Frías ML. Birth prevalence study of the Apert syndrome. Am J Med Genet. 1992;42:655–9.
47. Tolarova MM, Harris JA, Ordway DE, Vargervik K. Birth prevalence, mutation rate, sex ratio, parents' age, and ethnicity in Apert syndrome. Am J Med Genet. 1997;72:394–8.
48. Whitaker LA, Bartlett SP, Schut L, Bruce D. Craniosynostosis: an analysis of the timing, treatment, and complications in 164 consecutive patients. Plast Reconstr Surg. 1987;80(2):195–212.
49. Salomon JA, Vos T, Hogan DR, et al. Common values in assessing health outcomes: the disability weights for the Global Burden of Disease Study 2010. Lancet. 2012;380:2129–2143. https://doi.org/10.1016/S0140-6736(12)61680-8.
50. Renier D, Arnaud E, Cinalli G, Sebag G, Zerah M, Marchac D. Prognosis for mental function in Apert's syndrome. J Neurosurg. 1996;85:66–72.
51. David DJ, Anderson P, Flapper W, Syme-Grant J, Santoreneos S, Moore M. Apert syndrome: outcomes from the Australian craniofacial unit's birth

to maturity management protocol. J Craniofac Surg. 2016;27:1125–34.
52. Fernandes MB, Maximino LP, Perosa GB, Abramides DV, Passos-Bueno MR, Yacubian-Fernandes A. Apert and Crouzon syndromes—cognitive development, brain abnormalities, and molecular aspects. Am J Med Genet A. 2016;170:1532–7.
53. World Health Organization Department of Health Systems Financing. WHO guide to identifying the economic consequences of disease and injury. Geneva: World Health Organization (WHO); 2009.
54. OECD. Mortality risk valuation in environment, health and transport policies. OECD Publishing; 2012. https://doi.org/10.1787/9789264130807-en. Accessed 20 June 2024
55. Grimes CE, Quaife M, Kamara TB, Lavy CBD, Leather AJM, Bolkan HA. Macroeconomic costs of the unmet burden of surgical disease in Sierra Leone: a retrospective economic analysis. BMJ Open. 2018;8(3):e017824.
56. Hughes CD, Babigian A, McCormack S, Alkire BC, Wong A, Pap SA, Vincent JR, Meara JG, Castiglione C, Silverman R. The clinical and economic impact of a sustained program in global plastic surgery: valuing cleft care in resource-poor settings. Plast Reconstr J. 2012;130(1):87e–94e.
57. Nandoskar P, Coghlan P, Moore MH, Ximenes J, Moore EM, Karnon J, Watters DA. The economic value of the delivery of primary cleft surgery in Timor Leste 2000–2017. World J Surg. 2020;44(6):1699–705. https://doi.org/10.1007/s00268-020-05388-3.
58. Corlew DS, Alkire BC, Poenaru D, Meara JG, Shrime MG. Economic valuation of the impact of a large surgical charity using the value of lost welfare approach. BMJ Glob Health. 2016;1(4):e000059.
59. Poenaru D, Lin D, Corlew S. Economic valuation of the global burden of cleft disease averted by a large cleft charity. World J Surg. 2016;40(5):1053–9.
60. Saxton AT, Poenaru D, Ozgediz D, Ameh EA, Farmer D, Smith ER, Rice HE. Economic analysis of children's surgical care in low- and middle-income countries: a systematic review and analysis. PLoS One. 2016;11(10):e0165480. https://doi.org/10.1371/journal.pone.0165480.
61. Alkire BC, Shrime MG, Dare AJ, Vincent JR, Meara JG. Global economic consequences of selected surgical diseases: a modelling study. Lancet Glob Health. 2015;3(S2):S21–7.
62. Chung KY, Ho G, Erman A, Bielecki JM, Forrest CR, Sander B. A systematic review of the cost-effectiveness of cleft care in low- and middle-income countries: what is needed? Cleft Palate Craniofac J. 2022;60(12):1600–8.
63. Oda T, Pushman AG, Chung KC. Treatment of common congenital hand conditions. Plast Reconstr Surg. 2010;126(3):121e–33e.
64. Raposo-Amaral CE. Founding of the Brazilian Association of Apert Syndrome. J Craniofac Surg. 2018;29(6):1676. https://doi.org/10.1097/SCS.0000000000004758.
65. Lin Y, Pan IW, Harris DA, Luerssen TG, Lam S. The impact of insurance, race, and ethnicity on age at surgical intervention among children with nonsyndromic craniosynostosis. J Pediatr. 2015;166(5):1289–96. https://doi.org/10.1016/j.jpeds.2015.02.007.
66. Shweikeh F, Foulad D, Nuño M, Drazin D, Adamo MA. Differences in surgical outcomes for patients with craniosynostosis in the US: impact of socioeconomic variables and race. J Neurosurg. 2016;17(1):27–33. https://doi.org/10.3171/2015.4.PEDS14342.
67. Hashim PW, Patel A, Yang JF, Travieso R, Terner J, Losee JE, Pollack I, Jane J, Jane J, Kanev P, Mayes L, Duncan C, Bridgett DJ, Persing JA. The effects of whole-vault cranioplasty versus strip craniectomy on long-term neuropsychological outcomes in craniosynostosis. Plast Reconstr Surg. 2014;134(3):491–501.
68. Renier D, Lajeunie E, Arnaud E, Marchac D. Management of Craniosynostosis. Childs Nerv Syst. 2000;16(10–11):654–8. https://doi.org/10.1007/s003810000320.
69. Belouaer A, Cossu G, Al-Tayyari S, Bubenikova A, Caliman C, Agri F, Perez MH, Chanez V, Boegli Y, Mury C, Daniel RT, Messerer M. The enhanced recovery after surgery protocol for the surgical management of craniosynostosis: Lausanne experience. Neurosurg Focus. 2023;55(6):E14. https://doi.org/10.3171/2023.9.FOCUS23540.
70. Bonfield CM, Basem J, Cochrane DD, Singhal A, Steinbok P. Examining the need for routine intensive care admission after surgical repair of nonsyndromic craniosynostosis: a preliminary analysis. J Neurosurg. 2018;22(6):616–9. https://doi.org/10.3171/2018.6.PEDS18136.
71. Lin LO, McKenna RA, Zhang RS, Hoppe IC, Swanson JW, Bartlett SP, Taylor JA. A standardized perioperative clinical pathway for uncomplicated craniosynostosis repair is associated with reduced hospital resource utilization. J Craniofac Surg. 2019;30(1):105–9. https://doi.org/10.1097/SCS.0000000000004871.
72. Wolfswinkel EM, Howell LK, Fahradyan A, Azadgoli B, McComb JG, Urata MM. Is postoperative intensive care unit care necessary following cranial vault remodeling for sagittal synostosis? Plast Reconstr Surg. 2017;140(6):1235–9. https://doi.org/10.1097/PRS.0000000000003848.
73. Wu RT, Shultz BN, Gabrick KS, Abraham PF, Cabrejo R, Persing JA, Alperovich M. National longitudinal comparison of patients undergoing surgical management of craniosynostosis. J Craniofac Surg. 2018;29(7):1755–9. https://doi.org/10.1097/SCS.0000000000004775.
74. Dohlman JC, Prabhu SP, Staffa SJ, et al. Orbital and eyelid characteristics, strabismus, and intracranial pressure control in Apert children treated by endoscopic strip craniectomy versus fronto-orbital advancement. Plast Reconstr Surg Glob Open. 2023;11(5):e4937.
75. Riesel JN, Riordan CP, Hughes CD, et al. Endoscopic strip craniectomy with orthotic helmet-

ing for safe improvement of head growth in children with Apert syndrome. J Neurosurg Pediatr. 2022;29(6):659–66.
76. Fearon JA, Ditthakasem K, Harrison L, Herbert M. Thirty-year experience treating syndromic craniosynostosis: long-term outcomes following cranial expansions. Plast Reconstr Surg. 2024 Apr. [Online ahead of print]. https://doi.org/10.1097/PRS.0000000000011460.
77. The European Parliament and the Council of the European Union. Directive 2011/24/EU of the European Parliament and the Council of 9 March 2011. https://eur-lex.europa.eu/legal-content/EN/TXT/?uri=CELEX:32011L0024.
78. Global Burden of Disease Collaborative Network. Global Burden of Disease Study 2019 (GBD 2019) Disability Weights. Seattle, United States of America: Institute for Health Metrics and Evaluation (IHME), 2020.

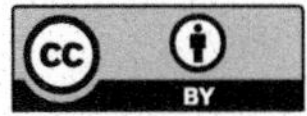

Global Health Policy and Advocacy

38

Ayla Gerk, Letícia Nunes Campos, Luiza Telles, Beatriz Laus Pereira Lima, and Shreenik Kundu

Introduction

Apert syndrome is a rare congenital disorder affecting approximately 1 in 65,000–88,000 live births. Characterized by craniosynostosis, midface hypoplasia, and syndactyly of the hands and feet, the syndrome typically results from pathogenic variants in the *FGFR2* gene [1, 2]. Due to the complexity of this syndrome, management requires early diagnosis, a coordinated, multidisciplinary approach to treatment, and long-term follow-up [3].

Despite advances in surgical techniques and interdisciplinary care models, patients with Apert syndrome continue to face significant barriers to accessing appropriate care [4, 5]. These barriers are more pronounced in low- and middle-income countries (LMICs), where health system limitations, provider shortages, and inequitable resource distribution hinder timely intervention. Delays in diagnosis and treatment can lead to preventable complications that adversely impact neurocognitive development, airway function, feeding, and overall quality of life [1, 6]. The social burden, often extending to entire families, is considerable, particularly in resource-limited settings where out-of-pocket expenses and lack of support services exacerbate vulnerabilities [7–10].

Rare diseases like Apert syndrome are frequently excluded from national and global health priorities despite the complex clinical needs and cumulative health care costs associated with these conditions [11]. Contributing factors include limited epidemiological data, diagnostic challenges, provider unfamiliarity, and stigma [12]. A general lack of public and political awareness compounds these issues, resulting in underinvestment in infrastructure, training, and policy frameworks to support care for rare diseases [12].

Apert syndrome exemplifies the broader systemic challenges of managing rare diseases in global health. These issues underscore the importance of integrating rare diseases into universal health coverage (UHC) agendas, strengthening health care services for affected individuals, and ensuring access to timely, quality-assured interventions. Structured, holistic care pathways are

A. Gerk (✉) · S. Kundu
Harvey E. Beardmore Division of Pediatric Surgery, The Montreal Children's Hospital, McGill University Health Centre, Montreal, QC, Canada

Faculty of Medicine and Health Sciences, McGill University, Montreal, QC, Canada

L. N. Campos
Faculdade de Ciências Médicas, Universidade de Pernambuco, Recife, Pernambuco, Brazil

Department of Clinical Research, Fundación SPINE, Buenos Aires, Argentina

L. Telles
Instituto de Educação Médica (IDOMED/Estácio), Vista Carioca Campus, Rio de Janeiro, RJ, Brazil

B. L. P. Lima
Universidade São Francisco, Campus Bragança Paulista, São Paulo, São Paulo, Brazil

J. G. Meara et al. (eds.), *Apert Syndrome*, https://doi.org/10.1007/978-3-032-12551-4_38

essential for enhancing outcomes and minimizing long-term costs to health care systems [6, 13].

This chapter explores the case for prioritizing Apert syndrome within global health, global surgery, and national health planning. It reviews the current global care landscape, examines structural inequities in access, and considers policy strategies, financing mechanisms, and ethical imperatives necessary to improve outcomes for patients with rare congenital diseases.

Apert Syndrome and Global Health: The Current Landscape

Like other rare diseases, Apert syndrome is associated with a prolonged and challenging diagnostic journey. Although its distinctive features may raise clinical suspicion at birth, definitive diagnosis requires a combination of physical examination, radiological imaging, and confirmation through molecular genetic testing [14, 15]. Given that the condition is rare, many health care professionals are unfamiliar with its presentation, which can lead to delays in diagnosis [16].

Timely access to specialized surgical teams is critical to the effective treatment of Apert syndrome. Timeliness is particularly important because surgical interventions must be coordinated with the child's growth and developmental milestones [17]. For example, correction of craniosynostosis typically occurs within the first year of life, while procedures such as jaw surgery and midline advancement are usually performed during childhood and adolescence [17]. The total number of surgeries varies significantly depending on symptom severity, access to health care, and individual clinical needs. Long-term follow-up studies report an average of approximately 10–15 surgical procedures per patient with Apert syndrome, includes, cranial vault surgeries, midfacial advancements, hand and foot syndactyly separations, orthognathic procedures, and secondary soft tissue revisions [6, 18–20].

Most low- and middle-income countries (LMICs) face significant barriers to the management of Apert syndrome and other forms of craniosynostosis. These include limited health care infrastructure, a shortage of trained professionals, and a lack of well-established referral systems [21]. The limited craniofacial centers established in LMICs are often located in major urban areas, making access difficult for patients living in rural or remote regions. In Brazil, for example, only 28 centers are accredited as references for treating craniofacial deformities, with the majority concentrated in the Southeast [22]. In contrast, high-income countries (HICs) tend to offer more comprehensive access to specialized care. For instance, 182 centers in the United States are certified by the Cleft Palate-Craniofacial Association. California has the most, with 22 centers, followed by Texas and New York, each with 13. However, some states, such as Wyoming and North Dakota, have no certified centers, illustrating that geographic disparities persist even in well-resourced settings [23]. This uneven distribution reflects broader fragmentation within health care systems, where coordination of long-term, multidisciplinary care remains a significant challenge. As a result, many patients miss critical windows for timely surgery and early neurodevelopmental interventions, leading to higher complication rates and reduced quality of life [21].

Social determinants of health such as poverty, education, geographic location, and cultural context critically influence access to care and long-term outcomes for individuals with Apert syndrome [24]. A study from a tertiary children's hospital in California found that children with craniosynostosis who had public insurance or lived in socioeconomically disadvantaged areas were significantly more likely to present late for surgical consultation [24]. Similarly, a review of 477 patients at a US academic medical center found that only 28% were referred to a craniofacial specialist within 3 months of birth. Delays were more common among children referred by non-pediatricians, those from minority backgrounds, and those with multiple suture involvement [25]. In Nigeria, a case study illustrated how early developmental challenges led to lifelong dependency, reduced educational attainment, and limited social relationships [10]. These findings underscore structural and social barriers to timely diagnosis, treatment, and access to care and highlight the negative effects of such barriers on quality of life.

Families of children with Apert syndrome face significant financial challenges due to the complexity and duration of required care. Although data specific to Apert syndrome are limited, research on other rare diseases shows that families often incur substantial out-of-pocket expenses [26]. These costs may include medical supplies, specialized therapies, and travel for treatment, many of which are not covered by insurance [26]. Indirect costs, such as lost income due to caregiving responsibilities, further compound the financial burden. For example, a study on Dravet syndrome reported that annual indirect costs average $81,582, mostly due to lost productivity [27]. In Brazil, families of children with rare conditions like cystic fibrosis and mucopolysaccharidosis reported income losses exceeding 100% of their earnings, with many resorting to obtaining loans or selling assets to fund treatment [28]. Given the ongoing nature of care in Apert syndrome, similar financial strain is likely. Addressing these economic burdens is essential to ensuring equitable access to care and improving long-term outcomes.

Beyond the burden on families, Apert syndrome also imposes significant costs on health systems. Treating a single patient often requires coordination among a multidisciplinary team, which may include plastic surgeons, neurosurgeons, pediatricians, hand surgeons, ophthalmologists, and speech therapists [18]. The syndrome's complexity demands substantial medical resources and ongoing monitoring to manage complications such as increased intracranial pressure, sleep apnea, and visual impairment [29, 30]. When these conditions remain untreated, the resulting complications can lead to increased long-term health care expenditures and strained public health systems. Further research is needed to quantify the full cost of managing Apert syndrome from a system-wide perspective to inform effective planning and resource allocation.

Apert syndrome exemplifies the multifaceted challenges that rare diseases pose to health systems around the world. From delays in diagnosis to the need for coordinated care and long-term support, individuals with Apert syndrome face a range of obstacles that affect their health, development, and quality of life. These challenges are especially pronounced in LMICs, where access to trained professionals and specialized centers is limited. At the same time, geographic and socioeconomic disparities persist, even in high-income settings. Families are often burdened by financial and emotional strain, while health care systems incur high long-term costs. Addressing these challenges requires comprehensive strategies that invest in infrastructure, professional training, policy development, and social support. A holistic approach integrating medical and social interventions is essential to ensure that individuals with Apert syndrome can lead full and healthy lives, regardless of their background or location.

The Evolution of Global Surgery and Neurosurgery

For decades, surgical care was considered a secondary or even tertiary concern within global health. Many considered surgery too costly, complex, and resource-intensive to warrant inclusion alongside primary care interventions such as vaccines or malaria prevention [31]. This perspective did not recognize that surgically treatable conditions account for 30% of the global burden of disease and that affordable management is achievable [32]. On June 29, 1980, Dr. Mahler, then director-general of the World Health Organization (WHO), highlighted the critical importance of surgical care in public health at the World Congress of the International College of Surgeons in Mexico, describing it as a stark reflection of health inequality [33]. However, this emphasis on surgical care did not gain traction, as reflected in comments made by Dr. Paul Farmer and Dr. Jim Kim in 2008 deeming surgery to be public health's "neglected stepchild" [34].

These discussions catalyzed an academic movement to establish surgery as an indivisible, indispensable component of health systems strengthening through robust publications and policy interventions. In 2015, three foundational documents were published: [1] volume one in the third edition of the World Bank's *Disease Control Priorities* entirely devoted to global surgery and addressing the significant barriers in LMICs; [2] the *Lancet* Commission on Global Surgery report (LCoGS), which provided scientific evidence on the global social and economic disparities in access to surgical care; and [3] World Health Commission Resolution 68.15, which politically committed Member States to enhance emergency and essential surgical care and anesthesia [31, 35, 36]. These texts provide a solid foundation for future discussions and strategies. In 2019, Dr. Tedros, WHO Director-General, stressed the importance of surgery in achieving UHC, urging countries to invest in this area [37].

In this context, global surgery has been defined as a multidisciplinary field that integrates education, research, clinical practice, and advocacy to enhance surgical and anesthetic care and promote health equity. Notably, global surgery focuses on addressing the needs of underserved populations and communities by adopting collaborative, cross-sectoral, and transnational strategies that bridge population-level interventions with individual patient care [31].

The LCoGS revealed that five billion people, over two-thirds of the world's population, lack access to safe, affordable, and timely surgical and anesthesia care [31]. The report estimated that 143 million additional surgical procedures are required annually in LMICs to meet essential health needs [31]. Moreover, each year 33 million individuals incur catastrophic health expenditures due to the costs associated with surgery [31]. Furthermore, the LCoGS emphasized that without immediate and consistent investment in expanding surgical services, LMICs would face ongoing economic losses [31]. From 2015 to 2030, these losses are projected to accumulate to a total of US$12.3 trillion (in 2010 US dollars, adjusted for purchasing power parity), primarily due to decreased productivity [31]. The report's findings reframed surgical care not as a luxury, but as a critical, inherent component of UHC. Importantly, the LCoGS introduced six core indicators, including surgical volume, workforce density, and perioperative mortality, that governments and health systems now use to benchmark progress (Fig. 38.1) [31].

The LCoGS introduced National Surgical, Obstetric, and Anesthesia Plans (NSOAPs), which are comprehensive policy frameworks that provide governments with a structured approach to strengthening surgical systems [38]. These plans are intentionally designed for integration into broader national health strategies. Aligned with WHO's health system building blocks, NSOAPs address six core components: infrastructure, service delivery, health information systems, workforce, financing, and governance [38, 39]. Over 40 countries across geographic regions are currently at various stages of developing NSOAPs. A compelling example emerged in Ecuador, where the NSOAP process was led and championed by Dr. Alfredo Borrero, a practicing neurosurgeon who was the country's vice president. In 2023, Ecuador became the first Latin American country to formally develop an NSOAP, a process performed in collaboration with Harvard Medical School's Program in Global Surgery and Social Change [40]. This partnership between political leadership and academic expertise underscores the importance of clinical credibility in advancing national reform, especially in specialized fields such as neurosurgery.

Amid the rise of global surgery, the field of global neurosurgery emerged. While both fields are driven by the same logic of health equity, global neurosurgery involves the urgency of highly time-sensitive and resource-dependent neurosurgical interventions. Neurosurgical conditions such as traumatic brain injury, hydrocephalus, neural tube defects, brain tumors, and stroke are among the leading causes of morbidity and mortality worldwide [41]. Nonetheless, many of these conditions remain untreated in LMICs due to lack of access. Approximately 22.6 million people worldwide require neurosurgical care each year, with 78% of this need concentrated in LMICs [42]. The situation is particularly dire in terms of workforce availability [43]. For example, Southern Africa has a density of 0.14 neurosurgeons per 100,000 population, followed by West Africa with 0.06, and East and Central

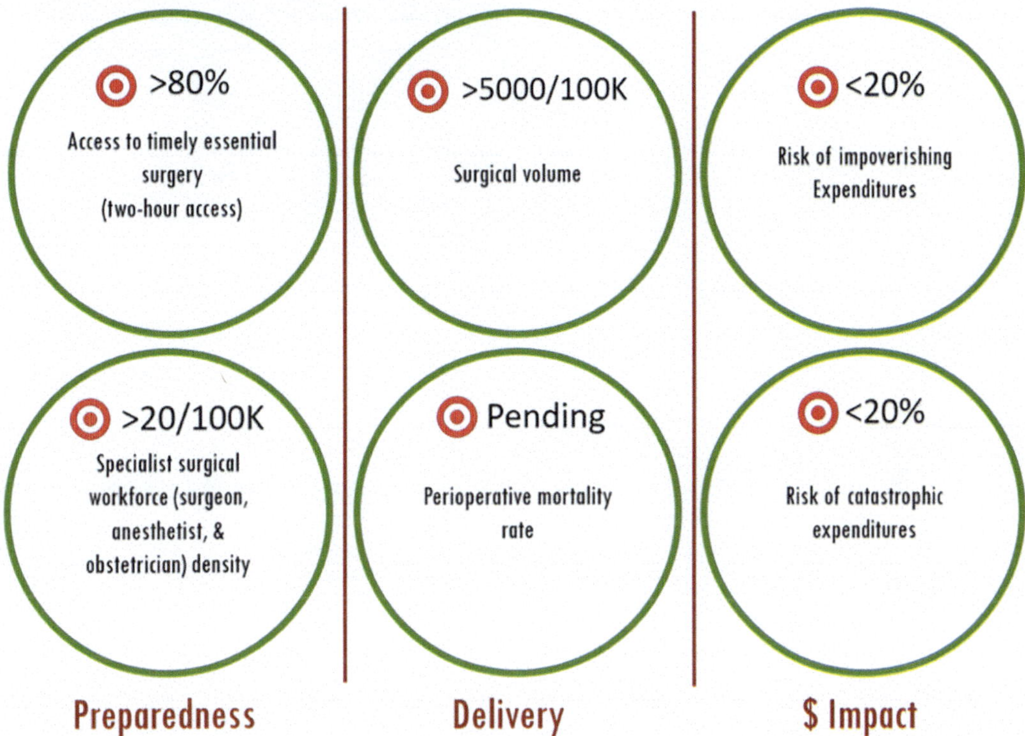

Fig. 38.1 The *Lancet* Commission on Global Surgery Indicators. The *Lancet* Commission on Global Surgery recommended that every country measure at least these six indicators to estimate the strength of its surgical system. (Source: https://blogs.worldbank.org/en/opendata/measuring-surgical-systems-new-paradigm-health-systems-strengthening)

Africa reporting just 0.04 per 100,000 [44]. These figures fall significantly short of the recommended minimum of one neurosurgeon per 100,000 population needed to meet basic neurosurgical care demands, as defined by the World Federation of Neurosurgical Societies (WFNS) (Fig. 38.2) [44]. An estimated 23,300 additional neurosurgeons are required globally to address more than five million essential neurosurgical cases that go untreated each year in LMICs [42].

System-level challenges such as shortages in the anesthesia workforce, insufficient data systems, limited access to postoperative critical care, and unreliable surgical equipment continue to compromise outcomes for patients requiring neurosurgical interventions [45, 46]. Even in facilities with trained personnel, the lack of functioning imaging technologies and inconsistent availability of essential surgical supplies, including implants and disposables, often leads to delays or suboptimal care. Moreover, the absence of robust national surgical registries in most LMICs hampers the ability to monitor surgical morbidity and mortality as well as to assess regional or socioeconomic disparities [47]. Beyond capacity building, there is a pressing need to prioritize patient and community empowerment, particularly regarding conditions that are frequently misunderstood or carry a significant stigma, such as craniosynostosis and neural tube defects [48].

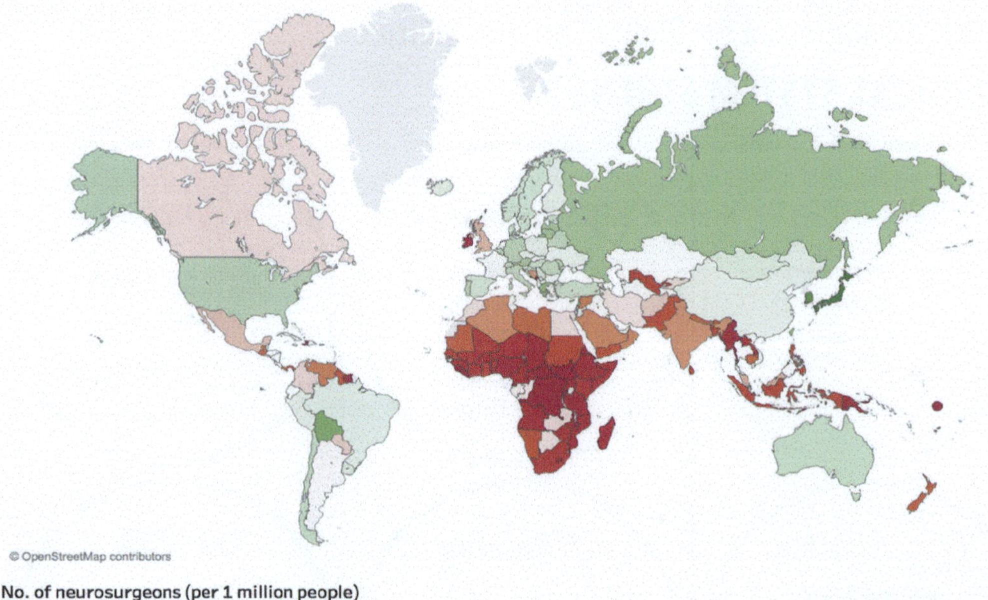

Fig. 38.2 Neurosurgeons per capita worldwide. Global map with relative densities of neurosurgeons per million population, with red indicating low densities and green indicating high densities. © OpenStreetMap contributors (http://www.openstreetmap.org/copyright). Figure is available in color online only. (Source: Mukhopadhyay et al. (2019). The global neurosurgical workforce: a mixed-methods assessment of density and growth. *Journal of Neurosurgery*, 130(4), 1142–1148. https://doi.org/10.3171/2018.10.JNS171723)

Established in 1955, WFNS has played a pivotal role in advancing neurosurgical capacity globally. The organization supports both short- and long-term capacity building via training centers in regional hubs including Rabat, Morocco and Recife, Brazil [49, 50]. Initiatives such as boot camps, virtual neuroanatomy modules, and spine surgery fellowships are increasingly accessible to surgeons from underserved regions [51].

Efforts by the global neurosurgical community to formulate strategic initiatives culminated with the Boston Declaration on Global Neurosurgery [52]. Unveiled on April 24, 2025, at the Edward M. Kennedy Institute in Boston, United States, this declaration represents a unified commitment to advancing neurosurgical care globally. Emphasizing the need for training, equipment, and responsive health systems, the declaration also highlights the importance of shifting protagonism to LMIC actors to ensure sustainable progress. The CURE Children's Hospital of Uganda, founded in 2001, reflects the leadership potential of LMIC actors. The hospital offers one of the most successful pediatric neurosurgery training programs in Africa and specializes in endoscopic treatment of hydrocephalus [53]. Its trainees have gone on to form or support existing neurosurgical units in more than a dozen countries. Similarly, the Asian Congress of Neurological Surgeons has fostered long-term mentorship and education through regional programs and collaborative initiatives [54]. While HIC-LMIC dynamics continue to evolve, progress has been made in promoting bilateral contributions to knowledge and capacity building. Institutions like the Barrow Neurological Institute in the United States have contributed through international observerships and visiting scholar programs, which enable visiting neurosurgeons to implement advanced skills and knowledge in their home countries and strengthen local systems. Through these initiatives, Barrow hosted over 60 scholars from 27 countries between July 2023 and February 2024 [55].

New models of collaboration have emerged to bridge the expertise gap. In tandem, academic institutions have expanded their role in global neurosurgery. For instance, Harvard Medical School's Program in Global Surgery and Social Change launched its Global Neurosurgery Initiative in 2018. This program conducts policy research, supports NSOAP integration, and advocates for increased investment in neurosurgical infrastructure [56]. InterSurgeon, an online global platform launched in 2018, connects neurosurgeons worldwide for case consultations, equipment sharing, and partnership development [57].

Despite these advances, challenges persist. Surgical care receives less than 2% of global health financing, divided among all subspecialties. Neurosurgery and craniofacial surgery are rarely included in national health benefit packages, a trend seen even in countries with NSOAPs. This exclusion has real-world consequences for patients, such as those with treatable brain tumors or congenital craniofacial conditions who are referred abroad, often at a catastrophic cost, or left untreated. For instance, India offers top-tier neurosurgical services in major cities, but accessibility to subpopulations residing in specific locales is often limited. Of the country's 1800 neurosurgeons, the vast majority are based in cities, leaving over 800 million rural residents with limited access and high out-of-pocket expenses [58, 59]. In Nigeria, a rural tertiary center serves five million people without access to computerized tomography (CT) or magnetic resonance imaging [58]. In Australia, rural patients often face long delays for transfers to urban centers [60]. In Canada, Indigenous and northern communities are severely impacted by inadequate resources, social problems, and challenges within the health care system [61]. In the United States, many rural hospitals have lost neurosurgical coverage altogether [62, 63]. These examples reflect a global failure to equitably integrate neurosurgery into health systems.

Notwithstanding, the trajectory of global surgery and neurosurgery is one of progress. Neurosurgical outreach programs are evolving from short-term missions to sustainable partnerships. New research is quantifying the cost-effectiveness of neurosurgical interventions, strengthening the case for their inclusion in UHC packages. As the global health community strives to achieve Sustainable Development Goal (SDG) 3, that of ensuring healthy lives and promoting well-being for all at all ages, surgical care must be viewed not as optional but as indispensable. Leaving surgical patients behind abandons the very principles of health equity. Ultimately, the recognition of surgery, and, by extension, neurosurgery and craniofacial surgery, as fundamental to public health is no longer a question of debate, but rather a matter of implementation, financing, and sustained political will.

National and Global Health Policy

Advancing care for individuals with Apert syndrome requires an understanding of the role of national and global health policy. Over the past decade, efforts to integrate rare diseases into health systems have gained traction, reaching a crucial milestone in 2019 with the United Nations' (UN) Political Declaration on UHC. For the first time, rare diseases were explicitly recognized as part of the global health agenda, as outlined in Resolution A/RES/74/2 [64–66]. This commitment was reaffirmed in September 2023 through a renewed Political Declaration at the UN General Assembly High-Level Meeting, which emphasized that achieving SDG 3.8-universal access to essential health services, medicines, and vaccines, requires the inclusion of individuals with rare diseases to truly leave no one behind [67].

Another key milestone occurred in 2019, when WHO formally included rare disease on its agenda during the 72nd World Health Assembly (WHA) [66, 68]. Building on this momentum, WHO advanced the rare-disease agenda through a resolution titled "Rare Diseases: A Global Health Priority for Equity and Inclusion," endorsed by its Executive Board in early 2025 [69]. Adopted at the 78th WHA in May 2025, the resolution marks a shift from recognition to implementation [69]. It urges Member States to adopt national strategies, invest in diagnostic and treatment infrastructure, and strengthen data systems, research capacity, and cross-sectoral collaboration.

During the 2010s, several countries began adopting national policies to address rare diseases, reflecting a growing political mandate [70]. The European Union (EU) stands out for its coordinated approach: all 28 Member States adopted a shared definition of rare diseases, fewer than 5 cases per 10,000 people, and operate under Regulation (EC) No. 141/2000, which promotes orphan drug development [71–73]. The European Project for Rare Disease National Plans (i.e., EUROPLAN), establishes clear priorities, timelines, and budgets to guide the development of national plans in countries across the EU [74]. These efforts are further supported by initiatives such as the European Reference Networks, the EU4Health program, and Horizon Europe funding, all aimed at improving early diagnosis, cross-border care, and equitable access to orphan medicines [75].

In contrast, Latin American policies on rare diseases remain heterogeneous [76]. Definitions vary across countries: Argentina, Chile, and Mexico follow the EU criteria, whereas Brazil defines rare diseases as those affecting fewer than 65 people per 100,000 population. Colombia uses a threshold of 1 in 5000, and Peru lacks a formal definition [71, 77]. Policy focus reflects similar divergence. Brazil's National Policy for Comprehensive Care for People with Rare Diseases emphasizes integration of rare diseases into the Unified Health System, the establishment of reference centers, and the development of clinical protocols [78]. Conversely, Chile's Ricarte Soto Law provides public funding for high-cost treatments, including some rare diseases, through general taxation [79]. Notably, Colombia's legislation prioritizes patient rights and the creation of a national registry, though implementation challenges remain [80]. Across the region, the lack of dedicated funding mechanisms constitutes a common barrier, which hinders cohesive and sustained policy efforts [78, 81].

In Asia, several countries have introduced policies for rare diseases [71]. China's experience, in particular, offers valuable insights. Since 2018, the government has published two editions of the *National Rare Diseases Catalog*, now listing 207 conditions. This initiative has helped establish a legal and institutional framework for managing rare diseases and protecting patient rights [82]. China also established a national collaborative network, comprising over 400 medical institutions, that facilitates coordinated referrals and telemedicine services [83]. To improve treatment access, the National Healthcare Security Administration has expanded its insurance catalog for seven consecutive years, covering more than 90 rare-disease medications. Moreover, the National Rare Diseases Registry System supports data collection for research and policymaking [84]. In India, the government has made significant progress in addressing rare diseases with the 2021 National Policy for Rare Diseases. This policy, which categorizes rare diseases according to treatment availability and costs, also includes strategies to facilitate early diagnosis, provide financial support, and establish regional centers of excellence [85]. Additionally, the bill promotes a digital platform for patient registries and encourages local drug development by simplifying regulations and providing financial incentives. Despite challenges such as high treatment costs and limited awareness, this policy represents a significant step forward in managing rare diseases in India [85].

Brazil has recently advanced efforts to support individuals with Apert syndrome through Bill No. 1943/2025 (Box 38.1). This bill proposes a legal framework authorizing the federal government to develop guidelines across seven areas: early diagnosis, specialized treatment, continuous multidisciplinary care, professional training, family support, scientific research, and public awareness [86]. The legislation also guarantees specific rights for individuals with Apert syndrome, including prioritized health care access, educational accommodations, streamlined pathways to specialized centers, and inclusive employment initiatives [86]. This bill reflects a growing commitment toward condition-specific legislation that integrates medical care, social inclusion, and human rights principles in rare-disease policy.

Box 38.1 Apert Syndrome Legislation
Brazil's Apert syndrome legislation, as proposed in Bill No. 1943/2025, outlines a legal framework for this syndrome and serves as a compelling example of condition-specific advocacy. Recently, a family with a child with Apert syndrome has propelled coordinated efforts in Brazil that have garnered national attention to the condition. In 2024, Brazil held its first national symposium focusing on syndromic and non-syndromic craniosynostosis, "Craniosynostosis Symposium: Comprehensive Care, Policy and Advocacy." [87] Bringing together diverse stakeholders, the event included hospitals, national and international collaborators, the vice president of Ecuador, the Brazilian Ministry of Health, patient organizations, and medical experts. The symposium catalyzed national dialogue, education, and media attention around Apert syndrome and rare craniofacial conditions that ultimately motivated this legislation [88]. This initiative demonstrates how targeted advocacy can enhance the visibility of a specific condition and prompt legislative reform.

Patient and Family Advocacy Organizations

The tireless efforts of patient and family advocacy organizations have driven much of the progress in rare-disease policy and care [74]. Across regions, these groups have influenced legislation, increased research funding, improved clinical care, and raised awareness of rare conditions [74]. Often grounded in personal experiences and a deep sense of urgency, these advocacy groups have elevated rare diseases from relative obscurity to matters of public health and human rights. Crucially, many of these movements have insisted on co-designing policies with health authorities to ensure that initiatives reflect real-world priorities such as timely diagnosis, coordinated care, and equitable access [89].

Several case studies across the Americas illustrate this influence. In the United States, the National Organization for Rare Disorders played a pivotal role in the passage of the Rare Diseases Act of 2002, which led to the establishment of the Office of Rare Diseases Research at the National Institutes of Health and the creation of the Rare Diseases Clinical Research Network [74, 90]. In Colombia, persistent advocacy by Fundación Enfermedades Huérfanas led to Law 1392 of 2010, recognizing rare diseases as a public health priority [80]. In Argentina, the Federation of Rare Diseases was instrumental in the adoption of Resolution 2329/2009, which launched the National Program for Uncommon Diseases [80].

Similarly, the European Organisation for Rare Diseases has coordinated national plans and launched the Rare Barometer Program. This patient-led platform informs EU-level policy. Moreover, Rare Diseases South Africa has led national awareness campaigns and collaborated with the government to include rare diseases in essential health services. In Asia, Japan's Ministry of Health, in collaboration with patient organizations, established the National Registry of Designated Intractable Diseases, which supports subsidized care and informs health policy through epidemiological data [91].

Effective policies for rare diseases depend on the active participation of advocacy groups in policy design [74]. Co-design ensures that policies are grounded in lived experience and address critical challenges such as diagnostic delays and fragmented services. For example, patient organizations in France played a significant role in the launch of the country's first National Plan for Rare Diseases in 2004, which emphasizes the importance of lifelong care and access to specialized centers. In Australia, over 70 advocacy groups were involved in shaping the 2020 National Strategic Action Plan for Rare Diseases, which formally integrated co-design principles into policy development.

Global Initiatives and Cross-sectoral Collaboration

Global initiatives have also advanced patient-centered policy strategies. In December 2019, Rare Diseases International (RDI), the global alliance for people living with rare diseases, signed a formal collaboration agreement with WHO. This partnership led to the establishment of the Collaborative Global Network for Rare Diseases (CGN4RD), a person-centered initiative designed to build local capacity, foster data sharing, and connect expert networks [66]. Comprising a global network and national and regional hubs, CGN4RD provides a structured framework for care coordination and policy development across countries. Additionally, WHO and RDI collaborated in developing the Operational Description of Rare Diseases, which provides a standardized framework to inform national planning and clinical practices.

Cross-sectoral collaboration plays an instrumental role in translating rare-disease policies into actionable initiatives, particularly in regions with limited resources. The Collaborative for Rare and Uncommon Diseases in the Caribbean and Latin America brings together stakeholders, patients, clinicians, researchers, and policymakers from over 20 countries to strengthen diagnosis, treatment, and advocacy efforts [92]. Similarly, Smile Train, the world's largest cleft-focused organization, operates in more than 95 countries by supporting local professionals with training and resource provision [93]. Lastly, the Canadian Organization for Rare Disorders collaborates with governments, researchers, and clinicians to develop and implement national strategies that enhance access to diagnosis and treatments for rare conditions [94].

Surgical System Strengthening as a Policy Response for Rare Diseases

Health systems must deliver integrated, multidisciplinary care to meet the complex and lifelong needs of individuals living with rare diseases. For instance, many of these conditions require timely access to specialized surgical interventions. However, essential services remain fragmented, inadequately funded, or unavailable in many countries. In settings where surgical care is not integrated into national health strategies, the needs of individuals with rare diseases may be further marginalized, leading to poorer health outcomes. Increasingly, coverage for surgery and rare diseases is being recognized as integral to achieving UHC, presenting a critical opportunity to address long-standing disparities [12, 31, 89, 95]. Incorporating care for rare diseases into national surgical system planning constitutes a key policy measure to advance equity and ensure no population is left behind.

Within this context, NSOAPs provide a structured policy framework to address the surgical needs of patients with rare diseases. These plans, led by governments and grounded in evidence and multistakeholder consensus, serve as comprehensive instruments to improve access to, delivery of, and financing of surgical care [96, 97]. Crucially, NSOAPs should be aligned with broader national health strategies to ensure political legitimacy and long-term integration into health systems. They guide reform across six key health system domains: infrastructure, workforce, service delivery, information management, financing, and governance [96]. To remain effective, NSOAPs must be treated as iterative policies, regularly reviewed and informed by reliable data. Annual evaluations, performance dashboards, and inclusive stakeholder consultations are essential for responsiveness and accountability [98]. Countries in all regions are currently at various stages of NSOAP development and implementation.

While comprehensive long-term evaluations are still underway, some nations have reported measurable progress in strengthening their surgical systems following the implementation of NSOAPs. For example, following NSOAP implementation from 2016 to 2020, Ethiopia experienced a significant increase in its surgical workforce density, rising from 0.35 to 5.19 specialists per 100,000 population. Initiatives like the Integrated Emergency Surgical Officer program and nurse–anesthetist training spurred this growth [39, 99]. Similarly, since the launch of Madagascar's NSOAP in 2019, the government has initiated the construction of 20 district hospitals to strengthen surgical capacity. In parallel, Madagascar established a training program, with support from the World Bank, to equip general practitioners with the skills necessary to perform essential surgical procedures. To date, 20 practitioners have been deployed to rural hospitals, with an additional 20 currently undergoing training [100].

Concerning rare-disease care, NSOAPs present strategic entry points for intervention (Fig. 38.3). These entry points can occur during NSOAP initial stages and situational analyses, through stakeholder engagement, priority setting, policy drafting, and the monitoring and evaluation phases. NSOAPs can offer a pathway to establish specialized surgical centers that concentrate expertise and resources for rare conditions. This integration of specialized surgical centers into larger health care centers is essential, as many syndromic and congenital conditions present early in life and require timely surgical intervention to prevent irreversible complications. In Apert syndrome, early craniotomy, typically performed at approximately six months of age, is crucial to prevent elevated intracranial pressure and associated cognitive impairments [4]. Subsequent surgeries, such as syndactyly release and midface advancement, are typically planned at specific developmental milestones to achieve the best functional and aesthetic outcomes [4]. Addressing complex conditions like Apert syndrome demands a coordinated, multidisciplinary approach. This process encompasses

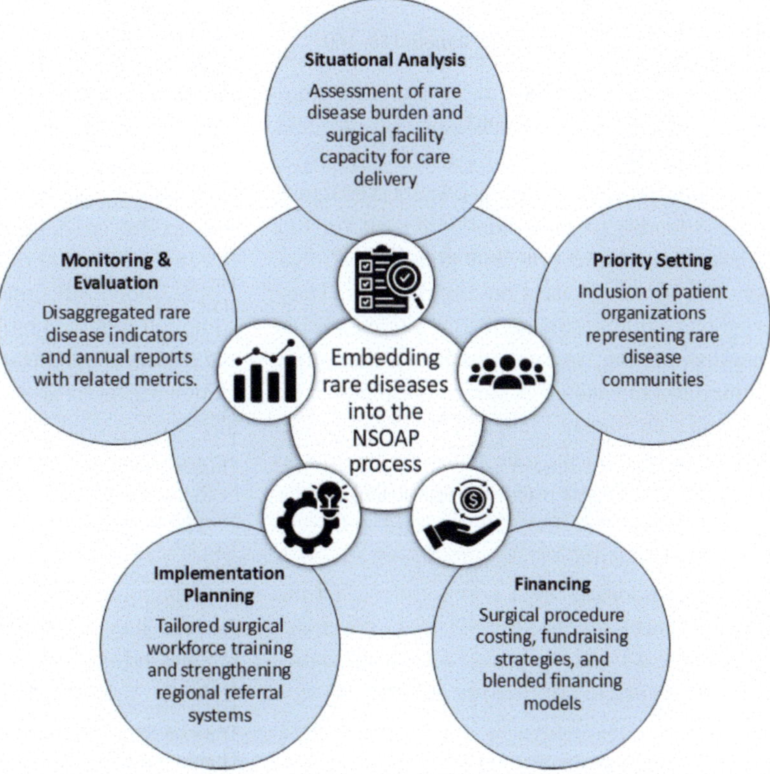

Fig. 38.3 Embedding rare diseases into the National Surgical, Obstetric, and Anesthesia Plan process. (Source: Figure was created by the authors inspired by the National Surgical, Obstetric, and Anesthesia Plan [NSOAP] framework, with modifications to reflect the specific needs and challenges of rare diseases [97])

early identification through prenatal ultrasound, preoperative planning, surgical intervention, rehabilitation, and psychosocial support [101–105]. Embedding these services within NSOAPs and financing them through packages of essential health service enhance their accessibility and sustainability.

NSOAPs can play a key role in promoting standardized, evidence-based care for rare diseases by supporting the development and dissemination of clinical guidelines. National rare-disease policies offer clear examples of this potential. In the decade following the 2014 enactment of Ordinance No. 199 in Brazil, the Ministry of Health published 63 clinical practice guidelines for rare diseases, covering conditions such as cystic fibrosis, myasthenia gravis, spinal muscular atrophy, and amyotrophic lateral sclerosis [106]. In France, the first National Plan for Rare Diseases (2005–2008) tasked the French National Authority for Health with developing national diagnostic and treatment protocols. By 2012, France had published 47 protocols, and the second National Plan introduced a streamlined process to accelerate their development using existing national and international guidelines [107].

Additionally, NSOAPs can strengthen health care workforce capacity by integrating rare-disease-specific training into existing curricula, organizing targeted workshops, and supporting continuing professional development. For example, the launch of Italy's national plan for rare diseases introduced pre- and postgraduate academic programs focused on rare diseases. These programs offer structured, multidisciplinary training across various medical specialties. Aiming to cultivate a "culture of suspicion," the initiatives encourage clinicians to consider rare diagnoses early in the care pathway, facilitating timely referrals and interventions [108]. In the United Kingdom, the 2021 Rare Diseases Framework identified increasing health care professional awareness as a core priority. To this end, the charity Medics4RareDiseases developed "Rare Disease 101," a free, accredited online course designed to improve the abilities of medical students and clinicians to recognize, diagnose, and manage rare conditions [109].

By enhancing health information systems, NSOAPs can improve the collection and analysis of surgical indicators, facilitating better-informed, data-driven policy decisions. Integrating rare-disease registries into these broader platforms for health data can further support ongoing monitoring and strategic planning. For instance, Brazil's national rare-disease registry presents an opportunity to align data collection with NSOAP objectives, thereby informing the development of surgical services. Similarly, France's *Banque Nationale de Données Maladies Rares*, which aggregates data from expert centers, and China's National Rare Diseases Registry System both demonstrate effective use of registries to advance rare-disease care within national health strategies [74, 110].

Despite their promise, implementing NSOAPs faces substantial challenges, particularly in sustainable financing [111]. Many plans remain donor-dependent, underfunded, or limited to pilot phases. Surgical care is often buried within general health budgets, leaving it vulnerable to political shifts and donor fatigue. Addressing this will require reimagining domestic and international financing strategies. Countries have begun exploring innovative models, including public–private partnerships (PPPs), targeted insurance schemes covering surgical procedures, and outcome-based contracts that link funding to measurable improvements in health care outcomes. Outcomes-based financing, in particular, can incentivize the delivery of quality care and ensure more efficient use of resources [112]. Although PPPs can mobilize additional resources and technical expertise, they demand careful regulation to align with public health objectives. Moreover, global co-financing mechanisms may be necessary to guarantee equitable access to high-cost surgical care for rare diseases [111].

The support of various funders can help overcome financial and operational challenges in implementing NSOAPs, particularly in addressing the surgical needs of rare diseases. These funders bring diverse resources, expertise, and strategic priorities that can be leveraged to strengthen surgical systems in LMICs (Table 38.1).

Table 38.1 Funder types and potential roles in supporting sustainable implementation of National Surgical, Obstetric, and Anesthesia Plans (NSOAPs)

Funder type	Examples	Role in supporting NSOAPs and rare diseases
Bilateral funders	United States Agency for International Development; United Kingdom foreign, Commonwealth & Development Office; *Deutsche Gesellschaft für Internationale Zusammenarbeit*	Provide financial and technical assistance focused on infrastructure development, surgical training, and capacity building in low- and middle-income countries
Multilateral organizations	World Health Organization; World Bank; Global Fund	Establish global and national health policies, fund surgical system strengthening, and set research priorities for surgery and rare diseases
Philanthropic foundations	Bill & Melinda Gates Foundation; Wellcome Trust; Chan Zuckerberg initiative	Invest in research, health innovation, capacity building, and initiatives promoting health equity, including genomic and surgical innovations
Synergistic partnerships	Cross-funder collaborations such as the Global Surgery 2030 agenda and the Global Financing Facility	Facilitate coordination among funders and stakeholders to align resources and strategies for the sustainable expansion of surgical care, including care for rare diseases
Catalytic surgical funds	Global surgery foundation's SURGfund	Support capacity-building projects that save lives and strengthen health systems, with a focus on maternal health, children's surgery, trauma, and cancer surgery
Rare-disease-specific initiatives	Novartis gene therapies; EveryLife foundation for Rare diseases	Develop and support access to treatments for rare diseases, Including gene therapies, And advocate for policy changes to improve care for rare-disease patients

NSOAPs provide a framework to integrate surgical care for rare diseases into national health systems. By supporting sustainable, data-driven health strategies and strengthening infrastructure, workforce, and service delivery, NSOAPs can improve access and outcomes for patients with complex needs, including those with rare conditions. Incorporating care for rare diseases into these plans promotes equity. While challenges in financing remain, engaging diverse funders and utilizing innovative models offer a pathway to ensure that no patient requiring surgical care is left behind.

Capacity Building for Apert Syndrome Care

Improving care for individuals with Apert syndrome in LMICs requires a comprehensive capacity-building strategy [113, 114]. While establishing specialized craniofacial centers remains a key strategic component, doing so is not always feasible in resource-limited settings. In these contexts, strengthening the infrastructure of existing hospital-based surgical capacity represents a more practical approach. Targeted investments in diagnostic imaging, fully equipped operating rooms, and enhanced postoperative care units can significantly improve treatment outcomes. Supporting this approach, a global study on cancer surgeries demonstrated that hospitals with essential facilities (e.g., ultrasound machines, CT scanners, and critical care units) achieved notably lower postoperative mortality rates, highlighting the critical role of infrastructure in surgical care [115].

Efforts to expand capacity in managing craniosynostosis should place particular emphasis on the availability of pediatric intensive care units (ICUs) and high-dependency units, given the pivotal role of structured postoperative monitoring in reducing complications and improving recovery outcomes [116]. A retrospective study involving 178 patients who underwent craniosynostosis surgery found that perioperative complications, such as bleeding, infection, and fever, were significantly associated with prolonged ICU stays, highlighting the need for close monitoring in specialized units [117].

Strengthening infrastructure is essential but insufficient to address the full scope of challenges related to Apert syndrome care in LMICs. The limited number of trained specialists, particularly in fields such as craniofacial surgery and pediatric neurosurgery, remains a major obstacle. Thus, expanding training opportunities in these areas is vital. Organizations such as Smile Train and the World Cleft Coalition have established programs that focus on training and supporting local surgeons in cleft and craniofacial surgery. These initiatives emphasize education, knowledge exchange, and capacity building to ensure sustainable and safe surgical care [93, 118]. Although these programs primarily focus on cleft conditions, they foster skills and infrastructure development that can be instrumental in managing more complex craniofacial anomalies, including craniosynostosis and Apert syndrome.

Additionally, establishing standardized, resource-appropriate clinical guidelines is critical for enhancing the management of Apert syndrome and craniosynostosis. Such protocols can support consistent diagnosis, timely referral, optimal surgical timing, and effective postoperative care in settings including hospitals without on-site craniofacial specialists. For instance, the updated Dutch guideline on craniosynostosis provides detailed recommendations for early diagnosis and intervention, helping prevent complications such as increased intracranial pressure [119]. Evidence also shows that implementing standardized perioperative and postoperative care protocols across hospitals reduces adverse events in pediatric cranial-vault reconstruction procedures, contributing to safer and more consistent surgical outcomes [120, 121]. Collectively, these guidelines help empower non-specialist clinicians, reduce variability in care, and improve overall treatment quality in diverse health care settings.

Access to specialized care in remote and underserved areas is another challenge that requires innovative solutions. Combining telemedicine with the development of regional referral networks can help overcome geographic and infrastructural barriers to care. For instance, Brazil's Unified Health System has implemented a remotely operated referral management system that improves access to specialist care while reducing unnecessary referrals [122]. In Ghana, three-dimensional (3-D) telemedicine technology allows multiple specialists to conduct virtual surgical consultations for patients in remote locations, minimizing the need for long-distance travel [122, 123]. Likewise, a cluster-randomized controlled trial in rural Alaska demonstrated that telemedicine referrals significantly enhanced access to specialty care for preschool children [124]. These examples demonstrate how integrating specialized centers into broader health networks through regional systems and telehealth can expand access to craniofacial care in underserved regions [125].

Empowering community health workers (CHWs) represents another important strategy in expanding care for Apert syndrome. Training can enable CHWs to identify early signs of Apert syndrome, support families, and facilitate navigation of health care systems. A study conducted in Brazil exemplifies this approach. In this study, 374 CHWs across 8 municipalities in the state of Rio Grande do Sul participated in an educational program focused on genetic diseases, with particular emphasis on mucopolysaccharidoses. The intervention significantly improved CHWs' knowledge, as evidenced by increased post-training test scores [126]. The authors concluded that CHWs play a fundamental role in identifying and preventing rare genetic diseases, emphasizing the need for continuous training strategies to empower these professionals in the field of rare genetic diseases [126].

Equally essential is the engagement of patient and family advocacy groups in the care process. These groups offer peer support, advocate for enhanced services, and promote culturally sensitive, patient-centered care. For example, the Brazilian Association of Apert Syndrome organizes events that bring families and health care professionals together to share experiences, discuss treatment strategies, and advocate for multidisciplinary care [127]. The second meeting of the Brazilian Association of Apert Syndrome, held in partnership with the *Sobrapar Crânio e Face Hospital*, focused on challenges and perspectives in treating Apert syndrome and other rare craniofacial conditions [127, 128]. Furthermore, organizations like Apert Brasil offer online platforms that allow families to connect, share resources, and support one another. These initiatives provide emotional and informational assistance, as well as contributing to the development of inclusive policies and practices that address the unique needs of individuals with craniofacial disorders [129]. Implementing monitoring and evaluation systems can enhance these efforts by tracking the effectiveness of capacity-building initiatives and ensuring they remain responsive to local contexts [129].

Building capacity for care of Apert syndrome in LMICs demands a multifaceted approach. Improving hospital infrastructure, expanding health care provider training, integrating telemedicine and advanced technologies, empowering CHWs, and involving patient and family groups are essential to bridging care gaps. Addressing these interconnected components can help reduce disparities and improve outcomes for children living with Apert syndrome.

Innovation and Digital Health

Despite advancements in biomedical science, many children with Apert syndrome face inequitable access to early diagnosis, accurate information, and timely surgical care. As previously discussed, patients in many settings face years of diagnostic delay and fragmented care pathways due to the absence of specialized teams, inadequate funding, knowledge gaps about rare diseases, limited access to advanced diagnostics such as CT imaging or genetic testing, and a lack of systemic support for referrals and follow-up care [130, 131]. These inequities stem not only from resource limitations, but also from the underdevelopment of care models for rare diseases. In response, a growing set of digital health innovations, including diagnostic tools and virtual training platforms powered by artificial intelligence (AI), is being developed and, in some contexts, implemented to support early diagnosis and expand surgical access for individuals with Apert syndrome and related conditions [130].

Digital platforms can support structured care for rare diseases (Fig. 38.4), even in decentralized health care systems, as exemplified by a nationally coordinated digital health initiative in Argentina. The Rare Diseases Community

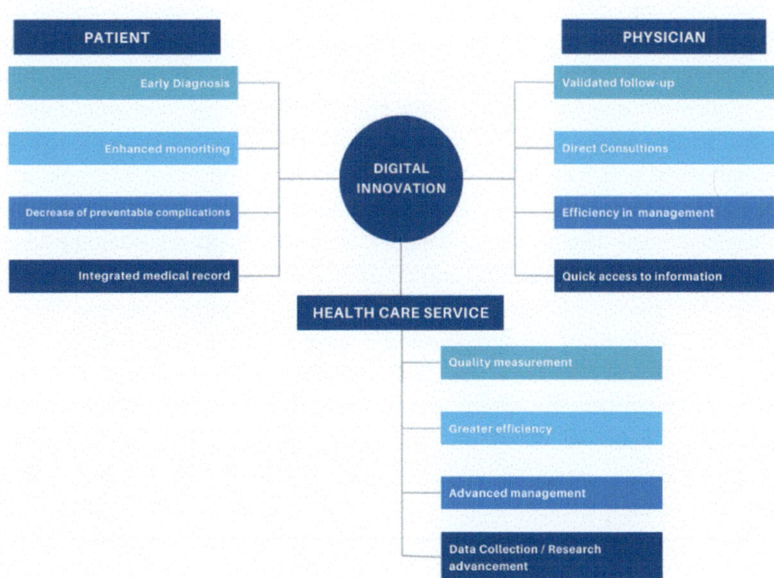

Fig. 38.4 Diagram of digital platform optimization of the patient journey and health care system management. (Source: Gerk et al. 2024; https://doi.org/10.1016/S2214-109X(24)00189-X [132])

(RDCom) platform connects patients and providers through a centralized interface that supports diagnosis, case tracking, and ongoing follow-up (Box 38.2) [132]. This digital ecosystem aims to reduce the time to diagnosis and facilitate multidisciplinary referrals, which are critical for patients with syndromic craniosynostosis.

Additionally, global data registries can yield epidemiological data that support evidence-based policies and program adoption for rare diseases. These registries are particularly valuable in addressing the challenges of low prevalence and fragmented information. For instance, WHO has enhanced the visibility of rare diseases by incorporating over 5500 conditions into the International Classification of Diseases (ICD)-11 system, facilitating standardized tracking and reporting across health systems [133, 134]. The European Platform on Rare Disease Registration addresses data fragmentation by unifying numerous national and regional registries [135]. The platform standardizes data collection and exchange, making registry data more discoverable and interoperable [136]. Similar initiatives like the European Rare Blood Disorders Platform and the Registry Hub for Rare Neuromuscular Diseases further exemplify efforts to promote interoperability among registries [137–139]. Moreover, the National Rare Disease Network (*Rede Nacional de Doenças Raras*, RARAS) in Brazil maps and monitors more than 250 specialized centers for rare diseases in the country [140]. By collecting data on infrastructure and workforce distribution, RARAS supports national planning and policy coordination. In parallel, the *Plataforma Integrada de Vigilância em Saúde* (i.e., Integrated Health Surveillance Platform) was developed to estimate the burden of craniosynostosis using demographic data from the Brazilian Institute of Geography and Statistics [141]. Preliminary findings from 2023 revealed that fewer than 60% of expected craniosynostosis cases were being recorded in public systems, highlighting the extent of underdiagnosis and missed surgical referrals [142].

In Africa, clinicians and researchers are developing continent-wide infrastructure and information management systems for rare diseases, which stand to benefit patients with Apert syndrome. The African Rare Disease Initiative (ARDI), supported by the U.S. National Institutes of Health, aims to harmonize registry systems, develop a mobile-first tracking application, and apply whole-genome sequencing to support diagnosis for at least 300 families across multiple countries [143]. ARDI emphasizes the leadership of African institutions in scientific research and data governance.

Box 38.2 Case Study: Rare Diseases Community (RDCom), A National Digital Platform for Rare-Disease Management in Argentina

RDCom has the aim to enable early diagnosis and structured follow-up of rare diseases through a centralized digital interface, improving patient–provider coordination and system-wide visibility. Interoperability with diagnostic tools and inclusion of decision-support algorithms offer a replicable model for managing complex syndromes like Apert through digital infrastructure.

In Senegal, neurologist Dr. Pedro Rodriguez Cruz has established a cohort of more than 1300 individuals with rare diseases through a partnership between community clinics and international genomic laboratories [144]. His work demonstrates the feasibility of decentralized data collection, biobanking, and family-based genetic counseling in West African settings. This approach could be adapted to support Apert syndrome diagnoses and related surgical planning in similar contexts.

In South Africa, several initiatives feature collaboration between the public health system and academia to improve diagnostic access and care coordination for individuals with rare conditions [66, 145]. An example is the establishment of the first rare diseases biobank on the African continent, which focuses primarily on collecting samples and information on rare congenital disorders [66]. These programs integrate digital tools, clinician training, and policy development to embed rare-disease care into UHC.

At the diagnostic level, AI is generating new possibilities for the early detection of syndromic craniofacial conditions. Clinical decision-support tools powered by deep learning facial recognition, such as Face2Gene, can accurately detect Apert syndrome from facial photographs [146–148]. Pilot studies in India and Africa suggest that even non-specialist providers can use this tool to flag potential syndromic cases in rural clinics [149, 150]. However, algorithmic bias remains a concern, as training datasets are mainly drawn from European and North American populations [151]. Ensuring these models reflect global phenotypic diversity is essential to avoid diagnostic disparities.

The use of virtual reality (VR) training is one of the most promising innovations in building surgical capacity. High-complexity craniofacial procedures, such as Le Fort III advancement and fronto-orbital remodeling, require anatomical expertise and procedural fluency. FundamentalVR, a simulation platform used in several LMIC training programs, allows residents to rehearse procedures, which could be expanded to include complex craniofacial procedures (Box 38.3) [152]. Laptop and mobile headset compatibility enables broader FundamentalVR accessibility in regions with limited infrastructure.

Box 38.3 Case Study: FundamentalVR, Immersive Surgical Training for Complex Pediatric Cases

FundamentalVR provides simulation modules for surgical procedures relevant to Apert syndrome, including cranial-vault remodeling and syndactyly release. The platform is currently being piloted in pediatric training programs in sub-Saharan Africa and Southeast Asia [153]. A meta-analysis conducted in 2025 found that surgical virtual reality training improved surgical performance, reduced operative times, and potentially improved patient outcomes.

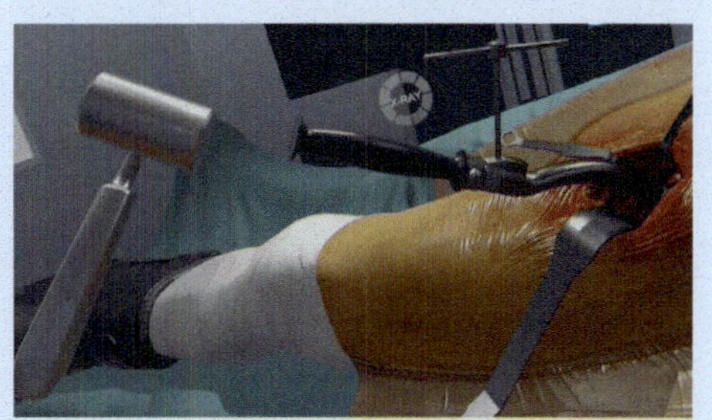

(Source: The FundamentalVR website [151])

Frugal innovation remains a critical approach in settings where medical imports are financially or logistically inaccessible. For example, biomedical engineers in Uganda and Brazil use open-source designs to print 3-D surgical guides and splints from recycled materials [154]. These locally adapted devices reduce surgical planning time and reduce costs by up to 80%. A study in Pakistan demonstrated that low-cost materials and open-source software can produce patient-specific cranial implants at a fraction of the conventional cost, thereby enhancing accessibility [155]. Similarly, craniofacial teams in India have used region-specific skull data to develop custom implants better suited to local populations [156, 157]. These solutions foster biomedical independence and ensure that device design accounts for cost-effective variations.

Sustainable care systems for rare diseases will require integration of digital innovation into national policies and training pathways. Five priorities emerge in this effort: (1) invest in interoperable registries using ICD-11 and Human Phenotype Ontology standards [158]; (2) establish mobile-first referral platforms to streamline patient navigation; (3) expand surgical training through hybrid VR and in-country mentorship; (4) incorporate rare diseases into national surgical plans; and (5) support South-led research, development, and implementation. These shifts are technologically feasible and necessary to achieve equitable access for people with Apert syndrome globally.

Table 38.2 Adaptable innovation initiatives for Apert syndrome surgical care in low- and middle-income countries

Stage	Innovation type	Worldwide examples
1. Early identification	Digital registries and artificial intelligence facial recognition	Rare diseases community (i.e., RDCom) (Argentina); *Plataforma Integrada de Vigilância em Saúde* (Brazil); Face2Gene pilots (India, Ghana); digital newborn screening (India, Sri Lanka)
2. Diagnosis and planning	Genomic sequencing and mobile tracking	African Rare Disease initiative (pan-Africa); Dr. Pedro Rodriguez Cruz (Senegal); Rare Disease biobank (Colombia); whole exome panels (India, Bangladesh)
3. Surgical capacity building	Virtual reality (VR) surgical simulation and open training tools	FundamentalVR; Osso VR (pilots in South Asia and East Africa); open-access craniofacial modules; in-country surgical bootcamps
4. Frugal biomedical innovation	Three-dimensional (3-D)-printed devices and local engineering	3-D-printed cranial molds (Uganda, Brazil); thermoplastic splints (India); blender-based planning (Latin America)
5. System integration	Policy platforms and national access networks	National Rare Disease Network (Brazil); Rare diseases access initiative (South Africa); national surgical plans (Ethiopia, Pakistan); Pan American Health Organization alignment tools

Innovation in rare surgical diseases cannot be separated from questions of justice, representation, and power. Tools such as RDCom, FundamentalVR, ARDI, and Face2Gene will only close gaps if they are adapted, governed, and sustained by the communities they are meant to serve. Apert syndrome exemplifies the need for a rare-disease agenda that is not only surgically sophisticated but also digitally enabled, inclusive, and globally equitable (Table 38.2).

Limited access to essential resources, accurate information, and appropriate care for Apert syndrome and other rare diseases further intensifies the burden on affected individuals and their families, particularly in LMICs [64, 159]. Equipping primary health centers to manage rare diseases is often unfeasible, and can be particularly challenging in these settings [160]. Therefore, scalable alternatives that enable accurate diagnosis, facilitate timely referral, and provide clear post-diagnostic guidance are critical [160]. Digital innovations, such as platforms that facilitate care coordination, improve reporting, and provide evidence-based information, offer adaptable models for LMICs. Addressing local needs and empowering regional champions can strengthen the integration of rare diseases into national health systems and advance more equitable care globally.

Ethical and Equity Considerations

As in other areas of global health, implementing initiatives for rare diseases such as Apert syndrome and other syndromic conditions raises complex ethical and equity-related challenges. Fundamental questions arise: who determines how limited health resources are allocated? Who leads rare-disease efforts? Who benefits from these interventions? How can we ensure that such investments do not reinforce existing disparities? Addressing these ethical considerations is a foundational step toward building equitable, community-driven global health policies that include and uplift individuals affected by rare diseases.

Understanding how scarce health resources are allocated is fundamental in addressing ethical considerations [161]. In many LMICs, budgets are already stretched to meet basic primary care needs. Surgical interventions for Apert syndrome, such as cranial-vault reconstruction, have a high upfront cost, and prioritizing these interventions can appear to divert funds from addressing more prevalent conditions. Yet, failing to invest in these specialized services perpetuates "diagnostic odysseys" and lifelong disability for affected children [64]. Transparent and participatory priority-setting mechanisms are essential to ensure that investments in rare diseases are balanced against broader health needs, thereby safeguarding distributive justice.

Another important ethical consideration is the tendency of top-down intervention design to overlook the real experiences of patients and caregivers. Families of children with rare conditions often feel excluded from intervention efforts, resulting in programs poorly aligned with local needs [162]. Embedding patient and family advocates in steering committees ensures that their concerns, needs, and preferences inform every stage of policies, programs, and projects [162]. Ireland's Rare Disease Research Partnership exemplifies such an approach. This initiative engaged patients, families, clinicians, and researchers in a co-designed process to identify and rank the top 15 research priorities for rare diseases, aiming to align national research agendas with the lived experiences and needs of the rare-disease community [163]. In Japan, the Commons Project established the "Evidence-Generating Commons" where stakeholders, collaborated through workshops to clarify patient difficulties, develop criteria for priority setting, and identify high-priority research topics [164].

Specific considerations must also be addressed in studies involving the collection of genomic and clinical data. While assembling such data can enhance diagnostic accuracy and inform personalized care strategies, it can generate apprehension about informed consent, data ownership, privacy, and equitable benefit-sharing. For instance, one study demonstrated that over 96% of 2800 patients' records could be uniquely identified using diagnosis codes, even after de-identification, highlighting the limitations of current privacy-protection methods and the potential for breaches of confidentiality [165]. Another study explored the perspectives of patients with rare diseases, informal caregivers, and health care professionals in Northern Portugal regarding the sharing of genomic data. The study revealed significant concerns among patients and caregivers about the lack of security and control over information access, as well as the extraction of information beyond research objectives [166]. These findings underscore that maintaining trust and integrity in research practices necessitates robust governance frameworks that address these concerns.

Including rare-disease patients in clinical trials can offer critical access to new treatments, but this practice raises ethical concerns about post-trial access. When a therapy proves beneficial, withdrawing it after the study may harm participants, especially those in low-resource settings where alternatives are unavailable. The Declaration of Helsinki emphasizes the ethical obligation to provide post-trial access to beneficial treatments for participants who responded positively during the study [167]. However, implementing this principle is complex. Challenges include determining whether the responsibility for providing treatment post-trial lies with sponsors, researchers, or health care systems and overcoming financial and logistical barriers, particularly in LMICs [168]. Additionally, unclear post-trial access policies can lead to inconsistent practices and ethical dilemmas, such as patients deteriorating if treatment is withdrawn. Comprehensive guidelines are necessary to address these challenges by clarifying responsibilities and ensuring continued access to effective therapies after trials, thereby prioritizing patient welfare and maintaining the integrity of clinical research [169].

Beyond research, innovation in rare diseases warrants reflection on ethical and equity considerations from conception to implementation. Innovation should be judged not only on its novelty or technical sophistication, but also on whether it reaches those who need it most and whether it helps reduce, rather than reinforce, health inequities [170]. Technologies like 3-D-printed cranial implants have potential for treating craniofacial conditions such as Apert syndrome. However, patent protections and high manufacturing costs can limit their accessibility in LMICs. To improve access, global frameworks must balance incentives for innovation and equitable distribution. Strategies such as patent pooling, where patent holders collectively license their intellectual property, could enhance access to essential technologies [171–173]. Value-based tiered pricing could also adjust costs to match a country's ability to pay, making life-saving technologies more affordable [171].

Moreover, we must challenge the idea that countries with fewer resources cannot adopt or sustain high-tech solutions. For example, Rwanda has successfully integrated drone delivery systems for blood and medical supplies through a partnership with Zipline [174]. This innovation has been scaled nationally, reducing delivery times in emergency situations. The success of this program proves that with adequate support, infrastructure, and local ownership, complex technologies can thrive in LMICs. The assumption that LMICs should always receive lower-tech or simplified solutions is neither fair nor ethical. Limiting access for LMICs based on such assumptions undermines their real potential. Frameworks should extend beyond promoting innovation to ensuring that innovations are accessible and ethical. Furthermore, we must leverage multistakeholder participation to build on facilitators and manage barriers efficiently.

Rare-disease collaborations have the potential to reproduce neocolonial dynamics, particularly when institutions from high-income countries (HICs) unilaterally shape research agendas, educational programs, guidelines, and models of care. Neocolonialism refers to using economic, cultural, and political influence to maintain control over less powerful nations through conditional aid and globalized structures of dependency [175]. As a result, LMICs often depend on research, resources, and treatments developed in HICs.

The persistence of short-term surgical missions, typically led by HIC teams, is one of the most visible forms of neocolonialism [176]. Although motivated by a desire to address urgent surgical needs, these missions can inadvertently foster dependence on external aid and disrupt local health care systems [177]. By operating outside existing health infrastructures, these missions may disrupt ongoing services, place additional strain on limited local resources, and diminish the leadership role of local professionals [178]. The absence of consistent follow-up care further compromises their impact, leaving local providers responsible for managing postoperative complications without adequate support [177, 179]. Additionally, these missions can perpetuate power imbalances by prioritizing external agendas over local needs. Thus, a shift toward sustainable, locally led models is crucial for strengthening health systems [178].

Public policies tailored to regional needs are essential in addressing these neocolonial roots [74]. Effective policies must be context-sensitive, incorporating each region's specific social, cultural, and economic realities. The principle of people-centered care is essential for healthcare systems [180]. In this regard, Germany's National Action Plan for People with Rare Diseases emphasizes coordinated care networks and patient involvement, aiming to improve medical care for rare-disease patients [181]. Similarly, Australia's Rare Diseases Strategic Framework incorporates stakeholder engagement to guide public health policy and practice toward "precision public health." [182]

Strengthening rare disease initiatives within global health requires more than technical solutions or expanded access to diagnostics; it necessitates a comprehensive approach that encompasses all aspects of care. Such an approach calls for a sustained commitment to ethical principles, equitable resource allocation, and the meaningful inclusion of affected communities in all stages of policy and program development. Transparent decision-making processes and context-sensitive approaches are pivotal to ensuring that efforts addressing rare diseases do not perpetuate existing inequities. By centering lived experiences and promoting inclusive governance, policies for rare diseases can contribute to more just and responsive health systems, especially in LMICs.

Conclusions and Vision for the Future

This chapter has examined the role of global health policy and advocacy in advancing care for Apert syndrome. Highlighting how a rare condition can reveal deeper flaws in health systems, the chapter underscores that rare diseases are not rare in their impact. Persistent delays in diagnosis, limited surgical capacity, and fragmented models of care reveal structural gaps that disproportionately affect children with rare congenital conditions. Thus, fully integrating rare diseases such as Apert syndrome into UHC and national surgical strategies, treating them as essential components, strengthens health systems.

Progress requires moving beyond short-term fixes toward sustainable investments that strengthen national infrastructure. This includes supporting multidisciplinary teams, expanding specialized surgical training, and conducting research tailored to the challenges of rare conditions in diverse settings. While digital health and simulation technologies are expanding access to care, their impact depends on implementing inclusive policies, equitable financing, and community-led approaches.

Strong data systems that track early diagnosis, timely surgery, and outcomes must be rooted in dignity and well-being to inform policy, guide funding decisions, and ensure accountability. Collaborative networks involving ministries of health, civil society, academic institutions, and affected communities can shift the focus from scarcity to shared strength. At the global level, cooperation across regions is essential, particularly through South–South partnerships that enable countries to share knowledge, coordinate responses, and drive innovation within their own contexts, thereby reducing their dependence on HICs.

Ultimately, improving surgical care for rare diseases is a matter of justice, affirming the right to health and the responsibility to provide lifesaving and life-enhancing care regardless of geography or diagnosis. Aligning rare-disease strategies with national surgical planning can help build integrated, people-centered systems that are both resilient and responsive to the needs of individuals with rare diseases. Apert syndrome provides a useful model for this integration, highlighting the need for robust policy, accurate and early diagnosis, coordinated multidisciplinary care, and long-term follow-up. Embedding these elements into national strategies ensures that future reforms reflect the lived experiences of patients and families.

References

1. Wenger TL, Hing AV, Evans KN. Apert syndrome. In: GeneReviews(®). Seattle (WA): University of Washington, Seattle; 1993.
2. Cohen MM Jr. Craniosynostoses: phenotypic/molecular correlations. Am J Med Genet. 1995;56(3):334–9.
3. Fadda MT, Ierardo G, Ladniak B, Di Giorgio G, Caporlingua A, Raponi I, et al. Treatment timing and multidisciplinary approach in Apert syndrome. Ann Stomatol (Roma). 2015 Apr;6(2):58–63.
4. Kumari K, Saleh I, Taslim S, Ahmad S, Hussain I, Munir Z, et al. Unraveling the complexity of apert syndrome: genetics, clinical insights, and future frontiers. Cureus. 2023 Oct;15(10):e47281.
5. Breik O, Mahindu A, Moore MH, Molloy CJ, Santoreneos S, David DJ. Apert syndrome: Surgical outcomes and perspectives. J Craniomaxillofac Surg. 2016 Sep;44(9):1238–45.
6. Karsonovich T, Patel BC. Apert syndrome. In: StatPearls. Treasure Island (FL): StatPearls Publishing; 2025.
7. Netherton J, Horton J, Stock NM, Shaw R, Noons P, Evans MJ. Psychological adjustment in Apert syndrome: parent and young person perspectives. Cleft Palate Craniofac J. 2023 Apr;60(4):461–73.
8. Saydam SZ, Çüçülayef D, Doğan TN, Crerand CE, Özek M. Social experiences of Turkish parents raising a child with Apert syndrome: A qualitative study. Cleft Palate Craniofac J. 2021 Mar;58(3):354–61.
9. Abdatam M, Nhungo CJ, Muhamba F, Mwanga AH, Akoko L, Mkony CA. Apert syndrome: a rare congenital anomaly and experience from a low-resource country: a case report and review of the literature. J Rare Dis [Internet]. 2025;4(1) https://doi.org/10.1007/s44162-024-00064-9.
10. Kana MA, Baduku TS, Bello-Manga H, Baduku AS. A 37-year-old Nigerian woman with Apert syndrome, medical and psychosocial perspectives: a case report. J Med Case Rep. 2018;12(1):126.

11. Nguengang Wakap S, Lambert DM, Olry A, Rodwell C, Gueydan C, Lanneau V, et al. Estimating cumulative point prevalence of rare diseases: analysis of the Orphanet database. Eur J Hum Genet. 2020 Feb;28(2):165–73.
12. Baynam G, Hartman AL, Letinturier MCV, Bolz-Johnson M, Carrion P, Grady AC, et al. Global health for rare diseases through primary care. Lancet Glob Health. 2024 Jul;12(7):e1192–9.
13. Tumienė B, Juozapavičiūtė A, Andriukaitis V. Rare diseases: still on the fringes of universal health coverage in Europe. Lancet Reg Health Eur. 2024;37(100783):100783.
14. Cacciaguerra G, Palermo M, Marino L, Rapisarda FAS, Pavone P, Falsaperla R, et al. The evolution of the role of imaging in the diagnosis of craniosynostosis: a narrative review. Children (Basel). 2021;8(9):727.
15. Zavala CA, Zima LA, Greives MR, Fletcher SA, Shah MN, Miller BA, et al. Can craniosynostosis be diagnosed on physical examination? A retrospective review. J Craniofac Surg. 2023;34(7):2046–50.
16. Apert syndrome [Internet]. [cited 2025 May 28]. Available from: https://rarediseases.info.nih.gov/diseases/5833/apert-syndrome
17. Mathijssen IMJ. Working Group Guideline Craniosynostosis. Updated guideline on treatment and management of craniosynostosis. J Craniofac Surg. 2021;32(1):371–450.
18. Allam KA, Wan DC, Khwanngern K, Kawamoto HK, Tanna N, Perry A, et al. Treatment of apert syndrome: a long-term follow-up study. Plast Reconstr Surg. 2011 Apr;127(4):1601–11.
19. Raposo-Amaral CE, Denadai R, de Oliveira YM, Ghizoni E, Raposo-Amaral CA. Apert syndrome management: changing treatment algorithm. J Craniofac Surg. 2020;31(3):648–52.
20. Tovetjärn R, Tarnow P, Maltese G, Fischer S, Sahlin PE, Kölby L. Children with Apert syndrome as adults: a follow-up study of 28 Scandinavian patients. Plast Reconstr Surg. 2012;130(4):572e–6e.
21. Wireko AA, Ahluwalia A, Ali SH, Shah MH, Aderinto N, Banerjee S, et al. Insights into craniosynostosis management in low- and middle-income countries: A narrative review of outcomes, shortcomings and paediatric neurosurgery capacity. SAGE Open Med. 2024;12:20503121241226891.
22. Almeida AMF d L, Chaves SCL, Santos CML, de Santana SF. Atenção à pessoa com fissura labiopalatina: proposta de modelização para avaliação de centros especializados, no Brasil. Saude Debate. 2017;41(spe):156–66.
23. Peck CJ, Parsaei Y, Lattanzi J, Gowda AU, Yang J, Lopez J, et al. The geographic availability of certified cleft care in the United States: A national geospatial analysis of 1-hour access to care. J Oral Maxillofac Surg. 2021;79(8):1733–42.
24. Jolibois MI, Roohani I, Moshal T, Lasky S, Urata M, Munabi NCO, et al. Sociodemographic factors associated with delayed presentation in craniosynostosis surgery at a tertiary children's hospital. Plast Reconstr Surg Glob Open. 2024;12(8):e6035.
25. Gandolfi BM, Sobol DL, Farjat AE, Allori AC, Muh CR, Marcus JR. Risk factors for delayed referral to a craniofacial specialist for treatment of craniosynostosis. J Pediatr. 2017;186:165–71.e2.
26. Buckle N, Doyle O, Kodate N, Kinch M, Somanadhan S. Caregiver-reported economic impacts of pediatric rare diseases-A scoping review. Healthcare (Basel). 2024;12(24):2578.
27. Whittington MD, Knupp KG, Vanderveen G, Kim C, Gammaitoni A, Campbell JD. The direct and indirect costs of Dravet syndrome. Epilepsy Behav. 2018;80:109–13.
28. Pinto M, Madureira A, Barros LB d P, Nascimento M, da Costa ACC, de Oliveira NV, et al. Complex care, high cost, and loss of income: frequent issues for families of children and adolescents with rare health conditions. Cad Saude Publica. 2019;35(9):e00180218.
29. de Jong T, Bannink N, Bredero-Boelhouwer HH, van Veelen MLC, Bartels MC, Hoeve LJ, et al. Long-term functional outcome in 167 patients with syndromic craniosynostosis; defining a syndrome-specific risk profile. J Plast Reconstr Aesthet Surg. 2010;63(10):1635–41.
30. Khong JJ, Anderson P, Gray TL, Hammerton M, Selva D, David D. Ophthalmic findings in Apert's syndrome after craniofacial surgery: twenty-nine years' experience. Ophthalmology. 2006;113(2):347–52.
31. Meara JG, Leather AJM, Hagander L, Alkire BC, Alonso N, Ameh EA, et al. Global surgery 2030: evidence and solutions for achieving health, welfare, and economic development. Am J Obstet Gynecol. 2015;213(3):338–40.
32. Shrime MG, Bickler SW, Alkire BC, Mock C. Global burden of surgical disease: an estimation from the provider perspective. Lancet Glob Health. 2015;3(Suppl 2):S8–9. https://doi.org/10.1016/S2214-109X(14)70384-5. https://www.thelancet.com/journals/langlo/article/PIIS2214-109X%2814%2970384-5/fulltext
33. Thee T. Address by Dr h. Mahler director-general of the world health organization [Internet]. [cited 2025 May 25]. Available from: https://cdn.who.int/media/docs/default-source/integrated-health-services-(ihs)/csy/surgical-care/mahler1980speech.pdf?sfvrsn=18072fa8_11
34. Farmer PE, Kim JY. Surgery and global health: a view from beyond the OR. World J Surg. 2008 Apr;32(4):533–6.
35. Price R, Makasa E, Hollands M. World Health assembly resolution WHA68.15: "strengthening emergency and essential surgical care and anesthesia as a component of universal health coverage", addressing the public health gaps arising from lack of safe, affordable and accessible surgical and anesthetic services. World J Surg. 2015 Sep;39(9):2115–25.

36. Debas HT, Donkor P, Gawande A, Jamison DT, Kruk ME, Mock CN, The International Bank for Reconstruction and Development/The World Bank. Essential surgery: disease control priorities, Third Edition. Washington (DC); 2015.
37. Pgssc H. WHO Director General Dr. Tedros Addressing the Global Surgery Community March 20, 2019 [Internet]. Youtube; 2019 [cited 2025 Jun 19]. Available from: https://www.youtube.com/watch?v=P1XLthxQs7g
38. Sonderman KA, Citron I, Mukhopadhyay S, Albutt K, Taylor K, Jumbam D, et al. Framework for developing a national surgical, obstetric and anaesthesia plan. BJS Open. 2019;3(5):722–32.
39. Gerk A, Campos LN, Telles L, Bustorff-Silva J, Schnitman G, Ferreira R, et al. Expansion of national surgical, obstetric, and anaesthesia plans in Latin America: can Brazil be next? Lancet Reg Health Am. 2024;37(100834):100834.
40. Hyman GY, Salamea JC, Gerk A, Kumar N, Wurdeman T, Park KB, et al. Ecuador's National Surgical Strengthening Plan: first in Latin America, provides hope for surgical care agenda. Rev Panam Salud Publica. 2024;48:e22.
41. Veerappan VR, Gabriel PJ, Shlobin NA, Marks K, Ooi SZY, Aukrust CG, et al. Global neurosurgery in the context of global public health practice, a literature review of case studies. World Neurosurg. 2022;165:20–6.
42. Dewan MC, Rattani A, Fieggen G, Arraez MA, Servadei F, Boop FA, et al. Global neurosurgery: the current capacity and deficit in the provision of essential neurosurgical care. Executive Summary of the Global Neurosurgery Initiative at the Program in Global Surgery and Social Change. J Neurosurg. 2019;130(4):1055–64.
43. Gupta S, Gal ZT, Athni TS, Calderon C, Callison WÉ, Dada OE, et al. Mapping the global neurosurgery workforce. Part 1: consultant neurosurgeon density. J Neurosurg. 2024;141(1):1–9.
44. Ukachukwu AEK, Still MEH, Seas A, von Isenburg M, Fieggen G, Malomo AO, et al. Fulfilling the specialist neurosurgical workforce needs in Africa: a systematic review and projection toward 2030. J Neurosurg. 2023;138(4):1102–13.
45. Shakir M, Shariq SF, Irshad HA, Khowaja AH, Tahir I, Rae AI, et al. Barriers to neurosurgical care of brain tumors in low- and middle-income countries: a systematic review of the service delivery challenges. World Neurosurg. 2024;187:211–22.e3.
46. Ariyo P, Trelles M, Helmand R, Amir Y, Hassani GH, Mftavyanka J, et al. Providing anesthesia care in resource-limited settings: A 6-year analysis of anesthesia services provided at Médecins Sans Frontières facilities. Anesthesiology. 2016;124(3):561–9.
47. Diehl T, Jaraczewski TJ, Ahmed KS, Khan MR, Harrison EM, Abebe BM, et al. Barriers and facilitators to collecting surgical outcome data in low- and middle-income countries: an international survey. Ann Surg Open. 2024;5(1):e384.
48. Shlobin NA, Ghotme KA, Arynchyna-Smith A, Gomez MG, Woodrow S, Blount J, et al. Neurosurgical advocacy in the prevention of neural tube defects: impacting global fortification policies through leadership, collaboration, and stakeholder engagement. Neurosurg Clin N Am. 2024;35(4):411–20.
49. World Federation of Neurosurgical Societies WFNS. Rabat Center Fellowship [Internet]. [cited 2025 May 23]. Available from: https://wfns.org/menu/50/rabat-center-fellowship?utm_source=chatgpt.com
50. World Federation of Neurosurgical Societies WFNS. Recife Reference Center for Training Young African Neurosurgeons (Portuguese speaking) [Internet]. [cited 2025 May 23]. Available from: https://wfns.org/training-centers/6/
51. World Federation of Neurosurgical Societies WFNS. Neurosurgical Education for Young Neurosurgeons [Internet]. [cited 2025 May 23]. Available from: https://wfns.org/newsletter/85?utm_source=chatgpt.com
52. Gupta S, Corley J, Ghotme KA, Nahed B, Drummond K, Hutchinson P, et al. The Boston declaration 2025: plan and pledges for progress in global neurosurgery. World Neurosurg. 2025;193:104–7.
53. Nambasi C. Empowering Medical Heroes: CURE Uganda's Neurosurgery Training Program (CURE Neuro) [Internet]. CURE Uganda -. Cure Uganda; 2024 [cited 2025 May 24]. Available from: https://uganda.cure.org/news/empowering-medical-heroes-cure-ugandas-neurosurgery-training-program-cure-neuro/
54. Asian Congress of Neurological Surgeons. Mission and Vision [Internet]. Asian Congress of Neurological Surgeons. [cited 2025 May 24]. Available from: https://asiancns.com/mission-and-vision/
55. Wachtel A. Barrow Global Neurosurgery [Internet]. Barrow Neurological Institute. 2024 [cited 2025 May 24]. Available from: https://www.barrowneuro.org/for-physicians-researchers/barrow-global/barrow-global-neurosurgery/
56. Global Neurosurgery Initiative [Internet]. pgssc. [cited 2025 May 24]. Available from: https://www.pgssc.org/gnsinitiative
57. InterSurgeon, Global Surgical partnerships [Internet]. InterSurgeon 2017 [cited 2025 May 24]. Available from: https://intersurgeon.org/
58. Upadhyayula PS, Yue JK, Yang J, Birk HS, Ciacci JD. The current state of rural neurosurgical practice: an international perspective. J Neurosci Rural Pract. 2018;9(1):123–31.
59. Ganapathy K. Neurosurgery in India: an overview. World Neurosurg. 2013;79(5–6):621–8.
60. Luck T, Treacy PJ, Mathieson M, Sandilands J, Weidlich S, Read D. Emergency neurosurgery in Darwin: still the generalist surgeons' responsibility. ANZ J Surg. 2015;85(9):610–4.

61. Salaheen Z, Moghaddamjou A, Fehlings M. Neurotrauma in indigenous populations of Canada-challenges and opportunities at a global level: a scoping review. World Neurosurg. 2022;167:213–21.e2.
62. Peterman N, Smith EJ, Liang E, Yeo E, Kaptur B, Naik A, et al. Geospatial evaluation of disparities in neurosurgical access in the United States. J Clin Neurosci. 2022;105:109–14.
63. Hunsaker JC, Herring L, Franklin S, Christensen KB, Chan B, Jensen RL. The path to neurosurgery: identifying obstacles to pursuing a medical career unique to rural high school students when compared with urban and suburban students. J Neurosurg. 2022;137(6):1866–71.
64. The Lancet Global Health. The landscape for rare diseases in 2024. Lancet Glob Health. 2024;12(3):e341.
65. Political declaration of the high-level meeting on universal health coverage. Session SF. General Assembly Distr.: General [Internet]. [cited 2025 May 17]. Available from: https://documents.un.org/doc/undoc/gen/n19/311/84/pdf/n1931184.pdf
66. Adachi T, El-Hattab AW, Jain R, Nogales Crespo KA, Quirland Lazo CI, Scarpa M, et al. Enhancing equitable access to rare disease diagnosis and treatment around the world: A review of evidence, policies, and challenges. Int J Environ Res Public Health [Internet]. 2023;20(6) https://doi.org/10.3390/ijerph20064732.
67. Political Declaration of the High-level Meeting on Universal Health Coverage "Universal health coverage: moving together to build a healthier world"[cited 2025 May 17]. Available from: https://www.un.org/pga/wp-content/uploads/sites/53/2019/07/FINAL-draft-UHC-Political-Declaration.pdf
68. Rare diseases feature for first time at World Health Assembly [Internet]. Rare Diseases International. 2019 [cited 2025 May 17]. Available from: https://www.rarediseasesinternational.org/rare-diseases-feature-for-first-time-at-world-health-assembly/
69. Rare diseases: a global health priority for equity and inclusion. World Health Organization (WHO) [Internet]. [cited 2025 May 17]. Available from: https://apps.who.int/gb/ebwha/pdf_files/EB156/B156_CONF2-en
70. Cortial L, Nguyen C, Julkowska D, Cocqueel-Tiran F, Moliner AM, Blin O, et al. Managing rare diseases: examples of national approaches in Europe, North America and East Asia. Rare Dis Orphan Drugs J. 2022;1:10.
71. Khosla N, Valdez R. A compilation of national plans, policies and government actions for rare diseases in 23 countries. Intractable Rare Dis Res. 2018;7(4):213–22.
72. Regulation (EC) No 141/2000 of the European Parliament and of the Council of 16 December 1999 on orphan medicinal products. Regulation - 141/2000 - EN - EUR-Lex [Internet]. [cited 2025 May 17]. Available from: https://eur-lex.europa.eu/eli/reg/2000/141/oj/eng
73. Hedley V, Bottarelli V, Weinman A, Taruscio D. Shaping national plans and strategies for rare diseases in Europe: past, present, and future. J Community Genet. 2021;12(2):207–16.
74. Dharssi S, Wong-Rieger D, Harold M, Terry S. Review of 11 national policies for rare diseases in the context of key patient needs. Orphanet J Rare Dis. 2017;12(1):63.
75. 2024 EU4Health Work Programme [Internet]. Public Health. [cited 2025 May 17]. Available from: https://health.ec.europa.eu/publications/2024-eu4health-work-programme_en
76. Wainstock D, Katz A. Advancing rare disease policy in Latin America: a call to action. Lancet Reg Health Am. 2023;18(100434):100434.
77. Dias AG, Daher A, Barrera Ortiz L, Carreño-Moreno S, Hafez HSR, Jansen AM, et al. Rarecare: A policy perspective on the burden of rare diseases on caregivers in Latin America. Front Public Health. 2023;11:1127713.
78. Félix TM, Oliveira BM de, Horovitz DDG. Building a National Policy for Rare Disease in Brazil. J Community Genet 2024 Sep 26;1–8.
79. Armijo N, Espinoza M, Zamorano P, Lahoz D, Yañez T, Balmaceda C. Analisis del proceso de Evaluación de Tecnologías Sanitarias del Sistema de Protección Financiera Para Diagnósticos y Tratamientos de Alto Costo en Chile (Ley Ricarte Soto). Value Health Reg Issues. 2022;(32):95–101.
80. Mayrides M, Ruiz de Castilla EM, Szelepski S. A civil society view of rare disease public policy in six Latin American countries. Orphanet J Rare Dis. 2020;15(1):60.
81. Lopes-Júnior LC, Ferraz VEF, Lima RAG, Schuab SIPC, Pessanha RM, Luz GS, et al. Health policies for rare disease patients: a scoping review. Int J Environ Res Public Health [Internet]. 2022;19(22) https://doi.org/10.3390/ijerph192215174.
82. Wang Y, Liu Y, Du G, Liu Y, Zeng Y. Epidemiology and distribution of 207 rare diseases in China: A systematic literature review. Intractable Rare Dis Res. 2024;13(2):73–88.
83. Ying Z, Gong L, Li C. An update on China's national policies regarding rare diseases. Intractable Rare Dis Res. 2021;10(3):148–53.
84. Guo J, Liu P, Chen L, Lv H, Li J, Yu W, et al. National Rare Diseases Registry System (NRDRS): China's first nation-wide rare diseases demographic analyses. Orphanet J Rare Dis. 2021;16(1):515.
85. Mishra S, Bhat D, Venkatesh MP. Navigating health policies and programs in India: exploring opportunities to improve rare disease management and orphan drug research. Orphanet J Rare Dis. 2024;19(1):446.
86. Conscientização da Síndrome de Apert. Portal da Câmara dos Deputados [Internet]. [cited 2025 May 17]. Available from: https://www.camara.leg.br/proposicoesWeb/fichadetramitacao?idProposicao=2501878

87. Craniosynostosis Symposium. HRAC-USP S. • 14 e 15/03/2024 (evento internacional presencial) [Internet]. HRAC-USP Bauru. [cited 2025 May 17]. Available from: https://hrac.usp.br/en/realizados/2024/craniosynostosis-symposium-2024/
88. Idealizado por pais de menino com síndrome rara, simpósio internacional reúne especialistas em doenças que causam anomalias no crânio [Internet]. G1. 2024 [cited 2025 May 24]. Available from: https://g1.globo.com/sp/bauru-marilia/noticia/2024/03/14/idealizado-por-pais-de-menino-com-sindrome-rara-simposio-internacional-reune-especialistas-em-doencas-que-causam-anomalias-no-cranio.ghtml
89. Chung CCY, Hong Kong Genome Project, Chu ATW, Chung BHY. Rare disease emerging as a global public health priority. Front Public Health 2022 10:1028545.
90. Rare Diseases Act of 2002. [cited 2025 May 18]. Available from: https://www.congress.gov/107/plaws/publ280/PLAW-107publ280.pdf
91. Kanatani Y, Tomita N, Sato Y, Eto A, Omoe H, Mizushima H. National registry of designated intractable diseases in Japan: present status and future prospects. Neurol Med Chir (Tokyo). 2017;57(1):1–7.
92. CEPCAL [Internet]. [cited 2025 May 17]. Available from: https://www.cepcal.org/
93. Smile Train Brasil. About [Internet]. [cited 2025 May 17]. Available from: https://www.smiletrainbrasil.com/en/about-us
94. CORD. About [Internet]. [cited 2025 May 17]. Available from: https://www.raredisorders.ca/about/about-cord
95. Roa L, Jumbam DT, Makasa E, Meara JG. Global surgery and the sustainable development goals. Br J Surg [Internet] 2019 Jan 8 [cited 2025 May 10];106(2):e44–52. Available from: https://academic.oup.com/bjs/article/106/2/e44-e52/6120762
96. Truché P, Shoman H, Reddy CL, Jumbam DT, Ashby J, Mazhiqi A, et al. Globalization of national surgical, obstetric and anesthesia plans: the critical link between health policy and action in global surgery. Glob Health. 2020;16(1):1.
97. UNITAR. National Surgical Obstetric Anesthesia Planning (NSOAP) Manual [Internet]. [cited 2025 Jun 19]. Available from: https://unitar.org/sustainable-development-goals/people/our-portfolio/programme-health-and-development/global-surgery/national-surgical-obstetric-anesthesia-planning-nsoap-manual
98. Katherine A, Isabelle C, Walter J, John M, Alexander P, Lina R, et al. National Surgical, Obstetric and Anaesthesia Planning Manual (2020 Edition). Sep 28 [cited 2022 Oct 7]; 2020. https://zenodo.org/record/3982869
99. Osebo C, Grushka J, Deckelbaum D, Razek T. Assessing Ethiopia's surgical capacity in light of global surgery 2030 initiatives: is there progress in the past decade? Surg Open Sci. 2024;28(19):70–9.
100. Ravelojaona V, Ma X, Samison MF, Rabemalala D, Ayala R, Ramamonjisoa A, et al. L'intégration des soins chirurgicaux et anesthésiques dans les soins de santé universels: un plan national pour le développement de la chirurgie à Madagascar. Can J Anaesth. 2023;70(7):1131–54.
101. Varlas VN, Epistatu D, Varlas RG. Emphasis on early prenatal diagnosis and perinatal outcomes analysis of Apert syndrome. Diagnostics (Basel). 2024;14(14):1480.
102. Mak ASL, Leung KY. Prenatal ultrasonography of craniofacial abnormalities. Ultrasonography. 2019;38(1):13–24.
103. Kang SG, Kang JK. Current and future perspectives in craniosynostosis. J Korean Neurosurg Soc. 2016;59(3):247–9.
104. Mathijssen IMJ. Guideline for care of patients with the diagnoses of craniosynostosis: working group on craniosynostosis: working group on craniosynostosis. J Craniofac Surg. 2015;26(6):1735–807.
105. Stock NM, Marik P, Magee L, Aspinall CL, Garcia L, Crerand C, et al. Facilitating positive psychosocial outcomes in craniofacial team care: strategies for medical providers. Cleft Palate Craniofac J. 2020;57(3):333–43.
106. Rare Diseases Clinical Practice Guidelines developed in the context of the Brazilian Public Health System in twelve years [Internet]. [cited 2025 May 23]. Available from: https://abstracts.cochrane.org/2024-prague-global-evidence-summit/rare-diseases-clinical-practice-guidelines-developed-context?utm_source=chatgpt.com
107. Kremp O, Dosquet P, Rath A. Professional clinical guidelines for rare diseases: methodology. Orphanet J Rare Dis. 2012;7(Suppl 2):A12.
108. Lenzi A, Basili S, Saiani L, Palese A, Limongelli G. Education in rare diseases. Where are we now? Recenti Prog Med. 2022;113(7):411–4.
109. Dunne TF, Jeffries D, Mckay L. Rare disease 101: an online resource teaching on over 7000 rare diseases in one short course. Orphanet J Rare Dis. 2024;19(1):275.
110. He J, Kang Q, Hu J, Song P, Jin C. China has officially released its first national list of rare diseases. Intractable Rare Dis Res. 2018;7(2):145–7.
111. Jumbam DT, Reddy CL, Meara JG, Makasa EM, Atun R. A financing strategy to expand surgical health care. Glob Health Sci Pract. 2023;11(3):e2100295.
112. Qin RX, Yoon S, Fowler ZG, Jayaram A, Stankey M, Samad L, et al. Financing surgical, obstetric, anaesthesia, and trauma care in the Asia-Pacific region: proceedings. BMC Proc. 2023;17(Suppl 5):10.
113. Ganske I, Khoshbin S, Katz JT. Teaching healthcare professionals to see. American journal of medical genetics Part C, Seminars in medical genetics [Internet]. 2021 Jun [cited 2025 May 28];187(2). Available from: https://pubmed.ncbi.nlm.nih.gov/33982871/
114. Monlleo IL, Mossey PA, Gil-da-Silva-Lopes VL. Evaluation of craniofacial care outside the

Brazilian reference network for craniofacial treatment. Cleft Palate-Craniofac J [Internet]. 2009 [cited 2025 May 28]; Available from: https://journals.sagepub.com/doi/10.1597/07-153.1
115. GlobalSurg Collaborative and NIHR Global Health Research Unit on Global Surgery. Effects of hospital facilities on patient outcomes after cancer surgery: an international, prospective, observational study. Lancet Glob Health. 2022;10(7):e1003–11.
116. Yöntem A, Aydın Y, Horoz ÖÖ, Yıldızdaş D, Ekinci F, Kılıç ŞS. Postoperative intensive care requirements of pediatric surgery patients. Turk J Pediatr Emerg Intensive Care Med. 2024;5:120–5.
117. Kalantar Hormozi A, Mahdavi N, Foroozanfar MM, Razavi SS, Mohajerani R, Eghbali A, et al. Effect of perioperative management on outcome of patients after craniosynostosis surgery. World J Plast Surg. 2017;6(1):48–53.
118. Kassam SN, Perry JL, Ayala R, Stieber E, Davies G, Hudson N, et al. World Cleft Coalition International Treatment Program Standards. The Cleft palate-craniofacial journal: official publication of the American Cleft Palate-Craniofacial Association [Internet]. 2020 Oct [cited 2025 May 28];57(10). Available from: https://pubmed.ncbi.nlm.nih.gov/32573279/
119. Faasse M, Mathijssen IMJ, ERN CRANIO Working Group on Craniosynostosis. Guideline on treatment and management of craniosynostosis: patient and family version. J Craniofac Surg 2023;34(1):418–433.
120. Battistelli EZ, Calabria O, Giani M, Moretto A, Cattaneo F, Alberio G, et al. Perioperative management and outcomes of pediatric craniosynostosis patients undergoing cranioplasty: a retrospective analysis. J Craniofac Surg [Internet] 2025 Jan [cited 2025 May 28];36(1). Available from: https://pubmed.ncbi.nlm.nih.gov/39724592/
121. Stricker PA, Goobie SM, Cladis FP, Haberkern CM, Meier PM, Reddy SK, et al. Perioperative outcomes and management in pediatric complex cranial vault reconstruction: a Multicenter Study from the Pediatric Craniofacial Collaborative Group. Anesthesiology [Internet]. 2017 Feb [cited 2025 May 28];126(2). Available from: https://pubmed.ncbi.nlm.nih.gov/27977460/
122. Gadenz SD, Basso J, Prbp de O, Sperling S, Zuanazzi MVD, Oliveira GG, et al. Telehealth to support referral management in a universal health system: a before-and-after study. BMC health services research [Internet]. 2021 Sep 25 [cited 2025 May 28];21(1). Available from: https://pubmed.ncbi.nlm.nih.gov/34563176/
123. Owolabi EO, Mac QT, Louw J, Davies JI, Chu KM. Telemedicine in Surgical Care in low- and Middle-Income Countries: A Scoping Review. World J Surg [Internet]. 2022 Aug [cited 2025 May 28];46(8). Available from: https://pubmed.ncbi.nlm.nih.gov/35428920/
124. Robler SK, Platt A, Turner EL, Gallo JJ, Labrique A, Hofstetter P, et al. Telemedicine referral to improve access to specialty care for preschool children in rural Alaska: A cluster-randomized controlled trial. Ear Hear [Internet] 2023 Nov [cited 2025 May 28];44(6). Available from: https://pubmed.ncbi.nlm.nih.gov/37226299/
125. Ahmed S, Chase LE, Wagnild J, Akhter N, Sturridge S, Clarke A, et al. Community health workers and health equity in low- and middle-income countries: systematic review and recommendations for policy and practice. Int J Equity Health 2022 ;21(1):1–30.
126. Pedrini DB, da Silva LP, Vieira TA, Giugliani R. Training of community health agents, a strategy for earlier recognition of mucopolysaccharidoses. J Community Genet. 2024;15(2):129–35.
127. A.B.S.A, ASSOCIAÇÃO BRASILEIRA DA SÍNDROME DE APERT [Internet]. [cited 2025 Jun 19]. Available from: https://absapert.com.br/
128. Encontro reúne especialistas da Saúde e famílias de crianças com doença rara craniofacial [Internet]. Hospital Sobrapar. 2025 [cited 2025 May 28]. Available from: https://sobrapar.org.br/encontro-sindrome-de-apert-campinas/
129. Apert Brasil [Internet]. Apert Brasil. [cited 2025 May 28]. Available from: https://apertbrasil.com.br/
130. Abdallah S, Sharifa M, I Kh Almadhoun MK, Khawar MM Sr, Shaikh U, Balabel KM, et al. The impact of artificial intelligence on optimizing diagnosis and treatment plans for rare genetic disorders. Cureus. 2023;15(10):e46860.
131. Huys SEF, Markus AF, Mommaerts MY. Obstacles for accessing customised craniofacial implants in low- and middle-income countries. J Oral Biol Craniofac Res. 2022;12(1):80–5.
132. Gerk A, Kundu S, Meara JG, Stegmann J. Digital solutions for rare diseases in global health. Lancet Glob Health. 2024 Jul;12(7):e1091.
133. Rare diseases [Internet]. [cited 2025 May 17]. Available from: https://www.who.int/standards/classifications/frequently-asked-questions/rare-diseases
134. Aymé S, Bellet B, Rath A. Rare diseases in ICD11: making rare diseases visible in health information systems through appropriate coding. Orphanet J Rare Dis. 2015;10(1):35.
135. ERDRI [Internet]. 2018 [cited 2025 May 18]. Available from: https://eu-rd-platform.jrc.ec.europa.eu/erdri_en
136. Aim of the Platform [Internet]. 2018 [cited 2025 May 17]. Available from: https://eu-rd-platform.jrc.ec.europa.eu/aim-of-the-platform_en
137. Registry Hub for Rare Neuromuscular Diseases [Internet]. European reference Network 2024 [cited 2025 May 17]. Available from: https://ern-euro-nmd.eu/reghub/
138. EuroBloodNet. European Rare Blood Disorders Platform [Internet]. EuroBloodNet. [cited 2025 May 17]. Available from: https://eurobloodnet.eu/enrol-first/

139. Home, ENROL Demo [Internet]. [cited 2025 May 18]. Available from: https://enrolplatform.eu/
140. de Oliveira BM, Bernardi FA, Baiochi JF, Neiva MB, Artifon M, Vergara AA, et al. Epidemiological characterization of rare diseases in Brazil: A retrospective study of the Brazilian Rare diseases network. Orphanet J Rare Dis. 2024;19(1):405.
141. Plataforma Integrada de Vigilância em Saúde, Ministério da Saúde [Internet]. [cited 2025 May 17]. Available from: http://plataforma.saude.gov.br/
142. Telles L, Lima BLP, Campos LN, Wagemaker S, Gerk A, Kim A, et al. The hidden burden of craniosynostosis in Brazil's Unified Health System: a 10-year retrospective analysis of the disease's diagnoses and surgical operations. J Craniofac Surg [Internet]. 2025 May 5.; Available from: https://doi.org/10.1097/SCS.0000000000011475
143. Ardi [Internet]. [cited 2025 May 17]. Available from: https://ardi.africa/en/about.html
144. Gelbard S. Rare diseases often go undiagnosed or untreated in parts of Africa. A project seeks to change that [Internet]. AP News 2025 [cited 2025 May 18]. Available from: https://apnews.com/article/senegal-genetic-diseases-africa-health-46790779474476d25eeef865ed0bf2a9
145. Malherbe H. Introducing the south African rare diseases access initiative. S Afr Med J. 2023;113(8):8.
146. Reiter AMV, Pantel JT, Danyel M, Horn D, Ott CE, Mensah MA. Validation of 3 computer-aided facial phenotyping tools (DeepGestalt, GestaltMatcher, and D-score): comparative diagnostic accuracy study. J Med Internet Res. 2024;26:e42904.
147. Pantel JT, Hajjir N, Danyel M, Elsner J, Abad-Perez AT, Hansen P, et al. Efficiency of computer-aided facial phenotyping (DeepGestalt) in individuals with and without a genetic syndrome: diagnostic accuracy study. J Med Internet Res. 2020;22(10):e19263.
148. Home [Internet]. Face2Gene. 2016 [cited 2025 May 18]. Available from: https://www.face2gene.com/
149. Narayanan DL, Ranganath P, Aggarwal S, Dalal A, Phadke SR, Mandal K. Computer-aided facial analysis in diagnosing dysmorphic syndromes in Indian children. Indian Pediatr. 2019;56(12):1017–9.
150. Arlt A, Knaus A, Hsieh TC, Klinkhammer H, Bhasin MA, Hustinx A, et al. Next-generation phenotyping in Nigerian children with Cornelia de Lange syndrome. Am J Med Genet A. 2024;194(9):e63641.
151. Liu C, Lee MK, Naqvi S, Hoskens H, Liu D, White JD, et al. Genome scans of facial features in East Africans and cross-population comparisons reveal novel associations. PLoS Genet. 2021;17(8):e1009695.
152. Fundamental Surgery [Internet]. Fundamental Surgery 2022 [cited 2025 May 18]. Available from: https://fundamentalsurgery.com/
153. Hutton D. Orbis, Fundamental VR team up to target training [Internet]. Ophthalmol Times 2024 [cited 2025 May 18]. Available from: https://www.ophthalmologytimes.com/view/orbis-fundamentalvr-team-up-to-target-training
154. Mahajan A, Hawkins A. Current implementation outcomes of digital surgical simulation in low- and middle-income countries: Scoping review. JMIR Med Educ. 2023;9:e23287.
155. Ashraf M, Choudhary N, Kamboh UA, Raza MA, Sultan KA, Ghulam N, et al. Early experience with patient-specific low-cost 3D-printed polymethylmethacrylate cranioplasty implants in a lower-middle-income-country: technical note and economic analysis. Surg Neurol Int. 2022;13(270):270.
156. Singh HN, Agrawal S, Kuthe AM. Design of customized implants and 3D printing of symmetric and asymmetric cranial cavities. J Mech Behav Biomed Mater. 2023;146(106061):106061.
157. Chaware SM, Bagaria V, Kuthe A. Application of the rapid prototyping technique to design a customized temporomandibular joint used to treat temporomandibular ankylosis. Indian J Plast Surg. 2009;42(1):85–93.
158. Rare diseases [Internet]. [cited 2025 May 17]. Available from: https://www.who.int/standards/classifications/frequently-asked-questions/rare-diseases#:~:text=ICD%2D11%20includes%20some%205500,Global%20Network%204%20Rare%20Diseases%22
159. Núñez-Samudio V, Arcos-Burgos M, Landires I. Rare diseases: democratising genetic testing in LMICs. Lancet. 2023;401(10385):1339–40.
160. Ferreira RL, do Nascimento IJB, de Almeida VIA, de Oliveira VRL, Marangne LG, Dos Santos Gameleira F, et al. The utilisation of primary health care system concepts positively impacts the assistance of patients with rare diseases despite limited knowledge and experience by health care professionals: A qualitative synopsis of the evidence including approximately 78 000 individuals. J Glob Health 2023;13:04030.
161. Adam T, Ralaidovy AH, Ross AL, Reeder JC, Swaminathan S. Tracking global resources and capacity for health research: time to reassess strategies and investment decisions. Health Res Policy Syst 2023;21(1):93.
162. Patel KB, Pfeifauf KD, Snyder-Warwick A. Family-centered pediatric plastic surgery care. Mo Med. 2021;118(2):124–9.
163. Somanadhan S, Nicholson E, Dorris E, Brinkley A, Kennan A, Treacy E, et al. Rare Disease Research Partnership (RAinDRoP): a collaborative approach to identify research priorities for rare diseases in Ireland. HRB Open Res. 2020;3:13.
164. Kogetsu A, Isono M, Aikyo T, Furuta J, Goto D, Hamakawa N, et al. Enhancing evidence-informed policymaking in medicine and healthcare: stakeholder involvement in the commons project for rare diseases in Japan. Res Involv Engagem. 2023;9(1):107.
165. Loukides G, Denny JC, Malin B. The disclosure of diagnosis codes can breach research participants' privacy. J Am Med Inform Assoc. 2010;17(3):322–7.

166. Amorim M, Silva S, Machado H, Teles EL, Baptista MJ, Maia T, et al. Benefits and risks of sharing genomic data for research: comparing the views of rare disease patients, informal carers and healthcare professionals. Int J Environ Res Public Health. 2022;19(14):8788.
167. Cho HL, Danis M, Grady C. Post-trial responsibilities beyond post-trial access. Lancet. 2018;391(10129):1478–9.
168. Mastroleo I. Post-trial obligations in the declaration of Helsinki 2013: classification, reconstruction and interpretation. Dev World Bioeth. 2016;16(2):80–90.
169. Mota JW, Hellmann F, Guedert JM, Verdi M, Bittencourt SC. Acesso a medicamentos Para doenças raras no pós-estudo: revisão integrativa. Rev Bioét. 2022;30(3):662–77.
170. Brock DW, Wikler D. Ethical issues in resource allocation, research, and new product development. In: Disease control priorities in developing countries. New York: Oxford University Press; 2006.
171. Chalkidou K, Claxton K, Silverman R, Yadav P. Value-based tiered pricing for universal health coverage: an idea worth revisiting. Gates Open Res. 2020;24(4):16.
172. Ragavan S, Vanni A. Can international patent law help mitigate cancer inequity in LMICs? AMA J Ethics. 2020;22(2):E102–11.
173. Burrone E, Gotham D, Gray A, de Joncheere K, Magrini N, Martei YM, et al. Patent pooling to increase access to essential medicines. Bull World Health Organ. 2019;97(8):575–7.
174. Nisingizwe MP, Ndishimye P, Swaibu K, Nshimiyimana L, Karame P, Dushimiyimana V, et al. Effect of unmanned aerial vehicle (drone) delivery on blood product delivery time and wastage in Rwanda: a retrospective, cross-sectional study and time series analysis. Lancet Glob Health. 2022;10(4):e564–9.
175. Seyi-Olajide JO, Brindle M, Faboya O, Sleemi A, Williams O, Ameh EA. Is neocolonialism existing in global surgery practice? An analysis of a web-based survey amongst global surgery practitioners. J Glob Health Rep. 2024;8:e2024016.
176. Ellis DI, Nakayama DK, Fitzgerald TN. Missions, humanitarianism, and the evolution of modern global surgery. Am Surg. 2021;87(5):681–5.
177. Chen S, Zolo Y, Ngulube L, Isiagi M, Maswime S. Global surgery and climate change: how global surgery can prioritise both the health of the planet and its people. BMC Surg. 2025;25(1):21.
178. Qin R, Alayande B, Okolo I, Khanyola J, Jumbam DT, Koea J, et al. Colonisation and its aftermath: reimagining global surgery. BMJ Glob Health. 2024;9(1):e014173.
179. Hyman GY, Jhunjhunwala R, Hanto DW. A cosmopolitan argument for temporary "diagonal" short-term surgical missions as a component of surgical systems strengthening. Glob Health Sci Pract. 2024;12(5):e2400046.
180. Integrated people-centred care [Internet]. [cited 2025 May 23]. Available from: https://www.who.int/health-topics/integrated-people-centered-care#tab=tab_1
181. Frank M, Eidt-Koch D, Aumann I, Reimann A, Wagner TOF, Graf von der Schulenburg JM. Maßnahmen zur Verbesserung der gesundheitlichen situation von Menschen mit seltenen Erkrankungen in Deutschland: Ein Vergleich mit dem Nationalen Aktionsplan. Bundesgesundheitsblatt Gesundheitsforschung Gesundheitsschutz. 2014;57(10):1216–23.
182. Baynam G, Bowman F, Lister K, Walker CE, Pachter N, Goldblatt J, et al. Improved diagnosis and care for rare diseases through implementation of precision public health framework. In: Adv Exp Med Biol, vol. 1031; 2017. p. 55–94.

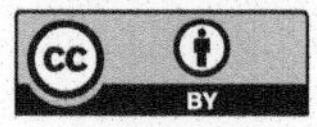

Index

J. G. Meara et al. (eds.), *Apert Syndrome*, https://doi.org/10.1007/978-3-032-12551-4

B

D

G

H

N

O

P

T

W

Y

Z